Treatment of Dystonia

Treatment of Dystonia

Edited by
Dirk Dressler
Hannover Medical School
Eckart Altenmüller
Institute of Music Physiology and Musicians' Medicine, Hannover, Germany
Joachim K. Krauss
Hannover Medical School

CAMBRIDGE
UNIVERSITY PRESS

CAMBRIDGE
UNIVERSITY PRESS

Shaftesbury Road, Cambridge CB2 8EA, United Kingdom

One Liberty Plaza, 20th Floor, New York, NY 10006, USA

477 Williamstown Road, Port Melbourne, VIC 3207, Australia

314–321, 3rd Floor, Plot 3, Splendor Forum, Jasola District Centre, New Delhi – 110025, India

103 Penang Road, #05–06/07, Visioncrest Commercial, Singapore 238467

Cambridge University Press is part of Cambridge University Press & Assessment, a department of the University of Cambridge.

We share the University's mission to contribute to society through the pursuit of education, learning and research at the highest international levels of excellence.

www.cambridge.org
Information on this title: www.cambridge.org/9781107132863

DOI: 10.1017/9781316459324

First published 2018

A catalogue record for this publication is available from the British Library

Library of Congress Cataloging-in-Publication data
Names: Dressler, Dirk, editor. | Altenmüller, Eckart, editor. | Krauss, Joachim K., editor.
Title: Treatment of dystonia / edited by Dirk Dressler, Eckart Altenmüller, Joachim K. Krauss.
Description: Cambridge; New York, NY: Cambridge University Press, 2018. |
Includes bibliographical references and index.
Identifiers: LCCN 2017046241 | ISBN 9781107132863 (hardback)
Subjects: | MESH: Dystonia
Classification: LCC RC935.D8 | NLM WL 390 | DDC 616.7/4–dc23
LC record available at https://lccn.loc.gov/2017046241

ISBN 978-1-107-13286-3 Hardback

Contents

Contributors

Jasper van Aalst
Department of Neurosurgery, MUMC+, Maastricht, the Netherlands

Alberto Albanese
Department of Neurology, Istituto Clinico Humanitas, Rozzano, Milano, Italy

Eckart Altenmüller
Institute of Music Physiology and Musicians' Medicine (IMMM), University of Music, Drama and Media, Hannover, Germany

Christian Amlang
Yale School of Medicine, Yale University, New Haven, CT, USA

Keyoumars Ashkan
Department of Neurology, Evelina London Children's Hospital, London, UK

Bettina Balint
Sobell Department of Motor Neuroscience and Movement Disorders, UCL Institute of Neurology, London, UK

Ausaf A. Bari
Division of Neurosurgery, University of Toronto, Toronto, Ontario, Canada

Hansjörg Bäzner
Department of Neurology, Katharinenhospital, Stuttgart, Germany

Jules G. Becher
Paediatric Rehabilitation, Department of Rehabilitation Medicine, VU University Medical Center, Amsterdam, the Netherlands

Kailash P. Bhatia
Sobell Department of Motor Neuroscience and Movement Disorders, UCL Institute of Neurology, London, UK

Hans Bigalke
Toxogen, Hannover, Germany

Christian Blahak
Department of Neurology and Neurogeriatry, Ortenau-Klinikum, Lahr, Germany

Jean-Pierre Bleton
Department of Neurology, Fondation Ophtalmologique Adolphe de Rothschild, Paris, France

Andrew Blitzer
New York Center for Voice and Swallowing Disorders, Head and Neck Surgical Group, St. Luke's Roosevelt Medical Center, New York, NY, USA

Saeed A. Bohlega
Department of Neurosciences, King Faisal Specialist Hospital & Research Centre, Riyadh, Saudi Arabia

Laura A. Bonouvrie
Paediatric Rehabilitation, Department of Rehabilitation Medicine, VU University Medical Center, Amsterdam, the Netherlands

Giovanni Broggi
Unit of Functional Neurosurgery, Fondazione IRCCS Istituto Neurologico 'Carlo Besta', Milan, Italy

Annemieke I. Buizer
Paediatric Rehabilitation, Department of Rehabilitation Medicine, VU University Medical Center, Amsterdam, the Netherlands

Gul Yalcin Cakmakli
Institute of Neurological Sciences and Psychiatry, Hacettepe University, Sihhiye, Ankara, Turkey

Matteo Caleo
CNR Neuroscience Institute, Pisa, Italy

Stefan J. Cano
Modus Outcomes, Letchworth Garden City, UK

Robert Chen
Division of Neurology, Department of Medicine, Toronto Western Hospital, University of Toronto, Toronto, Ontario, Canada

Sophie Cho
Human Motor Control Section, National Institute of Neurological Disorders and Stroke, National Institutes of Health, Bethesda, MD, USA

Laura Cif
Research Group on Movement Disorders in Children, Department of Neurosurgery, Gui de Chauliac University, Montpellier, France

Sophie Cleanthous
Modus Outcomes, Letchworth Garden City, UK

Carlo Colosimo
Department of Neurology, Santa Maria University Hospital, Terni, Italy

Cynthia L. Comella
Department of Neurological Sciences, Rush University Medical Center, Chicago, IL, USA

Roberto Cordella
Unit of Functional Neurosurgery, Fondazione IRCCS Istituto Neurologico 'Carlo Besta', Milan, Italy

Philippe Coubes
Research Group on Movement Disorders in Children, Department of Neurosurgery, Gui de Chauliac University, Montpellier, France

Aloysius Domingo
Institute of Neurogenetics, University of Lübeck, Lübeck, Germany

Joost van den Dool
Department of Neurology, University Medical Centre Groningen, Groningen, the Netherlands

Dirk Dressler
Movement Disorder Section, Department of Neurology, Hannover Medical School, Hannover, Germany

Roberto Eleopra
Neurological Unit I, IRCCS Fondazione Carlo Besta, Milan, Italy

Bulent Elibol
Faculty of Medicine, Department of Neurology, Hacettepe University, Sihhiye, Ankara, Turkey

Frank Erbguth
Department of Neurology, Nuremberg General Hospital, Paracelsus Medical University, Nuremberg, Germany

Roberto Erro
Sobell Department of Motor Neuroscience and Movement Disorders, UCL Institute of Neurology, London, UK

Glen Estrin
Dystonia Medical Research Foundation, Chicago, IL, USA

Sílvia Fàbregas-Molas
Institute of Art, Medicine and Physiology, Terrassa, Barcelona, Spain

Stanley Fahn
Department of Neurology, Columbia University College of Physicians & Surgeons, New York, NY, USA

Jessica Feeley
Dystonia Medical Research Foundation, Chicago, IL, USA

Keith Foster
Ipsen Bioinnovation Ltd, Abingdon, UK

Angelo Franzini
Unit of Functional Neurosurgery, Fondazione IRCCS Istituto Neurologico 'Carlo Besta', Milan, Italy

Karen Frei
Department of Neurology, Loma Linda University Medical Center, Loma Linda, CA, USA

Steven J. Frucht
NYU Langone Medical Center from Mount Sinai, New York, NY, USA

Shinichi Furuya
Musical Skill and Injury Center, Department of Information and Communication Sciences, Sophia University, Tokyo, Japan

Thomas Gasser
Department of Neurology, Eberhard Karls University, Tübingen, Germany

Robert E. Gross
Department of Neurosurgery, Emory University School of Medicine, Atlanta, GA, USA

Doreen Gruber
Department of Stereotactic Neurosurgery & Neurology, Otto-von-Guericke University Magdeburg, Germany

Mark Hallett
Human Motor Control Section, National Institute of Neurological Disorders and Stroke, National Institutes of Health, Bethesda, MD, USA

Tomoko Hanada
Department of Neurosurgery, Tokyo Women's Medical University, Tokyo, Japan

Daniela Hansen
Reta Lila Weston Institute of Neurological Studies, Department of Molecular Neuroscience and Queen Square Brain Bank, Institute of Neurology, UCL, London, UK

Gun-Marie Hariz
Department of Clinical Neuroscience, Umeå University, Umeå, Sweden

Marwan Hariz
Unit of Functional Neurosurgery, UCL Institute of Neurology, Queen Square, London, UK

Ellen J. Hess
Departments of Pharmacology and Neurology, Emory University, Atlanta, GA, USA

Janet Hieshetter
Dystonia Medical Research Foundation, Chicago, IL, USA

Shiro Horisawa
Department of Neurosurgery, Tokyo Women's Medical University, Tokyo, Japan

Paola Imbriani
Department of Systems Medicine, University of Rome 'Tor Vergata', Rome, Italy

Christos I. Ioannou
Institute of Music Physiology and Musicians' Medicine (IMMM), University of Music, Drama and Media, Hannover, Germany

Marjan Jahanshahi
Cognitive Motor Neuroscience Group, Sobell Department of Motor Neuroscience & Movement Disorders, UCL Institute of Neurology, National Hospital for Neurology & Neurosurgery, London, UK

Joseph Jankovic
Department of Neurology, Baylor College of Medicine, Baylor St. Luke's Medical Center, Houston, TX, USA

Beomseok Jeon
Department of Neurology, College of Medicine, Seoul National University Hospital, Seoul, Korea

Hyder A. Jinnah
Departments of Neurology, Human Genetics and Pediatrics, Emory University, Atlanta, GA, USA

Mandar Jog
Department of Clinical Neurological Sciences, Western University, London, Ontario, Canada

Eric A. Johnson
Department of Bacteriology, University of Wisconsin, Madison, WI, USA

Peter Kaňovský
Movement Disorders Center, Department of Neurology, Palacky University Medical School, Olomouc, Czech Republic

Barbara Illowsky Karp
National Institute of Neurological Disorders and Stroke, National Institutes of Health, Bethesda, MD, USA

Ryul Kim
Department of Neurology, Seoul National University Hospital, Seoul, Korea

Teresa Jacobson Kimberley
Department of Physical Therapy, School of Health and Rehabilitation Sciences, MGH Institute of Health Professions, Boston, MA, USA

Marianne King
Dystonia Specialist Nurse, Lancashire Teaching NHS Trust, Preston, Lancashire, UK

Christine Klein
Institute of Neurogenetics, University of Lübeck, Lübeck, Germany

Arne Knutzen
Department of Neurology, Christian-Albrechts-University Kiel, Kiel, Germany

Maria A. J. de Koning-Tijssen
Department of Neurology, University Medical Centre Groningen, Groningen, the Netherlands

Vladimir S. Kostić
Department of Neurology, Faculty of Medicine, University of Belgrade, Belgrade, Serbia

Anne Koy
Department of Pediatrics, University of Cologne, Cologne, Germany

Paul Krack
Division of Neurology, CHU Grenoble, Joseph Fourier University, Grenoble, France

Joachim K. Krauss
Department of Neurosurgery, Hannover Medical School, Hannover, Germany

Andrea A. Kühn
Movement Disorders and Neuromodulation Section, Charité, Humboldt University, Berlin, Germany

Andreas Kupsch
Department of Stereotactic Neurosurgery & Neurology, Otto-von-Guericke University Magdeburg, Germany

Zdravko Lacković
Laboratory of Molecular Neuropharmacology, Department of Pharmacology, University of Zagreb School of Medicine, Zagreb, Croatia

Stefania Lalli
Department of Neurology, Università Cattolica del Sacro Cuore, Milano, Italy

Anthony E. Lang
Division of Neurology, Toronto Western Hospital, University of Toronto, Toronto, Ontario, Canada

Rainer Laskawi
Department of Ear, Nose and Throat, University Medical Centre, Georg-August University, Göttingen, Germany

Andrè Lee
Department of Neurology, Klinikum Rechts der Isar, Technical University, Munich, Germany

Jean-Pierre Lin
Department of Neurology, Evelina London Children's Hospital, London, UK

Elan D. Louis
Departments of Neurology and Chronic Disease Epidemiology, Yale School of Medicine and Yale, School of Public Health, Yale University, New Haven, CT, USA

Andres M. Lozano
Division of Neurosurgery, Toronto Western Hospital, University of Toronto, Toronto, Ontario, Canada

Marta Maltese
Department of Systems Medicine, University of Rome 'Tor Vergata', Rome, Italy

Carine W. Maurer
Human Motor Control Section, National Institute of Neurological Disorders and Stroke, National Institutes of Health, Bethesda, MD, USA

Riccardo Mazzocchio
Department of Neurological and Neurosensory Sciences, University Hospital, Siena, Italy

Giuseppe Messina
Unit of Functional Neurosurgery, Fondazione IRCCS Istituto Neurologico 'Carlo Besta', Milan, Italy

Federico Micheli
Parkinson's Disease and Movement Disorders Unit, Department of Neurology, Hospital de Clínicas 'Jose de San Martin', University of Buenos Aires, Buenos Aires, Argentina

Kelly A. Mills
Movement Disorder and Neuromodulation Center, University of California San Francisco Medical Center, San Francisco, CA, USA

Akshitkumar M. Mistry
Department of Neurosurgery, Vanderbilt University Medical Center, Nashville, TN, USA

Cesare Montecucco
Department of Biomedical Sciences, University of Padova, Padova, Italy

Austen Peter Moore
The Walton Centre NHS Foundation Trust, Liverpool University, Liverpool, UK

Elena Moro
Division of Neurology, CHU Grenoble, Joseph Fourier University, Grenoble, France

Joseph S. Neimat
Department of Neurosurgery, Vanderbilt University Medical Center, Nashville, TN, USA

Alistair Newton
Dystonia Europe, Brussels, Belgium

Scott A. Norris
Department of Neurology, Washington University School of Medicine, St. Louis, MO, USA

Olga Orlova
I.M. Sechenov First Moscow State Medical University, Moscow, Russia

Jill L. Ostrem
Movement Disorder and Neuromodulation Center, University of California San Francisco Medical Center, San Francisco, CA, USA

Willem J. R. van Ouwerkerk
Department of Neurosurgery, VU University Medical Center, Amsterdam, the Netherlands

James Palmer
Department of Neurosurgery, Derriford Hospital, Plymouth, UK

Jung E. Park
Human Motor Control Section, National Institute of Neurological Disorders and Stroke, National Institutes of Health, Bethesda, MD, USA

Amande Pauls
Department of Neurology, University Hospital, Philipps University, Marburg, Germany

Ellen B. Penney
Department of Neurology, Yale School of Medicine and Yale School of Public Health, Yale University, New Haven, CT, USA

Joel S. Perlmutter
Departments of Radiology, Anatomy and Neurobiology, Occupational and Physical Therapy, Washington University, St. Louis, MO, USA

Heidrun Pickenbrock
Movement Disorders Section, Department of Neurology, Hannover Medical School, Hannover, Germany

Andy Pickett
Toxin Science Limited, Wrexham, UK

Zvezdan Pirtošek
Department of Neurology, University Medical Centre, Ljubljana, Slovenia

Antonio Pisani
Department of Systems Medicine, University of Rome 'Tor Vergata', Rome, Italy

Seth L. Pullman
Department of Neurology, Columbia University Medical Center, New York, NY, USA

Angelo Quartarone
Department of Neurosciences, University of Messina, Messina, Italy

René Reese
Department of Neurology, University of Rostock, Rostock, Germany

Maja Relja
Department of Neurology, University Hospital Centre, University of Zagreb School of Medicine, Zagreb, Croatia

Christian Riederer
Würzburg, Germany

Raymond L. Rosales
Department of Neurology and Psychiatry, Royal and Pontifical University of Santo Tomas and Hospital, Manila, Philippines

Ami R. Rosen
Department of Neurology, Emory University, Atlanta, GA, USA

Jaume Rosset-Llobet
Institute of Art, Medicine and Physiology, Terrassa, Barcelona, Spain

Ornella Rossetto
Department of Biomedical Sciences, University of Padova, Padova, Italy

Fereshte Adib Saberi
IAB – Interdisciplinary Working Group for Movement Disorders, Hamburg, Germany

Michel Sáenz-Farret
Hospital de Clínicas José de san Martín, University of Buenos Aires, Buenos Aires, Argentina

Christoph Schrader
Movement Disorders Section, Department of Neurology, Hannover Medical School, Hannover, Germany

Binit B. Shah
Department of Neurology, University of Virginia, Charlottesville, VA, USA

Christos Sidiropoulos
Parkinson's Disease and Movement Disorders Program, Henry Ford Hospital, West Bloomfield, MI, USA

Miriam Sklerov
Department of Neurology, Columbia University Medical Center, New York, NY, USA

Dan Soudant
Child Neurology, Department of Neurology, MUMC+, Maastricht, the Netherlands

Glenn T. Stebbins
Department of Neurological Sciences, Rush University Medical Center, Chicago, IL, USA

Thomas D. L. Steeves
Division of Neurology, Toronto Western Hospital, University of Toronto, Toronto, Ontario, Canada

Matthew A. Stern
Unit of Functional Neurosurgery, Fondazione IRCCS Istituto Neurologico 'Carlo Besta', Milan, Italy

Melanie Leigh D. Supnet
Department of Neurology and Psychiatry, Royal and Pontifical University of Santo Tomas and Hospital, Manila, Philippines

Christopher Tang
New York Center for Voice and Swallowing Disorders, Head and Neck Surgical Group, St. Luke's Roosevelt Medical Center, New York, NY, USA

Takaomi Taira
Department of Neurosurgery, Tokyo Women's Medical University, Tokyo, Japan

Nobuhiko Takeda
Department of Neurosurgery, Tokyo Women's Medical University, Tokyo, Japan

Onno Teernstra
Department of Neurosurgery, MUMC+, Maastricht, the Netherlands

Jan K. Teller
Dystonia Medical Research Foundation, Chicago, IL, USA

Mary Ann Thenganatt
Parkinson's Disease Center and Movement Disorders Clinic, Department of Neurology, Baylor College of Medicine, Houston, TX, USA

Lars Timmermann
Department of Neurology, University Hospital, Philipps University, Marburg, Germany

Daniel Truong
Parkinson's Disease and Movement Disorder Institute, Long Beach, CA, USA

R. Jeroen Vermeulen
Child Neurology, Department of Neurology, MUMC+, Maastricht, the Netherlands

Marie Vidailhet
Department of Neurology, AP-HP, Salpetriere Hopital, Sorbonne University – Pierre et Marie Curie University, Institut of Brain and Spine (ICM), Salpetriere, Paris, France

Jens Volkmann
Department of Neurology, University Hospital Würzburg, Würzburg, Germany

Uwe Walter
Department of Neurology, University of Rostock, Rostock, Germany

Thomas T. Warner
Reta Lila Weston Institute of Neurological Studies, Department of Molecular Neuroscience and Queen Square Brain Bank, Institute of Neurology, UCL, London, UK

Karoline Wenzel
Department of Neurology, Medical University Graz, Graz, Austria

Lena Zetterberg
Section of Physiotherapy, Department of Neuroscience, Uppsala University, Uppsala, Sweden

Kirsten E. Zeuner
Department of Neurology, Christian-Albrechts-University Kiel, Kiel, Germany

Ulf Ziemann
Department of Neurology & Stroke and Hertie Institute for Clinical Brain Research, Eberhard Karls University, Tübingen, Germany

Preface

Treatment of dystonia has been a challenge since the concept of dystonia was first formulated by C. David Marsden in London and Stanley Fahn in New York City. In the absence of causal treatment, multiple pharmacological, surgical, rehabilitative and experimental therapies have been brought up. With the advent of botulinum toxin therapy and deep brain stimulation, major advances have been achieved. Improved insight into the pathophysiologic and genetic bases of dystonia might provide guidelines for future therapies.

With all of this, treatment of dystonia is a multifactorial and multidisciplinary challenge. Providing an overview about available treatment options, describing synergistic effects and outlining strategies to approach this challenge is the goal of this book. It is based on the congress series 'International Congress on Treatment of Dystonia' taking place every three years in Hannover, Germany.

All chapters are grouped around several general topics. Each chapter can be read individually. Within the chapters, reference to other chapters of the book will be provided. Some overlap between chapters may occur. However, that will allow the reader to recognise nuanced differences in the way our authors interpret their topics.

We hope that we will provide the reader with a concise and up-to-date overview about the fascinating topic of treatment of dystonia.

Enjoy your reading as much as we enjoyed pulling together this book for you!

Dirk Dressler
Eckart Altenmüller
Joachim K. Krauss

Hannover, January 2018

Chapter 1

Development of the Concept of Dystonia as a Disease, a Syndrome and a Movement Phenomenology

Stanley Fahn

Origin of the Word 'Dystonia' and its Definition

The term dystonia was coined by Oppenheim (Oppenheim 1911; Klein & Fahn 2013) in his 1911 article describing four children with a condition not previously seen by him. Oppenheim called this syndrome by two different names: 'dystonia musculorum deformans' and 'dysbasia lordotica progressiva'. The first name relates to the spasms and to the postural deformities that develop in these children; the second name emphasises the dromedary gait and the progressive nature of the illness. Of importance, Oppenheim recognised this was an organic disorder and not one of psychogenic aetiology. Because of Oppenheim's fame worldwide as a leading neurologist, this disorder was recognised and neurologists began to use 'dystonia musculorum deformans'. Oppenheim coined the term dystonia to indicate that in this disorder there would be hypotonia on one occasion and tonic muscle spasms on another, usually but not exclusively elicited on volitional movements. Oppenheim also described twisted postures associated with muscle spasms that affected limbs and trunk; bizarre walking with bending and twisting of the torso; rapid, sometimes rhythmic jerking movements; and progression of symptoms, leading eventually to sustained fixed postural deformities. Whereas Oppenheim emphasised fluctuating muscle tone, none of the subsequent definitions of dystonia considered the presence of hypotonia very important. Rather, sustained and twisting movements were the dominant features that characterised a number of subsequent definitions of dystonia (Fahn 2011). In 1984, the Dystonia Medical Research Foundation established an ad hoc committee to develop an encompassing definition of 'dystonia' and a classification for the disorder. The committee consisted of (in alphabetical order): André Barbeau, Donald B. Calne, Stanley Fahn, C. David Marsden, John Menkes and G. Frederick Wooten. The committee met in February 1984 and proposed the following definition: 'Dystonia is a syndrome of sustained muscle contractions, frequently causing twisting and repetitive movements, or abnormal postures' (Fahn et al. 1987). This definition had been uniformly accepted until supplanted by the 2013 consensus definition (Albanese et al. 2013). This newer definition expanded the previous one from a single sentence into three sentences: 'Dystonia is a movement disorder characterized by sustained or intermittent muscle contractions causing abnormal, often repetitive, movements, postures, or both. Dystonic movements are typically patterned, twisting, and may be tremulous. Dystonia is often initiated or worsened by voluntary action and associated with overflow muscle activation.'

The Years Before Oppenheim

There were descriptions of dystonia prior to Oppenheim's publication, but since the term *dystonia* was not yet coined, different terminologies were used. For example, the focal dystonia of writer's cramp was recognised and called Schreibkrampf (Germany), crampe des écrivains (France) and scrivener's palsy (UK) (Pearce 2005). Blepharospasm was recognised, as well as the combination of cranial and cervical dystonia (Wood 1887; Meige 1910). In 1871, Hammond (Hammond 1871) coined the term 'athetosis' (Greek for 'without fixed position') for mobile spasms. Athetosis is now recognised as either writhing movements of dystonia or as a combination of dystonia with chorea. In 1893, Gowers (Gowers 1893) called generalised dystonia *tetanoid chorea* in a patient subsequently found to have Wilson's disease. Desterac (de Toulouse 1901) called cervical dystonia *spasmodic torticollis and functional spasms.* Leszynsky (1903) called the abnormal gait of dystonia a hysterical gait. Ramsay Hunt (1908) referred to generalised dystonia as myoclonia of the trunk, but after Oppenheim's paper, recognised it as dystonia (Hunt 1916). Schwalbe, a psychiatry trainee under Ziehen, reported on the Lewin family, calling it *maladie des tics and tonic cramps with hysterical symptoms* three years before Oppenheim's paper (Schwalbe 1908; Truong & Fahn 1988). This family was subsequently reported in at least eight different articles in the literature (summarised by Eldridge 1970).

The Years Immediately After Oppenheim's Publication

In the same year of Oppenheim's publication, Ziehen, the psychiatrist mentor of Schwalbe (Schwalbe 1908), also described the Lewin family; he called the condition *tonic torsion neurosis* (Ziehen 1911). Two Polish neurologists, Flatau and Sterling (Flatau & Sterling 1911), described their patients later that same year and rejected the notion of varying muscle tone as the distinguishing feature of dystonia in favour of the presence of twisting muscle spasms, calling it *progressive torsion spasm.* Flatau and Sterling also mentioned heredity as a factor in the disorder. The worldwide reputation of Oppenheim as an astute clinical neurologist helped in spreading knowledge about dystonia; immediately after his article was published, neurologists began publishing their own cases and preferred the name 'dystonia musculorum deformans' over the other offer of 'dysbasia lordotica progressiva' (Fraenkel 1912; Hunt 1916; Hallock & Frink 1917; Keschner 1918; Maas 1918; Mendel 1919; Abrahmson 1920; Frauenthal & Rosenheck 1920; Taylor 1920; Wechsler & Brock 1922). Mendel (1919) summarised all cases published up to 1919, and recognised the twisting nature of the movements and postures, suggested the term 'torsion dystonia', seeing it as a disease entity and distinguishing it from other abnormal movements (chorea, myoclonus, athetosis, hysteria).

Recognition of Secondary Dystonia, Leading to the Concept of Dystonia as a Syndrome Rather Than a Disease

In the year after Oppenheim's paper came the publication by Wilson of progressive lenticular degeneration (Wilson 1912), now known as Wilson's disease. Dystonia usually develops in this disorder. By the end of that decade came the pandemics of encephalitis lethargica, resulting often in postencephalitic parkinsonism and dystonia. In addition to these two dystonic disorders, many children with cerebral palsy manifested athetosis and dystonia. The realisation of symptomatic causes of dystonic movements and postures led to the belief by many that dystonia is a syndrome and not a specific disease entity. This concept was discussed by Wimmer at the Tenth International Neurological Reunion in Paris in 1929 (Wimmer 1929) and was widely accepted.

Resurrection of Dystonia as a Disease Entity and Not Just a Syndrome

Beginning in the 1920s and extending through the 1930s and early 1940s, dystonia was regarded as a manifestation of a number of disorders, that is, merely a clinical feature in disorders affecting the basal ganglia. Meynert (1871) first suggested that the basal ganglia were involved in disorders of abnormal movement. The concept of an *extrapyramidal system* and of *extrapyramidal diseases* was developed by Kinnier Wilson (1912, 1925). Wilson was referring to anatomical pathways related to the basal ganglia (extrapyramidal system) and the disorders that emanate from them when they are afflicted (extrapyramidal diseases). He emphasised that these disorders have three cardinal types of clinical phenomenology: variability of muscle tone (dystonia), involuntary movements and the seeming absence of true paralysis (Wilson 1925). Fahn (2011) subsequently explained the problems with using the term 'extrapyramidal'. (1) The basal ganglia have intimate connections with the pyramidal tract system and therefore the basal ganglia are not truly extrapyramidal. (2) There are other descending pathways through the spinal cord, such as vestibulospinal and reticulospinal pathways and technically these should also be called 'extrapyramidal', yet these are not related to the basal ganglia. (3) There are disorders of abnormal movement not associated with any basal ganglia pathology, such as myoclonus and ataxia, and therefore these would not fall under a term that originally referred to basal ganglia disorders. That is why Fahn coined the term *movement disorders* in 1968 to accommodate all conditions with abnormal movements (see Fahn 2011 for historical details).

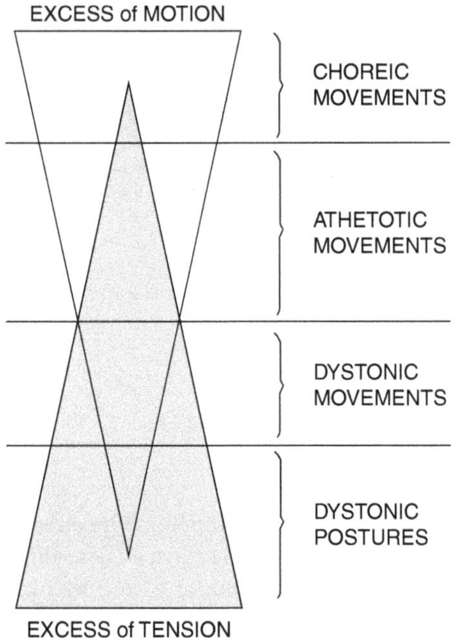

Figure 1.1 Figure from Herz (1944a) comparing excess tension and excess movement in different abnormal involuntary movements.

With this background of dystonia being regarded solely as a syndrome as its place in neurology at that time, Ernst Herz published a massive review of dystonia in a trilogy of back-go-back papers (Herz 1944a, 1944b, 1944c) describing his observations of dystonia, analysis of motion pictures of abnormal movement disorders and review of the literature. Among other contributions in these papers, Herz showed EMG samples of dystonic movements repeatedly showing simultaneous firing of agonist and antagonist muscles, whereas he demonstrated that in chorea there is only contractions of agonist muscles. Herz also compared dystonic movements and postures with athetosis and chorea by explaining their relationships to excess tension and excess movement (Figure 1.1). Herz concluded that in addition to dystonia being a manifestation of some disorders, and thus a syndrome, it can also be a specific disease entity. He said the diagnosis of 'dystonia' as a disease entity should be made only in cases with the following characteristics: (a) selective systemic symptoms in the form of dystonic movements and postures; and (b) gradual development, without recognisable aetiologic factors at the onset.

Herz emphasised that dystonic movements are slow, long-sustained turning movements; but he also mentioned the presence of rapid spasms sometimes seen in this disorder, calling them myoclonia and tic twitchings. For the more regular, rhythmic movements sometimes seen, he used the term *myorhythmia*. Today, myorhythmia has been used differently by different authors. Monrad-Krohn and Refsum (1958) and Masucci et al. (1984) used the term *myorhythmia* to label what is today called rhythmic myoclonias such as palatal myoclonus. But this use seems to have been abandoned today. Perhaps the most recent use of the term myorhythmia is for the slow-moving, repetitive, synchronous, rhythmic contractions in ocular, facial, masticatory and other muscles in Whipple disease, which have been called *oculofaciomasticatory myorhythmia* (Schwartz et al. 1986; Hausser-Hauw 1988; Tison et al. 1992).

The Definition of Dystonia Continued to Change Even After Herz's Contribution

Following Herz's massive review of dystonia in 1944 (Herz 1944a, 1944b, 1944c), neurologists accepted that dystonia can be a disease entity as well as a feature in several syndromes. But over time, different definitions for dystonia as an abnormal movement emerged. Denny-Brown, a respected neurologist and neurophysiologist, suggested dystonia should be applied to any posture with a fixed or relatively fixed attitude (Denny-Brown 1965). The problem with this definition is that it is too broad and could be applied to the fixed postures seen after hemiplegic strokes, for example. That is probably why Denny-Brown's definition never caught on. At the time the first international symposium on dystonia was convened in New York in 1975, Fahn and Eldridge proposed dystonic movements to be sustained, involuntary, twisting movements which could be fast or slow (Fahn & Eldridge 1976). These authors were troubled by the confusion caused by the term dystonia being used for both the movement phenomenology and the syndromes or disorders producing dystonic movements. Fahn and Eldridge therefore suggested that the term 'torsion dystonia' be used as the name for the disease entity, and 'dystonia' for the abnormal movements. But this separation never caught on and dystonia continued to be used for the movements and for the disease and syndrome.

At that first international symposium in 1975 another major advance was immediately accepted. This was C. David Marsden's analysis that dystonia does not need to be applied to just those people with generalised dystonia, but can be equally applied to focal and segmental dystonias (Marsden 1976). Marsden discussed in particular blepharospasm, oromandibular dystonia, writer's cramp, torticollis and axial dystonia. Prior to this paper, it was common to consider the focal and segmental dystonias as formes fruste, as was done in the epidemiology studies of Zeman and Dycken (Zeman & Dyken 1967). This symposium also contributed the publication by Lillian Lee and colleagues (1976) of X-linked recessive dystonia-parkinsonism found on the Island of Panay in the Philippines and the first English presentations of dopa-responsive dystonia by Masaya Segawa and colleagues (1976). At the symposium, Allen and Knopp (1976) presented a Caucasian family with this form of autosomal dominant dystonia.

The year after this international symposium, the first research-oriented foundation involved specifically with dystonia was established by the husband-and-wife team of Sam and Frances Belzberg from Vancouver, British Columbia in Canada, calling it the Dystonia Medical Research Foundation (DMRF). With an influx of funds from the Belzbergs, research grants were awarded to investigators with excellent grant applications. Two of the early concerns of the foundation were to have a uniformly accepted definition and classification of dystonia. As described above in the opening paragraph, an ad hoc committee was formed and it came up with the definition of 'Dystonia is a syndrome of sustained muscle contractions, frequently causing twisting and repetitive movements, or abnormal postures' (Fahn et al. 1987). This definition lasted until it was expanded in 2013 to 'Dystonia is a movement disorder characterized by sustained or intermittent muscle contractions causing abnormal, often repetitive, movements, postures, or both. Dystonic movements are typically patterned, twisting, and may be tremulous. Dystonia is often initiated or worsened by voluntary action and associated with overflow muscle activation', also presented in the opening paragraph above.

Classification Schemes for Dystonia

As the definition of dystonia has changed over time, the classification of dystonias has evolved as well. At the first international symposium on dystonia in 1975, Fahn and Eldridge (Fahn & Eldridge 1976) presented a classification based on aetiology, dividing the dystonias into idiopathic (familial and sporadic), secondary (heredodegenerative and environmental) and psychological (considered rare at that time). At the same symposium, Marsden et al. (1976) proposed a classification based on bodily distribution (focal, segmental and generalised). The ad hoc committee on definition and classification of dystonia formed by the DMRF met in 1984 (see above paragraph) and recommended a classification that included age at onset (because prognosis of dystonia was highly dependent on this factor), bodily distribution (expanded on the formulation of Marsden and colleagues (1976)) and aetiology. The triple parallel classification scheme was published by Fahn et al. a few years later (Fahn et al. 1987).

This parallel classification approach has been maintained but tweaked in subsequent attempts to improve the classification of dystonia. Fahn et al. (1998) added a new aetiologic category, dystonia-plus, to distinguish these non-degenerative dystonias that have an additional movement disorder component (e.g. parkinsonism and myoclonus) from primary dystonias (which are pure dystonia with the exception that tremor can be present). The dystonia-plus disorders include myoclonus-dystonia and dopa-responsive dystonia, among others. In 2011, a fifth aetiologic category was included to incorporate the dystonias seen as a component of other well-recognised movement disorders, such as Parkinson's disease, progressive supranuclear palsy, corticobasalganglionic degeneration, tics and the paroxysmal dyskinesias (Fahn et al. 2011).

The classification of dystonia received a major overhaul by the consensus committee in 2013 (Albanese et al. 2013), which classified dystonia into two major axes: Clinical Features and Aetiology. But the classification scheme is more complicated than just two major axes because there are five individual parallel classifications within Clinical Features and two parallel classifications within Aetiology, namely (1) neuropathology and (2) listing whether the disorder is inherited, acquired or idiopathic. Thus, there are actually seven parallel sections in this new classification scheme. Although more detailed than all previous classifications, the latest one avoids ambiguity and overlap when all seven categories are utilised (Albanese et al. 2013).

Other Developments in Dystonia

Over the 100 years since Oppenheim coined the term dystonia, there have been countless research studies that have shed light on epidemiology, pathology and genetics of dystonia. Each of these topics is too huge to cover in this chapter. Advances in therapy, particularly the application of botulinum toxin and the development of deep brain stimulation with specific targets to reduce dystonia, have been momentous and have provided much benefit for people with dystonia. Much remains to be done, however, and judging by past developments, the future holds great promise for exciting new advances in understanding and treating dystonia.

References

Abrahmson I. 1920. Presentation of case of familial dystonia musculorum of Oppenheim. *J Nerv Ment Dis* 51:451.

Albanese A, Bhatia K, Bressman SB, Delong MR, Fahn S, Fung VS, Hallett M, Jankovic J, Jinnah HA, Klein C, Lang AE, Mink JW, Teller JK. 2013. Phenomenology and classification of dystonia: a consensus update. *Mov Disord* 28:863–873.

Allen N, Knopp W. 1976. Hereditary parkinsonismdystonia with sustained control by L-dopa and anticholinergic medication. *Adv Neurol* 14:201–213.

de Toulouse Destarac. 1901. Torticolis spasmodique et spasmes fonctionnels. *Rev Neurol* 9:591–597.

Denny-Brown D. 1965. The nature of dystonia. *Bull NY Acad Med* 41:858–869.

Eldridge R. 1970. The torsion dystonias: literature review and genetic and clinical studies. *Neurology* 20(11), Part 2:1–78.

Fahn S. 2011. Classification of movement disorders. *Mov Disord* 26:947–957.

Fahn S, Eldridge R. 1976. Definition of dystonia and classification of the dystonic states. In: *Dystonia. Adv Neurol.* New York, Raven Press; 14:1–5.

Fahn S, Marsden CD, Calne DB. 1987. Classification and investigation of dystonia. In: Marsden CD, Fahn S (eds) *Movement Disorders 2.* London, Butterworths:332–358.

Fahn S, Bressman SB, Marsden CD. 1998. Classification of dystonia. In: Fahn S, Marsden CD, DeLong MR (eds) *Dystonia 3. Adv Neurol.* Philadelphia, Lippincott-Raven Pub.; 78:1–10.

Fahn S, Jankovic J, Hallett M. 2011. *Principles and Practice of Movement Disorders*, 2nd ed. Edinburgh, Saunders Elsevier, p. 267.

Flatau E, Sterling W. 1911. Progressiver Torsionspasmus bei Kindern. *Z Gesamte Neurol Psychiatr* 7:586–612.

Fraenkel J. 1912. Dysbasia lordotica progressiva, dystonia musculorum deformans – tortipelvis. *J Nerv Ment Dis* 39:361–374.

Frauenthal HW, Rosenheck C. 1920. Dystonia musculorum deformans with a report of a case. *J Nerv Ment Dis* 52:134.

Gowers WR. 1893. *A Manual of Diseases of the Nervous System*, 2nd ed. Philadelphia, Blakiston; 2:709–710.

Hallock FM, Frink HW. 1917. Case of dystonia musculorum. *J Nerv Ment Dis* 45:348.

Hammond WA. 1871. *A Treatise on Diseases of the Nervous System.* New York, D. Appleton.

Hausser-Hauw C, Roullet E, Robert R, Marteau R. 1988. Oculo-facio-skeletal myorhythmia as a cerebral complication of systemic Whipple's disease. *Mov Disord* 3:179–184.

Herz E. 1944a. Dystonia. I. Historical review: analysis of dystonic symptoms and physiologic mechanisms involved. *Arch Neurol Psychiatry* 51:305–318.

Herz E. 1944b. Dystonia. II. Clinical classification. *Arch Neurol Psychiat* 51:319–355.

Herz E. 1944c. Dystonia. III. Pathology and conclusions. *Arch Neurol Psychiat* 52:20–26.

Hunt JR. 1908. A case of myoclonia of the trunk muscles improved by psychophysical therapeutics. *J Nerv Ment Dis* 35:656–657.

Hunt JR. 1916. The progressive torsion spasm of childhood (dystonia musculorum deformans): a consideration of its nature and symptomatology. *JAMA* 67:1430–1437.

Keschner M. 1918. Dystonia musculorum deformans: report of a case and a review of the literature. *J Nerv Ment Dis* 47:103.

Klein C, Fahn S. 2013. Translation of Oppenheim's 1911 paper on dystonia. *Mov Disord* 28:851–862.

Lee LV, Pascasio FM, Fuentes FD, Viterbo GH. 1976. Torsion dystonia in Panay, Philippines. In: Eldrige R, Fahn S (eds) *Dystonia. Adv Neurol.* New York, Raven Press; 14:137–151.

Leszynsky W. 1903. Hysterical gait. *J Nerv Ment Dis* 30:33–34.

Maas O. 1918. Zur Kenntnis des Verlaufs der Dystonia musculorum deformans. *Neurol Zhl* 37:199.

Marsden CD. 1976. The problem of adult-onset idiopathic torsion dystonia and other isolated dyskinesias in adult life (including blepharospasm, oromandibular dystonia, dystonic writer's cramp, and torticollis, or axial dystonia). In: Eldrige R, Fahn S (eds) *Dystonia. Adv Neurol.* New York, Raven Press; 14:259–276.

Marsden CD, Harrison MJG, Bundey S. 1976. Natural history of idiopathic torsion dystonia. In: Eldrige R, Fahn S (eds) *Dystonia. Adv Neurol.* New York, Raven Press; 14:177–187.

Masucci EF, Kurtzke JF, Saini N. 1984. Myorhythmia: a widespread movement disorder – clinicopathological correlations. *Brain* 107:53–79.

Meige H. 1910. Les convulsion de le face, une forme clinique de convulsion faciale bilateral et mediane. *Rev Neurol* 21:437–443.

Mendel K. 1919. Torsiondystonie (Dystonia musculorum deformans, Torsionsspasmus). *Mschr Psychiat Neurol* 46:309–361.

Meynert T. 1871. Beiträge zur Differentialdiagnose des paralytischen Irrsinns. *Wiener Med Presse* 11:645–647.

Monrad-Krohn GH, Refsum S. 1958. *The Clinical Examination of the Nervous System.* 11th ed. New York, Paul B. Hoeber, p. 108.

Oppenheim H. 1911. Über eine eigenartige Krampfkrankheit des kindlichen und jugendlichen Alters (Dysbasia lordotica progressiva, Dystonia musculorum deformans). *Neurol Centrabl* 30:1090–1107.

Pearce JMS. 2005. A note on scrivener's palsy. *J Neurol Neurosurg Psych* 76:513.

Schwalbe W. 1908. Eine eigentümliche tonische Krampfform mit hysterischen Symptomen. Inaug Diss, Berlin, G. Schade.

Schwartz NA, Selhorst JB, Ochs AL, Beck RW, Campbell WW, Harris JK, Waters B, Velasco ME. 1986. Oculomasticatory myorhythmia: a unique movement disorder occurring in Whipple's disease. *Ann Neurol* 20:677–683.

Segawa M, Hosaka A, Miyagawa F, Nomura Y, Imai H. 1976. Hereditary progressive dystonia with marked diurnal fluctuation. In: Eldrige R, Fahn S (eds) *Dystonia. Adv Neurol.* New York, Raven Press; 14:215–233.

Taylor EW. 1920. Dystonia lenticularis (dystonia musculorum deformans). *Arch Neurol Psychia (Chic)* 4:417.

Tison F, Louvetgiendaj C, Henry P, Lagueny A, Gaujard E. 1992. Permanent bruxism as a manifestation of the oculo-facial syndrome related to systemic Whipple's disease. *Mov Disord* 7:82–85.

Truong DD, Fahn S. 1988. An early description of dystonia: translation of Schwalbe's thesis and information on his life. *Adv Neurol* 50:651–664.

Wechsler IS, Brock S. 1922. Dystonia Musculorum Deformans with especial reference to a myostatic form and the occurrence of decerebrate rigidity phenomena: a study of six cases. *Arch Neurol Psychiat* 8:538–552.

Wilson SAK. 1912. Progressive lenticular degeneration: a familial nervous system disease associated with cirrhosis of the liver. *Brain* 34:295–509.

Wilson SAK. 1925. The Croonian Lectures on some disorders of motility and of muscle tone, with special reference to the corpus striatum. Lecture I. *Lancet* 206(2):1–10.

Wimmer A. 1929. Le spasme de torsion. *Rev Neurol* 36:904–915.

Wood HC. 1887. *Nervous Diseases and their Diagnostics*. Philadelphia, Lippincott.

Zeman W, Dyken P. 1967. Dystonia musculorum deformans: clinical, genetic and pathoanatomical studies. *Psychiatr Neurol Neurochir* 70:77–121.

Ziehen T. 1911. Ein fall von tonischer Torsionsneurose. *Neurol Centrabl* 30:109–110.

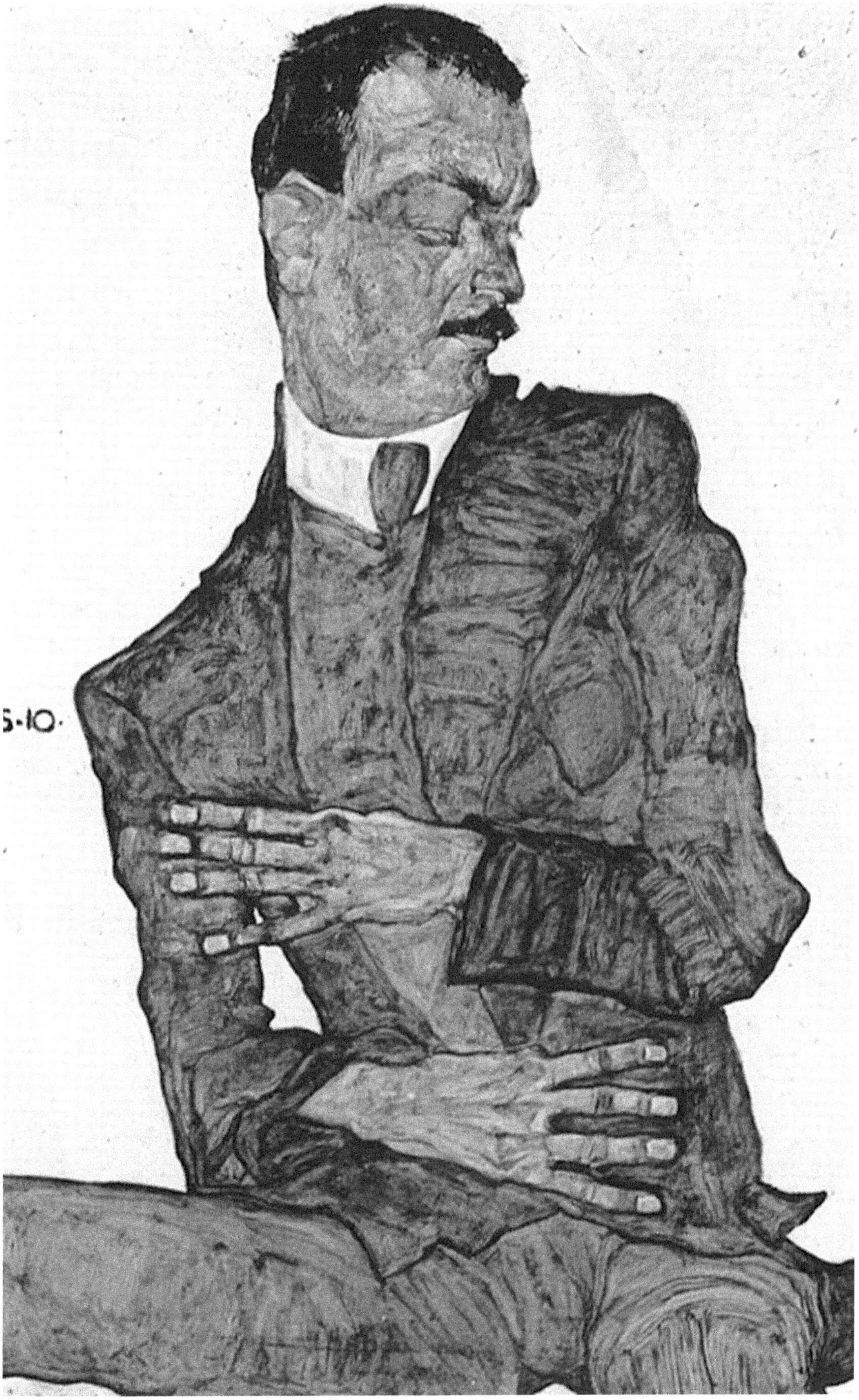
S·10·

Chapter 2

Classification of Dystonia

Alberto Albanese and Stefania Lalli

There has long been a need to update the classification of dystonia. This movement disorder has historically been considered at the same time a symptom and collection of syndromes. Knowledge about dystonias has greatly developed since the seminal description of *Dystonia musculorum deformans* by Oppenheim (Oppenheim 1911). In recent years, the phenomenology of dystonia has been defined and several new genetic forms have been described. The traditional concept of 'primary dystonia' encompassing both phenomenological and aetiological definitions was no longer tenable. In 2013 a new classification of dystonia was released after a two-year work based on consensus of dystonia experts (Albanese et al. 2013). We describe here the mainstay of the new classification and provide some critical comments for its implementation.

Historical View

The classification of dystonia syndromes has evolved over time, partly reflecting increased understanding of the various aetiologies and clinical presentations, and also varied opinions on the criteria used for grouping disorders together.

Since its first descriptions in the late nineteenth century there has been continuous debate about the nosologic classification and aetiology of dystonia syndromes. Although the first account of dystonia probably dates back to Gowers, it was Oppenheim who drew international attention to this new entity, by reporting four young patients (Oppenheim 1911). He coined the term 'dystonia musculorum deformans' to indicate that 'muscle tone was hypotonic at one occasion and in tonic muscle spasm at another, usually, but not exclusively, elicited upon voluntary movements'.

In June 1975, at the First International Dystonia Symposium, David Marsden proposed lumping together under the general heading of dystonia the focal forms of dystonia, already known as blepharospasm, Meige syndrome, torticollis and writer's cramp (Marsden 1976). In 1984, an ad hoc committee convened by the Dystonia Medical Research Foundation provided the first consensus definition of dystonia as follows: 'a syndrome consisting of sustained muscle contractions, frequently causing twisting and repetitive movements, or abnormal postures' (Fahn et al. 1987). This definition has been generally retained as the first general description for dystonia.

The classification of dystonia has evolved over time. Fahn and Eldridge (1976) first distinguished primary dystonia (with or without a hereditary pattern) from secondary dystonia (with other hereditary neurological conditions or due to known environmental cause), and psychological forms of dystonia. Subsequently, Fahn, Marsden and Calne proposed a classification of dystonia based on three axes: age at onset, distribution and aetiology (Fahn et al. 1987). The aetiological classification was later refined with the proposal of a dichotomous distinction between primary and secondary forms (Bressman 2004). The European Federation of Neurological Societies guidelines further distinguished the aetiology of dystonia syndromes as primary, heredodegenerative and secondary (or symptomatic) (Albanese et al. 2011).

While these clinical classifications were developed, a parallel classification system was developed based on discovery of new dystonia loci or genes, that were named DYTn (currently from DYT1 to DYT27) and listed in genetic databases (Klein 2014). The DYTn listing cannot be considered a classification system for dystonia, as it does not contain a comprehensive assemblage of all dystonia forms and is not helpful for clinical assessment.

Unsettled Issues With Earlier Classifications of Dystonia

The term 'primary' dystonia, although historically consistently used, carried some inherent implications. In dystonia, this term was most often used to describe phenotypes of relatively pure forms of dystonia, not associated with other neurological features and without evidence of pathological abnormalities. However, tremor occurs in a large proportion of patients with primary dystonia and there has been increasing recognition of associated neurological or psychiatric features indicating that the phenomenology is not purely motor. Bridging terms such as 'dystonia-plus' were introduced to acknowledge specific syndromes where dystonia predominated, combined with other neurological features, such as myoclonus or parkinsonism, in the absence of neuronal degeneration. Thus the category of 'primary' dystonia indicated at the same time isolated dystonia and no appreciable degeneration, whereas 'dystonia-plus' was employed for the coexistence of non-dystonic features (e.g. parkinsonism) and a degenerative nature of the condition.

The term 'secondary' dystonia also lacked clarity, as it was antithetical to primary and indicated non-isolated dystonia, a defined pathology or more generally a known aetiology. These varied meanings led to inconsistencies, with the term 'secondary dystonia' sometimes referring to any dystonia that is not primary, sometimes to any dystonia with a known cause, and sometimes only to acquired dystonias. Terms such as 'heredodegenerative' used in existing aetiological classification systems were problematic for many reasons. Some of the disorders typically positioned in this category were degenerative but not hereditary, such as sporadic Parkinson's disease. Other disorders were inherited, but there was no evidence for any degenerative process, such as Lesch–Nyhan disease. The 'heredodegenerative' label also did not appear applicable for the large group of neurodevelopmental disorders with dystonia, such as dystonic cerebral palsy.

The DYTn scheme was based historically on a sequentially numbered list of assigned genetic loci, rather than a classification system with an aetiological meaning. A further flaw with the DYTn nomenclature scheme was that it implied that disorders with a DYTn assignment were dystonic in nature. This is not necessarily the case. Disorders such as myoclonus-dystonia (DYT11) may be dominated by myoclonus, and have a DYTn designation because there is no locus naming convention for genetic myoclonus. Other disorders, such as Lubag (DYT3) and rapid-onset dystonia-parkinsonism (DYT12), in some patients may be dominated by parkinsonism rather than dystonia. The heterogeneous listing under the DYTn umbrella has uncertain value for exploring the biological bases for dystonia. Moreover, many disorders where dystonia is both a consistent and dominant feature of the clinical phenotype were described and given locus assignments before the DYTn convention was developed. As a result, these disorders lack DYTn designations. Examples of dystonic disorders laying outside the DYTn listing include Wilson's disease, Lesch–Nyhan disease, glutaric aciduria and deafness-dystonia syndrome.

New Definition and Current Classification

In May 2011 an international Consensus Committee was set up to provide a consensus on classification of dystonia as well as on terminology of dystonic disorders. Dystonia is now defined as:

> A movement disorder characterized by sustained or intermittent muscle contractions, causing abnormal, often repetitive, movements, postures or both. Dystonic movements are typically patterned, twisting and may be tremulous. Dystonia is often initiated or worsened by voluntary action and associated with overflow muscle activation.

This definition improves and expands the previous definition by summarising the relevant features of dystonia, particularly the combination of dystonic postures and dystonic movements, the tremulous nature of dystonic movements and the specific relationship of dystonia with voluntary movement. In most cases, dystonia combines abnormal movements and postures. Some forms of dystonia, such as blepharospasm and laryngeal dystonia, are not associated with postures, but are characterised by focal involuntary contractions that interfere with physiological opening or closing of the eyelids or the larynx.

The revised definition attempts to exclude such conditions that may mimic dystonia, which are also called 'pseudodystonias' (Fahn et al. 1998). In general, the pseudodystonias have a known or presumed cause that is thought to differ from the causes of the broader dystonia group. Some typical examples are: dystonic (tonic) tics, head tilt (vestibulopathy, trochlear nerve palsy), bent spine, camptocormia, scoliosis, atlanto-axial and shoulder subluxation, Arnold-Chiari malformation, congenital muscular torticollis, congenital Klippel-Feil syndrome and Sandifer syndrome (Albanese et al. 2013).

The new classification of dystonia has greatly innovated clinical usage. Two axes have been identified. Axis I depicts clinical features and provides a synthetic snapshot of the patient's clinical condition at a given moment. Axis II identifies aetiology based on anatomical alterations, or identified abnormalities.

Axis I: Clinical Features

This axis describes the patient's phenomenology at a given moment (Figure 2.1). Five descriptors are utilised in this axis: age at onset, body distribution, temporal pattern, coexistence of other movement disorders, and other neurological manifestations (Table 2.1).

Age at Onset

Classification by age is clinically important for both diagnostic testing and prognostic value. Dystonia that begins in childhood is more likely to have a discoverable cause, and to progress from focal to generalised. The new classification defines five age periods, from paediatric to adult: infancy (birth to two years); childhood (3–12 years); adolescence (13–20 years); early adulthood (21–40 years); late adulthood (40 years and older). Age at onset may give important clues to the underlying aetiology. Dystonia that emerges during the first year of life has a very high probability of being due to an inherited metabolic disorder with specific diagnostic implications and grave prognostic consequences. On the other hand, dystonia that emerges at 2–6 years of age might be more consistent with dystonic cerebral palsy, especially if it follows a period of developmental motor delay. Other dystonia syndromes, such as dopa-responsive dystonia, tend to emerge at 6–14 years of age. Finally, sporadic focal dystonia usually emerges after 50 years of age. In such context, several age categories focused on the most likely disorders occurring in each age group were proposed.

Body Distribution

Classification by body region is clinically important because of implications for diagnosis and therapy. For example, the diagnostic considerations in adult-onset focal dystonia are very different from those in young-onset generalised dystonia. Body regions involved by dystonia are the upper or lower cranial region, the cervical region, the larynx, the trunk, the upper or lower limbs. These different territories may be involved individually or in different combinations. The treatment of choice for focal and segmental dystonias involves botulinum neurotoxins, while for generalised dystonias more often involves

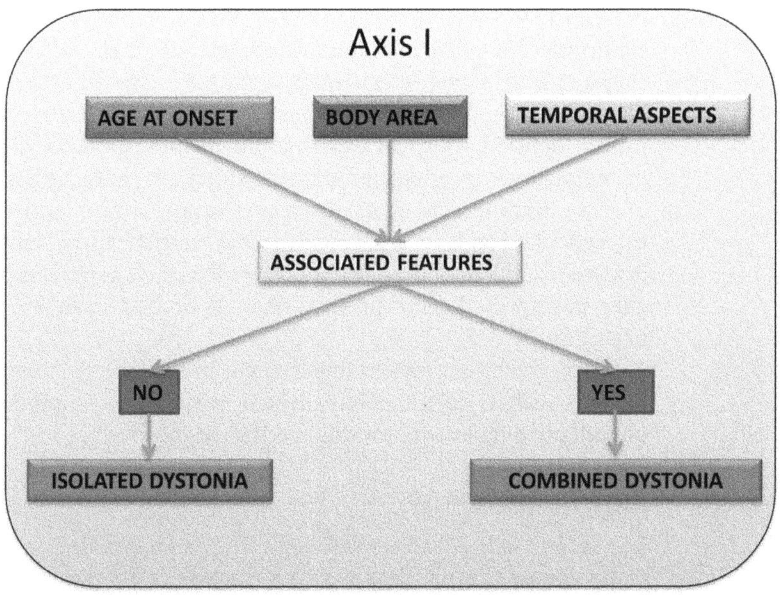

Figure 2.1 Axis I guides on the recognition of the phenomenology of dystonia and of the prevalent phenotypical pattern driving the search of a specific aetiology.

medications or surgery. Describing the body distribution has a relevant clinical value, including the possibility to evaluate spread of motor symptoms over time. The body distribution may change over time, typically with progression to the involvement of previously uninvolved sites.

Distribution is focal when only one body region is affected. Typical examples of focal forms are blepharospasm, oromandibular dystonia, cervical dystonia, laryngeal dystonia and writer's cramp. Cervical dystonia is considered a form of focal dystonia, although by convention the shoulder can be included as well as the neck.

In segmental distribution two or more contiguous body regions are affected. Typical examples of segmental forms are: cranial dystonia (blepharospasm with lower facial and jaw or tongue involvement) or bi-brachial dystonia.

Distribution is multifocal when two non-contiguous or more (contiguous or not) body regions are involved.

In generalised distribution the trunk and at least two other sites are involved. Generalised forms with leg involvement are distinguished from those without leg involvement.

In patients with hemidystonia, more body regions restricted to one body side are involved. Typical examples of hemidystonia are due to acquired brain lesions in the contralateral hemisphere.

Temporal Pattern

Dystonia phenomenology can evolve with disease progression or display momentary or daily variability in relation to voluntary actions, external triggers, compensatory phenomena, alleviating manoeuvres (gestes antagonistes) or psychological state. Variability allows separating dystonia that consistently occurs under the same conditions, be it task-specific, action-specific or spontaneous, from variable forms of dystonia (diurnal and paroxysmal). Paroxysmal dystonia should be distinguished from dystonia always triggered by the same activity or action (i.e. task-specific dystonia). In paroxysmal dystonia, the same trigger on different occasions might or might not induce an attack, whereas in action dystonia (including task-specific) the same motor activity will predictably induce dystonia. Paroxysmal dystonia typically lasts after the trigger has ended, while action (or task-specific) dystonia is no longer evident when the inducing action is completed. Disease course can be either static or progressive.

The variability can have four different patterns. Persistent: dystonia that persists to approximately the same extent throughout the day. Action-specific: dystonia that occurs only during a particular activity or task. Diurnal fluctuations: dystonia fluctuates during the day, with recognisable circadian variations in occurrence, severity and phenomenology. Paroxysmal: sudden self-limited episodes of dystonia usually induced by a trigger with return to pre-existing neurological state.

Associated Features

Current terminology classifies conditions where dystonia is the sole motor feature (apart from tremor) as 'isolated dystonia', while 'combined dystonia' refers to dystonias with other accompanying movement disorders.

Isolated or Combined Dystonia

Dystonia may occur in isolation or in combination with other movement disorders. The resulting syndromes may give rise to recognisable associations, such as isolated dystonia or dystonia with myoclonus, parkinsonism or other movement disorders, etc. Isolated dystonia encompasses many cases previously described as 'pure' or 'primary', whereas most patients previously classified under 'dystonia-plus' or 'heredodegenerative' would now be classified as having combined dystonia. Unlike previous classifications, in the new classification the term isolated or combined refers to the phenomenology, and does not carry implications about the underlying aetiology.

Table 2.1 Classification of dystonia

Axis I	
Clinical characteristics of dystonia	
• Age at onset	Infancy (birth to 2 years) Childhood (3–12 years) Adolescence (13–20 years) Early adulthood (21–40 years) Late adulthood (>40 years)
• Body distribution	Focal Segmental Multifocal Generalised (with or without leg involvement) Hemidystonia
• Temporal pattern	Disease course: Static Progressive Variability: Persistent Action-specific Diurnal Paroxysmal
Associated features	
• Isolated dystonia or combined with another movement disorder	Isolated dystonia Combined dystonia
• Occurrence of other neurological or systemic manifestations	List of co-occurring neurological manifestations
Axis II	
Aetiology	
• Nervous system pathology	Evidence of degeneration Evidence of structural (often static) lesions No evidence of degeneration or structural lesion
• Inherited or acquired	Inherited Autosomal dominant Autosomal recessive X-linked recessive Mitochondrial Acquired Perinatal brain injury Infection Drug Toxic Vascular Neoplastic Brain injury Psychogenic Idiopathic Sporadic Familial

Occurrence of Other Neurological or Systemic Manifestations

The presence or absence of other neurologic or systemic features is a vital component for characterising dystonia syndromes. A full history and examination are required to determine whether there are non-motor components of the syndrome. Of particular importance are ophthalmological symptoms or signs, which may suggest specific disorders. The presence of visual symptoms and dystonia mandate a formal ophthalmological examination to look for evidence of optic nerve or retinal abnormalities that are characteristic of some inherited metabolic diseases. Corneal abnormalities, in particular Kayser–Fleischer rings characteristic of Wilson's disease, can also be present. The presence of a supranuclear gaze palsy, whether vertical, horizontal or both, can be a useful clue.

Central nervous system involvement in addition to motor features such as cognitive impairment, psychiatric symptoms or epilepsy might drive towards specific diagnosis.

Axis II: Aetiology

The second axis addresses aetiology. This is an evolving area, to be updated regularly as new information is obtained. The aetiology of many forms of dystonia is still not fully understood. Two complementary characteristics may be useful for classification: identifiable anatomical changes and pattern of inheritance. Anatomical causes can be investigated using brain imaging or by pathology. Inheritance differentiates inherited from acquired conditions by means of metabolic, genetic or other tests.

Nervous System Pathology

Evidence of degeneration, either at the gross, microscopic or molecular level, provides a useful means to discriminate subgroups of dystonia into degenerative and non-degenerative forms. Degeneration is defined as a progressive structural abnormality, such as neuronal loss. Static lesions are non-progressive neurodevelopmental anomalies or acquired lesions. Alternatively, there may be no evidence of degeneration or structural lesion.

Inherited or Acquired Dystonia

Inherited (dystonia forms of proven genetic origin). The DYT classification is retained here as a useful list for designating subtypes, but not as a classification system. With the advances in genetic technologies such as exome and whole-genome sequencing, new genes underlying dystonia will be discovered and idiopathic dystonia types will be reclassified in inherited forms once new genes are recognised. A general overview of some phenotypes and genotypes underlying 'isolated' and 'combined' inherited dystonia syndromes is summarised in Figure 2.2.

Acquired Dystonia due to a known specific cause, such as perinatal brain injury, infection, drugs, toxic substances, vascular causes, neoplasms, brain injury, psychogenic or functional origin.

Idiopathic Unknown cause (sporadic or familial). Many cases of focal or segmental isolated dystonia with onset in adulthood fall into this category.

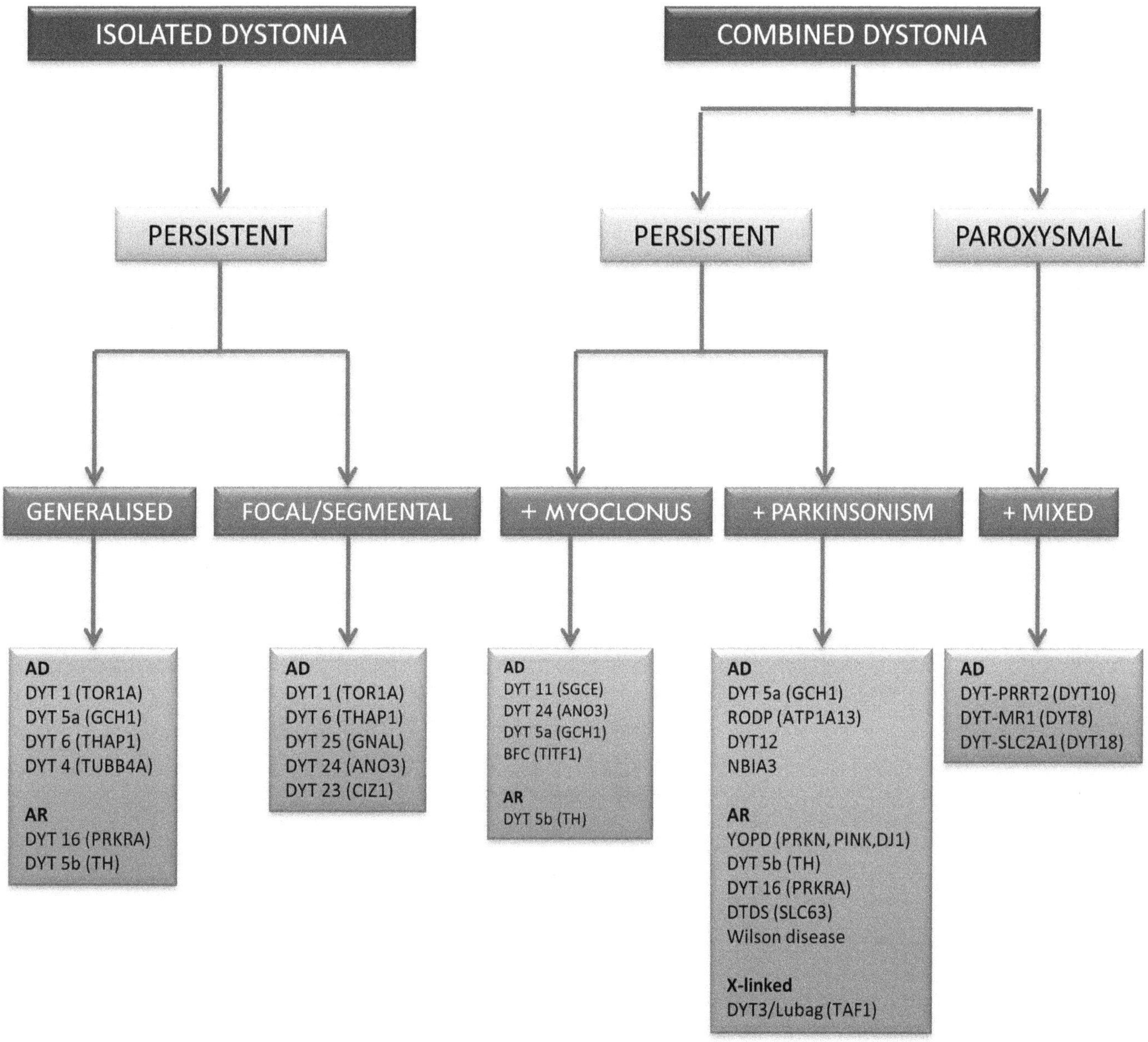

Figure 2.2 Overview of phenotypes and corresponding genotypes of hereditary forms of isolated and combined dystonia. Based on distribution of symptoms, dystonias can be further subdivided into isolated and combined (with other movement disorders) forms. According to the temporal pattern of the dystonia/dyskinesias, the latter are further grouped into persistent and paroxysmal. The paroxysmal forms of dystonia/dyskinesias present with a mixed pattern of hyperkinetic movement disorders (Klein 2014; Balint & Bhatia 2015). The underlying genes are given in parentheses. AD, autosomal dominant; AR, autosomal recessive; BHC, benign hereditary chorea; DTDS, dopamine transporter deficiency syndrome; RODP, rapid-onset dystonia-parkinsonism; YOPD, young-onset Parkinson's disease.

Conclusions

This new classification encompasses two axes, namely 'clinical characteristics' (Axis I) and 'aetiology' (Axis II). In this context, the clinical phenomenology (Axis I) could delineate a syndromic phenotypical pattern that will help in delineating dystonia aetiology (Figure 2.1).

The main changes from previous classifications are related to categories earlier determined by aetiology. The commonly used primary and secondary terms are not used in the new classification. Primary dystonia has been used either to refer to idiopathic dystonia or to name phenotypically isolated forms of dystonia, regardless of aetiology. For these reasons, the term 'primary' should be abandoned.

The recently proposed criteria may possibly meet resistance from the inertia of traditional habits and beliefs. However, these changes address numerous weaknesses in existing proposals for classification in a more clinically useful and biologically logical manner. Recently, a review of genetics of dystonias according to the clinical aspects of the new classification such as age at onset, if isolated or combined, and intermittent patterns has been published (Camargo et al. 2015).

In the systematic revision of the definition and classification, some issues were resolved only in part. First, the differentiation of pseudodystonia from dystonia needs further verification. The new definition should facilitate distinguishing true dystonia from look-alikes: once it is implemented in clinical practice, several pseudodystonias will be recognised to be different from true dystonia. Still, it may be possible that for the remaining forms better differentiation methods are required. Another, partially related, issue was where to place psychogenic dystonia in the aetiologic categorisation. Currently, it is listed among acquired forms, although psychogenic dystonia could be considered alternatively as a pseudodystonia. Another debated point was how to better characterise the presence of microscopic changes such as cell loss and degeneration. The development of molecular neuropathology will lead to the identification of more subtle features of neurodegenerative processes that may require improving the definition of neurodegeneration.

References

Albanese A, Asmus F, Bhatia KP, Elia AE, Elibol B, Filippini G, Gasser T, Krauss JK, Nardocci N, Newton A, Valls-Sole J. 2011. EFNS guidelines on diagnosis and treatment of primary dystonias. *Eur J Neurol* 18(1):5–18.

Albanese A, Bhatia K, Bressman SB, Delong MR, Fahn S, Fung VS, Hallett M, Jankovic J, Jinnah HA, Klein C, Lang AE, Mink JW, Teller JK. 2013. Phenomenology and classification of dystonia: a consensus update. *Mov Disord* 28(7):863–873.

Balint B, Bhatia KP. 2015. Isolated and combined dystonia syndromes: an update on new genes and their phenotypes. *Eur J Neurol* 22(4):610–617.

Bressman SB. 2004. Dystonia genotypes, phenotypes, and classification. *Adv Neurol* 94:101–107.

Camargo CH, Camargos ST, Cardoso FE, Teive HA. 2015. The genetics of the dystonias: a review based on the new classification of the dystonias. *Arq Neuropsiquiatr* 73(4):350–358.

Fahn S. 1988. Concept and classification of dystonia. *Adv Neurol* 50:1–8.

Fahn S, Eldridge R. 1976. Definition of dystonia and classification of the dystonic states. *Adv Neurol* 14:1–5.

Fahn S, Marsden C, Calne D. 1987. Classification and investigation of dystonia. In: *Movement Disorders 2*. Marsden CD and Fahn S, editors. London: Butterworths. 332–358.

Fahn S, Bressman SB, Marsden CD. 1998. Classification of dystonia. *Adv Neurol* 78:1–10.

Klein C. 2014. Genetics in dystonia. *Parkinsonism Relat Disord* 20 (Suppl. 1):S137–342.

Marsden CD. 1976. Dystonia: the spectrum of the disease. *Res Publ Assoc Res Nerv Ment Dis* 55:351–367.

Oppenheim H. 1911. Über eine eigenartige Krampfkrankheit des kindlichen und jugendlichen Alters (dysbasia lordotica progressiva, dystonia musculorum). *Neurol Zbl* 30:1090–1107.

Chapter 3

Primary or Idiopathic Dystonias ('Isolated Dystonia')

Bettina Balint, Roberto Erro and Kailash P. Bhatia

Dystonia is characterised by sustained or intermittent muscle contractions which cause abnormal, often repetitive, movements, postures, or both, or tremor, and which often worsen with action. The term has been used both to describe the hyperkinetic movement disorder itself and to encompass a group of disorders in which dystonia is only a sign, or part of a syndrome. Traditionally, we refer with 'primary or idiopathic dystonia' to conditions where the aetiology is either idiopathic or genetic, with absence of neurodegeneration. Clinically, this group is characterised by dystonia as the sole motor feature (apart from tremor) and the lack of other neurological signs. This definition largely overlaps with the new terminology 'isolated dystonia' according to the recent *consensus update on the definition, phenomenology, and classification of dystonia* (Albanese et al. 2013).

Table 3.1 Red flags cautioning against a diagnosis of primary dystonia

- History of perinatal birth injury
- Developmental delay
- Exposure to drugs (e.g. dopamine receptor blockers)
- Prominent bulbar involvement with tongue protrusion and dysphagia
- Unusual pattern with regard age at onset and distribution
- Sudden onset with rapid progression
- Hemidystonia
- Fixed dystonia
- Presence of other neurological or systemic signs

The Pattern of Primary Dystonia Defined by Age at Onset and Anatomical Distribution

The clinical spectrum of primary dystonia encompasses generalised forms as well as focal variants. In fact, there is a distinct pattern of distribution, which greatly depends on the age at onset. Deviation from this pattern, among other red flags (Table 3.1), should caution against primary dystonia as they suggest secondary or symptomatic dystonia (see Chapter 4).

Primary dystonia presenting at a young age (childhood/adolescence) usually starts in the lower limbs with in-turning of the feet and pigeon-toed walking, and subsequently spreads over the ensuing months to years, leading either to generalised dystonia in the majority of cases, or, less frequently, to segmental involvement. This is classically called the primary torsion dystonia, the archetype of which Oppenheim described in 1911 as 'dystonia musculorum deformans'. It became clear that most cases are due to DYT1 with *TOR1A* (Torsin1A) mutations, namely in-frame CAG deletions. This mutation has been shown to be responsible for ~80 per cent of all primary, early-onset dystonia in Ashkenazi Jewish populations and up to 50 per cent of primary, early-onset dystonia in non-Jewish populations (Bressman 2006). The inheritance follows an autosomal dominant pattern with reduced penetrance (30–40 per cent) (Bressman 2006). It was suggested that penetrance might be modified by genetic and extragenetic factors. With respect to genetic factors, it seems that the polymorphism 216H in cis or trans determines whether an individual may manifest or be protected (Risch et al. 2007). Some extragenetic factors, such as complications of vaginal delivery, possibly leading to mild perinatal asphyxia, have been associated with manifestation (Martino et al. 2013).

Rarely, primary dystonia can have a slightly later onset during adolescence and early adulthood, and start in the craniocervical, laryngeal or brachial areas before generalisation. In this scenario, particularly with prominent bulbar involvement with marked dysphonia, DYT6 with *THAP1* (thanatos associated protein domain containing, apoptosis associated protein 1) mutations are high on the list of the differential diagnosis (Fuchs et al. 2009; Xiromerisiou et al. 2012). A key question here is whether patients are able to eat, as dysphagia or oromandibular involvement with a tendency to push out food with the tongue are red flags for secondary causes (Schneider et al. 2006).

Overall, a later onset of dystonia, in middle or late adulthood, is usually associated with focal forms of dystonia and rarely has genetic underpinnings. These focal dystonias are 9–12 times more frequent than generalised dystonias (Nutt et al. 1988), and also follow a certain pattern in terms of age at onset and distribution.

Writer's cramp, defined as excessive involuntary muscle contractions leading to abnormal posturing on attempts to write, occurs more frequently in men and has a peak of onset at around 39 years of age (Sheehy et al. 1988). Patients often already have difficulty picking up or holding the pen; when writing, they hold the pen with excessive force and a dystonic posture of the hand and forearm (Figure 3.1a). Difficulties

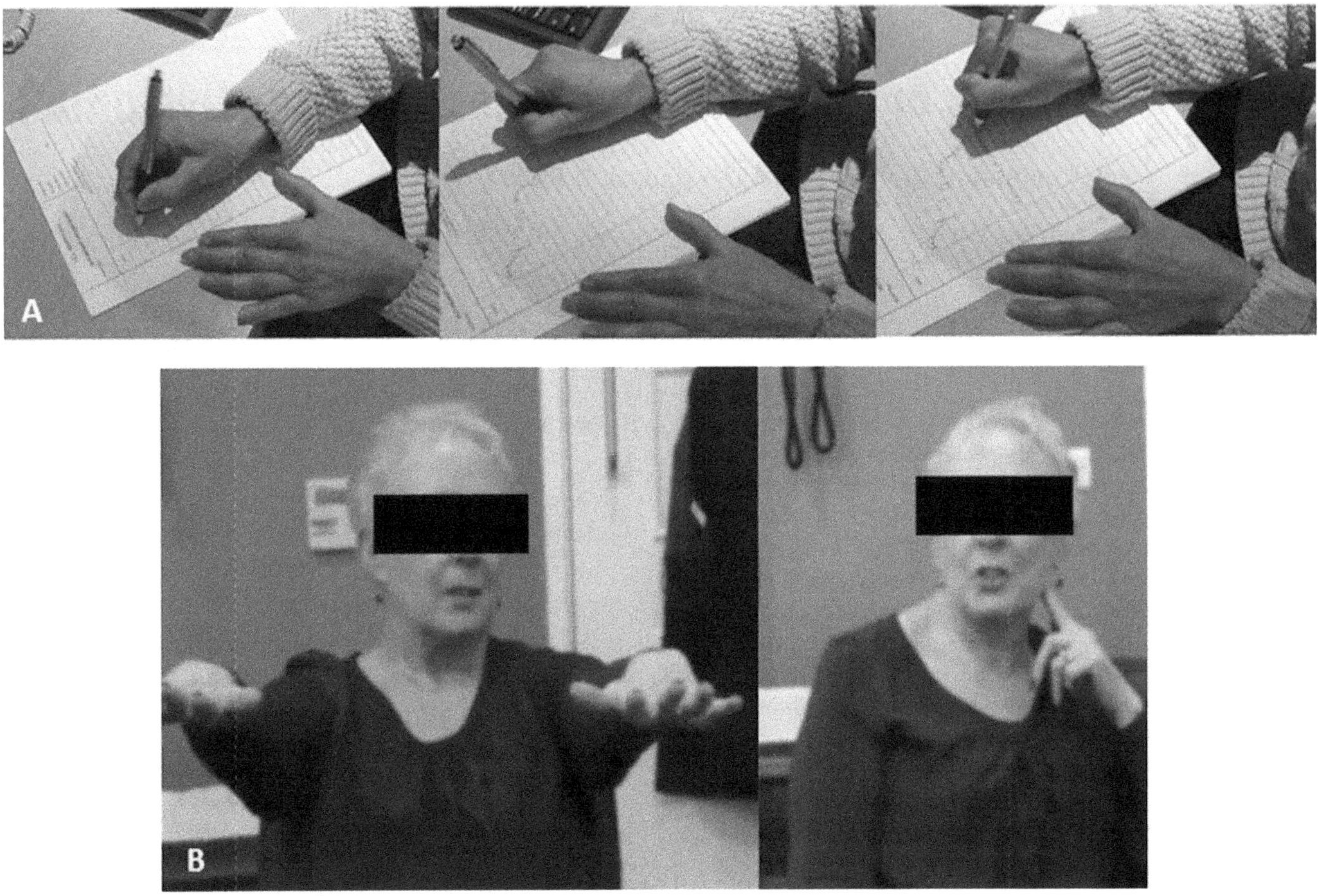

Figure 3.1 Examples of focal dystonia.
(a) Writer's cramp. The patient has progressive difficulties on attempting to write. Note the abnormal posturing of the right hand with a tight grip, and the inability to write in a straight line. To overcome the difficulties, the patient holds the pen in a different manner.
(b) Cervical dystonia with torticollis to the left. The patient uses a slight touch of the cheek as a sensory trick to correct her posture.

usually increase as writing continues. Sometimes the patients use a geste (like touching the affected hand with the other hand), a different way to hold the pen, or pens of different sizes, or even learn to write with the other hand to overcome these difficulties. However, in the latter group, a quarter develops writer's cramp in that extremity also. Often, during the further course, dystonia is not limited only to the task of writing itself, but becomes also obvious in other activities like using cutlery, brushing teeth, etc. Other craft or occupational cramps may occur wherever repetitive, frequent movements are performed; these have been described in typists, telegraphists, hairdressers and cigar rollers, among many others. A special chapter is dedicated to musician's dystonia (Chapter 44). Similarly, the lower limbs may be affected (e.g. dancers, sewing-machine workers), but this must be carefully differentiated from paroxysmal exercise-induced dystonia. Much rarer forms of focal idiopathic dystonias in this age group include axial dystonia affecting the trunk (mean age at onset 41, slight male preponderance) (Bhatia et al. 1997).

Cervical dystonia, in contrast, is the commonest form of dystonia, affecting mainly women in their fourth or fifth decade of life, with prevalence rates ranging from 89 up to 732 per 100 000 (Nutt et al. 1988; Müller et al. 2002). Onset is usually gradual, often with a pulling sensation and neck discomfort, which then evolves to persistent deviation of the neck. The most frequent form is torticollis, meaning abnormal posturing with the head turning to one side. Other variations are laterocollis (tilt to the side), retrocollis (neck extension) and antecollis (neck flexion); mixed forms also occur. Temporary remissions may occur, just as the overall pattern may change over time. The 'geste antagoniste', which patients often use to alleviate symptoms, refers to a light touch with the hand on the neck or the head, and, interestingly, just attempting the geste can often correct the abnormal posture (Figure 3.1b). Observing the geste is also a reassuring sign of primary dystonia for the clinician. Although generally considered a sporadic condition, there is now emerging evidence that many patients with cervical dystonia do have a family history, particularly those with tremulous cervical dystonia (Rubio-Agusti et al. 2013). A number of recent gene discoveries (see Bressman 2006) have confirmed this notion.

Dystonia affecting the cranial region occurs slightly later, namely around the sixth decade, but again with a female preponderance, and may present as blepharospasm, oromandibular dystonia, a combination of these ('Meige syndrome'), or laryngeal or laryngopharyngeal dystonia ('spasmodic dysphonia').

The first symptoms in patients with blepharospasm may be a feeling of discomfort in the eyes and abnormal sensitivity to bright light, before increased blinking and subsequent development of sustained paroxysms of eye closure. It remains a matter of discussion if ocular discomfort indeed represents ocular disease predisposing (possibly together with other contributing factors) to blepharospasm, or if these symptoms are part of the disorder itself. The spasms may initially be unilateral, but evolve then to bilateral affection, and are aggravated by fatigue, stress, reading and bright lights. Conversely, they improve with concentration, and are sometimes not obvious during the actual consultation. Therefore, constant blepharospasm is unusual and should evoke the thought of a functional disorder as differential diagnosis. Moreover, the inability to open the eyes can arise from so-called apraxia of eye opening, which is more often associated with degenerative disease. In contrast, patients with idiopathic blepharospam often use sensory tricks (e.g. touching the eyes, using glasses with a 'ptosis prop' or 'ptosis crutch').

Oromandibular dystonia can manifest as jaw opening, jaw protraction, jaw closing, lip pursing, tongue protrusion, and/or platysma overactivity. In most patients, this can produce difficulties chewing and speaking, and only rarely affects swallowing. Severe tongue protrusion and swallowing difficulties, however, are red flags pointing to secondary causes. Laryngeal dystonia may rarely occur in isolation, and affects a slightly younger age group than the other cranial dystonias, but more often it is part of a more widespread involvement. We distinguish two types, namely the adductor type with a strained voice and frequent pauses, which is much more frequent than the abductor type with a whispering/breathy quality. Laryngeal dystonia, as other dystonias, might be aggravated by anxiety and stress, and therefore mistaken as an expression of psychological issues.

Expanding the Phenotypic and Genotypic Spectrum: New Insights from Genetics

There are a number of newly described and rarer genetic forms of dystonia with onset ranging from childhood to adulthood and a distribution pattern deviating partly from the rule of thumb that early-onset dystonia starts in the legs.

For example, another autosomal dominant form of dystonia with onset from childhood to adulthood and focal or segmental is caused by DYT24 due to *ANO3* (anoctamin 3) mutations (Charlesworth et al. 2012). It is predominantly the upper body (cranial, laryngeal, arms) that is involved, and therefore the phenotypic spectrum ranges from tremulous cervical dystonia to presentation with isolated arm tremor.

Similarly, DYT25 due to dominantly inherited *GNAL* (guanine nucleotide-binding protein, alpha activating activity polypeptide, olfactory type Gα(olf)) mutations can cause childhood to adulthood onset of focal or segmental dystonia of the upper body, which rarely (~10 per cent) generalises (Fuchs et al. 2012). Again, patients might present with cervical dystonia, head or arm tremor, or spasmodic dysphonia.

In contrast, *CIZ1* (Cip1-interacting zinc finger protein 1) missense mutations were reported to cause cervical dystonia with age of onset varying between adolescence and late adulthood, and have been assigned to DYT23 (Xiao et al. 2012). However, this has not been replicated in other cohorts as several studies failed to detect clear pathogenic mutations (Dufke et al. 2015).

Two new genes for early onset, autosomal recessive, isolated dystonia have been described recently. Mutations in *HPCA* (hippocalcin) cause DYT2 dystonia, the phenotype of which consists of childhood to early adulthood onset of limb dystonia, and slow progression to generalised dystonia with predominant craniocervical involvement (Charlesworth et al. 2015).

The phenotype delineated so far for DYT27 due to *COL6A3* (Collagen, Type VI, alpha-3) mutations consists of a childhood to early adulthood onset with segmental dystonia mainly affecting the upper body, with predominantly craniocervical involvement and neck or hand being mostly the site of onset (Zech et al. 2015).

Table 3.2 provides an overview of genes causing isolated dystonia; altogether, however, it must be stressed that mutations of *ANO3* and *GNAL* are very rare, and that *CIZ1* mutations as a cause of dystonia await confirmation. Relevance and prevalence of the recessive genes *HPCA* and *COL6A3* will emerge with time.

Beyond the Motor Manifestation: The Non-Motor Features of Primary Dystonia

Although we define dystonia by its motor manifestation, there is growing evidence suggesting an important non-motor component to primary dystonia with clinical and pathophysiological implications. Such non-motor symptoms include abnormalities in specialised sensory and perceptual functions (temporal and special discrimination), as well as in neuropsychiatric and sleep domains (Stamelou et al. 2012).

Whereas overt sensory symptoms are not expected in primary dystonia, there is, however, the notion of mild sensory symptoms (discomfort in the neck prior to development of cervical dystonia, discomfort in the eyes before blepharospasm develops, and irritation of the throat in spasmodic dysphonia), and some patients explain their symptoms with an attempt to decrease them. The sensory trick, or geste antagoniste, is a hallmark feature in dystonia, tying in with experimental studies to suggest an alteration of sensory input and processing.

Depression appears to be a symptom of its own right in dystonia, rather than a mere reaction to the physical ailment. Psychiatric comorbidity can precede the actual motor symptoms by more than ten years, and seems not to correlate with the severity of dystonia per se. An open question in this regard is the notion of poor sleep quality, which may be part of the dystonia per se, or related to depression. This is likely to reflect on management, when impaired quality of life due to pain, depression and anxiety may influence the perceived benefit from treatments for motor symptoms. Besides, it may be that quality of life can be significantly improved by addressing the neuropsychiatric comorbidities.

Table 3.2 Identified genes in primary (isolated) dystonia: overview of genes causing isolated dystonia and the associated clinical phenotypes

DYT locus (gene)	Inheritance	Age of onset	Distribution	Clinical characteristics
DYT1 (*TOR1A*)	AD	Childhood	Generalised, rarely focal	Starting in the legs and spreading upwards; sparing of larynx and neck; can be jerky
DYT2 (*HPCA*)	ar	Childhood to early adulthood	Generalised, segmental	Onset with limb dystonia, slow progression to generalised or segmental dystonia with predominant craniocervical involvement
DYT4 (*TUBB4A*)	AD	Adolescence to early adulthood	Focal, segmental, generalised	Rare cause of isolated dystonia, prominent laryngeal ('whispering dysphonia') and oromandibular involvement; TUBB4A mutations present more often as the complex HABC spectrum
DYT6 (*THAP1*)	AD	Adolescence to early adulthood	Generalised > segmental	Rostrocaudal gradient with prominent laryngeal involvement
DYT23 (*CIZ11*)	AD	Adolescence to adulthood	Focal	(Tremulous) cervical dystonia; rare/awaiting confirmation
DYT24 (*ANO3*)	AD	Childhood to adulthood	Focal, segmental	Tremulous cervical dystonia; cranial, laryngeal, arm involvement; can present with isolated arm tremor, or as a jerky dystonia
DYT25 (*GNAL*)	AD	Childhood to adulthood	Focal, segmental, rarely generalised	Cervical dystonia; head or tremor; laryngeal dystonia; generalisation in 10 per cent; hyposmia in some cases
DYT27 (*COL6A3*)	ar	Childhood to early adulthood	Segmental	Mainly affecting the upper body, predominant craniocervical involvement; neck or hand being main sites of onset

Abbreviations: AD = autosomal dominant; ar = autosomal recessive; HBAC = hypomyelination with atrophy of the basal ganglia and the cerebellum.

In summary, primary dystonia follows a distinct pattern in terms of anatomical distribution in relation to age at onset. Idiopathic forms prevail overall, but an expanding spectrum of genotypes with mild variations of the described pattern is recognised (Figure 3.2). Whereas this is relevant for correct diagnosis, awareness of the non-motor features of dystonia, particularly the neuropsychiatric symptoms, is gaining importance for its management implications.

References

Albanese A, Bhatia K, Bressman SB, et al. 2013. Phenomenology and classification of dystonia: a consensus update. *Mov Disord* 28(7):863–873.

Bhatia KP, Quinn NP, Marsden CD. 1997. Clinical features and natural history of axial predominant adult onset primary dystonia. *J Neurol Neurosurg Psychiatry* 63(6):788–791.

Bressman S. 2006. Genetics of dystonia. *J Neural Transm Suppl* 70:489–495.

Charlesworth G, Plagnol V, Holmström KM, et al. 2012. Mutations in ANO3 cause dominant craniocervical dystonia: ion channel implicated in pathogenesis. *Am J Hum Genet* 91(6):1041–1050.

Charlesworth G, Angelova PR, Bartolome-Robledo F, et al. 2015. Mutations in HPCA cause autosomal-recessive primary isolated dystonia. *Am J Hum Genet* 96:657–665.

Dufke C, Hauser AK, Sturm M, Fluhr S, Wächter T, Leube B, Auburger G, Ott T, Bauer P, Gasser T, Grundmann K. 2015. Mutations in CIZ1 are not a major cause for dystonia in Germany. *Mov Disord* 30(5):740–743.

Fuchs T, Gavarini S, Saunders-Pullman R, Raymond D, Ehrlich ME, Bressman SB, et al. 2009. Mutations in the THAP1 gene are responsible for DYT6 primary torsion dystonia. *Nat Genet* 41:286–288.

Fuchs T, Saunders-Pullman R, Masuho I, et al. 2012. Mutations in GNAL cause primary torsion dystonia. *Nat Genet* 45(1):88–92.

Martino D, Gajos A, Gallo V, et al. 2013. Extragenetic factors and clinical penetrance of DYT1 dystonia: an exploratory study. *J Neurol* 260(4):1081–1086.

Müller J, Kiechl S, Wenning GK, et al. 2002. The prevalence of primary dystonia in the general community. *Neurology* 59(6):941–943.

Nutt JG, Muenter MD, Aronson A, Kurland LT, Melton LJ 3rd. 1988. Epidemiology of focal and generalized dystonia in Rochester, Minnesota. *Mov Disord* 3(3):188–194.

Risch NJ, Bressman SB, Senthil G, Ozelius LJ. 2007. Intragenic cis and trans modification of genetic susceptibility in DYT1 torsion dystonia. *Am J Hum Genet* 80(6):1188–1193.

Rubio-Agusti I, Pareés I, Kojovic M, Stamelou M, Saifee TA, Charlesworth G, Sheerin UM, Edwards MJ, Bhatia KP. 2013. Tremulous cervical dystonia is likely to be familial: clinical characteristics of a large cohort. *Parkinsonism Relat Disord* 19(6):634–638.

Schneider SA, Aggarwal A, Bhatt M, Dupont E, Tisch S, Limousin P, Lee P, Quinn N, Bhatia KP. 2006. Severe tongue protrusion dystonia: clinical syndromes and possible treatment. *Neurology* 67(6):940–943.

Sheehy MP, Rothwell JC, Marsden CD. 1988. Writer's cramp. *Adv Neurol* 50:457–472.

Stamelou M, Edwards MJ, Hallett M, Bhatia KP. 2012. The non-motor syndrome of primary dystonia: clinical and pathophysiological implications. *Brain* 135(Pt 6):1668–1681.

Xiao J, Uitti RJ, Zhao Y, et al. 2012. Mutations in CIZ1 cause adult onset primary cervical dystonia. *Ann Neurol* 71(4):458–469.

Xiromerisiou G, Houlden H, Scarmeas N, et al. 2012. THAP1 mutations and dystonia phenotypes: genotype phenotype correlations. *Mov Disord* 27(10):1290–1294.

Zech M, Lam DD, Francescatto L, et al. 2015. Recessive mutations in the a3 (VI) collagen gene COL6A3 cause early-onset isolated dystonia. *Am J Hum Genet* 96(6):883–893.

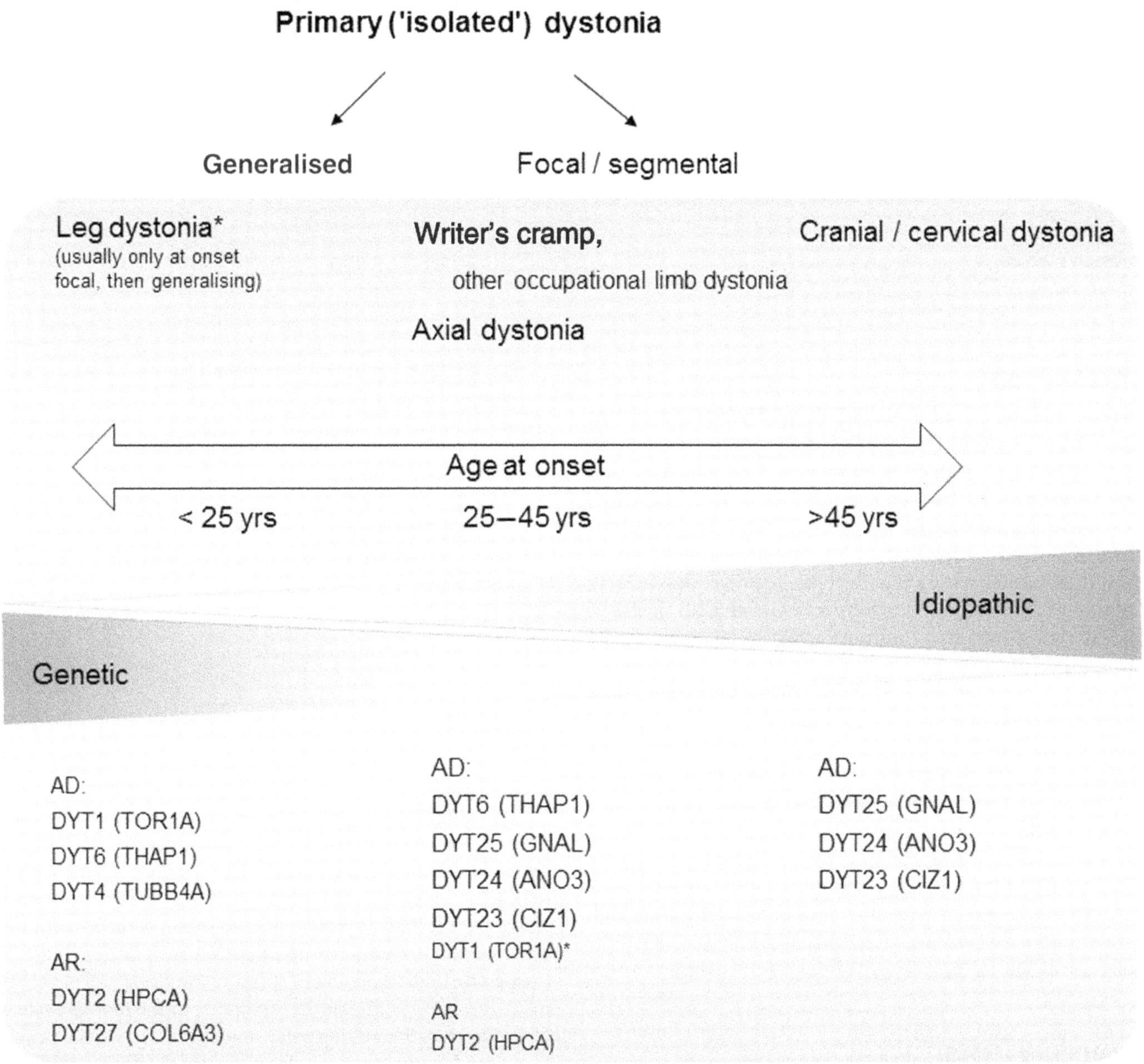

Figure 3.2 Primary dystonia follows a distinct pattern in terms of anatomical distribution in relation to age at onset. Idiopathic forms prevail overall, but an expanding spectrum of genotypes and phenotypes is recognised.

Chapter 4 Non-Primary Dystonias

Peter Kaňovský and Dirk Dressler

Introduction

Marsden and Fahn (Fahn et al. 1987; Fahn 1988) introduced four classification categories for dystonia based on their aetiology: **primary dystonia, secondary (symptomatic) dystonia, dystonia-plus syndromes** and **heredodegenerative dystonia.** In recent years, these original categories intermixed with the increasing evidence of the genetic, metabolic and environmental aetiologies of many diseases manifesting with dystonia (Asmus & Gasser 2010; Colosimo & Berardelli 2011; Dressler 2011; Fahn 2011). Today, there is a trend towards a clinico-pathological definition of only two groups: primary dystonias and non-primary (secondary) dystonias (Phukan et al. 2011). Non-primary dystonia consists of 'dystonia-plus syndromes' and 'symptomatic dystonia'. In 2010 Schneider and Bhatia tried to solve this taxonomical confusion by the identification of secondary dystonias on the basis of syndromic associations and clinical clues (Schneider & Bhatia 2010). They introduced the 'dystonic fingerprints', seminal clinical features suggestive of the secondary origin of dystonia (Table 4.1) together with a list of the most frequent syndromic associations (Table 4.2). Still, this concept might be seen as a most useful diagnostic tool. In this chapter, the current concept of 'split' aetiological classification is used (Table 4.3).

Secondary Dystonia

Pure secondary, i.e. symptomatic dystonias, are those caused by focal brain lesions (trauma, tumour, stroke, etc.), diffuse brain disorder, perinatal encephalopathy, infections, drugs or by direct impact of chemical agents. The most frequent movement disorder caused by focal brain lesions is dystonia – either focal, segmental or hemidystonia. Focal brain lesions may be localised in sensitive brain structures, including the striatum (particularly putamen), the pallidum, the thalamus (VPL nucleus of thalamus), the dorsolateral parietal cortex and the cerebellar hemispheres (Marsden et al. 1985; Schwartz et al. 1995; Kostič et al. 1996; Alarcon et al. 2001; Chuang et al. 2002). Putaminal lesions may cause pure hemidystonia; thalamic lesions may cause complex movement disorders with predominant limb dystonia (Lee et al. 1994). Dystonia may be part of the hemithalamic syndrome (hemiparesis, hemidystonia, hemiataxia, hemihypesthesia). Any focal brain lesion has to be suspected when contralateral body parts are affected. Even atypical lesions may produce dystonia such as multilevel brainstem lesions. Usually

Table 4.1 Features suggestive of secondary dystonia

Sudden onset and rapid progression
Hemidystonia
Cranial onset in childhood
Restriction to focal or segmental dystonia with childhood onset
Onset in legs in adults
Progression to generalised dystonia with adult onset
Prominent orobulbar involvement
Other neurological or systemic signs
Presence of painful spasms

the delay between the occurrence of the lesion and the onset of dystonia is weeks or months (Berardelli 1995). Longer delays make the diagnosis of secondary dystonia difficult.

Dystonia (together with true spasticity, rigidity and spasms) may be part of the spectrum of muscle hyperactivities seen in 'spastic conditions' (Dressler 2011) or 'spastic movement disorders' (Rosales et al. 2011) when pyramidal and extrapyramidal tracts are affected. Typically, here dystonia is tonic (with only rare fluctuations) and may be enhanced by the attempt to move the paretic limb. Dystonia in spastic conditions is probably the most common secondary dystonia due to the high prevalence of stroke as its underlying condition.

Secondary dystonia can also appear in the perinatal encephalopathy (perinatal cerebral injury, cerebral palsy), either isolated dystonia or as part of a spastic condition. Other names include 'athetoid cerebral palsy' and 'delayed onset dystonia' (Nelson 1996; Singer 1998; Fairhurst 2012).

Secondary dystonia may be caused by diffuse brain damage such as hypo- or hyperglycaemia and diffuse hypoxia, especially when regions with a high utilisation of oxygen and glucose such as the basal ganglia are affected (Johnston & Hoon 2000). Typically, the clinical presentation of diffuse brain damage is not monosymptomatic with dystonia, but rather complex with choreoathetosis, myoclonus and paresis. In some cases, dystonia may be progressive (Kostič et al. 1996; Venkatesan & Frucht 2006).

Dystonia may be caused by autoimmune conditions such as multiple sclerosis (Tranchant et al. 1995) and others (Janavz & Aminoff 1998; Baizabal-Carvallo & Jankovic 2012). It may also follow subacute sclerosing panencephalitis, Creutzfeld-Jakob disease, HIV-related encephalitis and neurosyphylis. It may arise as a post-infectious syndrome as in Japanese encephalitis,

Table 4.2 Syndromic associations and clinical clues in secondary dystonia

Clinical features	Differential diagnosis to consider
Dystonia with prominent oromandibular involvement	Drug-induced dystonia
	PKAN
	PLA2G6-associated neurodegeneration
	Neuroacanthocytosis
Dystonia and peripheral neuropathy	Neuroferritinopathy
	Lesch–Nyhan disease
	Niemann–Pick type C
	Metachromatic leukodystrophy
	Friedreich's ataxia
	Ataxia telangiectasia
Dystonia and eye movement disorders	Spinocerebellar ataxias (e.g. SCA3)
	Niemann–Pick type C
	Huntington's disease
	Ataxia telangiectasia
Dystonia and retinitis pigmentosa	PKAN
	GM2 gangliosidosis
Dystonia and deafness	Metachromatic leukodystrophy
	Mitochondrial disease
	Mohr–Tranebjaerg syndrome
	Woodhouse–Sakati syndrome
Dystonia and parkinsonism	Dopa-responsive dystonia
	Young-onset parkinsonism
	Wilson's disease
	Kufor–Rakeb disease
	PLA2G6-associated neurodegeneration
	Atypical parkinsonism (PSP, CBD, MSA)
Dystonia with progressive dementia	GM1, GM2 gangliosidosis
	Glutaric acidemia
	Huntington's disease
	Huntington's disease look-alike disorders

tick-borne European encephalitis and Reye syndrome (Alarcón et al. 2000; Maltête et al. 2006; Misra & Kalita 2010; Carroll & Sanchez-Ramos 2011; Netravathi et al. 2012; Hur & Hwang 2013; Tong et al. 2013).

There is a continued discussion on whether peripheral trauma may trigger dystonia (Jankovic 1994, 2001; Weiner 2001). More than ten years ago, the term 'reflex sympathetic dystrophy' was suggested for the complex disorder (dystonia, pain, amyotrophy) triggered by peripheral limb trauma (Serrano-Dueñas 2003). Today it is replaced by the nosological category 'regional pain syndrome' (Schott 2007; van Hilten et al. 2007; Maihofner et al. 2010). Dystonia in this syndrome may be progressive and devastating. Typically, it does not respond to botulinum toxin therapy. In severe cases it deserves surgical treatment, including amputation (Edwards et al. 2011; Hawley & Weiner 2011; van Rooijen et al. 2011).

Head trauma with small localised brain lesions may also be the cause of the secondary dystonia. It is usually caused by thalamic contusion. It presents with hemidystonia together

Table 4.3 Secondary dystonia classified according to underlying pathological process

I. Focal brain lesions
Vascular processes
Trauma
Tumour
Encephalitis
II. Diffuse brain damage
Impairment of neuronal energy metabolism
Ischaemia
Hypoxia
Mixed
Glucose
Impairment of systemic metabolism
Bilirubin
Calcium
Natrium
Increased intracranial pressure
Subdural haematoma
Normal pressure hydrocephalus
Drugs
Acute
Dopamine-blocking agents
Benzamides
Antihistamines
Dopamine agonists in Parkinson's disease
Tardive
Phenothiazines
Thioxanthenes
Butyrophenones
Diphenylbutyrylpiperidine
Dibenzazepine
Dibenzodiazepine
Thienobenzodiazepine
Substituted benzamides
Indolenes
Pyrimidinone
Tryicyclic antidepressants
Chemical agents
Mangenese
Copper
Methanol
Cyanide
Carbon monoxide
Ephedrone
Physical interactions
Electricity, radiation
Indirect central nervous effects
Peripheral trauma with reflex sympathetic dystrophy
Peripheral trauma without causalgia

with other signs of the hemithalamic syndrome (Pettigrew & Jankovic 1985; Lee et al. 1994).

Dystonia-Plus Syndromes

Dystonia-plus syndromes represent a heterogeneous group of diseases, where dystonia is accompanied by other neurological features. Gene mutations may be detected. At present, the following disorders are categorised as dystonia-plus syndromes: dopa-responsive dystonia (DRD), myoclonus-dystonia, rapid-onset dystonia-parkinsonism and DYT-16 dystonia-parkinsonism. In this chapter, only DRD and myoclonus-dystonia will be described. Syndromes connecting dystonia with parkinsonism are described in Chapter 6.

Dopa-Responsive Dystonia (DRD, DYT 5a/b)

Masaya Segawa was the first to recognise and describe this syndrome in Japanese children (Segawa et al. 1976). 'Dopa-responsive dystonia' is the term Nygaard introduced in 1988 (Nygaard et al. 1988). Alternatively, the term 'autosomal dominant GTP cyclohydrolase 1 deficiency' is used.

Dopa-responsive dystonia is a rare disorder best described by 'early-onset lower limb dystonia that can cause gait disorder, and has diurnal fluctuation pattern and promptly responds to L-DOPA treatment' (Nygaard et al. 1988). Dystonia is usually present in the early course of the disease and only later may parkinsonism develop. In adult-onset patients, dystonia and parkinsonism may develop together. Diurnal fluctuations are one of the pathognomic features of DRD, when symptoms worsen in the afternoon and are improved in the morning.

DRD is an inherited disorder. It may be caused by various gene defects with different penetrance. All known mutations affect the dopamine metabolism. The most frequent type of DRD, DYT-5a, is caused by the guanosine triphosphate cyclohydroxylase 1 gene defect on chromosome 14q22.1-q22.2 (Ichinose 1995). This type of DRD manifests in childhood, most frequently at the age of 5–7 years, although adult-onset variants have also been reported (Segawa et al. 2003). DYT-5 seems to have gender-differentiated penetration; females are more frequently affected than males. The typical initial clinical manifestation in childhood is asymmetric dystonia affecting one leg. Premotor symptoms may be non-specific, bothering the patient with leg stiffness, cramps or tiredness on exercise. Bilateral, often symmetric lower-limb dystonia and parkinsonism with predominant bradykinesia may develop later in the course of the disease. The diagnosis is usually made on the basis of disease history, clinical picture and response to an L-DOPA challenge (Nygaard 1993). Cerebral palsy may be a differential diagnosis in atypical cases. However, the progressive course of the disease and its typical L-DOPA responsiveness are clues. L-DOPA treatment works well in DRD in low doses and usually without any sign of tachyphylaxis.

Myoclonus-Dystonia (DYT11)

Also known as myoclonus-dystonia, myoclonic dystonia and dystonia-myoclonus, DYT11 is a rare autosomal dominant inherited disorder. The penetrance is incomplete and there is no gender difference. Its genetic basis is multiple mutations in the epsilon-sarcoglycan gene on the chromosome 7q21 (Zimprich et al. 2001). The typical manifestation is a jerky dystonia with predominant axial muscle involvement and some upper-limb involvement. Leg manifestations are rare. Psychiatric disorders may accompany the motor symptoms, such as anxiety, panic attacks, depression, obsessive-compulsive disorder and personality disorders (Klein 2003). DYT11 usually manifests in late childhood or early adulthood. Eighty per cent of affected individuals experienced the first symptoms before age 20. The course of DYT11 is usually mild and does not significantly affect the quality of life. Sometimes spontaneous remissions have been reported. DYT11 may be improved by low amounts of alcohol. This may help to confirm the diagnosis (Quinn 1996). Botulinum toxin therapy is successful. Valproate may also be helpful. In patients unresponsive to botulinum toxin therapy, deep brain stimulation may be considered.

Heredodegenerative Dystonia

In heredodegenerative forms, dystonia is only part of the clinical picture and is always accompanied by other neurological symptoms. In contrast to the dystonia-plus syndromes, dystonia in heredodegenerative dystonia is not the dominant symptom of the disease. However, heredodegenerative dystonia may start with dystonia as the sole initial symptom. Heredodegenerative dystonia is classified on the basis of the underlying pathological processes.

Heredodegenerative Dystonia in Mitochondriopathies

Mitochondriopathies are a group of disorders with an inherited gene defect in the mitochondrial DNA, which is only maternally inherited. In mitochondriopathies, mainly tissues with high energy consumption such as the muscles and the brain are affected. Probably dystonia is most often seen in Leigh's disease. Nevertheless, it may be present in any mitochondrial disorder (Finsterer 2008). Muscle biopsy provides a diagnostic clue in this condition. There is practically no cure for mitochondriopathies. Dystonia may be symptomatically treated by botulinum toxin therapy.

Heredodegenerative Dystonia in Inherited Metabolic Disorders

There are several conditions in which dystonia may form an important part of the clinical picture, such as Lesch–Nyhan syndrome (hyperuricaemia), Hartnup's disease, homocysteinaemia, methylmalonic acid disease and galactosemia. Lesch–Nyhan disease is a rare disorder, which – due to an X-linked recessive inheritance – affects only males. The metabolic defect causes hyperuricaemia and secondary hyperuricosuria. Dystonia in Lesch–Nyhan disease is usually localised in the head, forming a typical oromandibulolingual pattern. Self-mutilations in this body area due to dystonia are frequent in Lesch–Nyhan disease (Schneider et al. 2006). Diagnosis is based on the evidence of hyperuricaemia or results of genetic examination. Hartnup's disease is caused by impaired intestinal absorption and renal re-absorption of tryptophan and other neutral amino acids (Kraut & Sachs 2005). Dystonia might be a prominent feature. Other symptoms include ataxia, nystagmus and tremor. Psychiatric signs, such as hallucinations, are present in some cases. The first symptoms of this condition usually appear in childhood and early adulthood (Darras et al. 1989). The presence of increased amino acids levels in the urine confirms the diagnosis. Homocysteinaemia is an autosomal recessive disorder of the homocysteine metabolism with excessive homocysteine serum levels. Leading symptoms of this disease are bone deformities, homocysteinaemia (the normative data in laboratories may differ!) and homocystinuria. Dystonia may also be present (Berardelli et al. 1991). Methylmalonaemia or methylmalonic aciduria is also an autosomal recessive disorder. It presents with chronic metabolic acidemia and methylmalonic acid in the urine. Dystonia may occur together with chronic renal failure and thrombopenia and leukopenia (Wortmann et al. 2009). Galactosemia is, again, an autosomal recessive metabolic disease with increased serum levels of galactose. Symptoms include hepatomegaly, chronic renal failure and cataract together with prominent dystonia and other neurological symptoms (Rubio-Augusti et al. 2013).

Heredodegenerative Dystonia Caused by the Storage Disease

Accumulation of different toxic or noxious substances in body tissues can be caused by many gene defects, virtually all of them being autosomal recessive. The disposal of these substances can be limited to some body compartments or it may be diffuse. These rather rare disorders start in early or late childhood, but manifestation in adulthood may also occur, as in Wilson's disease. Somatic symptoms usually include hepatosplenomegaly and chronic renal failure. The neurological manifestations may vary from case to case and dystonia is very often present. *Wilson's disease*, also known as hepatolenticular degeneration, is caused by numerous gene defects on the short arm of chromosome 13 (Ala et al. 2007). In Wilson's disease, copper metabolism is impaired due to lack of ceruloplasmin, its serum transporting protein. Copper, then, is not excreted in the urine and accumulates in various body tissues, predominantly in the liver and the brain. Within the brain, maximum copper deposits are found in the basal ganglia. This is the cause of the predominant extrapyramidal symptoms including dystonia. Beside dystonia, tremor, chora, ataxia and epilepsy may be present. Additional psychiatric symptoms may often be present, including depression or psychosis. The diagnosis of Wilson's disease is based on increased serum and urine copper levels and on decreased serum level of ceruloplasmin. When in doubt, liver biopsy should be applied to confirm copper accumulation in the hepatocytes. Copper may also accumulate in the cornea and manifest as Keyser–Fleischer rings in practically all Wilson's patients. On magnetic resonance imaging the 'panda sign' in T2-weighted horizontal images of the brainstem is typical. Once considered, the diagnosis of Wilson's disease is not difficult to confirm. Chelation therapy with penicillamine or zinc can improve neurological symptoms almost completely. However, their chronic use may cause renal failure (Kitzberger et al. 2005). *GM1-gangliosidosis* is one of the lysosomal storage diseases. Lack of beta-galactosidase causes blockade of the lysosomal lipid metabolism. As a consequence, the GM1-ganglioside and other oligosaccharides accumulate in various tissues, including the brain. There are three types of GM1-gangliosidosis according to their manifestation age. In type 3, which usually appears in early adulthood, neurological symptoms may be predominant and include dystonia and parkinsonism (Inui et al. 1990). *Niemann–Pick disease* is also an autosomal recessive storage disease. Lysosomal accumulation of sphingomyelin in the liver, spleen, brain and bone marrow occurs in Niemann–Pick disease type A and type B. In type C, cholesterol and glycolipids are stored in lysosomes. Clinically apparent neurological symptoms are only present in type A and type C. Dystonia may occur only in type C, usually together with epilepsy, dementia and vertical gaze palsy (Shulman et al. 1995). Hepatosplenomegaly is a frequent finding. The disease manifests in childhood and diagnosis is made by the presence of hepatosplenomegaly and neurologic symptoms. It can be confirmed by bone marrow pathology (sea-blue histiocytes) and genetic testing. *Metachromatic dystrophy* is a disease in which sulphatides accumulate in lysosomes and myelin is destroyed in both peripheral and central nervous systems. The disease is caused by dysfunctional arylsuphatase A. The main neurological symptoms are dementia and polyneuropathy, which are relatively frequently accompanied by dystonia (Baumann et al. 2002). The disease manifestation may be in childhood and adulthood. Its course is often rapidly progressive. The diagnosis is based on brain MRI and confirmed by raised urine.

Other rare lysosomal storage diseases are the *neuronal ceroid lipofuscinosis* and *Gaucher's disease*, both manifesting with dystonia (Capablo et al. 2007). Diagnosis is based on raised palmitol protein thioesterase and beta-glucocerebrosidase in the leucocytes.

Mitochondrial storage diseases are caused by mitochondrial metabolite accumulation. They are all rare disorders and the *glutaric acidemia type 1* is probably the most frequently diagnosed one. The disease itself is caused by lack of glutaryl-coenzyme A dehydrogenase, which is needed for the metabolism of amino acids tryptophan, hydroxylysine and lysine. As a result, hydroxyglutaric acid and glutacemic acid accumulate in the brain and other tissues. In the brain, the basal ganglia are predominantly affected (Funk et al. 2005). Glutaric acidemia type 1 appears practically only in childhood. It manifests with athetosis or dystonia, which may be accompanied by spasticity and epilepsy. Diagnosis is based on the neurological symptoms and the course of the disease. It may be confirmed by reduced glutaryl-coenzyme A hydroxylase in fibroblasts and also by genetic testing. Glutaric acidemia type 1 is treatable by a low lysine diet, which usually stops progression, but remission never occurs.

Heredodegenerative Dystonia Caused by Nucleotide Repeat Diseases

Mostly overlooked, dystonia may occur in CAG repeat diseases. They are usually inherited in an autosomal dominant manner. Inheritance can be blurred due to the anticipation effect. *Huntington's disease* is probably the most frequent and most widely known CAG repeat disease. It is caused by a CAG repeat expansion in the 4q21-22 or 4p16.3 genes. The normal number of repeats is 29–35. A higher number indicates Huntington's disease. Age of manifestation and severity depend on the number of repeats. Huntington's disease usually manifests in middle age. However, onset before 30 years of age is not uncommon. In such cases, the clinical picture may resemble young-onset Parkinson's disease ('Westphal variant'). Nevertheless, Huntington's disease much more frequently manifests as slowly progressive chorea with cognitive decline often accompanied by psychosis and behavioural disorder. The pathological gene product is called huntingtin and accumulates widely within the brain, predominantly in the basal ganglia, namely the striatum. Dystonia may occur in the Westphal variant and in the further course of the disease (Post et al. 2013). The diagnosis of Huntington's disease is based on the typical clinical findings of progressive chorea, dementia, psychosis and behavioural disorder, accompanied by typical MRI findings with atrophy of the caudate head. It is confirmed by genetic testing. Treatment of Huntington's disease is symptomatic only and includes dopamine depletors, atypical neuroleptics and tetrabenazine. Botulinum toxin injections for dystonia were not effective. *Spinocerebellar ataxias* are a large group of autosomal dominant CAG repeat diseases. Currently, 38 gene loci (SCA1–SCA38) have been described. They manifest with a combined cerebellar and spinal cord syndrome, accompanied by a diverse mixture of symptoms originating from involvement of other systems. Dystonia may appear in SCA1, SCA3, SCA6, SCA7, SCA14, SCA15 and SCA17. Most frequently it occurs in SCA3 (Machado–Joseph disease in the older terminology) together with lower-body parkinsonism (Dressler 2011). *Dentato-rubro-pallido-Luysian atrophy* (DRPLA), another rare autosomal dominant CAG repeat disease, may occasionally manifest with dystonia (Hatano et al. 2003).

Dystonia as a Feature of Another Neurologic Diseases

Hallervorden–Spatz disease (pantothenate kinase-associated neurodegeneration, neurodegeneration with brain iron accumulation) is a rare degenerative disorder caused by a PKAN gene defect localised on gene locus 20p13. The disease usually manifests in childhood. However, adult-onset cases exist. In its typical form it manifests with oromandibulolingual and limb dystonia, sometimes also with torticollis (Gregory & Hayflick 2005). Parkinsonism and retinitis pigmentosa may accompany the clinical picture. The diagnosis is based on the clinical picture, childhood onset and typical brain MRI finding (eye-of-the-tiger sign). It is caused by iron accumulation in the pallidum. Only symptomatic treatment exists; dystonia has been treated with botulinum toxin injections with some effect (Dressler et al. 2001). Acanthocytosis is another possible feature of this disease. *Neuroacanthocytosis* is an autosomal recessive hereditary disorder, in which altered erythrocyte proteins are causing their conversion into acanthocytes. Focal facial, lingual and mandibular or segmental dystonia are accompanied by parkinsonism and polyneuropathy. Epilepsy may be also present (Bader et al. 2010). The disease manifests at a young age and its progression lasts 6–10 years. *Friedreich's ataxia* is the most common hereditary ataxia. Its prevalence is 1 per 30 000. In about 98 per cent of patients it manifests due to homozygosity for a GAA trinucleotide repeat expansion in intron 1 of FXN. This triplet expansion causes deficiency of frataxin, a small nuclear genome-encoded mitochondrial protein. Low frataxin levels lead to insufficient biosynthesis of iron–sulphur clusters that are required for mitochondrial electron transport and assembly of functional aconitase and iron dysmetabolism of the entire cell. The disease affects multiple sites in the central and peripheral nervous system, as well as a number of other organ systems, resulting in multiple signs and symptoms. Onset of this autosomal recessive condition is usually in the first two decades of life. Major clinical features include progressive ataxia, absent leg reflexes, increased plantar reflexes, peripheral sensory neuropathy and dystonia, usually in the form of torticollis or oromandibular or limb dystonia (Garcia-Ruiz et al. 2002). Visceral pathology includes the heart, resulting in cardiomyopathy, and the pancreas, resulting in diabetes mellitus. In *Parkinson's disease*, dystonia may occur in cases of DYT3 (X-linked dystonia-parkinsonism, Lubag) and DYT12 (rapid-onset dystonia-parkinsonism), both autosomal dominant neurodegenerative conditions described in another chapter. It may also occur in the initial or very early phase of idiopathic Parkinson's disease, usually in young female patients. Dystonia may present as torticollis, blepharospasm or task-specific hand dystonia. Painful foot dystonia may typically occur in young-onset Parkinson's disease. In late-stage Parkinson's disease a broad spectrum of dystonic symptoms may be present, either as painful off-dystonia of the foot or as 'start of dose', 'peak of dose' or 'end of dose' dystonia in the on-phase (Tolosa & Compta 2006). Whenever dystonia occurs in parkinsonism, the diagnosis of multiple system atrophy should be considered.

References

Ala A, Walker AP, Ashkan K, Dooley JS, Schilsky ML (2007) Wilson's disease. *Lancet* 369: 397–408.

Alarcón F, Duenas G, Cevallos N, Lees AJ (2000) Movement disorders in 30 patients with tuberculous meningitis. *Mov Disord* 15: 561–569.

Alarcón F, Tolosa E, Munoz E (2001) Focal limb dystonia in a patient with a cerebellar mass. *Arch Neurol* 58: 1125–1127.

Asmus F, Gasser T (2010) Dystonia-plus syndromes. *Eur J Neurol* 17 (Suppl. 1): 37–45.

Bader B, Walker RH, Vogel M, Prosiegel M, McIntosh J, Danek A (2010) Tongue protrusion and feeding dystonia: a hallmark of chorea-acanthocytosis. *Mov Disord* 25: 127–129.

Baizabal-Carvallo JF, Jankovic J (2012) Movement disorders in autoimmune diseases. *Mov Disord* 27: 935–946.

Baumann N, Turpin JC, Lefevre M, Colsch B (2002) Motor and psycho-cognitive clinical types in adult metachromatic leukodystrophy: genotype/phenotype relationships. *J Physiol Paris* 96: 301–306.

Berardelli A (1995) Symptomatic or secondary basal ganglia diseases and tardive dyskinesias. *Curr Opin Neurol* 8: 320–322.

Berardelli A, Thompson PD, Zaccagnini M, Giardini O, D'Eufemia P, Massoud R, Manfredi M (1991) Two sisters with generalised dystonia associated with homocystinuria. *Mov Disord* 6: 163–165.

Capablo JL, Franco R, de Cabezon AS, Alfonso P, Pocovi M, Giraldo P (2007) Neurologic improvements in a type 3 Gaucher disease patient treated with amiglucerase/amiglustat combination. *Epilepsia* 48: 1406–1407.

Carroll E, Sanchez-Ramos J (2011) Hyperkinetic movement disorders associated with HIV and other viral infections. *Hand Clin Neurol* 101: 323–334.

Chuang C, Fahn S, Frucht SJ (2002) The natural history and treatment of acquired hemidystonia: report of 33 cases and review of the literature. *J Neurol Neurosurg Psychiatry* 72: 59–67.

Colosimo C, Berardelli A (2011) Clinical phenomenology of dystonia. *Int Rev Neurobiol* 98: 509–523.

Darras BT, Ampola MG, Dietz WH, Gilmore HE (1989) Intermittent dystonia in Hartnup's disease. *Pediatr Neurol* 5: 118–120.

Dressler D (2011) Nonprimary dystonias. *Hand Clin Neurol* 101: 513–538.

Dressler D, Wittstock M, Benecke R (2001) Botulinum toxin for the treatment of jaw opening dystonia in Hallervorden–Spatz syndrome. *Eur Neurol* 45:287–288.

Edwards MJ, Alonso-Canovas A, Schrag A, Bloem BR, Thompson PD, Bhatia K (2011) Limb amputations in fixed dystonia: a form of body integrity disorder? *Mov Disord* 26: 1410–1414.

Fahn S (1988) Concept and classification of dystonia. *Adv Neurol* 50: 1–8.

Fahn S (2011) Classification of movement disorders. *Mov Disord* 26: 947–957.

Fahn S, Marsden CD, Calne DB (1987) Classification and investigations of dystonia. In: Marsden CD, Fahn S (Eds) *Movement Disorders 2*. London, Butterworths: 332–358.

Fairhurst C (2012) Cerebral palsy: the whys and hows. *Arch Dis Child Educ Pract Ed* 97: 122–131.

Finsterer J (2008) Leigh and Leigh-like syndrome in children and adults. *Pediatr Neurol* 39: 223–235.

Funk CB, Prasad AN, Frosk P, Sauer S, Kölker S, Greenberg CR, Del Bigio MR (2005) Neuropathological, biochemical and molecular findings in a glutaric acidemia type 1 cohort. *Brain* 128: 711–722.

Garcia-Ruiz PJ, Mayo D, Hernandez J, Cantarero S, Ayuso C (2002) Movement disorders in hereditary ataxias. *J Neurol Sci* 202: 59–64.

Gregory A, Hayflick SJ (2005) Neurodegeneration with brain iron accumulation. *Folia Neuropathol* 43: 286–296.

Hatano T, Okuma Y, Iijima M, Fujishima K, Goto K, Mizuno Y (2003) Cervical dystonia in dentatorubral-pallidoluysian atrophy. *Acta Neurol Scand* 308: 287–289.

Hawley JS, Weiner WJ (2011) Psychogenic dystonia and peripheral trauma. *Neurology* 77: 496–502.

Hur YJ, Hwang T (2013) Secondary paroxysmal dyskinesia associated with 2009 H1N1 infection. *Korean J Pediatr* 56: 42–44.

Inui K, Namba R, Ihara Y, Nobukuni K, Taniike M, Midorikawa M, Tsukamoto H, Okada S (1990) A case of chronic GM1 gangliosidosis presenting as dystonia: clinical and biochemical studies. *J Neurol* 237: 491–493.

Janavz LJ, Aminoff MJ (1998) Dystonia and chorea in acquired systemic disorders. *J Neurol Neurosurg Psychiatry* 65: 436–445.

Jankovic J (1994) Post-traumatic movement disorders: central and peripheral mechanisms. *Neurology* 44: 2006–2014.

Jankovic J (2001) Can peripheral trauma induce dystonia and other movement disorders? Yes! *Mov Disord* 16: 7–12.

Johnston MV, Hoon AH (2000) Possible mechanisms in infants for selective basal ganglia damage from asphyxia, kernicterus or mitochondrial encephalopathies. *J Child Neurol* 15: 588–591.

Kitzberger R, Madl C, Ferenci P (2005) Wilson disease. *Metab Brain Dis* 20: 295–302.

Klein C (2003) Myoclonus and myoclonus-dystonia. In: Pulst S (Ed.) *Genetics of Movement Disorders*. San Diego, CA, Academic Press: 449–469.

Kostic V, Svetel M, Kacar A (1996) Symptomatic dystonias associated with structural brain lesions: report of 16 cases. *Can J Neurol Sci* 23: 53–56.

Kraut JA, Sachs G (2005) Hartnup disorder: unraveling the mystery. *Trends Pharmacol Sci* 26: 53–55.

Lee MS, Rinne OJ, Ceballos-Baumann A, Thompson PD, Marsden CD (1994) Dystonia after head trauma. *Neurology* 44: 1374–1378.

Maihofner C, Seifert F, Markovic K (2010) Complex regional pain syndromes: new pathophysiological concepts and therapies. *Eur J Neurol* 17: 649–660.

Maltête D, Guyant-Maréchal L, Mihout B, Hannequin D (2006) Movement disorders and Creutzfeld-Jakob disease: a review. *Parkinsonism Relat Disord* 12: 65–71.

Marsden CD, Obeso J, Zarranz J, Lang AE (1985) The anatomical basis of symptomatic hemidystonia. *Brain* 108: 463–483.

Misra UK, Kalita J (2010) Overview: Japanese encephalitis. *Prog Neurobiol* 91: 108–120.

Netravathi M, Pal PK, Indira Devi B (2012) A clinical profile of 103 patients with secondary movement disorders: correlation of etiology with phenomenology. *Eur J Neurol* 19: 226–233.

Nygaard T (1993) Dopa-responsive dystonia: delineation of the clinical syndrome and clues to pathogenesis. *Adv Neurol* 60: 577–585.

Nygaard TG, Marsden CD, Duvoisin RC (1988) Dopa-responsive dystonia. *Adv Neurol* 50:377–384.

Pettigrew LC, Jankovic J (1985) Hemidystonia: a report of 22 patients and a review of the literature. *J Neurol Neurosurg Psychiatr* 48: 650–657.

Phukan J, Albanese A, Gasser T, Warner T (2011) Primary dystonia and dystonia-plus syndromes: clinical characteristics, diagnosis and pathogenesis. *Lancet Neurology* 10: 1074–1085.

Post B, van Belzen M, Marcelis C, Meijer FJ, Willemsen MA, van de Warrenburg BP (2013) Early onset dystonia and parkinsonism with abnormal globus pallidus signal in MRI: a diagnostic challlenge. *Mov Disord* 28: 2035–2036.

Quinn N (1996) Essential myoclonus and myoclonic dystonia. *Mov Disord* 11: 119–124.

Rosales RL, Kanovsky P, Fernandez HH (2011) What's the 'catch' in upper-limb post-stroke spasticity: expanding the role of botulinum toxin applications. *Parkinsonism Relat Disord* 17 (Suppl. 1): 3–10.

Rubio-Augusti I, Carecchio M, Bhatia KP, Kojovic M, Parees I, Chandrashekar HS, Footitt EJ, Burke D, Edwards MJ, Lachmann RH, Murphy E (2013) Movement disorders in adult patients with classical galactosemia. *Mov Disord* 28: 804–810.

Schneider SA, Bhatia KP (2010) Secondary dystonia: clinical clues and syndromic associations. *Eur J Neurol* 17 (Suppl. 1): 52–57.

Schneider SA, Aggarwal A, Bhatt M, Dupont E, Tisch S, Limousin P, Lee P, Quinn N, Bhatia KP (2006) Severe tongue protrusion dystonia: clinical syndromes and possible treatment. *Neurology* 67: 940–943.

Schott GD (2007) Peripherally-triggered CRPS and dystonia. *Pain* 130: 203–207.

Schwartz M, De Deyn PP, Van den Kerchove M, Pickut BA (1995) Cervical dystonia as a probable consequence of focal cerebral lesion. *Mov Disord* 10: 797–798.

Segawa M, Hosaka A, Miyagawa F, Nomura Y, Imai H (1976) Hereditary progressive dystonia with marked diurnal fluctuation. *Adv Neurol* 14: 215–233.

Segawa M, Nomura Y, Nishiyama N (2003) Autosomal dominant guanosine triphosphate cyclohydrolase I deficiency (Segawa disease). *Ann Neurol* 54: S32–45.

Serrano-Dueñas M (2003) Reflex sympathetic syndrome and peripheral dystonia. *Mov Disord* 18: 1212–1213.

Shulman LM, David NJ, Weiner WJ (1995) Psychosis as the initial manifestation of adult-onset Niemann–Pick disease type C. *Neurology* 45: 1739–1743.

Singer H (1998) Movement disorders in children. In: Tolosa E, Jankovic J (Eds) *Parkinson's Disease and Movement Disorders*, Philadelphia, PA, Lippincott, Williams and Wilkins: 739–754.

Tolosa E, Compta Y (2006) Dystonia in Parkinson's disease. *J Neurol* 253: 7–13.

Tong ML, Lin LR, Zhang HL, Huang SJ, Liu GL, Zheng WH, Su YH, Wu JY, Dong J, Liu LL, Yang TC (2013) Spectrum and characterization of movement disorders secondary to neurosyphilis. *Parkinsonism Relat Disord* 19: 441–445.

Tranchant C, Bhatia KP, Marsden CD (1995) Movement disorders in multiple sclerosis. *Mov Disord* 10: 418–423.

van Hilten JJ, Geraedts EJ, Marinus J (2007) Peripheral trauma and movement disorders. *Park Related Disord* 13 (Suppl. 3): S395–399.

van Roijen DE, Geraedts EJ, Marinus J, Jankovic J, van Hilten JJ (2011) Peripheral trauma and movement disorders: a systematic review of reported cases. *J Neurol Neurosurg Psychiatry* 82: 892–898.

Venkatesan A, Frucht S (2006) Movement disorders after resuscitation from cardiac arrest. *Neurol Clin* 24: 123–132.

Weiner W (2001) Can peripheral trauma induce dystonia? No! *Mov Disord* 16: 13–22.

Wortmann SB, Rodenburg RJ, Jonckheere A, de Vries MC, Huizing M, Heldt K, Van den Heuvel LP, Wendel U, Kluijtmans LA, Engelke UF, Wevers RA, Smeitink JA, Morava E (2009) Biochemical and genetic analysis of 3-methylglutatonic aciduria type IV: a diagnostic strategy. *Brain* 132: 136–146.

Zimprich A, Grabowski M, Asmus F, Naumann M, Berg D, Bertram M, Scheidtmann K, Kern P, Winkelmann J, Müller-Myhsok B, Riedel L, Bauer M, Müller T, Castro M, Meitinger T, Strom TM, Gasser T (2001) Mutation in the gene encoding epsilon-sarcoglykan cause myoclonus-dystonia syndrome. *Nat Genet* 29: 66–69.

Chapter 5

Epidemiology of Dystonia

Bulent Elibol and Gul Yalcin Cakmakli

Dystonia is known to be the third most common disorder in movement disorders clinics, following essential tremor and Parkinson's disease; however, there have been few systematic studies on the epidemiology of dystonia, with varying results (Defazio 2010). Considering the rapidly growing knowledge about the genetic basis of dystonia, alongside the availability of successful treatment options, there need to be more precise descriptive epidemiological data for rational planning of health services. Analytical epidemiology will also be complementary for better understanding of dystonia. In this chapter, we have reviewed the main studies, reviews and meta-analyses on prevalence and incidence estimates for primary dystonia, together with a summary of the reported genetic and environmental risk factors; in addition, we screened clinical series and reviews about the frequency of the main forms of secondary dystonia.

Prevalence and Incidence Studies for Primary Dystonia

Studying the epidemiology of primary dystonia has always been a challenge due to a number of limitations, such as difficulties in ascertainment and in using diagnostic criteria for this heterogeneous disorder, varying attitudes of treatment-seeking behaviour and the variability of study populations by age, sex and ethnic group (Defazio et al. 2004; Defazio 2010). Together with the methodological differences in study designs, all these limitations resulted in enormously wide ranges of estimated crude prevalence rates (CPR) in published studies: for primary early-onset dystonia ranging from 0.07 to 5.7/10^5, for primary late-onset dystonia from 3 to 732/10^5 (Defazio et al. 2004; Das et al. 2007; Defazio 2010; Steeves et al. 2012).

Differences in study design, such as service-based in mostly tertiary/quaternary clinics, or linkage of medical records in neurological and non-neurological services in a given area, and community-based studies lead to varying degrees of subject ascertainment. Studies based on treatment services have the advantage of more proper diagnosis, but may not include patients with mild symptoms/misdiagnoses, or the ones not seeking medical advice; therefore their results are usually in the low part of the range variability (Defazio et al. 2004; Defazio 2010). Family studies have proved these shortcomings by disclosing undiagnosed family members for up to one- to two-thirds of the index cases (Defazio 2010; Steeves et al. 2012). Community-based studies designed to overcome these problems are hard to perform, and they also have limitations in screening strategies for diagnosing dystonias with precision.

Primary Early-Onset Dystonia

Primary early-onset dystonia (PEOD) with symptom onset before age of 20 by definition commonly presents in one limb and then usually generalises. In the few available studies, prevalence estimates vary between 0.07 and 5.7/10^5 (Defazio et al. 2004; Das et al. 2007). The first large-scale record-linkage-based population study from Rochester and an older community-based study from China both detected the highest rates of 5/10^5 (Li et al. 1985; Nutt et al. 1988), very close to a more recent community-based study from India (5.7/10^5) (Table 5.1) (Das et al. 2007).

Considering the high frequency of the TOR1A gene in the Ashkenazi Jewish population, prevalence figures of PEOD are on the upper end of the variability in studies from Israel and New York, 2.4 and 5/10^5, respectively (Defazio et al. 2004). A record-linkage study from Northern England is also in the upper end, with 4/10^5 rate of PEOD (Butler et al. 2004), while results of the studies from Japan (n = 3; 0.07–0.4/10^5) (Defazio et al. 2004; Sugawara et al. 2006), Munich and Iceland (both 0.3/10^5) all stayed at the low end (Defazio et al. 2004; Steeves et al. 2012; Joensen 2016) (Table 5.1). The Rochester epidemiology project reported the only incidence estimate on PEOD as 0.2 per 10^5 person-year in 1988 (Nutt et al. 1988).

The underlying cause of PEOD is mainly genetic, but environmental factors are also considered in disease penetrance and expression, alongside genetic/epigenetic modifiers. GAG deletion in the TORIA gene is responsible for PEOD in almost 80 per cent of Ashkenazi Jewish and 16–53 per cent of non-Jewish patients, being more common in Slav, Polish and German populations and less common in Far East countries (Bressman 2007; Muller 2009). DYT6 (THAP1) mutations may account for up to 25 per cent of non-DYT1 familial PEOD cases in non-Jewish families, but probably for only a minority of PEOD cases (Bressman 2007; Muller 2009).

There are very scarce epidemiological data on the other forms of PEOD, because of their rarity. Among these, dopa-responsive dystonia is known to occur at 0.05–0.10/10^5, and paroxysmal kinesigenic dystonia in about one person in 150 000 (Muller 2009; Charlesworth & Bhatia 2013).

Table 5.1 Reported crude prevalence rates for primary dystonia per 100 000 (95% confidence interval)

City, country, years	Study design	Primary dystonia		BSP	Cervical	Upper limb	OM	Laryngeal
		Generalised	Focal/ segmental					
China, 1983 (Li et al. 1985)	Door-to-door	5 (1–15)	3 (0.4–11)/***	***	3 (0.4–11)	***	***	***
Assiut, Egypt, 1988–1990 (Defazio et al. 2004; Das et al. 2007)	Door-to-door	***	10 (2.6–24.3) /***	***	10	***	***	***
Tyrol, Italy, 2000 (Defazio et al. 2004; Das et al. 2007; Steeves et al. 2012)	Population sample	***	732 (319–1564)	–	–	–	–	–
Calcutta, India, 2007 (Das et al. 2007)	Door-to-door	5.72 (1.2–16.7)	38.2 (23.3–59)/ ***	5.7 (1.2–16.7)	3.8 (0.5–13.8)	21 (10.5–37.6)	***	***
Israel, 1949–1959 (Defazio et al. 2004; Defazio 2010)	Record-linkage	2.4 (1.2–4.3)	***/***	***	***	***	***	***
Rochester, USA, 1950–1982 (Nutt et al. 1988)	Record-linkage	3.4 (0.2–12.4)	29.5 (17.2–47.9)/***	1.7	8.9	6.9	6.9	5.2
Northern England, 1993–2002 (Butler et al. 2004)	Record-linkage	4 (1.1–10.1)	43 (30.6–56.9)	3.0 (2.4–7.3)	6.1 (5.1–6.4)	1.2	0.1	0.8
Iceland, 2005 (Joensen 2016)	Record-linkage	0.3 (0–1.9)	31.2/3.1	3.1	11.5	8	2.8	5.9
Yonago, Japan, 1988–1993 (Epidemiological Study of Dystonia in Europe (ESDE) Collaborative Group 2000; Defazio et al. 2004; Das et al. 2007)	Service-based	0.4 (0.01–2.3)	6.1 (3.4–10.1)/***	1.6[a]	2.9	***	1.6[a]	***
USA, 1990 (Defazio et al. 2004; Das et al. 2007)	Service-based	5 (3.9–6.3)	***	***	***	***	***	***
Puglia, Italy, 1987–1999 (Epidemiological Study of Dystonia in Europe (ESDE) Collaborative Group 2000; Defazio et al. 2004)	Service-based	***	13.3 (6.1–25.3)	13.3	***	***	***	***
Munich, Germany, 1996–1997 (Sugawara et al. 2006; Joensen 2016;)	Service-based	0.3 (0–0.6)	10.1(8.4–11.9)	3.1	5.4	0.38	0.23	1
Eight European countries, 1996–1997 (Epidemiological Study of Dystonia in Europe (ESDE) Collaborative Group 2000)	Service-based	***	11.7 (10.8–12.6)/ 1.5	3.6 (3.1–4.1)	5.7 (5.1–6.3)	1.4 (1.1–1.7)	***	0.7 (0.5–0.9)
Kyoto, Japan, 2000 (Defazio et al. 2004; Das et al. 2007; Joensen 2016)	Service-based	0.07 (0.002–0.4)	10.1 (8.4–11.8)	3.4 (3.6–6.5)	2.3 (1.6–3.3)	1.6 (1–2.3)	0.8 (0.3–1.4)	***
Belgrade, Yugoslavia, 2001 (Defazio et al. 2004; Joensen 2016)	Service-based	***	13.6 (11.6–15.9)	1.9 (1.2–2.8)	5.9 (4.6–7.5)	2.0 (1.2–2.8)	0.32	1.1 (0.6–2)
Foggia, Southern Italy, 2001–2002 (Defazio et al. 2004; Joensen 2016)	Service-based	***	12.7 (10.2–16.6)	5.9	4.4	2.4 (others)	-	-
Oslo, Norway, 1999–2002 (Defazio et al. 2004; Joensen 2016)	Service-based	***	25.4 (21.2–30.1)	4.7 (2.9–6.8)	13.0 (10–16.5)	2.4 (1.2–4.1)	0.8 (0.2–1.9)	2.8(1.5–4.5)
Akita, Japan, 2005 (Sugawara et al. 2006)	Service-based	0.68	14.4	10.4	2.8	1.1	***	***
Sardinia, Italy, 2006 (Steeves et al. 2012)	Service-based	***	3.2/***	3.2	***	***	***	***
Yonago, Japan, 2006 (Steeves et al. 2012)	Service-based	***	13.7 (9.1–18.3)/***	6.5[b] (3.3–9.7)	2.0 (0.2–3.8)	4.4 (1.8–7.0)	***	***
Faroe Islands, 2014 (Joensen 2016)	Service-based	***	60.2 (39.5–87.3)/***	0	47.8 (33.2–72.8)	8.3 (2.1–10.7)	2.1 (0–8.4)	2.1 (0–8.4)
Segovia, Spain, 1994 (Epidemiological Study of Dystonia in Europe (ESDE) Collaborative Group 2000; Joensen 2016)	N/A	***	27.9 (19.3–36.4)	16.3	3.4	6.1	***	2.0
Turku, Finland, 1996 (Epidemiological Study of Dystonia in Europe (ESDE) Collaborative Group 2000; Joensen 2016)	N/A	***	20.9 (16.8–25.6)	***	20.9(16.8–25.6)	***	***	***

Primary Late-Onset Dystonia

Primary late-onset dystonia (PLOD) is the most common form among primary dystonias. Age at onset is known to be the main determinant for patterns of body distribution and spread for most forms of primary dystonia (Defazio et al. 2004; Defazio 2010). PLOD (age at onset >20) presents either as focal (cervical, blepharospasm, oromandibular, limb or laryngeal) or segmental, but rarely as generalised forms. As seen in Table 5.1, most of the studies on focal and/or segmental PLOD are service (n = 13) or record-linkage based (n = 4), with only a few (n = 4) community-based studies, giving estimated CPRs from 3 to 732/10^5 (Defazio et al. 2004; Steeves et al. 2012; Joensen 2016). The highest outlier is from South Tirol, a population-based study performed by experts with stringent diagnostic criteria over a period of ten years in a small reference population over the age of 50, reporting a CPR of 732/10^5 with a very high 95 per cent CI (319–1564), raising the possibility of cluster-chance (Defazio 2010; Steeves et al. 2012). Interestingly, a very recent service-based study from the Faroe Islands disclosed the second highest rate of 60.2/10^5 (39.5–87.3), collected similarly in an extended period of almost 20 years. Prevalence rates over 25/10^5 are found in Caucasian populations of European descent, with the highest rates consistently among people of Scandinavian origin (Joensen 2016) (Table 5.1). However, the record-based ESDE study (European Study for Dystonia Epidemiology) from eight different European countries (Epidemiological Study of Dystonia in Europe (ESDE) Collaborative Group 2000), along with studies from Northern England, Germany and Serbia, pointed out more modest rates ranging between 12.9 and 15.2/10^5 (Butler et al. 2004; Defazio et al. 2004). In contrast, studies from other ethnicities (Japan and Egyptian studies, and Asian and African immigrants in an Oslo study) disclosed the lowest rates (6.1–10/10^5) (Defazio et al. 2004), with the exception of a community-based study from India (38.2/10^5) (Das et al. 2007). Such discrepancies may indicate varying genetic dispositions in different ethnic groups, or additional environmental factors, if not related to methodological shortcomings.

Cervical dystonia (CD) is the most common form among PLOD. In a recent analytical review, when service- and record-linkage-based studies were taken into account (eight from populations across Europe and four from Japan), the CPR of CD has been found to be between 2.8–18.3/10^5 (Defazio et al. 2013). A recent meta-analysis covering almost the same studies (together with two other service-based studies from Italy) revealed an overall CPR for CD of 4.98/10^5 (Steeves et al. 2012). This finding is close to the rate of 5.7/10^5 reported in the ESDE study (Epidemiological Study of Dystonia in Europe (ESDE) Collaborative Group 2000). As indicated in all studies and analytical reviews, these rates probably reflect only a portion of the accurate numbers in the community considering patients with mild symptoms or misdiagnoses. The few available community-based studies, on the other hand, differ in screening and assessment methods and may include selection bias for specific subtypes, as PLOD was represented only by CD cases (10/10^5) in an Egyptian study, while a similar door-to-door survey done in Calcutta, India, revealed a lower rate of 3.81/10^5 for CD in contrast to a much higher CPR for upper-limb dystonia (Defazio et al. 2004; Das et al. 2007). There are only two studies on incidence with estimated rates of 0.8 and 1.2 per 10^5 person-years (Nutt et al. 1988; Marras et al. 2007).

According to the few available studies providing age-adjusted prevalence rates, the CPR of CD showed an inverted U shape, with lower occurrence among the young and old (Epidemiological Study of Dystonia in Europe (ESDE) Collaborative Group 2000; Defazio et al. 2013). Gender distribution is comparably similar, with a female preponderance, ranging from 1.3 to 3.6:1, with an overall mean F:M ratio of 1.7:1 in most studied ethnic groups, except in the studies from Japan and Egypt (Defazio et al. 2013). CD was found to develop at earlier ages in males, suggesting differing risk factors affecting the phenotypic expression among genders (Defazio et al. 2013).

Blepharospasm (BSP) is the second most common form of PLOD, with a CPR varying between 1.6 and 13.3/10^5 with wide CIs (Table 5.1). The low-end rates are from the early studies in Rochester, USA, and in Yonago, Japan (1.7 and 1.6/10^5), while the high-end rates are from Puglia, southern Italy, and from Akita, Japan (13.3 and 10.4/10^5) (Epidemiological Study of Dystonia in Europe (ESDE) Collaborative Group 2000; Steeves et al. 2012; Joensen 2016). The Italian study included both focal and segmental BSP. When focal BSP was considered, the CPR of 7.4 was still much higher than in other European studies, depicting rates around 3.1–3.9/10^5, probably because patients were recruited also from ophthalmological services (Epidemiological Study of Dystonia in Europe (ESDE) Collaborative Group 2000; Steeves et al. 2012). The recently reported meta-analysis of these studies (pooling the data of six European, together with two Japanese studies) disclosed an overall rate of 4.2/10^5 (Steeves et al. 2012). As shown by most of these studies, the onset of BSP is frequently in the fifth and sixth decade, increasing steadily with advanced age. Women have much higher relative rates than men, as reported in the ESDE study (1.9:1) (Epidemiological Study of Dystonia in Europe (ESDE) Collaborative Group 2000).

Limb dystonia has been included in the available studies either as focal arm dystonia and/or as writer's cramp or other types of task-specific dystonia (taken together as upper-limb dystonia (ULD)). Lower-limb dystonia rarely occurs in isolation in PLOD. The CPR for ULD (usually as writer's cramp) is between 0.38–8.3/10^5 in reported service- and record-linkage-based studies from European populations (Epidemiological Study of Dystonia in Europe (ESDE) Collaborative Group 2000; Steeves et al. 2012; Joensen 2016). However, a much higher CPR was found in the only available community-based study from Calcutta, 21/10^5 for writer's cramp and 14.8/10^5 for writer's tremor (Das et al. 2007). These high rates might be explained by the screening procedure, but it may also be related to ethnic or environmental factors. Most of the studies reported a male preponderance with a F:M ratio of 0.7, in contrast to other subtypes of PLOD (Epidemiological Study of Dystonia in Europe (ESDE) Collaborative Group 2000; Steeves et al.

2012). Likewise, ULD cases are distinguished from others by their earlier mean age of onset (38.4 years vs 40.8 years for CD; 43.0 years for LD; and 55.7 years for oromandibular dystonia/ BSP) (Jinnah et al. 2013).

Other focal dystonias of adult onset, *oromandibular dystonia* (OMD), and *laryngeal dystonia* (LD) are relatively rare, compared to CD, BSP and ULD. Few studies reported wide ranges of CPRs: for OMD between 0.1 and 6.9/10^5 and for LD between 0.8 and 5.9/10^5 (Table 5.1) (Epidemiological Study of Dystonia in Europe (ESDE) Collaborative Group 2000; Steeves et al. 2012; Joensen 2016). If the results of a recent meta-analysis are taken into account, these numbers cluster at the lower end of variability around 0.52/10^5 for OMD and 1.54/10^5 for LD (Steeves et al. 2012). Gender distribution of both subtypes is clearly in favour of women by a F:M ratio of 2.0 for LD and 3.1 for OMD (Jinnah et al. 2013).

Studies on Risk Factors of Primary Late-Onset Dystonia

All family studies suggest genetic susceptibility of autosomal dominant inheritance with markedly reduced penetrance in PLOD, probably shared by different focal subtypes (Defazio 2010). Previous genetic studies disclosed a linkage to some loci and the possible contribution of known genes of PLOD (rarely TOR1A, but more often THAP1) (Jinnah et al. 2013). Recent search by newer molecular technologies introduced novel genes (TUBB4, CIZ1, GNAL and ANO3), which are putatively associated with different forms of PLOD (Jinnah et al. 2013). While mutations of CIZ1 and TUBB4 seem to be very rare, GNAL and ANO3 mutations are more frequent among familial PLOD with mostly craniocervical distribution (Jinnah et al. 2013).

Environmental risk factors for PLOD, investigated mainly by case-control studies, include neck trauma and scoliosis for CD, diseases of the anterior segment of the eye for BSP, sore throat for LD, and working or leisure activities requiring accurate and repetitive motor tasks for ULD, all indicating a role of peripheral injuries to related body parts (Defazio et al. 2013). Severe head trauma has been associated with different types of PLOD in one study (Defazio et al. 2013). Exposure time to sun might be an environmental risk for developing BSP, as shown by inverse association rates of BSP with latitude in previous studies (Molloy et al. 2016). On the other hand, coffee drinking seems to be a protective factor for BSP (Defazio et al. 2013). Overall, environmental factors appear to trigger or modify the development of PLOD in genetically susceptible individuals.

Another feature of PLOD is the varying degree of spread to adjacent body parts over time, which might also be determined by genetic/epigenetic and/or environmental risk factors. Among the PLODs, BSP has a greater risk of spread than CD and ULD, which is mainly evident during the first five years, with a decline afterwards; in CD and ULD spreading could often be seen later in the course (after 5–10 years) (Defazio 2010).

Prevalence of Secondary Dystonias

There are very few studies addressing the prevalence of non-primary dystonias in the community. Most data come from case series of tertiary or quaternary clinics and are open to bias. Although varying among centres, the relative frequency of non-primary dystonias is considered as 10–20 per cent of all dystonic syndromes (Dressler 2011). Among the most frequent causes of non-primary dystonias, tardive dystonia and dystonic cerebral palsy (dCP) are the most common. Even though the emergence of second-generation anti-psychotics (SGAs) might have decreased the incidence of tardive syndromes, first-generation anti-psychotics are still in use and SGAs are not free of this adverse effect. The prevalence rates for tardive dystonia varied considerably between 1.5 and 21 per cent of treated patients in a restricted number of relatively old studies (Dressler 2011). Data on the frequency of dCP can be drawn from studies of worldwide CP registers, reporting an increasing trend for the frequency of dCP, mainly occurring in children born at term accounting for 2 per 1000 live births (Himmelmann et al. 2009; Dressler 2011). The projection of these numbers to actual prevalence estimates for secondary dystonias, however, needs further epidemiological studies. In most of the reported studies on primary dystonias, the relative frequency of SDs has not been a specific point of interest, except by being exclusion criteria. Nevertheless, a service-based study from northern Japan reported the prevalence of drug-induced and other symptomatic dystonias (CP comprising 36 per cent of these cases) as 4.3/10^5 and 7.5/10^5, respectively (Sugawara et al. 2006). Interestingly, another community-based study from Calcutta revealed a higher total rate of secondary dystonia as 11.5/10^5 (with 4.2–25.0, 95 per cent CI) (Das et al. 2007).

Conclusions

Despite large variability of the results from available epidemiological studies, the CPR for primary dystonia clusters around 20/10^5 across populations of European descent (Epidemiological Study of Dystonia in Europe (ESDE) Collaborative Group 2000; Steeves et al. 2012; Joensen 2016), with a fairly stable ratio of early-onset vs late-onset cases as 1:10. Considering the problems of ascertainment, which is the shared reason of underestimates among all these studies, together with the secondary causes, the overall estimate for prevalence of dystonia may be expected to reach much higher numbers. Well-designed prospective studies over an extended period of time, covering large enough populations from different ethnicities, with the use of better clinical and/or genetic diagnostic tools may help to reveal more accurate CPR estimates to better understand and treat dystonia in the future.

References

Bressman SB. 2007. Genetics of dystonia: an overview. *Parkinsonism Relat Disord* 13 Suppl. 3:347–355.

Butler AG, Duffey PO, Hawthorne MR, Barnes MP. 2004. An epidemiologic survey of dystonia within the entire population of Northeast England over the past nine years. *Adv Neurol* 94:95–99.

Charlesworth G, Bhatia KP. 2013. Primary and secondary dystonic syndromes: an update. *Curr Opin Neurol* 26(4):406–412.

Das SK, Banerjee TK, Biswas A, Roy T, Raut DK, Chaudhuri A, Hazra A. 2007. Community survey of primary dystonia in the city of Kolkata, India. *Mov Disord* 22(14):2031–2036.

Defazio G. 2010. The epidemiology of primary dystonia: current evidence and perspectives. *Eur J Neurol* 17 Suppl. 1:9–14.

Defazio G, Abbruzzese G, Livrea P, Berardelli A. 2004. Epidemiology of primary dystonia. *Lancet Neurol* 3(11):673–678.

Defazio G, Jankovic J, Giel JL, Papapetropoulos S. 2013. Descriptive epidemiology of cervical dystonia. *Tremor Other Hyperkinet Mov (NY)* 3. doi:10.7916/D80C4TGJ

Dressler D. 2011. Nonprimary dystonias. *Handb Clin Neurol* 100:513–538.

Epidemiological Study of Dystonia in Europe (ESDE) Collaborative Group. 2000. A prevalence study of primary dystonia in eight European countries. *J Neurol* 247(10):787–792.

Himmelmann K, McManus V, Hagberg G, Uvebrant P, Krageloh-Mann I, Cans C, SCPE collaboration. 2009. Dyskinetic cerebral palsy in Europe: trends in prevalence and severity. *Arch Dis Child* 94(12):921–926.

Jinnah HA, Berardelli A, Comella C, Defazio G, Delong MR, Factor S, Galpern WR, Hallett M, Ludlow CL, Perlmutter JS, Rosen AR. 2013. The focal dystonias: current views and challenges for future research. *Mov Disord* 28(7):926–943.

Joensen P. 2016. High prevalence of primary focal dystonia in the Faroe Islands. *Acta Neurol Scand* 133(1):55–60.

Li SC, Schoenberg BS, Wang CC, Cheng XM, Rui DY, Bolis CL, Schoenberg DG. 1985. A prevalence survey of Parkinson's disease and other movement disorders in the People's Republic of China. *Arch Neurol* 42(7):655–657.

Marras C, Van den Eeden SK, Fross RD, Benedict-Albers KS, Klingman J, Leimpeter AD, Nelson LM, Risch N, Karter AJ, Bernstein AL, Tanner CM. 2007. Minimum incidence of primary cervical dystonia in a multiethnic health care population. *Neurology* 69(7):676–680.

Molloy A, Williams L, Kimmich O, Butler JS, Beiser I, McGovern E, O'Riordan S, Reilly RB, Walsh C, Hutchinson M. 2016. Sun exposure is an environmental factor for the development of blepharospasm. *J Neurol Neurosurg Psychiatry* 87(4):420–424.

Muller U. 2009. The monogenic primary dystonias. *Brain* 132(Pt 8):2005–2025.

Nutt JG, Muenter MD, Aronson A, Kurland LT, Melton LJ. 1988. Epidemiology of focal and generalized dystonia in Rochester, Minnesota. *Mov Disord* 3(3):188–194.

Steeves TD, Day L, Dykeman J, Jette N, Pringsheim T. 2012. The prevalence of primary dystonia: a systematic review and meta-analysis. *Mov Disord* 27(14):1789–1796.

Sugawara M, Watanabe S, Toyoshima I. 2006. Prevalence of dystonia in Akita prefecture in northern Japan. *Mov Disord* 21(7):1047–1049.

Chapter 6

The Motor Network Model for Dystonia

Hyder A. Jinnah and Ellen J. Hess

Introduction

The dystonias are a heterogeneous group of disorders defined by involuntary twisting or repetitive movements (Albanese et al. 2013). Unlike some other neurological disorders, the dystonias are not defined by a shared neuropathology. In fact, there are no obvious neuropathological correlates for most subtypes. However, the clinical manifestations likely arise from dysfunction of shared pathways of the nervous system involved in motor control.

Historically, dystonia was ascribed to dysfunction of basal ganglia circuits. However, more recent evidence has suggested a broader circuit that involves other regions, most notably the cerebellum. This evidence was first summarised in a comprehensive review covering basic neuroanatomical connections and evidence from human neuroimaging studies, neuropathology, physiology, cell biology and animal models (Neychev et al. 2011). The conclusion from this review was that the evidence was best accommodated by a motor network model in which several brain regions had a role. Since then, several additional reviews and commentaries have appeared addressing more specific features of the motor network model (Zoons et al. 2011; Avanzino & Abbruzzese 2012; Hendrix & Vitek 2012; Sadnicka et al. 2012; Filip et al. 2013; Lehericy et al. 2013; Prudente et al. 2014; Shakkottai 2014). The network appears to include the basal ganglia, cerebellum, sensorimotor cortex, thalamus, and probably other regions. These regions are all interconnected (Figure 6.1). How this network is disrupted to cause dystonia remains unknown, and several different mechanisms have been proposed (Prudente et al. 2014). It is possible that dystonia may arise from dysfunction of a single node in the network. It is also possible that dystonia requires simultaneous dysfunction of more than one node, or abnormal communication between the nodes. This review summarises evidence for each of these potential mechanisms.

Defining the anatomical substrates for dystonia traditionally has relied on classical neurological methods such as lesion studies and neuroimaging of affected individuals (Neychev et al. 2011). However, these sources of information provide only indirect information because demonstrating causality with these approaches in humans is rarely feasible. Here, we focus instead on selected examples from animal studies that provide proof of principle for different anatomical mechanisms underlying dystonia.

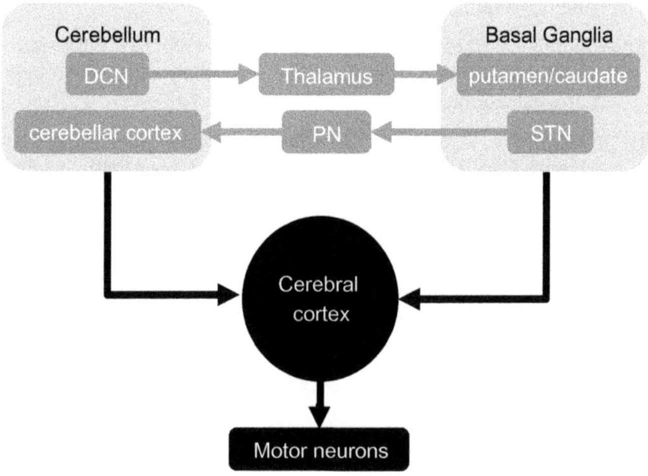

Figure 6.1 Traditional descriptions of major output pathways from the basal ganglia and cerebellum to the cerebral cortex are shown in black. Subcortical interconnections between these regions are shown in grey. Abbreviations: DCN, deep cerebellar nuclei; PN, pontine nuclei; STN, subthalamic nucleus.

Dystonia Caused by Dysfunction of a Single Node

Basal Ganglia Dystonias

There is good evidence that dysfunction originating in the basal ganglia can cause dystonia. One of the best examples is dopa-responsive dystonia, which most often arises from an inherited deficit in the synthesis of dopamine, an essential neurotransmitter in the basal ganglia (Kurian et al. 2011). It is most often caused by defects in GTP-cyclohydrolase, but less commonly arises from defects in sepiapterin reductase or tyrosine hydroxylase. Although each of these enzymes influences several neurotransmitters throughout the brain, the reversal of symptoms with levodopa points to an important role for dopamine.

Several genetic mouse models for dopa-responsive dystonia have been created by targeting the relevant enzymes (McDonald et al. 1988; Sato et al. 2008), but only one has dystonic symptoms that are reversed by levodopa (Rose et al. 2015). In this model, microinjection of levodopa into the striatum is sufficient to reverse symptoms, while microinjection of a precursor for norepinephrine does not. These results provide very strong evidence that it is selective dysfunction of dopamine transmission in the basal ganglia that causes dystonia. This model is not unique in implicating the basal ganglia as a source for dystonia. Other examples include rodent or primate models for tardive dystonia, or exposure to the striatal toxin 3-nitroproprionic acid (Wilson & Hess 2013).

Cerebellar Dystonias

There also is good evidence that dysfunction originating in the cerebellum can cause dystonia. In normal mice and rats, abnormal activation of the cerebellum with local microinjection of the glutamate agonist kainic acid in the cerebellum causes dystonic posturing (Pizoli et al. 2002; Alvarez-Fischer et al. 2012). These abnormal movements last for 1–2 hours, and animals have normal motor function afterwards, with no histological lesion of the cerebellum. The dystonic movements appear to be mediated by sustained activation of the AMPA subtype of glutamate receptors (Fan et al. 2012).

These results provide strong evidence that selective dysfunction of the cerebellum can trigger dystonia. This model is not unique in implicating the cerebellum as the source for dystonia. Other examples include rodent models with defects in calcium channels (Wilson & Hess 2013) and intracellular calcium processing (Hisatsune et al. 2013).

Other Possible Nodes

There is also evidence that isolated dysfunction of other anatomical regions may also cause dystonia, although the evidence is less abundant. For example, local pharmacological manipulations of several midbrain regions have been reported to cause abnormal movements resembling cervical dystonia in animals including the red nucleus (Walker et al. 1988), interstitial nucleus of Cajal (Klier et al. 2002) and superior colliculus (Holmes et al. 2012). These and other examples imply that dysfunction originating in a single node of the motor network can trigger dystonia, although they may ultimately operate through connections with other nodes.

Dystonia Caused by Dysfunction of More Than One Node

The Two-Hit Hypothesis

Simultaneous dysfunction of two nodes in the network can produce dystonia in a rat model of blepharospasm (Schicatano et al. 1997). In this model, rats with small lesions of the substantia nigra recover rapidly with no apparent motor deficits. Full recovery also is observed when the orbicularis oculi muscle is weakened by a minor crush injury to the nerve. However, the combination of these lesions in the same animal produces excessive eye blinking and orbicularis oculi spasms resembling blepharospasm. This model suggests that dystonia may sometimes arise from two separate but subclinical defects in different regions of the nervous system.

One Node Disrupts the Function of Another Node

Basal ganglia dysfunction traditionally is thought to result in motor dysfunction via thalamocortical pathways that ultimately link with motor neurons that cause movements. Similarly, dysfunction of the cerebellum traditionally is thought to result in abnormal movements through separate thalamocortical pathways to motor neurons. However, the basal ganglia and cerebellum have direct connections with each other, providing another pathway for motor dysfunction (Bostan & Strick 2010; Bostan et al. 2010). Abnormal signals from one of these regions could be transmitted to the second region, with motor dysfunction resulting from disrupted output of the second region.

In fact, this mechanism has been proposed for a mouse model of rapid-onset dystonia-parkinsonism. In this model, local blockade of sodium pumps with oubain in the cerebellum causes dystonia due to abnormal burst-firing of cerebellar Purkinje neurons (Chen et al. 2014; Fremont et al. 2014). Dystonia can be blocked either by severing the major outflow pathway of the cerebellum at the level of the deep cerebellar nuclei, or by severing a connection from the cerebellum to the basal ganglia at the level of the thalamic centromedian nucleus (Calderon et al. 2011). This result implies that dystonia in this model results from abnormal cerebellar activity that is transmitted first to the basal ganglia, and subsequently to motor output pathways.

Abnormal Communication Between Nodes

Another example of how communication between different nodes may influence dystonia comes from the tottering mouse mutant, which has paroxysmal dystonia associated with a point mutation affecting voltage-regulated calcium channels (Shirley et al. 2008). In humans, different mutations of the same channel cause multiple different disorders, including familial hemiplegic migraine, episodic ataxia type 2, spinocerebellar ataxia type 6, epilepsy, and focal or paroxysmal dystonia (Benarroch 2010; Rajakulendran et al. 2012).

In tottering mice, functional histochemical studies reveal selective activation of cerebellar pathways during dystonic attacks (Campbell & Hess 1998) and physiological studies reveal abnormal Purkinje neuron activity (Chen et al. 2009). Removal of abnormal cerebellar signals by surgical ablation (Neychev et al. 2008) or selective deletion of Purkinje neurons eliminates dystonic attacks in the tottering mutants (Campbell et al. 1999; Raike et al. 2013) In normal mice, selective introduction of the tottering mutation into cerebellar Purkinje neurons induces dystonia (Raike et al. 2013). These results provide strong evidence that dystonia originates from abnormal activity of Purkinje neurons in this model. However, the frequency and severity of dystonic attacks can be exaggerated by subclinical lesions of the basal ganglia with the neurotoxins 6-hydroxydopamine or quinolinic acid (Neychev et al. 2008). These results imply that the basal ganglia protects against dystonia in this model, by filtering out abnormal cerebellar signals.

Summary and Clinical Implications

There is good evidence from animals that different types of dystonia arise from different pathological mechanisms in a broader motor network. Although some of the strongest evidence comes from animal studies that cannot be directly replicated in humans, the observations establish biological proof-of-principle that dystonia may arise through different network mechanisms. Different subtypes of human dystonia may also arise from distinct nodes in the network, such as the basal ganglia or cerebellum. Other subtypes may arise from abnormal interactions among network nodes.

If this is also the case for humans, then clinical features may differ according to mechanism. There are many varying clinical manifestations of dystonia, such as mobile or tonic postures, continuous or intermittent movements, writhing or tremor-like movements, slow or fast movements, and others (Fahn 1984). It is feasible that these different manifestations reflect slightly different underlying mechanisms in the motor network. Although correlations between different subtypes of dystonia and their anatomical origins is currently lacking, one potential example is 'thalamic dystonia'. This subtype most often arises from focal lesions of the thalamus, and has been described as being characteristically very jerky and tremulous (Ghika et al. 1994; Kim 2001; Lehericy et al. 2001).

Another implication of different pathological mechanisms in the network is that optimum treatments for different subtypes may vary. For example, neuromodulation targeting the main outflow tract of the basal ganglia provides a remarkably effective treatment for certain types of dystonia, such as DYT1 dystonia (Vidailhet et al. 2012; Mills et al. 2014). Although this observation demonstrates that interrupting the network at this site can block dystonia, it does not imply that DYT1 dystonia is a 'basal ganglia dystonia'. Interestingly, neuromodulation directed to the same region provides little or no benefit for other types of dystonia, such as rapid-onset dystonia-parkinsonism. The reasons that neuromodulation does not work in this disorder remain unclear, but could imply that a different part of the motor network may need to be targeted. Thus deciphering the specific mechanisms by which the motor network is affected in different subtypes of dystonia has clear implications for surgical treatment strategies.

Acknowledgements

This work was supported in part by a grant to the Dystonia Coalition (U54 NS065701, TR000146) from the Office of Rare Diseases at the National Center for Advancing Translational Studies and the National Institute of Neurological Disorders and Stroke at the NIH.

References

Albanese A, Bhatia K, Bressman SB, DeLong MR, Fahn S, Fung VSC, Hallett M, Jankovic J, Jinnah HA, Klein C, Lang AE, Mink JW, Teller JK. 2013. Phenomenology and classification of dystonia: a consensus update. *Mov Disord* 28:863–873.

Alvarez-Fischer D, Grundmann M, Lu L, Samans B, Fritsch B, Moller JC, Schaefer MK, Hartmann A, Oertel WH, Bandmann O. 2012. Prolonged generalized dystonia after chronic cerebellar application of kainic acid. *Brain Res* 1464:82–88.

Avanzino L, Abbruzzese G. 2012. How does the cerebellum contribute to the pathophysiology of dystonia? *Basal Ganglia* 2:231–235.

Benarroch EE. 2010. Neuronal voltage-gated calcium channels: brief overview of their function and clinical implications in neurology. *Neurology* 74:1310–1315.

Bostan AC, Strick PL. 2010. The cerebellum and basal ganglia are interconnected. *Neuropsychol Rev* 20:261–270.

Bostan AC, Dum RP, Strick PL. 2010. The basal ganglia communicate with the cerebellum. *Proc Natl Acad Sci USA* 107:8452–8456.

Calderon DP, Fremont R, Kraenzlin F, Khodakhah K. 2011. The neural substrates of rapid-onset dystonia-parkinsonism. *Nat Neurosci* 14:357–365.

Campbell DB, Hess EJ. 1998. Cerebellar circuitry is activated during convulsive episodes in the tottering (tg/tg) mutant mouse. *Neurosci* 85:773–783.

Campbell DB, North JB, Hess EJ. 1999. Tottering mouse motor dysfunction is abolished on the Purkinje cell degeneration (pcd) mutant background. *Exp Neurol* 160:268–278.

Chen CH, Fremont R, Arteaga-Bracho EE, Khodakhah K. 2014. Short latency cerebellar modulation of the basal ganglia. *Nat Neurosci* 17:1767–1775.

Chen G, Popa LS, Wang X, Gao W, Barnes J, Hendrix CM, Hess EJ, Ebner TJ. 2009. Low-frequency oscillations in the cerebellar cortex of the tottering mouse. *J Neurophysiol* 101:234–245.

Fahn S. 1984. The varied clinical expressions of dystonia. *Neurol Clinics* 2:541–554.

Fan X, Hughes KE, Jinnah HA, Hess EJ. 2012. Selective and sustained AMPA receptor activation in cerebellum induces dystonia in mice. *J Pharmacol Exp Ther* 340:733–741.

Filip P, Lungu OV, Bares M. 2013. Dystonia and the cerebellum: a new field of interest in movement disorders? *Clin Neurophysiol* 124:1269–1274.

Fremont R, Calderon DP, Maleki S, Khodakhah K. 2014. Abnormal high-frequency burst firing of cerebellar neurons in rapid-onset dystonia-parkinsonism. *J Neurosci* 34:11723–11732.

Ghika J, Bogousslavsky J, Henderson J, Maeder P, Regli F. 1994. The 'jerky dystonic unsteady hand': a delayed motor syndrome in posterior thalamic infarctions. *J Neurol* 241:537–542.

Hendrix CM, Vitek JL. 2012. Toward a network model of dystonia. *Ann NY Acad Sci* 1265:46–55.

Hisatsune C, Miyamoto H, Hirono M, Yamaguchi N, Sugawara T, Ogawa N, Ebisui E, Ohshima T, Yamada M, Hensch TK, Hattori M, Mikoshiba K. 2013. IP3R1 deficiency in the cerebellum/brainstem causes basal ganglia-independent dystonia by triggering tonic Purkinje cell firings in mice. *Front Neural Circuits* 7:156.

Holmes AL, Forcelli PA, Desjardin JT, Decker AL, Teferra M, West EA, Malkova L, Gale K. 2012. Superior colliculus mediates cervical dystonia evoked by inhibition of the substantia nigra pars reticulata. *J Neurosci* 32: 13326–13332.

Kim JS. 2001. Delayed onset mixed involuntary movements after thalamic stroke. *Brain* 124:299–309.

Klier EM, Wang H, Constantin AG, Crawford JD. 2002. Midbrain control of three-dimensional head orientation. *Science* 295:1314–1316.

Kurian MA, Gissen P, Smith M, Heales S, Jr, Clayton PT. 2011. The monoamine neurotransmitter disorders: an expanding range of neurological syndromes. *Lancet Neurol* 10:721–733.

Lehericy S, Grand S, Pollak P, Poupon F, LeBas JF, Limousin P, Jedynak P, Marsault C, Agid Y, Vidailhet M. 2001. Clinical characteristics and topography of lesion in movement disorders due to thalamic lesions. *Neurology* 57:1055–1066.

Lehericy S, Tijssen MA, Vidailhet M, Kaji R, Meunier S. 2013. The anatomical basis of dystonia: current view using neuroimaging. *Mov Disord* 28:944–957.

McDonald JD, Cotton RGH, Jennings I, Ledley FD, Woo SLC, Bode VC. 1988. Biochemical defect of the hph-1 mouse mutant is a deficiency in GTP-cyclohydrolase activity. *J Neurochem* 50:655–657.

Mills KA, Starr PA, Ostrem JL. 2014. Neuromodulation for dystonia: target and patient selection. *Neurosurg Clin N Am* 25:59–75.

Neychev V, Fan X, Mitev VI, Hess EJ, Jinnah HA. 2008. The basal ganglia and cerebellum interact in the expression of dystonic movement. *Brain* 131:2499–2509.

Neychev VK, Gross R, Lehericy S, Hess EJ, Jinnah HA. 2011. The functional neuroanatomy of dystonia. *Neurobiol Dis* 42:185–201.

Pizoli CE, Jinnah HA, Billingsley ML, Hess EJ. 2002. Abnormal cerebellar signaling induces dystonia in mice. *J Neurosci* 22:7825–7833.

Prudente CN, Hess EJ, Jinnah HA. 2014. Dystonia as a network disorder: what is the role of the cerebellum? *Neuroscience* 260:23–35.

Raike RS, Weisz C, Hoebeek FE, Terzi MC, De Zeeuw CI, van den Maagdenberg AM, Jinnah HA, Hess EJ. 2013. Stress, caffeine and ethanol trigger transient neurological dysfunction through shared mechanisms in a mouse calcium channelopathy. *Neurobiol Dis* 50:151–159.

Rajakulendran S, Kaski D, Hanna MG. 2012. Neuronal P/Q-type calcium channel dysfunction in inherited disorders of the CNS. *Nat Rev Neurol* 8:86–96.

Rose SJ, Yu XY, Heinzer AK, Harrast P, Fan X, Raike RS, Thompson VB, Pare JF, Weinshenker D, Smith Y, Jinnah HA, Hess EJ. 2015. A new knock-in mouse model of L-DOPA responsive-dystonia. *Brain* 138:2987–3002.

Sadnicka A, Hoffland BS, Bhatia KP, van de Warrenburg BP, Edwards MJ. 2012. The cerebellum in dystonia: help or hindrance? *Clin Neurophysiol* 123:65–70.

Sato K, Sumi-Ichinose C, Kaji R, Ikemoto K, Nomura T, Nagatsu I, Ichinose H, Ito M, Sako W, Nagahiro S, Graybiel AM, Goto S. 2008. Differential involvement of striosome and matrix dopamine systems in a transgenic model of dopa-responsive dystonia. *Proc Natl Acad Sci USA* 105:12551–12556.

Schicatano EJ, Basso MA, Evinger C. 1997. Animal model explains the origins of the cranial dystonia benign essential blepharospasm. *J Neurophysiol* 77:2842–2846.

Shakkottai VG. 2014. Physiologic changes associated with cerebellar dystonia. *Cerebellum* 13(5):637–644.

Shirley TL, Rao LM, Hess EJ, Jinnah HA. 2008. Paroxysmal dyskinesias in mice. *Mov Disord* 23:259–264.

Vidailhet M, Jutras MF, Grabli D, Roze E. 2012. Deep brain stimulation for dystonia. *J Neurol Neurosurg Psychiatry* 84:1029–1040.

Walker JM, Matsumoto RR, Bowen WD, Gans DL, Jones KD, Walker FO. 1988. Evidence for a role of haloperidol-sensitive sigma opiate receptors in the motor effects of antipsychotic drugs. *Neurology* 38:961–965.

Wilson B, Hess EJ. 2013. Animal models for dystonia. *Mov Disord* 28:982–989.

Zoons E, Booij J, Nederveen AJ, Dijk JM, Tijssen MA. 2011. Structural, functional and molecular imaging of the brain in primary focal dystonia: a review. *Neuroimage* 56:1011–1020.

Chapter 7

Functional Imaging in Dystonia

Scott A. Norris and Joel S. Perlmutter

Overview

Idiopathic isolated dystonia is a heterogeneous disorder with regard to epidemiology, clinical characteristics, aetiology and response to therapy. Questions remain regarding the pathophysiology of idiopathic dystonia, largely due to lack of consistent anatomical data, biomarkers and animal models. The goal is to better understand pathologic correlations with dysfunction of brain regions, functional networks and receptor/neurotransmitter systems that may provide potential biomarkers of dysfunction and rationale for targets for new therapies. In this chapter, we will first discuss the commonly applied functional imaging techniques and then discuss applications to idiopathic and genetic forms of isolated dystonia. Functional neuroimaging already has consistently identified regional dysfunction in basal ganglia, cerebellum, sensorimotor cortex and thalamus. However, various inconsistencies mandate that we must emphasise the importance of cautions regarding potential methodological pitfalls and approaches to avoid them.

Functional Neuroimaging Techniques

Functional imaging includes measurement of brain function either in the 'resting state' or with activation by a task, drug or physiologic intervention. A variety of measures reflect brain function, including regional blood flow, metabolism, receptor binding or neurotransmitter activity. Molecular imaging methods including positron emission tomography (PET) and single photon emission computed tomography (SPECT) permit measurements of regional distribution of administered radioactivity that reflect various functions depending upon the administered radiopharmaceutical. Initially, these measures identified local changes in resting state measures of metabolism or blood flow that corresponded to specific clinical manifestations – an *in vivo* neuroimaging extension of the old clinical-pathologic correlation. The underlying assumption is that local flow or metabolism reflects local interneuronal activity or inputs into that brain region (Raichle 1987). More sophisticated analyses of such imaging data include identification of covariance networks – i.e. parts of the brain that seemed to have resting function measures that correlated with each other. Patterns of such covariance networks could be related to specific states or behaviours (Eidelberg et al. 1995).

One could apply these molecular imaging methods or MR (magnetic resonance)-based BOLD (blood oxygen level-dependent) measures to determine regional changes induced by various tasks, physiologic manoeuvres, drugs or non-physiologic stimulation. Such approaches provide a whole-brain view of responses to these 'activations' and how such responses change in disease states. One must interpret such changes in disease states with caution as altered performance in task-based studies between impaired and control groups could confound interpretation of brain responses – i.e. are brain responses altered by the disease state or by differences in performance and sensory feedback?

Although molecular imaging approaches permit only single or a few measures from each person for such correlational studies, the development of resting state functional magnetic resonance imaging (rs-fMRI) permits hundreds of measures from each participant, thereby allowing identification of resting state functional networks. These rs-fMRI techniques depend upon detection of BOLD signals that reflect the weighted ratio of oxyhaemoglobin (oxygenated and isomagnetic) and deoxyhaemoglobin (deoxygenated and paramagnetic). At rest, each voxel in the brain seemingly appears to have low-level noise, but closer inspection reveals that various networks of brain regions have varying BOLD signals that correlate with each other (Biswal et al. 1995). These correlation-based networks define resting state networks that may change in various disease states. The challenge in these types of studies has been the increasing evidence that rigorous quality control measures must be followed to avoid spurious and potentially non-reproducible results (Power et al. 2012).

Molecular imaging approaches measure specific binding sites for receptors or activity of various enzymes that may relate to neurotransmitter systems. These studies also can be either resting state or stimulation types. Resting state studies primarily attempt to identify regional changes in receptor or transmitters that correspond with a disease trait or state. Alternatively, physiologic, pharmacologic or electrical stimulation can potentially alter uptake or retention of specific radioligands. For example, amphetamine or a motor task can be employed to either displace or block retention of selected dopaminergic receptor radioligands. The change in retention of the radioligand reflects release of endogenous dopamine that competes for specific binding sites, thereby providing one measure of potential dopaminergic function.

Functional Imaging Data in Dystonia

Resting State Studies

Resting state PET studies of blepharospasm, cervical dystonia, and other dystonias including generalised, focal, multifocal and hemidystonia cause altered regional glucose metabolism in premotor, prefrontal and sensorimotor cortex, thalamus, basal ganglia, brainstem and cerebellum (Lehericy et al. 2013). Regional findings, however, vary considerably both within and across dystonia types. In blepharospasm, altered metabolism typically occurs in deeper subcortical structures (thalamus, brainstem, cerebellum) compared to cervical dystonia, and the other various dystonia types have altered metabolism in striatum, pallidum and cortical regions (for review, see Neychev et al. 2011; Zoons et al. 2011. Even within these specific forms of dystonia, reports vary with regard to involved regions. One potential confound is the lack of adequate descriptions of dystonic behaviour during the scans. Subtle movements can confound interpretation of findings by provoking regional metabolic or flow changes which also may reflect sensory processing. One blepharospasm study attempted to account for potential movement confounds by evaluating patients only following botulinum toxin injections that would reduce dystonia. This is a reasonable strategy assuming that botulinum injections do not alter brain function, but agreement on this point remains elusive. Multiple studies report alterations in the sensorimotor network, but potential behavioural confounds weaken the confidence of these findings.

Rather than limiting resting state analyses to identification of specific regional changes, principal component analyses can detect networks linked by a spatial covariance metabolic or flow pattern in the resting state. Networks of regions that co-vary can be identified and an individual score indicates the strength of the expression of this pattern. A dystonia-specific pattern in those with cervical dystonia or with TOR1A autosomal dominant dystonia includes posterior lenticular nucleus, cerebellum and supplemental motor areas. Non-manifesting carriers with TOR1A also have this pattern – demonstrating that behavioural confounds do not account for the findings. Similarly, manifesting carriers asleep also have the same pattern. Interestingly, non-manifesting carriers of the THAP1 genetic mutation have a different covariance pattern, including contributions from putamen, cerebellum, upper brainstem, thalamus and presupplemental regions that differ from manifesting carriers of THAP1 with a covariance pattern including presupplemental motor area, parietal association cortices, inferior cerebellar, brainstem and ventral thalamic regions. Note that these covariance patterns identify regions that vary together rather than regions that have specifically high or low metabolism. Nevertheless, together these studies suggest (1) some common metabolic regional involvement across the dystonias, (2) specific functional changes reflecting genetic aetiology, and (3) some distinct phenotype-specific metabolic effects.

Resting state fMRI studies in focal hand dystonia, cervical dystonia and writer's cramp reveal reduced functional connectivity involving the sensorimotor network, including supplemental motor area and premotor cortex as well as putamen (irrespective of the affected body region). Additional regions and networks were inconsistently altered across these dystonia types and may include thalamus, cerebellum, parietal cortex, globus pallidus pars externa and frontoparietal, executive control and primary visual networks (Karimi & Permutter 2015). A single study described voxel-wise analysis for the *amplitude* of low frequency fluctuations in a small group of those with blepharospasm rather than calculating correlations across regions, demonstrating increased amplitudes in the putamen, globus pallidus, insula and medial prefrontal cortex, and decreased amplitude in the somatosensory regions, thalami, cingulate cortex and cerebellum. However, two types of problems arise in these studies: methodological limitations and behavioural confounds. Common methodological concerns include quality assurance (i.e. motion correction) and adequacy of multiple comparison corrections. Motion confounds arise in two ways: frame to frame movement of the head or movement of the body with subsequent effects directly on regional BOLD signal (the behavioural confound) or disturbances in the magnetic field. Increasing evidence indicates that inadequate rigour in dealing with frame to frame movement can lead to spurious findings. Inadequate multiple comparison corrections also can lead to false-positive, unreproducible results. Family-wise error rate correction used in most studies for multiple comparisons occurs at the subject level only and may be inadequate. Only two of the aforementioned studies apply Bonferroni correction, but only at the group level across networks rather than a more stringent statistical option at the voxel level. However, this approach could be too conservative, leading to false negatives. Other approaches may be more appropriate, like Monte Carlo leave-one-out strategy or test–retest (relax multiple comparisons rigour in a first group to generate potential relevant findings and then test the reproducibility of these findings in a second group). To minimise movement confounds, one may study task-specific dystonias that occur only with a specific action and not at rest during a scan. Alternatively, some study resting state changes following therapeutic botulinum toxin injections to reduce unwanted movements, but results remain conflicting with partial restoration of altered functional connectivity in the sensorimotor, primary visual and prefrontal cortices and lentiform nuclei of those with cervical dystonia and no effect on connectivity in a task-specific form of dystonia, writer's cramp. Furthermore, some believe that botulinum injections into muscles also may directly affect brain function but this also remains unclear.

Task-Based Studies

Since many studies of resting state did not initially identify obvious regional abnormalities, investigators used task-related functional imaging to try to identify changes in an activated system that may not be present at rest. Task-related PET (FDG and [^{15}O]H_2O) and fMRI studies apply specific motor tasks during scan acquisition that elicit dystonia (e.g. writer's cramp, laryngeal dystonia, blepharospasm). These studies reveal common (but not consistent) alterations in sensorimotor processing regions, including primary sensorimotor cortex, premotor and sensory association areas, ipsilateral cerebellum, thalamus, and basal ganglia (Zoons et al. 2011). Across studies of the same dystonia type, there are numerous discrepancies in the regions affected, relative signal change, laterality, and relationships to severity and therapy. These discrepancies are also observed across studies of different types of dystonia. Even with careful observation of task performance, those with dystonia may employ different muscle engagement strategies that could coincide with different neural activation. Movement or sensory feedback secondary to the task may introduce brain state changes that do not reflect underlying pathophysiology, confounding interpretation of findings.

Tasks that do not induce dystonia (e.g. motor performance of a non-affected body region that does not produce dystonia or sensory stimulation) allow the study of activated brain regions or networks that may contribute to the underlying pathophysiology of dystonia without confounds related to motor and sensory feedback. For example, vibration-induced PET blood flow responses in the primary sensorimotor cortex were altered contralateral to stimulation in both affected and unaffected body regions in those with various forms of dystonia, including writer's cramp, blepharospasm, focal arm dystonia, cervical dystonia and typist's dystonia. Functional MRI revealed reduced separation (disorganisation) of the cortical hand representation during vibrotactile stimulation in idiopathic focal hand dystonia. Combined, these stimulation task studies indicate dysfunctional afferent inputs at multiple brain levels, including brain regions contralateral to unaffected body regions. Functional MRI alterations also occurred in parietal, cingulate, supplemental motor association and ipsilateral putamen during execution and imagined arm movements (non-dystonic movements in an unaffected body region) in those with cervical dystonia. While these imagined and sensory tasks demonstrate findings involving the sensorimotor network independent of overt dystonia, they may or may not have the same interpretation confounds, depending on whether the tasks elicit unintended motor responses (Lehericy et al. 2013).

Neurotransmitter Systems Studies

The first evidence of altered dopaminergic transmission in focal dystonia was reduced dopamine D2-like receptor binding in the putamen, measured by PET [^{18}F] spiperone (Perlmutter et al. 1997). Such changes may be somatotopically organised depending upon body part affected (Black et al. 2014). Numerous PET and SPECT studies in focal hand, cranial, cervical and inherited (TOR1A, DYT6, DYT11) dystonia replicated these findings. However, all of these studies used D2-like radioligands or those that were sensitive to endogenous dopamine concentrations. A recent study using N-methylbenperidol (NMB), a highly selective D2-receptor radioligand, did not identify reduced striatal uptake. The apparent discrepancy may reflect the high specificity of NMB for D2-specific dopamine receptors in contrast to other radioligands with little D2/D3 selectivity. Moreover, one commonly used D2-like radioligand [^{11}C] raclopride is particularly sensitive to endogenous dopamine levels. This sensitivity permits a strategy to quantify dopamine release by either a motor task or drug administration since the activation may cause striatal release of dopamine that could reduce the uptake or displace [^{11}C] raclopride. Application of this approach to those participants during tasks that do or do not provoke dystonic manifestations in those with either writer's cramp or laryngeal dystonia suggest possible divergent patterns of left striatal dopamine release during symptomatic (associated with decreased dopamine release) and asymptomatic (associated with increased dopamine release) tasks. These studies combined with prior reports suggest a somatotopic representation of reduced striatal dopamine. Potential limitations of many dopaminergic radioligand studies include inadequate specificity and potential confounds of endogenous striatal dopamine levels. Although such studies may identify a regional abnormality, the location of the receptor abnormality on pre- versus postsynaptic sites cannot be distinguished, nor do these studies address potential postsynaptic mechanisms that could affect receptor-mediated function.

While the majority of neurotransmitter imaging studies focus on dopamine transmission, there is limited evidence that the mechanisms of isolated idiopathic dystonia involve complex networks and neurotransmitter systems including gamma-aminobutyric acid (GABA) and acetylcholine (Ach). A recent PET study focusing on the GABAergic neurotransmitter systems revealed reduced [^{11}C]-flumazenil (a $GABA_A$ receptor antagonist) receptor affinity in the primary motor and premotor cortex, primary and secondary somatosensory cortex, and cingulate cortex in TOR1A carriers and those with isolated idiopathic dystonia. These data support prior MRI spectroscopy data and the hypotheses that dysfunctional neurotransmission contributes to disinhibition of the sensorimotor cortex. A single SPECT scan demonstrates reduced [^{123}I]iodobezovesamicol (a marker of acetylcholine receptors) striatal binding in those with cervical dystonia compared to controls. Future PET imaging studies would likely benefit from development and application of cholinergic radiotracers to investigate these pathways in dystonia.

Conclusions

Functional neuroimaging offers an important research tool to study regional network dysfunctions in dystonia. Great care must be taken when deciphering functional imaging data as many confounds influence results and interpretation. Regardless of inconsistencies across studies, common alterations of the sensorimotor networks including basal ganglia and cerebellum exist. Yet, functional imaging in isolation cannot discern whether altered network connections are causal, secondary or compensatory. However, functional imaging can identify regional or network dysfunction that permits greater depth of exploration perhaps best combined with other modalities including electrophysiology or structural imaging, like diffusion tensor imaging with MR. More specific radiopharmaceuticals also may permit more selective interpretation of underlying neurochemical pathophysiology. Either transmitter system-based approaches or more general regional or functional network imaging may provide targets for potential new interventions. Such targets of engagement can help to determine whether interventions reach the relevant degree of desired effect. This will bring a greater mechanistic rationale to therapeutic development.

Acknowledgements

This work was supported by grants from NIH (NS075321, NS41509, NS058714, NS065701), the Barnes Jewish Hospital Foundation (Elliot Stein Family Fund and Parkinson Disease Research Fund), the Dystonia Medical Research Foundation, the American Parkinson Disease Association Advanced Research Center at Washington University and the Murphy Fund for Neuroimaging of Dystonia.

References

Biswal B, Yetkin FZ, Haughton VM, Hyde JS. 1995. Functional connectivity in the motor cortex of resting human brain using echo-planar MRI. *Magn Reson Med* 34(4):537–541.

Black KJ, Snyder AZ, Mink JW, Tolia VN, Revilla FJ, Moerlein SM, Perlmutter JS. 2014. Spatial reorganization of putaminal dopamine D2-like receptors in cranial and hand dystonia. *PLoS One* 9(2):e88121.

Eidelberg D, Moeller JR, Ishikawa T, Dhawan V, Spetsieris P, Przedborski S, Fahn S. 1995. The metabolic topography of idiopathic torsion dystonia. *Brain* 118:1473–1484.

Karimi M, Perlmutter JS. 2015. The role of dopamine and dopaminergic pathways in dystonia: insights from neuroimaging. *Tremor Other Hyperkinet Mov (NY)* 5:280.

Lehericy S, Tijssen MA, Vidailhet M, Kaji R, Meunier S. 2013. The anatomical basis of dystonia: current view using neuroimaging. *Mov Disord* 28(7):944–957.

Neychev VK, Gross RE, Lehericy S, Hess EJ, Jinnah HA. 2011. The functional neuroanatomy of dystonia. *Neurobiol Dis* 42(2):185–201.

Perlmutter JS, Stambuk MK, Markham J, Black KJ, McGee-Minnich L, Jankovic J, Moerlein SM. 1997. Decreased [18F]spiperone binding in putamen in idiopathic focal dystonia. *J Neurosci* 17(2):843–850.

Power JD, Barnes KA, Snyder AZ, Schlaggar BL, Petersen SE. 2012. Spurious but systematic correlations in functional connectivity MRI networks arise from subject motion. *Neuroimage* 59(3):2142–2154.

Raichle M. 1987. Circulator and metabolic correlates of brain function in normal humans. In *Handbook of Physiology: The Nervous System*. Bethesda, MD: American Physiological Society, 643–674.

Zoons E, Booij J, Nederveen AJ, Dijk JM, Tijssen MA. 2011. Structural, functional and molecular imaging of the brain in primary focal dystonia: a review. *Neuroimage* 56(3):1011–1120.

Chapter 8

The Pathophysiology of Dystonia

Jung E. Park, Sophie Cho and Mark Hallett

Introduction

Dystonia is a neurological disorder characterised by involuntary muscle contractions leading to an excess of movements and abnormal postures (Quartarone & Hallett 2013; Balint & Bhatia 2014). Examples of other clinical features that are seen in this disorder include task specificity and overflow muscle activation including mirror dystonia (Albanese et al. 2013). The clinical spectrum can vary and other associated phenomenology such as tremor or myoclonus can co-occur (Kinugawa et al. 2009; Defazio et al. 2015). Dystonia can also vary in age of onset, temporal pattern and involved body parts (Albanese et al. 2013). It is presumed that both genetics and environmental factors play a role, as genetically susceptible individuals appear to develop focal dystonia with repetitive use of the body part or trauma as triggering factors (Sheehy & Marsden 1982; Hallett 2011).

The physiology of different types of dystonias is likely common to a certain extent, based on observations that patients can have more than one type of dystonia and different family members present with various types of dystonia. Investigations into the neurophysiology of dystonia have so far been mostly directed at the adult onset focal dystonias such as focal hand dystonia, blepharospasm and cervical dystonia. Efforts to analyse certain clinical features such as task specificity, mirror dystonia and overflow, as well as the responsiveness to specific therapeutic measures including gamma-aminobutyric acid (GABA)-ergic medications, repetitive transcranial magnetic stimulation (rTMS) and deep brain stimulation (DBS), are also ongoing. Future investigation of other types of dystonia will be necessary to fully understand the full range of the pathophysiology.

In this chapter, we review the pathophysiology of dystonia that is currently known, with an emphasis on the neurophysiology that has mostly been studied using transcranial magnetic stimulation (TMS) or functional brain imaging in patients with focal hand dystonia, cervical dystonia and isolated childhood-onset dystonia. There are several general abnormalities that appear to be present and play a role in the pathophysiology, including a loss of inhibition, sensory dysfunction and abnormal plasticity, which will be discussed in this chapter. Task specificity, an aspect of the disorder of which the neurophysiology has been studied with increasing interest, will also be discussed.

Loss of Inhibition

Previous studies have found evidence of deficient inhibition at multiple levels of the nervous system in patients with dystonia, including the cortex, brainstem and spinal cord (Hallett 2011). Whereas in healthy human subjects, various types of inhibition have been found, such as reciprocal inhibition (RI) of H reflexes, short intracortical inhibition (SICI), long intracortical inhibition (LICI), the cortical silent period (cSP), short-latency afferent inhibition (SAI), long-latency afferent inhibition (LAI) and surround inhibition, these have been found to be altered in patients with dystonia. Influences on the motor cortex coming from other brain areas including the premotor and parietal cortices, contralateral motor cortex and cerebellum that are found in healthy subjects also appear to be altered in patients with dystonia. These will now be discussed in more detail.

Deficient Reciprocal Inhibition of H Reflexes

RI, a measure of inhibition occurring at the spinal level, is quantified by the amount of H reflex attenuation following stimulation of Ia afferents from the antagonist muscle (Day et al. 1984). RI of H reflexes at rest is impaired in patients with focal hand dystonia (Chen et al. 1995), as well as in patients with cervical dystonia (Deuschl et al. 1992) and generalised dystonia (Tisch et al. 2006). In patients with writer's cramp, RI was impaired not only in the symptomatic hand, but in the asymptomatic hand as well. Furthermore, RI was found to be deficient in the clinically unaffected upper extremities in patients with cervical dystonia, indicating that there is a common disturbance of motor control mechanisms regardless of the type of dystonia (Deuschl et al. 1992). Importantly, while some electrophysiological findings such as intracortical inhibition (ICI) and cSP were found to be abnormal in non-manifesting DYT1 gene carriers, reciprocal inhibition has been reported to be normal (Edwards et al. 2003).

Loss of Short Intracortical Inhibition and Long Intracortical Inhibition

SICI is seen in healthy subjects with paired-pulse stimulation on the motor cortex, where an initial conditioning stimulus of subthreshold intensity is given prior to a test stimulus of suprathreshold intensity (Kujirai et al. 1993). At interstimulus intervals (ISIs) of less than about 5 ms, inhibition of the amplitude of the motor-evoked potential (MEP) is seen. SICI has been found to be reduced at rest and even further reduced in the movement initiation phase in patients with focal hand dystonia and DYT1 dystonia (Edwards et al. 2003; Beck et al. 2008). Patients with blepharospasm also appear to have deficient SICI (Sommer et al. 2002). However, in studies on patients with cervical dystonia, Segawa disease (DYT5) or myoclonus-dystonia (DYT11), SICI was found to be normal at rest (Hanajima et al. 2007; Sabine et al. 2008; van der Salm et al. 2009; Amadio et al. 2014).

LICI is another intracortical inhibitory influence seen in healthy subjects with paired-pulse stimulation on the motor cortex at intervals from 60 to 150 ms. To date, there are only a few reports of LICI in patients with dystonia. In patients with focal hand dystonia, LICI was found to be deficient on the symptomatic side only during voluntary muscle activation (Chen et al. 1997). In another investigation, LICI was found to be decreased at rest, but not during voluntary contraction of the affected hand in a group of patients with focal upper-limb dystonia and cervical dystonia (Espay et al. 2006).

Shortened Cortical Silent Period

The cSP is an interruption of ongoing electromyographic activity caused by TMS, lasting approximately 100–200 ms (Marsden et al. 1983). It is thought to originate from cortical inhibitory mechanisms, as well as spinal inhibitory mechanisms in the early part of the cSP (Chen et al. 1999). It may be mediated by $GABA_B$ receptors (Werhahn et al. 1999). Observations on the cSP in dystonia are conflicting. Studies have shown that the cSP is shortened in patients with focal hand dystonia, spasmodic dysphonia and cervical dystonia (Chen et al. 1997; Amadio et al. 2000; Samargia et al. 2014). Other studies have shown that the cSP is normal, task-specific or only abnormal on the symptomatic side (Chen et al. 1997; Stinear & Byblow 2005; Tinazzi et al. 2005).

Decreased Short-Latency Afferent Inhibition and Long-Latency Afferent Inhibition

Abnormal sensorimotor integration is also thought to underlie the physiology of dystonia (McDonnell et al. 2007). SAI and LAI are measures of sensorimotor integration, seen as a decrease of the MEP with delivery of a peripheral electrical stimulation to the hand of approximately 20 ms and 200 ms, respectively, prior to TMS of the contralateral motor cortex. They are thought to be mediated by GABA and cholinergic receptors (Di Lazzaro et al. 2000a, 2000b). Studies of SAI in patients with dystonia have shown mixed results, dependent on the state of the patient. SAI has been reported to be normal at rest in patients with focal hand dystonia (Abbruzzese et al. 2001; Kessler et al. 2005) and appears to be increased in these patients performing phasic movements, i.e. flexion of the second digit (Richardson et al. 2008). A trend towards less LAI in patients with focal hand dystonia at rest was seen, but no significant difference was found during phasic finger movement (Pirio Richardson et al. 2009), while another TMS study performed on patients at rest found deficient LAI in patients with focal hand dystonia, but intact LAI in patients with cervical dystonia (Abbruzzese et al. 2001).

Altered Influences on the Motor Cortex

Various brain regions are involved in the planning of movement, including the premotor, supplementary motor and posterior parietal cortices (Davare et al. 2008, 2010; Arai et al. 2012). In healthy human subjects, inhibitory influences on the primary motor cortex, including those from premotor cortices, contralateral motor area and cerebellum, have been reported. Healthy individuals in the resting state appear to have a resting premotor-to-motor inhibition that is modulated with grasp and different subregions of the premotor cortex appear to be involved in different types of grasp (Davare et al. 2006; Houdayer et al. 2012). Studies of the resting premotor influences in patients with focal hand dystonia have shown enhanced dorsal premotor-to-motor inhibition (Beck et al. 2009; Pirio Richardson et al. 2014), but other studies have reported a lack of ventral premotor-to-motor inhibition and decreased dorsal premotor-to-motor inhibition (Koch et al. 2008; Houdayer et al. 2012). Enhanced dorsal premotor-to-motor inhibition was also found in a recent study in patients with cervical dystonia (Pirio Richardson 2015).

Interhemispheric inhibition (IHI), the transcallosal influence between bilateral motor cortices that is seen in healthy individuals, was found to be abnormal in patients with writer's cramp at both short and long intervals (SIHI and LIHI) (Nelson et al. 2010). Writer's cramp patients were also found to show a trend for deficient IHI, but post hoc analysis revealed that only the subgroup of patients with mirror dystonia had a loss of IHI (Dickler et al. 2014). Therefore, it appeared that the impaired IHI in these patients is the mechanism responsible for the phenomenon of mirror dystonia.

Cerebellar inhibition (CBI) is seen in healthy subjects with stimulation of the cerebellum 5–7 ms prior to delivering a test pulse on the primary motor cortex (Ugawa et al. 1995). It is presumed that stimulation of the Purkinje cells occurs, which in turn inhibits deep cerebellar nuclei that reduces the tonic facilitation of the motor cortex. A study investigating the connections between the cerebellum and cortical circuits further found that CBI reduced SICI and increased intracortical facilitation (ICF) (Daskalakis et al. 2004). CBI has been reported to be deficient in patients with focal upper-limb dystonia (Brighina et al. 2009).

The motor cortex appears to receive facilitatory influences as well, coming from both ipsi- and contralateral parietal areas, as reported in healthy human subjects (Koch et al. 2007, 2009). This parieto-motor connectivity was shown to be reduced in patients with cervical dystonia, as well as those with writer's cramp (Delnooz et al. 2012; Porcacchia et al. 2014). Similar results have been reported in studies using functional brain imaging to probe the connectivity of the premotor–parietal circuit, which is considered to be involved in the writing network (Delnooz et al. 2012). Therefore, a decrease of facilitatory influences on the motor cortex may also play a role in the physiology of certain types of dystonia.

Loss of Surround Inhibition

Surround inhibition in the motor system is a functional process thought to underlie the selective execution of a desired movement, reflected by the decrease of corticospinal excitability of the surround muscles neighbouring the active muscles (Sohn & Hallett 2004). Suppression of MEP amplitude in the contralateral limb at interstimulus intervals of 35–70 ms was found with TMS following EMG onset in self-paced, voluntary finger movement in the ipsilateral M1 (Sohn et al. 2003). Inhibition of ipsilateral limb muscles not involved in the willed movement is also seen (Sohn & Hallett 2004). Surround inhibition appears to occur earlier and stronger in more complex tasks, peaking at 10 per cent of maximal force but lost at 40 per cent of maximal force (Beck et al. 2009; Beck & Hallett 2010). It has been reported to be deficient in patients with focal hand dystonia (Sohn & Hallett 2004; Beck et al. 2009), but a study on patients with cervical dystonia found intact surround inhibition in the asymptomatic body part (McDougall et al. 2015).

Despite efforts to characterise the processes contributing to surround inhibition, it is not clear what the responsible mechanisms are. Various processes including the cSP, LICI, ICF, SAI, LAI, IHI, dorsal premotor-to-motor inhibition, ventral premotor-to-motor inhibition and cerebellar inhibition have been investigated to determine their contribution to surround inhibition (Sohn & Hallett 2004; Richardson et al. 2008; Beck et al. 2009; Pirio Richardson et al. 2009; Houdayer et al. 2012; Poston et al. 2012). Most studies have concluded that these mechanisms do not seem to be contributory. On the other hand, mixed observations on SAI and SICI have been reported, as some studies have found these mechanisms to contribute to surround inhibition, while others have not (Sohn & Hallett 2004; Stinear & Byblow 2004; Voller et al. 2006; Beck et al. 2008; Kassavetis et al. 2011; Asmussen et al. 2014). In a recent study, surround inhibition was found with posterior-to-anterior current stimulation but not with anterior-to-posterior current. This might well imply that surround inhibition is due to intracortical circuits (Thirugnanasambandam et al. 2015).

Sensory Abnormalities

Another aspect of the pathophysiology of dystonia is abnormalities in sensory function and 'sensorimotor integration'. Clinically, motor problems are often preceded by subtle sensory symptoms in some patients; ill-defined bodily feelings (discomfort, pain or kinaesthetic sensations) are frequently reported weeks or months before dystonia develops and pain can be a component of dystonia. Some abnormalities can be brought out only by special testing. One type of abnormality is spatial and temporal discrimination. Patients with focal dystonia have difficulty in discriminating sensory stimuli in both spatial and temporal domains (Bara-Jimenez et al. 2000). Importantly, these abnormalities are present in unaffected body parts such as the unaffected hand in patients with focal hand dystonia (Scontrini et al. 2009). These sensory abnormalities have also been documented in some relatives of patients with inherited generalised dystonia (O'Dwyer et al. 2005). Kinaesthesia is also abnormal. The perceptual threshold for being able to identify the direction of a passive finger movement correctly was increased in patients with focal dystonia (Putzki et al. 2006). There are also abnormalities of the perception of vibratory tendon stimulation. Patients cannot match the movement of one elbow with the other one when the movement is produced by the tonic vibration reflex (Grunewald et al. 1997). Perception of the vibration-induced illusion of movement is abnormal for patients with different types of focal dystonia in multiple body joints (Yoneda et al. 2000). Similar to temporal discrimination abnormalities, a deficit of vibration-induced illusion was also identified in asymptomatic first-degree relatives of patients (Frima et al. 2008).

These alterations may be related to a deranged somatotopic representation in the sensory cortex as revealed by neurophysiological and neuroimaging studies. Abnormal somatotopy was demonstrated with somatosensory-evoked potential mapping with electroencephalography (Bara-Jimenez et al. 1998), magnetoencephalography (Meunier et al. 2001), functional magnetic resonance imaging (Butterworth et al. 2003; Nelson et al. 2009) and positron emission tomography (Catalan et al. 2012) (Figure 8.1). Not only were finger representation locations closer together than normal, but sometimes the representations were not in the correct order. These abnormalities are present on the unaffected side of patients with unilateral hand dystonia, and might even be more abnormal on the unaffected side (Meunier et al. 2001). One possible pathophysiological mechanism for these abnormalities could be a loss of lateral inhibition. Lateral inhibition can be demonstrated with a study of somatosensory-evoked potentials (SEPs) from the median and ulnar nerves. If the median and ulnar SEPs are produced together, the combined SEP is less than the sum of the two individual ones because of mutual inhibition. This is not shown in patients with focal hand dystonia (Tinazzi et al. 2000). The pathophysiology of the temporal discrimination abnormality was correlated to lack of inhibition of the P27 at the 5 ms interval using SEP recovery curves (Tamura et al. 2008). Therefore, it seems that the abnormality in sensory function might be similar to the abnormality in motor function; that is, a loss of short-latency inhibition.

Sensorimotor integration, which refers to how the sensory system interacts with the motor system, is also abnormal in dystonia. SAI and LAI are measures of sensorimotor integration as reviewed earlier in this chapter. The time course of this inhibition corresponds well with the timing of event-related synchronisation (ERS) after peripheral stimulation (Chen et al. 1999). Afferent peripheral feedback, therefore, might be a physiological mechanism for activating inhibitory ('gating') mechanisms at cortical or subcortical levels. SEP gating is a well-known phenomenon whereby SEPs are attenuated before and during movement (Starr & Cohen 1985). There may be two mechanisms of gating in SEP (Jones et al. 1989); peripheral gating is produced by interactions between an applied stimulus and movement-related afferent information, whereas central gating is produced by centrifugal modulation of sensory information for an appropriate movement. Theoretically, pre-movement gating of SEPs is thought to reflect central gating, while gating during active movement involves both peripheral and central gating. Murase et al. reported a lack of abnormal pre-movement gating of SEPs in writer's cramp (Murase et al. 2000), indicating that central gating of SEP is impaired in

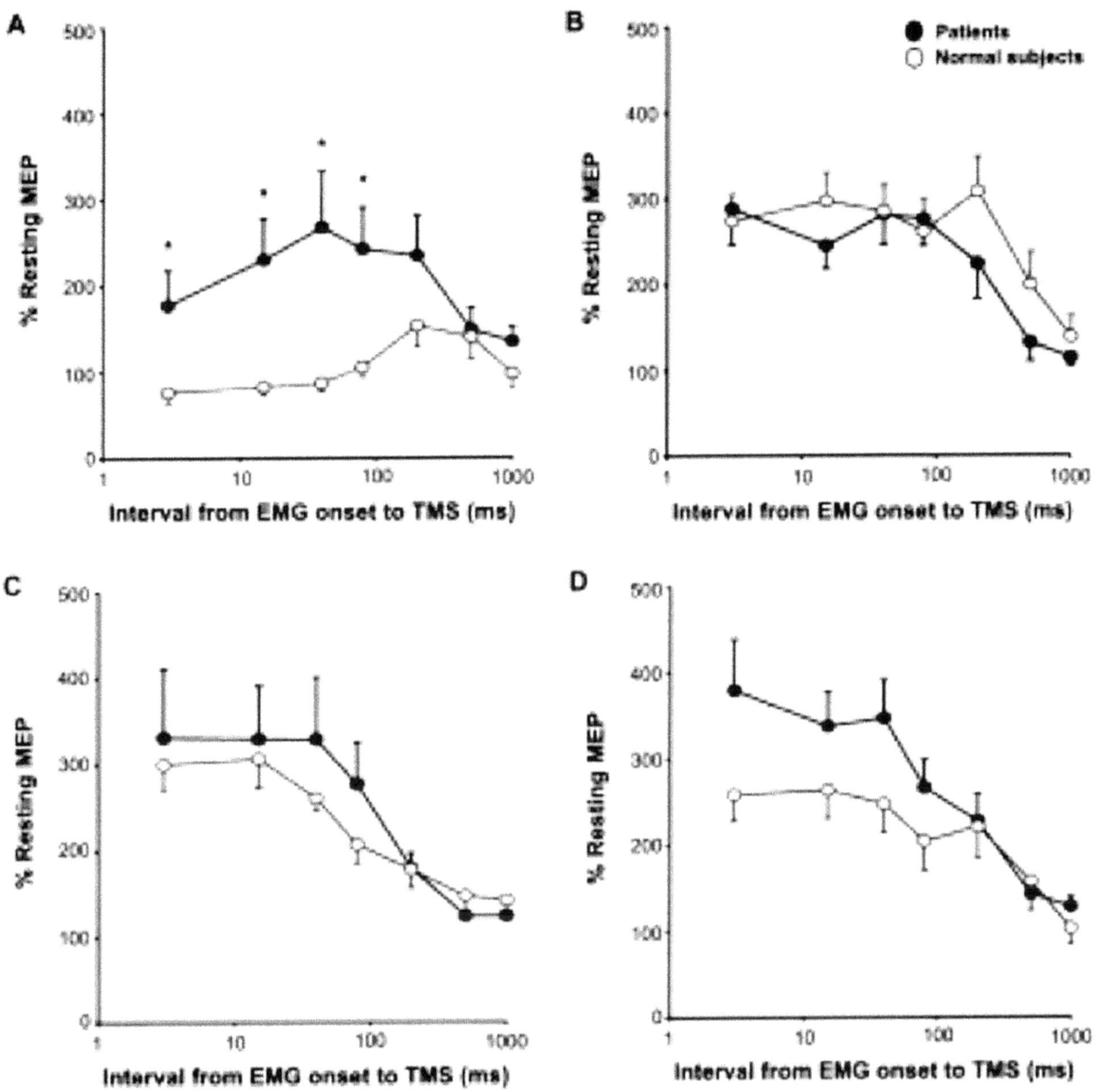

Figure 8.1 Motor-evoked potential (MEP) ratio of muscles at interstimulus intervals of 3, 15, 40, 80, 200, 500 and 1000 ms from electromyography (EMG) onset of flexor digitorum superficialis (FDS) to TMS, normalised to the MEP of the resting state. Asterisk denotes significant difference between the two groups ($p < 0.05$). (a) MEP amplitudes of abductor digiti minimi (ADM) are suppressed in healthy subjects but significantly enhanced in patients during flexion of the index finger. (b–d) MEP amplitudes of first dorsal interosseus (FDI), extensor indicis proprius (EIP) and FDS were enhanced in both groups, during and immediately after flexion of the index finger.

Figure taken from Sohn et al. (2004), with permission.

dystonia patients. The intriguing clinical phenomenon of the sensory trick is another indication of a sensory influence on the motor system, but its physiology is not understood (Ramos et al. 2014).

Abnormal Plasticity

Maladaptive plasticity appears to be an important feature for the pathogenesis of dystonia. A clear example is that typically hand dystonia is triggered by a period of intensive training of a particular movement (Quartarone et al. 2006; Roze et al. 2009). It seems likely that some abnormalities of plasticity may render some individuals susceptible to dystonia if plastic changes are pushed to their extreme by frequent repetition. This suggests a two-factor hypothesis: use-dependent environmental factors such as repetitive training and abnormal mechanisms of plasticity within sensorimotor loops.

A well-established approach to test plasticity in humans in a non-invasive way is paired associative stimulation (PAS). By using PAS, it has been demonstrated that both LTP-like and LTD-like facilitatory and inhibitory effects, respectively, are enhanced in writer's cramp patients on TMS-evoked MEPs (Quartarone et al. 2003). The data might be due to a failure of GABAergic mechanisms that are recruited during

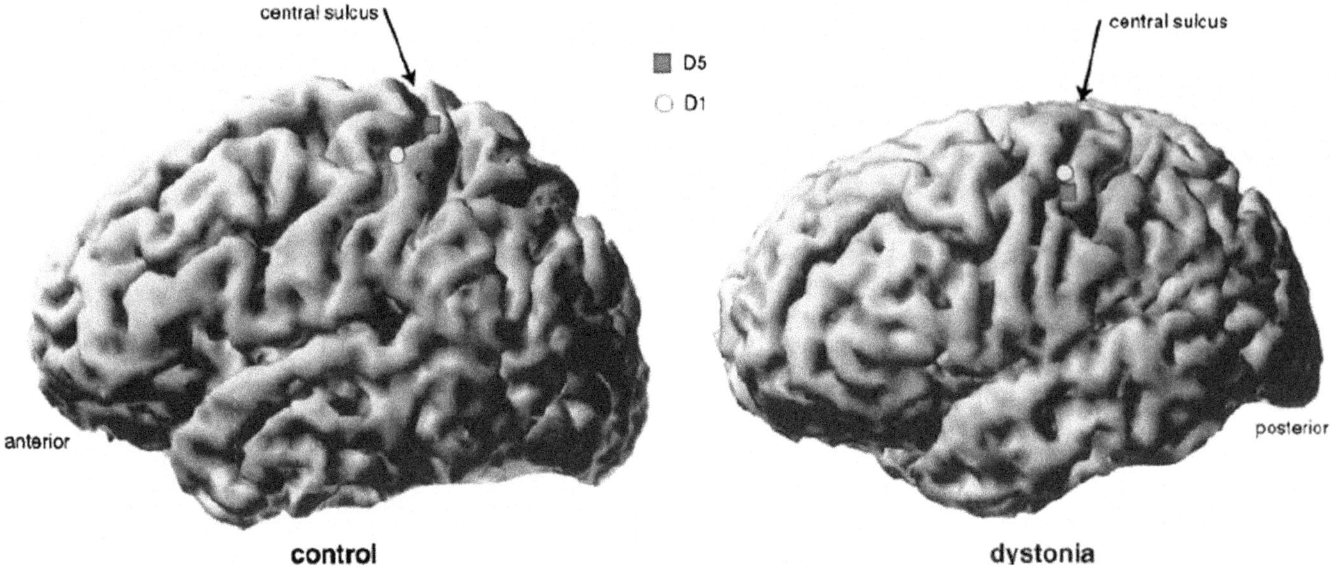

Figure 8.2 Three-dimensional reconstruction of the brain of a normal subject and a patient with hand dystonia. N20 source localisations for D1 and D5 are displayed. The normal cortical homuncular arrangement of the fingers is degraded in the patient.

Reproduced from Bara-Jimenez et al. (1998) with modification.

LTP-/LTD-like phenomena within sensory and motor cortices. An important feature of PAS-induced associative plasticity in healthy controls is somatotopic specificity as PAS after-effects are largely confined to the cortical target representation receiving the input (Stefan et al. 2000). Instead, in writer's cramp patients, PAS tends to change cortical excitability also of nearby muscle representations (Quartarone et al. 2003; Weise et al. 2006). This loss of spatial specificity by PAS appears to be related to the abnormality of surround inhibition that was mentioned earlier in this chapter. This abnormal plasticity is not confined to the neural circuits affected by dystonia, but is generalised across the entire sensorimotor system representing an endophenotypic trait of dystonia (Quartarone et al. 2008). Further evidence of abnormal plasticity of sensorimotor circuits is that cortical excitability probed by the somatosensory-evoked response P27 was abnormally enhanced by PAS in focal hand dystonia compared to healthy subjects (Tamura et al. 2009).

Homeostatic plasticity is an essential requirement of brain function so as to maintain overall synaptic weight in neuronal networks within a useful dynamic range (Turrigiano et al. 1998). Theoretically, without homeostasis, the positive-feedback nature of LTP could potentially trigger an uncontrolled increase in synaptic effectiveness, which could empower and destabilise neural circuits. Evidence in experimental models suggests that this can be prevented by making the amount of LTP dependent on the level of activity in postsynaptic neurons: the greater the ongoing activity, the less effective are processes leading to LTP, while processes leading to LTD are enhanced. Conversely, the lower the activity of the postsynaptic neurons, the more effective are processes that lead to LTP. Such 'synaptic scaling' is called homeostatic plasticity. Enhanced plasticity in dystonia might well be the result of a disruption of homeostatic plasticity within sensorimotor circuits. Homeostatic mechanisms have been studied by using a combined protocol where transcranial direct current stimulation (tDCS) primed the response of the motor cortex to a subsequent period of rTMS (Siebner et al. 2004). In healthy controls, preconditioning of the primary motor cortex with 10 minutes of anodal stimulation potentiated the inhibitory after-effects of 1 Hz rTMS while 10 minutes of cathodal stimulation increased the effect of facilitation. In patients with focal hand dystonia, the response to 1 Hz rTMS was unaffected by preconditioning with tDCS. In addition, the normal inhibitory effect of preconditioning with cathodal tDCS was absent (Quartarone et al. 2005). To what extent deficient homeostatic plasticity applies also to the behavioural level of practice-dependent plasticity induced by repetitive and highly stereotyped finger movements has also been addressed (Kang et al. 2011). The healthy subjects showed homeostatic suppression of practice-dependent plasticity after excitability-enhancing TMS protocol (PAS 25 ms). In patients with focal hand dystonia this homeostatic modulation was deficient and the magnitude of this deficiency correlated with clinical severity of the focal hand dystonia.

Task Specificity

Task specificity is an interesting phenomenon that patients with focal dystonia often exhibit. Frequent task-specific hand dystonias are writer's cramp and musician's cramp, such as pianist cramp. The effector, in these situations the hand, is normal (or close to normal) for all tasks except one. So the basic movement control mechanisms must be functioning reasonably well. Also, the motor programme for the task must be okay since other effectors, like the other hand, can carry out the motor programme. For writer's cramp, for example, writing is typically normal for the other hand and even for the affected limb if the writing is done with more proximal muscles, such as writing on a blackboard. Hence, the essence of the problem is the specific linkage of the one motor programme to one effector.

To figure out how a specific motor programme is linked to one effector in writing, an fMRI study was done in which healthy subjects performed writing, zigzagging and finger tapping with the right hand, left hand and right foot. It showed stronger activations in the left motor and premotor cortex, the left superior parietal cortex, anterior putamen and right cerebellum during right-hand writing. Also, an exploratory analysis showed that clusters in the left ventral premotor cortex and inferior and superior parietal cortices were only significantly active for right-hand writing (Horovitz et al. 2013). These areas were less active in writer's cramp (Gallea et al. 2016). These results suggest that movement parameters for writing are stored in secondary sensorimotor cortices of the extremity with which it is usually performed, that is, the dominant hand, including premotor and parietal cortices. Another positron emission tomography study looked at cerebral blood flow in patients with writer's cramp during various movement tasks including writing. During handwriting there was deficient activation in the premotor cortex in the patients compared with normal control participants. As the premotor cortex is one of the prominent areas for overlap between programme and effector, this might be a critical area for problems in patients.

Summary

There has been considerable progress in understanding the pathophysiology of dystonia. A possible mechanism that could explain most of the abnormalities is a deficiency in inhibitory interneurons. The loss of inhibition might be widespread, involving multiple levels of the central nervous system. Such a loss of inhibition could be a consequence of the abnormal genetic background in patients with dystonia and would predispose them to develop dystonia if there are other factors, such as repetitive activity in focal hand dystonia. If dystonia is characterised by a loss of inhibition, then augmenting inhibition might be helpful for treatment. Pharmacologic agents that have GABAergic actions are often useful in clinical practice. Physiological techniques to induce more inhibition have also been employed. DBS can be effective and it is interesting in this regard that there are improvements in physiological inhibition that correlate with clinical improvement (Tisch et al. 2006). Non-invasive neurostimulation to boost inhibition using TMS, tDCS or tACS are also being studied as potential therapeutic applications (Siebner et al. 1999; Huang 2010; Kanai et al. 2010; Benninger et al. 2011; Lalli et al. 2012).

References

Abbruzzese, G, R Marchese, A Buccolieri, B Gasparetto and C Trompetto (2001). Abnormalities of sensorimotor integration in focal dystonia: a transcranial magnetic stimulation study. *Brain* 124(Pt 3): 537–545.

Albanese, A, K Bhatia, SB Bressman, MR Delong, S Fahn, VS Fung, M Hallett, J Jankovic, HA Jinnah, C Klein, AE Lang, JW Mink and JK Teller (2013). Phenomenology and classification of dystonia: a consensus update. *Mov Disord* 28(7): 863–873.

Amadio, S, M Panizza, F Pisano, L Maderna, C Miscio, J Nilsson, MA Volonte, G Comi and G Galardi (2000). Transcranial magnetic stimulation and silent period in spasmodic torticollis. *Am J Phys Med Rehabil* 79(4): 361–368.

Amadio, S, E Houdayer, F Bianchi, H Tesfaghebriel Tekle, IP Urban, C Butera, R Guerriero, M Cursi, L Leocani, G Comi and U Del Carro (2014). Sensory tricks and brain excitability in cervical dystonia: a transcranial magnetic stimulation study. *Mov Disord* 29(9): 1185–1188.

Arai, N, MK Lu, Y Ugawa and U Ziemann (2012). Effective connectivity between human supplementary motor area and primary motor cortex: a paired-coil TMS study. *Exp Brain Res* 220(1): 79–87.

Asmussen, MJ, CM Zapallow, MF Jacobs, KG Lee, P Tsang and AJ Nelson (2014). Modulation of short-latency afferent inhibition depends on digit and task-relevance. *PLoS One* 9(8): e104807.

Balint, B and KP Bhatia (2014). Dystonia: an update on phenomenology, classification, pathogenesis and treatment. *Curr Opin Neurol* 27(4): 468–476.

Bara-Jimenez, W, MJ Catalan, M Hallett and C Gerloff (1998). Abnormal somatosensory homunculus in dystonia of the hand. *Ann Neurol* 44(5): 828–831.

Bara-Jimenez, W, P Shelton and M Hallett (2000). Spatial discrimination is abnormal in focal hand dystonia. *Neurology* 55(12): 1869–1873.

Beck, S and M Hallett (2010). Surround inhibition is modulated by task difficulty. *Clin Neurophysiol* 121(1): 98–103.

Beck, S, SP Richardson, EA Shamim, N Dang, M Schubert and M Hallett (2008). Short intracortical and surround inhibition are selectively reduced during movement initiation in focal hand dystonia. *J Neurosci* 28(41): 10363–10369.

Beck, S, E Houdayer, SP Richardson and M Hallett (2009a). The role of inhibition from the left dorsal premotor cortex in right-sided focal hand dystonia. *Brain Stimul* 2(4): 208–214.

Beck, S, M Schubert, SP Richardson and M Hallett (2009b). Surround inhibition depends on the force exerted and is abnormal in focal hand dystonia. *J Appl Physiol* 107(5): 1513–1518.

Benninger, DH, M Lomarev, G Lopez, N Pal, DA Luckenbaugh and M Hallett (2011). Transcranial direct current stimulation for the treatment of focal hand dystonia. *Mov Disord* 26(9): 1698–1702.

Brighina, F, M Romano, G Giglia, V Saia, A Puma, F Giglia and B Fierro (2009). Effects of cerebellar TMS on motor cortex of patients with focal dystonia: a preliminary report. *Exp Brain Res* 192(4): 651–656.

Butterworth, S, S Francis, E Kelly, F McGlone, R Bowtell and GV Sawle (2003). Abnormal cortical sensory activation in dystonia: an fMRI study. *Mov Disord* 18(6): 673–682.

Catalan, MJ, K Ishii, W Bara-Jimenez and M Hallett (2012). Reorganization of the human somatosensory cortex in hand dystonia. *J Mov Disord* 5(1): 5–8.

Chen, R, EM Wassermann, M Canos and M Hallett (1997). Impaired inhibition in writer's cramp during voluntary muscle activation. *Neurology* 49(4): 1054–1059.

Chen, R, B Corwell and M Hallett (1999a). Modulation of motor cortex excitability by median nerve and digit stimulation. *Exp Brain Res* 129(1): 77–86.

Chen, R, AM Lozano and P Ashby (1999b). Mechanism of the silent period following transcranial magnetic stimulation. Evidence from epidural recordings. *Exp Brain Res* 128(4): 539–542.

Chen, RS, CH Tsai and CS Lu (1995). Reciprocal inhibition in writer's cramp. *Mov Disord* 10(5): 556–561.

Daskalakis, ZJ, GO Paradiso, BK Christensen, PB Fitzgerald, C Gunraj and R Chen (2004). Exploring the connectivity between the cerebellum and motor cortex in humans. *J Physiol* 557(Pt 2): 689–700.

Davare, M, M Andres, G Cosnard, JL Thonnard and E Olivier (2006). Dissociating the role of ventral and dorsal premotor cortex in precision grasping. *J Neurosci* 26(8): 2260–2268.

Davare, M, R Lemon and E Olivier (2008). Selective modulation of interactions between ventral premotor cortex and primary motor cortex during precision grasping in humans. *J Physiol* 586(Pt 11): 2735–2742.

Davare, M, JC Rothwell and RN Lemon (2010). Causal connectivity between the human anterior intraparietal area and premotor cortex during grasp. *Curr Biol* 20(2): 176–181.

Day, BL, CD Marsden, JA Obeso and JC Rothwell (1984). Reciprocal inhibition between the muscles of the human forearm. *J Physiol* 349: 519–534.

Defazio, G, A Conte, AF Gigante, G Fabbrini and A Berardelli (2015). Is tremor in dystonia a phenotypic feature of dystonia? *Neurology* 84(10): 1053–1059.

Delnooz, CC, RC Helmich, I Toni and BP van de Warrenburg (2012). Reduced parietal connectivity with a premotor writing area in writer's cramp. *Mov Disord* 27(11): 1425–1431.

Deuschl, G, C Seifert, F Heinen, M Illert and CH Lucking (1992). Reciprocal inhibition of forearm flexor muscles in spasmodic torticollis. *J Neurol Sci* 113(1): 85–90.

Di Lazzaro, V, A Oliviero, M Meglio, B Cioni, G Tamburrini, P Tonali and JC Rothwell (2000a). Direct demonstration of the effect of lorazepam on the excitability of the human motor cortex. *Clin Neurophysiol* 111(5): 794–799.

Di Lazzaro, V, A Oliviero, P Profice, MA Pennisi, S Di Giovanni, G Zito, P Tonali and JC Rothwell (2000b). Muscarinic receptor blockade has differential effects on the excitability of intracortical circuits in the human motor cortex. *Exp Brain Res* 135(4): 455–461.

Edwards, MJ, YZ Huang, NW Wood, JC Rothwell and KP Bhatia (2003). Different patterns of electrophysiological deficits in manifesting and non-manifesting carriers of the DYT1 gene mutation. *Brain* 126(Pt 9): 2074–2080.

Espay, AJ, F Morgante, J Purzner, CA Gunraj, AE Lang and R Chen (2006). Cortical and spinal abnormalities in psychogenic dystonia. *Ann Neurol* 59(5): 825–834.

Frima, N, J Nasir and RA Grunewald (2008). Abnormal vibration-induced illusion of movement in idiopathic focal dystonia: an endophenotypic marker? *Mov Disord* 23(3): 373–377.

Gallea, C, SG Horovitz, M Najee-Ullah and M Hallett (2016). Impairment of a parteio-premotor network specialized for handwriting in writer's cramp. *Hum Brain Mapp* 37: 4363–4375.

Grunewald, RA, Y Yoneda, JM Shipman and HJ Sagar (1997). Idiopathic focal dystonia: a disorder of muscle spindle afferent processing? *Brain* 120 (Pt 12): 2179–2185.

Hallett, M (2011). Neurophysiology of dystonia: the role of inhibition. *Neurobiol Dis* 42(2): 177–184.

Hanajima, R, Y Nomura, M Segawa and Y Ugawa (2007). Intracortical inhibition of the motor cortex in Segawa disease (DYT5). *Neurology* 68(13): 1039–1044.

Horovitz, SG, C Gallea, M Najee-Ullah and M Hallett (2013). Functional anatomy of writing with the dominant hand. *PLoS One* 8(7): e67931.

Houdayer, E, S Beck, A Karabanov, B Poston and M Hallett (2012). The differential modulation of the ventral premotor–motor interaction during movement initiation is deficient in patients with focal hand dystonia. *Eur J Neurosci* 35(3): 478–485.

Huang, YZ (2010). The modulation of cortical motor circuits and spinal reflexes using theta burst stimulation in healthy and dystonic subjects. *Restor Neurol Neurosci* 28(4): 449–457.

Jones, SJ, JP Halonen and F Shawkat (1989). Centrifugal and centripetal mechanisms involved in the 'gating' of cortical SEPs during movement. *Electroencephalogr Clin Neurophysiol* 74(1): 36–45.

Kanai, R, W Paulus and V Walsh (2010). Transcranial alternating current stimulation (tACS) modulates cortical excitability as assessed by TMS-induced phosphene thresholds. *Clin Neurophysiol* 121(9): 1551–1554.

Kang, JS, C Terranova, R Hilker, A Quartarone and U Ziemann (2011). Deficient homeostatic regulation of practice-dependent plasticity in writer's cramp. *Cereb Cortex* 21(5): 1203–1212.

Kassavetis, P, BS Hoffland, TA Saifee, KP Bhatia, BP van de Warrenburg, JC Rothwell and MJ Edwards (2011). Cerebellar brain inhibition is decreased in active and surround muscles at the onset of voluntary movement. *Exp Brain Res* 209(3): 437–442.

Kessler, KR, D Ruge, TV Ilic and U Ziemann (2005). Short latency afferent inhibition and facilitation in patients with writer's cramp. *Mov Disord* 20(2): 238–242.

Kinugawa, K, M Vidailhet, F Clot, E Apartis, D Grabli and E Roze (2009). Myoclonus-dystonia: an update. *Mov Disord* 24(4): 479–489.

Koch, G, M Fernandez Del Olmo, B Cheeran, D Ruge, S Schippling, C Caltagirone and JC Rothwell (2007). Focal stimulation of the posterior parietal cortex increases the excitability of the ipsilateral motor cortex. *J Neurosci* 27(25): 6815–6822.

Koch, G, S Schneider, T Baumer, M Franca, A Munchau, B Cheeran, M Fernandez del Olmo, C Cordivari, E Rounis, C Caltagirone, K Bhatia and JC Rothwell (2008). Altered dorsal premotor–motor interhemispheric pathway activity in focal arm dystonia. *Mov Disord* 23(5): 660–668.

Koch, G, D Ruge, B Cheeran, M Fernandez Del Olmo, C Pecchioli, B Marconi, V Versace, E Lo Gerfo, S Torriero, M Oliveri, C Caltagirone and JC Rothwell (2009). TMS activation of interhemispheric pathways between the posterior parietal cortex and the contralateral motor cortex. *J Physiol* 587(Pt 17): 4281–4292.

Kujirai, T, MD Caramia, JC Rothwell, BL Day, PD Thompson, A Ferbert, S Wroe, P Asselman and CD Marsden (1993). Corticocortical inhibition in human motor cortex. *J Physiol* 471: 501–519.

Lalli, S, S Piacentini, A Franzini, A Panzacchi, C Cerami, G Messina, F Ferre, D Perani and A Albanese (2012). Epidural premotor cortical stimulation in primary focal dystonia: clinical and 18F-fluoro deoxyglucose positron emission tomography open study. *Mov Disord* 27(4): 533–538.

Marsden, CD, PA Merton and HB Morton (1983). Direct electrical stimulation of corticospinal pathways through the intact scalp in human subjects. *Adv Neurol* 39: 387–391.

McDonnell, MN, PD Thompson and MC Ridding (2007). The effect of cutaneous input on intracortical inhibition in focal task-specific dystonia. *Mov Disord* 22(9): 1286–1292.

McDougall, L, D Kiernan, ZH Kiss, O Suchowersky and TN Welsh (2015). Abnormal surround inhibition does not affect asymptomatic limbs in people with cervical dystonia. *Neurosci Lett* 14:7–11.

Meunier, S, L Garnero, A Ducorps, L Mazieres, S Lehericy, ST du Montcel, B Renault and M Vidailhet (2001). Human brain mapping in dystonia reveals both endophenotypic traits and adaptive reorganization. *Ann Neurol* 50(4): 521–527.

Murase, N, R Kaji, H Shimazu, M Katayama-Hirota, A Ikeda, N Kohara, J Kimura, H Shibasaki and JC Rothwell (2000). Abnormal premovement gating of somatosensory input in writer's cramp. *Brain* 123(Pt 9): 1813–1829.

Nelson, AJ, DT Blake and R Chen (2009). Digit-specific aberrations in the primary somatosensory cortex in writer's cramp. *Ann Neurol* 66(2): 146–154.

Nelson, AJ, T Hoque, C Gunraj, Z Ni and R Chen (2010). Impaired interhemispheric inhibition in writer's cramp. *Neurology* 75(5): 441–447.

O'Dwyer, JP, S O'Riordan, R Saunders-Pullman, SB Bressman, F Molloy, T Lynch and M Hutchinson (2005). Sensory abnormalities in unaffected relatives in familial adult-onset dystonia. *Neurology* 65(6): 938–940.

Pirio Richardson, S (2015). Enhanced dorsal premotor-motor inhibition in cervical dystonia. *Clin Neurophysiol* 126(7): 1387–1391.

Pirio Richardson, S, B Bliem, B Voller, N Dang and M Hallett (2009). Long-latency afferent inhibition during phasic finger movement in focal hand dystonia. *Exp Brain Res* 193(2): 173–179.

Pirio Richardson, S, S Beck, B Bliem and M Hallett (2014). Abnormal dorsal premotor–motor inhibition in writer's cramp. *Mov Disord* 29(6): 797–803.

Porcacchia, P, FJ Palomar, MT Caceres-Redondo, I Huertas-Fernandez, JF Martin-Rodriguez, F Carrillo, G Koch and P Mir (2014). Parieto-motor cortical dysfunction in primary cervical dystonia. *Brain Stimul* 7(5): 650–657.

Poston, B, SN Kukke, RW Paine, S Francis and M Hallett (2012). Cortical silent period duration and its implications for surround inhibition of a hand muscle. *Eur J Neurosci* 36(7): 2964–2971.

Putzki, N, P Stude, J Konczak, K Graf, HC Diener and M Maschke (2006). Kinesthesia is impaired in focal dystonia. *Mov Disord* 21(6): 754–760.

Quartarone, A and M Hallett (2013). Emerging concepts in the physiological basis of dystonia. *Mov Disord* 28(7): 958–967.

Quartarone, A, S Bagnato, V Rizzo, HR Siebner, V Dattola, A Scalfari, F Morgante, F Battaglia, M Romano and P Girlanda (2003). Abnormal associative plasticity of the human motor cortex in writer's cramp. *Brain* 126(Pt 12): 2586–2596.

Quartarone, A, V Rizzo, S Bagnato, F Morgante, A Sant'Angelo, M Romano, D Crupi, P Girlanda, JC Rothwell and HR Siebner (2005). Homeostatic-like plasticity of the primary motor hand area is impaired in focal hand dystonia. *Brain* 128(Pt 8): 1943–1950.

Quartarone, A, HR Siebner and JC Rothwell (2006). Task-specific hand dystonia: can too much plasticity be bad for you? *Trends Neurosci* 29(4): 192–199.

Quartarone, A, F Morgante, A Sant'Angelo, V Rizzo, S Bagnato, C Terranova, HR Siebner, A Berardelli and P Girlanda (2008). Abnormal plasticity of sensorimotor circuits extends beyond the affected body part in focal dystonia. *J Neurol Neurosurg Psychiatry* 79(9): 985–990.

Ramos, VF, BI Karp and M Hallett (2014). Tricks in dystonia: ordering the complexity. *J Neurol Neurosurg Psychiatry* 85(9): 987–993.

Richardson, SP, B Bliem, M Lomarev, E Shamim, N Dang and M Hallett (2008). Changes in short afferent inhibition during phasic movement in focal dystonia. *Muscle Nerve* 37(3): 358–363.

Roze, E, A Soumare, I Pironneau, S Sangla, VC de Cock, A Teixeira, A Astorquiza, C Bonnet, JP Bleton, M Vidailhet and A Elbaz (2009). Case-control study of writer's cramp. *Brain* 132(Pt 3): 756–764.

Sabine, M, L George, E Roze, E Apartis, JM Trocello and V Marie (2008). Cortical excitability in DYT-11 positive myoclonus dystonia. *Mov Disord* 23(5): 761–764.

Samargia, S, R Schmidt and TJ Kimberley (2014). Shortened cortical silent period in adductor spasmodic dysphonia: evidence for widespread cortical excitability. *Neurosci Lett* 560: 12–15.

Sattler, V, M Dickler, M Michaud, S Meunier and M Simonetta-Moreau (2014). Does abnormal interhemispheric inhibition play a role in mirror dystonia? *Mov Disord* 29(6): 787–796.

Scontrini, A, A Conte, G Defazio, M Fiorio, G Fabbrini, A Suppa, M Tinazzi and A Berardelli (2009). Somatosensory temporal discrimination in patients with primary focal dystonia. *J Neurol Neurosurg Psychiatry* 80(12): 1315–1319.

Sheehy, MP and CD Marsden (1982). Writers' cramp: a focal dystonia. *Brain* 105(Pt 3): 461–480.

Siebner, HR, JM Tormos, AO Ceballos-Baumann, C Auer, MD Catala, B Conrad and A Pascual-Leone (1999). Low-frequency repetitive transcranial magnetic stimulation of the motor cortex in writer's cramp. *Neurology* 52(3): 529–537.

Siebner, HR, N Lang, V Rizzo, MA Nitsche, W Paulus, RN Lemon and JC Rothwell (2004). Preconditioning of low-frequency repetitive transcranial magnetic stimulation with transcranial direct current stimulation: evidence for homeostatic plasticity in the human motor cortex. *J Neurosci* 24(13): 3379–3385.

Sohn, YH and M Hallett (2004a). Disturbed surround inhibition in focal hand dystonia. *Ann Neurol* 56(4): 595–599.

Sohn, YH and M Hallett (2004b). Surround inhibition in human motor system. *Exp Brain Res* 158(4): 397–404.

Sohn, YH, HY Jung, A Kaelin-Lang and M Hallett (2003). Excitability of the ipsilateral motor cortex during phasic voluntary hand movement. *Exp Brain Res* 148(2): 176–185.

Sommer, M, D Ruge, F Tergau, W Beuche, E Altenmuller and W Paulus (2002). Intracortical excitability in the hand motor representation in hand dystonia and blepharospasm. *Mov Disord* 17(5): 1017–1025.

Starr, A and LG Cohen (1985). 'Gating' of somatosensory evoked potentials begins before the onset of voluntary movement in man. *Brain Res* 348(1): 183–186.

Stefan, K, E Kunesch, LG Cohen, R Benecke and J Classen (2000). Induction of plasticity in the human motor cortex by paired associative stimulation. *Brain* 123(Pt 3): 572–584.

Stinear, CM and WD Byblow (2004). Impaired modulation of intracortical inhibition in focal hand dystonia. *Cereb Cortex* 14(5): 555–561.

Stinear, CM and WD Byblow (2005). Task-dependent modulation of silent period duration in focal hand dystonia. *Mov Disord* 20(9): 1143–1151.

Tamura, Y, M Matsuhashi, P Lin, B Ou, S Vorbach, R Kakigi and M Hallett (2008). Impaired intracortical inhibition in the primary somatosensory cortex in focal hand dystonia. *Mov Disord* 23(4): 558–565.

Tamura, Y, Y Ueki, P Lin, S Vorbach, T Mima, R Kakigi and M Hallett (2009). Disordered plasticity in the primary somatosensory cortex in focal hand dystonia. *Brain* 132(Pt 3): 749–755.

Thirugnanasambandam, N, R Khera, H Wang, SN Kukke and M Hallett (2015). Distinct interneuronal networks influence excitability of the surround during movement initiation. *J Neurophysiol* 114(2):1102–1108.

Tinazzi, M, A Priori, L Bertolasi, E Frasson, F Mauguiere and A Fiaschi (2000). Abnormal central integration of a dual somatosensory input in dystonia: evidence for sensory overflow. *Brain* 123 (Pt 1): 42–50.

Tinazzi, M, S Farina, M Edwards, G Moretto, D Restivo, A Fiaschi and A Berardelli (2005). Task-specific impairment of motor cortical excitation and inhibition in patients with writer's cramp. *Neurosci Lett* 378(1): 55–58.

Tisch, S, P Limousin, JC Rothwell, P Asselman, N Quinn, M Jahanshahi, KP Bhatia and M Hariz (2006a). Changes in blink reflex excitability after globus pallidus internus stimulation for dystonia. *Mov Disord* 21(10): 1650–1655.

Tisch, S, P Limousin, JC Rothwell, P Asselman, L Zrinzo, M Jahanshahi, KP Bhatia and MI Hariz (2006b). Changes in forearm reciprocal inhibition following pallidal stimulation for dystonia. *Neurology* 66(7): 1091–1093.

Turrigiano, GG, KR Leslie, NS Desai, LC Rutherford and SB Nelson (1998). Activity-dependent scaling of quantal amplitude in neocortical neurons. *Nature* 391(6670): 892–896.

Ugawa, Y, Y Uesaka, Y Terao, R Hanajima and I Kanazawa (1995). Magnetic stimulation over the cerebellum in humans. *Ann Neurol* 37(6): 703–713.

van der Salm, SM, AF van Rootselaar, EM Foncke, JH Koelman, LJ Bour, KP Bhatia, JC Rothwell and MA Tijssen (2009). Normal cortical excitability in myoclonus-dystonia: a TMS study. *Exp Neurol* 216(2): 300–305.

Voller, B, A St Clair Gibson, J Dambrosia, S Pirio Richardson, M Lomarev, N Dang and M Hallett (2006). Short-latency afferent inhibition during selective finger movement. *Exp Brain Res* 169(2): 226–231.

Weise, D, A Schramm, K Stefan, A Wolters, K Reiners, M Naumann and J Classen (2006). The two sides of associative plasticity in writer's cramp. *Brain* 129(Pt 10): 2709–2721.

Werhahn, KJ, E Kunesch, S Noachtar, R Benecke and J Classen (1999). Differential effects on motorcortical inhibition induced by blockade of GABA uptake in humans. *J Physiol* 517(Pt 2): 591–597.

Yoneda, Y, S Rome, HJ Sagar and RA Grunewald (2000). Abnormal perception of the tonic vibration reflex in idiopathic focal dystonia. *Eur J Neurol* 7(5): 529–533.

Chapter 9

Animal Models of Dystonia

Marta Maltese, Paola Imbriani and Antonio Pisani

Introduction

Dystonia is the third most common movement disorder, characterised by sustained muscle contractions, causing twisting repetitive movements and/or abnormal postures. Classification of different forms of dystonia is challenging and it has been recently a matter of revision (Albanese et al. 2013). Accordingly, dystonias can be subdivided based on either clinical characteristics (age at onset, body distribution, temporal features) or on aetiology (isolated or combined dystonia). In isolated dystonia, the dystonic symptoms can be a consequence of inherited genetic factors. In combined dystonia, the dystonic symptoms result from environmental factors, previous condition, brain injury or medications. In the past decade there has been much interest in developing animal models of dystonia, in an attempt to elucidate its pathogenesis and to promote the discovery of new therapeutic treatments. Multiple animal models of dystonia have now been generated, targeting different aspects of a very heterogeneous disorder. The animal models of dystonia may be organised into two major different groups: genetic models and phenotypic models. Genetic models of dystonia replicate genetic mutations found in human patients, providing a tool to investigate the role of mutated causative proteins at system and cellular level (Breakefield et al. 2008). Phenotypic models of dystonia mimic the dystonic phenotype observed in human patients through the injection of pharmacological compounds into specific brain areas (mainly striatum or cerebellum) or through brain injury, with the specific aim to detect brain regions or signalling pathways involved in dystonia. Here, we report the most commonly used animal models of dystonia.

Genetic Models of Dystonia

Different genetic forms of dystonia have been described. The identification of several mutations linked to dystonia onset lead to the development of multiple animal models extremely helpful to explore dystonia pathophysiology.

DYT1 Dystonia

DYT1 dystonia is a severe form of isolated, generalised and early onset (6–25 years of age) dystonia, inherited as an autosomal dominant trait, with a reduced penetrance (30–40 per cent). DYT1 dystonia is caused by a three base-pair deletion (ΔGAG mutation) in the DYT1/TOR1A gene, which encodes the ubiquitously expressed torsinA protein. TorsinA is a member of the AAA+ superfamily of ATPases, associated with a variety of cellular activities, including chaperone-mediated protein folding and vesicular trafficking. It is located predominantly within the lumen of the endoplasmic reticulum (ER) and in the nuclear envelope (NE) (Tanabe et al. 2009). Multiple DYT1 dystonia animal models have been generated, including both invertebrates and vertebrates.

Invertebrate Models of DYT1 Dystonia

Worms (*C. elegans*) and fruit flies (*D. melanogaster*) are extremely simple organisms, with a short-time generation and a well-defined nervous system. Hence, they represent very good model organisms to study specific gene functions and neurological diseases. *C. elegans* presents three torsin-related genes *tor-1*, *tor-2* and *ooc-5*, encoding for ATPases of AAA+ superfamilies. Overexpression of torsinA in *C. elegans* prevented neurodegeneration after 6-OHDA treatment in dopaminergic neurons. In contrast, expression of dystonia-associated mutant torsinA diminished neuroprotection against 6-OHDA. Additionally, *C. elegans* expressing variants of human torsinA mutations resulted in enhanced sensitivity to ER stress, suggesting the protective function of torsinA to maintain a homeostatic threshold against ER stress (Chen et al. 2010). In contrast with *C. elegans*, *D. melanogaster* contains only one torsin-related gene, torp4a, which shows a 34 per cent homology to human torsinA. By using RNA interference (RNAi) to analyse the function of torp4a in *D. melanogaster*, it has been reported that overexpression of torp4a prevented age-related degeneration in the fly retina. Conversely, down-regulation of torp4a led to increased and progressive retinal degeneration. In young flies' retinas, the authors found a correlation with a lysosome-related organelle, the pigment granule, suggesting that torp4a could play a role in transport or biogenesis of lysosome-related organelles (Muraro & Moffat 2006).

Together these invertebrate studies suggest a functional role for torsinA in managing chaperon-mediated protein folding, protecting from ER stress and maintaining intracellular homeostasis, which is altered in DYT1 dystonia.

Transgenic Rodent Models of DYT1 Dystonia

Several transgenic mouse lines overexpressing human mutated torsinA protein (ΔE-torsinA) have been generated, using different promoters in the mouse genome.

Shashidharan and coworkers generated a transgenic mouse model of DYT1 dystonia, by overexpressing human ΔE-torsinA protein through a neuron-specific enolase (NSE) promoter. These transgenic mice developed behavioural abnormalities, such as abnormal involuntary movements with dystonic-appearing and rapid bi-directional circling, coupled to a reduction in striatal dopamine levels (Shashidharan et al. 2005).

Grundmann and colleagues created a second line of transgenic mice, by using a murine prion protein promoter. These transgenic mice showed hyperactivity and decreased learning on the rotarod. Moreover, authors found that overexpressing both human wild-type and ΔE-torsinA induced inclusions formation, altered monoamine levels and NE impairments (Grundmann et al. 2007).

A third line of transgenic mice overexpressing human ΔE-torsinA was generated by Page and coworkers, specifically targeting transgene expression into midbrain dopaminergic neurons through a tyrosine hydroxylase (TH) promoter. Transgenic mice displayed motor abnormalities and altered dopamine (DA) release in response to cocaine, as a consequence of postsynaptic alterations in striatal DA transmission (Page et al. 2010).

Sharma and colleagues generated a DYT1 dystonia mouse model expressing a transgene encoding either the human ΔGAG mutant (hMT) or human wild-type (hWT) torsinA under the human cytomegalovirus (CMV) promoter (Sharma et al. 2005). Despite the absence of dystonic features, mice overexpressing hMT torsinA displayed a reduced ability to learn motor skills in an accelerating rotarod paradigm. Furthermore, hMT mice showed an increased striatal DA turnover, a defect in amphetamine-evoked DA release, and a compromised function of DA transporter (Balcioglu et al. 2007). The hMT mice have been extensively studied by means of electrophysiological techniques. Several lines of experimental evidence indicate a crucial role for the striatal cholinergic system in the pathophysiology of DYT1 dystonia. Physiologically, striatal cholinergic interneurons (ChIs) exhibit spontaneous tonic firing patterns, through which they release acetylcholine in the striatum without external synaptic input. Dopaminergic innervation from the substantia nigra pars compacta (SNpc) inhibits spontaneous tonic firing activity through the activation of D2 DA receptors located on ChIs, and consequently, acetylcholine release in the striatum. hMT mice exhibited an increased, rather than decreased, striatal cholinergic interneuron response after D2 DA receptor activation (Pisani et al. 2007). As a consequence, striatal medium spiny neurons (MSNs) showed significant abnormalities of long-term synaptic plasticity. Medium spiny neurons recorded from hMT mice displayed an increased long-term potentiation (LTP), but lacked both long-term depression (LTD) and synaptic depotentiation (SD) at corticostriatal synapses. Anticholinergic agents normalised striatal cholinergic signalling, fully restoring physiological synaptic plasticity in hMT mice (Martella et al. 2009). Such experimental evidence demonstrate that a 'loss of inhibition' characterises the impairment of synaptic plasticity.

In addition to mouse models, a transgenic rat has recently been generated by overexpressing human ΔE-torsinA under the human torsinA promoter. ΔETorA rats displayed a severely altered ultrastructure of the NE in different brain regions, as well as abnormal reflex responses beyond the motor phenotype. Furthermore, they exhibited severe abnormalities of striatal synaptic plasticity, consisting in the loss of LTD and SD, both restored by using M1 receptor antagonists (Grundmann et al. 2012).

Several transgenic rodent models of DYT1 dystonia have been generated. However, it should be recalled that different promoters, genetic backgrounds and changed insertion sites may induce non-physiological and ectopic protein expression, altering the experimental conditions in transgenic models.

Knock-In and Knock-Out Rodent Models of DYT1 Dystonia

TorsinA null (knock-out) and DYT1 ΔGAG knock-in mice were generated to investigate the cellular role of torsinA and the effect of the DYT1 mutation on torsinA function. DYT1 ΔGAG knock-in mice carry the trinucleotide deletion in the endogenous murine Tor1a gene, which is typically found in DYT1 patients. Both homozygous DYT1 ΔGAG knock-in (Tor1a $^{\Delta GAG/\Delta GAG}$) and torsinA knock-out (Tor1a $^{-/-}$) mice typically die within 48 hours after birth. Heterozygous DYT1 knock-in (Tor1a$^{+/\Delta GAG}$) mice had one normal Tor1a allele and the other with the distinctive ΔGAG mutation. Tor1a$^{+/\Delta GAG}$ mice showed deficient performance on the beam-walking test and hyperactivity in the open-field test. They also exhibited ubiquitin- and torsinA-containing aggregates in neurons of the pontine nuclei (Dang et al. 2005; Goodchild et al. 2005). Microdialysis studies revealed that baseline and amphetamine-stimulated DA release appeared to be lower in the caudoputamen of Tor1a$^{+/\Delta GAG}$ mice, compared to wild-type controls. Additionally, striatal D2 receptor binding and D2 receptor levels decreased in Tor1a$^{+/\Delta GAG}$ mice. Of interest, the alterations in striatal physiology found in Tor1a$^{+/\Delta GAG}$ mice resembled those described in hMT transgenic mice. Indeed, Tor1a$^{+/\Delta GAG}$ mice displayed a selective impairment of corticostriatal synaptic plasticity, whereas hippocampal LTP was normal. Striatal MSNs recorded from Tor1a$^{+/\Delta GAG}$ mice exhibited an increased LTP, whereas they failed to express LTD and SD. Competitive antagonists of M1 muscarinic receptors completely rescued synaptic plasticity deficits observed in Tor1a$^{+/\Delta GAG}$ mice. Moreover, cholinergic interneurons from Tor1a$^{+/\Delta GAG}$ mice displayed an abnormal excitatory response to D2R activation, further confirming an imbalance between dopaminergic and cholinergic striatal signalling (Martella et al. 2014).

Conditional Knock-Out Rodent Models of DYT1 Dystonia

Brain region-specific DYT1 conditional knock-out mice have been generated to understand how single brain regions or cell subtypes contribute to the pathophysiology of DYT1 dystonia. Yokoi and colleagues produced cerebral cortex-specific DYT1 conditional knock-out mice, which exhibited motor deficits and hyperactivity similar to those described in DYT1 heterozygous knock-in mice. Then, they generated striatum-specific DYT1 conditional knock-out mice (sKO), to selectively inactivate Dytl gene in the striatum. DYT1 sKO mice exhibited motor deficits and reduced striatal DA D2 receptor binding activity (Yokoi et al. 2011). Furthermore, Sciamanna and coworkers investigated a cholinergic neuron-specific DYT1 conditional knock-out mouse model. These animals do not have overt dystonia, but do have subtle motor abnormalities. Moreover, there are striking functional abnormalities of striatal cholinergic cells, with paradoxical excitation in response to D2 receptor activation and loss of muscarinic M2/M4 receptor inhibitory function (Sciamanna et al. 2009).

DYT5 Dopa-Responsive Dystonia

DYT5 dystonia, also known as dopa-responsive dystonia (DRD), is characterised by a generalised childhood-onset dystonia with diurnal fluctuations of symptoms and a dramatic response to L-dopa therapy. It is a dominantly inherited condition caused by mutations in the GTP cyclohydrolase 1 gene (GCH1). These mutations reduce the synthesis of BH4 (L-erythro-5,6,7,8-tetrahydrobiopterin), an essential cofactor for tyrosine hydroxylase (TH), the critical enzyme involved in dopamine biosynthesis. A transgenic mouse model for DRD has been generated to target selective dysfunction of TH activity in the striatum. Knock-out mutant mice developed abnormal movements and dystonic posture of the hindlimbs, related to a major depletion of TH labelling in the striatum (Sato et al. 2008).

DYT11 Dystonia

DYT11 myoclonus-dystonia (MD) is a movement disorder characterised by myoclonic jerks and dystonic movements that can be alleviated by alcohol. Additionally, it is often characterised by psychiatric symptoms, such as depression and anxiety disorders. It is caused by mutations in the maternally imprinted and paternally expressed SGCE gene, encoding the transmembrane glycoprotein ε-sarcoglycan. SGCE knock-out (SGCE KO) mice have been generated through the deletion of exon 4, resulting in a frame-shift mutation of SGCE gene. SGCE heterozygous knock-out mice exhibited myoclonus, balance impairments, motor-learning deficits in the beam-walking test, hyperactivity, anxiety and depression. SGCE KO mice also showed abnormal NEs in striatal MSNs and cerebellar Purkinje cells. Additionally, SGCE KO mice displayed significantly increased levels of striatal dopamine and its metabolites, but reduced striatal D2 receptor protein levels. Striatum-specific SGCE conditional KO (SGCE sKO) mice have been generated to dissect brain circuits involved in the pathogenesis of DYT11 dystonia. SGCE sKO mice exhibited motor deficits, but not myoclonus or nuclear envelope alterations, suggesting a direct correlation between the loss of ε-sarcoglycan function in the striatum and motor impairments observed in the complete SGCE KO mice (Yokoi et al. 2006).

DYT12 Dystonia

Rapid-onset dystonia-parkinsonism (DYT12) is inherited as an autosomal dominant disease with reduced penetrance. The phenotype is triggered by mental or physical stress. It is linked to dominant mutations in ATP1A3 gene, encoding the catalytic subunit (α3) of the Na^+/K^+ ATPase pump. Heterozygous mice carrying a point mutation in the Atp1a3 gene have been created. Heterozygous Atp1a3 KO mice showed an approximate 50 per cent reduction in α3 subunit expression, spatial learning impairments and hyperactivity. Conversely, they did not display motor deficits before the stress induction. After stress exposure, female Het mice showed dramatic motor deficits in the beam-walking and rotarod tests (DeAndrade et al. 2011). Finally, Calderon and coworkers induced the expression of rapid-onset dystonia-parkinsonism (DYT12) phenotype in mice through chronic bilateral perfusion of ouabain (ATP1a3 blocker) within the basal ganglia and the cerebellum (Wilson & Hess 2013).

Phenotypic Models of Dystonia

Toxins and drugs applied either systemically or in specific brain regions, such as basal ganglia and cerebellum, may induce the expression of dystonic phenotype in wild-type rodents. In adult C57Bl/6 mice, systemic subacute administration of 3-nitropropionic acid (3-NP) induced motor behavioural consequences consisting of hindlimb clasping, truncal dystonia, bradykinesia and impaired postural control. Histopathologically, there were discrete lesions of the dorsolateral striatum and a significant dopaminergic cell loss within the SNpc. In rats, a single systemic injection of 3-NP induced impairments of balance beam and rotarod motor tests, 24 h after injection. Systemic 3-NP increased NMDA receptor-dependent corticostriatal LTP over the same time period, although there was no evidence of striatal cell loss.

Conclusions

In the past decade, multiple animal models of dystonia have been generated. Genetic models offer the possibility to study specific gene functions and to analyse the pathophysiology of genetic dystonias. Conversely, phenotypic models of dystonia may prove useful to investigate behavioural phenotypes and neuronal circuits before and after brain damage. Although some conflicting elements emerged from different animal models of dystonia, some commonalities exist among the different models. The motor-learning impairment described in some models suggests an alteration of specific circuits and of synaptic plasticity processes. Second, several models display an alteration in striatal dopamine and acetylcholine signalling. Therefore, animal models, including invertebrates, represent a fundamental tool to investigate the pathophysiology of dystonia, independently from how closely the animal physiology may mimic the human condition. Rather, a useful animal model has to be considered according to its success in discovering new aspects and developing novel therapeutic strategies for the treatment of the disease.

References

Albanese A, Bhatia K, Bressman SB, et al. Phenomenology and classification of dystonia: a consensus update. *Mov Disord* 2013; 28: 863–873.

Balcioglu A, Kim MO, Sharma N, et al. Dopamine release is impaired in a mouse model of DYT1 dystonia. *J Neurochem* 2007; 102: 783–788.

Breakefield XO, Blood AJ, Li Y, et al. The pathophysiological basis of dystonias. *Nat Rev Neurosci* 2008; 9: 222–234.

Chen P, Burdette AJ, Porter JC, et al. The early-onset torsion dystonia-associated protein, torsinA, is a homeostatic regulator of endoplasmic reticulum stress response. *Hum Mol Genet* 2010; 19: 3502–3515.

Dang MT, Yokoi F, McNaught KS, et al. Generation and characterization of Dytl DeltaGAG knock-in mouse as a model for early-onset dystonia. *Exp Neurol* 2005; 196: 452–463.

DeAndrade MP, Yokoi F, van Groen T, et al. Characterization of Atp1a3 mutant mice as a model of rapid-onset dystonia with parkinsonism. *Behav Brain Res* 2011; 216: 659–665.

Goodchild RE, Kim CE, Dauer WT. Loss of the dystonia-associated protein torsinA selectively disrupts the neuronal nuclear envelope. *Neuron* 2005; 48: 923–932.

Grundmann K, Reischmann B, Vanhoutte G, et al. Overexpression of human wildtype torsinA and human DeltaGAG torsinA in a transgenic mouse model causes phenotypic abnormalities. *Neurobiol Dis* 2007; 27: 190–206.

Grundmann K, Glöckle N, Martella G, et al. Generation of a novel rodent model for DYT1 dystonia. *Neurobiol Dis* 2012; 47: 61–74.

Martella G, Tassone A, Sciamanna G, et al. Impairment of bidirectional synaptic plasticity in the striatum of a mouse model of DYT1 dystonia: role of endogenous acetylcholine. *Brain* 2009; 132: 2336–2349.

Martella G, Maltese M, Nisticò R, et al. Regional specificity of synaptic plasticity deficits in a knock-in mouse model of DYT1 dystonia. *Neurobiol Dis* 2014; 65: 124–132.

Muraro NI, Moffat KG. Down-regulation of torp4a, encoding the *Drosophila* homologue of torsinA, results in increased neuronal degeneration. *J Neurobiol* 2006; 66: 1338–1353.

Page ME, Bao L, Andre P, et al. Cell-autonomous alteration of dopaminergic transmission by wild type and mutant (DeltaE) TorsinA in transgenic mice. *Neurobiol Dis* 2010; 39: 318–326.

Pisani A, Bernardi G, Ding J, et al. Re-emergence of striatal cholinergic interneurons in movement disorders. *Trends Neurosci* 2007; 30: 545–553.

Sato K, Sumi-Ichinose C, Kaji R, et al. Differential involvement of striosome and matrix dopamine systems in a transgenic model of dopa-responsive dystonia. *Proc Natl Acad Sci USA* 2008; 105: 12551–12556.

Sciamanna G, Bonsi P, Tassone A, et al. Impaired striatal D2 receptor function leads to enhanced GABA transmission in a mouse model of DYT1 dystonia. *Neurobiol Dis* 2009; 34: 133–145.

Sharma N, Baxter MG, Petravicz J, et al. Impaired motor learning in mice expressing torsinA with the DYT1 dystonia mutation. *J Neurosci* 2005; 25: 5351–5355.

Shashidharan P, Sandu D, Potla U, et al. Transgenic mouse model of early-onset DYT1 dystonia. *Hum Mol Genet* 2005; 14: 125–133.

Tanabe LM, Kim CE, Alagem N, et al. Primary dystonia: molecules and mechanisms. *Nat Rev Neurol* 2009; 5: 598–609.

Wilson BK, Hess EJ. Animal models for dystonia. *Mov Disord* 2013; 28: 982–989.

Yokoi F, Dang MT, Li J, et al. Myoclonus, motor deficits, alterations in emotional responses and monoamine metabolism in epsilon-sarcoglycan deficient mice. *J Biochem* 2006; 140: 141–146.

Yokoi F, Dang MT, Li J, et al. Motor deficits and decreased striatal dopamine receptor 2 binding activity in the striatum-specific Dytl conditional knockout mice. *PLoS One* 2011; 6: e24539.

Chapter 10

Genetics of the Dystonias

Overview

Aloysius Domingo and Christine Klein

Introduction

The rise of next-generation sequencing in the past decade has revolutionised not only progress but also thought in the field of dystonia. As more genes causative for dystonic syndromes are discovered by this highly convenient and cost-effective method, we have also come to realise that genetic causes are not exclusive to familial forms, but may also account for the sporadic, more common presentations of dystonia. Rapid gene discovery in the last years has accelerated research into causative molecular mechanisms, pathways and networks. Although much has still to be clarified and confirmed in independent, multimodal investigations, work in genetics may be among the major breakthroughs in the field of dystonia in recent history. The availability of genetic testing for a wider set of genetic dystonias has also begun the translation of research findings into the clinical setting, while also necessitating knowledge of genetic forms among clinicians.

In this chapter, we include discussion on *DYT-TOR1A*, *DYT-THAP1* and *DYT-GNAL*, representing the isolated forms of dystonia, i.e. those where dystonia is the sole clinical manifestation. Briefly, we also review *DYT-GCH1* and *DYT-TH*, *DYT-ATP1A3*, and *DYT-SGCE*, to cover the most recognised combined forms of genetic dystonia, in which dystonia usually occurs in conjunction with another movement disorder. *DYT-TUBB4* is presented as an example of a complex phenotype, where the clinical spectrum includes features outside the realm of movement disorders and may include non-neurological syndromic manifestations. A systematic review of the complex dystonias is, however, beyond the scope of this chapter.

We will highlight for each isolated and combined form interesting genetic features, and, when possible, genotype–phenotype correlations. Although not meant to be definitive and diagnostic, a simplified classification algorithm based on inheritance, and genetic and phenotypic features, is presented (Figure 10.1). As previously noted, research in this field is growing rapidly and new information is available every few months. For example, in April 2015 novel genes for recessively inherited isolated dystonia (*HPCA* and *COL6A3*) have been described; these are awaiting confirmation in larger studies. Thus, the interested reader is encouraged to constantly and continuously check online resources (for example, GeneReviews at www.ncbi.nlm.nih.gov/books/NBK1155/) for new and up-to-date information. Lastly, this chapter covers the most common and well-reviewed forms of monogenic dystonia. Not covered are rare, complex forms, in which dystonia presents in combination with a variety of syndromic features.

Classification

The most well-known system of classifying the genetic dystonias is the *DYT* system of locus symbols. Originally devised to indicate chromosomal regions linked to presumably genetic forms where the causative gene has not yet been identified, the system has become misleading in many respects. The 'locus' *DYT2*, for example, lumps together families with early-onset autosomal recessive dystonia, although no common locus has been proposed. The *DYT14* and *DYT9* loci are redundant and represent a deletion of the *GCH1* gene and mutations in the *SLC2A1* gene, respectively. These genes have, however, already been identified in the *DYT5a* and *DYT18* loci. Lastly, *DYT* loci exist for unconfirmed or unreplicated reports of families with suspected genetic dystonias, as in *DYT7* and *DYT13*. It is for these reasons that experts advocate replacing *DYT* suffixes by gene names instead of numbers (i.e. *DYT-TOR1A* instead of *DYT1*) (Table 10.1) and allowing *DYT* symbols to be attached only to forms that have been sufficiently confirmed and replicated, in particular those where gene testing is already diagnostic for the condition (Marras et al. 2012).

Isolated Dystonia

DYT-TOR1A

Hermann Oppenheim may have been the first to describe a genetic form of dystonia when he wrote his treatise describing dystonia musculorum deformans in 1911. He was probably describing what we know today as early-onset dystonia due to TorsinA mutations (Klein & Fahn 2013). *DYT-TOR1A* is an early-onset, isolated, generalised dystonia, with an age at onset before 26 years, typically in a limb (Bressman et al. 2000) and usually sparing the craniocervical and trunk regions. Almost all cases are caused by a three base-pair (GAG) deletion in the *TOR1A* gene (Ozelius et al. 1997), inherited in an autosomal dominant fashion and most commonly described in the Ashkenazi Jewish population due to a founder effect. An interesting feature of *DYT-TOR1A* is reduced penetrance. Only about 30 per cent of mutation carriers will manifest symptoms and if these do not occur prior to 28 years of age, they

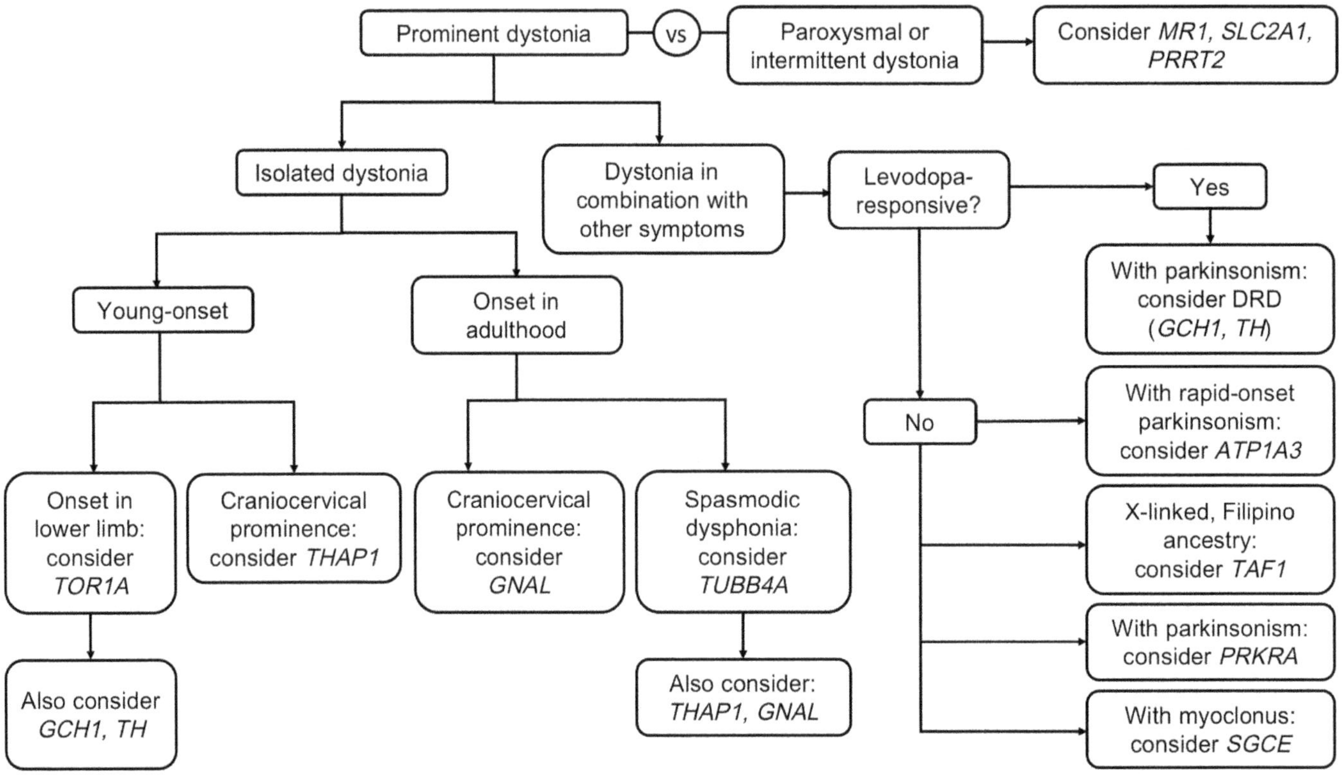

Figure 10.1 A simple classification algorithm is presented based on genetic and clinical features of the different monogenic dystonias. The algorithm is not meant to be definitive or diagnostic and recently discovered genes (i.e. those pending confirmation in larger studies) have been omitted.

will likely not occur for the rest of the mutation carrier's life. Furthermore, penetrance is modified by a 'protective mutation' occurring *in trans* (i.e. on the chromosome not carrying the GAG deletion). In mutation carriers that harbour this D2016H polymorphism in *TOR1A*, penetrance of the dystonic phenotype is further reduced to just 3 per cent (Risch et al. 2007).

DYT-THAP1

Like *DYT-TOR1A*, *DYT-THAP1* is also inherited in an autosomal dominant fashion, and healthy mutation carriers have also been described in many families (i.e. there is reduced penetrance). *DYT-THAP1* may manifest with features of focal and/or generalised – but always isolated – dystonia, usually with limb and cranial muscle involvement and speech involvement (Bressman et al. 2009). Mutations in the *THAP* domain-containing, apoptosis-associated protein 1 (*THAP1*) gene are causative (Fuchs et al. 2009), but unlike in *TOR1A*, many different missense and truncating mutations have been identified in *THAP1*. Also, while *DYT-THAP1* was first described in Amish Mennonites and although a founder mutation in *THAP1* exists in this population, recent studies indicate that isolated dystonia is rather genetically diverse in this ethnic isolate. Other genetic causes that have been identified include *DYT-TOR1A* and *DYT-GNAL* (Saunders-Pullman et al. 2014).

DYT-GNAL

Mutations in the guanine nucleotide-binding protein, alpha activating activity polypeptide, olfactory type (*GNAL*) gene cause adult-onset (age at onset is thirties to fifties) craniocervical dystonia (Fuchs et al. 2013), accounting for about 1 per cent of all cases of focal or segmental dystonia involving this region in one study (Kumar et al. 2014). Perhaps of significant clinical relevance is the observation that *GNAL* mutations occur in seemingly sporadic cases (in various populations) (Dobricic et al. 2014), making *DYT-GNAL* an important differential diagnosis in the most common form of isolated dystonia.

Other Genes Associated With Isolated Dystonia

Worthy of mention are some genes identified for isolated forms of dystonia, which remain to be replicated in larger, independent studies. Mutations in the *CIZ1* and *ANO3* genes have been proposed for adult-onset, primarily craniocervical dystonia (Charlesworth et al. 2013); however, sequence alterations in both genes have been found in variant databases (Lohmann & Klein 2013), arguing against their pathogenicity (MacArthur et al. 2014). *HPCA* has recently been proposed as one of the causative genes for the phenotype described in *DYT2*, i.e. recessively inherited isolated dystonia, due to homozygous and compound heterozygous mutations identified in the gene in two independent families (Charlesworth et al. 2015). Lastly, recessive mutations in the *COL6A3* gene are also thought to cause isolated, segmental dystonia that is primarily craniocervical (Zech et al. 2015). Sequencing of these genes in phenotypically consistent cases is currently recommended only on a research (and not diagnostic) basis, and also in an effort to replicate the original results and discover more families or cases harbouring the same mutations.

Table 10.1 Monogenic dystonias

Gene/locus	Clinical disorder	Inheritance	OMIM number	*DYT* symbol	Related reference
		Isolated dystonias			
TOR1A	Early-onset, generalised dystonia (Oppenheim dystonia)	Autosomal dominant	128100	DYT1	Ozelius et al., 1997
THAP1	Adolescent-onset dystonia, most prominent in the upper body regions	Autosomal dominant	602629	DYT6	Fuchs et al., 2009
GNAL	Adult-onset segmental craniocervical dystonia	Autosomal dominant	615073	DYT25	Fuchs et al., 2013
No single locus, HPCA*	Early-onset, isolated dystonia with prominent craniocervical symptoms	Autosomal recessive	224500	DYT2	Charlesworth et al., 2015
COL6A3*	Early-onset, isolated dystonia with prominent craniocervical symptoms	Autosomal recessive	120250	DYT27	Zech et al., 2015
		Combined dystonias			
GCH1	Dopa-responsive dystonia (Segawa disease)	Autosomal dominant	128230	DYT5a, DYT14	Segawa et al., 1976
TH	Dopa-responsive dystonia	Autosomal recessive	605407	DYT5b	Lüdecke et al., 1995
ATP1A3	Rapid-onset dystonia-parkinsonism	Autosomal dominant	128235	DYT12	de Carvalho Aguiar et al., 2004
PRKRA	Young-onset dystonia-parkinsonism	Autosomal recessive	612067	DYT16	Camargos et al., 2008
SGCE, RELN*	Myoclonus-dystonia	Autosomal dominant	159900	DYT11	Zimprich et al., 2001
KCTD17*	Non-alcohol-responsive myoclonus-dystonia with prominent dystonia	Autosomal dominant	616386	DYT26	Mencacci et al., 2015
TAF1*	X-linked dystonia-parkinsonism (Lubag disease)	X-linked recessive	314250	DYT3	Nolte et al., 2003; Makino et al., 2007
		Complex dystonia			
TUBB4	Isolated whispering dystonia in original family, complex dystonia in H-ABC syndrome	Autosomal dominant	128101	DYT4	Lohmann et al., 2013
		Paroxysmal dyskinesias (may present with dystonia)			
MR1	Paroxysmal non-kinesigenic dyskinesia	Autosomal dominant	118800	DYT8, DYT20?	Rainier et al., 2004
SLC2A1	Paroxysmal exertion-induced dyskinesia	Autosomal dominant	601042	DYT9, DYT18	Weber et al., 2001
PRRT2	Paroxysmal kinesigenic dyskinesia	Autosomal dominant	128200	DYT10, DYT19?	Chen et al., 2011
		Unconfirmed and unreplicated loci			
9q34, CIZ1	Adult-onset craniocervical dystonia	Autosomal dominant	614860	DYT23	Xiao et al., 2012
11p, ANO3	Adult-onset craniocervical dystonia	Autosomal dominant	615034	DYT24	Charlesworth et al., 2012
18p	Adult-onset focal dystonia	Autosomal dominant	602124	DYT7	Leube et al., 1996
1p36	Multifocal dystonia	Autosomal dominant	607671	DYT13	Valente et al., 2001
18p11	Myoclonus-dystonia	Autosomal dominant	607488	DYT15	Grimes et al., 2001
20q13	Isolated dystonia	Autosomal recessive	612406	DYT17	Chouery et al., 2008
2q14-21	Adult-onset mixed dystonia with generalisation	Autosomal dominant	614588	DYT21	Norgren et al., 2011
?	Reserved but not published		none	DYT22	none

* genes awaiting confirmation in larger genetic or functional studies

Combined Dystonia

DYT-TH and DYT-GCH1

Dopa-responsive dystonia (DRD) is characterised by childhood-onset dystonia that responds dramatically to levodopa therapy and exhibits marked diurnal fluctuation (Segawa et al. 1976). Parkinsonism is a common feature, especially in late stages, and may rarely be the only sign. The penetrance in women is twice that in males. Autosomal recessive DRD is associated with mutations in the tyrosine hydroxylase (*TH*) gene and the more frequent autosomal dominant form is caused by mutations in the GTP cyclohydrolase 1 (*GCH1*) gene. Despite gene testing being widely available and withstanding the exquisite treatability of the disease, there is considerable diagnostic delay in diagnosis. Many mutation carriers display residual dystonic or parkinsonian as well other motor (i.e. restless legs syndrome) and non-motor symptoms with levodopa therapy, likely as a result of diagnostic and therapeutic delay (Tadic et al. 2012).

DYT-ATP1A3, Alternating Hemiplegia and CAPOS Syndrome, DYT-PRKRA

Rapid-onset dystonia-parkinsonism (RDP) with an abrupt onset within hours to weeks, occurring in response to physical or emotional stress, is inherited in an autosomal dominant fashion with reduced penetrance and is associated with mutations in the *ATP1A3* gene (de Carvalho Aguiar et al. 2004). The spectrum of phenotypes associated with mutations in *ATP1A3* includes other neurologic conditions; alternating hemiplegia of childhood (*AHC*) and *CAPOS* syndrome (cerebellar ataxia, areflexia, pes cavus, optic atrophy and sensorineural hearing loss) are also linked with *ATP1A3* mutations (Sweney et al. 2015). Rapid-onset dystonia-parkinsonism usually presents in adolescence or early adulthood, while *AHC* and *CAPOS* syndrome are diseases of infants and children. The young-onset generalised dystonia in *DYT/PARK-PRKRA* is usually accompanied by parkinsonism (hence the addition of PARK in the proposed nomenclature), is recessively inherited and caused by mutations in the *PRKRA* gene (Camargos et al. 2008).

DYT-SGCE

Myoclonus-dystonia (MD) is characterised by myoclonus in combination with dystonia (usually cervical dystonia or writer's cramp), with onset typically in childhood or early adolescence. Symptoms dramatically but transiently improve with alcohol intake. MD is inherited as an autosomal dominant trait and is caused by loss-of-function mutations in the epsilon-sarcoglycan (*SGCE*) gene (Zimprich et al. 2001). Reduced penetrance upon maternal transmission of the disease allele is caused by maternal genomic imprinting (Müller et al. 2002). *SGCE* mutations, however, cannot account for more than half of cases of familial and sporadic MD. Recently, mutations in the *RELN* (Groen et al. 2015a) and *CACNA1B* (Groen et al. 2015b) genes have been proposed to contribute to this genetic heterogeneity. However, the relevance of *CACNA1B* variants is under debate (Mencacci et al. 2015a). Mutations in *KCTD17* have also been recently proposed to account for *SGCE*-negative cases of MD, where dystonia is prominent and progressive and where the symptoms are not responsive to alcohol (Mencacci et al. 2015b).

DYT-TUBB4

Mutations in the tubulin beta 4 (*TUBB4*) gene were linked to whispering and spasmodic dysphonia in the original Australian family where the gene was first found (Lohmann et al. 2013). A dystonic 'hobby horse gait' was also characteristic. Interestingly, *TUBB4* mutations have now also been found in cases of hypomyelination with atrophy of the basal ganglia and cerebellum (H-ABC) (Simons et al. 2013), a leukoencephalic disorder with grossly abnormal neuroimaging. Thus, *TUBB4* (as *ATP1A3*) may exemplify pleiotropy, in which phenotypically different conditions are caused by mutations in the same gene. The presentation of isolated dystonia in the original *DYT4* family may represent an exception rather than the rule.

Other Combined Dystonias

X-linked dystonia-parkinsonism (XDP) also combines dystonia and parkinsonism, and is so far described only in individuals of Filipino descent and is unequivocally thought to be caused by several mutations occurring in the vicinity of the *TAF1* gene (Domingo et al. 2015, 2016). Patients present in adulthood with focal or segmental dystonia. The dystonia subsequently generalises and patients develop parkinsonism, which dominates the disease picture in the second decade. Interestingly, XDP is unique among the dystonias in that overt neurodegeneration has been observed in autopsied specimens.

Mutations in *PRRT2, MR1* and *SLC2A1* underlie dyskinetic/dystonic disorders with highly variable paroxysmal symptoms, including heterogeneous dystonic presentations (Waln & Jankovic 2015). They are thus better classified under the paroxysmal hyperkinetic movement disorders. However, as seen in Table 10.1, these syndromes were previously assigned *DYT* symbols due to the presence of variable dystonic features in the original patients.

Implications for Diagnosis and Therapy

Although molecular therapy for dystonia – in the context of gene replacement or gene knock-out therapy – is neither available nor tested in humans, the recognition and accurate diagnosis of a genetic form may also have therapeutic implications. The establishment of a final genetic diagnosis is in itself helpful in alleviating uncertainty and patient anxiety. It is a viable alternative against a costly and drawn-out 'diagnostic odyssey', which patients with complicated disorders usually have to endure (Lohmann & Klein 2014). For some dystonias, i.e. dopa-responsive dystonia *(DYT-TH, DYT-GCH1)*, the genetic diagnosis may even lead to appropriate therapy. For others, identification of the correct genetic form guides treatment options and sets expectations. *DYT-TOR1A*, for example, has been shown to have exemplary long-term response to deep brain stimulation. Meanwhile, the results for *DYT-THAP1* are less consistent (Brüggemann et al. 2015). Importantly, genetic testing in neurologic conditions should always be guided by accurate interpretation and appropriate genetic counselling, especially in dystonia, where many novel genes have yet to be confirmed to be truly pathogenic (Domingo et al. 2016).

Conclusions

Genetic dystonias are characterised by both genetic and clinical heterogeneity (even in seemingly homogeneous populations), making rigid definitions of syndromes incomprehensive and – sometimes – false. The reader is encouraged to keep an open mind when diagnosing genetic dystonia, as some 'new' and complex phenotypes may in fact be due to already-known causes (as we have seen for *GCH1/TH-DRD*) and vice versa: new genes are being identified rapidly for classic presentations (i.e. isolated craniocervical dystonia). Dystonia indeed has many faces and this certainly includes the genetic forms.

References

Bressman SB, Sabatti C, Raymond D, de Leon D, Klein C, Kramer PL, Brin MF, Fahn S, Breakefield X, Ozelius LJ (2000) The DYT1 phenotype and guidelines for diagnostic testing. *Neurology* 54, 1746–1752.

Bressman SB, Raymond D, Fuchs T, Heiman GA, Ozelius LJ, Saunders-Pullman R (2009) Mutations in THAP1 (DYT6) in early-onset dystonia: a genetic screening study. *Lancet Neurol* 8, 441–446.

Brüggemann N, Kühn A, Schneider SA, Kamm C, Wolters A, Krause P, Steigerwald F, Wittstock, M, Lozano AM, Hamani C (2015) Short- and long-term outcome of chronic pallidal neurostimulation in monogenic isolated dystonia. *Neurology* 84, 895–903.

Camargos S, Scholz S, Simon-Sanchez J, Paisan-Ruiz C, Lewis P, Hernandez D, Ding J, Gibbs JR, Cookson MR, Bras J (2008) DYT16, a novel young-onset dystonia-parkinsonism disorder: identification of a segregating mutation in the stress-response protein PRKRA. *Lancet Neurol* 7, 207–215.

Charlesworth G, Bhatia KP, Wood NW (2013) The genetics of dystonia: new twists in an old tale. *Brain* 136, 2017–2037.

Charlesworth G, Angelova PR, Bartolome-Robledo F, Ryten M, Trabzuni D, Stamelou M, Abramov AY, Bhatia KP, Wood NW (2015) Mutations in HPCA cause autosomal-recessive primary isolated dystonia. *Am J Hum Genet* 96, 657–665.

de Carvalho Aguiar P, Sweadner KJ, Penniston JT, Zaremba J, Liu L, Caton M, Linazasoro G, Borg M, Tijssen MAJ, Bressman SB (2004) Mutations in the Na+/K+ -ATPase alpha3 gene ATP1A3 are associated with rapid-onset dystonia parkinsonism. *Neuron* 43, 169–175.

Dobricic V, Kresojevic N, Westenberger A, Svetel M, Tomic A, Ralic V, Petrovic I, Lukic MJ, Lohmann K, Novakovic I (2014) De novo mutation in the GNAL gene causing seemingly sporadic dystonia in a Serbian patient. *Mov Disord* 29, 1190–1193.

Domingo A, Westenberger A, Lee LV, Brænne I, Liu T, Vater I, Rosales R, Jamora RD, Pasco PM, Cutiongco-dela Paz EM (2015) New insights into the genetics of X-linked dystonia-parkinsonism (XDP, DYT3). *Eur J Hum Genet* 23, 1334–1340.

Domingo A, Amar D, Grütz K, Lee LV, Rosales R, Brüggemann N, Jamora RD, Cutiongco-Dela Paz E, Rolfs A, Dressler D (2016a) Evidence of TAF1 dysfunction in peripheral models of X-linked dystonia-parkinsonism. *Cell Mol Life Sci* 73, 3205–3215.

Domingo A, Erro R, Lohmann K (2016b) Novel dystonia genes: clues on disease mechanisms and the complexities of high-throughput sequencing. *Mov Disord* 31, 471–477.

Fuchs T, Saunders-Pullman R, Masuhol, Luciano MS, Raymond D, Factor S, Lang AE, Liang T-W, Trosch RM, White S (2013) Mutations in GNAL cause primary torsion dystonia. *Nat Genet* 45, 88–92.

Fuchs T, Gavarini S, Saunders-Pullman R, Raymond D, Ehrlich ME, Bressman SB, Ozelius LJ (2009) Mutations in the THAP1 gene are responsible for DYT6 primary torsion dystonia. *Nat Genet* 41, 286–288.

Groen JL, Andrade A, Ritz K, Jalalzadeh H, Haagmans M, Bradley TEJ, Jongejan A, Verbeek DS, Nurnberg P, Denome S (2015a) CACNA1B mutation is linked to unique myoclonus-dystonia syndrome. *Hum Mol Genet* 24, 987–993.

Groen JL, Ritz K, Jalalzadeh H, van der Salm SMA, Jongejan A, Mook OR, Haagmans MA, Zwinderman AH, Motazacker MM, Hennekam RC (2015b) RELN rare variants in myoclonus-dystonia. *Mov Disord* 30, 415–419.

Klein C, Fahn S (2013) Translation of Oppenheim's 1911 paper on dystonia. *Mov Disord* 28, 851–862.

Kumar KR, Lohmann K, Masuho I, Miyamoto R, Ferbert A, Lohnau T, Kasten M, Hagenah J, Bruggemann N, Graf J (2014) Mutations in GNAL: a novel cause of craniocervical dystonia. *JAMA Neurol* 71, 490–494.

Lohmann K, Klein C (2013) Genetics of dystonia: what's known? What's new? What's next? *Mov Disord* 28, 899–905.

Lohmann K, Klein C (2014) Next generation sequencing and the future of genetic diagnosis. *Neurotherapeutics* 11, 699–707.

Lohmann K, Wilcox RA, Winkler S, Ramirez A, Rakovic A, Park J-S, Arns B, Lohnau T, Groen J, Kasten M (2013) Whispering dysphonia (DYT4 dystonia) is caused by a mutation in the TUBB4 gene. *Ann Neurol* 73, 537–545.

MacArthur DG, Manolio TA, Dimmock DP, Rehm HL, Shendure J, Abecasis GR, Adams DR, Altman RB, Antonarakis SE, Ashley EA (2014) Guidelines for investigating causality of sequence variants in human disease. *Nature* 508, 469–476.

Marras C, Lohmann K, Lang A, Klein C (2012) Fixing the broken system of genetic locus symbols: Parkinson disease and dystonia as examples. *Neurology* 78, 1016–1024.

Mencacci NE, R'bibo L, Bandres-Ciga S, Carecchio M, Zorzi G, Nardocci N, Garavaglia B, Batla A, Bhatia KP, Pittman AM (2015a) The *CACNA1B* R1389H variant is not associated with myoclonus-dystonia in a large European multicentric cohort. *Hum Mol Genet* 10.1093/hmg/ddv255.

Mencacci NE, Rubio-Agusti I, Zdebik A, Asmus F, Ludtmann MHR, Ryten M, Plagnol V, Hauser A-K, Bandres-Ciga S, Bettencourt C (2015b) A missense mutation in KCTD17 causes autosomal dominant myoclonus-dystonia. *Am J Hum Genet* 96, 938–947.

Müller B, Hedrich K, Kock N, Dragasevic N, Svetel M, Garrels J, Landt O, Nitschke M, Pramstaller PP, Reik W (2002) Evidence that paternal expression of the epsilon-sarcoglycan gene accounts for reduced penetrance in myoclonus-dystonia. *Am J Hum Genet* 71, 1303–1311.

Ozelius LJ, Hewett JW, Page CE, Bressman SB, Kramer PL, Shalish C, de Leon D, Brin MF, Raymond D, Corey DP (1997) The early-onset torsion dystonia gene (DYT1) encodes an ATP-binding protein. *Nat Genet* 17, 40–48.

Risch NJ, Bressman SB, Senthil G, Ozelius LJ (2007) Intragenic cis and trans modification of genetic susceptibility in DYT1 torsion dystonia. *Am J Hum Genet* 80, 1188–1193.

Saunders-Pullman R, Fuchs T, San Luciano M, Raymond D, Brashear A, Ortega R, Deik A, Ozelius LJ, Bressman SB (2014) Heterogeneity in primary dystonia: lessons from THAP1, GNAL, and TOR1A in Amish-Mennonites. *Mov Disord* 29, 812–818.

Segawa M, Hosaka A, Miyagawa F, Nomura Y, Imai H (1976) Hereditary progressive dystonia with marked diurnal fluctuation. *Adv Neurol* 14, 215–233.

Simons C, Wolf NI, McNeil N, Caldovic L, Devaney JM, Takanohashi A, Crawford J, Ru K, Grimmond SM, Miller D (2013) A de novo mutation in the beta-tubulin gene TUBB4A results in the leukoencephalopathy hypomyelination with atrophy of the basal ganglia and cerebellum. *Am J Hum Genet* 92, 767–773.

Sweney MT, Newcomb TM, Swoboda KJ (2015) The expanding spectrum of neurological phenotypes in children with ATP1A3 mutations, alternating hemiplegia of childhood, rapid-onset dystonia-parkinsonism, CAPOS and beyond. *Pediatr Neurol* 52, 56–64.

Tadic V, Kasten M, Brüggemann N, Stiller S, Hagenah J, Klein C (2012) Dopa-responsive dystonia revisited: diagnostic delay, residual signs, and nonmotor signs. *Arch Neurol* 69, 1558–1562.

Waln O, Jankovic J (2015) Paroxysmal movement disorders. *Neurol Clin* 33, 137–152.

Zech M, Lam DD, Francescatto L, Schormair B, Salminen AV, Jochim A, Wieland T, Lichtner P, Peters A, Gieger C (2015) Recessive mutations in the alpha3 (VI) collagen gene COL6A3 cause early-onset isolated dystonia. *Am J Hum Genet* 96, 883–893.

Zimprich A, Grabowski M, Asmus F, Naumann M, Berg D, Bertram M, Scheidtmann K, Kern P, Winkelmann J, Muller-Myhsok B (2001) Mutations in the gene encoding epsilon-sarcoglycan cause myoclonus-dystonia syndrome. *Nat Genet* 29, 66–69.

Chapter 11

Dystonia

From Genomics to Proteomics and Beyond

Thomas T. Warner and Daniela Hansen

The dystonias are a group of hyperkinetic movement disorders whose principal cause is neuron dysfunction at one or more interconnected nodes of the motor system. The study of genes and proteins which cause familial dystonia provides critical information about the cellular pathways involved in this dysfunction which disrupts the motor pathways at systems level. In recent years, study of the increasing number of DYT genes has implicated a number of cell functions which appear to be involved in the pathogenesis of dystonia (Ledoux et al. 2013). This review will focus on recent advances in genetic dystonias with relevance to neuronal function and highlight areas that may be developed into potential novel therapeutic strategies from the study of DYT1 dystonia.

Genomics

To date, more than 20 monogenic inherited dystonias and dystonia-related disorders (DYT1–DYT25) have been reported in Online Mendelian Inheritance in Man (OMIM). The known genetic forms include all monogenic inheritance patterns (autosomal dominant, autosomal recessive and X-linked) (Xiao et al. 2014).

DYT1

Dystonia associated with DYT1 gene encoding the protein torsinA is the best characterised and the best studied in terms of pathogenesis. DYT1 is transmitted as an autosomal dominant trait with a penetrance of about 30 per cent (Albanese et al. 2013).

In 1997, an in-frame three base-pair deletion (ΔGAG, ΔE) in the TORA gene encoding the AAA+ protein torsinA was discovered as the cause of DYT1 dystonia. While best described in Ashkenazi Jews, the DYT1 mutation has arisen *de novo* several times in diverse populations. Mutation carriers who do not develop dystonia by their early twenties often remain symptom-free for life (Dauer 2014).

Despite the incomplete penetrance, 2-deoxyglucose studies show that all carriers exhibit abnormal brain metabolism, with increased metabolic activity in the cerebellum, putamen/globus pallidus and supplementary motor cortex. The factors that determine conversion from subclinical 'endophenotype' to overt disease remain unknown. Possible genetic modifiers of the torsinA pathway include torsinB, which has redundant functions, and other torsinA-interacting proteins, including lamina-associated polypeptide (LAP1), luminal domain-like LAP1 (LULL1) and printor. LAP1 and torsinB function with torsinA to maintain normal nuclear membrane morphology (Tanabe et al. 2012).

DYT3

DYT3, caused by mutations affecting expression of TAF1, is the only known X-linked form of dystonia and the only known 'DYT' with documented neurodegeneration. Endemic in the Philippines, it is characterised by a combination of dystonia and parkinsonism (Klein et al. 1993).

DYT4

DYT4 describes autosomal dominantly inherited whispering dysphonia with generalised dystonia with a characteristic hobby horse ataxic gait caused by mutation of the β-tubulin (TUBB4a) gene (Hersheson et al. 2013).

DYT5

Most cases of dopa-responsive dystonia (DRD) are autosomal dominant and caused by mutations in the GCH1 gene, encoding the enzyme GTP cyclohydrolase 1 (Camargo et al. 2015). Autosomal recessive forms of DRD caused by mutations in genes for tyrosine hydroxylase and sepiapterin reductase are described (Klein et al. 1993; Camargo et al. 2015).

DYT6

DYT6 dystonia is an autosomal dominant syndrome with about 60 per cent penetrance. Mutations in the THAP1 gene encoding the transcription factor thanatos-associated protein 1 have been identified (Dauer 2014). Currently over 60 different missense and truncating THAP1 pathogenic variants have been reported (Klein et al. 1993).

DYT11

Myoclonus-dystonia, DYT11, is a rare autosomal dominant movement disorder with variable penetrance. The myoclonic jerks often improve with alcohol. The DYT11 gene encodes the glycoprotein ε-sarcoglycan (Camargo et al. 2015).

DYT12

Rapid-onset dystonia-parkinsonism (RDP) is an autosomal dominant condition. The gene responsible for the disease, DYT12/ATP1A3, encodes the Na^+/K^+-ATPase α3 (ATP1A3), a catalytic subunit of the sodium pump (Camargo et al. 2015).

DYT23

A recent study identified a CIZ1 (c790A>G, p.S264G) mutation in a large Caucasian pedigree with late-onset primary cervical dystonia. CIZ1 encodes Cip1-interacting zinc finger protein 1, a DNA replication factor expressed in the human brain (Ledoux et al. 2013). To date, replication of the pathogenicity of this gene in further kindreds is lacking.

DYT24

Anoctamin 3 (ANO3) is believed to act as a calcium-gated chloride channel and is highly expressed in human neurons. A putative mutation in ANO3 gene was identified in an autosomal dominant family with craniocervical dystonia (Ledoux et al. 2013).

DYT25

Mutations in GNAL are associated with craniocervical dystonia that can generalise. GNAL encodes the stimulatory alpha subunit, Gαolf (Fuchs et al. 2013).

Proteomics and Cell Biology of DYT1 Dystonia

TorsinA Function

The DYT1 gene and its protein torsinA have been studied in more detail than any other DYT locus. Study of torsinA in cell and animal models has shed light on potential pathogenic pathways and networks, making it an exemplar for genetic forms of dystonia. A unique feature of these dystonias is the absence of neurodegeneration, implying that they are a result of neuronal dysfunction and not death.

Torsin ATPases belong to the widespread AAA+ family of ATPases, which typically function as oligomers and use hydrolysis of ATP for many diverse cellular functions, including protein trafficking, membrane fusion, protein folding and degradation (Rose et al. 2015). They are the only AAA+ ATPases to reside in the endoplasmic reticulum (ER) and contiguous nuclear envelope (NE) in mammalian cells. TorsinA is expressed in high levels in the nervous system. Overexpression of torsinA ΔE in cultured cells leads to whorled membrane inclusions derived from the NE (Hewett et al. 2000). Blebbing of the inner nuclear membrane is also seen in neurons of torsinA knock-out mice, torsinA ΔE homozygous knock-in mice and mice in which torsinA ΔE knock-in allele is expressed on a knock-out background, suggesting it is a loss-of-function mutation (Goodchild et al. 2005). Neurons may be susceptible to loss of function as they express torsinA at high levels compared to other members of the torsin family, which therefore may not be able to compensate for torsinA loss of function.

Protein, cell-based and animal models have implicated four broad categories of pathogenic cell mechanisms (Rose et al. 2015):

1. Molecular chaperone/protein quality control including involvement of the ER-associated protein degradation (ERAD) pathway.
2. Vesicle/protein trafficking with evidence to support a role in modulating synaptic vesicle cycling at the presynaptic terminal.
3. Cellular architecture with interaction with a variety of structural proteins including kinesin light chain 1, nuclear lamins, nesprin-3 and vimentin.
4. Nuclear envelope vesiculation/trafficking with evidence suggesting torsinA involvement in a nuclear transport pathway involving vesiculation of the NE, which may participate in quality control by exporting misfolded proteins to the ER. This would require the need for membrane-spanning adaptor proteins such as LAP1 and LULL1, which are known to interact with torsinA.

The NE and DYT1 Dystonia

It is increasingly clear that interaction of both LAP1 and LULL1 are key for the binding, activation and folding of torsinA (Rose et al. 2015). The key torsinA mutations lie at the predicted torsin–cofactor interface, again supporting a loss-of-function effect. These adaptors are likely to play an important role in the recent finding in transgenic animals that torsinA is a key regulator for control of neuronal nuclear membrane budding during a specific developmental window which is disrupted by torsinA loss of function, and can be moderated by torsinB (Tanabe et al. 2016).

The hypothesis is that early neurodevelopmental disruption of NE budding by mutant torsinA, with persisting budding which affects neuronal migration, lays down the network susceptibility to dystonia. One area of study for potential anatomy of this susceptibility has been identified in multiple mouse models of DYT1 dystonia and implicates dysfunction of striatal cholinergic interneurons (Eskow Jaunarajs et al. 2015). Paradoxical excitation of cholinergic interneurons in the presence of dopamine D2 receptor agonists and impairment of striatal synaptic plasticity was observed, which were improved after administration of M1 receptor antagonists. It was suggested that this may represent a common dystonia endophenotype.

Lipid Metabolism

A recent report studying torsin function in *Drosophila* found that torsin AAA+ proteins regulate cellular lipid metabolism, and identified a relationship between human torsinA localised in the inner NE, rapid expansion of the nuclear membranes and increased membrane lipid levels (Grillet et al. 2016). In addition, *Drosophila* torsin regulates lipid metabolism via the lipin phosphatidic acid phosphatase enzyme. These findings need to be replicated in human and mouse models, but may provide mechanisms linking the ER, NM and developmental disturbances seen.

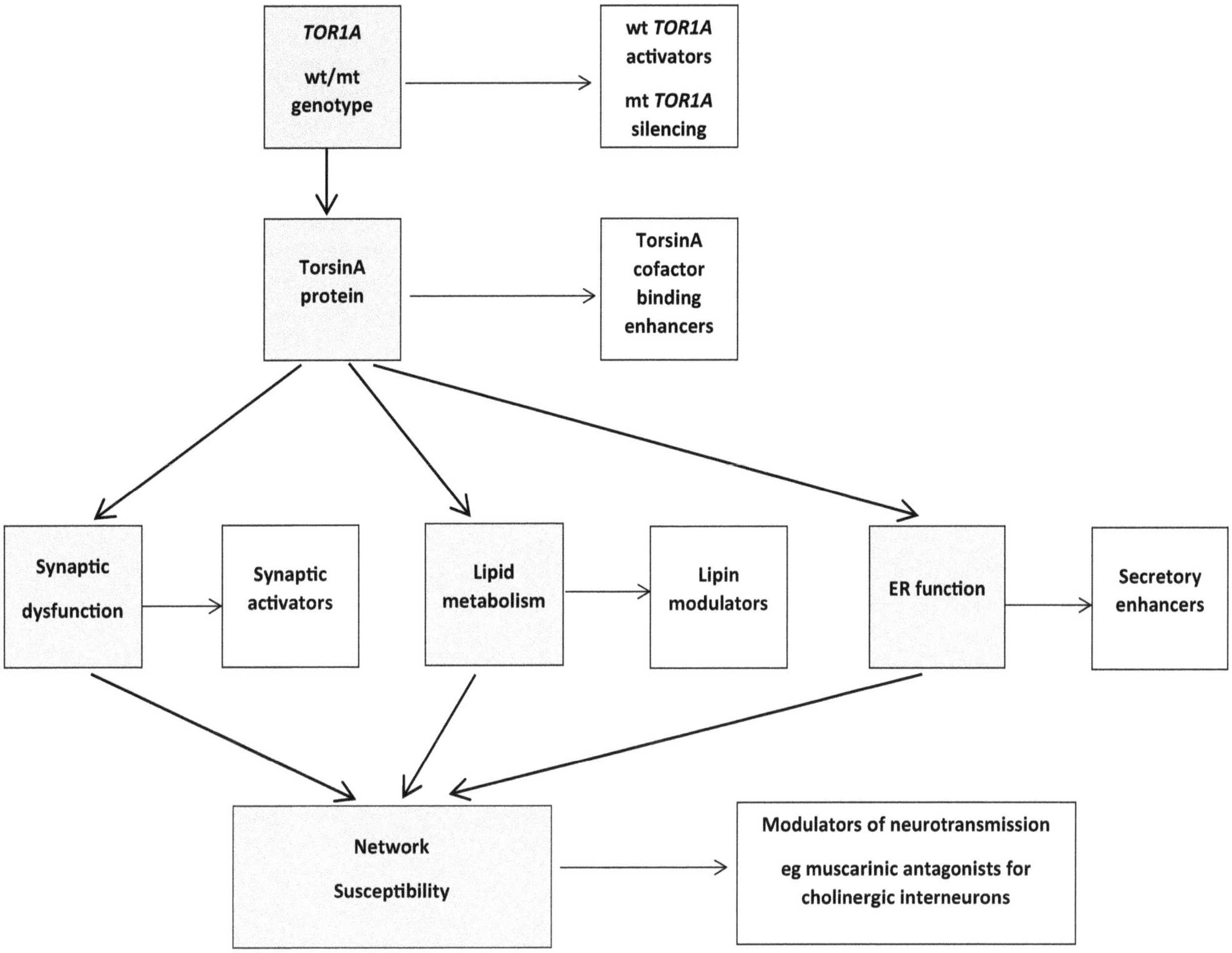

Figure 11.1 Molecular approach to novel DYT1 dystonia therapeutics. Shaded boxes represent potential pathogenic mechanisms. Unshaded boxes depict possible therapeutic strategies.

The Future and Novel Therapeutics

Figure 11.1 summarises potentially tractable pathways/mechanisms based on study of DYT1 dystonia. Early work involved demonstration of the potential for mutant allele torsinA silencing, the use of an assay of ER secretory function in nematodes, and reversal of synaptic vesicle cycling deficits by expression of specific SNARE proteins (Cao et al. 2010; Granata et al. 2011).

However, these may be focusing on downstream effects of a more basic mechanistic problem. Thus a strategy to strengthen the association of torsinA and its cofactors, potentially through use of small molecules, or use of molecular activators of torsin ATPase of the wild-type torsinA allele could compensate for the abnormalities identified. In view of the recent work on lipid metabolism, modification of lipin activity may be worth further investigation. Finally, exploration of targeted muscarinic cholinergic receptor antagonists could address issues related to network susceptibility and excess plasticity.

References

Albanese A, Bhatia K, Bressman SB, Delong MR, Fahn S, Fung VS, Hallett M, Jankovic J, Jinnah HA, Klein C, Lang AE, Mink JW, Teller JK. 2013. Phenomenology and classification of dystonia: a consensus update. *Mov Disord* 28(7):863–873.

Camargo CH, Camargos ST, Cardoso FE, Teive HA. 2015. The genetics of the dystonias: a review based on the new classification of the dystonias. *Arq Neuropsiquiatr* 73(4):350–358.

Cao S, Hewett JW, Yokoi F, Lu J, Buckley AC, Burdette AJ, Chen P, Nery FC, Li Y, Breakefield XO, Caldwell GA, Caldwell KA. 2010. Chemical enhancement of torsinA function in cell and animal models of torsion dystonia. *Dis Model Mech* 3(5–6): 386–396.

Dauer W. 2014. Inherited isolated dystonia: clinical genetics and gene function. *Neurotherapeutics* 11(4):807–816.

Eskow Jaunarajs KL, Bonsi P, Chesselet MF, Standaert DG, Pisani A. 2015. Striatal cholinergic dysfunction as a unifying theme in the pathophysiology of dystonia. *Prog Neurobiol* 127–128:91–107.

Fuchs T, Saunders-Pullman R, Masuho I, Luciano MS, Raymond D, Factor S, Lang AE, Liang TW, Trosch RM, White S, Ainehsazan E, Herve D, Sharma N, Ehrlich ME, Martemyanov KA, Bressman SB, Ozelius LJ. 2013. Mutations in GNAL cause primary torsion dystonia. *Nat Genet* 45(1):88–92.

Goodchild RE, Kim CE, Dauer WT. 2005. Loss of the dystonia-associated protein torsinA selectively disrupts the neuronal nuclear envelope. *Neuron* 48(6):923–932.

Granata A, Koo SJ, Haucke V, Schiavo G, Warner TT. 2011. CSN complex controls the stability of selected synaptic proteins via a torsinA-dependent process. *EMBO J* 30(1):181–193.

Grillet M, Dominguez Gonzalez B, Sicart A, Pottler M, Cascalho A, Billion K, Hernandez Diaz S, Swerts J, Naismith TV, Gounko NV, Verstreken P, Hanson PI, Goodchild RE. 2016. Torsins are essential regulators of cellular lipid metabolism. *Dev Cell* 38(3):235–247.

Hersheson J, Mencacci NE, Davis M, MacDonald N, Trabzuni D, Ryten M, Pittman A, Paudel R, Kara E, Fawcett K, Plagnol V, Bhatia KP, Medlar AJ, Stanescu HC, Hardy J, Kleta R, Wood NW, Houlden H. 2013. Mutations in the autoregulatory domain of beta-tubulin 4a cause hereditary dystonia. *Ann Neurol* 73(4):546–553.

Hewett J, Gonzalez-Agosti C, Slater D, Ziefer P, Li S, Bergeron D, Jacoby DJ, Ozelius LJ, Ramesh V, Breakefield XO. 2000. Mutant torsinA, responsible for early-onset torsion dystonia, forms membrane inclusions in cultured neural cells. *Hum Mol Genet* 9(9):1403–1413.

Klein C, Marras C, Munchau A. 1993. Dystonia overview. In: *GeneReviews(R)*. Pagon RA, Adam MP, Ardinger HH, Wallace SE, Amemiya A, Bean LJH, Bird TD, Ledbetter N, Mefford HC, Smith RJH, editors. Seattle, WA: University of Washington.

Ledoux MS, Dauer WT, Warner TT. 2013. Emerging common molecular pathways for primary dystonia. *Mov Disord* 28(7):968–981.

Rose AE, Brown RS, Schlieker C. 2015. Torsins: not your typical AAA+ ATPases. *Crit Rev Biochem Mol Biol* 50(6):532–549.

Tanabe LM, Martin C, Dauer WT. 2012. Genetic background modulates the phenotype of a mouse model of DYT1 dystonia. *PLoS One* 7(2):e32245.

Tanabe LM, Liang CC, Dauer WT. 2016. Neuronal nuclear membrane budding occurs during a developmental window modulated by torsin paralogs. *Cell Rep* 16(12):3322–3333.

Xiao J, Vemula SR, LeDoux MS. 2014. Recent advances in the genetics of dystonia. *Curr Neurol Neurosci Rep* 14(8):462.

Chapter 12

Dystonia and Tremor

Ellen B. Penney and Elan D. Louis

Introduction

Tremor associated with dystonia was described by Oppenheim in his seminal 1911 description of four patients with generalised dystonia (Klein & Fahn 2013). Very little emphasis, however, was placed on tremor in dystonia until the 1990s, when it became increasingly recognised that there is significant clinical overlap between the tremor in patients with dystonia and that of patients with essential tremor (ET). It became evident both that patients with tremor were frequently being misclassified, and that there may be an underlying pathophysiological connection between dystonia and ET. Focus was therefore placed on characterising tremor in patients with dystonia and identifying clinical features that could differentiate dystonic tremor from ET. This research, however, is still in its infancy and the clinical and pathophysiological connection between dystonia and ET is keenly debated. In this chapter, we review our current understanding of the prevalence and characteristics of tremor in patients with dystonia and discuss the possible relation to ET.

Prevalence of Tremor in Patients With Dystonia

Numerous case series have examined the prevalence of tremor in patients with dystonia and report tremor in anywhere from 11 to 87 per cent (Defazio & Fabbrini 2015). These studies have generally been small, examined heterogeneous patient populations with different types of dystonia, and used a range of different criteria for identifying tremor. Additionally, many of these studies were retrospective chart reviews, and may have underestimated the prevalence of tremor. It is therefore difficult to draw firm conclusions from these studies, even when taken in aggregate.

Recently, two large studies were published that prospectively examined patients with adult-onset idiopathic dystonia to establish the prevalence of tremor (Defazio et al. 2013; Erro et al. 2014). These two studies, however, reported disparate results. The study by Defazio and colleagues (Defazio et al. 2013) examined 429 Italian patients with dystonia, finding tremor in 16.7 per cent, with no patients exhibiting rest tremor. Erro and colleagues (Erro et al. 2014) studied 473 patients from the United Kingdom and identified tremor in 55.4 per cent, with rest tremor in 12.1 per cent. Both series found that patients with tremor had longer disease duration than patients without tremor, and that patients with segmental/multifocal dystonia were more likely to have tremor than patients with focal dystonia. In patients with focal dystonia, tremor was most common in those with cervical dystonia and tremor was more common in the region affected by the dystonia than in unaffected regions. Therefore, at least some of the discrepancies between these two studies could be a function of the longer disease duration in the Erro series, and the higher prevalence of blepharospasm in the Defazio series. The Defazio series tried to examine the onset of tremor in relation to the dystonia and found that in 82 per cent of patients the tremor appeared after the dystonia. In patients with tremor onset before dystonia, ~30 per cent reportedly had tremor for more than ten years before onset of dystonia. Although this information needs to be viewed with some caution, as it was based in part on patient recall, it suggests that tremor may be the presenting symptom or sign in up to 18 per cent of patients who later develop dystonic movements/postures, and that in a minority of patients tremor may predate the dystonic movements/postures by many years.

Very few studies have explored the prevalence of tremor in patients with familial, childhood-onset generalised dystonia. Several studies describing families with the DYT1 mutation report tremor in these patients (Lebre et al. 1999; Nomura et al. 2000), but other reports of DYT1 patients do not mention tremor. It is possible that tremor is a common feature in DYT1 patients but was simply not characterised in all studies. Another explanation, however, is that tremor is only seen in some DYT1 families and that tremor in these families is due to specific genetic modifiers. Recently, mutations in ANO3, a predicted Ca^{2+}-gated chloride channel, have been reported in several families in which all effected members have a combination of dystonic movements/postures and pronounced tremor often involving the head, voice and hands (Charlesworth et al. 2012). This indicates that tremor may be a fundamental manifestation of some genetically specific types of dystonia. Further descriptions of patients with known genetic mutations would help to improve our understanding of the genetic underpinnings of tremor in patients with dystonia.

Characteristics of Tremor in Patients With Dystonia

Tremor in patients with dystonia has been characterised as either 'dystonic tremor' (DT) occurring in a body region with dystonic movements/postures (such as head tremor in cervical dystonia or writer's tremor with a limb dystonia), or 'tremor associated with dystonia' (TAWD), which occurs in a region unaffected by dystonic movements/postures (Deuschl et al. 1998; Defazio & Fabbrini 2015). Both tremor types are usually postural and may have a kinetic component or, in some cases, be task-specific (Defazio et al. 2013; Erro et al. 2014). More recently, what on the surface resembles a rest tremor has been reported in patients with dystonia, and this tremor is usually described as unilateral or asymmetric (Erro et al. 2014). Dystonic tremor has classically been described as irregular, jerky and occurring in bursts or flurries (Jedynak et al. 1991; Deuschl et al. 1998). It may exhibit larger amplitude towards the direction of the dystonic movement and a 'null point' at which tremor amplitude is reduced when the limb is allowed to take the dystonic posture. These classic dystonic features, however, are not always present, particularly in TAWD. Several neurophysiological studies have examined hand tremor in patients with cervical dystonia and typically find a low-amplitude postural tremor with a frequency of ~6–8 Hz, which may be slower and of larger amplitude with movement (Deuschl et al. 1997; Shaikh et al. 2008). This tremor may therefore be clinically indistinguishable from that seen in patients with ET.

Dystonia versus Essential Tremor

Difficulties Distinguishing the Two in Clinical Settings

As noted above, it may be difficult to distinguish the tremor of ET from that of dystonia. Efforts to identify features that can differentiate between the tremor of ET and tremor in dystonia have had some limited success. The best clinical evidence exists for head tremor. ET typically starts in the hands and then spreads to the head and voice. Population-based and clinic-based series indicate that isolated head tremor almost never occurs in ET (Louis & Dogu 2009). Furthermore, head tremor in patients with cervical dystonia persists in 68 per cent of patients when supine, whereas in ET supine head tremor only occurs in 8 per cent of patients (Agnew et al. 2012).

Differentiating features for upper extremity tremor have been more difficult to elucidate. As noted above, dystonic limb tremor is often an irregular, jerky tremor with a directional preponderance (see DT above), but these features are not always seen (see TAWD above). Neurophysiological studies have identified some possible subtle differences between ET tremor and dystonic tremor, including higher average amplitudes in ET and greater irregularity in dystonia (Shaikh et al. 2008). However, there is significant overlap in the neurophysiological features of these two populations, so this alone cannot easily be used to diagnose individual patients.

Pathophysiological Relationship Between the Two Diseases?

ET family studies have reported a high prevalence of dystonia in family members (Jankovic et al. 1997; Louis et al. 2013). Patients with long-standing ET may eventually develop dystonic movements/postures. These observations support the concept that ET and dystonia may be pathophysiologically related diseases. As reviewed below, this could be a feature of cerebellar involvement in both, although this remains to be determined.

There is significant evidence that ET involves pathophysiological changes in the cerebellum. Functional magnetic resonance imaging (fMRI) and positron emission tomography (PET) studies have shown increased activity and blood flow in the cerebellum of patients with ET (Passamonti et al. 2012). Structural imaging studies demonstrate reduced cerebellar volume in ET patients (Passamonti et al. 2012). Postmortem analysis has revealed cerebellar Purkinje cell pathology, including abnormal dendritic arbours, axon swellings and reduced Purkinje cell counts, suggesting that ET may be a Purkinje cell disorder eventually leading to neurodegeneration (Louis 2016).

Dystonia has classically been considered a basal ganglia disorder but increasing evidence suggests that it is a network disorder involving multiple structures, including the cerebellum (Neychev et al. 2011). Space-occupying posterior fossa mass lesions may be associated with dystonia, and PET studies have shown increased cerebellar activity and blood flow in patients with dystonia (Neychev et al. 2011). The tottering mutant mouse (Cacna1a mutation) is a model of human paroxysmal dystonia and has abnormal cerebellar Purkinje cell activity early in the dystonic attacks (Neychev et al. 2011). In the tottering mouse and an unrelated rat model of dystonia, removal of the cerebellum abolishes the dystonia (Neychev et al. 2011). Furthermore, the phenotype of the tottering mouse may depend specifically on Purkinje cell function since Purkinje cell degeneration eliminates dystonia in this model (Neychev et al. 2011). One small neuropathological study of six patients with cervical dystonia identified patchy Purkinje cell loss and axonal swellings (Prudente et al. 2013).

Treatment of Tremor in Dystonia

There is relatively limited information regarding treatment of tremor in dystonia. A review of papers published up to 2013 identified only 13 articles on the use of oral medications, and seven studies on botulinum neurotoxin (BoNT) treatment for tremor in dystonia (Fasano et al. 2014). None of these studies was controlled and most used no formal assessment tool. All of the studies on oral medications were small, containing 1–22 patients (median three). The most commonly studied oral medications were anticholinergic agents, beta-blockers and benzodiazepines. In total, 16 patients were treated with anticholinergic agents and approximately two-thirds reported mild to moderate subjective improvement with treatment. Propranolol was beneficial in seven of nine patients with focal dystonia and arm tremor, but was ineffective in ten patients with head/jaw tremor. Benzodiazepines produced at least mild improvement in nine of eleven patients. The evidence is slightly stronger supporting the use of BoNT. These studies were larger and in total more than 300 patients with dystonic head/voice tremor treated with BoNT have been described in the literature. All of these studies reported an improvement in tremor after BoNT treatment.

None of the large dystonia deep brain stimulation (DBS) trials studied tremor, but 20 smaller studies, including a total of 44 patients, have reported improvement of dystonic tremor in patients treated with DBS or ablation (Fasano et al. 2014; Pauls et al. 2014). These studies were all small and most included a single patient, but in general the studies reported moderate to marked improvement of tremor after surgery. Tremor improvement has been reported with DBS of the globus pallidus internus, thalamic ventralis intermedius nucleus, ventrolateral thalamic nucleus, and subthalamic nucleus or surrounding white matter. The small number of studies with small sample sizes makes it difficult to quantify the effect of DBS treatment or determine whether a specific target region is more effective than any other.

Conclusion

The study of tremor in patients with dystonia is a relatively new field and has only been actively researched over the last several decades. Our understanding of tremor in patients with dystonia is, therefore, not surprisingly still in its infancy. Additional research is needed focusing on everything from basic questions regarding the prevalence of tremor in dystonia and the clinical features associated with it, to complex questions regarding the pathophysiology of the process and effective treatments. By advancing our knowledge of tremor in dystonia, we would also enhance our understanding of related diseases, particularly ET.

References

Agnew A, Frucht SJ, Louis ED. 2012. Supine head tremor: a clinical comparison of essential tremor and spasmodic torticollis patients. *J Neurol Neurosurg Psychiatry* 83(2):179–181.

Charlesworth G, Plagnol V, Holmström KM, Bras J, Sheerin UM, Preza E, et al. 2012. Mutations in ANO3 cause dominant craniocervical dystonia: ion channel implicated in pathogenesis. *Am J Hum Genet* 91(6):1041–1050.

Defazio G, Fabbrini G. 2015. Is tremor in dystonia a phenotypic feature of dystonia? *Neurology* 84(10):1053–1059.

Defazio G, Gigante AF, Abbruzzese G, Bentivoglio AR, Colosimo C, Esposito M, et al. 2013. Tremor in primary adult-onset dystonia: prevalence and associated clinical features. *J Neurol Neurosurg Psychiatry* 84(4):404–408.

Deuschl G, Heinen F, Guschlbauer B, Schneider S, Glocker FX, Lücking CH. 1997. Hand tremor in patients with spasmodic torticollis. *Mov Disord* 12(4):547–552.

Deuschl G, Bain P, Brin M, Quinn N, Rothwell J. 1998. Consensus statement of the Movement Disorder Society on tremor. *Mov Disord* 13(S3):2–23.

Erro R, Rubio-Agusti I, Saifee TA, Cordivari C, Ganos C, Batla A, et al. 2014. Rest and other types of tremor in adult-onset primary dystonia. *J Neurol Neurosurg Psychiatry* 85(9):965–968.

Fasano A, Bove F, Lang AE. 2014. The treatment of dystonic tremor: a systematic review. *J Neurol Neurosurg Psychiatry* 85(7):759–769.

Jankovic J, Beach J, Patel PI. 1997. Familial essential tremor in 4 kindreds. *Arch Neurol* 54:289–294.

Jedynak CP, Bonnet AM, Agid Y. 1991. Tremor and idiopathic dystonia. *Mov Disord* 6(3):230–236.

Klein C, Fahn S. 2013. Translation of Oppenheim's 1911 paper on dystonia. *Mov Disord* 28(7):851–862.

Lebre AS, Durr A, Jedynak P, Ponsot G, Vidailhet M, Agid Y, et al. 1999. DYT1 mutation in French families with idiopathic torsion dystonia. *Brain* 122(1):41–5.

Louis ED. 2016. Essential tremor: a common disorder of Purkinje neurons? *Neurosci* 22: 108–118.

Louis ED, Dogu O. 2009. Isolated head tremor: part of the clincal spectrum of essential tremor? Data from population-based and clinic-based case samples. *Mov Disord* 24(15):2281–2285.

Louis ED, Hernandez N, Alcalay RN, Dennis J. 2013. Prevalence and features of unreported dystonia in a family study of 'pure' essential tremor. *Park Relat Disord* 19(3):359–362.

Neychev VK, Gross RE, Lehéricy S, Hess EJ, Jinnah HA. 2011. The functional neuroanatomy of dystonia. *Neurobiol Dis* [Internet] 42(2):185–201. Available from: http://dx.doi.org/10.1016/j.nbd.2011.01.026

Nomura Y, Ikeuchi T, Tsuji S, Segawa M. 2000. Two phenotypes and anticipation observed in Japanese cases with early onset torsion dystonia (DYT1): pathophysiological consideration. *Brain Dev* 22 Suppl 1:S92–S101.

Passamonti L, Cerasa A, Quattrone A. 2012. Neuroimaging of essential tremor: what is the evidence for cerebellar involvement? *Tremor Other Hyperkinet Mov (NY)* 2:1–11.

Pauls KAM, Hammesfahr S, Moro E, Moore AP, Binder E, El Majdoub F, et al. 2014. Deep brain stimulation in the ventrolateral thalamus/subthalamic area in dystonia with head tremor. *Mov Disord* 29(7):953–959.

Prudente CN, Pardo CA, Xiao J, Hanfelt J, Hess EJ, LeDoux MS, et al. 2013. Neuropathology of cervical dystonia. *Exp Neurol* 241(1):95–104.

Shaikh AG, Jinnah HA, Tripp RM, Optican LM, Ramat S, Lenz F, et al. 2008. Irregularity distinguishes limb tremor in cervical dystonia from essential tremor. *J Neurol Neurosurg Psychiatry* 79(2):187–189.

Chapter 13

Posttraumatic Dystonia

Karen Frei and Daniel Truong

In a small number of patients, trauma precedes the onset of dystonia. Significant head trauma is a well-recognised precipitating factor. However, it has been increasingly recognised that peripheral trauma can also cause dystonia. This chapter will review dystonia resulting from both head injury (central) and peripheral trauma.

Central Trauma

Most of the time, significant head trauma is thought to be the precipitating event resulting in dystonia. Posttraumatic movement disorders secondary to severe head injury occur in 22.6 per cent of patients. Dystonia, one of the posttraumatic movement disorders, occurs less commonly than tremor, comprising 4.1 per cent of posttraumatic movement disorder cases (Krauss et al. 1996). Hemidystonia and focal dystonia are the most common forms of posttraumatic dystonia resulting from head trauma (Krauss et al. 1992). There are reports of focal dystonia including cervical dystonia which can occur alone or along with the hemidystonia. Reports of bilateral dystonia have been published. Axial dystonia involving the neck and trunk has been reported following closed head trauma with encephalomalacia involving the head of the caudate nucleus (Jabbari et al. 1992). However, posttraumatic hemidystonia accounts for only 7–9 per cent of all hemidystonia cases (Lee et al. 1994). In a study of 22 hemidystonia patients, 73 per cent of the patients had prior hemiparesis or basal ganglia lesions on imaging studies, but only eight were attributed to trauma (Jankovic 1994).

Posttraumatic dystonia occurs in a delayed manner after head injury, with the onset noted to be from one day to six years following the initial head injury (Krauss & Jankovic 2002). Hemiparesis often precedes the development of dystonia following head injury. As plegia resolves, the dystonia tends to appear. Dystonia begins focally starting in the previously hemiplegic limb and tends to spread from two to five years after onset until stabilisation of symptoms. Focal dystonia can spread to become segmental and then hemidystonia. Rarely will it continue to spread and develop into generalised dystonia. Also, dystonia tends to start distally and spread proximally. Dystonia may begin in the fingers or hand and spread to the proximal arm or to the ipsilateral foot and toes. This progression of dystonia is similar to that which occurs following stroke or after anoxic events. Occasionally spontaneous improvement occurs.

The length of delay in onset of posttraumatic dystonia was not found to correlate with the severity of head injury or the duration of the initial hemiplegia. The interval between head trauma and the onset of dystonia appeared to be longer for those with head injury occurring at a younger age (Scott & Jankovic 1996).

As the development of dystonia does not occur in every case of head injury with structural lesions on MRI, some risk factors have been proposed for the development of posttraumatic dystonia. Lee et al. (1994) proposed three risk factors: younger age at time of head trauma; severity of head trauma and duration of hemiplegia; and anatomic locations of lesions on brain imaging. There also may be an individual susceptibility towards the development of posttraumatic dystonia.

Structural lesions are usually found on brain MRI and most commonly the lesions are located in the basal ganglia – the contralateral caudate, putamen and thalamus. There have been cases reported of upper brainstem or superior cerebellar peduncle lesions, however. The presence of generalised cerebral oedema and/or focal lesions on initial head CT is associated with the development of posttraumatic dystonia. There are reports of lesions occurring in the lenticular or thalamic regions seen on brain imaging after the onset of dystonia. Lesions in the basal ganglia and thalamus suggest damage to the putamino-pallido-thalamic neuronal circuit in the course of dystonia development (Lee et al. 1994).

Medical treatment for trauma-induced dystonia is usually ineffective. Medications including propranolol, tetrabenazine, baclofen, levodopa and carbamazepine have been tried but not found to be beneficial. Anticholinergics and clonazepam may have a mild beneficial effect. Botulinum toxin injections are used as first-line treatment in these cases. Response to these injections is variable. Alternative treatments include stereotactic lesions in the globus pallidus, deep brain stimulation (DBS) or intrathecal baclofen. Secondary forms of dystonia such as posttraumatic dystonia do not appear to respond to DBS as well as primary generalised dystonia. Response to DBS with leads placed in the globus pallidus appears to be variable and may be related to degree or size of damage to the basal ganglia. A case of GPi DBS has been successful in treating posttraumatic hemidystonia for four years (Loher et al. 2000).

Peripheral Trauma

Less severe, peripheral trauma has been associated with the development of dystonia. In fact, Gowers in 1888 suggested that peripheral trauma as well as central trauma may cause movement disorders. The role of peripheral trauma is controversial in part due to challenges in associating it with the development of dystonia. Recall bias, secondary gain and legal ramifications all present challenges to the confirmation of peripheral trauma-induced dystonia. Because of these problems, criteria have been adopted to help define peripheral trauma-induced dystonia (Truong et al. 1991). The injury must be severe enough to cause local symptoms for at least two weeks. The onset of the dystonia should be within days up to one year after the injury and the onset of the movement disorder must be anatomically related to the site of the injury (Jankovic 1994).

Using these criteria to define peripheral trauma-induced dystonia, several differences from idiopathic dystonia have been noted. Causalgia, also known as reflex sympathetic dystrophy or complex regional pain syndrome (CRPS), is associated with peripheral trauma-induced dystonia. Some dystonic postures are 'fixed' and immobile and may persist during sleep. Posttraumatic dystonia does not tend to respond to sensory tricks (Truong et al. 1991).

Probably the most common form of peripheral trauma-induced dystonia is cervical dystonia following whiplash or other neck injury. Several reports described this entity in published case series (Truong et al. 1991; Goldman & Ahlskog 1993; Tarsy 1998; Sa et al. 2003; Frei et al. 2004; O'Riordan & Hutchinson 2004). There appears to be some distinction between peripheral trauma-induced cervical dystonia and idiopathic cervical dystonia. The characteristics of peripheral trauma induced-dystonia were first pointed out by Truong (Truong et al. 1991) and later further clarified in their follow-up paper (Frei et al. 2004). There is limited cervical range of motion with fixed posture, lack of response to sensory tricks, persistence of symptoms during sleep, lack of improvement of symptoms after sleep, poor response to botulinum toxin injections and dominance of laterocollis. Severe pain appears to be a major factor in these cases.

Several case reports can be found in the literature regarding peripheral trauma associated with the development of blepharospasm and focal shoulder or hand dystonia (Jankovic 1994). Oromandibular dystonia has been reported following dental procedures. Location of the injury tends to dictate the type of dystonia that develops.

Peripheral trauma appears to be a rare cause of dystonia with only a small number of patients developing dystonia in the setting of a large number of traumatic events. There may be a predisposition towards the development of dystonia with inciting trauma. A family history of essential tremor or dystonia, perinatal injury and prior exposure to dopamine receptor-blocking drugs may represent risk factors for the development of posttraumatic dystonia (Jankovic 1994).

There have been a few theories proposed to explain the pathophysiology of peripheral trauma-induced dystonia. Peripheral trauma may alter the sensory input and induce central cortical and subcortical reorganisation, which could account for the development of dystonia. Alteration of the sensory cortex has been proposed to be the mechanism for the development of writer's cramp or occupational dystonia involving repetitive use. It is also possible that trauma may cause dystonia by triggering or accelerating the progression of pre-existing subclinical disease. Because this form of dystonia may be more closely related to structural causes of dystonia such as the pseudodystonia that develops in atlantoaxial subluxation, it is possible that the onset of physical trauma with localised pain in the context of critical psychological factors may lead to contracture and guarding of the musculature presenting as dystonia (Sa et al. 2003).

Medications tend to be ineffective and negative trials with trihexyphenidyl, baclofen, levodopa and benzodiazepines have been reported. Steroids may be helpful with the associated reflex sympathetic dystrophy. Botulinum toxin injections have sometimes been effective (Frei et al. 2004).

References

Frei KP, Pathak M, Jenkins S, Truong DD. 2004. Natural history of posttraumatic cervical dystonia. *Mov Disord* 19(12):1492–1498.

Goldman S, Ahlskog JE. 1993. Posttraumatic cervical dystonia. *Mayo Clin Proc* 68(5):443–448.

Jabbari B, Paul J, Scherokman B, Van Dam B. 1992. Posttraumatic segmental axial dystonia. *Mov Disord* 7(1):78–81.

Jankovic J. 1994. Post-traumatic movement disorders: central and peripheral mechanisms. *Neurology* 44(11):2006–2014.

Krauss JK, Jankovic J. 2002. Head injury and posttraumatic movement disorders. *Neurosurgery* 50(5):927–939; discussion 939–940.

Krauss JK, Mohadjer M, Braus DF, Wakhloo AK, Nobbe F, Mundinger F. 1992. Dystonia following head trauma: a report of nine patients and review of the literature. *Mov Disord* 7(3):263–272.

Krauss JK, Trankle R, Kopp KH. 1996. Post-traumatic movement disorders in survivors of severe head injury. *Neurology* 47(6):1488–1492.

Lee MS, Rinne JO, Ceballos-Baumann A, Thompson PD, Marsden CD. 1994. Dystonia after head trauma. *Neurology* 44(8):1374–1378.

Loher TJ, Hasdemir MG, Burgunder JM, Krauss JK. 2000. Long-term follow-up study of chronic globus pallidus internus stimulation for posttraumatic hemidystonia. *J Neurosurg* 92(3):457–460.

O'Riordan S, Hutchinson M. 2004. Cervical dystonia following peripheral trauma: a case-control study. *J Neurol* 251(2):150–155.

Sa DS, Mailis-Gagnon A, Nicholson K, Lang AE. 2003. Posttraumatic painful torticollis. *Mov Disord* 18(12):1482–1491.

Scott BL, Jankovic J. 1996. Delayed-onset progressive movement disorders after static brain lesions. *Neurology* 46(1):68–74.

Tarsy D. 1998. Comparison of acute- and delayed-onset posttraumatic cervical dystonia. *Mov Disord* 13(3):481–485.

Truong DD, Dubinsky R, Hermanowicz N, Olson WL, Silverman B, Koller WC. 1991. Posttraumatic torticollis. *Arch Neurol* 48(2):221–223.

Chapter 14

Non-Motor Symptoms in Dystonia

Marjan Jahanshahi

Dystonia can make performance of simple daily activities difficult. In generalised dystonia and some focal dystonias the visible disfiguring nature of the condition can have a negative impact on the patients' self-esteem and social participation (Jahanshahi 2005). Dystonia negatively impacts quality of life (QoL) (Ben-Shlomo et al. 2002; Page et al. 2007) and most domains of QoL are poorer than in the general population and in other chronic disorders such as Parkinson's disease or multiple sclerosis (Camfield et al. 2002). Depression and anxiety are among the major determinants of QoL in dystonia (Ben-Shlomo et al. 2002; Page et al. 2007). A review of the literature on cognitive dysfunction and psychiatric comorbidity in a range of dystonic disorders highlights that both are common in most types of dystonia and likely to have a major influence on the QoL of the patients and should therefore be targeted in the clinical management of the disorder.

Cognitive Function in Dystonia

The main findings in relation to cognitive function in idiopathic and various types of inherited dystonia are summarised in Table 14.1.

Cognitive deficits are not considered part of the clinical presentation or disease progression in idiopathic dystonia or generalised dystonia associated with the DYT1 gene. Studies of cognitive function in idiopathic dystonia or generalised dystonia associated with the DYT1 gene have been previously reviewed (Jahanshahi et al. 2003; Torkamani & Jahanshahi 2014). Despite considerable heterogeneity across the samples of these studies in terms of the exact type and extent of dystonia, a number of conclusions can be drawn from this evidence.

First, global and main domains of cognitive function such as IQ, memory and language are not impaired. Second, the neuropsychological studies have revealed isolated deficits in specific aspects of cognition, including visuo-spatial function relating to egocentric space, impaired semantic fluency and dual-task performance, greater susceptibility to retroactive interference, deficits in set-shifting, in sustained attention and in working memory. For example, two recent studies have reported deficits on set-shifting in a computerised version of the Wisconsin Card Sorting test in patients with blepharospasm (Lange et al. 2016a, 2016b). Also from meta-analysis of the results of six studies of cognition which assessed performance on the Wisconsin Card Sorting test in dystonia patients, it has been concluded that dystonia impairs concept formation and set-shifting on this task (Lange et al. 2016b). Most of these isolated and specific deficits reported across studies of cognition in idiopathic or DYT1 dystonia relate to executive function and may reflect fronto-striatal dysfunction. Third, more 'experimental' studies have reported deficits in praxis in cervical dystonia (CD), slower mental rotation of hands but not feet in writer's cramp and deficits in explicit sequence learning in both manifesting and non-manifesting carriers of the DYT1 gene (for details of studies, see Torkamani & Jahanshahi 2014).

Nevertheless, it is likely that the presence or absence of neuropsychiatric symptoms, particularly depression and anxiety, that are common in dystonia and the anticholinergic and benzodiazepine medication used to treat dystonia can independently of the movement disorder be associated with/result in cognitive impairment, and thus may be important confounding influences on cognition in dystonia. Also, as previously suggested (Jahanshahi et al. 2003), some of these deficits such as the impaired dual-task performance or deficits in attention may be related to the patients' attempts to control their dystonia during cognitive testing. In support of this proposal, it has been shown that improvement of blepharospasm following botulinum toxin injections was associated with significant improvement on a test of sustained attention (Allam et al. 2007).

To date, very few imaging studies with cognitive tasks have been completed in dystonia. One such recent study (Zeuner et al. 2016) revealed that during reward-based probabilistic reversal learning, patients with writer's cramp showed greater activation of the dorsal anterior cingulate following negative feedback compared to controls, suggesting problems with integration of reinforcement information during decision making in these patients.

The picture is different in most forms of inherited or heredodegenerative dystonias which are commonly associated with cognitive deficits. This evidence has also been previously reviewed, providing all the relevant references (Torkamani & Jahanshahi 2014).

Cognition in X-linked dystonia-parkinsonism (DYT3) has been investigated in a single case prior to (Howe et al. 2009) and after (Kemmotsu et al. 2011) treatment with deep brain stimulation (DBS). The patient had performance and verbal IQs in the borderline and low-average ranges respectively, as well as impairment in memory, visuo-spatial function, language and executive functioning which improved to an extent

Table 14.1 Summary of findings of cognitive function in idiopathic dystonia and various types of inherited or heredodegenerative dystonia

Type of dystonia	Cognitive function affected
Idiopathic focal or segmental dystonia or generalised DYT1	Isolated deficits in sustained attention, set-shifting, semantic fluency, dual-task performance, visuo-spatial function and egocentric space, praxis, mental rotation of hands, explicit sequence learning.
X-Linked dystonia parkinsonism (DYT3)	67-year-old man had performance and verbal IQs in the borderline and low-average ranges respectively and impaired memory, visuo-spatial function, language and executive function.
Dopa-responsive dystonia (DYT5)	Normal IQ only in those treated with levodopa from early age, otherwise IQ in borderline to extremely low range, concentration and verbal memory deficits in some cases, improvement of concept formation and set-shifting with levodopa treatment.
Myoclonus-dystonia (DYT11)	Some studies reported no cognitive deficits, others documented deficits in verbal learning and memory, processing speed, or semantic verbal fluency.
Rapid-onset dystonia parkinsonism (DYT12)	Developmental delay, intellectual, linguistic and psychomotor delay part of phenotype of alternating hemiplegia of childhood, with cognitive deficits more evident with increasing age. Impairment of verbal and non-verbal memory, verbal fluency and executive function.
Pantothenate kinase-associated neurodegeneration	Variability in cognitive function, ranging from 'normal' to 'severely impaired', with dementia noted in cases with PKAN mutation, rates of dementia ranging from 10 to 30 per cent of cases. 'Fronto-striatal' dysfunction revealed by neuropsychological assessment.
Lesch–Nyhan disease	Original description considered mental retardation as a feature, but some attenuated variant cases with IQs in the borderline or low-average range described since. In one cohort, 67 per cent had learning difficulties but 15 per cent had IQs in the normal range. A 'dose relationship' between the level of hypoxanthine-guanine phosphoribosyltransferase enzyme deficiency and severity of cognitive impairment. Progressive decline in cognition.
Wilson's disease	Original description included cognitive decline. Some noted the cognitive profile to fit subcortical dementia, others consider dementia to be less common and a feature of the terminal stages. Deficits in attention, visuo-spatial perception and reasoning, memory and learning, verbal and abstract reasoning and construction in symptomatic cases but not in asymptomatic carriers. Extent of cognitive impairment does not correlate with severity of neurological symptoms or level of copper toxicity. Treatment with penicillamine and zinc also had a positive impact on cognitive function.

after withdrawal of anticholinergic medication. Twenty-seven months after DBS surgery, mild improvement on the Mattis Dementia Rating scale and generally stable cognitive status comparable to preoperative levels were reported.

In dopa-responsive dystonia (DYT5), the main focus has been on assessment of IQ. The evidence suggests normal IQ in patients treated with levodopa from an early age; otherwise patients with dopa-responsive dystonia have IQs in the borderline to extremely low range. Levodopa treatment also improves concept formation and set-shifting on the Wisconsin Card Sorting test. Deficits in concentration and verbal memory have also been reported in a retrospective examination of case reports.

Studies examining cognition in families with one or more individuals with myoclonus-dystonia (DYT11) have provided mixed evidence. Some studies have reported deficits in verbal learning and memory and processing speed (Doheny et al. 2002) or semantic verbal fluency (van Tricht et al. 2012); others have not found any evidence of cognitive dysfunction on neuropsychological assessment (Foncke et al. 2009).

In rapid-onset dystonia-parkinsonism (DYT12), developmental delay, intellectual, linguistic and psychomotor delay are part of the phenotype of alternating hemiplegia of childhood and the cognitive deficits become more evident with increasing age. Impairment of verbal and non-verbal memory, verbal fluency and executive function have also been documented.

Cognitive impairment is considered part of the presentation of pantothenate kinase-associated neurodegeneration (PKAN) and the five siblings first described had dementia. However, variability in cognitive function, ranging from 'normal' to 'severely impaired' is also evident. Documented rates of dementia have ranged from 10 to 30 per cent of cases with PKAN. A profile of 'fronto-striatal' dysfunction has also been revealed by neuropsychological assessment.

When Lesch–Nyhan disease (LND) was first described, mental retardation was considered a feature of the disease. However, some attenuated variant LND cases with IQs in the borderline or low-average range have been described since. In the largest cohort to date, 67 per cent had learning difficulties but 15 per cent had IQs in the normal range. A 'dose relationship' between the level of hypoxanthine-guanine phosphoribosyltransferase enzyme deficiency and severity of cognitive impairment has been reported. Standardised neuropsychological assessment is difficult as many of the patients with LND have severe motor disability and speech impairment. Longitudinal investigation has revealed a progressive decline in line with developmental disabilities.

Kinnier Wilson's original description of the disorder that bears his name included cognitive decline. Some have noted that cognitive dysfunction in Wilson's disease fits the profile of subcortical dementia, while others consider dementia to be less common and a feature of the terminal stages of the illness. Deficits in attention, visuo-spatial perception and reasoning, memory and learning, verbal and abstract reasoning and construction have been reported in symptomatic cases but not observed in asymptomatic carriers. The extent of cognitive impairment does not correlate with the severity of the neurological symptoms or the level of copper toxicity. Nevertheless, treatment of Wilson's disease with penicillamine and zinc also had a positive impact on cognitive function.

Psychiatric Manifestations of Dystonia

A large literature on psychiatric manifestations in dystonia exists, most of it focused on idiopathic focal or segmental dystonias and particularly on CD. These studies differ in their methodology. While some have used the structured clinical interview or the international composite diagnostic interview and applied criteria from the *Diagnostic Statistical Manual* (DSM) to define psychiatric disorders in dystonia; others have relied on validated self-report measures such as the Beck Depression Inventory, Beck Anxiety Inventory and Yale Brown Obsessive Compulsive Scale. The sample sizes across these studies range from single case reports to large-scale investigations. The studies also differ in terms of whether disease or healthy control groups were included. Key information about whether the dystonia patients were taking psychoactive medication for treatment of their motor symptoms or psychiatric problems at the time of study is missing from most reports. Despite these methodological limitations, there is now consistent evidence for elevated rates of psychiatric disorder, particularly depression, anxiety and obsessive compulsive disorder (OCD) in dystonia, which can in some cases precede the onset of the movement disorder (Jahanshahi 2005; Torkamani & Jahanshahi 2014).

There is abundant evidence of high rates of psychiatric disorder, particularly depression and anxiety, in CD. In one study, 66 per cent of CD patients fulfilled the criteria for at least one diagnosis of current or lifetime psychiatric disorder (Wenzel et al. 1998). Lifetime prevalence of anxiety was reported in 34 per cent, with panic disorder being the most frequent type of anxiety disorder, affecting 30 per cent of the sample. Major depressive disorder affected 25 per cent and OCD was found in 7 per cent. Of the patients in this sample, 43 per cent experienced psychiatric symptoms before the onset of their dystonia. In another study, 116 CD patients were compared to a representative German sample (Gündel et al. 2001). Both lifetime and current rates of mood and anxiety disorders were significantly elevated in patients relative to the general population, with lifetime mood disorders in 54 per cent, anxiety disorders in 84 per cent, of which 71 per cent had social phobias. Current social phobia showed a ten-fold increase in CD, while current mood disorders were increased 2.4 times, and all lifetime psychiatric morbidity was increased 2.6 times in CD compared to the general population. Elsewhere, 70 patients with CD and 16 with blepharospasm were assessed and compared to a population-based sample ($N = 3943$) (Lencer et al. 2009). Compared to the population-based sample, the dystonia patients had a 4.5-fold increased chance of a psychiatric disorder, and their lifetime prevalence of psychiatric or personality disorder was 71 per cent. Mood and anxiety disorders in 68 per cent (Fabbrini et al. 2010) and a current or lifetime psychiatric diagnosis in 71 per cent have been reported in blepharospasm (Wenzel et al. 2000), with depression and phobias being the most common diagnoses. Similarly, the rates of depression and anxiety have also been reported to be significantly higher in patients with spasmodic dysphonia than matched healthy controls, with rates of 39 per cent (Cannito 1991). Findings in relation to patients with focal hand dystonia are inconsistent. One study reported OCD in 13 per cent, recurrent depression in 18 per cent and anxiety disorders in 26 per cent of their sample with focal hand dystonia (Voon et al. 2010); another study with a smaller sample did not find any mood or anxiety disorders and only one patient had OCD and another adjustment disorder (Fabbrini et al. 2010). The differences between the two studies may relate to the first including patients with musician's dystonia, for whom higher rates of social phobia and specific phobias has been documented by others (Altenmüller & Jabusch 2010); the second study focused on writer's cramp.

OCD is associated with most types of dystonia. An investigation of OCD in 76 patients with primary focal dystonia found that 20 per cent of the sample met DSM-IV criteria for OCD and 4 per cent for obsessive compulsive spectrum disorders (Cavallaro et al. 2002). The rates of OCD in blepharospasm range from 3.6 per cent (Fabbrini et al. 2010) to 67 per cent (Munhoz et al. 2005). Despite the widely differing rates, the results are consistent in so far as suggesting that while these rates are significantly higher than healthy controls, they are similar to disease control groups such as patients with hemifacial spasm. The differing rates may partly result from the use of different assessment tools (self-report measures versus psychiatric interviews). Nevertheless, high rates of OCD in focal

Table 14.2 Summary of findings of psychiatric morbidity in idiopathic dystonia and various types of inherited or heredodegenerative dystonia

Type of dystonia	Most common types of psychiatric disorder
Idiopathic focal or segmental dystonia or generalised DYT1	Depression, anxiety, OCD, sleep disturbance
X-Linked dystonia-parkinsonism (DYT3)	Depression, anxiety and apathy only after DBS surgery but not preoperatively
Dopa-responsive dystonia (DYT5)	Depression, anxiety, OCD, sleep disturbance
Myoclonus-dystonia (DYT11)	Depression and anxiety in manifesting and non-manifesting DYT11 carriers, higher in former group. Whether higher rates of OCD and alcohol abuse inconsistent across studies
Rapid-onset dystonia-parkinsonism (DYT12)	Mood and anxiety disorder, OCD and alcohol dependence, psychosis
Pantothenate kinase-associated neurodegeneration	Depression, OCD, tic disorder, psychosis
Lesch–Nyhan disease	Self-injurious behaviour, aggression
Wilson's disease	Depression, bipolar disorder, incongruous behaviour

dystonias, particularly blepharospasm and CD, seem fairly well established.

There is evidence for the association of major recurrent depression with the DYT1 GAG deletion. In a study of 96 symptomatic manifesting carriers (MCs) of the DYT1 mutation with generalised dystonia, 60 asymptomatic MCs and 65 non-manifesting carriers (NMCs), it was found that risk of recurrent major depressive disorder (MDD) was increased in both MC groups compared to NMCs. The mutation carriers had an earlier age of onset of recurrent MDD than did NMCs. The groups did not differ in other affective disorders. The severity of dystonia was not associated with the risk of recurrent MDD. It was concluded that the psychiatric expression of DYT1 appears to be limited to recurrent early-onset MDD, as carriers were not at increased risk for other affective disorders and that MDD is associated with the DYT1 mutation independently of motor manifestations of dystonia (Heiman et al. 2004). A later study by the same investigators on the same sample (Heiman et al. 2007) found no significant differences between the three groups in terms of OCD. Therefore, unlike early-onset MDD, no association was found with OCD and the DYT1 gene.

Prior to DBS surgery, there was no significant depression or apathy in a patient with X-linked dystonia-parkinsonism (Howe et al. 2009), although moderate depression, increased levels of apathy and some anxiety were documented after surgery (Kemmotsu et al. 2011).

In DRD, psychiatric abnormalities were not noted in the original description. Subsequent studies have, however, revealed high rates of depression, anxiety, OCD and sleep disturbance ranging from 10 to 55 per cent (van Hove et al. 2006; Tadic et al. 2012).

In myoclonus-dystonia, while higher rates of depression and/or anxiety disorder in the MCs than the NMCs have been documented (Doheny et al. 2002; Saunders-Pullman et al. 2002; van Tricht et al. 2012), there is less consensus across these studies regarding whether rates of OCD and alcohol abuse are also elevated. The question of whether or not the severity of myoclonus and dystonia are significantly correlated with anxiety and depression, alcohol abuse or OCD for the MCs is also inconsistently supported across these studies, which influences the interpretation of these psychiatric symptoms as reactive or an expression of the DYT11 mutation.

In rapid-onset dystonia-parkinsonism, mood and anxiety disorder, OCD and alcohol dependence and psychosis have been documented in MCs and also in NMCs (Barbano et al. 2012; Brashear et al. 2012).

A range of psychiatric disorders, including depression, OCD, tic disorders and psychosis, have been reported in PKAN (Marelli et al. 2005).

Self-injurious behaviour was included in the original descriptions of Lesch–Nyhan disease. These self-injurious behaviours range from biting of lips and fingers to poking the eyes with a finger and catching hands or feet in the wheelchair or its sharp parts, which can be severe enough to result in amputation, infection or blindness. These patients can also display aggressive behaviours and motor stereotypies.

Wilson's disease has been associated with a range of psychiatric symptoms including depression, bipolar disorder and incongruous behaviour which occur in about 18–50 per cent of patients and seem to be more common in children than adult patients (Dening & Berrios 1990; Akil & Brewer 1995; Shanmugiah et al. 2008).

A number of the investigations included disease control groups and therefore allow comparison of the nature and rates of psychiatric disorders in dystonia with other chronic disorders. A clear pattern does not emerge from the existing evidence. While one set of studies suggests that rates of psychiatric comorbidity, particularly depression and anxiety, are significantly higher and often twice the rates in disease control groups such as hemifacial spasm (e.g. Fabbrini et al. 2010), others do not find any such differences in rates of OCD or depression between dystonia and other physical or neurological disorders (e.g. Munhoz et al. 2005). Still others suggest that rates of depression and anxiety are significantly higher in Parkinson's disease than in dystonia, while OCD may be somewhat higher in dystonia than in Parkinson's disease (Dias et al. 2011). Clearly, the type of disease control group (e.g. involving basal ganglia dysfunction or not; involving disfigurement or not) and the specific assessment approach used (structured interview versus rating scale or self-report measure) are factors that are likely to have influenced results across studies.

Psychiatric disorder in dystonia can either have a biological basis and be primary or be secondary to the onset and experience of living with a disfiguring and disabling disease. Existing evidence supports both the primary and secondary nature of psychiatric disorder in dystonia. Several lines of evidence support the primary nature of psychiatric disorder in dystonia. First, in a proportion of cases the onset of psychiatric disorder precedes the development of dystonia (Wenzel et al. 1998; Lencer et al. 2009; Fabbrini et al. 2010). Second, the rates of recurrent major depressive disorder were higher and with earlier age of onset in both manifesting and non-manifesting DYT1 carriers than non-carriers (Heiman et al. 2004). Other evidence supports the secondary aetiology of psychiatric disorders in dystonia. First, some reported that depression and anxiety are significantly associated with dystonia severity (Lewis et al. 2008). Others have found that perceived disfigurement, body image dissatisfaction, negative body concept, pain, functional disability, satisfaction with social support and use of maladaptive or depressive coping strategies, and life events prior to dystonia onset were among the key predictors of depression in CD (Jahanshahi 1991; Gündel et al. 2001; Lewis et al. 2008). Second, in a two-year longitudinal study of CD, 25 per cent of the sample were depressed at both assessment points and more importantly changes in mood and disability closely tracked changes in the severity of CD over the follow-up period (Jahanshahi & Marsden 1990). Third, depression and anxiety show significant improvement when dystonia improves with botulinum toxin injections (e.g. Jahanshahi & Marsden 1992) or DBS (e.g. Halbig et al. 2005). It is likely that both the primary and secondary routes to the aetiology of psychiatric disorders are valid in dystonia.

Sleep

In CD, none of the standard sleep variables obtained from polysomnography were different from age-matched controls (Lobbezoo et al. 1996a). However, relative to healthy controls, impaired sleep quality is more common in CD (Avanzino et al. 2010; Paus et al. 2011; Eichenseer et al. 2014), even after controlling for depression, anxiety and benzodiazepine use and gender and age-matching with controls (Eichenseer et al. 2014). Excessive daytime sleepiness was not different in CD and controls (Avanzino et al. 2010; Paus et al. 2011; Eichenseer et al. 2014).

In blepharospasm and ormandibular dystonia, reduction of slow and REM sleep and impairment of sleep efficiency and quality of sleep have been reported (Avanzino et al. 2010; Paus et al. 2011), although excessive daytime sleepiness was no higher than controls (Avanzino et al. 2010; Paus et al. 2011). While abnormal dystonic movements gradually reduced from wakefulness to non-REM and REM sleep, they did not disappear completely.

Polysomnographic studies in primary and secondary generalised dystonia and control participants have reported occasional occurrence of involuntary movements observed during wakefulness during stage 1 sleep or after awakening or lightening of sleep but not in the deeper stages of sleep (Fish et al. 1990). They did not find any evidence of abnormal sleep spindles in primary torsion dystonia (Fish et al. 1990) and axial atonia was maintained during REM sleep in dystonia (Fish et al. 1990). In contrast, an earlier study also using polysomnography reported abnormalities including overabundance of stage 2 sleep, a characteristic pattern of spindle activity, increased latency to sleep and reduced sleep efficiency in 25 cases from the literature and four cases examined by the investigators (Jankel et al. 1983). CD is improved by a supine position during sleep.

Pain

Pain is a common experience in CD, reported by 75 per cent (Kutvonen et al. 1997), and negatively impacts daily activities and quality of life (Page et al. 2007). Pain and other non-motor signs such as fatigue and perceived self-efficacy accounted for 46 per cent of the variance in functional disability in CD (Zetterberg et al. 2012). In CD, experience of pain in the head and neck area may reflect lower pain thresholds (Lobbezoo et al. 1996b), somatosensory changes (Tinazzi et al. 2004) or relate to the head deviation and muscle co-contractions, although no correlations between severity of motor signs or degenerative changes on neck X-rays and pain were found (Kutvonen et al. 1997). Cervical pain intensity is reduced by sleep (Lobbezoo et al. 1996a, 1996b).

Sensory Features

Of relevance to the idea that deficits in sensorimotor integration are a feature of dystonia, increased temporal and spatial discrimination thresholds (the ability to distinguish two stimuli delivered close in time or spatial position as being distinct) has been documented in various forms of dystonia (Tinazzi et al. 2004). Temporal and spatial discrimination abnormalities have been shown in the unaffected body parts of dystonia patients as well as in their non-manifesting relatives (Molloy et al. 2003; O'Dwyer et al. 2005), suggesting relevance as a primary endophenotypic deficit. These results together with MEG evidence for altered somatotopic organisation of the sensory cortex in patients with focal hand dystonia (Meunier et al. 2001) suggest that deficits in sensorimotor integration are a feature of dystonia. The 'geste antagoniste', a form of sensory trick present in many focal dystonias, whereby for example a light touch to the side of the face or head relieves CD, has also been considered as evidence for the importance of sensorimotor integration in dystonia. Imaging has shown that use of the geste antagoniste is associated with reduction of the overactivity in the supplementary motor area and primary sensorimotor cortex and increased activation of parietal cortex in cervical dystonia (Naumann et al. 2000).

Conclusions

Dystonia is a movement disorder with prominent non-motor signs. Non-motor signs such as depression and anxiety have a major influence on the quality of life in dystonia (Ben-Shlomo et al. 2002; Page et al. 2007), which makes it essential for these non-motor signs to be the focus of clinical management in dystonia alongside the movement disorder. Successful treatment of dystonia with botulinum toxin or deep brain stimulation improves depression, pain and quality of life (Jahanshahi et al. 2011) and produces no major adverse effect on cognition (Halbig et al. 2005; Jahanshahi et al. 2014).

References

Akil M, Brewer GJ. 1995. Psychiatric and behavioral abnormalities in Wilson's disease. *Adv Neurol* 65:171–178.

Allam N, Frank JE, Pereira C, Tomaz C. 2007. Sustained attention in cranial dystonia patients treated with botulinum toxin. *Acta Neurol Scand* 116:196–200.

Altenmüller E, Jabusch HC. 2010. Focal dystonia in musicians: phenomenology, pathophysiology and triggering factors. *Eur J Neurol* 17 (Suppl. 1):31–36.

Avanzino, L, Martiono, D, Marches, R, et al. 2010. Quality of sleep in primary focal dystonia: a case-control study. *Eur J Neurol*, 17:576–581.

Barbano RL, Hill DF, Snively BM, Light LS, et al. 2012. New triggers and non-motor findings in a family with rapid-onset dystonia-parkinsonism. *Parkinsonism Relat Disord* 18:737–741.

Ben-Shlomo Y, Camfield L, Warner T, Epidemiological Study of Dytonia in Europe (ESDE) Collaborative Group. 2002. What are the determinants of quality of life in people with cervical dystonia. *J Neurol Neurosurg Psychiatry* 72:608–614.

Brashear A, Cook FM, Hill DF, et al. 2012. Psychiatric disorders in rapid-onset dystonia parkinsonism. *Neurology* 79:1168–1173.

Camfield L, Ben-Shlomo Y, Warner T, Epidemiological Study of Dytonia in Europe Collaborative Group. 2002. Impact of cervical dystonia on quality of life. *Mov Disord* 17:838–841.

Cannito MP. 1991. Emotional considerations in spasmodic dysphonia: psychometric quantification. *J Communicat Disord* 24:313–329.

Cavallaro R, Galardi G, Cavallini MC, et al. 2002. Obsessive compulsive disorder among idiopathic focal dystonia patients: an epidemiological and family study. *Biol Psychiatry* 52:356–361.

Dening TR, Berrios GE. 1990. Wilson's disease: a longitudinal study of psychiatric symptoms. *Biol Psychiatry* 28:255–265.

Dias FM, Kummer A, Doyle FC, Harsányi E, Cardoso F, Fontenelle LF, Teixeira AL. 2011. Psychiatric disorders in primary focal dystonia and in Parkinson's disease. *Neuropsychiatr Dis Treat* 7:111–116.

Doheny DO, Brin MF, Morrison CE, et al. 2002. Phenotypic features of myoclonus-dystonia in three kindreds. *Neurology* 59:1187–1196.

Eichenseer SR, Stebbins GT, Comella CL. 2014. Beyond a motor disorder: a prospective evaluation of sleep quality in cervical dystonia. *Parkinsonism Rel Disord* 20:405–408.

Fabbrini G, Berardelli I, Moretti G, Pasquini M, Bloise M, Colosimo C, et al. 2010. Psychiatric disorders in adult-onset focal dystonia: a case-control study. *Mov Disord* 25: 459–456.

Fish DR, Allen PJ, Sawyers D, Marsden CD. 1990. Sleep spindles in torsion dystonia. *Arch Neurol* 47:216–218.

Foncke EM, Cath D, Zwinderman K, Smit J, Schmand B, Tijssen M. 2009. Is psychopathology part of the phenotypic spectrum of myoclonus-dystonia? A study of a large Dutch M-D family. *Cogn Behav Neurol* 22: 27–33.

Gündel H, Wolf A, Xidara V, Busch R, Ceballos-Baumann AO. 2001. Social phobia in spasmodic torticollis. *J Neurol Neurosurg Psychiatry* 71:499–504.

Halbig TD, Gruber D, Kopp UA, Schneider GH, Trottenberg T, Kupsch A. 2005. Pallidal stimulation in dystonia: effects on cognition, mood, and quality of life. *J Neurol Neurosurg Psychiatry* 76:1713–1716.

Heiman GA, Ottman R, Saunders-Pullman RJ, et al. 2004. Increased risk for recurrent major depression in DYT1 dystonia mutation carriers. *Neurology* 63:631–637.

Heiman GA, Ottman R, Saunders-Pullman RJ, et al. 2007. Obsessive compulsive disorder is not a clinical manifestation of the DYT1 dystonia gene. *Am J Med Genet B Neuropsychiatr Genet* 144B:361–364.

Howe LL, Kellison IL, Fernandez HH, Okun MS, Bowers D. 2009. Neuropsychological profile of a Filipino gentleman with X-linked dystonia-parkinsonism: a case report of Lubag disease. *Clinical Neuropsychology* 23(1):100–117.

Jahanshahi M. 1991. Psychosocial correlates of depression in torticollis. *J Psychos Res* 35:1–15.

Jahanshahi M. 2005. Behavioural and psychiatric manifestations in dystonia. In K Anderson, W Weiner, A Lang (eds) *Behavioural Neurology of Movement Disorders, 2nd Edition*, Adv Neurol, 96, Philadelphia, PA: Lippincott Williams & Wilkins, pp. 291–319.

Jahanshahi M, Marsden D. 1990. A longitudinal follow-up study of depression, disability and body concept in torticollis. *Behav Neurol* 3:233–246.

Jahanshahi M, Marsden CD. 1992. Psychological functioning before and after treatment of torticollis with botulinum toxin. *J Neurol Neurosurg Psychiatry* 55(3):229–231.

Jahanshahi M, Rowe J, Fuller R. 2003. Cognitive executive function in dystonia. *Movement Disord* 18: 1470–1481.

Jahanshahi M, Czernecki V, Zurowski AM. 2011. Neuropsychological, neuropsychiatric, and quality of life issues in DBS for dystonia. *Mov Disord* 26 (Suppl. 1):S63–S78.

Jahanshahi M, Torkamani M, Beigi M, Wilkinson L, Page D, Madeley L, Bhatia K, Hariz M, Zrinzo L, Limousin P, Ruge D, Tisch S. 2014. Pallidal stimulation for primary generalised dystonia: effect on cognition, mood and quality of life. *J Neurol* 261(1):164–173. doi: 10.1007/s00415-013-7161-2.

Jankel WR, Allen RP, Niedermeyer E, Kalsher MJ. 1983. Polysomnographic findings in dystonia musculorum deformas. *Sleep* 6:261–265.

Kemmotsu N, Price CC, Oyama G, Okun MS, Foote KD, Howe LL, Bowers D. 2011. Pre- and post-GPi DBS neuropsychological profiles in a case of X-linked dystonia-Parkinsonism. *Clinic Neuropsychol* 25(1): 141–159.

Kutvonen O, Dastidar P, Nurmikko T. 1997. Pain in spasmodic torticollis. *Pain* 69:279–286.

Lange F, Seer C, Salchow C, Dengler R, Dressler D, Kopp B. 2016a. Meta-analytical and electrophysiological evidence for executive dysfunction in primary dystonia. *Cortex* 82:133–146.

Lange F, Seer C, Dengler R, Dressler D, Kopp B. 2016b. Cognitive flexibility in primary dystonia. *J Int Neuropsychol Soc* 22:662–670.

Lencer R, Steinlechner S, Stahlberg J, Rehling H, Orth M, Baeumer T, Rumpf HJ, Meyer C, Klein C, Muenchau A, Hagenah J. 2009. Primary focal dystonia: evidence for distinct neuropsychiatric and personality profiles. *J Neurol Neurosurg Psychiatry* 80:1176–1179.

Lewis L, Butler A, Jahanshahi M. 2008. Depression in focal, segmental and generalized dystonia. *J Neurol* 255:1750–1755.

Lobbezoo F, Thu Thon M, Remillard G, et al. 1996a. Relationship between sleep, neck muscle activity, and pain in cervical dystonia. *Can J Neurol Sci* 23:285–290.

Lobbezoo F, Tanguay R, Thon MT, Lavigne GJ. 1996b. Pain: perception in idiopathic cervical dystonia (spasmodic torticollis). *Pain* 67:483–491.

Marelli C, Piacentini S, Garavaglia B, Girotti F, Albanese A. 2005. Clinical and neuropsychological correlates in two brothers with pantothenate kinase-associated neurodegeneration. *Mov Disord* 20:208–212.

Meunier S, Garnero L, Ducorps A, Mazieres L, Lehericy S, du Montcel ST, et al. 2001. Human brain mapping in dystonia reveals both endophenotypic traits and adaptive reorganization. *Ann Neurol* 50:521–527.

Molloy FM, Carr TD, Zeuner KE, Dambrosia JM, Hallett M. 2003. Abnormalities of spatial discrimination in focal and generalized dystonia. *Brain* 126: 2175–2182.

Munhoz RP, Teive HA, Della Coletta MV, Germiniani FM, Iwamoto FM, Camargo CH, Werneck LC. 2005. Frequency of obsessive and compulsive symptoms in patients with blepharospasm and hemifacial spasm. *Arq Neuropsiquiatr* 63:213–216.

Naumann M, Magyar-Lehmann S, Reiners K, Erbguth F, Leenders KL. 2000. Sensory tricks in cervical dystonia: perceptual dysbalance of parietal cortex modulates frontal motor programming. *Ann Neurol* 47:322–328.

O'Dwyer JP, O'Riordan S, Saunders-Pullman R, Bressman SB, Molloy F, Lynch T, et al. 2005. Sensory abnormalities in unaffected relatives in familial adult-onset dystonia. *Neurology* 65:938–940.

Page D, Butler A, Jahanshahi M. 2007. Quality of life in focal, segmental, and generalized dystonia. *Mov Disord* 22:341–347.

Paus, S., Gross, J., Moll-Muller, M et al. 2011. Impaired sleep quality and restless leg syndrome in idiopathic focal dystonia: a controlled study. *J Neurol* 258:1835–1840.

Saunders-Pullman R, Shriberg J, Heiman G, et al. 2002. Myoclonus dystonia: possible association with obsessive-compulsive disorder and alcohol dependence. *Neurology* 58:242–245.

Shanmugiah A, Sinha S, Taly AB, Prashanth LK, Tomar M, Arunodaya GR, Reddy JY. 2008. Psychiatric manifestations in Wilson's disease: a cross-sectional analysis. *J Neuropsychiatry Clin Neurosci* 20:81–85.

Tadic V, Kasten M, Brüggemann N, Stiller S, Hagenah J, Klein C. 2012. Dopa-responsive dystonia revisited: diagnostic delay, residual signs, and nonmotor signs. *Arch Neurol* 69(12):1558–1562.

Tinazzi M, Fiorio M, Bertolasi L, Aglioti SM. 2004. Timing of tactile and visuotactile events is impaired in patients with cervical dystonia. *J Neurol* 251:85–90.

Torkamani M, Jahanshahi M. 2014. Neuropsychological and neuropsychiatric features of dystonia and the impact of medical and surgical treatment. In A Troster (ed.) *Clinical Neuropsychology and Cognitive Neurology of Parkinson's Disease and Other Movement Disorders,* Oxford: Oxford University Press.

van Hove JLK, Steyaert J, Matthijs G, et al. 2006. Expanded motor and psychiatric phenotype in autosomal dominant Segawa syndrome due to GTP cyclohydrolase deficiency. *J Neurol Neurosurg Psychiatry* 77:18–23.

van Tricht MJV, Dreissen, YEM, Cath D, et al. 2012. Cognition and psychopathology in myoclonus-dystonia. *J Neurol Neurosurg Psychiatry* 83:814–820.

Voon V, Butler TR, Ekanayake V, Gallea C, Ameli R, Murphy DL, et al. 2010. Psychiatric symptoms associated with focal hand dystonia. *Mov Disord* 25:2249–2252.

Wenzel T, Schnider P, Wimmer A, Steinhoff N, Moraru E, Auff E. 1998. Psychiatric comorbidity in patients with spasmodic torticollis. *J Psychosom Res* 44:687–690.

Wenzel T, Schnider P, Griengl H, Birner P, Nepp J, Auff E. 2000. Psychiatric disorders in patients with blepharospasm: a reactive pattern? *J Psychosom Res* 48:589–591.

Zetterberg L, Lindmark B, Söderlund A, Åsenlöf P. 2012. Self-perceived non-motor aspects of cervical dystonia and their association with disability. *J Rehabil Med* 44:950–954.

Zeuner KE, Knutzen A, Granert O, Sablowsky S, Götz J, Wolff S, Jansen O, Dressler D, Schneider SA, Klein C, Deuschl G, van Eimeren T, Witt K. 2016. Altered brain activation in a reversal learning task unmasks adaptive changes in cognitive control in writer's cramp. *Neuroimage Clin* 10:63–70.

Chapter 15

Scales for Assessment of Dystonia

Cynthia L. Comella and Glenn T. Stebbins

The selection of a rating scale to assess disease severity is one of the crucial elements in designing a clinical trial of a therapeutic intervention. A useful scale is one that is designed to measure a particular disorder, which demonstrates validity, reliability and reproducibility. The scale should be sensitive, or responsive, to change in the disorder secondary to intervention. Finally, the rating scale should be efficient and practical in a clinical setting. The World Health Organization (WHO) developed a model to standardise disease outcomes into four categories: pathology, impairment, disability and handicap. The second of these, impairment, refers to the functional consequence of a disease process, reflecting organ dysfunctions or abnormalities of body structure. Current dystonia rating scales have primarily been assessed for their clinimetric properties relative to impairment (motor abnormalities). A recent comprehensive review of the rating scales for focal and generalised dystonia was published by a taskforce as a part of the Movement Disorders Committee on Rating Scales Development (Albanese et al. 2013) (Table 15.1).

In the development of a comprehensive rating scale, a frequently utilised approach is the Delphi method (Taylor et al. 2008). This methodology includes experts in various aspects of the disorder, and provides a listing of pertinent domains and disease characteristics that are ranked in order of importance. This process is repeated until there is agreement among experts that the items cover the important aspects of the disorder. It is an iterative process, in which there is a progressive reduction in items from the item pool and a preliminary scale is constructed. The items included in the preliminary scale can then be evaluated through cognitive pretesting (Willis 2006). Cognitive pretesting involves interviewing a small number of both examiners (raters) and respondents (ratees) to assess task difficulty for each item. This process evaluates respondent interest, attention span and comfort, with all questions involving patient or caregiver input for the response and can assist in identifying problems of logical structure in items that could affect understanding. After modifications suggested by the cognitive pretesting are made, the scale is developed.

Once the scale is developed, it undergoes psychometric testing for reliability and validity. The scale is tested in a large number of subjects (approximately ten subjects for each item in the scale). Reliability testing should assess internal consistency, test–retest reliability, inter-rater reliability and intra-rater reliability. The internal consistency of a scale, usually measured with Cronbach's alpha, assesses whether the scale 'hangs together' by testing to correlation between each half of the scale across all permutations of halves. The individual contribution of each item to the scale is assessed through the item-to-total correlation and items that do not contribute, or that decrease Cronbach's alpha, can be considered for removal from the scale. Test–retest reliability assesses if the scale is stable in its measurement across a short delay in administration. Inter- and intra-rater reliability assess if the scale produces similar results when used by the different raters (inter-rater) or the same rater (intra-rater) in similar settings.

The validity of a scale is the extent to which it measures what it is supposed to measure. There are three major components of validity: content and face validity, construct validity and criterion validity. Content and face validity represent the extent to which the domains of a rating scale assess the condition being rated. Content validity is often established during the Delphi process, where the panellists rate each item for its importance to the target condition. These rankings can be used to create a content validity ratio (CVR) of the scale. Construct validity is an important measure of a rating scale's validity and is usually assessed through factor analyses. This type of analysis identifies the underlying structure of the rating scale and groups those items that measure a particular aspect of the disorder into clusters or factors. The factor structure should be logical and consistent with the identified domains that the scale is purported to measure. A valid scale adequately measures the features of the disorder, and criterion validity assesses this by correlating the rating scale results with an independent measure (the 'gold standard'). Responsiveness of the scale refers to the ability to detect change in the disorder, and the minimal clinically relevant change is a measure of the meaningful changes (Stebbins 2012).

Rating Scales for Dystonia

Dystonia is a dynamic disorder manifested by involuntary, abnormal sustained postures that change in severity based on posture, activity and sensory input. Dystonia is categorised by body distribution into focal (involving a single body area), segmental (involvement of two or more contiguous body areas) and generalised (involving at least one leg, the trunk and some other body area). Dystonia rating scales, likewise, have been specifically developed to assess these categories of dystonia,

Table 15.1 Rating scales classification (modified from Albanese et al. 2013)

Dystonia	Scale	Status
Generalised dystonia	**Fahn–Marsden Dystonia Rating Scale**	**Recommended**
	Unified Dystonia Rating Scale	Suggested
	Global Dystonia Rating Scale	Suggested
Blepharospasm	**Blepharospasm Disability Index (BSDI)**	**Recommended**
	Jankovic Rating Scale	Suggested
	Blepharospasm Disability Scale	Suggested
Blepharospasm and cervical dystonia	**Craniocervical Dystonia Questionnaire (CDQ-24)**	**Recommended**
Cervical dystonia	**Toronto Western Spasmodic Torticollis Scale**	**Recommended**
	Cervical Dystonia Impact Scale (CDIP-58)	**Recommended**
	Functional Disability Questionnaire	Suggested
	Tsui Scale	Suggested
Oromandibular dystonia	Oromandibular Dystonia Questionnaire	Suggested
Spasmodic dysphonia (laryngeal dystonia)	**Voice Handicap Index**	**Recommended**
	Vocal Performance Questionnaire	**Recommended**
	Unified Spasmodic Dysphonia Rating Scale	Suggested
	Voice Handicap Index 10	Suggested
Arm dystonia	Arm Dystonia Disability Scale	Suggested

Recommended: (1) applied to dystonia; (2) used by more than one group; (3) clinimetric studies show reliability, validity and sensitivity to change.
Suggested: Meets criteria 1 and one other criteria.

with separate scales for generalised dystonia and for each body region affected.

The changeable quality of dystonia has made the development of reliable rating scales problematic, and has necessitated the development of standardised examination protocols that include dystonia-activating manoeuvres, such as writing, chewing and speaking. The state-dependent character of dystonia has resulted in the addition of items that are intended to capture the effects of sensory inputs or to measure the duration of time that dystonia is present during the examination. Most rating scales additionally provide a uniform examination protocol to ensure consistent and complete assessments of the patients.

Fahn–Marsden Scale, VDRS and GDS

In an early manuscript, Fahn developed rating scales for each of the classes of dystonia, including the Fahn–Marsden Scale for primary dystonia (Fahn 1989). The Fahn–Marsden dystonia rating scale (F-M) has been a standard instrument used to assess the severity of generalised dystonia (Burke et al. 1985). The global scale has two parts: a movement scale based on the motor features of dystonia, and a disability scale based on the patient's subjective impairment in activities of daily living. The movement scale has two separate factors assessing nine body regions (eyes, mouth, speech and swallowing, neck, bilateral arms and legs, and trunk). The factors include a severity factor that measures the intensity of movement and is tailored to each body area, and a provoking factor that assesses the circumstances of rest or activity that elicit the dystonia in each area. The final score for each body area is the product of the two factors, with the exception of eyes, mouth and neck, which are further multiplied by 0.5. The maximal score of the F-M movement scale is 120. The disability scale assesses a variety of functions (speech, handwriting, feeding, eating/swallowing, hygiene, dressing and walking) rated from 0 (normal) to 4 (severe), with a maximal score of 30. The psychometric properties of the F-M have been assessed in one study using ten patients and four raters. This study demonstrated good to excellent inter-rater agreement and validity as assessed by a good correlation of the movement scale with the global dystonia severity scale and the dystonia disability scale. A subsequent study assessing the F-M in 100 patients using 25 dystonia experts showed good to excellent agreement for the total score, but only fair agreement (weighted kappa of 0.37–0.62) for dystonia in the eyes, jaw and face (Comella et al. 2003). The F-M has been used widely, particularly to assess the effects of deep brain stimulation (DBS) in adults and children with generalised dystonia.

The Unified Dystonia Rating Scale (UDRS) was developed in 1997 at a consensus conference of dystonia experts, and was intended to address the potential limitations of the F-M scale by subdividing body regions and separately assessing a duration factor measuring time dystonia was present during the examination. This scale rates 14 body regions for dystonia severity and duration, with each scored from 0 to 4. The total score for the UDRS is 112. Similar to the F-M, testing in a large number of dystonia patients showed good to excellent inter-rater agreement, with the lowest agreement for face, eyes, jaws and speech.

The Global Dystonia Rating scale (GDS) was designed to rate dystonia in 14 body areas using a 0 (no dystonia) to 10 (worst possible dystonia) rating. Interestingly, this scale likewise demonstrated good to excellent inter-rater agreement.

The F-M, UDRS and GDS have not been tested for clinical responsiveness to therapeutic interventions or reproducibility. The F-M has been used frequently as an outcome for pharmacological and surgical studies of generalised dystonia. The UDRS has been used as a measure of efficacy following surgical interventions. The GDS has been used as a screening tool for dystonia severity. Although applicable to generalised dystonia, these scales are not considered useful for focal dystonia. Each focal dystonia is assessed using a scale developed for that particular dystonia.

Cervical Dystonia Rating Scales

The instruments used to assess the severity of cervical dystonia, a common focal dystonia involving the neck, are numerous and include objective and subjective rating scales and quantitative measures (Tsui et al. 1988; Greene et al. 1990; Consky & Lang 1994; Lindeboom et al. 1996). Several clinical rating scales have been developed, including the Columbia Torticollis Scale, the Tsui Scale and the Toronto Western Spasmodic Torticollis Scale (TWSTRS) (Tsui et al. 1988; Greene et al. 1990; Consky & Lang 1994; Tarsy 1997). The TWSTRS is currently the most widely utilised. The TWSTRS consists of three subscales: motor severity, activities of daily living and pain. The motor severity scale is a ten-item rater assessment that evaluates the severity of head posture in several axes of movement (turning, tilting, anterocollis, retrocollis, shoulder elevation), the effect of sensory tricks, range of motion, and duration that dystonia is present during the examination. The TWSTRS subsection for motor severity has been evaluated for inter-rater reliability and validity (Consky & Lang 1994), and a teaching tape has been developed to ensure consistency across raters for multicentre trials (Comella et al. 1997). The TWSTRS has been used extensively in clinical trials of pharmacological and surgical interventions. However, deficiencies in the TWSTRS have been identified, including the lack of an item for head tremor and inconsistent scaling for each item (Jost et al. 2013). The TWSTRS has undergone revisions to remedy these deficiencies and is part of the ongoing work to develop a Comprehensive Cervical Dystonia Rating Scale that will capture both motor and non-motor features of cervical dystonia (Comella et al. 2015).

The Cervical Dystonia Impact Profile (CDIP) is a self-administered scale that assesses the impact of cervical dystonia on quality of life (Cano et al. 2004, 2006). This scale includes 58 items that are grouped into eight subscales. Following a mathematical programme, the eight subscale scores are then transformed to a single scale between 0 and 100. The CDIP has demonstrated reliability and validity and has been shown to be responsive to change following botulinum toxin treatments (Cano et al. 2006).

Other Focal Dystonia Rating Scales

Rating scales for blepharospasm have been recently developed. The Blepharospasm Disability Index (BSDI) is a six-item rating scale completed by the patient which rates ability to do daily activities. This scale has demonstrated reliability but requires additional clinimetric testing for validity and sensitivity to change. The Jankovic Rating Scale (JRS) assesses the severity and frequency of blepharospasm. Both severity and frequency are rated 0–4 (Jankovic et al. 2009). Patient report is needed to complete the scale. There is a correlation between the BDSI and the JRS, but clinimetric properties have not yet been adequately evaluated. A recently developed rating scale for blepharospasm, the Blepharospasm Severity Scale, was developed using a modified Delphi method. This scale includes an intensity rating consisting of four items, and a frequency rating with two items. The scale was found to have good internal consistency and acceptable inter-rater and intra-rater reliability (Defazio et al. 2015).

Scales to assess the severity of limb dystonia and occupational dystonia (writer's cramp, musician's dystonia) have been particularly problematic. Most studies use patient-derived assessments or electrophysiological tests. The writer's cramp rating scale (WCRS) and arm dystonia disability scale (ADDS) (Fahn 1989; Wissel et al. 1996) have been used but never tested for clinimetric properties. For many limb and occupational dystonias, customised rating scales are developed that are specifically tailored to evaluate the particular task affected by the dystonia (Zeuner et al. 2007).

There is currently a need for rating scale development and clinimetric testing for many additional focal and occupational dystonias. Developing and validating such measures contribute to the accurate diagnosis of dystonias, the monitoring of interventions and the development of new therapies to treat this disease.

References

Albanese A, Sorbo FD, Comella C, Jinnah HA, Mink JW, Post B, Vidailhet M, Volkmann J, Warner TT, Leentjens AF, Martinez-Martin P, Stebbins GT, Goetz CG, Schrag A. 2013. Dystonia rating scales: critique and recommendations. *Mov Disord* 28(7):874–883.

Burke RE, Fahn S, Marsden CD, Bressman SB, Moskowitz C, Friedman J. 1985. Validity and reliability of a rating scale for the primary torsion dystonias. *Neurology* 35(1):73–77.

Cano SJ, Warner TT, Linacre JM, Bhatia KP, Thompson AJ, Fitzpatrick R, Hobart JC. 2004. Capturing the true burden of dystonia on patients: the cervical dystonia impact profile (CDIP-58). *Neurology* 63(9):1629–1633.

Cano SJ, Hobart JC, Edwards M, Fitzpatrick R, Bhatia K, Thompson AJ, Warner TT. 2006. CDIP-58 can measure the impact of botulinum toxin treatment in cervical dystonia. *Neurology* 67(12):2230–2232.

Comella CL, Stebbins GT, Goetz CG, Chmura TA, Bressman SB, Lang AE. 1997. Teaching tape for the motor section of the Toronto Western Spasmodic Torticollis Scale. *Mov Disord* 12(4):570–575.

Comella CL, Leurgans S, Wuu J, Stebbins GT, Chmura T, Dystonia Study Group. 2003. Rating scales for dystonia: a multicenter assessment. *Mov Disord* 18(3):303–312.

Comella CL, Fox SH, Bhatia KP, Perlmutter JS, Jinnah HA, Zurowski M, McDonald WM, Marsh L, Rosen AR, Waliczek T, Wright LJ, Galpern WR, Stebbins GT. 2015. Development of the comprehensive cervical dystonia rating scale: methodology. *Mov Disord Clin Pract* 2(2):135–141.

Consky E, Lang AE. 1994. Clinical assessments of patients with cervical dystonia. In: *Therapy with Botulinum Toxin (Neurological Disease and Therapy)*. Jankovic J, Hallett M, editors. New York: Marcel Dekker.

Defazio G, Hallett M, Jinnah HA, Stebbins GT, Gigante AF, Ferrazzano G, Conte A, Fabbrini G, Berardelli A. 2015. Development and validation of a clinical scale for rating the severity of blepharospasm. *Mov Disord* 30(4):525–530.

Fahn S. 1989. Assessment of the primary dystonias. In: *Quantification of Neurologic Deficit*. Munsat T, editor. London: Butterworths.

Greene P, Kang U, Fahn S, Brin M, Moskowitz C, Flaster E. 1990. Double-blind, placebo-controlled trial of botulinum toxin injections for the treatment of spasmodic torticollis. *Neurology* 40(8):1213–1218.

Jankovic J, Kenney C, Grafe S, Goertelmeyer R, Comes G. 2009. Relationship between various clinical outcome assessments in patients with blepharospasm. *Mov Disord* 24(3):407–413.

Jost WH, Hefter H, Stenner A, Reichel G. 2013. Rating scales for cervical dystonia: a critical evaluation of tools for outcome assessment of botulinum toxin therapy. *J Neural Transm (Vienna)* 120(3):487–496.

Lindeboom R, de Haan RJ, Aramideh M, Brans JW, Speelman JD. 1996. Treatment outcomes in cervical dystonia: a clinimetric study. *Mov Disord* 11(4):371–376.

Stebbins GT. 2012. Clinical rating scale development. In: *Rating Scales in Parkinson's Disease: Clinical Practice and Research*. Sampaio C, Goetz CG, Schrag A, editors. Oxford: Oxford University Press.

Tarsy D. 1997. Comparison of clinical rating scales in treatment of cervical dystonia with botulinum toxin. *Mov Disord* 12(1):100–102.

Taylor WJ, Schumacher HR, Jr, Baraf HS, Chapman P, Stamp L, Doherty M, McQueen F, Dalbeth N, Schlesinger N, Furst DE, Vazquez-Mellado J, Becker MA, Kavanaugh A, Louthrenoo W, Bardin T, Khanna D, Simon LS, Yamanaka H, Choi HK, Zeng X, Strand V, Grainger R, Clegg D, Singh JA, Diaz-Torne C, Boers M, Gow P, Barskova VG. 2008. A modified Delphi exercise to determine the extent of consensus with OMERACT outcome domains for studies of acute and chronic gout. *Ann Rheum Dis* 67(6):888–891.

Tsui JK, Eisen A, Calne DB. 1988. Botulinum toxin in spasmodic torticollis. *Adv Neurol* 50:593–597.

Willis G. 2006. Cognitive interviewing as a tool for improving the informed consent process. *J Empir Res Hum Res Ethics* 1(1):9–24.

Wissel J, Kabus C, Wenzel R, Klepsch S, Schwarz U, Nebe A, Schelosky L, Scholz U, Poewe W. 1996. Botulinum toxin in writer's cramp: objective response evaluation in 31 patients. *J Neurol Neurosurg Psychiatry* 61(2):172–175.

Zeuner KE, Peller M, Knutzen A, Holler I, Munchau A, Hallett M, Deuschl G, Siebner HR. 2007. How to assess motor impairment in writer's cramp. *Mov Disord* 22(8):1102–1109.

Section I | Basics

Chapter 16

Theories Behind Dystonia Scale Development

Sophie Cleanthous and Stefan J. Cano

Clinical Outcome Assessments

Clinical outcome assessments (COAs) are increasingly used to assess health outcomes in dystonia research and practice (Albanese et al. 2013). As health outcomes cannot be measured directly using diagnostic blood tests or imaging, COAs include rating scales to quantify them (Food and Drug Administration 2013). COAs can differ in structure (single items to multi-domain scales), specificity (e.g. generic across conditions, disease or site/body part specific), responder (e.g. clinician, patient, observer/proxy) as well as type of response scale (e.g. Likert scale, checklist or visual analogue scale) (Food and Drug Organisation 2009). Nevertheless, COAs have a common quality, which is the subjective judgement present each time a responder (whether it is the patient, carer or clinician) is asked to choose the response option that best describes a particular item.

As scores derived from COAs are used to make decisions about the state of disease and treatment in dystonia, it is important that they are fit for purpose (Food and Drug Administration 2013). COAs should specifically and comprehensively capture the health outcome under measurement, i.e. the concept of interest (COI), in the context of use (COU) (Food and Drug Administration 2013). Further, it is essential to evaluate the extent to which summing scores derived from subjective judgement leads to valid measurement. This is achieved through the discipline of psychometrics (Food and Drug Organisation 2009).

Psychometric Theories

Currently, there are three main psychometric approaches grounded in different types of measurement theories: Classical Test Theory (CTT), Rasch Measurement Theory (RMT) and Item Response Theory (IRT) (Hobart & Cano 2009; Cano & Hobart 2011).

Classical Test Theory

Health outcome research is currently dominated by CTT. This approach is associated with the widely recognised properties of reliability, validity and ability to detect change which constitute the recommended criteria for COA assessment of both scientific (Aaronson et al. 2002) and regulatory bodies (Food and Drug Organisation 2009). CTT is grounded in Steven's definition of measurement – 'the assignment of numerals to objects or events according to some rule' – which differs from the classical definition of measurement used in the natural sciences (i.e. the numerical estimation and expression of the magnitude of one quantity relative to another) (Stevens 1946). CTT proposes that in measurement a person's observed score is the sum of their true and error scores (Box 16.1) and psychometric evaluation examines raw scores without weighing or standardisation against assumptions underlying this measurement theory (Novick 1966).

Box 16.1 Classical Test Theory

$$O = T + E$$

Where the observed score (O) is the person's manifest score on a scale. The true score (T) is the person's 'real' score. This is unobservable (a theoretical value) because of the associated measurement error – the error score (E).

CTT has a fundamental drawback (Andrich 1988), which is that the true score is unobservable and theoretical; consequently, the observed score cannot be tested or falsified. Therefore, CTT psychometric criteria can easily be met. In practice, this results in four main limitations of the approach: (1) measurement using ordinal rather than interval scores; (2) scale properties (e.g. reliability) being sample-dependent; (3) measurement (responder total scores) being scale-dependent, prohibiting individual assessment; and (4) a lack of item scaling prohibiting the creation of a clinically meaningful measurement continuum comprising items of higher and lower difficulty (Rasch 1960; McDowell & Newell 1987; Andrich 1988).

Rasch Measurement Theory

More recently the modern psychometric paradigms of RMT (Rasch 1960; Andrich 1988) and IRT have been used in COA psychometric evaluation. These 'modern test theories' can be traced back to Thurstone's measurement requirements, including interval scaling and measurement invariance, which are more in line with the requirements of measurement in the natural sciences. In the middle of the last century, Georg Rasch, a Danish mathematician, argued that social measurement should conform to invariant comparison, like physical measurement. On this basis, the simple logistic model (the 'Rasch

Box 16.2 Rasch Model

$$Pr\{x_{ni}|\beta_n,\delta_i\}=\frac{e^{x_{ni}(\beta_n-\delta_i)}}{1+e^{(\beta_n-\delta_i)}}$$

where $x_{ni}\in[0,1]$; β_n and δ_i are the measurements of person n and item i, respectively, upon the same latent trait, and e is the natural logarithm constant (2.718).

model'; Box 16.2) was originally proposed to describe reading ability (Rasch 1960).

The Rasch model proposes that the probability of response to an item is a logistic function of the relative difference between a person's ability and the item's difficulty. Applying the Rasch model, RMT defines how a set of items should perform to generate reliable and valid measurements, and RMT analysis examines the extent to which the observed raw data 'fit' predictions expected by the Rasch model (Andrich 1988; Hobart & Cano 2009).

Assessing the difference between the expected and observed scores indicates the degree to which summing the COA items approximates rigorous measurement. Guttman probabilistic scaling is used to estimate expected scores and a variety of investigations (graphical and numerical) are conducted to evaluate measurement properties of a COA, including scale-to-sample targeting, adequacy of type and kind of response options, item and person fit, item bias and stability between subgroups (Hobart & Cano 2009).

Item Response Theory

IRT (Lord & Novick 1968) also utilises logistic models in an attempt to describe measurement as the relationship between a person's ability and his/her response to an item. However, unlike the RMT, the IRT proposes additional parameters in an attempt to explain observed data that fail to satisfy the criteria of the single (one-parameter) logistic model (Hobart & Cano 2009). Two-parameter models (Box 16.3a) include an item discrimination parameter and three-parameter models (Box 16.3b) include a guessing parameter (Waller 1976; Lumsden 1977). As such, despite their similarities, the IRT becomes a statistical modelling paradigm aiming to find the best model to fit the data, whereas the RMT is a diagnostic paradigm aiming to find the strongest items and identify measurement anomalies (Andrich 2004; Cano & Hobart 2011).

Comparison of CTT and RMT

In comparison to CTT, modern psychometric evaluation benefits from the ability to rigorously verify measurement properties of COAs using testable theories. RMT specifically addresses all the CTT limitations described above as (1) interval-level measurement can be constructed from raw ordinal data; (2) item and person parameter estimates are provided that are free of sample and scale distribution; (3) item scaling allows for item subsets to be used; and (4) measurement is suitable for individual as well as group comparisons. Nevertheless, the theory

Box 16.3 IRT Models

$$Pr\{x_{ni}|\beta_n,\delta_i,\alpha_i\}=\frac{e^{x_{ni}[\alpha_i(\beta_n-\delta_i)]}}{1+e^{[\alpha_i(\beta_n-\delta_i)]}} \quad (a)$$

$$\Pr\{x_{ni}\,|\beta_n,\delta_i,\alpha_i,c_i\}=c_i+(1+c_i)+\frac{e^{x_{ni}[\alpha_i(\beta_n-\delta_i)]}}{1+e^{[\alpha_i(\beta_n-\delta_i)]}} \quad (b)$$

(a) is the basic 2P model, which is equivalent to the equation in Box 16.2, with the addition of α_i, which represents the slope of item ι (discrimination). The basic 3P model is shown in (b). In this instance, the additional c_i represents a constant describing the lower asymptote due to guessing for item ι.

and application of modern psychometrics is more complex, challenging their popularity and application so far in health measurement (Hobart & Cano 2009; Cano & Hobart 2011).

Content Validity

Regardless of the psychometric paradigm of choice, it is essential to comprehensively define the COI that a COA purports to measure; in other words, to establish content validity. Supporting every COA with an empirically derived conceptual framework ensures that its items are appropriate and comprehensive relative to the COI in the specific COU (McDowell & Newell 1987; Food and Drug Organisation 2009). Guidelines suggest that conceptual frameworks are vital and should be developed using an iterative qualitative methodology and the direct input of the patient population and clinical experts of the condition under measurement. Content validity is fundamental and cannot be rectified by subsequent measurement properties and should not be ignored by scale developers (Food and Drug Organisation 2009).

COAs and Dystonia Research

A systematic review of COAs used across different types of dystonia concluded that more than one-third did not fulfil the validity, reliability and responsiveness criteria (Albanese et al. 2013), replicating earlier unfavourable findings in cervical dystonia, primarily with regards to responsiveness (Cano et al. 2004a; Jost et al. 2013). Nevertheless, some existing COAs have been developed using more comprehensive methodology, such as the Cervical Dystonia Impact Profile (CDIP-58) (Cano et al. 2004b). The CDIP-58 was developed and validated using a step-wise and comprehensive approach involving an exploration of the COI in the COU using patient interviews, expert opinion and literature findings leading to a large item pool generation followed by two postal surveys in independent CD samples and using rigorous RMT techniques to form and evaluate CDIP-58 scales (Cano et al. 2004b). CDIP-58 has been shown to be reliable and valid and able to detect change after botulinum neurotoxins therapy (Cano et al. 2008; Albanese et al. 2013).

Conclusions

As the assessment of dystonia increasingly relies on health outcomes and less so on traditional parameters of clinical morbidity and mortality, COAs play an increasingly central role in research and practice. Developing and evaluating COAs using a comprehensive psychometric methodology is crucial for these to be fit for purpose and provide clinically meaningful and interpretable data. RMT offers a rigorous psychometric methodology for developing and evaluating COAs (Hobart & Cano 2009; Cano & Hobart 2011).

References

Aaronson N, Alonso J, Burnam A, Lohr KN, Patrick DL, Perrin E, Stein RE. 2002. Assessing health status and quality-of-life instruments: attributes and review criteria. *Qual Life Res* 11(3):193–205.

Albanese A, Sorbo FD, Comella C, Jinnah HA, Mink JW, Post B, Vidailhet M, Volkmann J, Warner TT, Leentjens AF, Martinez-Martin P, Stebbins GT, Goetz CG, Schrag A. 2013. Dystonia rating scales: critique and recommendations. *Mov Disord* 28(7):874–883.

Andrich D. 1988. *Rasch Models for Measurement.* Beverly Hills, CA: Sage Publications.

Andrich D. 2004. Controversy and the Rasch model: a characteristic of incompatible paradigms? *Med Care* 42(Suppl. 1):I7–I16.

Cano SJ, Hobart JC. 2011. The problem with health measurement. *Patient Prefer Adherence* 5:279–290.

Cano SJ, Hobart JC, Fitzpatrick R, Bhatia K, Thompson AJ, Warner TT. 2004a. Patient-based outcomes of cervical dystonia: a review of rating scales. *Mov Disord* 19(9):1054–1059.

Cano SJ, Warner TT, Linacre JM, Bhatia KP, Thompson AJ, Fitzpatrick R, Hobart JC. 2004b. Capturing the true burden of dystonia on patients: the Cervical Dystonia Impact Profile (CDIP-58). *Neurology* 63(9):1629–1633.

Cano SJ, Warner TT, Thompson AJ, Bhatia KP, Fitzpatrick R, Hobart JC. 2008. The Cervical Dystonia Impact Profile (CDIP-58): can a Rasch developed patient reported outcome measure satisfy traditional psychometric criteria? *Health Qual Life Outcomes* 6:58.

Food and Drug Administration. 2013. Qualification of Clinical Outcome Assessments (COAs); www.fda.gov/Drugs/DevelopmentApprovalProcess/DrugDevelopmentTools QualificationProgram/ucm284077.htm

Food and Drug Organisation. 2009. Patient-reported outcome measures: use in medical product development to support labelling claims; www.fda.gov/downloads/Drugs/Guidances/UCM193282.pdf

Hobart J, Cano S. 2009. Improving the evaluation of therapeutic interventions in multiple sclerosis: the role of new psychometric methods. *Health Technol Assess* 13(12):iii, ix–x, 1–177.

Jost WH, Hefter H, Stenner A, Reichel G. 2013. Rating scales for cervical dystonia: a critical evaluation of tools for outcome assessment of botulinum toxin therapy. *J Neural Transm* 120(3):487–496.

Lord FM, Novick MR. 1968. *Statistical Theories of Mental Test Scores.* Reading, MA: Addison-Wesley.

Lumsden J. 1977. Person reliability. *Appl Psychol Meas* 1: 477–482.

McDowell I, Newell C. 1987. *Measuring Health: A Guide to Rating Scales and Questionnaires.* Oxford: Oxford University Press.

Novick MR. 1966. The axioms and principal results of Classical Test Theory. *J Math Psychol*; 3:1–18.

Rasch G. 1960. *Probabilistic Models for Some Intelligence and Attainment Tests.* Copenhagen: Danish Institute for Education Research.

Stevens SS. 1946. On the theory of scales of measurement. *Science* 103(2684):677–680.

Waller M. 1976. *Estimating Parameters in the Rasch Model: Removing the Effects of Random Guessing.* Princeton, NJ: Educational Testing Service.

Chapter 17

Linking Allied Health Professionals and Physicians

The IAB Model

Fereshte Adib Saberi and Dirk Dressler

Introduction

Increasing complexity of diagnostics and therapeutics in movement disorders requires interdisciplinary collaboration involving numerous health professionals and medical specialists. Coordinating all professions involved is challenging for many reasons: different educational backgrounds produce different terminologies, different classification systems, different explanatory models, different views and different approaches. General lack of quantitative measurements and classification systems and lack of evidence-based evaluation further inhibits the flow of information. General deterioration of communication skills favours individual rather than cooperative collaboration structures. IAB – Interdisciplinary Working Group for Movement Disorders – wants to establish a platform for communication and collaboration to improve patient care in movement disorders. Its structure is shown in Figure 17.1.

IAB Regional Groups

IAB's activities started in 2006 with a regional group to promote and to optimise multidisciplinary therapy of movement disorders in Hamburg, Germany (Adib Saberi & Dressler 2011). More than 25 physiotherapists, occupational therapists, speech therapists, nurse specialists, physicians and invited guests meet regularly, once every three months. The meetings cover specific topics including presentation of common movement disorders, classification and quantification systems, case studies and political and educational discussions. While the topics are selected to represent a curriculum providing a broad view over a large number of topics, the meetings themselves are based on group interaction with sufficient time for discussions. In the meantime, additional IAB Regional Groups were founded in other regions of Germany covering the Hannover, Cologne and Berlin regions. Special subgroups for Parkinson's assistants and for the transition phase from paediatric to adult neurology were founded out of the IAB Regional Groups. IAB acquired the rights on the Hannover Video Club, a well-established lecture series with meetings four times a year featuring national and international movement disorder specialists.

IAB Website

The IAB website can be found at www/iabnetz.de. It gives an overview about IAB and its activities. The calendar of events features those organised by IAB and its members, as well as events of general interest. It gives links to related organisations, both nationally and internationally, including the International Neurotoxin Association, the Movement Disorders Society, the International Association of Parkinsonism and Related Disorders, Symtox, ParkinsonNet, Dystonia Europe and Dystonia Medical Research Foundation. It provides a list of IAB members so that movement disorder specialists in the IAB covered regions can be identified easily. The IAB website features the IAB products and gives details about the newly started IAB Academy. A news section provides news relevant to IAB members and public visitors. A job section informs about jobs offered and jobs searched. Selected scientific publications can be found in the publication section. The website also offers the opportunity to register for all upcoming IAB meetings and IAB Academy courses.

IAB Publication Arm

The IAB publication arm produces various printed materials. The Communication Calendar is a tool to synchronise botulinum toxin therapy and physiotherapy in patients suffering from spasticity (Figure 17.2) (Adib Saberi et al. 2012). It is accompanied by an instruction manual. An evaluation study run by Hannover Medical School showed satisfactory results (Adib Saberi et al. 2015). The Communication Form connects different therapists involved in the treatment of a patient with a movement disorder. It is based on the International Classification of Functioning, Disability and Health (ICF) and the Goal Attainment Scale (GAS) (Adib Saberi et al. 2011). It is easy to use and was readily adopted by all IAB members. The Treatment Calendar monitors the dynamics of the botulinum toxin therapy in between injection series. It is based on a self-assessment scale. For use in cervical dystonia it was evaluated as the Dystonia Discomfort Scale (DDS) (Dressler et al. 2014). A patient book on botulinum toxin therapy explains the basic properties of botulinum toxin and all its major indications. The recently acquired Heiligendamm Video Productions has produced educational videos on movement disorders and their treatments for the last ten years.

IAB Academy

The newly started IAB Academy is focused on offering educational courses for all movement disorder therapists. It has

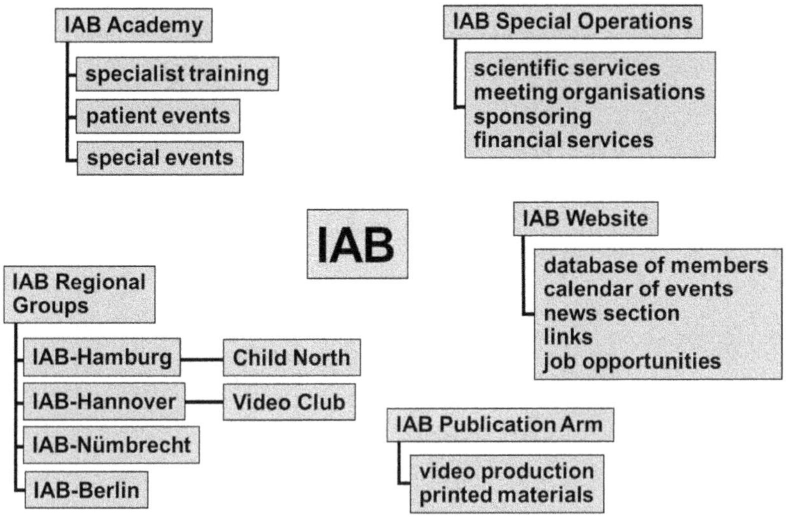

Figure 17.1 Structure of IAB – Interdisciplinary Working Group for Movement Disorders.

developed formalised postgraduate training to obtain protected and patented qualification as a movement disorders therapist according to the IAB concept (MDT-IAB). It is addressed to all therapists in the field of movement disorders. The qualification can be obtained through in-service training. Support can be requested from national German institutions. If attended besides regular employment it usually takes about one year to complete all necessary courses. Additionally, the IAB Academy offers CME-accredited lectures and events that may be open to patients and relatives as well. On special occasions the IAB Academy forms taskforces to organise consensus meetings and to publish consensus statements (Dressler et al. 2015; Dressler et al. 2016).

IAB Special Operations

IAB Special Operations is a provider for all services in the field of movement disorders, including scientific services, meeting organisations, sponsoring and financial services. IAB Special Operations wants to assist with all organisational problems in the field of movement disorders.

IAB Scientific Advisory Board

The multidisciplinary IAB Scientific Advisory Board consists of acknowledged movement disorders specialists, members of patient groups and professionals in law and business administration. It gives advice to the IAB organisations and helps with the specific skills of its members.

Outlook

IAB's stability over more than nine years and its expansion into more regions and other activities documents the demand for interdisciplinarity in diagnosis and treatment of movement disorders. Improving interdisciplinary collaboration, promoting education and developing methods to standardise diagnosis and to measure therapeutic effects can improve the quality of movement disorder diagnoses and treatment. Standards developed by IAB can help to maintain general therapeutic standards and thus protect both patient rights and the rights and interests of movement disorder therapists in an increasingly difficult environment. IAB has started to provide material for users outside Germany. Together with partners it may spread to other European countries.

References

Adib Saberi F, Dressler D (2011) Interdisciplinary Special Interest Groups (ISIG) for optimizing multimodal therapy of movement disorders. *Mov Disord* 26 (Suppl. 2):S47–S47.

Adib Saberi F, Pickenbrock H, Dressler D (2011) Communication calendar for botulinum toxin therapy of spasticity in an outpatient setting. In: *7th International Conference on Basic and Therapeutic Aspects of Botulinum and Tetanus Toxins*. Santa Fe, NM.

Adib Saberi F, Pickenbrock H, Dressler D (2012) Communication form for optimizing multimodal therapy of movement disorders. *Mov Disord* 27 (Suppl. 1):S292–S293.

Adib Saberi F, Pickenbrock HM, Dressler D (2015) The ComCal to facilitate the communication between physicians and physiotherapists in botulinum neurotoxin therapy of spasticity. *Toxicon* 93 (Suppl.): S55.

Dressler D, Kupsch A, Seitzinger A, Paus S (2014) The dystonia discomfort scale (DDS): a novel instrument to monitor the temporal profile of botulinum toxin therapy in cervical dystonia. *Eur J Neurol* 21:459–462.

Dressler D, Berweck S, Chatzikalfas A, Ebke M, Frank B, Hesse S, Huber M, Krauss JK, Mücke K-H, Nolte A, Oelmann H-D, Schönle PW, Schmutzler M, Pickenbrock H, Van der Ven C, Veelken N, Vogel M, Vogt T, Adib Saberi F (2015) Intrathecal baclofen therapy in Germany: proceedings of the IAB-Interdisciplinary Working Group for Movement Disorders consensus meeting. *J Neural Transm* 122:1573–1579.

Dressler D, Altenmueller E, Bhidayasiri R, Boholega S, Chana P, Chung TM, Frucht S, Garcia-Ruiz PJ, Kaelin A, Kaji R, Kanovsky P, Laskawi R, Micheli F, Orlova O, Relja M, Rosales R, Slawek J, Timerbaeva S, Warner TT, Adib Saberi F (2016) Strategies for treatment of dystonia. *J Neural Transm* 123:251–258.

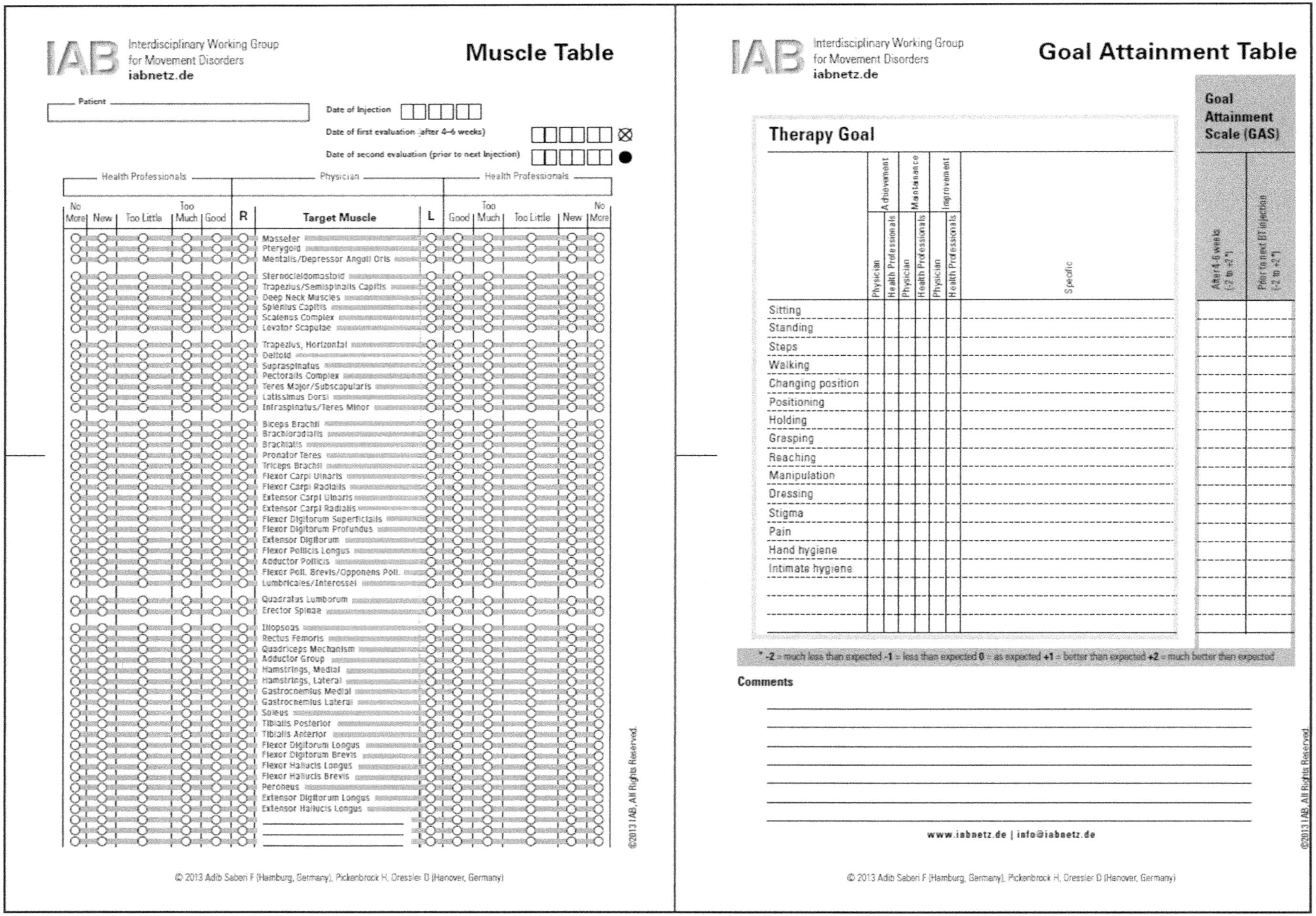

Figure 17.2 The Communication Calendar (CC) for improvement of interdisciplinary treatment of spasticity, linking physicians using botulinum toxin therapy and physiotherapists.

Chapter 18

The Role and Responsibility of the Dystonia Specialist Nurse

Marianne King

A dystonia specialist nurse (DSN) is a qualified Registered General Nurse (RGN) preferably with a BSc honours degree, with neurological experience and a special interest in this condition. This role came about when a nurse in the North East of England wanted to prove that a specialist nurse could give as effective a treatment with botulinum toxin (BT) therapy in an outreach setting as a consultant in a hospital environment (Barnes & Whittaker 2001). Their conclusions were that a DSN not only delivers safe and effective care, but also is financially viable and patient-friendly, and patients often preferred the outreach service:

> Thousands of patients in the UK suffering from long term conditions are helped by specialist nurses in many conditions. These type of health care professionals provide a level of care and support they could not do without. (RCN 2010)

A DSN, like any other specialist nurse, is dedicated to a particular area of nursing. Dystonia is a long-term incurable neurological condition needing complex management. A structured approach is necessary as each patient presents differently and disability fluctuates from person to person (Bowling 1997). Dystonia can cause a profound deterioration in a person's individual health together with severe social or financial difficulties. In the absence of cure or prevention, dystonia needs well-coordinated case management, liaising with other healthcare professionals where necessary. Historically, dystonia has been poorly managed due to lack of knowledge of the disease. It is therefore paramount for the DSN to raise public awareness of dystonia.

A specialist in this field delivers direct patient care, educates patients on symptom management and supports both patients and their caregivers. According to the Royal College of Nursing (Royal College of Nursing 2010), specialist nurses can prevent hospitalisation by providing as much information as possible and having the knowledge to explain to the patients their symptoms and treatments, and supporting them as much as possible. By providing a more holistic approach, patients are able to manage their own condition better. DSNs provide better access to the service as the nurse develops her/his own caseload, which leads to a service suited to the patient's condition. Patients are seen in a more timely manner, as the DSN's time is not as restricted as that of the consultant, who sees an array of neurological conditions. DSN clinics generally have fewer patients. Therefore there is scope to talk to patients, especially to those with complicated or psychological issues. DSNs also have the capacity to expedite appointments for patients where necessary. This leads to a decrease in complaints as the patients are being seen as and when needed, and when recommended by BT therapy guidelines. This also ensures optimum BT therapy outcome (Jankovic 2004).

DSNs take a leading role in ensuring that the best care possible is provided for their patients. Providing direct patient care, educating patients, caregivers and other healthcare professionals improves self-awareness. They understand and listen to their patients, providing a friendly, holistic and more approachable path to treatment. The patients are able to contact the DSN via phone to answer any questions they may have. This impacts on other healthcare professionals, such as consultants, GPs and casualty, freeing up their time to see more complicated or urgent cases. With the current government guidelines, a specialist nurse role helps to meet targets. Specialist nurses have also proven to reduce dropout rates as patients have continuity of care and regular organised appointments.

DSNs can provide care at the point of need by providing community-based care either in primary care trusts, general practitioner surgeries, community care homes or sometimes in the patient's own home.

The Dystonia Society UK reports:

> Botulinum toxin injections can be effectively provided through outreach services based in local community hospitals and health centres. In rural areas, outreach services address an important patient need. 35% of patients currently have a round trip travel time of more than 2 hours to their injection centre and, among this group, 55% report travel as a problem. The problem of travel is exacerbated by the fact that many patients are elderly – the average age of someone receiving botulinum injections is 60 years with 23% of patients over 70 years (Dystonia Society UK 2014).

Therefore, if the nurse travels to outreach clinics, rather than the patient to a regional centre by hospital transport, it could save the commissioners up to 45 per cent of the price of a hospital outpatient appointment; in other words, the further a patient travels by hospital transport the more it costs the commissioners (Dystonia Society UK 2014).

DSNs need to have extensive knowledge of their subject and of neurology in general. They need to be up to date with current issues, as patients' knowledge has improved through use of the internet and through patient organisations. DSNs should keep up to date by attending national and international conferences; they should network and reflect on their practice. Within these networking days, teaching packs are discussed, as well as problems for which solutions are often found. By networking, competencies, benchmarks, pathways, protocols and standards can be formalised and updated. These guidelines are often multi-professional, including general practitioners, patients, consultants, specialist nurses, patient organisations and other healthcare professionals. By using a shared care model, guidelines are patient-focused, current and safe, and so enhance quality. Shared care protocols or pathways are key developments and ensure that others have up-to-date information on the disease. There have been numerous anecdotal incidents of success with subjective appraisal of outcomes, including better relationships, team harmony, fewer conflicts, job satisfaction, better communication and improved professional growth (Peterson & Allen 1986; Jones & Ortiz 1989; McDonough 1996; cited in Anthony 2014). It is therefore the responsibility of the specialist nurse to be involved and to challenge poor-quality and out-of-date guidelines.

With the Nursing and Midwifery Council (NMC) code of conduct being revalidated in 2015, all registered nurses will have to demonstrate their fitness to practice. 'Every contact, action and decision made by a nurse is governed by core professional standards and principles. The standards by which nurses practice are key to the quality of the service provided' (NMC 2015).

A specialist nurse needs the skills to analyse data, leading to the ability to implement evidence-based care. This includes auditing the service to monitor and improve practice, ensuring what should be done is being carried out. Audits can also highlight areas needing improvements, such as developments of outreach clinics, more information or a friendlier waiting area, to name a few. By liaising with patient organisations such as the Dystonia Society UK, information can be delivered to patients. Many DSNs attend local meetings delivered by the Dystonia Society UK, which involves seeing patients outside the hospital environment.

In conclusion, specialist nurses, as highlighted in many reviews, are an asset to any service. They provide holistic care to each person individually. A patient with a personal nurse giving information, support and ensuring continuity of care appears to have an enhanced outcome as compared to those who have not. DSNs, with their extended knowledge, provide high levels of good judgement and make decisions with discretion. They ensure government targets are met and patients are given the treatment when and how they deserve. This can only lead to improved use of NHS resources in an already overstretched system.

References

Anthony M (2004). Shared governance models: the theory, practice, and evidence. *Online J Issues Nurs* 9(1). Available: www.nursingworld.org/MainMenuCategories/ANAMarketplace/ANAPeriodicals/OJIN/TableofContents/Volume92004/No1Jan04/SharedGovernanceModels.aspx.

Barnes MJ, Whittaker J (2001). Botulinum toxin for people with dystonia treated by an outreach nurse practitioner: a comparative study between home and clinic treatment service. *Eur J Neurol* 8:19–21.

Bowling A (1997). Measuring Health: A Review of Quality of Life Measurement Scale. 2nd edition. Buckingham: Open University Press.

Dystonia Society UK (2014). A guide to dystonia best practice. Available: www.dystonia.org.uk/pdf/Professional Research/GoodPracticeGuide(amendedNov2011).pdf.

Jankovic J (2004). Treatment of cervical dystonia with botulinum toxin. *Mov Disord* 19:109–115.

Jones, LS, Ortiz M (1989). Increasing nursing autonomy and recognition through shared governance. *Nurs Adm Q* 13(4):11–16.

McDonough KJ (1996). A shared governance system more structured than substance. *J Nurs Admin* 20:14–19.

NMC (Nursing and Midwifery Council) (2015). Professional staff quality services. Available: www.nmc-uk.org.

Peterson ME, Allen DG (1986). Shared governance: a strategy for transforming organizations, part 2. *J Nurs Admin* 16(2):11–16.

Royal College of Nursing (2010). Changing lives saving money. Available: www.rcn.org.

Chapter 19

History of Dystonia Treatments

Frank Erbguth

Introduction

Dystonia has a short scientific history in medicine. No conclusive aetiological concepts existed until the early twentieth century, and treatments were mainly of a symptomatic nature. Thereafter, along with organic aetiological concepts, agents focusing on neurotransmission were used for symptomatic treatment; psychologically oriented aetiological concepts prompted psychotherapeutic approaches, claiming causal therapeutic effect.

Spectrum of Dystonia Treatments from the Past Until Today

The development of therapeutic options in dystonic movement disorders has consisted of the approaches summarised in Table 19.1.

Treatments in the Nineteenth and Early Twentieth Centuries

The phenomenology of different forms of focal dystonia, such as blepharospasm, torticollis, oromandibular dystonia and writer's cramp was described in the nineteenth century by various authors, including Johann Heinrich Kopp (Kopp 1836), William Richard Gowers (Gowers 1888) and Henry Meige (Meige & Feindel 1902) as 'cramps' or 'occupational spasms'. While these publications hardly mentioned treatment strategies, Rene Cruchet (Cruchet 1907) presented in 1907 a book focusing on treatment of spasmodic torticollis in which he described across 836 pages numerous case reports with a variety of treatment options (Figure 19.1).

Along with the textbooks on clinical neurology at this time (e.g. Wilhelm Erb (Erb 1874) or Hermann Oppenheim (Oppenheim 1894), these case reports and series reports suggested the following treatments for dystonia:

- electric stimulation of the involved muscles and/or their antagonists (Figure 19.2);
- mechanical correction by bandages (Figure 19.3);
- orthopaedic surgery (e.g. achillotenotomy) for joint contractures;
- devices using imitation sensory tricks, which were identified as disease modifying (Figure 19.4);
- physiotherapy to suppress the dystonic-involved muscles and to strengthen their antagonists;
- medications with relaxing properties or with influence on neurotransmission such as bromine, atropine, scopolamine;
- hypnosis, suggestion therapy and psychological support in cases of supposed 'mental' focal dystonia;
- immobilisation and retraining in occupational dystonia (e.g. writer's cramp).

Generalised dystonia was described in the early twentieth century by two landmark papers: Walter Schwalbe from Berlin described in his doctoral thesis from 1908 the familial nature of generalised dystonia disorders in three siblings of the Jewish family Lewy ('A peculiar presentation of tonic spasms with hysterical symptoms') (Schwalbe 1908); and the German neurologist Hermann Oppenheim introduced the term 'dystonia' in 1911 in his description of generalised dystonia in four young patients

Table 19.1 Spectrum of dystonia treatments

Peripheral mechanical measures	Corrections of dystonic muscular overactivity and subsequent abnormal movements and postures by orthotic devices (e.g. ribbons, casts, splints), peripheral muscle and nerve surgery, electrotherapy, physiotherapy and chemodenervation with botulinum toxin
Psychological treatments and systemic relaxation therapies	Therapies focusing on the supposed psychological background of dystonia (non-specific psychotherapy, psychoanalysis, hypnosis, relaxation therapy, psychological counselling and support groups)
Pharmacological treatments	Medications focusing on either the peripheral (nerve, muscle) or central nervous overexcitation and neurotransmitter disturbances (narcotics, tranquillisers, (anticholinergics, dopaminergics, dopamine receptor antagonists, GABA-receptor antagonists)
Treatments using 'sensory trick circuits'	Feedback-training, sensory stimulation therapies
(Stereotactic) brain surgery	Thalamotomy, pallidotomy, deep brain stimulation

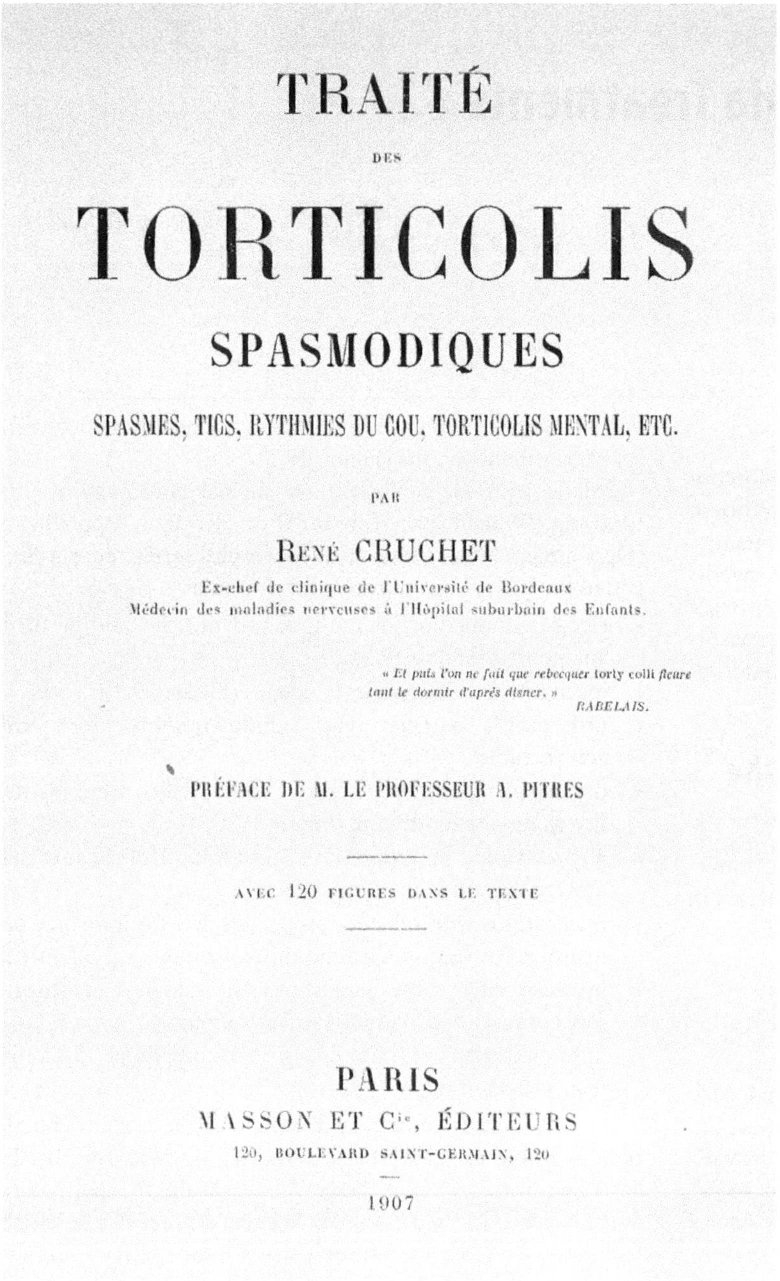
TRAITÉ

DES

TORTICOLIS

SPASMODIQUES

SPASMES, TICS, RYTHMIES DU COU, TORTICOLIS MENTAL, ETC.

PAR

RENÉ CRUCHET

Ex-chef de clinique de l'Université de Bordeaux
Médecin des maladies nerveuses à l'Hôpital suburbain des Enfants.

« Et puis l'on ne fait que rebecquer torty colli fleure tant le dormir d'après disner. »
RABELAIS.

PRÉFACE DE M. LE PROFESSEUR A. PITRES

AVEC 120 FIGURES DANS LE TEXTE

PARIS
MASSON ET Cie, ÉDITEURS
120, BOULEVARD SAINT-GERMAIN, 120

1907

Figure 19.1 Title page of Cruchet's book on treatment of spasmodic torticollis.

('About a peculiar cramping sickness in children and adolescents (dysbasia lordotica progressiva, dystonia musculorum deformans)' (Oppenheim 1911). In their publications, Schwalbe and Oppenheim described anecdotally several treatment trials in their patients, such as suggestion, hypnosis, casts, splints, orthopaedic surgery and various medications, which all had no or only temporary effect. Among the medications used, atropine was considered to have a certain positive effect on the cramps. However, both pioneers of the scientific perception of generalised dystonia made no explicit therapeutic suggestions at all.

Psychotherapy and Psychoanalysis

After the early twentieth century, neurological interest in dystonia dropped for decades; psychiatry, especially under the strong psychoanalytic influence of the period, avidly offered Freudian hypotheses of conversion disorder to explain the bizarre contorted and disfiguring postures of focal and generalised dystonia. Accordingly, psychoanalytic sessions and conflict uncovering psychotherapy were recommended as first-line therapy of dystonia and were the preferred treatment options of focal dystonia till the 1970s (Paterson & Lond 1945; Mitscherlich 1971).

Oral Medications

Pharmacologic treatment of dystonia has focused on medications influencing both central and peripheral pharmacology, though these were often only modestly effective and frequently caused significant adverse effects.

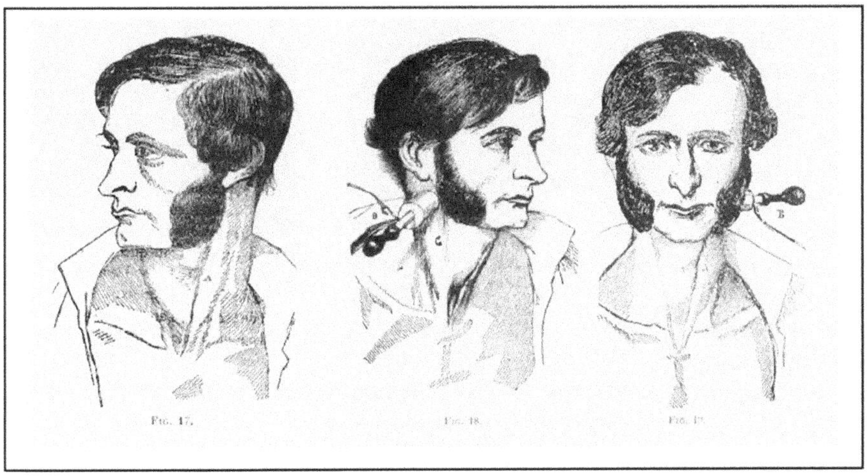

Figure 19.2 Electrotherapy in rotatory spasmodic torticollis to the right (left) with stimulation of the antagonistic right (middle) and the overactive left (right) sternocleidomastoid muscle.

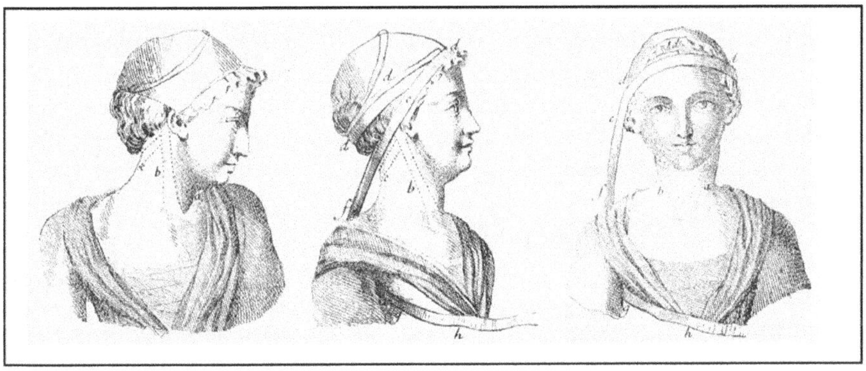

Figure 19.3 Effective correction of rotatory spasmodic torticollis to the left (left) by an application of a metallic ribbon (middle and right).

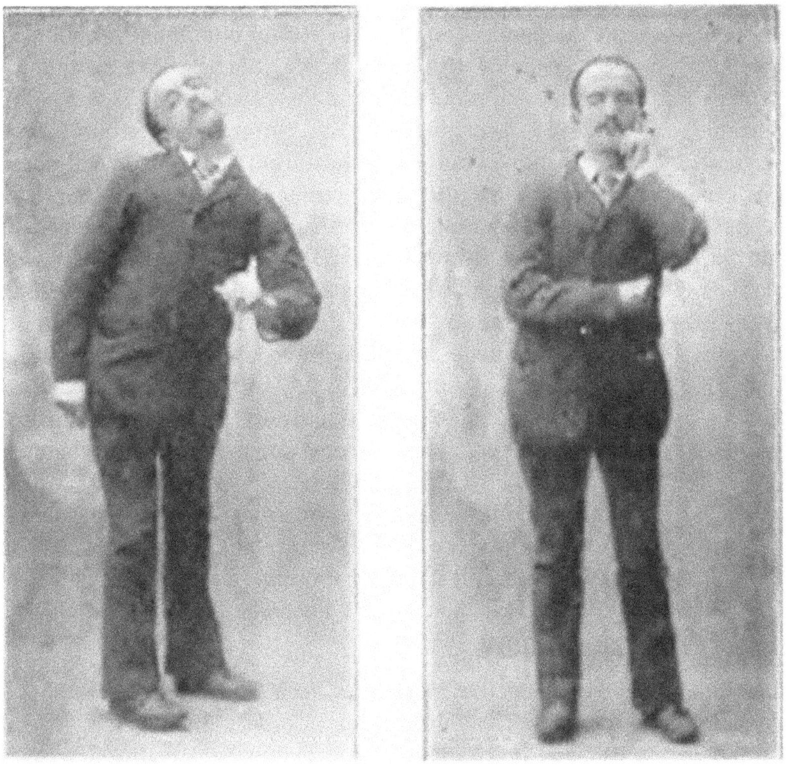

Figure 19.4 Effective correction of segmental dystonia by a sensory trick gesture.

In advancement of historical **anticholinergic treatments** with atropine and scopolamine, oral administration of trihexyphenidyl was studied and preferred for dystonia treatment (Burke et al. 1986). Other anticholinergic agents have been used with variable success, including benztropine, biperiden, procyclidine and orphenadrine (Cloud & Jinnah 2010). The presynaptic GABA receptor agonist **baclofen**, which primarily is used to treat spasticity, has been used for oral treatment of generalised dystonia – particularly in children. The substance has also been applied intrathecally and intraventricularly for treatment of generalised dystonia refractory to oral medication (Cloud & Jinnah 2010). **Levodopa**, which is effective and safe in dopa-responsive dystonia, was used to treat other generalised dystonia with contradictory results. Other dopaminergic agents including bromocriptine, apomorphine and lisuride have been studied for dystonia treatment with inconclusive results. **Dopamine receptor antagonists** such as classic (e.g. haloperidol) and atypical (e.g. clozapine, quetiapine, risperidone) antipsychotics showed inconclusive data; coupled with their side-effect profile these have generally been discouraged in dystonia treatment. The **dopamine depletor** tetrabenazine has been found to be effective for the treatment of a variety of hyperkinetic movement disorders, including chorea, tics, tardive dyskinesia, myoclonus, and also in focal and generalised dystonia. **Benzodiazepines** are often used in dystonia, of which clonazepam is the most frequently used in various forms. Multiple **other drugs** have been used to treat dystonia in small, open trials. These agents include oral and intravenous lidocaine, riluzole, lithium, antiepileptic drugs, tizanidine and nabilone (Cloud & Jinnah 2010).

Muscle Surgery and Peripheral Denervations

Myotomy of the sternocleidomastoid muscle was introduced in the nineteenth century; however, this procedure showed poor long-term results. Selective denervation of branches of the accessory nerve in cervical dystonia was one of the preferred procedures, before botulinum toxin entered and dominated the therapy, showing good results in 80 per cent of cases (Bertrand 1993). Denervation of branches of the facial nerve was performed in patients with blepharospasm. However, the treatment severely affected eye closure (Figure 19.5). In analogy to the concept of vascular compression in trigeminal neuralgia, hemifacial spasm and vestibular paroxysm and its treatment by Janneta's microvascular decompression, this operation was also performed in patients with spasmodic torticollis (Jho & Jannetta 1995).

Physical and Occupational Therapy

Physical and occupational therapy are the oldest concepts of dystonia treatments, focusing on centrally and peripheral mediated improvement of symptoms, sometimes maximising the use of sensory tricks to ameliorate dystonic activity. In advancement of historical ideas of immobilising muscles involved in dystonia, sensorimotor retuning, also known as constraint-induced movement therapy, may be useful in hand dystonia, e.g. writer's cramp and musician's dystonia. The technique

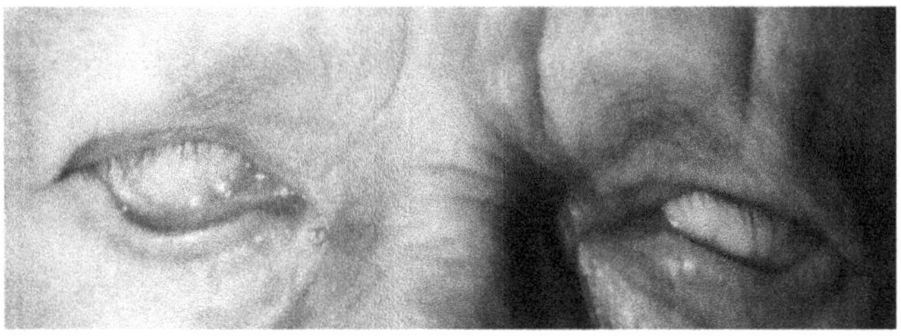

Figure 19.5 Patient with blepharospasm with severe Bell's phenomenon after surgical denervation of facial nerve branches innervating the orbicularis oculi muscle.

consists of splinting the non-dystonic fingers, thereby forcing the dystonic finger to work in concert with the other fingers to complete the desired task (Cloud & Jinnah 2010).

The Therapeutic Breakthrough: Botulinum Toxin and Deep Brain Stimulation

The treatment armamentarium in dystonia has dramatically changed over the last 30 years, first with the introduction of botulinum toxin injections for the treatment of focal dystonia and then with the advent of deep brain surgery for generalised dystonia.

Botulinum Toxin

The idea for the use of botulinum toxin was first expressed by the German poet and physician Justinus Kerner in 1822 (Erbguth & Naumann 1999). One hundred and fifty years later his idea was realised and implemented by the ophthalmologist Alan B. Scott in San Francisco, based on preparatory work of the botulinum toxin experts Daniel B. Drachman, Edward Schantz, Arnold Burgen, Eric Johnson and others (Scott 1994). With the publication of 67 successful botulinum toxin injections in patients with strabismus by Alan B. Scott, botulinum toxin was established as a novel therapeutic agent (Scott 1980). By the 1980s, Scott and many other groups injected the US type A preparation of botulinum toxin (initially named Oculinum®, later Botox®) for the treatment of blepharospasm, cervical, laryngeal, oromandibular and hand dystonia. Simultaneously, a British type A preparation (Dysport®) was effectively used for the treatment of all forms of focal dystonia. A German type A preparation (Xeomin®) free of the complexing botulinum toxin proteins, and therefore considered not to generate antibodies, was launched in 2005. A toxin B product named Neurobloc®/Myobloc™ was registered in 2000. Additional Asian type A preparations come from the Lanzhou Institute of Biological Products in China (Hengli®, Prosigne®), where the manufacturing expertise came from Yinchun Wang, a former collaborator of Edward Schantz, and from the Medy-Tox Company in South Korea (Neuronox®).

Brain Surgery

The use of ablative procedures, such as pallidotomy and thalamotomy, to treat movement disorders, including dystonia, dates back to the 1940s (Cloud & Jinnah 2010). Though these procedures can be effective in treating different types of dystonia, they have largely been replaced by deep brain stimulation. Dystonia has been treated effectively with deep brain stimulation in the internal segment of the globus pallidus since the late 1990s. Initial trials focused on primary generalised dystonia until recently; sham-controlled trials have shown efficacy in cervical dystonia (Kupsch et al. 2006; Volkmann et al. 2014).

References

Bertrand CM (1993) Selective peripheral denervation for spasmodic torticollis: surgical technique, results, and observations in 260 cases. *Surg Neurol* 40:96–103.

Burke RE, Fahn S, Marsden CD (1986) Torsion dystonia: a double-blind, prospective trial of high-dosage trihexyphenidyl. *Neurology* 36:160–164.

Cloud LJ, Jinnah HA (2010) Treatment strategies for dystonia. *Expert Opin Pharmacother* 11:5–15.

Cruchet R (1907) *Traité des torticolis spasmodiques, spasmes, tics, rythmes du cou, torticolis mental, etc.* Masson, Paris.

Erb W (1874) *Handbuch der Krankheiten des Nervensystems.* Vogel, Leipzig.

Erbguth FJ, Naumann M (1999) Historical aspects of botulinum toxin: Justinus Kerner (1786–1862) and the 'sausage poison'. *Neurology* 53:1850–1853.

Gowers WR (1888) *A Manual of Diseases of the Nervous System.* J and A Churchill, London.

Jho HD, Jannetta PJ (1995) Microvascular decompression for spasmodic torticollis. *Acta Neurochir (Wien)* 134:21–26.

Kopp JH (1836) *Denkwürdigkeiten in der ärztlichen Praxis.* Hermann, Frankfurt.

Kupsch A, Benecke R, Müller J, Trottenberg T, Schneider GH, Poewe W, Eisner W, Wolters A, Müller JU, Deuschl G, Pinsker MO, Skogseid IM, Roeste GK, Vollmer-Haase J, Brentrup A, Krause M, Tronnier V, Schnitzler A, Voges J, Nikkhah G, Vesper J, Naumann M, Volkmann J, Deep-Brain Stimulation for Dystonia Study Group (2006) Pallidal deep-brain stimulation in primary generalized or segmental dystonia. *N Engl J Med* 355:1978–1990.

Meige H, Feindel E (1902) *Les tics et leur traitmant.* Masson, Paris.

Mitscherlich M (1971) Spasmodic torticollis. *Psychother Psychosom* 19:62–75.

Oppenheim H (1894) *Lehrbuch der Nervenkrankheiten für Ärzte und Studierende.* Karger, Berlin.

Oppenheim H (1911) Über eine eigenartige Krampfkrankheit des kindlichen und jugendlichen Alters (Dysbasia lordotica progressiva, Dystonia musculorum deformans). *Neurol Centrabl* 30:1090–1107.

Paterson MT, Lond MB (1945) Spasmodic torticollis: results of psychotherapy in 21 cases. *Lancet* 246:556–559.

Schwalbe W (1908) Eine eigentümliche tonische Krampfform mit hysterischen Symptomen. Inaugural Diss. G. Schade, Berlin.

Scott AB (1980) Botulinum toxin injection into extraocular muscles as an alternative to strabismus surgery. *Ophthalmology* 87:1044–1049.

Scott AB (1994) Foreword. In: Jankovic J, Hallett M (eds) *Therapy with Botulinum Toxin.* Marcel Dekker, New York, pp. vii–ix.

Volkmann J, Mueller J, Deuschl G, Kühn AA, Krauss JK, Poewe W, Timmermann L, Falk D, Kupsch A, Kivi A, Schneider GH, Schnitzler A, Südmeyer M, Voges J, Wolters A, Wittstock M, Müller JU, Hering S, Eisner W, Vesper J, Prokop T, Pinsker M, Schrader C, Kloss M, Kiening K, Boetzel K, Mehrkens J, Skogseid IM, Ramm-Pettersen J, Kemmler G, Bhatia KP, Vitek JL, Benecke R, DBS Study Group for Dystonia (2014) Pallidal neurostimulation in patients with medication-refractory cervical dystonia: a randomised, sham-controlled trial. *Lancet Neurol* 13:875–884.

Chapter 20

Dystonia in Arts and Artists

Hansjörg Bäzner and Christian Riederer

Introduction

In the 1970s, the British neurologist C. David Marsden gathered under the heading of dystonias many disparate entities, such as writer's cramp, torticollis and blepharospasm (Marsden 1976a). Additionally, he drew attention to representations of dystonic conditions in arts when he referred to a sixteenth-century painting of a yawning man by the Flemish Renaissance painter Pieter Brueghel the Elder (1525–1569), and even proposed the term 'Brueghel's syndrome' as an eponym for the blepharospasm–oromandibular dystonia syndrome (Marsden 1976b). Similar depictions of deformations, spasms and convulsions can be found in all art forms, including literature, painting and sculpture. These works were not primarily created to illustrate medical conditions and do not always show pathological conditions, but they often record morbid characteristics that the artists noticed and observed.

Recent additions to the literature on abnormal postures in art include the publications of Garcia-Ruiz and colleagues, who investigated drawings and sculptures from the ancient Egypt and Moche civilisations, as well as contemporary artworks (Garcia-Ruiz et al. 2015), a report on facial dystonia in a drawing by Giovanni Agostino da Lodi from the early sixteenth century (Bono et al. 2015) and the evaluation of neurologic and dystonic conditions in the famous 'Cantigas de Santa Maria', a vast illustrated collection of monophonic songs from the thirteenth century (Gondim et al. 2015).

While most neurologists will confirm that a walk through large art collections may educe associations with various neurological diseases, including dystonia, many artists were simply intrigued by abnormal human body postures. Most did not mean to feature a disease or dystonia at all, so that any observation in this context must be interpreted with caution.

Distorted Bodies and Extremities

The medical history of dystonia in a narrower sense is relatively young, but artworks include evidence of the existence of its peculiar symptoms long before they were discussed by medical writers. For example, a sketch by the Italian Baroque painter Baldassare Franceschini (Volterrano) in the Musée du Louvre in Paris, 'Il gobbo Trafedi' ('the hunchback Trafedi'; around 1663), shows a hunchbacked dwarf, a servant in the Medici household, leaning on a balustrade and exhibiting a dystonic leg posture. Similarly, the painting 'El pie varo' ('The club-foot'; 1642) by Spanish artist Jose de Ribera (1591–1652), also housed in the Louvre, shows a picturesque young beggar who carries a crutch across his shoulder and holds a piece of paper in his hand to incite people to charitable donations (Figure 20.1). His

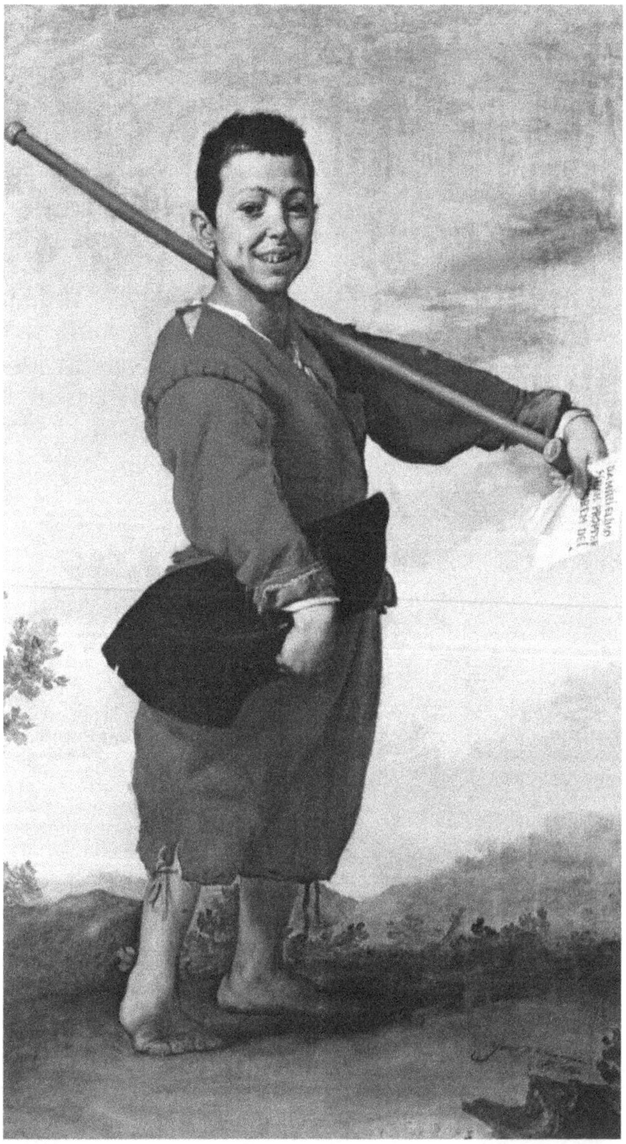

Figure 20.1 'El patizambo (The clubfooted boy)' from Jose de Ribera, 1642.

right foot and ankle have the form of a club foot, leaving room for speculation on the causes of the deformation.

Another fine example of the similarity between artistic and scientific depictions of dystonic conditions is the painting 'The crippled boy', an early work by the Spanish artist José Gallegos y Arnosa (1857–1917). The posture of this boy with ripped trousers and a crutch in his left hand, perhaps begging, strikingly resembles the appearance of a young boy included in Hermann Oppenheim's famous 1911 treatise on 'dystonia musculorum deformans' that was pivotal in popularising the term 'dystonia' (Oppenheim 1911).

Similarly, good representations of dystonic hands were provided by Edouard Castres (1838–1902) in his 'Porteuse d'eau au bord du Nil' ('Water-carrier on the Nile') and by Piero della Francesca (1415–1492) in his painting of St. Chiare (Clare) d'Assisi (around 1460–1470). The masterful Isenheim altarpiece by the German Matthias Grünewald (sixteenth century) also includes representations of deformed extremities, sometimes interpreted as the result of ergotism, which was epidemic in the late Middle Ages (Garcia de Yébenes & Garcia de Yébenes 1991). Dystonic conditions are also present in the engravings of the baroque French printmaker Jacques Callot (1592–1635). A less known but convincing example of a dystonic foot is included in the engravings by Louis Basile Carré de Montgeron (1686–1754) of 'la demoiselle Fourcroy' (1732), representative of a series of miraculous faith healings in France known as the 'Convulsionnaires of Saint-Médard' (De Montgeron 1741). As this story is relatively unknown, we cite the 1864 report by Robert Dale Owen in *The Atlantic Monthly* in 1864 (Owen 1864):

> The Demoiselle Fourcroy, alleged to have been suddenly cured, on the fourteenth of April, 1732, by means of these convulsions, of a confirmed anchylosis, which had deformed her left foot, and which the physicians had pronounced incurable, thus describes, in her deposition, her sensations: 'They caused me to take wine in which was some earth from the tomb of M. de Paris, and I immediately engaged in prayer .... 'Almost at the same moment I was seized with a great shuddering, and soon after with a violent agitation of the members, which caused my whole body to jerk into the air, and gave me a force I had never before possessed, so that the united strength of several persons present could scarcely restrain me. After a time, in the course of these violent convulsive movements, I lost all consciousness. As soon as they passed off, I recovered my senses, and felt a sensation of tranquility and internal peace, such as I had never experienced before.'

Not all depictions of dystonia were focused on illustrating morbid conditions, so they should be interpreted with caution. A good example is the artist Egon Schiele (1890–1918), whose oeuvre contains, at first glance, clear examples of cervical dystonia, Meige (or Brueghel) syndrome and generalised dystonia. Schiele was a leading Austrian expressionist painter who, as the protégé of Gustav Klimt, strongly influenced the Viennese artistic scene during the early twentieth century. His depiction of his own body in self-portraits in a twisted, contorted, dystonia-like pose, together with contemporary photographs that capture the artist in dystonic postures, have raised questions about whether he suffered dystonia. According to an excellent recent article, there are, however, no grounds to accept this hypothesis (Erbguth 2010). Schiele's concept of distorted and at times bizarre body postures reflected, in fact, a confluence of the expressionist formal style of displaying extroverted emotions and psychological conflicts with the emerging interest in Vienna's art scene and intellectual circles with photographs of patients with movement disorders. There are reliable indications, for instance, that Schiele was familiar with the images of psychiatric and neurological disorders published in the 'Iconographie Photographique de la Salpêtrière' and the later 'Nouvelle Iconographie de la Salpêtrière', including hysterical and dystonic postures. Further, he was an admirer of expressionist performing artists such as the dancers Erwin Dom Osen and Moa. The brevity of Schiele's life adds to the popular fantasy of the outlaw who lived fast and died young. Quite remarkably, photographs of Schiele on his deathbed show him in a posture suggestive of head and neck dystonia.

Segmental Dystonia in the Arts

The dystonic condition 'torticollis' (wry neck) has a remarkable history. For example, François Rabelais (1483–1553) uses the term in several chapters of his monumental novel, *La vie de Gargantua et de Pantagruel*' (1532–1564). In a closer medical context, the Dutch surgeon Nicolaes Tulp (1593–1674), well known from his depiction in Rembrandt's 'De anatomische les van Dr. Nicolaes Tulp' ('The anatomy lesson of Dr. Nicolaes Tulp'; 1632), referred to spasmodic torticollis and proposed a surgical treatment ('curatio obstipi capitis') by dissecting the sternocleidomastoid muscle in his 'Observationes medicae' of 1652 (Tulp 1652; Figure 20.2).

In the nineteenth century, scientific interest in the condition increased dramatically, driven particularly by contributions from the Salpêtrière Hospital in Paris. Much has been already written about the contributions to artistic depictions of parkinsonism by Paul Richer (1849–1933), Jean Martin Charcot's laboratory chief and professor at the École nationale supérieure des Beaux-Arts in Paris, but his drawings and sketches of dystonic conditions are also remarkable. Influenced by Charcot's research into hysteria, he published the monograph *Paralysies et contractures hystériques* in 1892, featuring a vast number of scientific drawings, as well as references to a grotesque relief on the campanile of the church Santa Maria Formosa in Venice (Richer 1892).

Further noteworthy examples of medical depictions of torticollis are found in the publications of the prominent French neurologist Édouard Brissaud (1852–1909), who coined the term 'torticollis mental' and provided photographs of his patients in 1894 (Brissaud 1893–1894). Such photographical documentation was not entirely new. An excellent photograph of a patient with torticollis was included in the 1872 edition of the *Revue photographique des hopitaux de Paris* (Bourneville & Demontméja 1872).

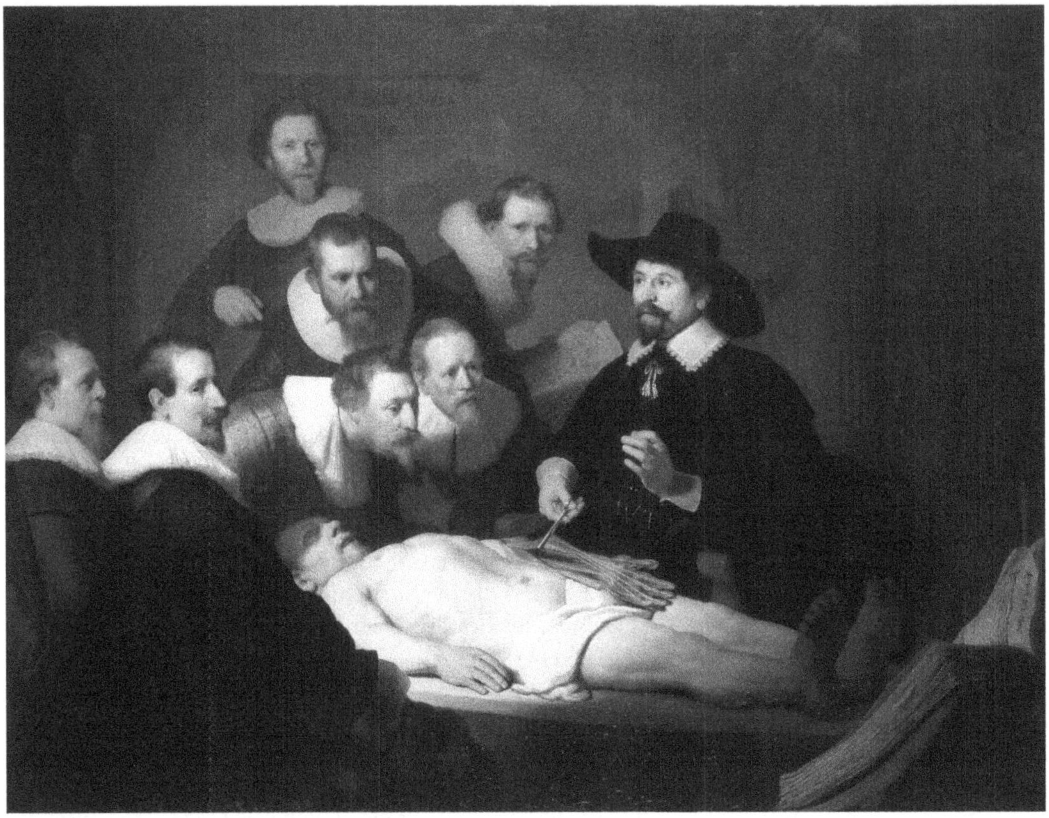

Figure 20.2 'The anatomy lesson of Dr. Nicolaes Tulp', Rembrandt van Rijn, 1632.

A noteworthy sculptural representation of torticollis was produced by the Romanian artist Constantin Brâncuşi (1876–1957), whose sculpture 'Souffrance' or 'Le Supplice II' ('Suffering', 'Torture'; 1952) is a bust of a young boy with an obviously painful cervical deformation (Garcia Ruiz & Martinez Castrillo 2009). Also intriguing are the artworks of the German-Austrian sculptor Franz Xaver Messerschmidt (1736–1783), the production of whose series of 69 busts, the so-called 'character heads', was presumably inspired by his close friend, the Viennese doctor and miracle healer Franz Anton Mesmer (1734–1815) (Husslein-Arco 2013). Two heads feature facial convulsions, one being a yawing man (Figure 20.3) and the other a man with clear eyestrain (Figure 20.4). The yawning head resembles Caravaggio's 'Medusa' (1596), as well as Brueghel's 'De Gaper' from the mid-sixteenth century.

Dystonia in Artists

Two subtypes of focal dystonia are of particular interest when discussing the artists themselves: writer's cramp and musician's dystonia. The Italian physician Bernardino Ramazzini (1633–1714) identified writer's cramp as an occupational disorder in professional writers in his landmark oeuvre *De morbis artificium diatribe* (1700) (Ramazzini 1700). One famous sufferer in recent times was the famous physician and missionary Albert Schweitzer (1875–1965), who tried to cope with these muscle cramps by slowing down his handwriting, using special pens or holding pens in a way to allow him to write more clearly (Tacik et al. 2012). More than 300 years ago, artists such as Lucas Ciamberlanus (born around 1580) and Johann Christoph Albrecht (active 1692–1725), among others, documented the appropriate manner for holding a pen or a quill. This does not establish that writer's cramp was known by these authors, but may reflect continuous discussion about writing techniques that are most comfortable and less likely to induce fatigue or cramp.

Musician's dystonia, on the other hand, most commonly affects the hand, causing fingers to curl under or to jut out inappropriately. It occurs not only among pianists but also among string and woodwind players, guitarists and percussionists. In addition, brass and woodwind players are susceptible to embouchure dystonia, which may cause the lips to tremble or the jaw to lock, or to otherwise affect the face, mouth and tongue. The manner in which body, arm and hand are positioned for piano playing has certainly changed in recent centuries, but this was already an important matter in Victor Haddoff's illustrations from 1782, in which he compared correct and incorrect positions at the piano.

The most famous historical example of an artist with focal dystonia was the German pianist Robert Schumann (1810–1856), one of the most prominent composers of the early romantic period. He displayed extraordinary skills at the piano early in adolescence and planned a career as a concert pianist. After initial success, increasing technical difficulties hampered his progress in the years 1831 and 1832. He noted in his diary: '2 hours finger exercises – Toccata 10 times – finger exercises 6 times – variations 20 times myself – and it still didn't

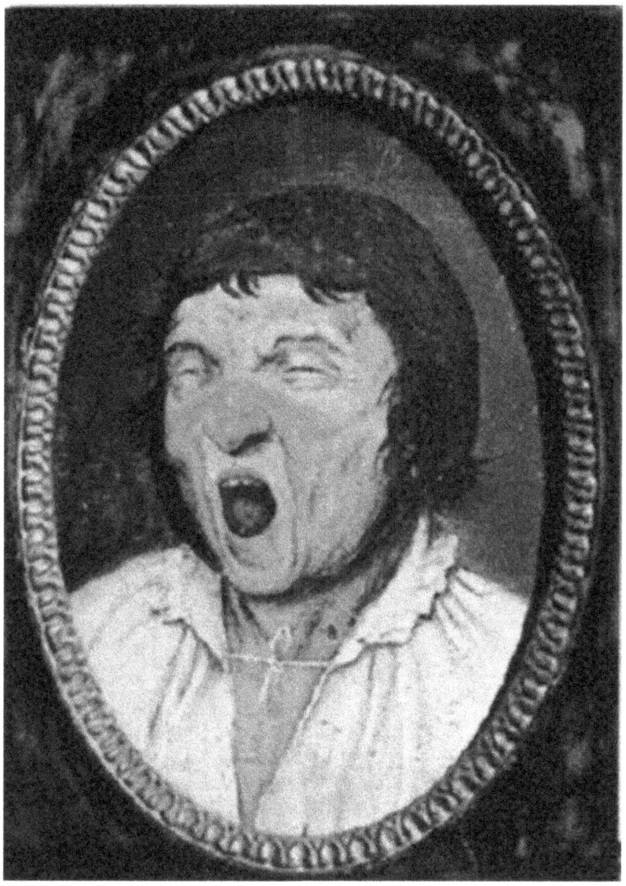

Figure 20.3 'De Gaper' (Yawning Man), Pieter Bruegel the Elder, Musées royaux des Beaux-Arts de Belgique, Brussels, Belgium.

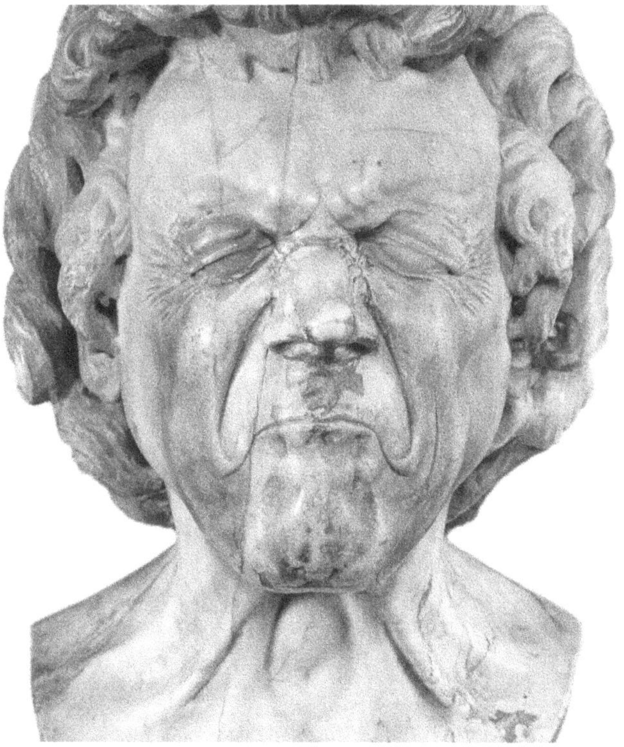

Figure 20.4 'Character Head' by Franz Xaver Messerschmidt (1736–1783), Belvedere, Vienna, Austria.

work with the Alexander variations in the evening – frustration over this – extreme frustration (January 4, 1830)'. As has been excellently explored by Eckart Altenmüller (Altenmüller & Jabusch 2010), he developed a task-specific loss of voluntary control of the middle finger of his right hand. By means of a finger-stretching device ('Cigarrenmechanik') Schumann tried to relieve his situation. In parallel, he composed his 'Toccata' (opus 7), a piano work that allowed a high-level virtuoso performance without requiring the middle finger of the right hand. However, from 1833 he almost completely ceased playing written scores, but continued to improvise at the piano. It seems apparent that Schumann suffered a focal, task-specific dystonia of the right hand, now referred to as pianist's cramp.

The American pianist Leon Fleisher (born 1928) also suffers from focal dystonia. He has been very successfully treated with botulinum toxin injections and was able to return to the concert podium to perform highly acclaimed recitals and to record respected CDs, as documented in the acclaimed documentary *Two Hands*. Citing a 2007 article by Oliver Sacks in *Reader's Digest 2007*:

> At the end of our visit that day at my home, Fleisher agreed to play something on my piano, a beautiful old 1894 Bechstein concert grand that I had grown up with – my father's piano. Fleisher sat at the piano and carefully, tenderly stretched each finger. Then, with his arms and hands almost flat across the keyboard, he started to play. He played a piano transcription of the Bach cantata 'Sheep May Safely Graze', as arranged for piano by Egon Petri. Never, I thought, had this piano been played by such a master. I had the feeling that Fleisher had sized up the piano's character within seconds that he had matched his playing to the instrument, to bring out its greatest potential. Fleisher seemed to distill the beauty, drop by drop, like an alchemist, into flowing notes of an almost unbearable beauty. (Sacks 2007)

References

Altenmüller E, Jabusch HC. 2010. Focal dystonia in musicians: phenomenology, pathophysiology, triggering factors, and treatment. *Med Probl Perform Art* 25:3–9.

Bono F, Morelli M, Quattrone A. 2015. Facial dystonia as depicted in art in the time of Leonardo da Vinci. *Lancet Neurol* 14:351. doi: 10.1016/S1474-4422(15)70012-8.

Bourneville DM, Demontméja A. 1872. *Revue photographique des hopitaux de Paris*. Paris. Delahaye.

Brissaud E. 1893–1894. *Vingt-quatrième leçon. Tics et spasmes cloniques de la face. Leçons sur les maladies nerveuses: La Salpêtrière*. Paris. Masson.

Carre De Montgeron, LB. 1741. *Continuation Des Demonstrations De Miracles Operes a L'intercession De M. De Paris & Autres Appelans. Observations Sur L'oeuvre Des Convulsions et Sur L'etat Des Convulsionnaires*. Tome Second.

Erbguth FJ. 2010. Egon Schiele and dystonia. *Front Neurol Neurosci* 27:46–60.

García de Yébenes J, García de Yébenes P. 1991. Dystonia in the painting of Matias Grunewald: epidemic ergotism in the late middle ages. *Arch Neurobiol (Madr)* 54:37–40.

Garcia Ruiz PJ, Martinez Castrillo JC. 2009. Cervical dystonia and Constantin Brancusi. *Mov Disord* 24:1849–1850.

Garcia-Ruiz PJ, Slawek J, Sitek EJ, Martinez Castrillo JC. 2015. Art and dystonia. *J Neurol Sci* 356:49–54.

Gondim Fde A, Griesbach SH, Thomas FP. 2015. Neuropsychiatric phenomena in the medieval text Cantigas de Santa Maria. *Neurology* 84(19):1991–1996.

Husslein-Arco A (ed.). 2013. *Franz Xaver Messerschmidt-Charakterköpfe*. Wien. Belvedere.

Marsden CD. 1976a. The problem of adult-onset idiopathic torsion dystonia and other isolated dyskinesias in adult life (including blepharospasm, oromandibular dystonia, dystonic writer's cramp, and torticollis, or axial dystonia). *Adv Neurol* 14:259–276.

Marsden CD. 1976b. Blepharospasm-oromandibular dystonia syndrome (Brueghel's syndrome): a variant of adult-onset torsion dystonia? *J Neurol Neurosurg Psychiatry* 39:1204–1209.

Oppenheim H. 1911. Über eine eigenartige Krampfkrankheit des kindlichen und jugendlichen Alters (Dysbasia lordotica progressiva, Dystonia musculorum deformans). *Neurologisches Centralblatt* 30:1090–1107.

Owen, RD. 1864. The Convulsionists of Saint-Medard. *The Atlantic Monthly* February–March.

Ramazzini B. 1700. *De morbis artificum diatriba*. Modena. Antonii Capponi.

Richer P. 1892. *Paralysies et contractures hystériques*. Paris. Octave Doin.

Sacks O. 2007. Hand delivered: how a top musician overcame the crudest crises of all. *Reader's Digest* (November): 69–72.

Tacik P, Schrader C, Weber E, Dressler D. 2012. Albert Schweitzer: a patient with writer's cramp. *Parkinsonism Relat Disord* 18:453–457.

Tulp N. 1652. *Observationes medicae* (2nd edition). Amsterdam. Ludovicum Elzeviriu.

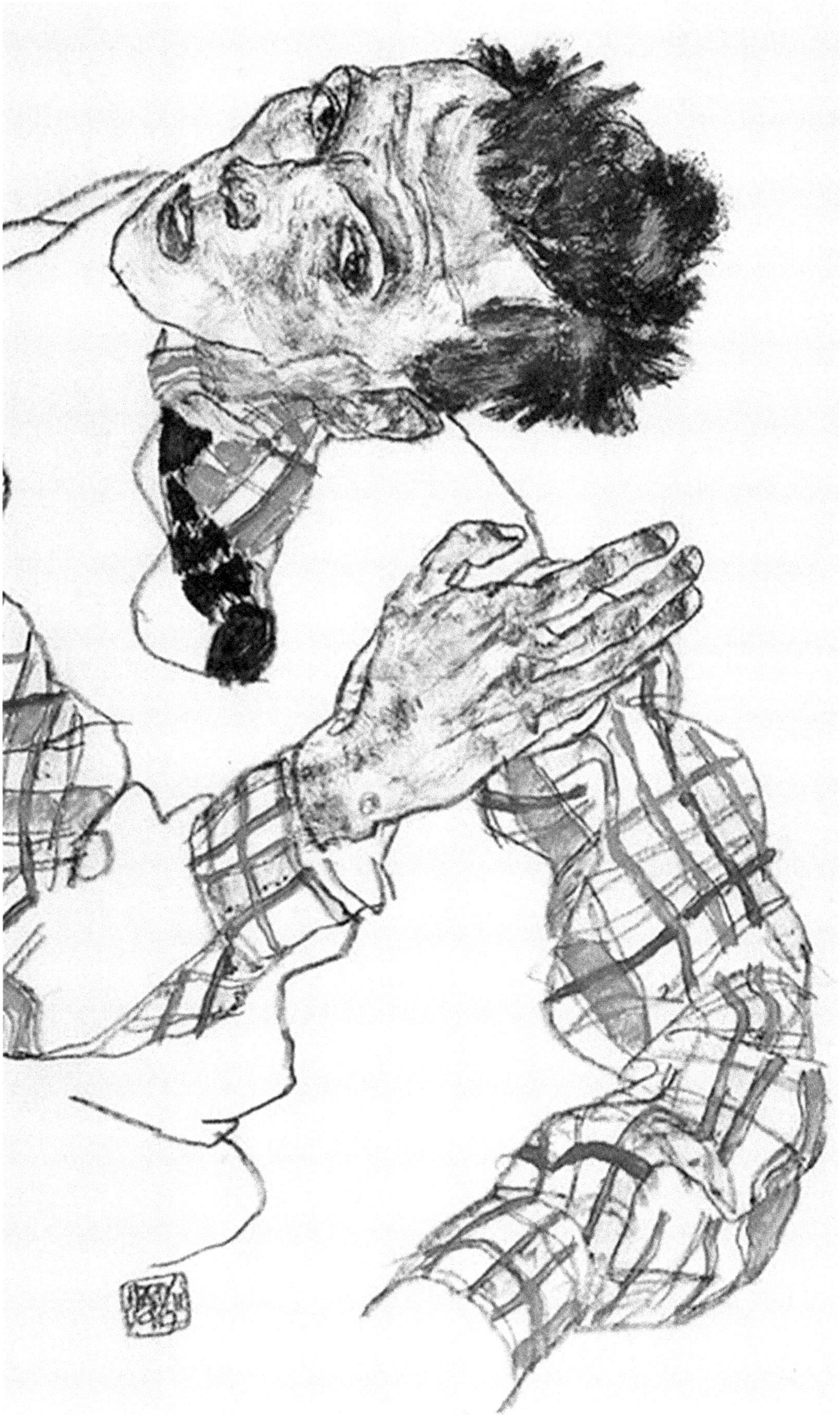

Chapter 21

The Global Market for Botulinum Toxin

Andy Pickett*

There is little doubt that botulinum toxin (BoNT) has been one of the most successful and enduring products ever developed in the world of pharmaceuticals. Since the first publication from Alan Scott, in the 1970s (Scott et al. 1973), use of the BoNT products in the worlds of both therapeutic and aesthetic treatments has grown year-on-year. For products that were first licenced in the late 1980s, nearly 30 years ago, their use has widened, not faded. Their applicability to bringing real benefit to patients in a multitude of ways and improving the quality of life of countless people cannot be overstated. Although not life-saving, the BoNT products are now a mainstay of many areas of neurology, urology and pain treatment. New uses are being identified on a regular basis and shown clinically to be of important value in patient treatments.

The financial size of the BoNT market is notoriously difficult to determine. While accurate data are kept for therapeutic usage, no equivalent data exist for the aesthetic market. Estimates in the order of $2 billion are currently available, growing to $20 billion in a decade. But in fact the potential financial returns could be described as limitless, given the number of new uses being highlighted.

In the beginning there were two products – Oculinum® and Dysport®. Oculinum®, pioneered by Alan Scott through his company Oculinum Inc., started life on the west coast of the United States at the Smith-Kettlewell Institute. Dysport®, pioneered through doctors and the Centre for Applied Microbiology and Research, was born in the United Kingdom after several UK doctors had trained with Alan Scott and realised the huge potential of such a product to treat difficult diseases, such as strabismus, which only had surgical interventions until then (Elston & Russell 1985). Oculinum® was purchased by Allergan soon after licensing in the United States and became Botox®. The background to Oculinum® has been described recently (Pickett 2013). Botox® became firmly established in the United States and, shortly afterwards, Europe and the rest of the world. Dysport® did not reach the United States until 2009, for many reasons that have not yet been described, but this gave a virtual monopoly to Allergan for many years and enabled that brand to become world-dominant.

Both of these first-generation serotype A products contain the active neurotoxin complexed with a range of other natural accessory proteins, often termed neurotoxin-associated proteins (NAPs). Despite much commercial argument over many years between companies, these NAPs have been found to clearly separate from the active BoNT upon reconstitution in the vial, before injection (Eisele et al. 2011) and have no known role for the pharmaceutical action of the products. In addition, no detrimental effects have been identified to date in having them present. This is of course contrary to the role that NAPs have when toxin is ingested as a food poison (Fujinaga et al. 2013).

After the initial years of the two type A products, many years were to pass before another BoNT product became available. What is not realised or often discussed was that another serotype, type F, went into clinical testing in several countries long before the advent of the type B product Neurobloc (Pickett 2015). Several publications exist on the use of type F but, with a comparably very short duration of action, the product was never to see commercialisation. Indeed, Neurobloc® has also not generally been a successful product due mainly to the high doses required and the formation of immunoresistance through prolonged use in many patients. The reason why serotype B BoNT is required in such high doses has only recently been identified and is due to inefficiencies in one of the receptors specifically in man. The product has been bought and sold several times by the owning companies in its history.

In the early 2000s a new serotype A product emerged from work in Germany and the company Merz. Their product, Xeomin, was developed outside of Merz to start with, but then first licenced in Germany in 2005. Xeomin® has slowly become available in many other countries. The product has distinguishing properties of being complex-protein free and, with a high concentration of the stabiliser human serum albumin, has been granted storage under qualified room temperature conditions (<25 °C). As such, Xeomin® could be considered a second-generation BoNT after the initial, complexed type A products.

The three main products, Botox®, Dysport® and Xeomin®, dominate the world market. However, other products have slowly emerged in certain countries and have steadily gained

* Disclosures: Andy Pickett is Director and Founder of Toxin Science Limited, UK; Adjunct Professor at the Botulinum Research Center, IAS, USA; and Senior Programme Leader & Scientific Expert, Neurotoxins, Galderma Aesthetic and Corrective Global Business Unit. The opinions and views expressed are those of the author and Toxin Science Limited only.

Table 21.1 Botulinum toxin products from Asia, current as of end 2015 (©Toxin Science Limited, 2015)

Product™	Company	Country	Bacterial production strain	Process	u/vial [product specific]	Excipients (in vial)
BTXA/Prosigne/ Redux/Lantox/ Lanzox	Lanzhou Institute of Biological Products/Hugh Source International	China	Hall	Crystallisation, dialysis	50/100 u	5 mg gelatin 25 mg dextran 25 mg sucrose
Meditoxin/ Neuronox/Siax/ Botulift/Cunox	MedyTox Inc.	South Korea	Hall	Acid precipitations, dialysis	50/100/200 u	0.5 mg HSA 0.9 mg NaCl
Innotox	MedyTox Inc.	South Korea	Hall	Unknown	25/50 u	No human serum albumin or animal products
Botulax/Zentox/ Regenox	Hugel Pharma	South Korea	CBFC26	Protamine sulphate DEAE sepharose chromatography	50/100/200 u	0.5 mg HSA 0.9 mg NaCl
Nabota/Evosyal (DWP 450)	Daewoong Pharmaceutical Co. Ltd	South Korea	Hall	High-Pure Technology® (patented)	100 u	0.5 mg HSA 0.9 mg NaCl

Table 21.2 New local botulinum toxin products currently available, end 2015 (©Toxin Science Limited, 2015)

Product™	Company	Country	u/vial (product specific)	Excipients (in vial)
Masport	Masoondarou Company	Iran	500 u	0.5 mg HSA 2.5 mg lactose
Relatox/Relatoks	Microgen Company	Russia	50/100 u	Gelatine
BOTOgenie	Bio-Med Pvt. Ltd	India	50/100 u	5 mg lactose
BTXA	Intas Pharmaceuticals Ltd	India	100 u	Unknown

market positions in many places, with the notable exceptions of Europe and the United States, where they are unavailable. Four of these products have come from Asia, three from South Korea alone (Tables 21.1 and 21.2).

The oldest of these Asian BoNTs is CBTXA from Lanzhou Institute in China (since 1997). This product is unique in the world in using both dextran and gelatine as stabilisers instead of the traditional HSA found in all but one of the other products. The presence of these stabilisers carries a degree of risk for the product that is not the case with all the other BoNTs, namely the possibility of anaphylactic shock to the gelatine (Kamin et al. 2006). Significant side-effects have been reported for this Chinese product (Careta et al. 2015).

The three Korean BoNT products have been developed, as stated by those companies, as 'copies' of Botox®. Their formulations are similar or the same as Botox® but the manufacturing processes are different and use different strains of the production organisms (Kim 2014). Clinical trials of these products have slowly been published and often show that the potency units of the products are different to each other. Often, head-to-head aesthetic clinical trials at the same dosage as Botox® have shown significant differences in results. This only serves to emphasise the statement, included on prescribing information and product literature worldwide, that the potency units of each product are specific to that product and are not interchangeable. This is amply demonstrated by studies that use apparently 'equal' units of two different products yet the results of one are superior/inferior to the other included in the clinical testing.

In addition to the Asian toxins now available, there are other, regional products that have limited use in various countries. Typical examples are shown in Table 21.3. There are virtually no clinical data published as yet for these products. Very limited information is available from the company websites. Sometimes, a video of specific product use is posted on YouTube (e.g. www.youtube.com/watch?v=Osd4TGEIGma, accessed 10 November 2015). There is no information available as to exactly why these regional products have been developed, but the main reason is believed to be to provide a much cheaper alternative to the main branded products through local manufacture.

One area of work that is directed specifically towards the aesthetic areas of treatment is the development of so-called 'topical' toxin products. A number of companies have been working in this area for many years (Table 21.3), the most notable being the Californian company Revance, which has been active in the field since 2002. Published data on their RT001 product has shown its limited efficacy for treatment of specific facial areas (Glogau 2012). In addition, the transport mechanism for the BoNT across the dermal layers is highly inefficient, given the very high doses of active BoNT that are needed to gain effect. The company has been the subject of much speculation and share price movements in response to their publication of data over the years, but the certainty that a topical aesthetic BoNT

Table 21.3 Development of topical botulinum toxin products worldwide, 2015 (©Toxin Science Limited, 2015)

Company	Country	Product name	Technology	Clinical data published
Revance	United States	RT001-RTT150	TransMTS®	Yes
Transdermal Corp.	Canada	CosmeTox	InParT (mixed micelles/ ionic nanoparticles)	Yes
Anterios	United States	ANT-1207 lotion	Unknown	No
Malvern Cosmeceutics Ltd	United Kingdom	MCL005-2 gel	Unknown	No

will reach the market and, most importantly, be a useful and efficacious product over years has yet to be determined. Other companies publicising their work on topical toxins have yet to provide any substantial clinical trial data.

Finally, the area of modified BoNT molecules with new or enhanced properties has been in vogue for a number of years. The company Syntaxin, now owned by Ipsen, spun out of the Centre for Applied Microbiology and Research, has been the most notable in the field, with publications in the area now going back 20 years. The main molecules under consideration are termed targeted secretion inhibitors (TSIs) and use modified BoNT molecules to retarget their activity to different cell types where normally BoNT is not active (Masuyer et al. 2014). Molecules from Syntaxin are currently in early clinical studies, but the doses of these modified molecules needed to obtain effects are considerably higher than the native BoNT. As such, subjects such as the development of immunogenic responses will feature more heavily than for the native molecules.

From early beginnings of very few products, the global market for BoNT has grown significantly and now encompasses a range of products, both global and local, together with considerable research and development on new products for specific, targeted uses. The future of BoNT is therefore as bright today as in the very first years of availability, now over 30 years ago.

References

Careta, MF, L Delgado and R Patriota, 2015. Report of allergic reaction after application of botulinum toxin. *Aesthet Surg J.* 35: NP102–NP105.

Eisele, KH, K Fink, M Vey and HV Taylor, 2011. Studies on the dissociation of botulinum neurotoxin type A complexes. *Toxicon.* 57: 555–565.

Elston, JS and RW Russell, 1985. Effect of treatment with botulinum toxin on neurogenic blepharospasm. *Br Med J (Clin Res Ed).* 290: 1857–1859.

Fujinaga, Y, Y Sugawara and T Matsumura, 2013. Uptake of botulinum neurotoxin in the intestine. *Curr Top Microbiol Immunol.* 364: 45–59.

Glogau, R, A Blitzer, F Brandt, M Kane, GD Monheit and JM Waugh, 2012. Results of a randomized, double-blind, placebo-controlled study to evaluate the efficacy and safety of a botulinum toxin type A topical gel for the treatment of moderate-to-severe lateral canthal lines. *J Drugs Dermatol.* 11: 38–45.

Kamin, W, P Staubach, B Klar-Hlawatsch and M Knuf, 2006. Anaphylaxis after vaccination due to hypersensitivity to gelatin. *Klin Padiatr.* 218: 92–94.

Kim, BJ, HH Kwon, SY Park, et al., 2014. Double-blind, randomized non-inferiority trial of a novel botulinum toxin A processed from the strain CBFC26, compared with onabotulinumtoxin A in the treatment of glabellar lines. *J Eur Acad Dermatol Venereol.* 28: 1761–1767.

Masuyer, G, JA Chaddock, KA Foster and KR Acharya, 2014. Engineered botulinum neurotoxins as new therapeutics. *Annu Rev Pharmacol Toxicol.* 54: 27–51.

Pickett, A, 2013. Historical aspects of botulinum toxin used clinically: part I – is that the right serotype? *The Botulinum J.* 2: 176.

Pickett, A, 2015. Historical aspects of botulinum toxin used clinically: part II: overcoming resistance. *The Botulinum J.* doi: https://doi.org/10.1504/TBJ.2015.078134.

Scott, AB, A Rosenbaum and CC Collins, 1973. Pharmacologic weakening of extraocular muscles. *Invest Ophthalmol.* 12: 924–927.

Chapter 22

Molecular Mechanisms of Botulinum Toxin

Ornella Rossetto and Cesare Montecucco*

Introduction

Different bacterial species of the genus *Clostridium* carry genes that encode for one or more of the more than 40 presently known botulinum neurotoxins (BoNTs) isoforms. They are grouped into seven different serotypes abbreviated BoNT/A to /G followed by an Arabic number to distinguish subtypes (Hill & Smith 2013; Rossetto et al. 2014). They act on cholinergic nerve terminals and cause inhibition of neurotransmission with ensuing flaccid paralysis and autonomic dysfunctions that are typical of botulism. The major form of botulism in the adult is *foodborne botulism*, which occurs upon the ingestion of BoNT-contaminated food; the toxins must survive the proteolytic environment of the gastrointestinal tract to reach the intestine, where they are adsorbed (Johnson & Montecucco 2008). Epidemiologic data and *in vitro* characterisation showed that only serotypes A, B, E and, rarely, F cause human botulism, whereas serotypes C and D are prevalent in bird and cattle botulisms (Smith & Sugiyama 1988).

In neurotoxigenic *Clostridia*, the BoNT gene is always situated next to the non-toxic, non-haemagglutinin gene, which encodes a non-toxic, non-haemagglutinin protein that adopts a similar fold, forming with BoNT a heterodimer resembling interlocking hands (Gu et al. 2012). The bont/ntnh genes are in close proximity to genes encoding several haemagglutinin components (HAs) or orfX proteins. These proteins associate with the BoNT/NTNH heterodimer, giving rise to large oligomers termed progenitor toxin complexes (PTC) (Lee et al. 2013). BoNT and NTNH are associated in a 1:1 stoichiometry, and their extensive protein–protein contacts effectively decreases BoNT exposure to external damaging agents, whereas HA components have no direct contact with neurotoxin. HAs form three arms that project outward from NTNH and have the main role of facilitating intestinal trans-epithelial absorption of BoNT and thus promoting internalisation of the toxin into the bloodstream (Lee et al. 2013; Simpson 2013). *C. botulinum* type A1 can produce several complexes known as LL (19S), L (16S) and M (12S), which range from 900 to 300 kDa, depending on the association of BoNT/A with different numbers of the components mentioned above. In the complex, the proteins are not covalently linked but their association occurs in bacterial cultures and naturally contaminated food. The complex is stable at acidic pH, but dissociates above neutral pH (pH ≥7) (Eisele et al. 2011). The BoNT/A1 formulations used for clinical application are either purified neurotoxin complex (Botox or onabotulinumtoxinA and Dysport/abobotulinumtoxinA) or the BoNT molecule alone (Xeomin or incobotulinumtoxinA).

The definition of the crystal structure of progenitor toxin complex of BoNT is one of the main achievements in BoNT research, together with the identification of many toxin subtypes within each serotype. Their number has dramatically grown, reaching several dozens of BoNTs in a few years, and many others are predicted to be discovered (Montecucco & Rasotto 2015). Despite the existence of a high number of toxin variants, all BoNTs are structurally similar and consist of two chains linked by a unique disulphide bond: a light chain or metalloprotease domain (abbreviated L, 50 kDa) and a heavy chain (abbreviated H, 100 kDa) linked by a single interchain disulphide bond. The H chain consists of a membrane translocation domain (abbreviated HN, 50 kDa) and a HC receptor binding domain which is structurally divided into two domains: HC-N (25 kDa) and HC-C (25 kDa) (Lacy et al. 1998). Such a structure is functionally correlated to the four steps of the mode of BoNTs intoxication of nerve terminals, which are: (1) binding to nerve terminals mediated by HC-C; (2) internalisation into small synaptic vesicles (SV); (3) translocation of the L chain across the synaptic vesicle membrane mediated by HN; and (4) cleavage of SNARE proteins mediated by the L chain (Lacy et al. 1998; Binz & Rummel 2009; Rossetto et al. 2014). BoNTs are a marvel of protein design whose unique biological properties have led them to become not only the most potent toxins known, but also highly effective and successful therapeutic agents for the treatment of a wide variety of human neuroperipheral syndromes (Montal 2010). The increased understanding of the detailed structures of the different toxins combined with an improved understanding of their unique biological properties, i.e. different binding partners, different trafficking, different substrates and exclusive enzyme–substrate interactions, will open up a huge opportunity to identify new therapeutic BoNTs with improved features

* The authors' research is supported by grants from the Fondazione CARIPARO Project 'Synaptic Functions and Role of Glial Cells in Brain and Muscle Diseases', by the Italian Ministry of Defence (Progetto PNRM – NIB), by the 'Axonomics Project' of the Provincia Autonoma di Trento to CM and by grant from the University of Padova (Progetto PRIN) to OR.

with respect to the neurotoxins presently available on the market or to be exploited for new clinical applications.

At the same time, it is surprising that despite a great variability within their primary structure, BoNTs have been evolved to use a highly similar mechanism to block nerve terminals. This offers the possibility to rationally design new molecules capable of inhibiting BoNTs, independently from their antigenic properties.

Mechanisms of Action

BoNTs first recognise and bind to cholinergic motor neurons with high affinity and specificity, and then enter the cells where they can release a potent enzyme. Recent reviews have described in detail a step-by-step analysis of the mode of action of BoNTs (Simpson 2013; Rossetto et al. 2014). Here we provide a brief update on the main recent achievements regarding the molecular mechanism of BoNT intoxication, with particular focus on how the new information could help the search for toxin inhibitors for overriding the paralytic action of BoNTs.

Neurospecific Binding

To selectively target the presynaptic membrane of peripheral nerve terminals, BoNTs have evolved a double receptor binding mode, via the C-terminal part of the HC domain (HC-C), based on the interaction with a polysialoganglioside (PSG) and a protein receptor in the lumen of SVs. The latter has been defined in molecular details for BoNT/B, BoNT/G and the chimeric BoNT/DC, which bind segment 40–60 of the luminal domain of the synaptic vesicle protein synaptotagmin (Syt) and for BoNT/A and BoNT/E, which bind to two different segments of the fourth luminal loop of the SV transmembrane protein SV2 (for a complete list of references see Rummel 2013; Rossetto et al. 2014). The dual binding interaction with PSG and SV receptors increases the strength of BoNT interactions with the membrane as it is the product of the two binding affinities (Montecucco 1986) and mediates the ensuing endocytosis inside the lumen of synaptic vesicles.

Entry Into the Nerve Terminal

After binding to the presynaptic receptors, BoNTs enter into the nerve terminal. BoNT/A1 was recently visualised predominantly inside synaptic vesicles within the mouse neuromuscular junction in the number of 1–2 toxin molecules per vesicle, which correlates with the number of SV2 receptors in the SV membrane (Colasante et al. 2013). This finding also correlates with the early observation by Hughes and Whaler (1962) that binding and internalisation of this BoNT is activity-dependent and provides the morphological demonstration that BoNTs exploit the SV cycle as 'Trojan horses' to enter motor neuron terminals *in vivo*. However, it has been shown that BoNT/A1, especially at high doses, can exploit alternative trafficking pathways, which may direct the neurotoxin to an endosomal compartment and then to axonal carriers targeted for retrograde transport (Antonucci et al. 2008; Restani et al. 2012). Therefore, the consolidated dogma that the effects of BoNTs remain restricted to the peripheral nervous system is now confuted by a substantial body of experimental evidence in favour of the fact that peripherally applied BoNT/A can directly affect central circuits. A more detailed understanding of these central effects of BoNTs will provide valuable information for present and future uses of these neurotoxins in clinical practice (Mazzocchio & Caleo 2015).

Membrane Translocation

In order to reach their intracellular targets in the cytosol of nerve cells, the catalytically active L domain must be translocated from the SV lumen into the cytosol. The low pH inside the SV lumen induces a concerted structural change of the L domain, of the HN domain and of membrane lipids, leading to insertion of both the L and the HN domain into the membrane. An ion translocation channel is thus formed that chaperones the passage of the partially unfolded L from the lumenal to the cytosolic side of the SV membrane (Montal 2010; Rossetto et al. 2014; Pirazzini et al. 2016). L remains attached to the SV until the interchain disulphide bond is reduced. This is the final step of its membrane translocation (Fischer & Montal 2007; Pirazzini et al. 2013). A pharmacologic approach has led to the identification of the NADPH–thioredoxin reductase (TrxR)–thioredoxin (Trx) system being responsible for the cytosolic release of L in the cytosol (Pirazzini et al. 2013, 2014). Importantly, inhibitors of TrxR and Trx prevent neuronal intoxication by BoNT, attenuate its neuroparalytic action, and, when administered to mice prior to BoNT exposure, prolong time to death and decrease the death frequency (Pirazzini et al. 2014). These studies have shown for the first time *in vivo* that the reduction of the single interchain disulphide bond is a key and general event in nerve intoxication of all BoNTs, and that the TrxR–Trx system is a target for drug discovery to prevent and treat botulism, regardless of the serotype or subtype causing intoxication.

Enzymatic Activity of BoNT L Chains and Duration of Neuroparalysis

Once released in the cytosol of the nerve terminal, the L chain of the BoNTs displays its metalloproteolytic activity and cleaves one of the three SNARE proteins: the L chain of BoNT/B, /D, /F and /G cleave VAMP at different peptide bonds, BoNT/A and /E cleave SNAP25, while BoNT/C is the only one capable of cleaving two substrates, SNAP25 and Syntaxin (Binz 2013; Pantano & Montecucco 2013). SNAREs form a heterotrimeric complex that constitutes the core of the neuroexocytosis nanomachine and their proteolysis impairs its assembly and/or function (Pantano & Montecucco 2014). Substrate-specific binding combined with sequence variations proximal to the active site in the L chains determine serotype specificity (Montal 2010; Binz 2013; Rossetto et al. 2014). At the present time, the substrates of only a minority of the BoNT subtypes have been determined. In addition, the turnover rate of these enzymes inside the nerve terminal is not known *in vivo*, a parameter that has a profound effect on the performance of the L metalloprotease in terms of the onset of paralysis. Regarding BoNT/A, which is the serotype associated with the most severe human botulism and the most commonly used serotype for clinical purposes, ten different subtypes have been identified so far (Rossetto et al. 2014) and the analyses of several of these subtypes have revealed distinct characteristics, ranging from differences in cell entry and enzyme kinetics to differences in potency in mice and cell-model specific potency. A recent *in vivo* study showed that BoNT/A2 results in a faster onset of local paralysis than BoNT/A1, 3, 4 and 5, whereas BoNT/A3 results in significantly faster recovery of motor neuron deficiency after local injection (Pellett et al. 2015).

There is a substantial consensus that the duration of BoNT-induced neuroparalysis corresponds to the lifetime of the L chain within the nerve terminal. In other words, as long as there are L molecule(s) there is SNARE cleavage and corresponding blockade of neurotransmitter release. Different BoNTs have a different duration of action: from the 3–4 months of BoNT/A1 to the few weeks of BoNT/E1 in human skeletal muscles (Eleopra et al. 2004). However, it is becoming evident that other factors come into play in the duration of action of BoNT/A1 and BoNT/C (Pantano & Montecucco 2014) and that muscle and Schwann cells are determinants of the shorter duration of action of BoNT/A1 and BoNT/B at skeletal nerve terminals where a process of sprouting occurs with respect to their much longer duration at cholinergic autonomic terminals where sprouting does not take place (Rossetto et al. 2015).

Conclusions

Thanks to advances of genetic and molecular methods, the existence of many BoNT variants has been demonstrated in recent years. The presence of many BoNTs endowed with different immunogenic properties but very similar cellular and molecular mechanisms of action calls for an intensification of the current studies aimed at identifying inhibitors of specific steps of BoNT neuron intoxication and very promising results have been recently achieved in this field. At the same time, this multitude of novel BoNTs provides a real goldmine of potential novel therapeutics endowed with improved properties with respect to those of existing BoNTs. Moreover, there is a growing line of research that aims at changing the binding specificity and affinity and the duration of BoNT action in order to obtain tailor-made therapeutics and more sophisticated tools to be used in cell biology studies (Masuyer et al. 2014).

References

Antonucci F, Rossi C, Gianfranceschi L, Rossetto O, Caleo M (2008) Long-distance retrograde effects of botulinum neurotoxin. *A J Neurosci* 28:3689–96.

Binz T (2013) Clostridial neurotoxin light chains: devices for SNARE cleavage mediated blockade of neurotransmission. *Curr Top Microbiol Immunol* 364:139–157.

Binz T, Rummel A (2009) Cell entry strategy of clostridial neurotoxins. *J Neurochem* 109:1584–1595.

Colasante C, Rossetto O, Morbiato L, Pirazzini M, Molgó J, Montecucco C (2013) Botulinum neurotoxin type A is internalized and translocated from small synaptic vesicles at the neuromuscular junction. *Mol Neurobiol* 48:120–127.

Eisele KH, Fink K, Vey M, Taylor HV (2011) Studies on the dissociation of botulinum neurotoxin type A complexes. *Toxicon* 57:555–565.

Eleopra R, Tugnoli V, Quatrale R, Rossetto O, Montecucco C (2004) Different types of botulinum toxin in humans. *Mov Disord* 8:S53–S59.

Fischer A, Montal M (2007) Crucial role of the disulfide bridge between botulinum neurotoxin light and heavy chains in protease translocation across membranes. *J Biol Chem* 282: 29604–29611.

Gu, S, Rumpel S, Zhou J, Strotmeier J, Bigalke H, Perry K, Shoemaker CB, Rummel A, Jin R (2012) Botulinum neurotoxin is shielded by NTNHA in an interlocked complex. *Science* 335:977–981.

Hill KK, Smith TJ (2013) Genetic diversity within *Clostridium botulinum* serotypes, botulinum neurotoxin gene clusters and toxin subtypes. *Curr Top Microbiol Immunol* 364:1–20.

Hughes R, Whaler BC (1962) Influence of nerve-ending activity and of drugs on the rate of paralysis of rat diaphragm preparations by *Cl. botulinum* type A toxin. *J Physiol* 160:221–233.

Johnson EA, Montecucco C (2008) Botulism. *Handb Clin Neurol* 91:333–368.

Lacy DB, Tepp W, Cohen A, DasGupta BR, Stevens RC (1998) Crystal structure of botulinum neurotoxin type A and implications for toxicity. *Nat Struct Biol* 5:898–902.

Lee K, Gu S, Jin L, Le TT, Cheng LW, Strotmeier J, Kruel AM, Yao G, Perry K, Rummel A, Jin R (2013) Structure of a bimodular botulinum neurotoxin complex provides insights into its oral toxicity. *PLoS Pathog* 9:e1003690.

Masuyer G, Chaddock JA, Foster KA, Acharya KR (2014) Engineered botulinum neurotoxins as new therapeutics. *Annu Rev Pharmacol Toxicol* 54: 27–51.

Mazzocchio R, Caleo M (2015) More than at the neuromuscular synapse: actions of botulinum neurotoxin A in the central nervous system. *Neuroscientist* 21:44–61.

Montal M (2010) Botulinum neurotoxin: a marvel of protein design. *Annu Rev Biochem* 79:591–617.

Montecucco C (1986) How do tetanus and botulinum toxins bind to neuronal membranes? *Trends Biochem Sci* 11:314–317.

Montecucco C, Rasotto MB (2015) On botulinum neurotoxin variability. *MBio* 6:e02131-14.

Pantano S, Montecucco C (2014) The blockade of the neurotransmitter release apparatus by botulinum neurotoxins. *Cell Mol Life Sci* 71:793–811.

Pellett S, Tepp WH, Whitemarsh RC, Bradshaw M, Johnson EA (2015) In vivo onset and duration of action varies for botulinum neurotoxin A subtypes 1–5. *Toxicon* 107(Pt A):37–42.

Pirazzini M, Bordin F, Rossetto O, Shone CC, Binz T, Montecucco C (2013) The thioredoxin reductase–thioredoxin system is involved in the entry of tetanus and botulinum neurotoxins in the cytosol of nerve terminals. *FEBS Lett* 587:150–155.

Pirazzini M, Azarnia Tehran D, Zanetti G, Megighian A, Scorzeto M, Fillo S, Shone CC, Binz T, Rossetto O, Lista F, Montecucco C (2014) Thioredoxin and its reductase are present on synaptic vesicles, and their inhibition prevents the paralysis induced by botulinum neurotoxins. *Cell Rep* 8:1870–1878.

Pirazzini M, Azarnia Tehran D, Leka O, Zanetti G, Rossetto O, Montecucco C (2016) On the translocation of botulinum and tetanus neurotoxins across the membrane of acidic intracellular compartments. *Biochim Biophys Acta* 1858:467–474.

Restani L, Giribaldi F, Manich M, Bercsenyi K, Menendez G, Rossetto O, Caleo M, Schiavo G (2012) Botulinum neurotoxins A and E undergo retrograde axonal transport in primary motor neurons. *PLoS Pathog* 8:e1003087.

Rossetto O, Pirazzini M, Montecucco C (2014) Botulinum neurotoxins: genetic, structural and mechanistic insights. *Nat Rev Microbiol* 12:535–549.

Rossetto O, Pirazzini M, Montecucco C (2015) Current gaps in basic science knowledge of botulinum neurotoxin biological actions. *Toxicon* 107(Pt A):59–63.

Rummel A (2013) Double receptor anchorage of botulinum neurotoxins accounts for their exquisite neurospecificity. *Curr Top Microbiol Immunol* 364:61–90.

Simpson L (2013) The life history of a botulinum toxin molecule. *Toxicon* 68:40–59.

Smith LD, Sugiyama H (1988) *Botulism: The Organism, its Toxins, the Disease.* Springfield, IL: C.C. Thomas Publisher.

Chapter 23

Indirect Central Nervous System Effects of Botulinum Toxin

Melanie Leigh D. Supnet and Raymond L. Rosales

Introduction

Botulinum neurotoxin Perhaps it is an anti-thesis of a thinking that BoNT has not only purely peripheral effects, but that there are indirect central effects. This chapter posits that indirect (i.e. central modulation) BoNT effects may be more tenable, given the contemporary evidences.

BoNT, among other applications in movement disorders, has been proven effective and safe for the treatment of dystonia and spasticity. Withstanding the test of time of over 20 years, the peripherally mediated chemodenervation by local injection with BoNT is hinged on its blockade of presynaptic docking proteins along cholinergic terminals. In dystonia specifically, the goal of BoNT treatment is to achieve a balance between weakness sufficient to reduce dystonia, but insufficient to interfere with function. Previous electrophysiological and functional imaging studies attest that the clinical effect of BoNT in dystonia is assumed to be also accompanied by dynamic changes at multiple levels of the sensorimotor network, from the neuromuscular junction, spinal cord, brainstem and to the cerebral cortex (Kanovský et al. 2011).

While recent animal studies (Caleo et al. 2009) suggest direct central or trans-synaptic BoNT effects, the daunting issue remains whether, indeed, these elegant pre-clinical data would translate to clinically meaningful advantage or adverse impacts. However, the largely unresolved occurrence of neuromuscular jitters in uninjected muscles (e.g. opposite limb or another body region, following single-fibre electromyography) far from BoNT-injected sites will not favour an indirect central effect, given an *in vivo* production of unstable and abnormal neuromuscular junction potentials. This phenomenon observed in pre-clinical and dystonia studies (Rosales et al. 2006) is best understood as either a systemic toxin migration or a trans-synaptic spread (Figure 23.1).

Thus, this chapter aims to highlight the indirect central nervous system (CNS) effects of BoNT from peripherally mediated mechanisms. We shall therefore attempt to summarise the intriguing functional changes produced in the sensory afferents arriving at the spinal cord, brainstem and cerebral cortex, induced by BoNT, as we allude to both dystonia and spasticity.

Direct Muscle Effects of BoNT Therapy

BoNT has the ability to remain relatively localised at the injection site, which contributes to its remarkable record for safety and clinical efficacy. The neurotoxin injected into skeletal muscles disrupts neurotransmission of cholinergically mediated extrafusal and intrafusal muscles via cleavage of presynaptic vesicle fusion proteins; SNAP25 for BoNT type A and synaptobrevin for BoNT type B, both being used in clinics. In effect, muscle denervation and a transient reinnervation pattern ensues until the original neuromuscular junctional transmission is re-established after approximately 12 weeks (Pickett & Rosales 2011). As seen in biopsied spastic muscles, BoNT-injected muscles show larger average fibre area, increased capillary density, increased central nucleation, increased percentage of fibres expressing both fast and slow myosin heavy chain isoforms, including an increased expression of developing MHC isoforms. Together with denervation, all these intrinsic muscle responses indicate a degeneration–regeneration cycle that may postulate a beneficial BoNT effect to functional recovery (Ward & Lieber 2009). In denervation of fusimotor endings, BoNT (whether type A or B) can lead to a reduction of the spindle input to the alpha motor neurons, critical in maintaining tonic myotatic reflexes. Thus, the relief with BoNT injection in dystonia may not only be due to muscle weakening, but may also be due to a decrease in the tonic myotatic reflex from modulation of spindle afferences (Rosales et al. 1996). The local passive mechanical effects of muscle weakening and relaxation may also indirectly impinge on the relevant tendon and joint with their corresponding afferent inputs (see Box 23.1).

BoNT Effects Beyond the Injection Site

The Spinal Cord Circuitry

Animal studies demonstrated a retrograde BoNT transport after injection in a muscle. It then reaches the corresponding spinal hemisegment and induces physiological changes at the level of the alpha-motor neurons and other ventral horn cells (Habermann et al. 1974). BoNT, directly applied into the ventral root, exerts a central action on the cholinergic transmission of Renshaw cells, hence inhibition of the Ia inhibitory interneurons (Hagenah et al. 1977).

The effects of BoNT on spinal cord mechanisms have been studied using F-waves, H-reflexes and reciprocal inhibition of the H-reflex. An increase in the F-wave and in the F-wave/M-wave ratio was observed in healthy subjects (Hamjian et al. 1994), suggesting an enhanced alpha-motor neuron excitability

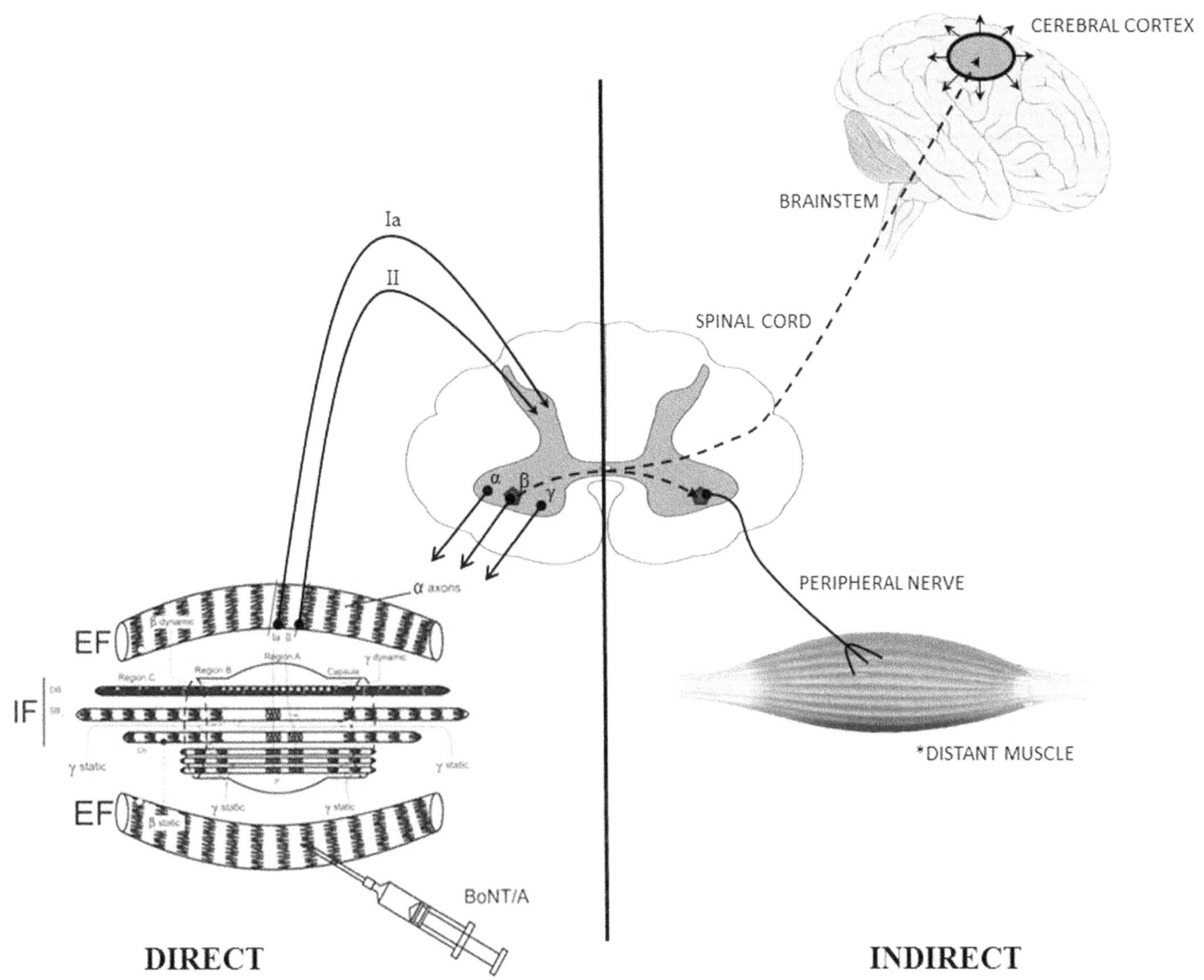

Figure 23.1 Botulinum toxin therapy effects at the peripheral segmental and supra-segmental levels.

Box 23.1

1. **Muscles:**
   - **Extrafusal**; direct chemodenervation
   - **Intrafusal**: direct chemodenervation
   - **Distant muscles:** subclinical, unless in high doses
   - **Vasculature**: neuromotor sympathetic tone
2. **Corresponding tendons and joints:**
   - Secondary effects on Golgi tendon organs and joint receptors
3. **Segmental/spinal:**
   - Sensory modulation from muscle afferents-fusimotor reflexes
4. **Supraspinal:**
   - Modulation of central sensorimotor programmes, including subcortical/cortical effects

after BoNT injection. Changes in F-waves have been observed in patients with focal dystonia, again suggesting excitability changes in the alpha-motor neurons (Wohlfarth et al. 2001). Discrepant results have been observed in studies using H-reflex and reciprocal inhibition between agonist and antagonist muscles (Priori et al. 1995). In a study involving patients with idiopathic segmental forearm dystonia, an increase of the second phase of reciprocal inhibition (defective phase in dystonic patients) was observed after BoNT injection. It is possible that BoNT can transiently restore presynaptic inhibition between forearm antagonist muscles. Differences in the afferent feedback from the affected muscles in these different clinical conditions could be the underlying factor in the different results, as were observed in spastic children, based on improvement of Hmax:Mmax ratios (Fascarelli et al. 2011).

BoNT seems to indirectly alter the excitability of spinal cord circuitry in humans by acting on the presynaptic intrafusal neuromuscular junction and decreasing spindle afferent input to the spinal cord. This effect leads to an increase in the presynaptic inhibition of flexor muscle afferents. An indirect action is in keeping with the experimental evidence of a fusimotor denervation after BoNT intramuscular injection in animals (Rosales et al. 1996). The significance of fusimotor influences in dystonia is hinged on the following factors. (1) Due to dystonic co-contractions, the muscle spindles are in constant change, requiring a brisk reprogramming of circuitry. (2) In contrast to isolated contractions, co-contractions that occur in dystonia may also induce a greater fusimotor drive to contracting muscles. (3) At the spinal level, the overall fusimotor-driven inflow from Ia & II afferents during voluntary contraction has an 'autogenic' excitatory effect. (4) The fusimotor reflexes are 'task-dependent' – only active when subjects are performing an appropriate motor task. Thus, their role seem to be more towards setting the background operating level of fusimotor drive than in moment-to-moment control of movement (Pierrot-Deseilligny and Burke 2005).

One way to highlight the possible role of BoNT injection in reducing muscle afferent feedback may be gleaned in the case of writer's cramp, wherein abnormalities in the descending control of spinal inhibitory interneurons could alter the balance between the reflex inhibition and facilitation of the gamma motor neurons. In this scenario, there will be an enhanced sensitivity of the tonic vibration reflex (TVR) (Kaji et al. 2010). In a group of patients with focal hand dystonia, modelled with application of the TVR, the maximal M-wave (Mmax) ratio before and after BoNT injections, the maximal voluntary contraction (MVC) and the TVR were measured. The TVR ratio was significantly more depressed and remained depressed for a long time compared to the Mmax and MVC ratios (Rosales et al. 2011). This interesting result could not be explained on the basis of concomitant denervation of extrafusal fibres alone. Besides acting on extrafusal fibres, BoNT injection could change the afferent inflow from the vibrated muscle by acting on the fusimotor synapses as well and changing the reflex activation of intrafusal muscle fibres during vibration. The denervation of intrafusal muscle fibres may have a special sensitivity to suppress the TVR after BoNT injection, suggesting that this effect may contribute to its clinical benefits. The same group of investigators found a similar reduction of TVR in patients with post-stroke upper-limb spasticity (Rosales et al. 2011). The significant decrease of the TVR was only observed in those patients who retain some degree of strength and active movement, suggesting that the BoNT action on the injected muscles is directly related to the reduction of muscle spindles firing after the blockade of intrafusal fibres. Likewise, muscle afferent block with lidocaine–ethanol combination, purportedly affecting mainly the muscle spindles, does induce relief of spasms when injected in dystonias (Conte et al. 2010).

The Effects on Brainstem Mechanisms

The possible effect of BoNT injections on brainstem mechanisms has been investigated mainly by studying changes in the excitability of brainstem reflexes in patients with cranial dystonia. Brainstem circuits can easily be studied by blink reflex technique. Recent studies by Conte and colleagues (Conte et al. 2010) did not show changes in the blink reflex recovery cycle after BoNT treatment of patients with blepharospasm. Another study done by Zeuner and colleagues (Zeuner et al. 2010) inducing time-specific plasticity in the blink reflex with the application of high-frequency stimulation protocols also did not show any change in recovery curves of the blink reflex after BoNT injections. Thus, it appears that, to date, tenable evidence of BoNT influence on brainstem excitability networks are lacking. A study by Ce and colleagues (Ce 2000) using brainstem auditory-evoked responses (BAER) to observe changes in the specific circuitry in patients with craniocervical dystonia and hemifacial spasm treated with BoNT, found it did not induce changes in BAER.

The Effects on Cortical Mechanisms

Possible BoNT-induced changes to functional cortical organisation were investigated using various neurophysiological techniques. In healthy humans injected with BoNT to the extensor digitorum brevis muscle and studied with motor-evoked potentials and cortical silent periods, the cortical excitability can be modified and maintained for three months post-injection (Kim et al. 2006). Among cases with focal hand dystonia, a study was conducted employing long-latency reflexes (LLRs), which have been successfully used to test afferent sensory and efferent motor pathways travelling via the cortex (Naumann & Reiners 1997). A significant reduction in the amplitude of the late (LLR2) component, which is believed to be of cortical origin (cortical generator involving the supplementary area), was observed on the clinically affected side after BoNT treatment. The finding suggests that BoNT injections can modify the afferent input coming from the injected muscles and modulate the abnormal central motor pattern involved in focal dystonia (Palomar et al. 2012).

Somatosensory-evoked potentials (SEPs) is another way of studying the influence of the afferent peripheral inputs on the cortex. Kanovsky and colleagues (Kanovsky et al. 1998) recorded SEPs before and after treatment with BoNT for cervical dystonia. There was a significant reduction in the amplitude of the P22/N30 precentral component (recorded contralaterally to the direction of head deviation) paralleling the clinical improvement in head position. The SEP precentral component seems to reflect the activation of a functional cortical–subcortical–cortical loop (including the basal ganglia as well as the premotor and supplementary motor areas). The authors postulated that their findings might reflect changes in precentral cortex excitability secondary to BoNT-induced modulation of spindle afferent inputs. An improvement in the cortical SEPs with associated reduction of spasticity was observed in a study performed in children with spastic diplegic cerebral palsy (Fascarelli et al. 2011). A central reorganisation of the affected muscles after BoNT injections can be directly related to the improvement in the amplitude of SEPs after BoNT.

There is evidence of changes in cortical organisation of different areas after BoNT injections. In a study by Byrnes and colleagues (Byrnes et al. 1998), transcranial magnetic stimulation (TMS) was used to map the topography of primary motor cortex projections of upper-limb muscles in patients with writer's cramp during sustained isometric contraction. BoNT treatment induced a clinical improvement of focal hand dystonia with a temporal reversal of cortical map abnormalities. This study suggested that changes in the primary motor cortex of dystonic patients might be secondary to abnormal afferent inputs that BoNT may transiently normalise. A reversible reorganisation of the hand motor cortical representation after BoNT injections was also found by the same investigators among patients with cervical dystonia and primary writing tremor (Byrnes et al. 1998).

Possible changes in the pattern of cortical activation induced by BoNT injection have been investigated with the use of positron emission tomography (PET). PET activation studies show an overactivity of striatum and non-primary motor areas and an underactivity of the primary motor cortex in cases of dystonia and during voluntary movements (Ceballos et al. 1997). Increased activation in the parietal cortex and caudal supplementary motor area producing significant improvement in handwriting after BoNT injections were noted in patients with focal hand dystonia. These results suggest cortical reorganisation secondary to deafferentation of alpha-motor neurons or changes in motor strategy. Functional MRI studies done in patients with hemiplegia and chronic distal arm spasticity after ischaemic stroke affecting the motor cortex have also shown cortical changes after the use of BoNT (Senkarova et al. 2010). A significant correlation was found between the clinical improvement and the decrease of activation of the posterior cingulate/precuneus regions after BoNT injection. This associative area seems to have an increased activation after a motor stroke and the authors suggest that changes in the cortical reorganisation after BoNT treatment could produce more focused activation of areas affected by stroke. The BoNT effect could also lead to a decreased activation of the previously enhanced areas.

Brain plasticity is another concept relevant to the potential targets of BoNT. In particular, transient deafferentation can result in short-term plasticity. Changes in a peripheral feedback or its central integration play a major role in the pathophysiology of movement disorder. It is possible that long-term clinical benefits of BoNT treatment could also reflect plastic changes in motor cortex output after the reorganisation of the entire synaptic circuitry. Changes in cortical plasticity have recently been reported in patients with cervical dystonia after BoNT treatment (Kojovic et al. 2011).

Human studies nevertheless support the idea that BoNT injected at therapeutic doses induces spinal or cortical effects by indirectly inducing brain changes. This occurs by plastic rearrangement subsequent to denervation or alterations in sensory input.

Clinical Context

BoNT as applied in focal dystonia and upper/lower spasticity has achieved Grade-A recommendations from various interest groups. The recommendations are based on robust clinical trials (level-A studies) that feature BoNT's clinical efficacy, paired with safety, across indications. Optimised efficacy of BoNT is largely hinged on proper technique, accurate muscle selection and targeting, correct dosing and dilutions, among others.

In the case of dystonia, BoNT is akin to a 'sensory trick' via mechanoreceptors, that potentially abolish or reduce the overactive muscles (Rosales & Dressler 2010). The sensorimotor networks that become disordered in dystonia are targeted by BoNT in their dual local effects (i.e. extrafusal and intrafusal muscles), as well as their indirect segmental and suprasegmental modulation (see Figure 23.1).

Although the aetiopathogenesis of dystonia and spasticity differ, both conditions overlap as regard the co-contractions of muscles, overactivity of extrafusal and intrafusal muscles, changes in site and visco-elastic properties of intrinsic muscles, occurrence of varying degrees of pain, and segmental and suprasegmental compensatory circuitry changes (Rosales 2012). Both at the peripheral level and at the higher levels, the role of BoNT injection in dystonia is apparent. BoNT remains an efficacious regimen in dystonia as it may alter inputs to the motor programmes, allow reprogramming of central circuitry from a peripheral approach and serve as an early intervention to circumvent compensatory changes like posturing, and the possible contribution of the pain (Rosales 2012).

In the case of spasticity, BoNT is directed towards blocking active muscles that alter motor control, and its effect can be enhanced by electrical stimulation of the peripheral nerve (Eleopra et al. 1998), instrumental targeting (Picelli et al. 2014) and neurorehabilitation (Yamada et al. 2014). The effect of BoNT along pain networks is another interesting phenomenon, and which is hinged on either an indirect modulation or unclear direct effects (Aoki 2005). In the clinics, the muscle weakening effect of BoNT appears to be perhaps mechanistically different from its pain reduction effect. Such occurrences have been alluded to in both dystonia and spasticity, wherein pain may appear reduced in otherwise still active injected muscles (Rosales et al. 2012).

Conclusion

BoNT may potentially affect central circuits by at least three mechanisms, which are (see Figure 23.1 and Box 23.1): (1) BoNT-mediated blockade of gamma-motor endings with consequent reduction of spindle afferent input from the injected muscle; (2) plastic changes following BoNT-mediated blockade of neuromuscular transmission. Theoretically, two sites of plasticity can be envisaged following blockade of neuromuscular transmission – one regarding the motor neurons and the other concerning the target muscle. Indeed there is evidence for rearrangement at both sides. (3) Retrograde transport and trancytosis of BoNT following uptake at the neuromuscular junction. Co-contraction occurs in both dystonia and spasticity, and this abnormality in motor control, whether from changes in cortical excitability and intracortical inhibition or as part of the upper motor neuron syndrome, can be modified by BoNT through local changes and central modulation of segmental and suprasegmental circuitries. In effect, BoNT may aid in restoring the balance of sensorimotor control, and may optimise neuromotor relearning with physiotherapy.

References

Aoki KR (2005). Review of a proposed mechanism for the antinociceptive action of botulinum toxin type A. *Neurotoxicol* 26:785–793.

Byrnes ML, Thickbroom GW, Wilson SA, Sacco P, Shipman JM, Stell R (1998). The corticomotor representation of upper limb muscles in writer's cramp and changes following botulinum toxin injection. *Brain* 121:977–988.

Caleo M, Antonucci F, Restani L, Mazzocchio R (2009). A re-appraisal of the central effects of botulinum toxin type A: by what mechanism? *J Neurochem* 109: 15–24.

Ce, P (2000). Central effects of botulinum toxin: study of brainstem auditory evoked potentials. *Eur J Neurol* 7: 747.

Ceballos-Baumann AO, Sheean G, Passingham RE, Marsden CD, Brooks DJ (1997). Botulinum toxin does not reverse the cortical dysfunction associated with writer's cramp: a PET study. *Brain* 120:571–582.

Conte A, Fabbrini G, Belvisi D, Marsili K, Di Stasio F, Berardelli A (2010). Electrical activation of the orbicularis oculi muscle does not increase the effectiveness of botulinum toxin type A in patients with blepharospasm. *Eur J Neurol* 17:449–455.

Eleopra R, Tugnoli V, De Grandis D, Montecucco C (1998). Different time courses of recovery after poisoning with botulinum neurotoxin serotypes A and E in humans. *Neurosci Lett* 256: 135–138.

Fascarelli F, Di Rosa G, Bisozzi E, Castelli E, Santilli V (2011). Neurophysiological changes induced by the botulinum toxin type A injection in children with cerebral palsy. *Eur J Paediat Neurol* 15: 59–64.

Habermann E (1974). ^{125}I labeled neurotoxin from *Clostridium botulinum* A: preparation, binding to synaptomoses and ascent to spinal cord. *Naunyn Schmiedebergs Arch Pharmacol* 281: 47–56.

Hagenah R, Bebecke R, Wiegand H (1977). Effect of type A botulinum toxin on the cholinergic transmission at the spinal Renshaw cells and on the inhibitory action at Ia inhibitory interneurons. *Arch Pharmal* 299: 267–272.

Hamjian JA, Walker F (1994). Serial neurophysiological studies of intramuscular botulinum-A toxins in human. *Muscle Nerve* 17: 1385–1392.

Kaji R, Rosako Y, Suyama K, Maeda T, Uechi Y, Iwasaki M (2010). Botulinum toxin type A in post-stroke upper limb spasticity. *Curr Med Res Opin* 26:1983–1992.

Kanovský P, Rosales RL (2011). Debunking the pathophysiological puzzle of dystonia: with special reference to botulinum toxin therapy. *Parkinsonism Relat Disord* 17: S11–S14.

Kim DY, Oh BM, Paik NJ (2006). Central effect of botulinum toxin A in humans. *Int J Neurosci* 116(6): 667–680.

Kojovic M, Caronni A, Bologna M, Bhatia K, Rothwell J, Edwards M (2011). Botulinum toxin injections reduce associative plasticity in patients with primary dystonia. *Movement Disord* 26(7): 1282–1289.

Naumann M, Reiners R (1997). Long-latency reflexes of hand muscles in idiopathic focal dystonia and their modification by botulinum toxin. *Brain* 120: 409–416.

Palomar F, Mir P (2012). Neurophysiological changes after intramuscular injection of botulinum toxin. *Clinic Neurophysiol* 123: 54–60.

Picelli A, Lobba D, Midiri A, Prandi P, Melotti C, Baldessarelli S, Smania N (2014). Botulinum toxin injection into the forearm muscles for wrist and fingers spastic overactivity in adults with chronic stroke: a randomized controlled trial comparing three injection techniques. *Clin Rehabil* 28(3): 232–242.

Pickett A, Rosales RL (2011). New trends in the science of botulinum toxin-A as applied in dystonia. *Int J Neurosci* 121: 22–34.

Pierrot-Deseilligny E, Burke D. (2005). *The Circuitry of the Human Spinal Cord: Its Role in Motor Control and Movement Disorders.* Cambridge: Cambridge University Press.

Priori A, Berardelli A, Mercuri B, Manfredi M (1995). Physiological effects produced by botulinum toxin treatment of upper limb dystonia: changes in reciprocal inhibition between forearm muscles. *Brain* 118:801–807.

Rosales RL (2012). Dystonia, spasticity and botulinum toxin therapy: rationale, evidences and clinical context. In: RL Rosales (Ed.), *Dystonia: The Many Facets.* Croatia: Intech Open Access Publishers.

Rosales RL, Dressler D (2010). On muscle spindles, dystonia and botulinum toxin. *Eur J Neurol* 17 (Suppl. 1): 71–80.

Rosales RL, Arimura K, Takenaga S, Osame M (1996). Extrafusal and intrafusal muscle effects in experimental botulinum toxin-A injection. *Muscle Nerve* 19: 488–496.

Rosales RL, Dressler D, Bigalke H (2006). Pharmacologic differences between botulinum toxins. *Eur J Neurol* 13: 2–10.

Rosales RL, Delos Santos MM, Ng AR, Teleg R, Dantes M, Lee LV, Fernandez HH (2011a). The broadening application of chemodenervation in X-linked dystonia-parkinsonism (part I): muscle afferent block versus botulinum toxin-A in cervical and limb dystonias. *Int J Neurosci* 121: 35–43.

Rosales RL, Kanovsky P, Fernandez HH (2011b). What's the 'catch' in upper-limb post-stroke spasticity: expanding the role of botulinum toxin applications. *Parkinsonism Relat Disord* 17: S3–S10.

Rosales RL, Kong KH, Goh KJ, Kumthornthip W, Mok VCT, Delgado-De Los Santos MM, Chua KSG, Abdullah SJF, Zakine B, Maisonob P, Magis A, Wong KSL (2012). Botulinum toxin injection for hypertonicity of the upper extremity within 12 weeks after stroke: a randomized controlled trial. *Neurorehabil Neural Repair* 26(7): 812–821.

Senkarova Z, Hlustik P, Otruba P, Herzig R, Kanovsky P (2010). Modulation of cortical activity in patients suffering from upper arm spasticity following stroke and treated with botulinum toxin A: an fMRI study. *J Neuroimaging* 20: 9–15.

Ward SR, Lieber RL (2009). Biological and mechanical pathologies in spastic skeletal muscle: the functional implications of therapeutic toxins. In: J Jankovic (Ed.), *Botulinum Toxin: Therapeutic Clinical Practice and Science.* Philadelphia, PA: Saunders.

Wohlfarth K, Schubert M, Rothe B, Elek J, Dengler R (2001). Remote F-wave changes after local botulinum toxin application. *Clin Neurophysiol* 112: 636–640.

Yamada N, Kakuda W, Kondo T, Mitani S, Shimizu M, Abo M (2014). Local muscle injection of botulinum toxin type A synergistically improves the beneficial effects of repetitive transcranial magnetic stimulation and intensive occupational therapy in post-stroke patients with spastic upper limb hemiparesis. *Eur Neurol* 72: 290–298.

Zeuner KE, Knutzen A, Al-Ali A, Hallett M, Deuschl G, Bergmann TO (2010). Associative stimulation of the supraorbital nerve fails to induce timing-specific plasticity in the human blink reflex. *PLoS One* 5:13602–13614.

Chapter 24

Direct Central Nervous System Effects of Botulinum Neurotoxin

Matteo Caleo and Riccardo Mazzocchio*

Introduction

Abundant evidence indicates that administration of botulinum neurotoxin type A (BoNT/A) triggers changes at the level of the central nervous system (CNS). This central reorganisation has been demonstrated using a series of physiological techniques in humans (Marchand-Pauvert et al. 2013; Mazzocchio & Caleo 2015) and biochemical and physiological assays in animals (Antonucci et al. 2008; Restani et al. 2012a; Koizumi et al. 2014; Matak & Lackovic 2014; Rossetto et al. 2015). In this chapter, we review the data supporting a direct central action of this neurotoxin mediated by long-range axonal transport, followed by a process of cell-to-cell transfer (referred to as transcytosis) by which the neurotoxin gains access to second-order neurons in the CNS. Several pathogens exploit this trafficking route to reach the CNS (Salinas et al. 2010). In addition to BoNT/A, also botulinum neurotoxin B (BoNT/B) may exert transynaptic effects following axonal transport (Ramachandran et al. 2015).

Long-Distance Retrograde Effects of BoNT/A in Animal Models

Direct evidence for retrograde trafficking of BoNT/A has been obtained in spinal cord motor neurons (Restani et al. 2012a) and hippocampal neurons (Wang et al. 2015; Bomba-Warczak et al. 2016) cultured in microfluidic devices. Following administration of fluorescently labelled toxin to the axon terminals, imaging of the axon channels revealed a retrograde flow of BoNT/A-containing carriers. These carriers move at an average speed of about 1 micron/sec and are prevalently non-acidic, as shown by lack of colocalisation with Lysotracker (Restani et al. 2012a; Wang et al. 2015). Evidence suggests that at least a fraction of the retrogradely transported BoNT/A remains catalytically active, as shown by cleavage of the BoNT/A substrate, the synaptic protein SNAP-25, in the somatodendritic compartment (Restani et al. 2012a; Wang et al. 2015; Bomba-Warczak et al. 2016). Importantly, cleavage of SNAP-25 has been demonstrated *in vivo* in the facial nucleus and spinal cord, after delivery of BoNT/A to the whisker pad and hindlimb muscles, respectively (Antonucci et al. 2008; Restani et al. 2012a; Koizumi et al. 2014). This retrograde propagation of SNAP-25 cleavage is blocked by application of colchicine, a microtubule depolymerising agent, indicating a key role for microtubule-based axonal transport (Antonucci et al. 2008).

To perform its actions at the level of central circuits, BoNT/A should (1) be transported in a catalytically active form, (2) undergo transcytosis into afferent synapses and (3) exert functional effects (i.e. blockade of neurotransmission) at these distant synapses. Experimental evidence has been obtained for each of these steps, using the rat visual pathway as a model system. In particular, studies have been conducted on the long-range, unidirectional projections connecting the retina with the superior colliculus/optic tectum via retinal ganglion cell fibres. In this model system, delivery of BoNT/A to the tectum results in appearance of BoNT/A-truncated SNAP-25 in the retina within three days (Antonucci et al. 2008; Restani et al. 2012b).

(1) One crucial question is whether this distant SNAP-25 cleavage depends upon BoNT/A catalytic activity within the retina, or is simply due to retrograde transfer of the BoNT/A-altered SNAP-25 generated at the tectal terminals. To demonstrate retrograde transfer of the active toxin, the optic nerve was transected three days after BoNT/A delivery to the tectum to prevent any further transport and BoNT/E was injected in the retina to cleave BoNT/A-altered SNAP-25 into a smaller 22 kDa fragment (Antonucci et al. 2008). At the completion of BoNT/E effects, there was a return of BoNT/A-truncated SNAP-25 in the retina, demonstrating the transfer of the catalytic activity of BoNT/A from the tectum to retinal cells (Antonucci et al. 2008).

(2) The issue of transcytosis was addressed by analysing the neuronal populations expressing BoNT/A-cleaved SNAP-25 within the retina after tectal delivery of BoNT/A. Particularly robust staining for BoNT/A-truncated SNAP-25 was found in the cholinergic cells impinging onto retinal ganglion cells (Antonucci et al. 2008; Restani et al. 2012b). Thus, BoNT/A appears to reach specific classes of second-order neurons via a transcytosis process. The reasons for this cholinergic cell specificity are not completely understood but might be due to the fact that

* We thank Dr Laura Restani for fruitful discussions on the topics covered in this review. This work was supported by Fondazione Pisa (grant #158/2011).

these terminals express high levels of SV2C, one of the high-affinity protein receptors for BoNT/A (Antonucci et al. 2008).

(3) To examine whether cholinergic synapses containing cleaved SNAP-25 are functionally impaired, calcium imaging was performed to quantify 'retinal waves', i.e. activity bursts that propagate within the retina and are driven by acetylcholine release, thus providing a readout of cholinergic neurotransmission (Restani et al. 2012b). The results were clear in indicating a depression of wave frequency (indicative of cholinergic dysfunction) in retinas from animals injected with BoNT/A into the tectum. Retrograde BoNT/A caused also a significant enlargement of presynaptic terminals in the retina, with accumulation of synaptic vesicles that are unable to fuse with the plasma membrane to release their neurotransmitter (Restani et al. 2012b). Altogether, these data converge to indicate inhibition of neuroexocytosis in intoxicated synapses distant to BoNT/A inoculation.

A similar scenario may be envisaged for motor neurons, even if there is currently no information on the central synapses that are affected following BoNT/A retrograde transport and transcytosis. Unlike tetanus neurotoxin, BoNT/A might preferentially target excitatory synapses in the CNS (Verderio et al. 2004). This effect would predict a reduction in the motor neuron firing rate that has been indeed verified experimentally in the animal (Moreno-Lopez et al. 1997). This dampened discharge is bound to impair Renshaw cell inhibition via reduced input through the motor neuron recurrent collaterals (Figure 24.1). Recurrent inhibition could also be reduced via an action of the toxin at the cholinergic synapse between motor neuron collaterals and Renshaw cells. In the case of upper cranial motor neurons, recurrent collaterals are lacking but a reduction of motor neuron excitability through transcytosis and block of presynaptic excitatory terminals may combine with the peripheral blockade (Figure 24.1), allowing for clinical benefits even when the neuromuscular blockade is over.

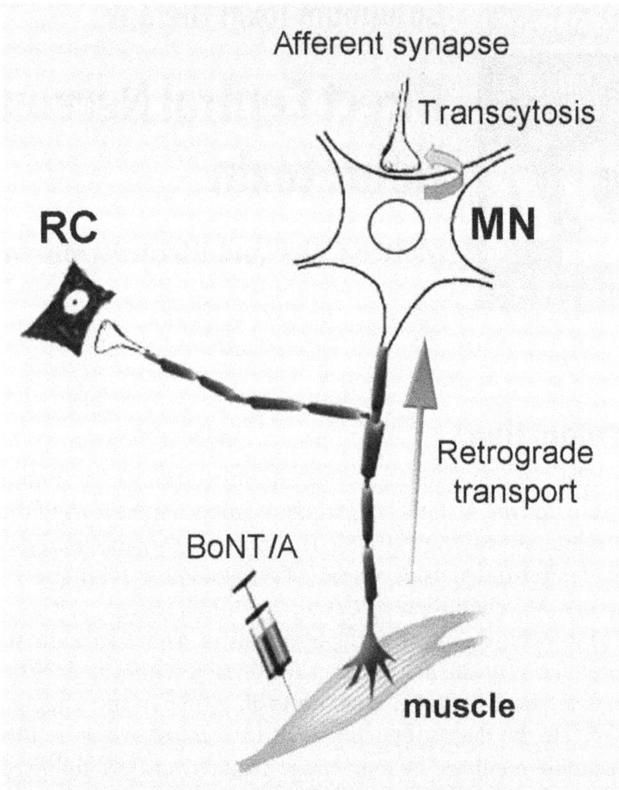

Figure 24.1 Mechanisms underlying direct central effects of botulinum neurotoxin type A (BoNT/A). BoNT/A injected intramuscularly acts mainly at the neuromuscular junction but at least a fraction of the catalytically active toxin undergoes retrograde axonal transport to the motor neuron (MN) and transcytosis into afferent synapses. Reduced motor neuron discharges result in decreased input to Renshaw cells (RC), thus dampening recurrent inhibition. Reduced inputs to the motor neuron may also combine with the peripheral blockade of neurotransmission.

Central Effects of BoNT/A in Human Patients

There are several central actions of BoNT/A (summarised below) that give rise to meaningful clinical changes, and may be explained with direct central effects on either recurrent inhibitory networks or motor neuron excitability.

A central effect of BoNT/A in patients with spasticity is a reduction in the heteronymous recurrent inhibition from the peripherally injected soleus muscle to the non-injected quadriceps muscle (Marchand-Pauvert et al. 2013). This may be explained either via blockade of the cholinergic synapse between motor neuron recurrent collaterals and Renshaw cells, or through an action on excitatory spinal synapses with a direct reduction of motor neuron activity (Mazzocchio & Caleo 2015). Functionally, the down-regulation of activity in the Renshaw cell extensive network releases the reciprocal Ia inhibition (by reduced Renshaw cell inhibition of the inhibitory Ia interneurons) from the injected agonist to the antagonist, resulting in improved locomotor synchrony because of less ankle muscle co-contraction after BoNT/A (Aymard et al. 2013) and decouples motor neuron pools located at different segmental levels linking limb muscle groups in abnormal synergies (Mazzocchio & Caleo 2015). As shown for spasticity, the release of the reciprocal Ia inhibition and the decoupling of the motor neuron pools following BoNT/A-induced reduction in the activity of the Renshaw cell network may also be particularly relevant in limb dystonia, a condition characterised by a dysfunction in the pattern of agonist/antagonist coordinated activity and overflow into muscles not involved in the task (Hallett 2011).

Patients with upper-limb dystonia exhibit reduced presynaptic inhibition of Ia terminals between flexor and extensor forearm muscles. Presynaptic inhibition is restored to normal levels after injection of BoNT/A in the wrist flexors of these patients (Priori et al. 1995). It is thought that lesser muscle afferent input from the wrist flexor (the injected muscle) could decrease the presynaptic gating on the extensor Ia terminals, resulting in a larger presynaptic inhibition of the Ia afferents from the wrist flexors (Priori et al. 1995). However, the dominant group I peripheral input to the interneurons mediating reciprocal inhibition between wrist muscles is not Ia, but Ib, in origin. In addition, there is multi-convergence on several interneurons of proprioceptive and cutaneous volleys from forearm flexors (involved in exploratory hand movements and grasp) and proprioceptive input from extensors and proximal muscles (involved in the postural adjustments of the wrist), suggesting that the control of wrist posture during hand movements may be mediated through different kinds of interneurons, such as non-reciprocal group I interneurons, group II interneurons and, in particular, propriospinal-like interneurons controlling the activity of many upper limb motor neurons. Indeed, in writer's cramp, a focal hand dystonia in which abnormal postures only occur during writing, activity in propriospinal neurones is affected on the dystonic side, while spinal group I excitation is not modified (Marchand-Pauvert & Iglesias 2008). Thus, the mechanisms for a direct central effect could be mainly through the Renshaw network, as documented in spastic subjects. An action, through retrograde axonal transport and transcytosis, on the excitatory propriospinal-like interneuron terminals onto forearm motor neurons could be envisaged, but it has yet to be demonstrated.

Trapezius and dorsal neck motor neurons also give and receive recurrent inhibition. Recurrent inhibitory connections within the neck segments C3 and C4 are distributed to a variety of motor neuron species and extend at least to the adjacent segment. As elsewhere in the spinal cord, (1) homonymous axons are the most effective; (2) recurrent inhibition occurs between synergists (splenius elicits the strongest recurrent inhibition but receives the least) and is most effective on motor neurons located at the same level (e.g. from semispinalis capitis to splenius); and (3) recurrent inhibition extends beyond synergist connections (e.g. from splenius to levator scapulae). However, it is not possible to extend the comparison to correlation with reciprocal inhibition, as there is no evidence that Ia reciprocal inhibition occurs among neck motor neurons (Brink & Suzuki 1987). Since recurrent inhibition is a prominent feature of the spinal organisation controlling neck muscles, modulation of its activity through BoNT/A central effects could improve control of head movements in cervical dystonia by disentangling abnormal muscle coupling in the neck.

In cranial dystonia, an argument against possible central effects is that the enhanced recovery cycle of the blink reflex is not influenced after BoNT/A treatment of blepharospasm (Valls-Sole et al. 1991). However, this may indicate that there is little influence of muscular afferents upon the excitability of brainstem interneurons either because muscle spindles are lacking or because the blink reflex loop is only in part representative of the control of eyelid closure (Matsuo et al. 2014). On the other hand, mechanisms for a central direct effect could be retrograde axonal transport and transynaptic effect on terminals impinging onto cranial motor neurons, as demonstrated in the animal (Pastor et al. 1997). This could decrease motor neuron firing (Moreno-Lopez et al. 1997), thus adding a second level of motor neuron inhibition in the CNS. Indeed, several data challenge the view that the improvements seen in focal dystonias after treatment with BoNT/A are only the result of the local weakness at the injected muscles:

1. In the case of blepharospasm, a late improvement, continuing over weeks, is present at a time when EMG fibrillation potentials from orbicularis oculi muscle have disappeared and the amplitude of the facial CMAP has almost recovered (Valls-Sole et al. 1991). Similarly, patients with arm dystonia may enjoy a clinical beneficial effect of BoNT/A treatment months after the local weakness disappears (Priori et al. 1995).
2. Adjacent, but not injected, muscles around the eyes, such as the lower facial muscles, can also show a reduction in muscle spasms (Giladi 1997).
3. Besides a reduction of the spasm intensity, a reduction of the spasm frequency has been reported in patients with blepharospasm (Valls-Sole et al. 1991) and jerky torticollis (Giladi 1997). This effect is difficult to explain on the basis of muscle paresis alone.
4. BoNT/A treatment also effectively alleviates some annoying sensory symptoms of the dystonias such as tension and tenderness at the neck in spasmodic torticollis, as well as ocular irritation, burning or light hypersensitivity in patients with blepharospasm (Giladi 1997). This supports an effect of BoNT/A also on central sensory aspects of the dystonias.

References

Antonucci F, Rossi C, Gianfranceschi L, Rossetto O, Caleo M (2008). Long-distance retrograde effects of botulinum neurotoxin A. *J Neurosci* 28:3689–3696.

Aymard C, Giboin LS, Lackmy-Vallee A, Marchand-Pauvert V (2013). Spinal plasticity in stroke patients after botulinum neurotoxin A injection in ankle plantar flexors. *Physiol Rep* 1:e00173.

Bomba-Warczak E, Vevea JD, Brittain JM, Figueroa-Bernier A, Tepp WH, Johnson EA, Yeh FL, Chapman ER (2016). Interneuronal transfer and distal action of tetanus toxin and botulinum neurotoxins A and D in central neurons. *Cell Rep* 16:1974–1987.

Brink EE, Suzuki I (1987). Recurrent inhibitory connexions among neck motoneurones in the cat. *J Physiol* 383:301–326.

Giladi N (1997). The mechanism of action of botulinum toxin type A in focal dystonia is most probably through its dual effect on efferent (motor) and afferent pathways at the injected site. *J Neurol Sci* 152:132–135.

Hallett M (2011). Neurophysiology of dystonia: the role of inhibition. *Neurobiol Dis* 42:177–184.

Koizumi H, Goto S, Okita S, Morigaki R, Akaike N, Torii Y, Harakawa T, Ginnaga A, Kaji R (2014). Spinal central effects of peripherally applied botulinum neurotoxin A in comparison between its subtypes A1 and A2. *Front Neurol* 5:98.

Marchand-Pauvert V, Iglesias C (2008). Properties of human spinal interneurones: normal and dystonic control. *J Physiol* 586:1247–1256.

Marchand-Pauvert V, Aymard C, Giboin LS, Dominici F, Rossi A, Mazzocchio R (2013). Beyond muscular effects: depression of spinal recurrent inhibition after botulinum neurotoxin A. *J Physiol* 591:1017–1029.

Matak I, Lackovic Z (2014). Botulinum toxin A, brain and pain. *Prog Neurobiol* 119–120:39–59.

Matsuo K, Ban R, Ban M, Yuzuriha S (2014). Trigeminal proprioception evoked by strong stretching of the mechanoreceptors in

Muller's muscle induces reflex contraction of the orbital orbicularis oculi slow-twitch muscle fibers. *Eplasty* 14:e30.

Mazzocchio R, Caleo M (2015). More than at the neuromuscular synapse: actions of botulinum neurotoxin A in the central nervous system. *Neuroscientist* 21:44–61.

Moreno-Lopez B, Pastor AM, de la Cruz RR, Delgado-Garcia JM (1997). Dose-dependent, central effects of botulinum neurotoxin type A: a pilot study in the alert behaving cat. *Neurology* 48:456–464.

Pastor AM, Moreno-Lopez B, De La Cruz RR, Delgado-Garcia JM (1997). Effects of botulinum neurotoxin type A on abducens motoneurons in the cat: ultrastructural and synaptic alterations. *Neuroscience* 81:457–478.

Priori A, Berardelli A, Mercuri B, Manfredi M (1995). Physiological effects produced by botulinum toxin treatment of upper limb dystonia: changes in reciprocal inhibition between forearm muscles. *Brain* 118 (Pt 3):801–807.

Ramachandran R, Lam C, Yaksh TL (2015). Botulinum toxin in migraine: role of transport in trigemino-somatic and trigeminovascular afferents. *Neurobiol Dis* 79:111–122.

Restani L, Giribaldi F, Manich M, Bercsenyi K, Menendez G, Rossetto O, Caleo M, Schiavo G (2012a). Botulinum neurotoxins A and E undergo retrograde axonal transport in primary motor neurons. *PLoS Pathog* 8:e1003087.

Restani L, Novelli E, Bottari D, Leone P, Barone I, Galli-Resta L, Strettoi E, Caleo M (2012b). Botulinum neurotoxin A impairs neurotransmission following retrograde transynaptic transport. *Traffic* 13:1083–1089.

Rossetto O, Pirazzini M, Montecucco C (2015). Current gaps in basic science knowledge of botulinum neurotoxin biological actions. *Toxicon* 107(Pt A):59–63.

Salinas S, Schiavo G, Kremer EJ (2010). A hitchhiker's guide to the nervous system: the complex journey of viruses and toxins. *Nat Rev Microbiol* 8:645–655.

Valls-Sole J, Tolosa ES, Ribera G (1991). Neurophysiological observations on the effects of botulinum toxin treatment in patients with dystonic blepharospasm. *J Neurol Neurosurg Psychiatry* 54:310–313.

Verderio C, Pozzi D, Pravettoni E, Inverardi F, Schenk U, Coco S, Proux-Gillardeaux V, Galli T, Rossetto O, Frassoni C, Matteoli M (2004). SNAP-25 modulation of calcium dynamics underlies differences in GABAergic and glutamatergic responsiveness to depolarization. *Neuron* 41:599–610.

Wang T, Martin S, Papadopulos A, Harper CB, Mavlyutov TA, Niranjan D, Glass NR, Cooper-White JJ, Sibarita JB, Choquet D, Davletov B, Meunier FA (2015). Control of autophagosome axonal retrograde flux by presynaptic activity unveiled using botulinum neurotoxin type A. *J Neurosci* 35:6179–6194.

Chapter 25

Analgesic Effects of Botulinum Toxins

Zdravko Lacković and Maja Relja

Introduction

The light chain of botulinum toxin (BT) molecule shows zinc metalloprotease activity. Inside the cell, BT type A (BT-A) cleaves synaptosomal-associated protein (SNAP-25; 25 kDa) while BT type B (BT-B) and some other clinical less-important subtypes cleave vesicle-associated membrane protein (VAMP). Proteins SNAP-25 and VAMP are parts of the soluble n-ethylmaleimide-sensitive factor attachment receptor (SNARE) family, necessary for vesicular release of neurotransmitters. Cleavage of the SNARE proteins particularly inhibits the release of acetylcholine and results in muscle weakness and – in higher doses (botulism) – paralysis. Application of small non-toxic doses of BT is widely used to achieve long-lasting relaxation of targeted muscles (Matak & Lacković 2014).

Classical symptoms of botulism have led to the assumption that the BT action is selective for cholinergic transmission only. However, in line with the ubiquitous role of SNAREs, BT-A blocks the neurotransmitter release of most neurotransmitters (Matak & Lacković 2014). Moreover, BT might have some actions independent of SNAP-25 (Matak & Lacković 2015). In addition to neuromuscular disorders, there has been increased interest in the use of BT to treat a variety of medical conditions refractory to conventional treatment, ranging from pain to psychiatric disorders and premature ejaculation. The analgesic effect of BT is currently widely investigated. The approved indications are chronic migraine and dystonia (frequently associated with pain) (Matak & Lacković 2014). BT-A's reduction of pain hypersensitivity and allodynia lasting several months makes this a unique antinociceptive drug.

There are currently over 20 commercial preparations of BT (Matak & Lacković 2014). There are no international standards and the potency units are specific to each BT product. Therefore, the FDA approved new ('generic') names for different BT products registered in the United States, including onabotulinumtoxinA (Allergan, Botox®), abobotulinumtoxinA (Ipsen, Dysport®), incobotulinumtoxinA (Merz, Xeomin®) and rimabotulinumtoxinB for BT-B (Solstice Neurosciences, Neurobloc®/Myobloc®). There are some pharmacokinetic differences between different preparations, but all of them block neurotransmitter release with different molecular targets for BT-A and BT-B. Recently, the Dressler group compared the efficacy of Botox® and Xeomin® to that of Dysport® in long-term treatment of blepharospasm (Kollewe et al. 2015). No significant difference was found apart from the potency labelling. Accordingly, in this chapter we do not distinguish between different brands of BT-A, only shortly describing the differences between BT-A and BT-B.

Discovery of BT-A's Antinociceptive Activity

As early as the 1980s, it was observed that BT-A reduces the pain associated with neuromuscular hyperactivity disorders such as cervical dystonia (Tsui et al. 1986). However, it was believed that this is a consequence of decreased muscle hyperactivity (Matak & Lacković 2014). Hyperactive muscles might compress small blood vessels and induce ischaemia that 'leads to the release of bradykinin and sensitisation or excitation of nociceptors. BT is a causal therapy in these cases because it stops the excessive ACh release' (Mense 2004). Though, it was found that pain relief does not always occur simultaneously with the paretic BT effect and sometimes it lasts longer than the neuromuscular effect (Relja & Klepac 2002; Matak & Lacković 2014). In a double-blind dose–response study in our clinical department we (MR) observed that BT-A's effect on pain in cervical dystonia occurred after one week, while the beneficial effect on motor function started after two weeks. Moreover, we observed that the BT dose inducing antinociceptive effects (50 MU) was lower than the dose required for motor improvement (100–150 MU) (Relja & Klepac 2002).

Current Clinical Development

Independently from pain associated with muscle hyperactivity, the antinociceptive BT effect was reported in types of chronic pain not primarily associated with muscular hyperactivity, like migraine, tension-type headache or different types of neuropathic pain (Relja et al. 2007; Matak & Lacković 2014; Intiso et al. 2015; Table 25.1). Thus, it is accepted that BT-A's effects on pain are mediated by its direct effects on peripheral sensory nerve endings.

Migraine. Results of large (1384 patients) multicentric phase III research evaluating migraine prophylaxis therapy (PREEMPT) studies (Dodick et al. 2010) showed that BT-A treatment reduced the number of migraine attacks per month, suggesting that it may be used as a prophylactic treatment of chronic migraine. Consequently, the FDA approved onabotulinumtoxinA for the treatment of chronic migraine. There have

Table 25.1 Systemic reviews and meta-analyses of botulinum toxin type A's (BT-A) efficacy in different pain conditions

Type of pain (reference)	Type of research settings	Outcome conclusions
Shoulder pain (Singh & Fitzgerald 2011)	Systemic review Six randomised controlled trials, 164 patients	Promising, but more studies are needed
Shoulder pain (Wu et al. 2015)	Systematic review and meta-analysis	Compared with steroid or placebo injection BT improves pain score and range of motion
Trigeminal neuralgia (Hu et al. 2013)	Systemic review Six studies,101 patients	Promising, but randomised controlled double-blinded studies are lacking
Low-back pain and sciatica (Waseem et al. 2010)	Systemic review Three randomised trials, 123 patients	Heterogeneity of the studies prevented meta-analysis
Subacute/chronic neck pain (Langevin et al. 2011)	Nine controlled trials 503 participants	Not clinically important or a significant benefit of BT-A
Myofascial pain syndromes in adults (Soares et al. 2012)	Four studies 233 participants	Inconclusive evidence
Subpectoral breast implants (Winocour et al. 2014)	Systemic review Seven clinical trials on 427 women	Promising, but lacks methodological rigour
Benign masseter muscle hypertrophy (Fedorowicz et al. 2013)	23 full text articles analysed	No randomised clinical trials or controlled clinical trials

been many comments and additional studies. We (MR) participated in the PREEMPT-1 and PREEMPT-2 studies. In general, the efficacy and safety of BT-A therapy in migraine is considered well established.

Cervical Dystonia. Different degrees of pain in the cervical region are reported by more than 60 per cent of patients and the pain intensity is directly related to disease severity. BT is currently considered the treatment of choice for cervical dystonia and can lead to an improvement in pain and dystonic symptoms in up to 90 per cent of patients (Camargo et al. 2015).

Apart from chronic migraine and dystonia, BT is used off-label in neurology, urology, orthopaedics, etc. Intiso and coworkers (Intiso et al. 2015) reviewed pain complicating frequent disorders of the central and peripheral nervous system such as spinal cord injury, post-stroke shoulder pain, painful diabetic neuropathy, posttraumatic neuralgia, phantom limb pain, etc.

Gaps in Clinical Research

Results of some clinical studies with BT-A are contradictory, such as its effects on myofacial pain (Göbel et al. 2006) or tension-type headache (Matak & Lacković 2014). Results of systemic reviews are also inconclusive (Table 25.1). The reason for this may be the lack of standardised guidelines for BT-A application, dosage and appropriate definition of study primary outcomes. Here are some examples of uncertainty concerning doses to be used:

In a trial on 34 patients with benign prostatic hyperplasia, efficacy and safety of both BT-A 100 and 200 MU doses were similar (Arnouk et al. 2012).

In a randomised double-blind placebo-controlled trial of 84 patients with classical trigeminal neuralgia, beneficial effect of BT-A was found. However, efficacy between a 25 MU dose and three times higher dose (75 MU) was similar (Zhang et al. 2014).

In 68 patients with post-stroke arm spasticity, half of the recommended BT-A dose had a satisfactory effect (Agafonova & Khasanova 2014).

In axillary hyperhidrosis, BT is considered the treatment of choice, but its dosing varies widely. In a prospective double-blind intra-individual side-to-side comparison study, 51 patients with symmetric axillary hyperhidrosis were treated with 100 MU or 50 MU unilaterally or bilaterally. Ninety per cent of the patients reported the overall therapeutic effect as 'excellent' independently of the site of injection or the dose used. Authors suggested that the therapeutic effect saturates at 50 MU, but lower doses were not investigated (Dressler & Adib Saberi 2013).

In a randomised trial the effect of 1500, 3000 and 5000 MU in 27 children with cerebral palsy and refractory sialorrhoea was investigated; 3000 MU BT-B injected into the salivary glands significantly improved the frequency and severity of sialorrhoea in children with cerebral palsy. The lower dose was ineffective and the higher dose produced more side-effects with no greater benefit (Basciani et al. 2011).

Controversies About BT's Mechanism of Action: Is It Peripheral or Central?

The analgesic effect of BT-A has been linked to the blockade of peripheral release of neurotransmitters in the animal model of formalin-induced pain (Cui et al. 2004). It was assumed that the biochemical mechanism remains the same between BT-A's effect on the motor nerve or peripheral sensory nerve: enzymatic blockade of neurotransmitter release. BT-A was found to block the release of glutamate in the periphery as well as c-Fos expression centrally (Cui et al. 2004). These observations were interpreted by Aoki and others, proposing that BT-A blocks peripheral sensitisation and indirectly reduces central sensitisation (Matak & Lacković 2015).

Beside the indirect evidence from *in vivo* or *ex vivo* experiments, the inhibitory effect of BT-A on glutamate release *in vivo* up to now was found only in two experiments: formalin-induced pain in rats (Cui et al. 2004) and in a recent *in vivo* experiment on 12 healthy volunteers. Volunteers were pretreated with BT-A (10 MU) on the volar forearm and dermal microdialysis was applied to collect interstitial samples before and after the application of a capsaicin patch (8 per cent) and mild heat (40 °C/60 min) to provoke glutamate release, pain and vasodilation. The provoked pain intensity as well as glutamate release was lower in the BT-A-pretreated arm. However, the reduction in pain was not correlated with glutamate level, and the origin of this endogenous glutamate is unknown (Bittencourt da Silva et al. 2014).

Although direct evidence for the peripheral mechanism of BT actions is weak, this view constituted a 'dogma' in BT research for many years (Matak & Lacković 2014). Obviously, it was easier to accept that BT acts on pain principally in the same way as on the muscular system. And, apparently, there was some concern that the new point of action can possibly bring new and unwanted effects. As Currà and Berardelli (Currà & Berardelli 2009) point out, BT 'injected locally has also been considered safe because no evidence showed that the toxin acts also at distant sites'.

In 2005, we (ZL) found that pretreatment with BT-A significantly reduced or completely abolished the enhanced sensitivity to mechanical and thermal stimuli provoked by peripheral carrageenan or capsaicin injections in rats (Bach-Rojecky & Lacković 2005; Matak & Lacković 2014). However, in contrast to observation by Cui and coworkers (Cui et al. 2004) with formalin, we found no effect of BT on the carrageenan-induced paw oedema. We hypothesised that the mechanism of the antinociceptive action of BT-A might be much more complex than the suggested inhibition of transmitter release in the periphery. In a more detailed study, BT had no effect on the size of carrageenan-induced paw oedema measured as paw volume and weight, the capsaicin-induced extravasations of plasma proteins labelled by Evans blue or by direct histological examination of inflamed tissue (Bach-Rojecky & Lacković 2009). Accordingly, we assumed that the mechanism of antinociceptive and anti-inflammatory effect of BT-A is not the same as previously suggested, and that a new mechanism should be researched.

Intracerebroventricular application of BT-A or BT-B reduced the second phase of the formalin test similarly as peripheral administration, demonstrating that BT-A may act not only peripherally (Matak & Lacković 2014).

Several observations from our laboratory indicate that BT-A has a central mechanism of action:

Using the model of unilateral injection of acidic saline solution into the gastrocnemius muscle as an animal model of bilateral muscle hyperalgesia, we found that BT-A subcutaneously injected into ipsilateral hindpaw abolished hyperalgesia bilaterally. We additionally observed the bilateral antinociceptive effect after unilateral application of BT-A in rats with streptozotocin-induced diabetic neuropathy, as it had been reported previously in plaxitel-induced neuropathy (Matak & Lacković 2014).

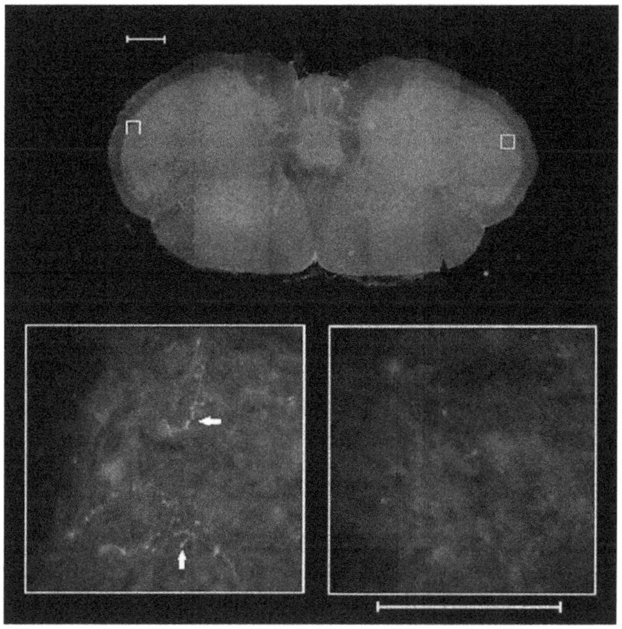

Figure 25.1 After peripheral application of botulinum toxin type A (BT-A) (5 MU/kg) in rat whisker pad, enzymatic activity of BT-A could be found in nerve elements in ipsilateral trigeminal nucleus caudalis. Cleaved SNAP-25 immunofluorescent staining (arrows) in ipsilateral trigeminal nucleus caudalis of the caudal medulla coronal section. Details of the method are described previously (48–51). Low magnification = 500 m scale bar, high magnification = 100 m.

Courtesy of Ivica Matak.

Prevention of axonal transport by colchicine inhibits the BT-A analgesic action in different pain models, demonstrating the central mechanism of the antinociceptive effect of BT-A (Matak & Lacković 2014).

Immunohistochemical detection of BT-A-cleaved SNAP-25 ($SNAP\text{-}25_{197}$) in the trigeminal nucleus caudalis (Figure 25.1) and lumbar dorsal horn after peripheral injection of BT-A, demonstrating that enzymatically active BT-A is transported to the central nervous system, where it alters the nociceptive neurotransmission (Matak & Lacković 2014).

The occurrence of cleaved SNAP-25 in trigeminal nucleus and BT-A's antinociceptive activity in formalin-induced orofacial pain were prevented by denervation with capsaicin, suggesting altered nociceptive transmission at the central synapse of primary afferents. The association of BT-A with capsaicin-sensitive TRPV1-expressing neurons might be associated with observed selectivity of BT-A's action only in certain types of pain (Matak & Lacković 2014).

Specificity of Botulinum Toxin Type B

BT-B (rimabotulinumtoxinB, Neurobloc®/MyoBloc®) was (by a few months) the first FDA-approved treatment for cervical dystonia in the United States. In contrast to BT-A cleaving SNAP-25, BT-B cleaves VAMP. Since both proteins are part of the

SNARE complex necessary for neurotransmitter exocytosis, similar effects could be expected. BT-A has the longest half-life followed by BT types C, B, F and E (Matak & Lacković 2014). BT-A produced muscle weakness in mice at several times lower doses than BT-B and the duration of its effect was longer (30 vs 14 days) (Aoki 2002). Intraplantar BT-B (1 MU) given unilaterally into the hindpaw of mice ipsilaterally decreased (Marino et al. 2014):

- formalin-evoked flinching;
- capsaicin-evoked plasma extravasation in the hindpaw;
- intraplantar formalin-evoked dorsal horn substance P release and neuronal activation (c-Fos);
- ipsilateral dorsal root ganglion cleaved VAMP, substance P release and activation of c-Fos.

Accordingly, BT-B after unilateral intraplantar delivery is taken up by the peripheral terminal and transported to the ipsilateral sensory ganglia to cleave VAMP. It is acting presynaptically to block release from the spinal peptidergic terminal.

Dressler and coworkers (Dressler & Benecke 2003; Dressler & Eleopra 2006; Kollewe et al. 2015) used BT-B to treat cervical dystonia, hyperhidrosis, spastic conditions, cerebral palsy, hemifacial spasm, bladder dysfunction, spasmodic dysphonia, sialorrhoea, anal fissures, piriformis syndrome, various pain conditions and cosmetic applications. Generally, its therapeutic effects are comparable to BT-A. However, BT-B produced substantially more anticholinergic adverse effects (Dressler & Benecke 2003).

Is Botulinum Toxin Analgesic? Lessons from Preclinical Research

In contrast to most conventional analgesics in experimental animals, BT has no effect on acute pain, with an important and protective function. In contrast to that, BT shows selective activity on longer-lasting pain assumed to be associated with development of central sensitisation. The classical formalin test could be the best example. The formalin test for nociception in the rat paw causes a reproducible biphasic response. The first phase is characterised by extensive licking (0–15 min), caused by the direct stimulation of nociceptors by formalin. The second phase of extensive licking (15–60 min) is a result of the released inflammatory mediators probably caused by peripheral and central sensitisation. BT-A prevents only the second inflammatory phase (Cui et al. 2004; Bach-Rojecky & Lacković 2005; Bach-Rojecky & Lacković 2009).

In addition to formalin, BT-A in rodents abolishes capsaicin- and carrageenan-induced pain, neuropathic pain induced by ligature of the sciatic nerve or the infraorbital branch of the trigeminal nerve, streptozotocin-induced diabetic neuropathy postsurgical hyperalgesia and generalised abdominal pain (Bach-Rojecky & Lackovic 2009; Matak & Lacković 2014). How is pain measured in animals? Usually, we measure movement responses to additional painful stimuli (usually mechanical or thermal). Thus, what is measured is not 'basic' or 'tonic' chronic pain but rather a reaction to the additional pain; supersensitivity including allodynia. In all pain models investigated up to now we see the beneficial effect of BT on pain supersensitivity and allodynia (especially if we are using Von Frey filaments). That should be taken into account when comparing results of animal experiments with those of humans.

References

Agafonova NV, Khasanova DR (2014) [The use of different doses of botulotoxin A in the treatment of early arm poststroke spasticity]. [Article in Russian] *Zh Nevrol Psikhiatr Im S S Korsakova* 114: 68–71.

Aoki R (2002) Botulinum neurotoxin serotypes A and B preparations have different safety margins in preclinical models of muscle weakening efficacy and systemic safety. *Toxicon* 40: 923–928.

Arnouk R, Suzuki Bellucci C, Benatuil Stull R, de Bessa J, Malave C, Gomes C (2012) Botulinum neurotoxin type A for the treatment of benign prostatic hyperplasia: randomized study comparing two doses. *Sci World J* 2012: 463574.

Bach-Rojecky L, Lacković Z (2005) Antinociceptive effect of botulinum toxin type A in rat model of carrageenan and capsaicin induced pain. *Croat Med J* 46: 201–208.

Bach-Rojecky L, Lacković Z (2009) Central origin of the antinociceptive action of botulinum toxin type A. *Pharmacol Biochem Behav* 94(2): 234–238. doi: 10.1016/j.pbb.2009.08.012.

Basciani M, DiRienzo F, Fontana A, Copetti M, Pellegrini F, Intiso D (2011) Botulinum toxin type B for sialorrhoea in children with cerebral palsy: a randomized trial comparing three doses. *Dev Med Child Neurol* 53: 559–564.

Bittencourt da Silva L, Karshenas A, Bach F, Rasmussen S, Arendt-Nielsen L, Gazerani P (2014) Blockade of glutamate release by botulinum neurotoxin type A in humans: a dermal microdialysis study. *Pain Res Manag* 19: 126–132.

Camargo C, Cattai L, Teive H (2015) Pain relief in cervical dystonia with botulinum toxin treatment. *Toxins* (Basel) 7: 2321–2335.

Cui M, Khanijou S, Rubino J, Aoki K (2004) Subcutaneous administration of botulinum toxin A reduces formalin-induced pain. *Pain* 107: 125–133.

Currà A, Berardelli A (2009) Do the unintended actions of botulinum toxin at distant sites have clinical implications? *Neurology* 72:1095–1099.

Dodick D, Turkel C, DeGryse R, Aurora S, Silberstein S, Lipton R, Diener H, Brin MF, PREEMPT Chronic Migraine Study Group (2010) OnabotulinumtoxinA for treatment of chronic migraine: pooled results from the double-blind randomized placebo-controlled phases of the PREEMPT clinical program. *Headache* 50: 921–936.

Dressler D, Adib Saberi F (2013) Towards a dose optimisation of botulinum toxin therapy for axillary hyperhidrosis: comparison of different Botox doses. *J Neural Transm* 120: 1565–1567.

Dressler D, Benecke R (2003) Autonomic side effects of botulinum toxin type B treatment of cervical dystonia and hyperhidrosis. *Eur Neurol* 49: 34–38.

Dressler D, Eleopra R (2006) Clinical use of non-A botulinum toxins: botulinum toxin type B. *Neurotox Res* 9: 121–125.

Fedorowicz Z, van Zuuren E, Schoones J (2013) Botulinum toxin for masseter hypertrophy. *Cochrane Database of Systematic Reviews* 9(9): CD007510.

Göbel H, Heinze A, Reiche G, Hefter H, Benecke R, Dysport Myofascial Pain Study Group (2006) Efficacy and safety of a single botulinum type A toxin complex treatment (Dysport) for the relief of upper back myofascial pain syndrome: results from a randomized double-blind placebo-controlled multicentre study. *Pain* 125: 82–88.

Hu Y, Guan X, Fan L, Li M, Liao Y, Nie Z, Jin L (2013) Therapeutic efficacy and safety of botulinum toxin type A in trigeminal neuralgia: a systematic review. *J Headache Pain* 14: 72.

Intiso D, Basciani M, Santamato A, Intiso M, Di Rienzo F (2015) Botulinum toxin type A for the treatment of neuropathic pain in neuro-rehabilitation. *Toxins* 7: 2454–2480.

Kollewe K, Mohammadi B, Köhler S, Pickenbrock H, Dengler R, Dressler D (2015) Blepharospasm: long-term treatment with either Botox® Xeomin® or Dysport®. *J Neural Transm* 122: 427–431.

Langevin P, Peloso PM, Lowcock J, Nolan M, Weber J, Gross A, Roberts J, Goldsmith CH, Graham N, Burnie SJ, Haines T (2011) Botulinum toxin for subacute/chronic neck pain. *Cochrane Database Syst Rev* 7: CD008626.

Marino MJ, Terashima T, Steinauer JJ, Eddinger KA, Yaksh TL, Xu Q (2014) Botulinum toxin B in the sensory afferent: transmitter release spinal activation and pain behavior. *Pain* 155: 674–684.

Matak I, Lacković Z (2014) Botulinum toxin A brain and pain. *Prog Neurobiol* 119–120: 39–59.

Matak I, Lacković Z (2015) Botulinum neurotoxin type A: actions beyond SNAP-25. *Toxicology* 335: 79–84.

Mense S (2004) Neurobiological basis for the use of botulinum toxin in pain therapy. *J Neurol* 251(Suppl. 1): 1–7.

Relja M, Klepac N (2002) Different doses of botulinum toxin A and pain responsiveness in cervical dystonia. *Neurology* 58: A474.

Relja M, Poole AC, Schoenen J, Pascual J, Lei X, Thompson C, European BoNTA Headache Study Group (2007) A multicentre double-blind randomized placebo-controlled parallel group study of multiple treatments of botulinum toxin type A (BoNTA) for the prophylaxis of episodic migraine headaches. *Cephalalgia* 27: 492–503.

Singh JA, Fitzgerald PM (2011) Botulinum toxin for shoulder pain: a Cochrane systematic review. *J Rheumatol* 38(3): 409–418.

Soares A, Andriolo RB, Atallah AN, da Silva EM (2012) Botulinum toxin for myofascial pain syndromes in adults. *Cochrane Database Syst Rev* 4: CD007533.

Tsui JK, Eisen A, Stoessl AJ, Calne S, Calne DB (1986) Double-blind study of botulinum toxin in spasmodic torticollis. *Lancet* 2: 245–247.

Waseem Z, Boulias C, Gordon A, Ismail F, Sheean G, Furlan AD (2010) Botulinum toxin injections for low-back pain and sciatica. *Cochrane Database Syst Rev* 1: CD008257.

Winocour S, Murad MH, Bidgoli-Moghaddam M, Jacobson SR, Bite U, Saint-Cyr M, Tran NV, Lemaine V (2014) Systematic review of the use of botulinum toxin type A with subpectoral breast implants. *J Plast Reconstr Aesthet Surg* 67: 34–41.

Wu T, Fu Y, Song HX, Ye Y, Dong Y, Li JH (2015) Effectiveness of botulinum toxin for shoulder pain treatment: a systematic review and meta-analysis. *Arch Phys Med Rehabil* 16(15).

Zhang H, Lian Y, Ma Y, Chen Y, He C, Xie N, Wu C (2014) Two doses of botulinum toxin type A for the treatment of trigeminal neuralgia: observation of therapeutic effect from a randomized double-blind placebo-controlled trial. *J Headache Pain* 15: 65.

Chapter 26

Manufacture of Commercial Botulinum Neurotoxins for Human Treatment

Eric A. Johnson

General Background

Botulinum neurotoxins are produced by neurotoxigenic *Clostridia* (Hatheway & Johnson 1998). Botulinum neurotoxin is a *c.*150 kDa protein which in its toxic form consists of a dichain molecule comprised of a heavy chain (*c.*100 kDa) and light chain (*c.*50 kDa) linked by a single disulphide bond and non-covalent interactions (Sugiyama 1980; DasGupta 1989). There are seven serotypes of botulinum neurotoxin (A–G) defined on the basis of specific antibody neutralisation by homologous antisera. There are also toxin isotypes ('subtypes') defined by genetic sequence, including more than ten each of A (A1–A10) and B (B1–B10) (Hill et al. 2015). Currently, serotype A1 and to a lesser extent serotype B1 are used for human treatment and are commercially manufactured. A recent review describes aspects of the manufacture of Botox® and Dysport® (Pickett 2014).

Depending on the strain of *Clostridium botulinum*, serotype and subtype of botulinum neurotoxins, and production conditions, the neurotoxins are produced in cultures as a component of protein complexes, in which non-toxic proteins and ribonucleic acids associate with the active botulinum neurotoxin component (Schantz & Johnson 1992). The primary non-toxic proteins known to exist in the purified complexes are a molecule termed non-toxic-non-haemagglutinin (NTNH) and haemagglutinin (HA) protein derivatives of various sizes (Sakaguchi 1982). The complexes were initially characterised in the 1940s by their sedimentation properties in the ultracentrifuge and by diffusion studies (Schantz & Johnson 1992), and later by chromatographic and electrophoretic methods (DasGupta 1989; Malizio et al. 2000). There are four basic botulinum toxin complexes defined by their size, protein composition and physiochemical properties. *Clostridium botulinum* type A production strains synthesise complexes of *c.*900 kDa (LL, 19S), *c.*550 kDa (L, 16S), *c.*300 kDa (M, 12S) and botulinum neurotoxin (150 kDa, 7S). The type A1 LL complex and purified botulinum neurotoxin have mainly been used for human treatments. The LL complex consists of neurotoxin molecules non-covalently associated with five non-toxic proteins that are visualised by SDS-PAGE (Figure 26.1). The non-toxic proteins impart stabilisation to the neurotoxin during production, purification and finishing. *C. botulinum* type B produces the L and M complexes, but not the large LL complex found in type A. To achieve full toxicity, the 150 kDa precursor neurotoxin polypeptide must be cleaved to the dichain form.

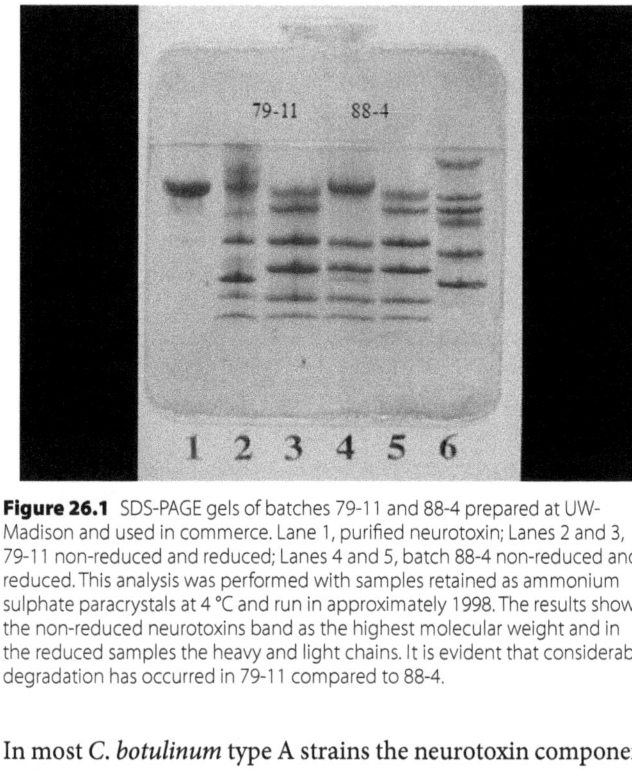

Figure 26.1 SDS-PAGE gels of batches 79-11 and 88-4 prepared at UW-Madison and used in commerce. Lane 1, purified neurotoxin; Lanes 2 and 3, 79-11 non-reduced and reduced; Lanes 4 and 5, batch 88-4 non-reduced and reduced. This analysis was performed with samples retained as ammonium sulphate paracrystals at 4 °C and run in approximately 1998. The results show the non-reduced neurotoxins band as the highest molecular weight and in the reduced samples the heavy and light chains. It is evident that considerable degradation has occurred in 79-11 compared to 88-4.

In most *C. botulinum* type A strains the neurotoxin component of 150 kDa is activated nearly completely by inherent proteases produced in the cultures, while in most type B strains the 150 kDa is only partially activated (15–30 per cent) to the dichain form and activation by processing can be used to achieve maximum toxicity during manufacture.

Safety Precautions

Since botulinum neurotoxin is the most potent toxin known to humankind, safety measures are paramount in its manufacture. The Centers for Disease Control and Prevention (CDC) recommends Biosafety Level 3 primary containment and personnel precautions for facilities producing large (numerous milligram) quantities of the toxins. In 1997 in the United States, *C. botulinum* cultures and toxins were included in a group of Select Agents whose inventory, transfer and laboratory inspections are controlled by the CDC. To ensure safety of personnel, appropriate resources including a biosafety manual, spill control and other standard operating procedures (SOPs) must be accessible in the laboratory. All personnel must be trained in these procedures as well as in safe laboratory practices. Appropriate personal protective equipment including lab coats, eye protection and gloves are required by persons who handle botulinum toxin. When performing steps where aerosols may be created (such as centrifugation), special precautions need to be taken. Botulinum toxin should be handled in sealed, unbreakable containers and manipulated in a Class II or III biological safety cabinet.

Early Developments of Botulinum Toxin for Human Treatment

The conceptual and experimental frameworks of botulinum toxin as a drug have been reviewed (Schantz & Johnson 1992; Wortzman & Pickett 2009). The conceptual prediction of botulinum toxins for human treatment was speculated by Kerner in Germany in the early 1800s, but the realisation and application of botulinum toxin for human treatment originated at Fort Detrick in the United States in the 1940s (Schantz & Johnson 1992). The first tangible breakthroughs occurred in the 1950s and 1960s when Edward J. Schantz produced botulinum 'crystalline' toxin, the LL (900 kDa) complex at Fort Detrick, Maryland, and provided preparations to Daniel Drachman at Johns Hopkins University for studies of its effects on nerve-muscle tissues in chicks (Drachman 1971; Johnson 1999). Drachman's research group elegantly showed that botulinum toxin from Schantz caused atrophy in chicken leg muscles with a long duration. Drachman, Burgen and colleagues showed that the primary mechanism of botulinum neurotoxin was the blockade of acetylcholine at the neuromuscular junction in motor neurons (Burgen et al. 1949; Drachman 1971).

During this development period in the 1960s and 1970s, Drachman was contacted by Alan B. Scott at the Smith Kettlewell Eye Research Institute, who wanted to evaluate botulinum toxin for the treatment of strabismus by manipulation of agonist and antagonist muscles affecting eye alignment. By virtue of these communications Scott contacted Schantz, who supplied crystalline botulinum toxin type A for monkey and later human studies. Scott's remarkable work on strabismus was published in 1973 and 1981 (Scott et al. 1973; Scott 1981, 1989) and an Investigational New Drug application for strabismus correction was filed in 1977. In December 1989 the Food and Drug Administration (FDA) licenced botulinum toxin type A (Oculinum®, Batch 79-11) as an orphan drug for the treatment of strabismus, hemifacial spasm and blepharospasm.

In 1988–1991 Allergan acquired the materials, technology and knowhow from Oculinum® and the University of Wisconsin and somehow attained the trademark Botox, although this term had been used by researchers for many years. Schantz and myself retroactively provided a manufacturing description to the FDA for the production and purification of Botox 79-11 and we are designated on the first FDA Master Batch Record for Botox® as a drug for human treatment. At this time, the FDA approved botulinum toxins on a batch basis and did not require demonstration of consistency, process validation and extensive preclinical development as chemistry, manufacturing and control (CMC) for batches as is presently mandated. During production of many batches we found variations in batch quality in terms of potency; certain batches, such as 88-4, were superior to 79-11. Several batches were produced at the University of Wisconsin and sent to Scott, and two were eventually used in commerce, 79-11 in the United States and 88-4 in Europe. Although the contracts with Allergan only involved 79-11, Allergan acquired and used 88-4 in Europe with sales of hundreds of millions of dollars. Upon request, Allergan refused to return 88-4 and other batches or provide any retribution to the University of Wisconsin where these batches were produced and qualified. Allergan also acquired the production strain *Clostridium botulinum* Hall'Schautz'hype from Scott without the permission of the University of Wisconsin.

During the 1980s and early 1990s Scott also collaborated with several physicians for treatment of a number of neurological disorders including dystonias, spasticity and aesthetic treatments. Scott was the pivotal physician who helped guide others in the wider application of botulinum toxin type A in many disorders, estimated to comprise more than 100 indications. Most of these syndromes have been used off-label in small groups of humans, and clinical trials and registration will be needed to safely and efficaciously use botulinum toxin for new indications.

Following the approval of Botox® in 1989, Dysport® was approved in 1990–1991 and used in the United Kingdom and eventually in other countries for human treatment. Following the commercial success of Botox® and Dysport®, several other botulinum products have been developed and approved in the United States, including Xeomin® and Myobloc®. Additional botulinum toxin products have been developed and used in certain countries and are expanding in their use worldwide. Several other botulinum toxin products are in preclinical development and clinical trials. Nevertheless, Botox®, being the innovator product, is the dominant botulinum toxin worldwide, accounting for 70–80 per cent of the global market.

An important aspect of the Investigational New Drug application progression and eventual FDA approval of Oculinum® was that Scott needed a consistent and uniform supply of high-quality crystalline botulinum toxin type A. Schantz and I worked together in establishing properties to define the quality of Oculinum® (later Botox®) (Schantz & Johnson 1992). During this period we produced many batches of toxin and we realised that the production and purification conditions could result in variations in toxin properties, particularly the specific toxicity (units per nanogram of protein) (Schantz & Johnson 1992). The differences in properties and quality of botulinum toxins resulting during manufacture can have deleterious effects in human treatment (Borodic et al. 1996). Procedures to assure product consistency, stabilisation with human serum albumin, drying and lyophilisation, potency and safety were developed. The primary criteria for quality evaluation of a batch of crystalline botulinum toxin type A were a specific toxicity of ≥30 U/ng ± 20 per cent, a 260/278 nm spectroscopic ratio less than 0.60 (indicating less than 0.1 per cent of nucleic acids) and the characteristic protein banding pattern by SDS-PAGE. At the time, these criteria were satisfactory to meet FDA specifications and served as the basis for approval of Botox®. Approval requirements have advanced to much more rigorous criteria and approval is not granted for single batches by the FDA.

There have been considerable efforts in the development of non-native botulinum toxin products. Several companies have devoted large research efforts to recombinant botulinum toxins and chimeric constructs, but these have certain limitations and have not yet been approved for commercial use in humans. Certain companies have also considered the development of biosimilars as approved botulinum toxin products, but biosimilars present considerable challenges as botulinum toxin is a large and complex molecule. Nonetheless, several additional companies are now producing botulinum neurotoxin A1 as an injectable. The development of subtypes other than A1 and B1 with different pharmacological properties are also being explored.

Critical Properties of Botulinum Toxin Manufactured for Human Use

Certain properties of botulinum toxin are of paramount importance for human use and must be achieved during manufacturing. Being a biologic, differences in chemical and biologic properties are observed during manufacture and an important goal for the active pharmaceutical ingredient is consistency of the product.

Potency

The most important property of botulinum toxin is potency of the manufactured toxin, because higher specific toxicities (MU/ng of botulinum toxin preparation) require lower quantities for injection and decrease unwanted side-effects, including resistance to botulinum toxin, the formation of neutralising antibodies and 'spread' of botulinum toxin to neighbouring tissues and systemically. Botulinum toxin potency is defined in toxicity units (MU), where 1 MU represents the LD_{50} for a botulinum toxin preparation determined in a quantal intraperitoneal mouse bioassay (Schantz & Johnson 1992). The mouse bioassay is the 'gold standard' method and has merit in requiring all steps in the intoxication process (toxin binding, internalisation, release of the L chain into the nerve cytosol and cleavage of SNARE substrates). However, the mouse bioassay has an inherent variability of 15–25 per cent in units among labs. Furthermore, in the current regulatory environment, different companies are permitted to use their own individual assay protocols instead of a preferred international standardised assay using a defined botulinum toxin standard. The disparity in the mouse bioassay promulgates variability in specific toxicity and active MU in the finished product. Thus, it is not currently feasible to directly compare the potency of botulinum commercial products based on animal studies and in limited human studies. This variation among products has also led to the need for injection of different units of specific products for many indications. The discrepancy in MU among commercial products is exemplified by Dysport®, in which it is generally accepted that three LD_{50} units of Dysport® are equivalent to one LD_{50} unit of Botox® for most indications. The reasons for this are not clear and may be due to the different assay conditions or more likely to differences in the botulinum neurotoxin compositions in the two products.

As with other biological drug products, there have been advances in assays of botulinum toxins. The mouse hemidiaphragm assay has been advocated in certain countries in Europe. However, this assay is tedious and still requires the use of numerous animals. A promising and FDA-approved assay for API and approved for Botox® and Xeomin® are neuronal cell-based assays, which require all four steps in intoxication (Rossetto et al. 2014) and has much less variability than the mouse bioassay (*c.*10 per cent). The use of animals is not necessary once the assay is validated since neuronal cell lines are used. Other assays such as cleavage of SNARE substrates, ELISA and other *in vitro* assays are useful for monitoring toxin activities during manufacturing or in clinical samples, but are not suitable for determination of potency for the API since they measure only limited steps in the intoxication process or rely solely on binding to antibodies.

As a background of potency of manufactured products, the specific toxicity of purified botulinum neurotoxins type A1 and B1 are generally 1–3 × 10^8 LD_{50} per mg, or 7–10 pg of neurotoxin per U. As expected, the complexes that contain non-toxic proteins in addition to neurotoxin have lower specific toxicities due to the extra protein load. Fresh preparations of LL complex produced by Schantz and myself possessed ≥3 × 10^7 LD_{50} per mg (≥30 U/ng) (Schantz & Johnson 1992). On ageing and handling, this specific toxicity of some batches, including the FDA-approved batch 79-11, decreased from 30 to 3 MU/ng, indicating a 90 per cent decrease in activity with the consequence of considerable inactive toxin being injected into humans. Such degradation is inherent in many biologic pharmaceuticals. The injection of low potency of 79-11 resulted in a relatively high incidence of antibody formation in humans. In 1997 a new batch of botulinum toxin complex was prepared by Allergan and referred to as 'new' Botox®, with a higher specific toxicity and accordingly reduced antibody formation in patients. Since biologics undergo some inactivation on long-term storage, it is desirable to periodically prepare fresh batches of high potency for clinical use.

The protein load in finished product (drug substance) of current batches of Botox® has been reported to be 5 ng per 100 MU vial or about 20 MU/ng, indicating that some toxicity is lost during manufacturing and finishing. Ipsen has reported that 4.35 ng of botulinum toxin complex is present in a 500 MU vial, giving a specific toxicity of about 143 Dysport® MU/ng of toxin complex (though 12.5 ng per vial was reported earlier). The specific toxicity of the Dysport® product is uncommonly high compared to LL type A complexes purified by several independent laboratories. Considering the reported high Dysport®-specific potency, either the composition contains considerable free neurotoxin as well as complexes of LL, L and M, but this is not supported by SDS-PAGE gel visualisation. Moreover, it has been reported that a Dysport® commercial toxin preparation contained the contaminants flagellin, clp protease and toll-like receptor proteins (Panjwani et al. 2008), which has not been observed in other botulinum toxin products. The presence of these contaminants brings into question the degree of Dysport® purification.

Purified neurotoxin (150 kDa) is currently being manufactured by various companies. My laboratory initially developed and patented purified neurotoxin for pharmaceutical use (Johnson et al. 1986), but this product development failed and never reached commercialisation, in my view mainly due to the inability of the commercial sponsor and the Wisconsin Alumni Research Foundation to obtain manufacturing process validation, adequate Chemistry and Manufacturing Control (CMC) data, and filing of a Biologics Licensing Agreement and New Drug Application after more than ten years of efforts. The development of purified neurotoxin as an Active Pharmaceutical Agreement was followed later by researchers at Merz Pharmaceuticals, who produced a successful botulinum neurotoxin product that entered commercial use (Frevert 2015). Purified neurotoxin has a specific toxicity of 200–300 MU/ng and thus a 100 MU vial would contain 0.3–0.5 ng of active toxin. In practice, close to 1 ng is added per vial since some potency loss occurs on drying and finishing of the product. There is a dearth of data on the consistency of units per vial of commercial botulinum products. Although vials are labelled with a given unit quantity, e.g. 100 MU per vial, the variation allowed by the FDA is 80–115 MU per vial. Thus, there can be a 15–20 per cent variation in units per vial, which confounds the evaluation of products in the clinical setting and in clinical trials. There is a need for a comprehensive published study of the comparative variation in units per vial of approved products.

Protein and Nucleic Acid Composition of Botulinum Toxins

The protein composition and nucleic acid contamination are also important factors in botulinum toxin quality. Botulinum toxins exist naturally as protein complexes and contain ribonucleic acid. Determination of the protein pattern and nucleic acid content is important for evaluation of toxin purity and quality. Botulinum toxin associates with ribonucleic acid during formation in clostridial cells, and this can be removed by ethanol precipitation or anion exchange chromatography, depending on the purification strategy. For the LL complex, six bands are observed on SDS-PAGE under non-reducing conditions and seven under reducing conditions (Figure 26.1). The bands consist of botulinum neurotoxin (*c.*150 kDA), NTNH (*c.*140 kDa) and haemagglutinins (*c.*50, 33, 20 and 17 kDA). The haemagglutinins are derived in native cultures from a single HA polypeptide by proteolytic processing.

The highest purified commercial preparation is that of the former 'Purtox' and also of Xeomin®, which contain only the neurotoxin component without the complexing proteins. Other companies are also developing products consisting of only the neurotoxin without complexing proteins. The purification of the BoNTs without the complexing proteins lowers the protein load injected into patients and may help to avoid unwanted reactions possibly imparted by NTNH and haemagglutinins. Although the overall protein load is reduced, the quantity of neurotoxin injected is unchanged compared to the respective complexes to elicit the paralytic effect. The injection of only the neurotoxin with associated lower protein load has been speculated to reduce antigenicity, but this does not seem likely since the units of active toxin in the complex and purified botulinum neurotoxin per unit are equivalent.

Formulation

The different commercial products contain various excipients. Botox®, Dysport® and Xeomin® contain different levels of human serum albumin (HSA), which is integral in stabilising the product during dilution, filling and drying. There has been concern that the use of human proteins as an excipient could lead to injection of human viruses or prions, but long-term use has not shown any pathologic consequences. Still, the presence of human protein may have negative connotations for an injectable drug. Consequently, some companies are developing non-human-based excipients such as soy proteins, peptides and organic polymers.

Critical Steps in Manufacturing and Approval of Botulinum Toxin for Commercial Use

Overview

The manufacture of botulinum toxin for commercial use follows certain critical steps, assessment of toxin properties, clinical trials and regulatory approval. Manufacture falls under the general area of CMC. This includes the manufacturing facility, process equipment, materials used, the manufacturing process, the personnel involved, the chemistry of the product including characterisation and proof of identity and stability, quality assurance release, documentation and training required (Geigert 2013). CMC regulatory compliance requires that all manufacturing processes are carried out within regulatory agencies' requirements and expectations. Guidance documents from the FDA, the European Agency for the Evaluation of Medicinal Products (EMEA), the Clinical Trials Directive and the International Conference on Harmonization (ICH) are helpful in developing and assessing key issues in manufacturing. Process development, CMC and manufacture have been described for biologics (Geigert 2013).

The following are the main steps and considerations in botulinum toxin manufacture, with emphasis on microbiological and botulinum toxin properties. Other important aspects of manufacture compliance, including facilities, equipment validation, personnel, training and records, clinical trials and necessary submissions are beyond the scope of this chapter. Manufacturing for human use requires quality controls and appropriate in-process controls and is carried out under appropriate good manufacturing processes (GMPs). During manufacturing development, it is extremely important to have preclinical meetings with regulatory agencies encompassing areas of Investigational New Drug Application (INDA), CMC and for filing of a Biologics Licence Application (BLA) and New Drug Application (NDA). It is also of paramount importance to consult with the regulatory agencies before implementing any changes in manufacturing, which generally requires scrupulous comparability protocols and testing, with potential well-recognised consequences that the inability to rectify changes of the site of manufacture or changes in the manufacturing process may result in product rejection.

Strain of *C. botulinum* for Master and Working Cell Banks and for Toxin Production

At the heart of the manufacturing process is the *C. botulinum* for botulinum toxin manufacture. Different companies have reported the use of individual strains, most having been isolated by Ivan C. Hall, although some companies use strains from different sources. There are many 'Hall A' strains and these differ in important properties. Moreover, the strains initially derived from Ivan Hall have been stored in media containing meat and other animal proteins, which has been a concern for possible transmission of prions or certain viruses. Certain companies have isolated new strains of *C. botulinum* type A for manufacture without being grown or stored in media containing animal protein. Also, certain companies have proposed maintenance of strains in media not containing animal proteins, particularly soy-based media. The *C. botulinum* strain used for manufacturing is characterised for purity by agar plating and testing of physiological properties, particularly botulinum toxin production. The *C. botulinum* production strain is also analysed for the presence of transmissible genetic elements including plasmids and phage. The master and working seed banks need to be genetically characterised by typing (e.g. pulsed field gel electrophoresis) or ideally by whole genome sequencing. The master cell bank should be maintained for long periods and the manufacturer should avoid the frequent preparation of new master cell banks except when potential deleterious conditions are encountered, such as critical deviations in the required temperature control or transfer of the production of the strain to a different manufacturing facility. The strain used by Schantz (Hall A Schantz; Hall A-*hyper*) for initial batches of Botox was apparently originally isolated by Ivan Hall, but the production at Fort Detrick was obtained from J. Howard Mueller at Harvard Medical School (Schantz & Johnson 1992). This strain developed at Fort Detrick is unusual compared to most other *C. botulinum* type A strains as it not known to form endospores and produces high quantities of botulinum toxin type A1 ($1–3 \times 10^6$ LD_{50}s per ml of culture medium). This strain was acquired by Allergan from the University of Wisconsin through Alan Scott, and Allergan attempted to patent the strain as a proprietary Allergan strain but the patent was later abandoned as its source was clearly Schantz at UW-Madison. Initially, Porton Down used a strain NCTC 2916 which was stored in Robertson's meat broth (Hambleton et al. 1981), but this strain was later abandoned when it became clear it possessed a BoNT/A gene cluster and an inactive 'silent' type B gene cluster (Hutson et al. 1996). The strain for production of Dysport® has been termed 'Hall A' and 'proprietary' (Wortzman & Pickett 2009), but its properties and genome sequence have not been publicly disclosed. Botulinum toxin type B has also been developed as a commercial product (Brashear 2001). The Beans or Okra B strain are used, which are good toxin producers. There are certain disadvantages in manufacture with type B, in that botulinum neurotoxin from *C. botulinum* type B strains attain only about 15–30 per cent activation to the active dichain form in the native cultures.

Culture Medium

The culture medium is used for growth and storage of master and seed cultures, as well as for toxin production in reactors. The master and seed cultures are generally prepared by harvesting cells in the active growth phase and storing with a cryoprotectant (e.g. glycerol) at –80 °C. The culture medium is critical for maximum and consistent toxin titres, activation to the dichain form and efficient flocculation with acid as the initial step in purification and minimisation of contaminants in the final product. Crystalline type A toxin (Schantz & Johnson 1992) is produced in a medium consisting of a casein digest, yeast extract and glucose at initial pH 7.3. The most critical component is the casein digest and it usually is necessary to screen different lots to obtain maximum growth, toxin formation, autolysis flocculation with acid, and recovery of botulinum toxin from the acid mud. Growth occurs during the first 1–2 days and this is followed by near complete autolysis of the culture during days 2–4. In *C. botulinum* type A Schantz, the toxin is completely (>95 per cent) activated to the dichain form by the organism's proteases.

Fermentation Parameters

In the commercial setting, botulinum toxin is produced in stirred tank bioreactors with minimum agitation to avoid the introduction of air and to maximise the ability of *C. botulinum* to harbour cell–cell interaction and possibly quorum sensing to maximise toxin production. Some companies use nitrogen sparging to help maintain anaerobic conditions. Growth can be assayed *in situ* by removal of culture samples and potentially by gas analysis related to production. Contamination is rare, but if it occurs will result in an unwanted bio-burden in the product. Other monitoring tests are pH, temperature, nutrient utilisation and fermentation products, including organic acids and alcohols which can be determined *in situ*. Most importantly, the titre of botulinum toxin during the fermentation must be monitored.

Purification of Botulinum Toxins for Human Treatment

During the 1940s when purification procedures were first being developed, column chromatography was in its infancy and was not used in botulinum toxin purification. The first step in nearly all serotypes of botulinum toxins is acid precipitation, initially noticed by Snipe and Sommer in 1928. On acid addition white flocks form that precipitate by gravity or can be recovered by centrifugation (Schantz & Johnson 1992). The method used at Fort Detrick employed an initial acid precipitation, a second series of precipitations in aqueous media, precipitation in 15 per cent ethanol at –5 °C and finally very slow crystallisation of the botulinum toxin complex over several days to approximately 0.9 M ammonium sulphate (Schantz & Johnson 1992). This procedure was used for the initial batches of Oculinum® and Botox®. Generally, about 150–200 mg of the LL (19S) complex can be obtained from 10 litres of culture medium and on purification about 10–15 mg of botulinum neurotoxin. The pKa of the LL complex is about 5.6 and its concentration can be determined using an extinction coefficient (absorbency of 1.65 for 1 mg of toxin per ml in a 1 cm light path). The pKa of purified neurotoxin has been reported to be in the range of 6.06–6.4, with an average of pKa of 6.1. The LL complex is stable for many years when precipitated from the culture medium to pH 3.5 with sulphuric acid. Purified neurotoxin is stable from several months to more than three years, depending on the concentration of toxin (usually 0.2 mg) and in 10 mM sodium phosphate buffer, pH7.0 + 0.15 M sodium chloride. The purification process is designed to eliminate microbial/spore contaminants, nucleic acid contamination and unwanted antigenic materials such as non-toxin bacterial proteins. In today's regulatory environment it is essential to show production and purification process validation. Generally, process validation is performed during the manufacture of phase II and III clinical materials. Process validation requires the production of at least three consecutive batches of drug product with consistent properties.

Although the initial Oculinum® (Botox®) batches were made by acid precipitation, ethanol precipitation and formation of paracrystals in *c.*0.9 M ammonium sulphate, currently most companies utilise acid precipitation and chromatographic methods to purify the complexes, as well as purified neurotoxin. The general scheme is as follows. After approximately four days of incubation, acid precipitation is used to flocculate and concentrate the toxin complex from the culture fluid. The precipitated toxin complex ('mud') is stable at lower pHs of *c.*3.5 for years. The toxin complex is solubilised in sodium phosphate buffer and re-precipitated with ammonium sulphate. The toxin complex is purified and the nucleic acids are removed by cation ion exchange chromatography at an acidic pH. The neurotoxin is separated from the complex proteins by chromatography at about pH 7.9 on DEAE-Sephadex A-50 (Malizio et al. 2000). Trace contaminates are removed by a second chromatography on a cation exchange column. For high purification, gel filtration or affinity purification using immobilised *p*-aminophenyl β-D-thiogalactopyranoside have been used. The biological activity can be roughly estimated by the intravenous (IV) time to death method or preferably the intraperitoneal (IP) endpoint dilution method (Schantz & Johnson 1992; Malizio et al. 2000). The best storage method for botulinum neurotoxin is dependent on the end use of the material. Neurotoxin standards with stabilising protein added have been kept for years at room temperature with no appreciable loss of activity. Ammonium sulphate precipitated botulinum neurotoxin can be stored at 4 °C for several weeks. However, within a month, SDS-PAGE will show some breakdown products of the toxin. The neurotoxin can also be stored at freezing temperatures with 50 per cent glycerol as a cryoprotectant for several months to years. Since the LL complex is very stable, purifying the neurotoxin from the complex as required has been used.

Botulinum toxin in liquid suspension or solution is prone to inactivation by aggregation and likely other degradation reactions, including proteolysis by exogenous proteases, autocatalytic degradation, deamidation and oxidation. Aggregation is the most prevalent cause of denaturation and occurs during agitation, sparging with gas and other manipulations. Aggregation is particularly of concern at alkaline pHs and on dilution to low concentrations of pg to ng per ml. Aggregation can be prevented by diluting with a buffered solution at ≤pH 6.8 containing another protein such as HSA.

Finishing

The purified API needs to be formulated with excipients and dispensed into vials for drying. Some companies have marketed liquid formulations, but a low pH of *c.*5.5 is used, which can lead to discomfort during human injections. Preparation of the toxin for dispensing as a drug requires dilution in a suitable diluent for retention of toxicity, filtration for sterility and drying. Dilution to ng per ml of botulinum toxin requires an excipient for retention of activity. HSA is commonly used at various concentrations. Generally, the higher levels of HSA provide best protection on storage and may also prevent 'spread' of toxin on injection. Drying conditions and the fill volume of the vials are important for retention of toxicity. At a small fill volume of 0.1 ml, the toxin solution can be prepared by flash drying as is performed with Botox®, while at higher fill volumes such as 0.5 ml lyophilisation is usually required for maximum recovery. Up to 30 per cent loss can occur during drying and freeze-drying; optimisation of drying conditions is essential.

CMC Analyses of Botulinum Toxin During Toxin Production and in the Drug Substance and Drug Product

Since the minimal characterisation of Oculinum® (Botox®) in the late 1980s, approval of the API currently requires much more detailed characterisation. Guidance for biologic manufacturing is outlined in several FDA and ICH documents. Important facets include the following characterisations.

Characterisation of the Production Strain

The *C. botulinum* strain used for manufacturing is characterised for its purity by agar plating and testing of physiological properties, including carbon and nitrogen source utilisation and toxin production. The *C. botulinum* production strain is also analysed for the presence of transmissible genetic elements including plasmids and phage. The master and working seed banks need to be genetically characterised by typing (e.g. pulsed field gel electrophoresis) or ideally by whole genome sequencing. The master cell bank should be maintained for long periods and the manufacturer should avoid the frequent preparation of new master cell banks except when potential deleterious conditions are encountered, such as critical deviations in the required temperature control or transfer of the production of the strain to a different manufacturing facility.

Process Validation and Demonstration of Consistency of Toxin Lots

Currently, the FDA does not approve botulinum toxin products by single batches and requires process validation and proof in consistency of production. Process validation is a comprehensive and extensive process, requiring API consistency of at least three consecutive batches. In addition, the manufacturer is generally required to make at least one batch per year to further support consistency of product.

Testing of Drug Substance Drug Product

Extensive testing is essential to demonstrate the safety, purity, biochemical properties and potency of the botulinum toxin product. These general areas include QC stability tests, QC release tests, product characterisation and extensive analytical tests. Guidance documents are available from regulatory agencies as well as documentation of previously approved botulinum toxin products. Drug substance used for preparation of the final drug product must possess expected purity, potency, uniform product without degradation forms, free from any undesired bio-burden and meticulous chemical characterisation. Currently, the chemical characterisation usually requires quantitative electrophoretic analysis, amino acid sequencing, mass spectroscopy and other protein characterisation methods.

Release Specifications

Release criteria include sterility, identity, purity, potency testing, absence of endotoxin and absence of any bio-burden. The drug product must be stored and transported under carefully defined conditions and used within the shelf life.

Preparation of BLA/NDA Submission

A detailed and complete description of the manufacturing process is necessary for market approval submission. The CMC information to be included in the BLA/NDA dossier has been described for various biological products (Geigert) and in FDA guidance documents.

Summary

Botulinum toxin has become a vital drug for treatment of dystonias and myriad neurological disorders. The manufacture and purification of botulinum toxin products is at the core of the quality of the material injected into humans. Schantz and colleagues initially developed the manufacture of botulinum toxin for humans at Fort Detrick, Maryland. Alan Scott performed pioneering critical experiments with botulinum toxin in monkeys and eventually in humans. He was also involved in assessment of various batches produced by Schantz and myself and for development of optimal formulation parameters. Currently, there are several commercial botulinum toxin products available and more are in development. The current development and approval of botulinum toxins for human use must be performed in a CDC-approved facility under good manufacturing process conditions with essential quality control and Chemistry and Manufacturing Control requirements. The approval of an Investigational Drug Application, Biologic Licence Application and a New Drug Application has advanced to rigorously controlled manufacturing procedures and testing. Currently, botulinum toxin commercial products vary in composition and optimal potency. Individual botulinum toxin products are currently assayed and characterised by different procedures by individual companies. Ideally, as this field further advances, the botulinum toxin industry will use standardised assay and detection methods leading to an in-depth comparison and understanding of the commercial products for human treatment. Advances in pharmaceutical future botulinum toxins will eventually entail the use of new subtypes and hybrid and chimeric compositions of matter for optimised treatment results in humans.

References

Borodic G, Johnson EA, Goodnough MC, Schantz EJ (1996) Botulinum toxin therapy, immunologic resistance, and problems with available materials. *Neurology* 46: 26–29.

Brashear A (2001) Botulinum toxin type B: a new injectable treatment for cervical dystonia. *Expert Opin Invest Drugs* 10: 2191–2199.

Burgen ASV, Dickens F, Zatman LF (1949) The action of botulinum toxin on the neuro-muscular junction. *J Physiol* 109: 10–24.

DasGupta BR (1989) The structure of botulinum neurotoxin. In: Simpson LL, ed., *Botulinum Neurotoxin and Tetanus Toxin*. San Diego, ca, Academic Press, pp. 53–67.

Drachman DB (1971) Botulinum toxin as a tool for research on the nervous system. In: Simpson LL, ed., *Neuropoisons: Their Pathophysiological Actions. Vol. 1. Poisons of Animal Origin*. New York, Plenum Press, pp. 325–347.

Frevert J (2015) Pharmaceutical, biological, and clinical properties of botulinum neurotoxin type A products. *Drugs R D* 15: 1–9.

Geigert J (2013) *The Challenge of CMC Regulatory Compliance for Biopharmaceuticals*. New York, Springer-Verlag.

Hambleton P, Capel B, Bailey N, Heron N, Crooks A, Melling J, Tse C-K, Dolly JO (1981) Production, purification and toxoiding of *Clostridium botulinum* type A toxin. In: Lewis GE, ed., *Biomedical Aspects of Botulism*. New York, Academic Press, pp. 247–260.

Hatheway CL, Johnson EA (1998) *Clostridium*: the spore-bearing anaerobes. In: Collier L, Balows A, Sussman M, eds, *Topley and Wilson's Microbiology and Microbial Infections*, ninth edition, *Vol. 2: Systematic Bacteriology*. London, Arnold, pp. 731–782.

Hill KK, Xie G, Foley BT, Smith TJ (2015) Genetic diversity within the botulinum neurotoxin-producing bacteria and their neurotoxins. *Toxicon* 107 (Pt A): 2–8.

Hutson RA, Zhou Y, Johnson EA, Sugiyama H, Hatheway CL (1996) Genetic characterization of *Clostridium botulinum* type A containing silent B neurotoxin gene sequences. *J Biol Chem* 271: 10786–10792.

Johnson EA (1999) Clostridial toxins as therapeutic agents: benefits of nature's most toxic proteins. *Ann Rev Microbiol* 53: 551–575.

Malizio CJ, Goodnough MC, Johnson EA (2000) Purification of *Clostridium botulinum* type A neurotoxin. In: Holst O, ed., *Bacterial Toxins: Methods and Protocols*. New Jersey, Humana Press.

Panjwani N, O'Keefe RO, Pickett A (2008) Biochemical, functional and potency characteristics of type A botulinum toxin in clinical use. *The Botulinum J* 1: 153–166.

Pickett A (2014) Botulinum toxin as a clinical product: manufacture and pharmacology. In: Foster KA, ed., *Clinical Applications of Botulinum Neurotoxin*. New York, Springer, pp. 7–49.

Rossetto O, Pirazzini M, Montecucco C (2014) Botulinum neurotoxins: genetic, structural and mechanistic insights. *Nat Rev Microbiol* 12: 535–549.

Sakaguchi G (1982) *Clostridium botulinum* toxins. *Pharmacol Ther* 19: 165–194.

Schantz EJ, Johnson EA (1992) Properties and use of botulinum toxin and other microbial neurotoxins in medicine. *Microbiol Rev* 56: 80–92.

Scott AB (1981) Botulinum toxin injection of eye muscles to correct strabismus. *Trans Am Ophtthalmol Soc* 79: 734–770.

Scott AB (1989) Clostridial toxins as therapeutic agents. In: Simpson LL, ed., *Botulinum Neurotoxin and Tetanus Toxin*. San Diego, CA, Academic Press, pp. 399–412.

Scott AB, Rosenbaum A, Collins CC (1973) Pharmacologic weakening of extraocular muscles. *Invest Opthamol* 12: 924–927.

Sugiyama H (1980) *Clostridium botulinum* neurotoxin. *Microbiol Rev* 44: 419–448.

Wortzman MS, Pickett A (2009) The science and manufacturing behind botulinum neurotoxin type A-ABO in clinical use. *Aesthet Surg J* 29: S34–S42.

Chapter 27

Pharmacology of Botulinum Toxins

Dirk Dressler and Keith Foster

Introduction

Botulinum toxin (BT) drugs consist of a complex mixture of substances, which differ between BT products (Table 27.1). Pharmacologically and therapeutically, the most important difference is the botulinum neurotoxin (BNT) serotype used. BNT types A and B are commercially available as BT drugs, whereas BNT types E, C and F, so far, have been tried in humans on an experimental basis only. BNT types A and B have different affinities for the motor system (Peng et al. 2012; Strotmeier et al. 2012) and the autonomic nervous system (Dressler & Benecke 2003). It is only the BNT that binds to and enters presynaptic nerve terminals. In regard to action at the nerve terminal, therefore, other components of the BT are not involved. Formulation differences may, however, influence therapeutic properties. An acidic buffer system may increase injection site pain, as in rimabotulinumtoxinB. Gelatine stabilisation, as in Hengli®, may cause allergic reactions. Differences in protein content may affect tissue perfusion and antigenicity. BT drugs are neither identical nor generic. Some of their differences matter therapeutically, others may not.

Structure and Nomenclature

As shown in Figure 27.1, BT drugs consist of the BT component and excipients. Excipients may include lactose, sucrose, NaCl and human serum albumin for stabilisation purposes and buffer systems for pH calibration. The BT component is formed by BNT and by non-toxic proteins also known as complexing proteins. Different BT types may be identified as BT-A, BT-B, BT-C, BT-D, BT-E, BT-F and BT-G, and their BNT as BNT-A, BNT-B, etc.

BNT are dichain proteins consisting of a heavy chain with a molecular weight of 100 kD and a light chain with a molecular weight of 50 kD. The dichain BNT is formed from a single chain progenitor toxin by proteolysis. The two chains are connected by a single disulphide bridge that is essential for BNT's biological activity, making BT sensitive to various environmental factors.

BNT is produced by various species of *Clostridia* as a complex with various complexing proteins to form BT. The identity of the complexing proteins and the stoichiometry of the complex varies between the serotypes and with *Clostridial* strain. It is also affected by the medium used for bacterial growth and the methods employed to purify the BT. In incobotulinumtoxinA the complexing proteins are removed during the manufacturing process so that BNT is the only BT component in this BT drug, with a molecular weight of 150 kD. Other BT drugs contain different complexing protein compositions so that their total molecular weight differs from that of BNT-A. BT-A is produced in three different complex sizes: M (300 kD), L (500 kD) and LL (900 kD). The precise nature of the complex present in many commercial BT products has not been published.

Mode of Action

When BT is injected into a target tissue, BNT selectively binds to receptors located on cholinergic nerve terminals. BNT has a dual receptor mechanism that underpins both its selectivity for and potency at peripheral nerve terminals. Initially BNT binds to polysialo-gangliosides that are abundant on the outer leaflet of presynaptic membranes (Rummel 2013). Ganglioside binding enables an initial capture and concentration of BNT on the presynaptic membrane, facilitating binding to the protein receptor.

One of the major breakthroughs in recent years has been the elucidation of the BNT protein receptors. BNT binds to one of two classes of protein receptor, synaptotagmin (Syt) or synaptic vesicle glycoprotein 2 (SV2), in a serotype-specific manner (Rummel 2013). Both Syt and SV2 are synaptic vesicle membrane proteins, and the BNT binding site is to a luminal domain located on the inside of the synaptic vesicle. Binding requires vesicle fusion at the presynaptic membrane and exposure of the luminal protein domains on the cell surface. It has been known for many years that BNT uptake is activity-dependent and that this can influence clinical effect (Hallett 2015). The requirement for binding to the intraluminal domain of a synaptic vesicle membrane protein provides a mechanistic understanding of this.

Following internalisation into the recycling synaptic vesicle, acidification of the vesicle leads to a conformational change in the BNT and translocation of the light chain into the neuronal cytosol (Beard 2014). BNT light chains are zinc-dependent metalloproteases that selectively cleave proteins essential for synaptic vesicle docking and fusion at the presynaptic membrane, SNARE (**s**oluble **N**-ethylmaleimide-sensitive fusion **a**ttachment protein **re**ceptor) proteins (Pellizzari et al. 1999). Different BNTs cleave different SNARE proteins at unique peptide bonds. BNT-A, BNT-C and BNT-E cleave SNAP-25,

Table 27.1 Properties of different botulinum toxin drugs

	Botox®	**Dysport®**	**Xeomin®**	**NeuroBloc® Myobloc®**
Alternative names	Vistabel® Botox® Cosmetic	Azzalure®	Bocouture® Xeomin® Cosmetic	
Non-proprietary names	OnabotulinumtoxinA	AbobotulinumtoxinA	IncobotulinumtoxinA	RimabotulinumtoxinB
Manufacturer	Allergan plc Dublin Ireland	Ipsen Pharma Boulgne Bilancourt France	Merz Pharmaceuticals Frankfurt/M Germany	US WorldMeds Louisville, KY USA
Pharmaceutical preparation	Powder	Powder	Powder	Ready-to-use solution 5000 MU-U/ml
Storage conditions	Below 8 °C	Below 8 °C	Below 25 °C	Below 8 °C
Shelf life	36 months	24 months	36 months	24 months
Botulinum toxin type	A	A	A	B
Clostridium botulinum strain	Hall A	Hall A	Hall A	Bean B
SNARE target	SNAP-25	SNAP-25	SNAP-25	VAMP
Purification process	Precipitation and crystallisation	Precipitation and chromatography	Precipitation and chromatography	Precipitation and chromatography
Stabilisation	Vacuum drying	Freeze-drying (lyophilisate)	Vacuum drying	pH-reduction
Excipients (standard vial)	Human serum albumin 500 ug/vial NaCl 900 ug/vial buffer system	Human serum albumin 125 ug/vial Lactose 2500 ug/vial buffer system	Human serum albumin 1 mg/vial Sucrose 4.7 mg/vial buffer system	Human serum albumin 0.5 mg/ml Disodium succinate 0.01 M Sodium chloride 0.1 M H_2O Hydrochloric acid
Biological activity – Standard vial	100 MU-A/vial	500 MU-I/vial	100 MU-M/vial	10.0 kMU-U/vial
Biological activity – Alternative vials	50 MU-A/vial 200 MU-A/vial	300 MU-I/vial	50 MU-M/vial	1.0 kMU-U/vial 2.5 kMU-U/vial

MU-A: mouse unit in the Allergan mouse lethality assay.
MU-U: mouse unit in the US WorldMeds mouse lethality assay.
MU-I: mouse unit in the Ipsen mouse lethality assay.
MU-M: mouse unit in the Merz mouse lethality assay.

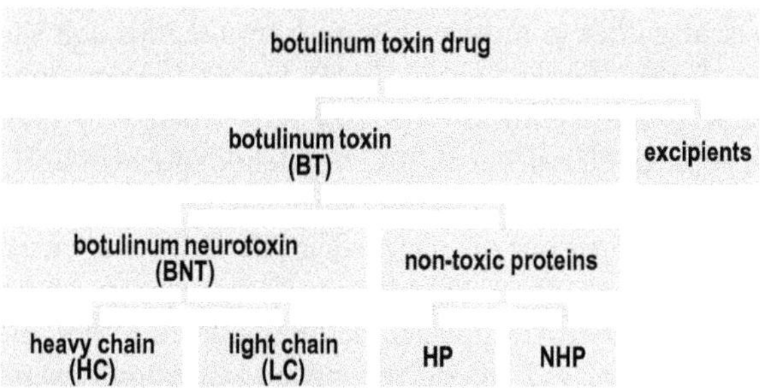

Figure 27.1 Contents of botulinum toxin drugs.
HP: haemagglutinating protein
NHP: non-haemagglutinating protein

BNT-B, BNT-D, BNT-F and BNT-G cleave VAMP (vesicle-associated membrane protein = synaptobrevin) and BNT-C also cleaves syntaxin.

Cleavage of SNARE proteins prevents formation of a complex between SNARE proteins at the presynaptic membrane (SNAP-25 and syntaxin) and VAMP in the synaptic vesicle membrane (Schiavo et al. 2000). Without formation of this complex, the vesicle cannot fuse with the presynaptic membrane and release of neurotransmitter is inhibited. Entry of BNT into presynaptic terminals of peripheral motor neurons therefore inhibits acetylcholine release, resulting in flaccid muscle paralysis, which is the predominant pharmacological effect underpinning many of its therapeutic uses. Depending on the target tissue, BT blocks not only cholinergic neuromuscular transmission, but also cholinergic autonomic innervation of sweat glands, tear glands, salivary glands and smooth muscles.

BNT inhibition of neurotransmitter release is very prolonged. This is as a result of survival of the light chain within the terminal, continuing to cleave SNARE protein and prevent vesicle fusion. Eventually vesicle fusion is regained, neurotransmitter release is restored and function resumes. The duration of inhibition of neurotransmitter release differs between BNT serotypes and between categories of neuron. BNT-A is the longest-acting serotype, with a duration at the human neuromuscular junction of around three months; at the other extreme is BNT-E with a duration at the same target of 3–4 weeks (Eleopra et al. 1998). The precise mechanism underpinning the long duration of effect of BNT and its eventual cessation is not fully understood, but is a feature of the intracellular light chain and its cleavage of SNARE protein (Tsai et al. 2014). The prolonged activity of BNT-A is an important aspect of the therapeutic benefit of BT-A products.

When BNT-A blocks the cholinergic synapse, the neuron forms new synapses replacing its original ones – a process known as sprouting. Originally it was thought that sprouting is responsible for the termination of BNT action. Recently, however, it became clear that sprouting is a temporary recovery process only and that the original synapses are eventually regenerated and the sprouts are removed (de Paiva et al. 1999).

Given that BNT prevents synaptic transmission only temporarily, and that structural neuronal changes or functional neuronal impairment other than the synaptic blockade cannot be detected, we suggested classifying BNT not as a neurotoxin, but as a temporary neuromodulator (Brin et al. 2004).

First BT effects can be detected after intramuscular injection within 2–3 days, depending on the detection methods used. BT reaches its maximal effect after about two weeks, remains there for about 2.5 months and then gradually starts to decline. BT injections into glandular tissue can exert prolonged effects of up to 6–9 months.

BT action features a dose–effect correlation (Dressler & Rothwell 2000). It can be used for patient-based antibody testing (Dressler et al. 2000). Additionally, a dose–duration correlation can be described (Keller 2006). Both correlations are valid only within certain limits. They can be used for comparison of different BT drugs and for modelling of optimal BT dosing. When the dose–duration correlation is not considered together with the dose–effect correlation, comparison of BT drugs becomes inaccurate. For comprehensive drug comparison, adverse effect profiles also need to be considered.

Apart from a direct action upon the striate muscle, BNT can act upon the muscle spindle organ, reducing its centripetal information traffic (Dressler et al. 1993; Filippi et al. 1993; Rosales et al. 1996). Whether this muscle afferent blockade is relevant to BT's therapeutic action remains unclear (Kaji et al. 1995a, 1995b).

In addition to the blockade of the acetylcholine secretion, animal experiments indicate BT induces blockade of transmitters involved in pain perception, pain transmission and pain processing, including substance P, glutamate, calcitonin gene-related peptide (CGRP) and noradrenaline (Foster 2004). There are numerous clinical studies on the use of BT to treat chronic pain (Jabbari & Machado 2014). Recent studies indicate that cranial BT injections can successfully reduce chronic migraine (Aurora et al. 2014; Kollewe et al. 2016).

Biological Activity of BT Drugs

The biological activity of therapeutic BT preparations is measured in mouse units (MU) in the mouse lethality assay, 1 MU being the amount of BT which kills 50 per cent of the BT-intoxicated mice. Mouse units therefore describe a biological activity and can correspond to different mass units according to the amount of inactivated BT contained within the preparation in addition to the active BT. The activity assays used by the manufacturers are performed differently, meaning that the activity labelling of the different BT drugs cannot be compared (Wohlfahrt et al. 2009) and should not be used to calculate dose ratios (Brin et al. 2014).

The potency labelling of different BT types also cannot be compared directly. The motor effects of Botox® and Myobloc®/NeuroBloc® seem to be comparable on a 1:40 ratio, whereas for treatment of autonomic disorders this conversion ratio could be different (Dressler et al. 2002). Overall, BT-B has relatively stronger autonomic and relatively weaker motor effects as compared to BT-A (Dressler & Benecke 2003).

Recently, cell-based assays were developed to replace the mouse lethality assay (Fernández-Salas et al. 2012; Johnson et al. 2013), offering the possibility to manufacture BT drugs without the need to sacrifice large numbers of mice.

Safety Aspects and Adverse Effects

When patients with chronic disorders are treated with a symptomatic therapy, issues of long-term safety become relevant. Since BT therapy was introduced in the late 1980s, large numbers of patients have been exposed to BT, many with high doses over prolonged periods of time. However, none of these patients has experienced additional long-term adverse effects. The broad therapeutic window and strong local effects provide BT drugs with an excellent adverse effects profile. Adverse effects are inherent to the therapeutic principle itself, being linked to the mode of action of BNT. They can be classified as local or systemic. Local adverse effects are caused by diffusion of BNT from the target tissue into adjacent tissues. Systemic adverse effects occur in tissues distant from the injection site and are due to BNT spread within the blood circulation. Despite its almost complete binding to the cholinergic nerve terminal, small amounts of BNT can be distributed with the blood circulation. This systemic spread can be detected by an increased neuromuscular jitter in muscles distant from the injection site (Lange et al. 1987; Girlanda et al. 1992). For BNT-A, systemic spread may become clinically relevant only when very high doses are applied (Dressler et al. 2015). Systemic spread of BNT-B is substantially higher and autonomic adverse effects occur frequently even when low or intermediate BT-B doses are used (Dressler & Benecke 2003). BT adverse effects occur in a typical time window after BT application, usually starting after one week and lasting for 1–2 weeks. Severity and duration depend on the dose applied. Although BT can produce numerous indirect central nervous system effects, direct ones beyond the alpha motor neuron have not been described after clinical intramuscular injection. BT transport through the blood–brain barrier is not possible due to BT's molecular size, and central nervous system adverse effects have not been reported so far. Central activity of BNT following intramuscular injection has recently been reported in animal models, potentially linked to retrograde neuronal transport of the BNT (Antonucci et al. 2008; Mazzocchio & Caleo 2015). These reports rely on extremely sensitive detection of the light chain activity via cleavage of the

SNARE protein, however, and as such it is difficult to judge the quantitative or clinical relevance of the observation. This is an area of BNT pharmacology that requires further study to understand its physiological or clinical relevance.

Outlook

BT drugs are highly potent drugs with a unique and intriguing mechanism of action. With the advent of new BT drugs, comparative studies will become more interesting. Using the two main elements of BT drugs, the specific binding ability of the heavy chain and the specific cleavage ability of the light chain, BT drugs may be used far beyond current indications.

References

Antonucci F, Rossi C, Gianfranceschi L, Rossetto O, Caleo M (2008) Long-distance retrograde effects of botulinum neurotoxin. *A J Neurosci* 28:3689–3696.

Aurora SK, Dodick DW, Diener HC, DeGryse RE, Turkel CC, Lipton RB, Silberstein SD (2014) OnabotulinumtoxinA for chronic migraine: efficacy, safety, and tolerability in patients who received all five treatment cycles in the PREEMPT clinical program. *Acta Neurol Scand* 129:61–70.

Beard M (2014) Translocation, entry into the cell. In: Foster KA (ed.) *Molecular Aspects of Botulinum Neurotoxin*. New York: Springer; pp151–170.

Brin MF, Dressler D, Aoki R (2004) Pharmacology of botulinum toxin therapy. In: Jankovic J, Comella C, Brin MF (eds) *Dystonia: Etiology, Clinical Features, and Treatment*. Philadelphia, PA: Lippincott Williams & Wilkins; pp93–112.

Brin MF, James C, Maltman J (2014) Botulinum toxin type A products are not interchangeable: a review of the evidence. *Biologics* 8:227–241.

de Paiva A, Meunier FA, Molgo J, Aoki KR, Dolly JO (1999) Functional repair of motor endplates after botulinum neurotoxin type A poisoning: biphasic switch of synaptic activity between nerve sprouts and their parent terminals. *Proc Natl Acad Sci USA* 96:3200–3205.

Dressler D, Benecke R (2003) Autonomic side effects of botulinum toxin type B treatment of cervical dystonia and hyperhidrosis. *Eur Neurol* 49:34–38.

Dressler D, Rothwell JC (2000) Electromyographic quantification of the paralysing effect of botulinum toxin. *Eur Neurol* 43:13–16.

Dressler D, Eckert J, Kukowski B, Meyer BU (1993) Somatosensorisch Evozierte Potentiale bei Schreibkrampf: Normalisierung pathologischer Befunde unter Botulinum Toxin Therapie. *Z EEG EMG* 24:191.

Dressler D, Rothwell JC, Bigalke H (2000) The sternocleidomastoid test: an in-vivo assay to investigate botulinum toxin antibody formation in man. *J Neurol* 247:630–632.

Dressler D, Adib Saberi F, Benecke R (2002) Botulinum toxin type B for treatment of axillar hyperhidrosis. *J Neurol* 249:1729–1732.

Dressler D, Saberi FA, Kollewe K, Schrader C (2015) Safety aspects of incobotulinumtoxinA high-dose therapy. *J Neural Transm* 122:327–333.

Eleopra R, Tugnoli V, Rossetto O, De Grandis D, Montecucco C (1998) Different time courses of recovery after poisoning with botulinum neurotoxin serotypes A and E in humans. *Neurosci Letts* 256:135–138.

Fernández-Salas E, Wang J, Molina Y, Nelson JB, Jacky BP, Aoki KR (2012) Botulinum neurotoxin serotype A specific cell-based potency assay to replace the mouse bioassay. *PLoS One* 7:e49516.

Filippi GM, Errico P, Santarelli R, Bagolini B, Manni E (1993) Botulinum A toxin effects on rat jaw muscle spindles. *Acta Otolaryngol* 113:400–404.

Foster KA (2004) The analgesic potential of clostridial neurotoxin derivatives. *Expert Opin Investig Drugs* 13:1437–1443.

Girlanda P, Vita G, Nicolosi C, Milone S, Messina C (1992) Botulinum toxin therapy: distant effects on neuromuscular transmission and autonomic nervous system. *J Neurol Neurosurg Psychiatry* 55:844–845.

Hallett M (2015) Explanation of timing of botulinum neurotoxin effects, onset, duration, and clinical ways of influencing them. *Toxicon* 107:64–67.

Jabbari B, Machado DG (2014) Clinical use of botulinum neurotoxins: pain. In: Foster KA (ed.) *Clinical Applications of Botulinum Neurotoxin*. New York: Springer; pp153–176.

Johnson EA, Pellett S, Whitemarsh RCM, Tepp WH (2013) Compositions and methods for toxigenicity testing. International Patent Application PCT/US2012/057825.

Kaji R, Kohara N, Katayama M, Kubori T, Mezaki T, Shibasaki H, Kimura J (1995a) Muscle afferent block by intramuscular injection of lidocaine for the treatment of writer's cramp. *Muscle Nerve* 18:234–235.

Kaji R, Rothwell JC, Katayama M, Ikeda T, Kubori T, Kohara N, Mezaki T, Shibasaki H, Kimura J (1995b) Tonic vibration reflex and muscle afferent block in writer's cramp. *Ann Neurol* 38:155–162.

Keller JE (2006) Recovery from botulinum neurotoxin poisoning in vivo. *Neurosci* 139:629–637.

Kollewe K, Escher C, Fathi D, Wulff DU, Paracka L, Mohammadi B, Karst M, Dressler D (2016) Long-term treatment of chronic migraine with onabotulinumtoxinA: efficacy, quality of life and tolerability in a real-life setting. *J Neural Transm* 123:533–540.

Lange DJ, Brin MF, Warner CL, Fahn S, Lovelace RE (1987) Distant effects of local injection of botulinum toxin. *Muscle Nerve* 10:552–555.

Mazzocchio R, Caleo M (2015) More than at the neuromuscular synapse: actions of botulinum neurotoxin A in the central nervous system. *Neuroscientist* 21:44–61.

Pellizzari R, Rossetto O, Schiavo G, Montecucco C (1999) Tetanus and botulinum neurotoxins: mechanism of action and therapeutic uses. *Philos Trans R Soc Lond B Biol Sci* 354:259–268.

Peng L, Tepp WH, Pitkin RM, Johnson EA, Stenmark P, Dong M (2012) Botulinum neurotoxin D-C uses synaptotagmin I and II as receptors, and human synaptotagmin II is not an effective receptor for type B, D-C and G toxins. *J Cell Sci* 125:3233–3242.

Rosales RL, Arimura K, Takenaga S, Osame M (1996) Extrafusal and intrafusal muscle effects in experimental botulinum toxin-A injection. *Muscle Nerve* 19:488–496.

Rummel A (2013) Double receptor anchorage of botulinum neurotoxins accounts for their exquisite neurospecificity. *Curr Top Microbiol Immunol* 364:61–90.

Schiavo G, Matteoli M, Montecucco C (2000) Neurotoxins affecting neuroexocytosis. *Physiol Rev* 80:717–766.

Strotmeier J, Willjes G, Binz T, Rummel A (2012) Human synaptotagmin-II is not a high affinity receptor for botulinum neurotoxin B and G: increased therapeutic dosage and immunogenicity. *FEBS Lett* 586:310–313.

Tsai YC, Moller BE, Adler M, Oyler GA (2014) Molecular basis for persistence of botulinum neurotoxin: the role of intracellular protein degradation pathways. In: Foster KA (ed.) *Molecular Aspects of Botulinum Neurotoxin*. New York: Springer; pp191–206.

Wohlfahrt K, Sycha T, Ranoux D, Naver H, Caird D (2009) Dose equivalence of two commercial preparations of botulinum neurotoxin type A: time for a reassessment? *Curr Med Res Opin* 25:1573–1584.

Chapter 28

Immunology of Botulinum Toxin Therapy

Dirk Dressler and Hans Bigalke

Introduction

As botulinum toxin (BT) drugs mainly consist of proteins, antigenicity was an issue since they were introduced as a new treatment option. Initially, it was thought that minute BT quantities and long re-exposition intervals would protect against antibody formation (Biglan et al. 1986; Gonnering 1988). In the early 1990s, however, the first cases of formation of antibodies against BT (BTAB) and antibody-induced therapy failure (ABTF) occurred and studies on risk factors for ABTF were performed. When the first BT type B drug and the first BT drug free of complexing proteins were introduced antigenicity was discussed, again. Most recently, new antigenicity data suggest re-evaluating treatment algorithms with respect to maximal BT doses and minimal interinjection intervals.

Looking at the actual ABTF frequency under the currently applied safety precautions, BT antigenicity may seem a minor problem. However, considering the potential to improve BT therapy by lifting these restrictions makes it worthwhile to discuss antigenicity of BT therapy.

With a considerable number of new BT drugs currently being developed, monitoring their antigenicity during the developmental phase and after they are applied in a large number of patients is another challenge.

Definitions

Table 28.1 summarises the most important definitions and abbreviations necessary to discuss BT antigenicity (Dressler 2004b).

Composition of BT Drugs

BT drugs consist of botulinum neurotoxin (BNT), complexing proteins (CP, also sometimes called accessory proteins) and excipients. Excipients may vary among the different BT drugs on the market (Dressler & Foster in press). They include human serum albumin and buffer systems in onabotulinumtoxinA, abobotulinumtoxinA, incobotulinumtoxinA and rimabotulinumtoxinB, NaCl in onabotulinumtoxinA, lactose in abobotulinumtoxinA, sucrose in incobotulinumtoxinA and H_2O and disodium succinate in rimabotulinumtoxinB. The BT component contains all protein constituents and consists of BNT and CP. CPs are protein aggregates consisting of non-toxic non-haemagglutinin protein (NTNHA) of around 130 kD and haemagglutinin proteins (HA) of around 50 kD. Depending on the BT type, BNT and CP form different protein aggregates. In BT type A, BNT and CP form three protein aggregates: small aggregates of around 280 kD, medium aggregates of around 600

Table 28.1 Definitions and abbreviations according to Dressler (2004b)

Term	Abbreviation	Definition
Therapy failure	TF	BT therapy effect less than expected
Subjective therapy failure	Subjective TF	Therapy failure as reported by the patient
Objective therapy failure	Objective TF	Therapy failure as judged by the injector
Complete therapy failure	Complete TF	Complete lack of BT therapeutic effects and/or BT adverse effects
Partial therapy failure	Partial TF	Reduced BT therapeutic effects (duration and/or extent) and/or BT adverse effects
Primary therapy failure	Primary TF	Reduced BT effect starting with therapy initiation
Secondary therapy failure	Secondary TF	Reduced BT effect starting after several injection series
Antibody-induced therapy failure	ABTF	Reduced BT therapeutic effects and/or reduced BT adverse effects caused by BT antibodies
Botulinum toxin antibodies	BTAB	Antibodies directed against botulinum neurotoxin or complexing proteins
Neutralising antibodies	Neutralising BTAB	BT antibodies directed against functionally relevant botulinum neurotoxin epitopes
Non-neutralising antibodies	Non-neutralising BTAB	BT antibodies directed against complexing proteins or functionally irrelevant botulinum neurotoxin epitopes
Relevant antibody titre	Relevant BTAB titres	BT antibody titres sufficient to reduce BT efficacy
Non-relevant antibody titre	Non-relevant BTAB titres	BT antibody titres insufficient to reduce BT efficacy

kD and large aggregates of around 900 kD (Frevert & Dressler 2010; Rossetto et al. 2014). The CP composition varies among the different BT type A drugs. In incobotulinumtoxinA all CP have been removed during the manufacturing process. BTAB may be formed against each of these proteins. When they are directed against therapeutically relevant BNT epitopes they are called neutralising BTAB and may reduce BT's effects. When they are directed against therapeutically non-relevant BNT epitopes or against CP they are called non-neutralising BTAB and do not interfere with BT's effects.

Antigen–Antibody Reaction

BTAB belong to the IgG isotype. They are produced by plasma cells and memory B cells and stay in tissues and in the serum. BTAB and BNT are related in a functional balance. Low BTAB titres inactivate only small amounts of BNT, thus reducing BT's effects only marginally. High BTAB titres, however, can inactivate large amounts of BNT, thus completely blocking BT's effects. Increasing the amount of BT administered may compensate for low to intermediate BTAB titres (Dressler et al. 2002). Compensating for high BTAB titres has not been tried yet, but may bear a substantial risk of further stimulating BTAB formation. To judge the clinical relevance of BTAB with respect to therapy failure, BTAB titres need to be measured quantitatively and the test used needs to be disclosed.

Dynamics of BTAB Formation

ABTF is secondary therapy failure. Screening of serum samples in blood banks does not indicate the existence of pre-formed BTAB (Bigalke, personal communication). Even botulism does not seem to produce lasting BTAB titres. ABTF usually develops 2–3 years after initiation of BT therapy. After four years of BT therapy occurrence of ABTF seems to be rare (Dressler 2004b). Exceptionally, only a few exposures may be sufficient to stimulate BTAB formation and to induce complete ABTF (Dressler 2000b, 2004a; Dressler et al. 2010). Before complete ABTF manifests, partial ABTF usually occurs and produces reduced extent and/or reduced duration of BT effects. Figure 28.1 shows an example of a typical patient with the development of ABTF (Dressler 2004b). Persistence of BTAB after cessation of BT application varies (Dressler & Bigalke 2002). Within four years about half of the BTAB titres may drop to clinically irrelevant titres, while the other half persist (Dressler & Bigalke 2002). Some of them may eventually drop; some, however, persist thereafter, potentially permanently.

Frequency of ABTF

The exact frequency of ABTF could only be determined if a specified group of patients would be followed up throughout a relevant period of time. This, however, has never been done so far. Therefore, all figures regarding ABTF frequency are estimates. ABTF frequency for focal dystonias is in the range of 1–5 per cent. They have not been reported for non-focal dystonias. Antigenicity differences between onabotulinumtoxinA and abobotulinumtoxinA have not been found. ABTF

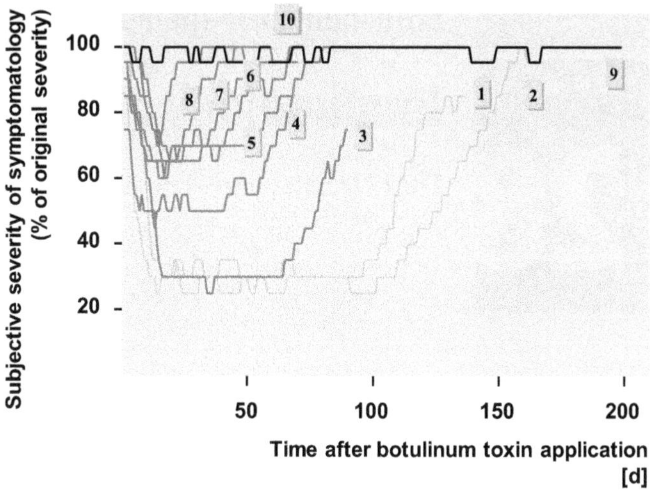

Figure 28.1 Development of antibody-induced therapy failure in a patient receiving botulinum toxin therapy.
Source: Dressler (2000a).

frequency in rimabotulinumtoxinB is substantially higher. In cervical dystonia it is in the order of 40 per cent (Dressler et al. 2003). Whether this is caused by the specific preparation of rimabotulinumtoxinB or by an intrinsically higher antigenicity of BT type B remains unclear. In patients with exclusive incobotulinumtoxinA treatment ABTF has not been detected so far, despite its worldwide use for more than a decade in various indications.

Risk Factors for BTAB Formation

Risk factors for ABTF were studied in the early 1990s (Greene et al. 1994; Jankovic & Schwartz 1995; Dressler & Dirnberger 2000). They include BT doses given at each injection series (single doses), latencies between subsequent injection series (interinjection intervals) and booster injections, i.e. BT injections with interinjection intervals of less than two weeks. The cumulative BT dose could be excluded as a risk factor. Effects of gender and age were not found (Dressler & Dirnberger 2000). All of these findings are based on group comparisons with group sizes of well under 30 patients. Therefore, the exact kind of correlation (linear, exponential, threshold effects, etc.) between the risk factor and ABTF frequency could not be determined, thus leaving these findings largely irrelevant for clinical practice.

BTAB Testing

BTAB testing can be performed with structural tests such as ELISA (Dressler et al. 2014b) and radioimmunoprecipitation assays (Dressler et al. 2001). Structural BTAB tests are mainly used as screening tests. Whether the detected BTAB are neutralising needs to be confirmed by functional tests. However, a recently developed ELISA test for BTAB detection (Dressler et al. 2014b) can be adjusted not only to produce highly sensitive results but also highly specific results. Functional BTAB tests can be based on any biological function sensitive to BT. Usually they are based on test animal lethality, i.e. a mixture of skeletal muscle paresis and autonomic dysfunction. This so-called mouse lethality assay or mouse protection assay is time-consuming, expensive and exposes large numbers of mice to prolonged agony. However, it is still considered the gold standard. The mouse diaphragm assay or hemidiaphragm assay is a functional *ex vivo* test with superior quality features able to replace the mouse lethality assay (Dressler et al. 2000). Human functional tests include the extensor digitorum brevis test (Kessler & Benecke 1997), the frowning or frontalis test (Hanna & Jankovic 1998), the sternocleidomastoideus test (Dressler et al. 2000b) and various sweat tests (Birklein et al. 2002; Voller et al. 2004). These tests are performed directly on the patient with suspected BTAF. Most patient-based tests are not quantitative and not quality tested. Especially the frowning test and also the extensor digitorum brevis test may produce unreliable results as they are not based on dose–effect curves.

Frequent Mistakes in Interpreting Antibody-Induced Therapy Failure

Interpretation of ABTF is complicated. Testing of BTAB has to be performed with tests that are quality-assessed with respect to their sensitivity, specificity and reliability to limit false-positive or false-negative results. Still, most BTAB tests are lacking a sufficient quality assessment. BTAB tests have to produce quantitative results. Thresholds for positive test readings are debatable. Low titres are usually functionally irrelevant. Only substantial BTAB titres can produce clinically detectable effects. Principal limitations of BTAB tests have to be known: ELISA tests with sufficient sensitivity may be used to screen large numbers of sera at moderate costs; the presence of non-neutralising BTAB in positive sera has to be excluded by subsequent confirmation tests such as the mouse lethality assay or the mouse diaphragm assay. All conclusions about antigenicity of BT drugs or treatment algorithms have to take into account the dynamics of BTAB formation, as only sufficient exposure times guarantee objective results. Assuming presence of BTAB based on the analysis of the clinical response to BT alone is unacceptable, as most cases of therapy failure are not caused by BTAB, but by suboptimal injection schemes or by unfavourable subtypes of the treated condition.

Strategies to Manage ABTF

BTAB may or may not drop after cessation of BT therapy (Dressler & Bigalke 2002). Even if they drop, latencies are far too long to be compatible with an effective BT therapy. BT dosage increase can overcome ABTF when it is partial and when BTAB titres are low (Dressler et al. 2002). However, the risk of further stimulating BTAB formation remains. BTAB reduction or inactivation by intravenous immunoglobulin application does not seem to work (Dressler et al. 2000a). Extraction of BTAB by plasmapheresis is principally possible, but impractical (Naumann et al. 1998). Specific immunoadsorption may be theoretically possible, but problems including BNT washout from the immunoadsorption column need to be solved first. Immunosuppressants such as mycophenolate may prevent reoccurrence of previously dropped BTAB titres (Duane et al. 2000). Replacing the BT drug that induced BTAB formation by a BT drug derived from a different BT type can overcome ABTF. When BT type B is given in patients with BT type A ABTF, normal therapeutic effects can be regained (Dressler et al. 2003). However, 40 per cent of these patients may develop BT type B ABTF within a few applications (Dressler et al. 2003). The opposite crossover effect has not been reported so far. BT type F has been tried to overcome BT type A ABTF on an experimental basis only, as it is not available commercially (Greene & Fahn 1993). Exchanges between BT drugs of the same BT type are not effective since BT antibodies are cross-reactive for all BT drugs of the same BT type. Once ABTF has occurred, BT therapy should be switched to an alternative BT type. If ABTF to the alternative BT occurs, conventional treatment options should be considered (Dressler et al. 2015). Since conventional treatment options are in most cases of limited efficacy, deep brain stimulation often remains the only realistic alternative. Prevention of ABTF is of paramount interest.

Treatment Algorithms to Prevent BTAB

According to the risk factors for BTAB formation, BT drugs should be dosed in principle as low as possible and should be applied with the longest possible interinjection intervals. However, this approach is limited by the need for therapeutic efficacy. Recent studies show that BT drugs can be tolerated without ABTF in higher doses (Dressler et al. 2014a) and in shorter interinjection intervals (Dressler & Adib Saberi 2016) than previously thought. However, both studies are based on the application of incobotulinumtoxinA only. Conventional BT drugs need to be studied for this purpose. As long as no other experience is available, booster injections – i.e. BT injections with interinjection intervals of less than two weeks – should be avoided. In any case, BT drugs with the lowest available antigenicity should be used. With no published reports on ABTF after ten years of international usage in a wide spectrum of indications, incobotulinumtoxinA seems to be the drug of choice (Dressler 2012).

References

Biglan AW, Gonnering R, Lockhart LB, Rabin B, Fuerste FH (1986) Absence of antibody production in patients treated with botulinum A toxin. *Am J Ophthalmol* 101:232–235.

Birklein F, Walther D, Bigalke H, Winterholler M, Erbguth F (2002) Sudomotor testing predicts the presence of neutralizing botulinum A toxin antibodies. *Ann Neurol* 52:68–73.

Dressler D (2000a) *Botulinum Toxin Therapy*. Stuttgart: Thieme Verlag.

Dressler D (2000b) Complete secondary botulinum toxin therapy failure in blepharospasm. *J Neurol* 247:809–810.

Dressler D (2004a) New formulation of BOTOX®: complete antibody-induced therapy failure in hemifacial spasm. *J Neurol* 251:360.

Dressler D (2004b) Clinical presentation and management of antibody-induced failure of botulinum toxin therapy. *Mov Disord* 19 (Suppl. 8):S92–S100.

Dressler D (2012) Five-year experience with incobotulinumtoxinA (Xeomin®): the first botulinum toxin drug free of complexing proteins. *Eur J Neurol* 19:385–389.

Dressler D, Adib Saberi F (2016) Immunological safety of incobotulinumtoxinA (Xeomin®) therapy with reduced interinjection intervals. *J Neural Transm* 122:327–333.

Dressler D, Bigalke H (2002) Botulinum toxin antibody titres after cessation of botulinum toxin therapy. *Mov Disord* 17:170–173.

Dressler D, Dirnberger G (2000) Botulinum toxin therapy: risk factors for therapy failure. *Mov Disord* 15 (Suppl. 2):51.

Dressler D, Foster K (in press) Pharmacology of botulinum toxins. In: Dressler D, Altenmüller E, Krauss JK (eds) *Treatment of Dystonia*. Cambridge: Cambridge University Press.

Dressler D, Zettl U, Bigalke H, Benecke R (2000a) Can intravenous immunoglobulin improve antibody mediated botulinum toxin therapy failure? *Mov Disord* 15:1279–1281.

Dressler D, Dirnberger G, Bhatia K, Quinn NP, Irmer A, Bigalke H, Marsden CD (2000b) Botulinum toxin antibody testing: comparison between the mouse diaphragm bioassay and the mouse lethality bioassay. *Mov Disord* 15:973–976.

Dressler D, Bigalke H, Rothwell JC (2000c) The sternocleidomastoid test: an in-vivo assay to investigate botulinum toxin antibody formation in man. *J Neurol* 247:630–632.

Dressler D, Muenchau A, Bhatia KP, Quinn NP, Bigalke H (2002) Antibody induced botulinum toxin therapy failure: can it be overcome by increased botulinum toxin doses? *Eur Neurol* 47:118–121.

Dressler D, Benecke R, Bigalke H (2003) Botulinum toxin type B (NeuroBloc®) in patients with botulinum toxin type A antibody-induced therapy failure. *J Neurol* 250:967–969.

Dressler D, Wohlfahrt K, Meyer-Rogge E, Wiest L, Bigalke H (2010) Antibody-induced failure of botulinum toxin a therapy in cosmetic indications. *Dermatol Surg* 36 (Suppl. 4):2182–2187.

Dressler D, Adib Saberi F, Kollewe K, Schrader C (2014a) Safety aspects of incobotulinumtoxinA high dose therapy. *J Neural Transm* 122:327–333.

Dressler D, Gessler F, Tacik P, Bigalke H (2014b) An enzyme-linked immunosorbent assay for detection of botulinum toxin-antibodies. *Mov Disord* 29:1322–1324.

Dressler D, Altenmueller E, Bhidayasiri R, Bohlega S, Chana P, Chung TM, Frucht S, Garcia-Ruiz PJ, Kaelin A, Kaji R, Kanovsky P, Laskawi R, Micheli F, Orlova O, Relja M, Rosales R, Slawek J, Timerbaeva S, Warner TT, Saberi FA (2015) Strategies for treatment of dystonia. *J Neural Transm* (epub ahead of printing).

Duane DD, Monroe J, Morris RE (2000) Mycophenolate in the prevention of recurrent neutralizing botulinum toxin A antibodies in cervical dystonia. *Mov Disord* 15:365–366.

Frevert J, Dressler D (2010) Complexing proteins in botulinum toxin type A drugs: a help or a hindrance? *Biologics* 4:325–332.

Gonnering RS (1988) Negative antibody response to long-term treatment of facial spasm with botulinum toxin. *Am J Ophthalmol* 105:313–315.

Greene PE, Fahn S (1993) Use of botulinum toxin type F injections to treat torticollis in patients with immunity to botulinum toxin type A. *Mov Disord* 8:479–483.

Greene P, Fahn S, Diamond B (1994) Development of resistance to botulinum toxin type A in patients with torticollis. *Mov Disord* 9:213–217.

Hanna PA, Jankovic J (1998) Mouse bioassay versus Western blot assay for botulinum toxin antibodies: correlation with clinical response. *Neurology* 50:1624–1629.

Jankovic J, Schwartz K (1995) Response and immunoresistance to botulinum toxin injections. *Neurology* 45:1743–1746.

Kessler KR, Benecke R (1997) The EBD test: a clinical test for the detection of antibodies to botulinum toxin type A. *Mov Disord* 12:95–99.

Naumann M, Toyka KV, Mansouri Taleghani B, Ahmadpour J, Reiners K, Bigalke H (1998) Depletion of neutralising antibodies resensitises a secondary non-responder to botulinum A neurotoxin. *J Neurol Neurosurg Psychiat* 65:924–927.

Rossetto O, Pirazzini M, Montecucco C (2014) Botulinum neurotoxins: genetic, structural and mechanistic insights. *Nat Rev Microbiol* 12:535–549.

Voller B, Moraru E, Auff E, Benesch M, Poewe W, Wissel J, Müller J, Entner T, Bigalke H, Schnider P (2004) Ninhydrin sweat test: a simple method for detecting antibodies neutralizing botulinum toxin type A. *Mov Disord* 19:943–947.

Chapter 29

Use of Non-A/Non-B Botulinum Toxins

Roberto Eleopra

Introduction

Clostridium botulinum produces seven different neurotoxins, abbreviated from BoNT/A to BoNT/G (Rossetto et al. 2014). Human botulism has been used to decide which serotypes should be tested as therapeutic agents (Johnson & Montecucco 2008). Epidemiologic data suggest that serotypes A, B, E, F and G cause human botulism in adults, while only few papers report human outbreaks of types C and D. Animal species vary extensively in their sensitivity to BoNT serotypes (Smith & Sugiyama 1988) and determination of the susceptibility of humans to the various toxin serotypes is remarkable, because of the large application of BoNT/A and /B to the therapy of human diseases (Hallett 2000; Jankovic 2004). So, in clinical practice the use of non-A or non-B BoNT serotypes might be proposed in cases of an immune response to BoNT/A or when different mechanisms of action and different durations are required to improve the clinical management. In humans, few data about comparative dose–response characteristics of the seven toxin serotypes exist, and the mechanism responsible for the different time-courses of the different toxins are unclear (Rossetto et al. 2014). This chapter summarises the characteristics of the non-A/non-B BoNT serotypes in humans, except for BoNT/G where there are no human data available.

Botulinum Neurotoxin Serotype C (BoNT/C)

BoNT/C cleaves both SNAP-25 and syntaxin, making it unique among BoNTs. This double target specificity suggests it could be a valuable alternative to the use of BoNT/A. Coffield et al. (1997) confirm an effect of BoNT/C in surgically excised human muscle and these experimental results offer compelling evidence that isolated human tissue is sensitive to it. We were the first to report the great potential of BoNT/C injection in humans (Eleopra et al. 1997) and also to compare several serotypes in human muscles (Eleopra et al. 2004). In these papers the source of BoNT/C was reported as Wako Chemicals, while it was purified from strain NCTC 8264. Before testing BoNT/C in dystonia, we compared BoNT/C and BoNT/A in the mouse hemidiaphragm assay. Later, we tested low dosages in the extensor digitorum brevis (EDB) muscle (Eleopra et al. 1997) and in the abductor digiti minimi muscle (ADM) against BoNT/A (Eleopra et al. 2006) with similar effects. We also tested human BoNT/C safety by the Motor Unit Number Estimation (MUNE) technique, not revealing motor neuron decrease after application (Eleopra et al. 2002). Based on these data, a few BoNT-naïve patients with focal dystonia were treated with BoNT/C. All showed a good clinical response. Four blepharospasm patients and ten torticollis patients received BoNT/C, with results similar to BoNT/A (Eleopra et al. 1997, 2004, 2006). Even as only a few dystonia patients were treated with BoNT/C, clinical improvement was good and lasted for a maximal 30 days, with slow recovery after about eight weeks. None of the patients treated reported any significant adverse reactions. In conclusion, these preliminary studies demonstrate that BoNT/C is a safe and valid therapy for dystonia and a useful alternative to BoNT/A.

Botulinum Neurotoxin Serotype D (BoNT/D)

BoNT/D is the most powerful of all BoNTs in animals. It cleaves VAMP but it is considered not to be active in isolated human pyramidalis muscles (Coffield et al. 1997). In contrast, a recent review by Anderson et al. (2009) reported that BoNT/D is active in human intercostal muscles. Recently, we have investigated BoNT/D's action in mice and in humans *in vivo* by a quantitative neurophysiological assessment of the skeletal neuromuscular paralysis (Eleopra et al. 2013). This investigation shows that BoNT/D is very active in mice and rats, but poorly effective in humans as BoNT/D 10 MU produced only a slight EDB inhibition after one week. Higher doses may produce stronger effects. In conclusion, no definite clinical data about BoNT/D therapy in humans are available.

Botulinum Neurotoxin Serotype E (BoNT/E)

Like BoNT/A, BoNT/E cleaves SNAP-25, also producing inhibition of acetylcholine release. Recovery time is similar to that of BoNT/A. In our preclinical study in humans (Eleopra et al. 1998) we assessed simultaneous injections of BoNT/A and BoNT/E in two opposite body sides. Eleven patients with idiopathic blepharospasm (BS) received BoNT/A 3 MU and BoNT/E 3 MU in opposite EDBs. Subsequently, seven BS patients received a combination of BoNT/A 4 MU + BoNT/E 2 MU in one EDB and BoNT/E 4 MU + BoNT/A 2 MU in the opposite EDB (Eleopra et al. 1998). In both experiments, target muscles receiving BoNT/E recovered faster than those treated with BoNT/A ($p < 0.001$). Patients receiving the BoNT/A and BoNT/E mixtures recovered with a time-course similar to BoNT/E and clearly faster than that observed with BoNT/A alone. Concluding, BoNT/E has an effect in humans but shows fast and complete recovery. Therefore, BoNT/E may only be used when shorter effects are required.

Botulinum Neurotoxin Serotype F (BoNT/F)

BoNT/F demonstrates specificity for vesicle-associated membrane proteins (VAMP, synaptobrevin) and was the first non-A serotype used in humans as an alternative to BoNT/A. Initially, BoNT/F was used in patients with antibodies against BoNT/A and was reported in 1992 in two patients with torticollis, one with oromandibular dystonia and one with stuttering (Ludlow et al. 1992; Greene & Fahn 1993). Greene and Fahn (1993) proposed that BoNT/F may also be helpful in clinical situations where short effects are required, when faster and brief muscle spasm relief is desired or a predictive test for operations is necessary. BoNT/F in *de novo* dystonia patients seems to produce shorter effects and seems to require higher doses as compared to BoNT/A (Greene & Fahn 1996; Chen et al. 1998). In 1999, Mezaki and colleagues (1999) injected BoNT/A or BoNT/F in the orbicularis oculi of blepharospasm patients and 1:1 mixture of both in the contralateral orbilcularis oculi. They compared the peak effect and the action duration in a double-blind controlled study and concluded that the duration of action of the mixture was longer than by BoNT/F alone and shorter than by BoNT/A alone. They used a combination of two different BoNT serotypes in order to evaluate possible additive neuromuscular blocking effects. In conclusion, BoNT/F is a valid alternative to BoNT/A only when short effects are required. Higher BoNT/F dosage may produce a subjectively better and longer response, although it is shorter than that of BoNT/A. Immunogenicity of BoNT/F in long-term treatments is still unknown.

References

Anderson J, Williams PT, Katos AM, et al. 2009. Botulinum toxins. In Gupta RC, ed., *Handbook of Toxicology of Chemical Warfare Agents*. Amsterdam: Elsevier BV: 407–432.

Chen R, Karp BI, Hallett M. 1998. Botulinum toxin type F for treatment of dystonia: long-term experience. *Neurology* 51:1494–1496.

Coffield JA, Bakry N, Zhang RD, et al. 1997. In vitro characterization of botulinum toxin types A, C and D action on human tissues: combined electrophysiologic, pharmacologic and molecular biologic approaches. *J Pharmacol Exp Ther* 280:1489–1498.

Eleopra R, Tugnoli V, Rossetto O, et al. 1997. Botulinum neurotoxin serotype C: a novel effective botulinum toxin therapy in human. *Neurosci Lett* 224: 91–94.

Eleopra R, Tugnoli V, Rossetto O, et al. 1998. Different time courses of recovery after poisoning with botulinum neurotoxin serotypes A and E in humans. *Neurosci Lett* 256: 135–138.

Eleopra R, Tugnoli V, Quatrale R, et al. 2002. Botulinum neurotoxin serotypes A and C do not affect motor units survival in humans: an electrophysiological study by motor units counting. *Clin Neurophysiol* 113: 1258–1264.

Eleopra R, Tugnoli V, Quatrale R, et al. 2004. Different types of botulinum toxin in humans. *Mov Disord* 19 (Suppl. 8):S53–S59.

Eleopra R, Tugnoli V, Quatrale R, et al. 2006. Clinical use of non-A botulinum toxins: botulinum toxin type C and botulinum toxin type F. *Neurotox Res* 9:127–131.

Eleopra R, Montecucco C, Devigili G, et al. 2013. Botulinum neurotoxin serotype D is poorly effective in humans: an in vivo electrophysiological study. *Clin Neurophysiol* 124: 999–1004.

Greene PE, Fahn S. 1993. Use of botulinum toxin type F injections to treat torticollis in patients with immunity to botulinum toxin type A. *Mov Disord* 8:479–483.

Greene PE, Fahn S. 1996. Response to botulinum toxin F in seronegative botulinum toxin A-resistant patients. *Mov Disord* 11:181–184.

Hallett M. 2000. How does botulinum toxin work? *Ann Neurol* 48:7–8.

Jankovic J. 2004. Botulinum toxin in clinical practice. *J Neurol Neurosurg Psychiat* 75:951–957.

Johnson EA, Montecucco C. 2008. Botulism. In: Engel AG, ed., *Neuromuscular Junction Disorders: Handbook of Clinical Neurology*. Amsterdam: Elsevier: 333–368.

Ludlow CL, Hallett M, Rhew K, et al. 1992. Therapeutic use of type F botulinum toxin. *N Engl J Med* 326:349–350.

Mezaki T, Kaji R, Brin MF, et al. 1999. Combined use of type A and F botulinum toxins for blepharospasm: a double-blind controlled trial. *Mov Disord* 14:1017–1020.

Rossetto O, Pirazzini M, Montecucco C. 2014. Botulinum neurotoxins: genetic, structural and mechanistic insights. *Nature* 12:535–549.

Smith LD, Sugiyama H. 1988. *Botulism: The Organism, its Toxins, the Disease*. Springfield, IL: C.C. Thomas Publ.

Chapter 30

Clinical Muscular Anatomy for the Botulinum Toxin Injector

Mandar Jog and Robert Chen

Introduction

The success of botulinum toxin (BT) injections is largely dependent on the appropriate localisation and targeting of the affected muscles. Although issues such as dilution, needle length, nature of the clinical syndrome such as stroke versus dystonia all contribute to the variability of injection response, the need to understand the functional anatomy, including the surface anatomy, cannot be overstated.

In this review we will focus on the key muscles and syndromes that are seen by a clinical practice and develop the anatomical approach to targeting appropriate muscles for each of the syndromes. The selected muscles will be reviewed individually, including structure and surface localisation. The anatomical aspects, including the cadaveric and surface anatomy, will be discussed. This approach will be different than a traditional textbook of anatomy, of which there are many. Since the review relies on already well-known anatomical atlases, there will not be any exhaustive references. The authors will attempt to provide clinical pearls for the injector as appropriate throughout.

The review will be divided into four sections. The first section will cover the face and jaw muscles. The second section will concentrate on those muscles and syndromes that affect the neck. The third and fourth sections will concentrate on the upper and lower limbs.

Muscles of the Face

Muscles of the face are different than most other body muscles as they are inserted into other muscles as compared to between bones. Hence the action of these muscles is complex since the movement/size/action of one muscle can impact that of another that originates or inserts into it.

Orbicularis Oculi

The orbicularis oculi muscle is supplied by the temporal and zygomatic branches of the facial nerve and has two parts: the palpebral portion on the eyelid and the orbital portion, which is circumferential. The pretarsal portion of the orbicularis oculi is along the eyelid and also includes the levators of the eyelid, which must be avoided from being injected; the preseptal portion, which is under the eyebrow; and then the orbital portion, which is circumferential. Both orbital as well as palpebral orbicularis oculi narrows the palpebral fissure, and is thus an antagonist to the levator muscles that elevate the eyes. The palpebral part is responsible for the blinking reflex and hence those patients that simply have excessive blinking require injection of the palpebral portion of the orbicularis oculi, often in the upper lid. Those that have more forced closure along with the corrugator as well as procerus muscles may require injection in the orbital portion.

Corrugator Supercilii

The corrugator supercilii muscle is an angular muscle that is contiguous with the orbital portion of the orbicularis oculi muscle. The corrugator supercilii muscle, located above the eyebrow, is supplied by the temporal branches of the facial nerve. Together with the procerus, the corrugator supercilii draws down the middle part of the eyebrow, thereby causing deep frown lines over the roof of the nose

Frontalis

The frontalis muscle is contiguous with the procerus, goes all the way up into the scalp and also is contiguous with the orbicularis oculi orbital portion. The muscle is part of a large muscle complex that goes all the way back over the scalp to the occipital area. However, the frontal belly of the frontalis muscle, also supplied by the facial nerve, is contiguous medially to the procerus muscle and down below with the orbital portion of orbicularis oculi, as well as the corrugator supercilii muscle. The frontalis muscle is involved in wrinkling of the forehead. Although divided between the two sides of the head, the frontalis muscle generally works together, such that the forehead wrinkles are produced simultaneously. Hence those patients that require injections generally require injections on both sides if wrinkling of the forehead is a predominant clinical problem.

Procerus

The procerus muscle is a triangular muscle. It is involved in elevation of the eyebrow, but also in patients that have blepharospasm, the procerus muscle will be hyper-contractile. For those patients that have full eye closure with sustained contraction of the eyes, we inject the procerus muscle as well. The injection of the procerus is done in a couple of spots, generally close to the eyebrow.

Depressor Supercilii

The depressor supercilii has its origin on the medial orbital rim, near the lacrimal bone, and inserts on the medial aspect of the bony orbit, just below the corrugator supercilii. This muscle aids pulling down the medial portion of the eyelid along with the corrugator.

Zygomaticus Major

The muscle arises from the zygomatic arch and inserts into the corner of the mouth, immediately next to the levator of the lip. This muscle lifts the corner of the mouth. It is injected at the origin of the muscle at the zygomatic arch to avoid injections into the lip levators. The needle is kept almost superficial since the muscle is thin and is injected midway along a line connecting the top of the pinna to the corner of the mouth.

Risorius

This muscle arises from the fascia of the parotid gland and inserts into the orbicularis oris, essentially as a superficial cutaneous muscle that pulls the corner of the mouth sideways. This generates a 'false smile'. It is innervated by the facial nerve and is injected halfway along a straight line connecting the lower portion of the pinna to the corner of the mouth

Nasalis

The nasalis muscle is supplied by the buccal branches of the facial nerve. There are two parts to the nasalis muscle. The alar part, which is the outer portion or the external part of the nasalis muscle, widens the nasal openings or the external nares and flares the nostrils. It is generally this alar part that is injected in patients that have hemifacial spasm or crinkling of the nose opening of their nostrils. The transverse part is responsible for narrowing the nares and slightly lowering the tip of the nose, and is generally not injected.

Levator Angularis Oris/Levator Labii Superioris/ Levator Labii Superioris Alaeque Nasi

The levator angularis oris muscle is part of the triad that moves and elevates the lip, including levator labii superioris alaeque nasi, levator labii superioris itself and levator angularis oris. It is supplied by the zygomatic branches of the facial or the seventh nerve. Again, these muscles are generally not injected because they produce a drooping of the lip not advisable for most patients. However, if one were to inject the superficial muscle, the location of injection is about a centimetre off from the corner of the lip. As per its name, the levator angularis oris is at an angle of approximately 35–40 degrees from the straight position between the corners of the lip to the eye. The injection is again done superficially, with the needle puncturing approximately 1–2 mm into the corner of the crease along the cheek border.

The levator labii superioris itself is at the corner of the mouth. This muscle, along with the alaeque nasi, lifts the angle of the mouth. Injection of this muscle is also uncommon because, again, botulinum toxin injected into this muscle will produce drooping of the lip. However, if there is substantial elevation of the lip, the muscle can be injected again at a 30-degree angle.

Levator labii superioris alaeque nasi is generally not injected. However, if one does wish to inject this muscle it is because the corner of the mouth is pulled towards the nostril. Owing to its origin on the nasal wing, it raises the lateral margin of the nares. This function is supported also with nasalis, allowing the nasal cavity to be opened. It is responsible for producing this crease in the face. The injection again is done superficially, in low doses, yet the injection is not subcutaneous. Unlike the orbicularis oculi, the injection angle has to be slightly higher, not parallel to the skin. The injection is done approximately 30 degrees from the face.

Mentalis

The mentalis muscle is a fairly large muscle bounded by the orbicularis oris above and the depressor labii inferioris on the sides. This muscle is also supplied by the mandibular branch of the facial or the seventh cranial nerve. The action of this muscle as a chin muscle is to pull down the lower lip, along with the depressor angularis oris. The mentalis muscle is superficial and is injected on either side. The muscle produces an elevation of the chin and is injected superficially at an angle of approximately 45 degrees, with the needle puncturing only 1–2 mm, as with all other facial muscles.

Depressor Angularis Oris

Depressor angularis oris is a muscle that will pull down the angle of the lip. This muscle is generally not injected because it produces significant impairment of a patient's ability to smile. Along with the levator complex, the depressor angularis oris is therefore generally avoided. However, if this muscle is to be injected for a dystonia that pulls down the lip then the injection is done approximately parallel to the face, with the needle puncturing 1–2 mm into the skin. The muscle is triangular and fairly superficial, and is easy to inject. The muscle is supplied by the marginal mandibular branch of the facial nerve. This muscle draws the corners of the mouth downwards and hence smooths out the nasal labial fold, producing bilaterally a lip-down action.

Depressor Labii Inferiorus

This muscle arises diagonally from the mandible, and inserts with the orbicularis oris muscle superiorally. Below, depressor labii is continuous with the fibres of the platysma muscle and this muscle assists in the pulling down of the lip. In this way, it works along with the depressor angularis oris and orbicularis oris muscles.

Orbicularis Oris

The orbicularis oris muscle is involved in all actions of movement of the lips. The muscle is supplied by the buccal branches as well as the marginal mandibular branches of the facial nerve.

From anatomical perspectives, the orbicularis oris muscle is divided by action and by location into two parts. The marginal part goes all the way around the lips, at the bottom and at the top. The marginal part is responsible for the pouting response, pursing the lips forward and out. Hence those patients that have a pout or a protrusion of the lips require injections generally superficially in four such sites or six sites distributed across the marginal portion of the orbicularis oris muscle. However, the second component of orbicularis oris is the labial or also circumferential part that goes along the vermillion border of the lips. Unlike the marginal part, which is involved in pouting, the labial part of the orbicularis oris muscle pulls the lips back in a smile, pursing the lips such that they curve inwards. Those patients that have pulling of the corners of the lip, with lip borders going inwards as opposed to pouting, require injection of the orbicularis oris muscle again in four or six sites along the vermillion border, avoiding the marginal orbicularis oris muscle.

Masseter

The masseter muscle along with the medial pterygoid and temporalis is a strong muscle involved in closing the jaw and independently can also protrude and retract the jaw slightly. The location of the muscle is approximately two fingers in front of the angle of the jaw. Injection has to be done superficially since a lot of vessels run through this region. The needle angle is generally from the front or from the back approximately 30–45 degrees, with the needle puncturing 0.5–1 cm into the masseter muscle.

Medial Pterygoid

The medial pterygoid muscle, unlike all of the other facial muscles, is actually innervated by the trigeminal nerve, the mandibular branch. The medial pterygoid is involved in closure of the jaw. The muscle a large muscle inside the angle of the jaw, hence closing the jaw forcefully. The muscle is involved in jaw closure along with temporalis and masseter. In order to inject the medial pterygoid muscle, there are two approaches. The first approach requires EMG guidance, with injection from the angle of the jaw vertically up into the medial pterygoid muscle. You can see the probe coming through in the medial pterygoid from this angle of injection. The muscle is essentially vertically up with the needle, but does require EMG guidance. The other approach is through the mouth, with the needle pointing upwards and laterally such that the medial pterygoid muscle is approached so. This injection technique does not require EMG guidance because you can feel the muscle by inserting your finger inside the mouth and towards the outer part of the tooth line in the superior portion.

Lateral Pterygoid

The lateral pterygoid muscle goes from the upper part of the angle of the jaw deep inside the mouth. This muscle is involved in the opening and slight protrusion of the jaw, and along with the medial pterygoid muscle and the ipsilateral and contralateral pterygoid muscles is also involved in sideways motion of the jaw. The lateral pterygoid muscle is supplied by the mandibular nerve, which is a component of the trigeminal nerve. For the injection of the lateral pterygoid muscles, one has to put the needle through the mandibular notch, generally using EMG guidance. The needle goes in approximately three-quarters of an inch, but one has to be careful not to go too deep as the muscle is perpendicular to the needle itself and hence it is quite possible to go right through the muscle and potentially into the other deeper muscles of the mouth, even missing the lateral pterygoid entirely.

Digastric

There are two bellies of this muscle, but only the anterior belly is injected. The posterior belly is attached to the mastoid notch on the inferior surface of the skull. It is innervated by the facial nerve. The anterior belly arises from the inside of the lower border of the mandible, the digastric fossa, and passes downward and backward. It is innervated by the trigeminal nerve. The tendon in the middle joins the two bellies. The digastric opens the jaw along with the lateral pterygoid, and is injected superficially as it is a small muscle, approximately 1 cm lateral to the midline of the jaw.

Tongue

The tongue itself is a complex group of muscles that are difficult to differentiate. The superior longitudinal muscle of the tip of the tongue, the inferior longitudinal muscle at the tip of the tongue, the transverse muscles that go deep along the margins of the tongue outside, and then finally of course the genioglossus, which makes up the entirety of the muscle bulk. The tongue is involved with protrusion, curling, lifting up, among other movements. However, injection of the tongue is predominantly in the belly of the genioglossus. There are two ways to inject the tongue. The first would be to go from below the midline of the jaw, laterally, directly into the tongue. This may require EMG guidance because the needle has to traverse a long distance. However, it is equally easy to have the tongue protruded and the injections done just beyond the midline to avoid the major blood vessels. However, the major venous structures of the tongue are actually below and hence if we stay away from the bottom and go through the top of the tongue, the injections are a lot easier. Generally, the injections of the genioglossus or the tongue muscle are for protrusion of the tongue involved in lingual dystonia.

Parotid Gland

The parotid gland is located right at the angle of the jaw. The gland is behind the masseter muscle and is divided into two lobes: the upper and the lower part. Injection of the parotid gland for sialorrhoea needs therefore to be done in two locations: superior to the angle of the jaw and inferiorly. Again, since major vascular and nerve bundles run through the parotid gland, injection should be done posteriorly as far as possible in these two locations, above the angle and below. The needle should be fairly superficial since the gland is palpable, and the needle should not go deeper than approximately 2–3 mm into the gland above and below the parotid gland.

Muscles of the Neck

Splenius Capitis

The splenius capitis muscle is supplied by the primary branches of the spinal nerves C3, 4 and 5. The muscle goes backwards and down towards the spinous processes. When both splenius capitis muscles are active on the two sides of the neck, the neck will extend. When one side of the splenius capitis is active, the neck will flex laterally and rotate ipsilaterally. Injection of the splenius capitis muscle is generally directed in multiple sites approximately one thumb behind the sternocleidomastoid insertion and one thumb directed outwards such that if you put your thumb behind the ear and rotate it, the needle can go on the outside of the thumb. Larger doses are then divided in either one spot above and below, and more anteriorly as well as posteriorly, or injections can be given at the border of the trapezius and semispinalis capitis.

Sternocleidomastoid

The sternocleidomastoid muscle has both the sternal head and a clavicular head that fans the superior portion of the clavicle. The muscle is innervated by the eleventh or accessory cranial nerve. The muscle has two main actions. First, in isolation the muscle can turn the head contralaterally and hence is involved in the typical torticollis along with the splenius capitis muscle, which is on the side of the turn. In addition, in lateral collis, since the sternocleidomastoid goes all the way back, the muscle when active along with ipsilateral splenius capitis as well as levator scapulae and the other elevators of the shoulder can produce a lateral collis. The injection of the muscle is generally done such that the needle is pointing anteriorly, potentially avoiding the side-effect of dysphagia.

Levator Scapulae

The levator scapulae muscle, going all the way down to the angle of the scapula at the top, is innervated by the dorsal scapular nerve as well as the ventral ramii from the C3, 4 and 5 nerve roots. This muscle elevates the shoulder blade and can even prevent it from being pulled down. For patients that have torticollis with shoulder elevation, levator scapulae muscle may need to be injected. The relationship of this muscle is such that the splenius capitis muscle is above it, the sternocleidomastoid muscle is anterior and angled towards the clavicle, and hence the injection of this particular muscle requires one to first localise the splenius capitis muscle by one thumb behind the ear, rotating the thumb for the splenius capitis muscle, followed by which another thumb below is the levator scapulae. It is also possible to inject the levator scapulae muscle below the angle of the upper part of the trapezius.

Platysma

Platysma, which is a very thin superficial muscle, is innervated by the cervical branches of the facial nerve. As a cutaneous muscle, it stretches the skin from the jaw or the mandible all the way to the collarbone or the clavicle. Because it is a very thin muscle, injections should be done parallel to the line of the skin as compared to perforating through. The muscle belly is thin enough that even 1 mm or more of needle protrusion will perforate through. Hence, the injection of the platysma is done similar to the orbicularis oculi, where superficial blebs are created during the injection in multiple spots. The platysma may be involved in jaw opening along with the lateral pterygoid and the digastric muscle.

Scalenus Medius

The scalene muscle complex, consisting of the anterior, middle and posterior scalene muscles, is innervated by the direct branches of the cervical and brachial plexus from C4 up to C8 nerve roots. The anterior and the middle scalenes raise the first rib, and the posterior second rib when the cervical vertebrae are in the locked position. Hence patients that have significant laterocollis with the neck tilted to one side with significant elevation also of the shoulder will require injection not only of the splenius capitus, potentially the sternocleidomastoid, levator scapulae, but also of the scalene muscle complex. However, due to the anatomical restrictions, it is generally not possible for us to access certainly the anterior and definitely the posterior scalene muscles. Hence the injection is almost always universally done in the scalenus medius. The injection should be done parallel to the shoulder to avoid going deep to perforate the muscle, since the apex of the lung is not too far away.

Trapezius

The trapezius muscle is a large fan-shaped muscle that traverses all the way down to the edge of the scapula, along both sides. The trapezius is divided into three parts: the ascending or lower fibres, the transverse or middle fibres, and the descending or upper fibres that go along the shoulder to the edge of the scapula. The lower or ascending part of the trapezius muscle is supplied by the accessory or the eleventh cranial nerve. These lower fibres are involved with pulling down the scapula, with simultaneous contraction of the lower and upper fibres producing a lateral rotation of the scapula. The medial portion of the trapezius muscle will pull the head backwards, and along with semispinalis capitis is injected in patients that have retrocaput. The lower portion should be injected in those that manifest more of a retrocollis. However, the trapezius muscle also spans all the way out to the humerus and therefore is involved in shoulder elevation. In addition to this, the trapezius muscle can bring the borders of the scapula together and elevate them. However, in most neck dystonias, one does not inject the lower portion of the trapezius muscle and injections are concentrated and superficially distributed along the outer lateral portion of the trapezius for shoulder elevation and superficially in the midline in numerous spots for retrocollis. The needle only penetrates approximately 0.5 mm into the trapezius since the muscle is superficial. The muscle is contiguous and therefore divided dosing is best.

Semispinalis Capitis

This muscle is deep to the splenius capitis and trapezius muscles, and is involved in pulling the neck back into a retrocaput.

It begins along the transverse processes of the first six cervical vertebrae and inserts into the occipital bone. It is innervated by the cervical nerves. It can be injected just below the occipital protuberance for the retrocaput positioning, making sure that the needle is through the trapezius.

Muscles of the Upper Limb

Biceps Brachii

The biceps brachii muscle has two heads and is supplied by the musculocutaneous nerve from C5 and C6 nerve roots. It flexes and supinates the forearm at the elbow joint. This dual action of flexion as well as supination of the elbow is maximised when the elbow is at 90 degrees. The bicep muscle is a big and thick muscle but has tendinous portions in the top of both heads. Injection of the bicep muscle should be done in approximately the middle portion of the upper arm, usually with multiple injection sites.

Infraspinatus

The infraspinatus muscle sits below the spine of the scapula. It is a large fan-like muscle innervated by the suprascapular nerve C5–C6. It is a major lateral rotator of the arm, especially when the arm is actually abducted. It may be injected in patients with truncal or cervical dystonia who have lateral rotation of the shoulder. The injection of this muscle is easy since it can be injected with multiple injections below the spine. The injection will go through the trapezius muscles.

Pectoralis Major

The pectoralis major muscle is a large muscle innervated by the medial pectoral nerve. The muscle has a clavicular component and a sternal component, and attaches to the seventh rib below. It is involved in adduction and internal rotation of the arm. The muscle bulk is easy to palpate to the lateral and superior aspect of the nipple area. Injections are usually distributed in several spots in the muscle.

Rhomboid Major

Rhomboid major is supplied by the dorsal scapular nerve, going from the spinous processes of the first to the fifth thoracic vertebrae to the medial border of the scapula. The rhomboids are involved in elevating the scapula and retracting it towards the spine. The rhomboids are not usually injected for cervical dystonia, but may be injected for pain or for those patients with truncal dystonia who have pulling of the scapula towards the midline.

Supraspinatus

The muscle is innervated by the suprascapular nerve C4–C6, and sits above the spinous processes of the scapula. The supraspinatus muscle is involved in the first 10–15 degrees of abduction of the shoulder. Medial to it is the levator scapulae muscle, the rhomboids, and below the spine of the scapula is the infraspinatus. Injection of the supraspinatus muscle for patients who have excessive abduction of the shoulder would require injections to go through the trapezius muscle. Injections can be given in multiple spots. EMG is required for this localisation to avoid injections of the trapezius muscle.

Teres Major

The muscle is supplied by the thoraco-dorsal nerve, C5, 6 and 7. It is a large muscle that originates in the posterior aspect of the inferior angle of the scapula and inserts into the crest of the lesser tubercle of the humerus, allowing it to adduct and medially rotate the arm. Therefore, in conditions where the arm is adducted to the chest wall, muscles such as pectoralis major and teres major may be injected. The muscle is injected approximately three fingers above the angle of the inferior portion of the scapula, where it can be easily palpated, the needle penetrating approximately 1 cm.

Triceps Brachii

The triceps muscle is the main extensor of the elbow joint and is supplied by the radial nerve, the C6–C8 branches. EMG guidance is not required and all three heads of the triceps can be injected by palpation and activation of the triceps muscle by extension of the elbow joint. Since the muscle is large and the predominant belly is in the upper half of the arm, injections can be divided into three or four sites. The needle goes approximately 1 cm into the muscle, with the patient extending the elbow joint.

Brachioradialis

The muscle is supplied by the radial nerve C5 and C6 roots. The main belly is in the proximal one-third of the muscle, followed by a tendinous aponeurosis that goes all the way down. The muscle is a predominant flexor of the elbow and allows the forearm to return from extreme supination or pronation to a midline position. The muscle is injected approximately two fingers below the olecranon process. The muscle is easily palpated with the elbow flexed.

Extensor Carpi Radialis

The extensor carpi radialis longus and brevis are supplied by the radial nerve, the C6 and C7 branches. The main action of these muscles is to extend the wrist joint but also cause radial deviation along with the flexor carpi radialis muscle. With the forearm pronated, the injection site is generally 4–6 cm below the lateral epicondyle. With the fingers flexed and wrist extended, the muscle can be easily palpated. The extensor digitorum communis for the second digit, which is on the ulnar side, should be palpated to avoid injection in this muscle. Under EMG guidance, it should be checked that there is activation of the muscle with wrist extension but not with extension of the second digit.

Extensor Carpi Ulnaris

The extensor carpi ulnaris extends and causes ulnar deviation of the wrist, and is supplied by the radial nerve, roots C6–C8.

With the forearm pronated, it is on the ulnar side of extensor digitorum communis. The muscle is fairly superficial and the needle should be inserted about 0.5 cm. This muscle is injected one-third of the distance from the elbow to the wrist, along the shaft of the ulna. The muscle can be activated by extension of the wrist with the fingers flexed. EMG guidance is required and extension of digits four and five should be checked to avoid injection of the extensor digitorum communis for these digits, which may cause finger weakness.

Extensor Digitorum

Extensor digitorum communis is supplied by the radial nerve, C6–C8 roots. Its main belly is in the proximal one-third or one-half of the muscle followed by the extensor expansion, that then splits the tendons into those that go to the individual fingers digits 2–4. It is the main extender of the finger. With the forearm pronated, the muscle is located about one-third of the way from the elbow to the wrist, on the ulnar side of the extensor carpi radialis muscle. The individual fascicles for each finger can be easily palpated with extension of each finger and can be injected separately. The muscle is fairly superficial and the needle should be inserted approximately 0.5–1 cm under EMG guidance. The doses used are usually low because weakness of the finger extensor often causes functional disability.

Extensor Indicis

This muscle predominantly extends the index finger. Although the tendon of the muscle goes to the radial of the wrist, the belly of the muscle is on the ulnar portion. The muscle is innervated by the deep branches of the radial nerve, made up of roots C6–C8. Extensor indicis works along with the tendon from the extensor digitorum communis to extend the index finger. Injection is done with the forearm pronated from the ulnar side approximately two finger breadths (1.5–2 cm) above and slightly radial to the styloid process. EMG guidance is required.

Extensor Pollicis Longus

The extensor pollicis longus, which sits next to the extensor indicis on the ulnar side and extensor pollicis brevis on the radial side, inserts in the distal phalanx of the thumb. It extends the thumb and is also involved in thumb abduction. It is supplied by the deep branches of the radial nerve, roots C6–C8. With the forearm pronated, the muscle is located approximately four finger breadths above the styloid process of the ulnar. The muscle is superficial and one only needs to go approximately 0.5–1 cm for localisation.

Flexor Carpi Radialis

The flexor carpi radialis muscle is located on the medial side or the ulnar side rather than the radial side of the forearm. It is supplied by the C6–C8 roots that make up the median nerve. The flexor carpi radialis muscle flexes the wrist as its predominant action, but can also abduct the hand, causing a radial deviation along with extensor carpi radialis. Localising the medial epicondyle and the biceps tendon, the muscle is approximately four finger breadths below the midpoint, with the needle puncturing approximately 0.5–1 cm under EMG guidance. The distal part of this muscle is tendinous, and therefore the proximal one-third is the best site for injection. The flexor digitorum superficialis is close to this muscle. Too deep an injection has the chance of hitting the pronator teres.

Flexor Carpi Ulnaris

The flexor carpi ulnaris muscle is supplied by the C7 to T1 roots that make up the ulnar nerve. The main action is to flex the wrist but also to ulnar deviate or adduct the wrist along with its extensor counterpart. The main belly of the muscle is in the proximal half to the middle part of the forearm along the ulnar side. Palpating the shaft of the ulna from the olecranon process approximately halfway, the muscle is approximately two fingers along the forearm. The muscle is activated by bending the wrist with the muscle easily palpated. The flexor carpi ulnaris is superficial, and the needle should be kept superficial, approximately 0.5–1 cm. Inserting the needle too deep will result in injection of the flexor digitorum profundus. Injections can be divided into two or three sites, and EMG guidance is required.

Flexor Digitorum Profundus

The lateral half of this muscle is supplied by the median nerve, and specifically the anterior interosseous branch made up of roots C8 and T1. The medial half of flexor digitorum profundus is supplied by the ulnar nerve. The main action of flexor digitorum profundus is to flex the metacarpophalangeal joints of fingers two through five. This muscle is the exclusive flexor of the distal interphalangeal joints. It is a powerful flexor when the wrist is extended. This muscle is localised by placing the little finger on the olecranon, followed by the other fingers above it. When the fingers are placed along the shaft of the ulna, flexor digitorum profundus is injected along the edge of the ulna above the fingers. The ulnar innervated flexor digitorum profundus is more superficial, approximately 1.5–2 cm, while the median innervated portion is deeper. Injection of flexor digitorum profundus is not done through the upper compartment or the flexor part of the forearm, but from the medial side such that flexor carpi ulnaris is avoided, generally with the patient having their elbow flexed and supinated. Like all forearm muscles, the injections must be done under EMG guidance. If the needle is not deep enough, it may hit the flexor carpi ulnaris.

Flexor Digitorum Superficialis

The flexor digitorum superficialis is a complex muscle to inject. The flexor carpi radialis is above, ulnaris is on the ulnar side and digitorum profundus is below. The localisation of the major belly of flexor digitorum superficialis is done with the injector's wrist placed upon the wrist of the patient, with the index finger being the location of the most ideal spot of injection of the flexor digitorum superficialis. However, this muscle is complicated in that the fascicles of the second and the fifth digit are below the third and the fourth. In addition, the fascicle that moves the index finger is further distal as compared to the third and fourth. Hence, injection of flexor digitorum superficialis requires that the injector knows this orientation. In order to inject the third and the fourth digit, the location pointed out earlier is ideal. However, in order to inject either the fifth digit or the second digit, generally one has to move farther distal and has to definitely go deeper because the third and the fourth digits would otherwise be injected. Under EMG guidance, each finger is flexed individually and injection is performed only when the injector is sure that the needle is in the appropriate component of the flexor digitorum superficialis.

Flexor Pollicis Longus

The flexor pollicis longus muscle is on the radial side of the forearm. It is supplied by the median nerve, specifically the anterior interosseous branch. It inserts on the volar aspect of the distal phalanx of the thumb to flex the thumb. This is the predominant and in fact the exclusive flexor of the interphalangeal joint of the thumb. The injection of this muscle is done at approximately the middle of a line from the biceps to the head of the radius. The muscle is fairly superficial and therefore injection of the needle, done under EMG guidance, should be approximately 1–1.5 cm deep while the distal phalanx is flexed. The muscle can be palpated here fairly easily when the thumb is flexed at the distal phalanx. One to three injections in divided doses can be given.

Pronator Quadratus

The pronator quadratus muscle is innervated by the C6 to T1 roots that make up the anterior interosseous branch of the median nerve. It is involved in the pronation of the forearm along with the pronator teres. The injection site is approximately 2–3 fingers between a line connecting the radial and ulnar ends. The injection is deep through the interosseous membrane and has to be done under EMG guidance. The patient can be asked to activate the muscle by pronating the forearm with the needle in the muscle. The muscle is flat and fairly large, and therefore it is easy to penetrate.

Pronator Teres

The pronator teres muscle, which is supplied by the median nerve roots C6 and possibly C7, is involved in the pronation of the forearm; it is located approximately two finger breadths below the midpoint between the biceps tendon and the medial epicondyle. The pronator teres is best injected under EMG guidance with the needle pointing at approximately 90 degrees to the arm partially pronated and the injection being 0.5–1 cm below the skin surface at maximum.

Supinator

This muscle is innervated by roots C5 and C6, which make up the posterior interosseous branch of the radial nerve. It is the strongest supinator of the elbow when it is extended. In addition, the supinator is aided by the biceps brachii muscle for providing supination. Hence in patients that require injection for problematic supination, it is advisable to inject both the biceps as well as the supinator. To locate this muscle, one needs to palpate the tendon of the biceps muscle, and the supinator is approximately three fingers below along the radial surface. The injections are done at an angle of approximately 45 degrees with the arm resting in this position. EMG guidance is essential as one will pass through the extensor digitorum communis approximately 1 cm through the skin. The muscle may, however, be somewhat deeper and one has to avoid injecting the extensor digitorum communis in order to prevent finger extension weakness.

Abductor Pollicis Brevis

Abductor pollicis, supplied by the ulnar nerve roots C8 to T1, is an abductor of the thumb, pulling it towards the palm. This muscle is also involved in opposing the thumb. The injection is relatively easy as there are no other muscles in the area. With the thumb somewhat abducted, the muscle can be grasped in the hand and injected straight, approximately 1–2 mm into the abductor pollicis.

Flexor Pollicis Brevis

Flexor pollicis brevis is also supplied by the median nerve. The main action is to flex the proximal phalanx of the thumb. The two heads of the muscle are located superficially and deep, one below the other. These two heads can be injected by following a line between the ulnar aspect metacarpal joint and the metacarpophalangeal joint under EMG guidance, with the needle superficial and pointed perpendicular in the midline of the thenar eminence. The superficial head is approximately 0.5–1 cm deep and approximately 1.5–2 cm deep for the deeper head.

Lumbricals

Lumbricals one and two are supplied by the median nerve, while lumbricals three and four are supplied by the ulnar nerve. The lumbricals flex the metacarpophalangeal joints of all of these four fingers, and also extend the respective proximal interphalangeal joints. For example, while writing in patients with writer's cramp, the lumbricals may be active and could require injection. The lumbricals are on the radial or the lateral side of the tendons of the flexor digitorum superficialis. The lumbricals are injected just below the head of the metacarpals, superficially in the hand, approximately 2–3 mm into the palm. Each lumbrical has to be injected individually. One has to be careful injecting the first lumbrical because if the needle is inserted too deeply, it will hit the adductor pollicis. A line drawn along the heads of the metacarpals will allow the injector to get an approximate idea as to where the lumbricals need to be injected. Generally all four lumbricals may require injection if the hand is affected, especially in spasticity.

Opponens Pollicis

Opponens pollicis, a fairly large muscle supplied by the median nerve and roots C7 to T1, is responsible for opposing the thumb to the little finger. Along with the flexion, abduction and internal rotation of the thumb, this allows the dexterous task of putting our thumb and little finger together. The muscle is located lateral and slightly below the abductor pollicis brevis. The injection of this muscle, however, is from the outside or the radial side, below the abductor pollicis brevis. The needle is inserted approximately 0.5–1 cm horizontally into the thenar eminence with the thumb relaxed.

Muscles of the Lower Limb

Biceps Femoris

The biceps femoris muscle is long with a short head, supplied by the sciatic nerve. It extends the hip joint, rotates the thigh laterally and flexes the knee. Since it is big and powerful, it can also rotate the knee laterally. The injection of the biceps muscle can be divided into the long and the short head, but a line can be drawn from the head of the fibula to the ischial tuberosity where the muscle originates. Injections can be given in multiple spots along the length of the muscle in the middle part of the thigh. It is a superficial muscle and can be easily palpated. EMG may be helpful, especially when injecting the short head. The injections are approximately 2–3 cm deep.

Gluteus Maximus

The muscle is supplied by the inferior gluteal nerves from roots L5 to S2. It brings the trunk from a flexed to an upright position to stabilise the trunk and prevent it from tilting forward. It also extends the hip joint. The muscle is large and easy to inject, the lower curvature of the buttocks laterally off the midline. The injections can be divided into two or three different locations.

Gluteus Medius

The gluteus medius muscle, supplied by the superior gluteal nerve made up of L4, 5 and S1 roots, abducts the femur at the hip joint, rotating the thigh medially. During walking, this muscle makes sure the pelvis does not drop towards the opposite side, drawing it towards the weight-bearing leg. This allows the other leg to swing freely when walking. The gluteus medius muscle is injected on the lateral side approximately 3–4 cm below the greater trochanter and near the top of the iliac crest. Several injection sites can be used.

Gracilis

The gracilis muscle is a long and thin muscle. It is also supplied, like the other adductors, by the obturator nerve and hence its main action remains that of adduction. However, this muscle traverses all the way down to the tibia, beginning also at the pubic tubricle along with the other adductors. The muscle also adducts the hip joint along with the other major adductors. The muscle is palpated fairly easily along its tract and the injection technique requires one to draw a line from the pubic tubricle to the medial condyle of the femur. The injection is given approximately midway along that tract by having the patient adduct the thigh when the gracilis muscle can be palpated. It is a superficial muscle and therefore the injection can be perpendicular to the leg, approximately 1 cm deep. Again, since it is a thin muscle, electromyographic guidance may be required.

Iliopsoas

The iliopsoas muscle has two components: the iliacus, supplied by the femoral nerve, and the psoas or psoas major, supplied by L2, 3 and 4. The muscle goes deep inside into the abdomen and hence most of the injections that one would do from the surface are in the iliacus and not the psoas. The iliacus muscle curves around the crest, coming down past the femoral artery. The main action of the muscle is to balance the hip on the femur, especially when the femur is fixed. It flexes the leg at the hip joint. Injection of the iliacus portion of the iliopsoas muscle requires one to palpate the femoral artery. The injection point is lateral to the femoral artery, generally 2–3 cm deep. EMG guidance is generally required, with the patient flexing the hip joint.

Piriformis

Next to the gluteus minimis muscle are a group of four muscles made up of the piriformis with the sciatic nerve underneath, obturator externus, and the superior and inferior gemelli. All of these muscles laterally rotate the thigh. The piriformis is supplied by the nerve to piriformis and hence this muscle may be injected for those conditions that result in the piriformis syndrome.

Quadriceps Femoris

The quadriceps femoris muscle complex is made up of the rectus femoris, vastus lateralis, vastus intermedius and vastus medialis. It is innervated by the femoral nerve from L2–L4 roots. This muscle complex flexes the hip joint and extends the knee joint. The injection of each of these muscles is relatively easy due to the large bulk of the muscle. The rectus femoris is a thin and fairly superficial muscle, and hence the injections can be spread in the middle part of the thigh in 2–4 sites at approximately 1 cm. Injection of the vastus intermedius muscle has to go deeper, approximately 3–4 cm, to hit the muscle belly. Vastus lateralis is injected laterally through the tendinous sheet of tensor facia lata, while vastus medialis is injected approximately two fingers medial to the rectus femoris from the medial side.

Semimembranosus

The semimembranosus muscle is supplied by the tibial portion of the sciatic nerve. Together with the other muscles of the hamstrings, such as the biceps femoris and semitendinosus, the muscle flexes the knee joint in a strong fashion and also extends the hip joint, and allows propulsion during walking. Its trajectory goes from the ischial tuberosity to the medial portion of the femur. Along that line, the injection can be divided into several spots in the middle of the thigh. The muscle is generally easily palpated. It is medial to the biceps femoris and is reasonably superficial. Injections can be given 1–2 cm, or even up to 3–4 cm deep.

Semitendinosus

The semitendinosus muscle, just like semimembranosus, is part of the hamstring complex. It is easily seen and palpated, and is supplied by the tibial portion of the sciatic nerve. It extends the hip joint, allowing the leg that is weight-bearing to propulse forward. It also flexes the knee joint, and the injection site is similar to semimembranosus, with a line from the ischial tuberosity down to the knee joint. Along this line, injections can be given in several spots, with the biceps femoris to the lateral side and semimembranosus to the medial side. The muscle is palpable and superficial, and hence injections can be given 1–2 cm or up to 3–4 cm deep.

Gastrocnemius

The gastrocnemius muscle is supplied by the tibial nerve from nerve roots S1 and S2. Its main action is to plantarflex the ankle joint and flex the knee joint. It plays a vital role in producing propulsion, as one rolls from the heel to toe during ambulation. It can be injected easily by simply palpating the muscle. The injection sites should be approximately one-third of the way from the knee joint. Injections have to be divided between the medial and lateral bellies in multiple sites. It should be noted that the distal portion or the lower portion is the Achilles tendon, and the soleus muscle is below. Hence the injection of the gastrocnemius muscle should be done high up. The muscle is superficial, and therefore injections can be given at 1–3 cm deep.

Soleus

The soleus, which is below the gastrocnemius, is supplied by the tibial nerve branches S1 and S2. This muscle is important in plantarflexion of the ankle and also in flexing the knee joint. It is especially important for maintaining an upright position, preventing the ankle joint from collapsing during ambulation. Since this muscle is deeper but farther down the leg from the gastrocnemius, the easiest way to inject this muscle is either medially below the gastrocnemius, approximately one-third of the way from the Achilles tendon or the heel, or directly through the tendinous portion of the gastrocnemius. Injections approximately 2–5 cm through the tendinous portion of the gastrocnemius will hit the soleus. Multiple injections should be performed as this is a large muscle. EMG guidance can be helpful.

Tibialis Posterior

The tibialis posterior muscle is a difficult muscle to inject from behind. Its tendon runs beneath the sole of the foot; in fact, the easiest access to the tibialis posterior is to go along the margin of the tibial bone, approximately one-third of the way up from the medial epicondyle. The edge of the tibial bone can be palpated, and the needle is inserted under EMG. Injections are therefore somewhat deep, and can be divided into two or three spots, making sure under EMG guidance that you have the proper localisation by getting the patient to plantarflex the foot, and making sure that you are not in the flexors of the toe. The injections therefore are deep, approximately 3–4 cm at approximately 45 degrees to the tibial bone. A technique would be to roll off the edge of the tibial bone with your needle, first touching the bone, and then going medial to that and deeper, such that the landmarks are clear.

Tibialis Posterior

This muscle is along the posterior surface of the tibia. It is involved in inversion and plantarflexion of the foot. The tendon of the muscle runs beneath the heel and sole of the foot. Since the flexor digitorum longus and flexor hallucis longus are superficial to the tibialis posterior, one will have to pass through these muscles to inject the tibialis posterior. The easiest technique to inject the tibialis posterior is to follow the mid-portion of the tibia. The needle can be rolled off that particular portion of the bone and tibialis posterior is then injected in this particular spot. The muscle has a fairly thick belly, and injections can be distributed in two or three sites in the middle portion of the leg, just off the tibia. One has to be careful not to go beyond approximately 1 cm, as other deeper muscles of the foot are present underneath. The tibialis posterior is the first muscle to be encountered off of the tibia. Electromyography is extremely helpful in the injection of this muscle.

Adductor Brevis

The muscle is supplied by the obturator nerve and L2–L4 nerve roots. Along with the other adductors, it adducts the thigh at the hip joint. It is just above the adductor longus muscle. It is easily palpated by first finding the pubic tubercle and going approximately 7–10 cm below. Since the muscle inserts itself along the femur, just like the adductor longus, the muscle is injected superficially. The injection depth is about 4–5 cm.

Adductor Longus

This muscle is supplied by the obturator nerve from roots L2–L4. The muscle begins at the pubic tubercle, and goes along the femur. The main action of the adductor longus is to bring the knee inwards towards the midline. The adduction is maximal when the hip joint is flexed. The easiest way to inject this muscle is to palpate the pubic tubercle and go approximately 5–10 cm into this area. Injection is done with the hip slightly externally rotated with hip adduction to activate the muscle. The injection depth is approximately 2–4 cm since the muscle is superficial and visible.

Adductor Magnus

The adductor magnus muscle is the largest muscle of the adductor complex, which includes the adductor longus, brevis and gracilis. This muscle is supplied not only by the obturator nerve, but also by the sciatic nerve. It is the major adductor of the hip joint. The injection of the muscle is slightly more medial, and towards the inside, as compared to the gracilis or the adductor longus and brevis muscle. The patient has the thigh externally rotated in a lying or sitting position. The injection sites are distributed throughout the large muscle, approximately two-thirds of the way from the pubic tubercle to the medial condyle along the medial surface of the thigh. The injection is fairly superficial, approximately 1–4 cm deep.

Abductor Hallucis

The abductor hallucis muscle is supplied by the medial plantar nerves from root S1 and S2. Its main action is to abduct the big toe. It also allows flexion of the corresponding metatarsal phalangeal joint. The muscle is injected superficially along the medial side of the foot, approximately one finger below the navicular bone. Since the belly of the muscle is generally more posterior, it is advisable to keep the injections closer to the heel rather than forward. Injection depth is about 0.5 cm.

Extensor Digitorum Brevis

The extensor digitorum brevis is supplied by the deep peroneal nerve. Along with extensor digitorum longus, its predominant action is to extend the second to fourth toe. The muscle is palpable and is activated by extension of the toes. The needle is kept superficial and one or two injection sites is enough. The depth of the injection is 0.5–1 cm.

Extensor Digitorum Longus

Extensor digitorum longus is the predominant muscle that extends the toes. It is supplied by the deep peroneal nerve and is close to the extensor hallucis longus. It has a superior border to the tibialis anterior. It also spans the gap between the tibia and the fibula. The injection of the muscle is done approximately halfway between the ankle and the knee, above the line joining the lateral and medial epicondyle. If the injection is too proximal, one will hit the tibialis anterior. The muscle generally should be injected using EMG guidance, although it is fairly superficial. The injection depth is 0.5–1.5 cm and injections can be divided into several spots.

Extensor Hallucis Longus

The muscle is supplied by the deep peroneal nerve from roots L5 and S1, and is the only real extensor of the big toe. The muscle is fairly superficial, and along the lateral border of the anterior portion of the tibia. The muscle can be palpated by having the patient extend the big toe. The tibialis anterior is very close, and therefore, it is advisable to stay away from the bottom portion of the tibialis anterior in order to inject the extensor hallucis longus. The muscle is approximately four fingers above the medial and lateral epicondyle line, being lower and deeper than that for the extensor digitorum longus at 1–2 cm deep, and the muscle is injected in one or two spots along the lateral edge of the tibia.

Flexor Digitorum Brevis

The muscle is supplied by the medial plantar nerve. With the flexor digitorum longus, it flexes the toes. The injection site is the aponeurosis in the middle of the arch of the foot. Injection can be done at the midpoint of a line between the middle toe to the calcaneus. Injections can be given in 1–3 sites with a depth of about 1 cm. The injections are often painful.

Flexor Digitorum Longus

The muscle is innervated by the tibial nerve L5, S1 and S2. Its main action is to flex the toes. This muscle is important during ambulation for lifting off of the toes. Curling of the toes as it occurs in patients with dystonia requires injection of the flexor digitorum longus. The injection site is between halfway and the bottom third of the tibial shaft. The muscle is superficial to the tibialis posterior, and if the needle is too deep the tibialis posterior will be injected. Injection depth is 1.5–2 cm, with injections divided into several sites. EMG guidance or stimulation is required.

Flexor Hallucis Longus

The flexor hallucis longus is supplied by the tibial nerve and is located close to the flexor digitorum longus. It flexes the distal phalanx of the great toe, allowing the flexion of the foot and the ankle to be coordinated with toe flexion. It can be injected medial to the Achilles tendon about four finger breadths above the medial epicondyle or, alternatively, between one-half to the bottom third of the tibial shaft with the needle directed laterally. If the injection is too deep, the tibialis posterior may be injected. If it is too medial, the flexor digitorum longus may be injected. The injection depth is 1.5–3 cm. EMG or stimulation should be used.

Chapter 31

Ultrasound Guidance for Botulinum Toxin Application

Uwe Walter and Dirk Dressler

Principle of Ultrasonography

Ultrasonography (US) allows a simple, non-invasive, real-time visualisation of muscles and their surrounding structures. It can visualise the entire procedure of BT application. Other imaging modalities, including X-ray or magnetic tomography, are expensive and time-consuming, may include exposure to radiation and image availability is delayed. US-guided intramuscular BT injections were first described by Japanese neurologists and soon afterwards propagated by German neuropaediatricians (Mezaki et al. 2000; Berweck et al. 2002). With adequate anatomical knowledge, US localisation of muscles is straightforward. Needle-tracking skills can be trained by practising on cadavers, gel phantoms, meat preparations, etc. (Boon et al. 2011). There is an increasing number of US workshops, online US courses and mobile app-based learning programs (Walter & Dressler 2014). In principle, all contemporary US machines can be used if equipped with an appropriate linear-array transducer. The applied US frequency determines the image resolution and the penetration depth. Superficial and small target muscles in the arm require optimal resolution and therefore higher US frequencies of about 13.0 MHz (10.0–18.0 MHz). Profound and large target muscles in the neck, trunk and leg require higher penetration depth and are therefore best visualised with lower US frequencies of about 7.5 MHz (5.0–10.0 MHz) (Peetrons 2002). For optimal imaging geometrics, a rectangular probe position with only moderate pressure on the underlying tissue is recommended. Normal muscles can be identified easily on US by their 'starry night' appearance on transverse sections and pennate appearance on longitudinal sections, by the identification of their origin and insertion and their diameter changes on contraction (Peetrons 2002; Boon et al. 2011). Muscle tissue normally has a low echogenicity which is increased by fibrotic processes and by infiltration of fat tissue, which may be caused by various neuromuscular disorders. Individual muscle fibres cannot be distinguished from each other by US. Muscle fibres are organised in grouped bundles (fascicles) surrounded by fibroadipose tissue called perimysium. Hyperechogenic perimysium can be distinguished from muscle fascicles with diameters of more than 2 mm. The highly echogenic epimysium allows distinguishing muscles from each other (Peetrons 2002; Walter & Dressler 2014). Unlike normal muscle tissue, the dermis and epidermis are highly echogenic, whereas the subcutaneous fatty tissue has a medium echogenicity (Figure 31.1). Periosteum and compacta are highly echogenic, while the spongiosa is of low echogenicity due to US attenuation behind the compacta. Tendons are of high echogenicity, which typically decreases when the US transducer is angulated. This decrease of echogenicity can be used to discriminate tendons from nerves. Larger nerves are typically seen with highly echogenic myelin sheaths and less echogenic nerve fibres (Figure 31.1). Vessel lumina are of low echogenicity and blood flow inside vessels can be visualised by applying colour-coded Doppler-US.

Ultrasonography for BT Application

BT injections are usually performed with 20 mm/27-gauge or 40 mm/27-gauge needles. For profound muscles 80 mm/23-gauge or 120 mm/25-gauge needles may be used (Walter & Dressler 2014). Special injection needles optimised for US imaging have become available (Figure 31.2). Skin disinfection should be performed with non-alcoholic agents since alcohol may harm the US transducer surface. The injection needle is inserted adjacent to the US transducer. Bacteriostatic ultrasound gel is available, but regular ultrasound gel appears also to be safe. In principle, there are two techniques of US-guided needle insertion with respect to the US imaging plane: the in-plane technique with whole-needle path displayed within the imaging plane; and the off-plane technique with only the needle tip displayed within the imaging plane. Moreover, if a US transducer equipped with a needle guide holder is used together with biopsy software, guide lines in the live US image show the expected course of the needle through the tissue (Kopf et al. 2011). The 'freehand' off-plane technique without external needle guide is sufficient for most superficial (depth <3 cm) US-guided BT injections. For this, the US transducer should be placed in a way that the target structure is displayed in the centre of the US screen (Figures 31.1, 31.3). Then the midpoint of the transducer length corresponds to the location of the target structure and can be used as a landmark for needle insertion (Walter & Dressler 2014). If necessary, a wooden stick or the needle cap can be pressed towards the skin at the planned insertion site, with pressure movements visible on US, to confirm correct targeting prior to needle insertion. The inserted needle is displayed with high echogenicity, with its intensity depending on the needle diameter. With the off-plane technique, gentle movements of the needle are helpful to detect the needle tip.

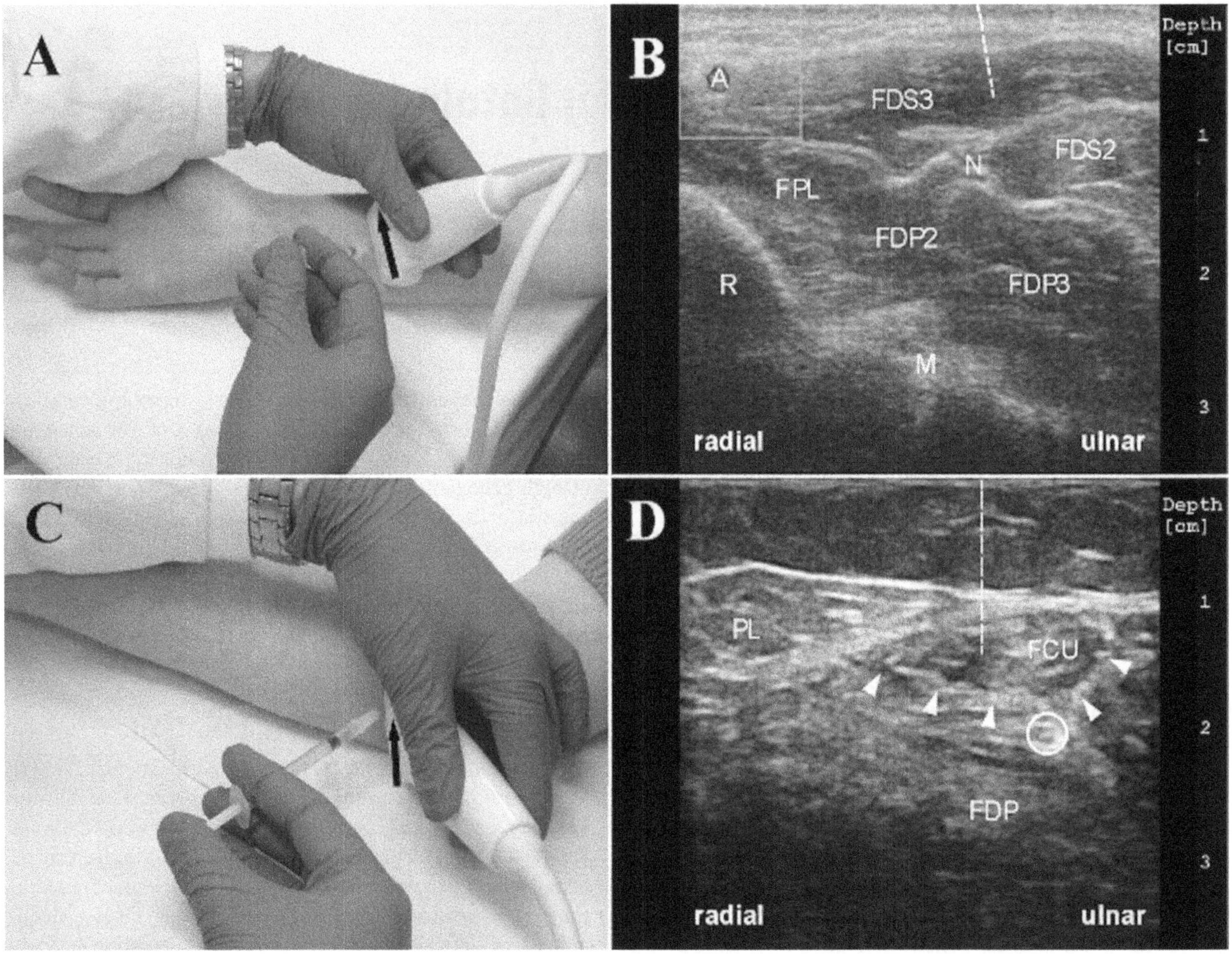

Figure 31.1 Ultrasonography (US) of the volar forearm for guiding BT injection in patients with writer's cramp. (a) Position of US transducer and syringe (off-plane injection technique) for guiding BT injection into the third flexor digitorum superficialis muscle. The arrow indicates the orientation of the transducer (arrow head corresponding to left side of the US image shown in (b)). (b) US image showing the flexor digitorum superficialis (FDS), flexor digitorum profundus (FDP) and flexor pollicis longus (FPL) muscles, the radial artery (A), the median nerve (N), the radius (R) and the membrana interossea (M). Note that the second and third FDS (but not the FDP) muscles are paradoxically 'exchanged' in anatomic order, which may cause needle displacement if using techniques other than US guidance. The dashed line indicates the off-plane path of the injection needle. (c) Position of US transducer and syringe (off-plane injection technique) for guiding BT injection into the flexor carpi ulnaris muscle. The arrow indicates the orientation of the transducer (arrow head corresponding to left side of US image shown in (d)). (d) US image showing the flexor carpi ulnaris (FCU, indicated by triangles; circle: ulnar nerve), palmaris longus (PL) and flexor digitorum profundus (FDP) muscles. The dashed line indicates the off-plane path of the injection needle. A small depot of injected BT solution is visible with low echogenicity in the centre of the FCU muscle.

The injected BT solution usually presents as a mildly echogenic depot with a local volume effect (Figure 31.1). Visualisation of the injected BT solution can also be used to correct the needle position before injecting the entire volume. Filing of at least one US image of the needle position within the target tissue is recommended (Hobson-Webb & Boon 2013). Alternatively, or in addition, a US image showing the injected BT volume within the target tissue may be filed (Walter & Dressler 2014).

US-Guided BT Application in Dystonia

Table 31.1 categorises the usefulness of US guidance in various potential target muscles. In some cranial and cervical muscle groups, US guidance is not (pterygoid) or only hardly (mimic, pharyngeal, laryngeal) feasible. Supra- and infrahyoid muscles can be visualised with US (Gervasio et al. 2010). However, guided BT injection is rarely necessary. US guidance is feasible for lateral and dorsal neck muscles, axial muscles, shoulder muscles, proximal and distal arm muscles, intrinsic hand muscles and leg muscles. For some muscles (e.g. longus colli, obliquus capitis inferior, forearm muscles) US visualisation may protect sensitive structures (nerves, large vessels) adjacent to the target muscles (Figure 31.1) (Fujimoto et al. 2012). Distinct thin, unselectively activated muscles (e.g. infrahyoid, longissimus capitis) can only be targeted with US guidance (Figure 31.3) (Walter & Dressler 2014). Adverse effects such as dysphagia occurring after BT injections into the sternocleidomastoid muscle can be reduced by switching from EMG guidance to US guidance (Hong et al. 2012). However, conventional BT application into the upper third of the sternocleidomastoid

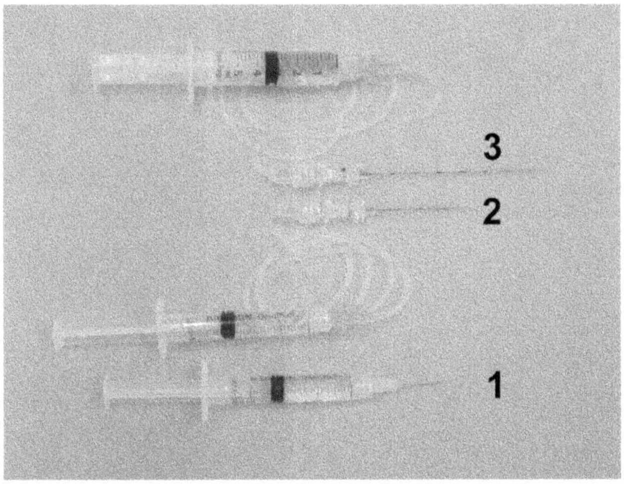

Figure 31.2 Injection needles typically used for US-guided BT injection. (1) Standard needle for superficial targets (20 mm/27-gauge); (2) midsize needle customised for optimal US visualisation (40 mm/24-gauge); (3) long needle customised for optimal US visualisation (80 mm/22-gauge).

muscle may have the same effect (Walter & Dressler 2014). Small prospective randomised studies have compared US guidance with active EMG guidance and manual application in forearm and leg muscles in adults with post-stroke spasticity and demonstrated superiority of both US guidance and active EMG guidance (Picelli et al. 2012, 2014). Studies comparing US-guided and manual BT application in dystonia are scarce. A pilot study applying multimodal-imaging (including US) guided BT application showed favourable treatment effects in patients with cervical dystonia (Lee et al. 2009). A recent study demonstrated favourable outcome for patients with cervical dystonia if treated with US-guided BT injection combined with orthopaedic joint brace rather than with conventional BT injection combined with orthopaedic brace (Huang et al. 2015). Active EMG guidance, US guidance or a combination of both have been found to be most helpful when targeting the forearm muscles, especially for task-related dystonia (Lim et al. 2011). In many of our patients with writer's cramp, the BT dose could be reduced when switching from manual application to US guidance (Walter & Dressler 2014). Additional time for US guidance compared to the manual approach is reasonable if applied only in selected patients. Patients likely to benefit from US guidance include those with suboptimal treatment results under conventional manual BT application, patients with alterations in joint or muscle anatomy, patients with deep and thin cervical target muscles, especially the scalene, longissimus capitis and obliquus capitis inferior muscles, or when single finger flexors or extensors in task-related dystonia are to be injected (Walter & Dressler 2014; Schramm et al. 2015).

References

Berweck S, Feldkamp A, Francke A, Nehles J, Schwerin A, Heinen F (2002) Sonography-guided injection of botulinum toxin A in children with cerebral palsy. *Neuropediatrics* 33:221–223.

Boon AJ, Oney-Marlow TM, Murthy NS, Harper CM, McNamara TR, Smith J (2011) Accuracy of electromyography needle placement in cadavers: non-guided vs. ultrasound guided. *Muscle Nerve* 44:45–49.

Fujimoto H, Mezaki T, Yokoe M, Mochizuki H (2012) Sonographic guidance provides a low-risk approach to the longus colli muscle. *Mov Disord* 27:928–929.

Gervasio A, Mujahed I, Biasio A, Alessi S (2010) Ultrasound anatomy of the neck: the infrahyoid region. *J Ultrasound* 13:85–89.

Hobson-Webb LD, Boon AJ (2013) Reporting the results of diagnostic neuromuscular ultrasound: an educational report. *Muscle Nerve* 47:608–610.

Hong JS, Sathe GG, Niyonkuru C, Munin MC (2012) Elimination of dysphagia using ultrasound guidance for botulinum toxin injections in cervical dystonia. *Muscle Nerve* 46:535–539.

Huang L, Chen HX, Ding XD, Xiao HQ, Wang W, Wang H (2015) Efficacy analysis of ultrasound-guided local injection of botulinum toxin type A treatment with orthopedic joint brace in patients with cervical dystonia. *Eur Rev Med Pharmacol Sci* 19:1989–1993.

Kopf H, Mostbeck GH, Loizides A, Gruber H (2011) Ultrasound-guided interventions at peripheral nerves: diagnostic and therapeutic indications. *Ultraschall Med* 32:440–456.

Lee IH, Yoon YC, Sung DH, Kwon JW, Jung JY (2009) Initial experience with imaging-guided intramuscular botulinum toxin injection in patients with idiopathic cervical dystonia. *AJR Am J Roentgenol* 192:996–1001.

Lim EC, Quek AM, Seet RC (2011) Accurate targeting of botulinum toxin injections: how to and why. *Parkinsonism Relat Disord* 17 (Suppl. 1):S34–39.

Mezaki T, Matsumoto S, Sakamoto T, Mizutani K, Kaji R (2000) Cervical echomyography in cervical dystonia and its application to the monitoring for muscle afferent block (MAB). *Rinsho Shinkeigaku* 40:689–693.

Peetrons P (2002) Ultrasound of muscles. *Eur Radiol* 12:35–43.

Picelli A, Tamburin S, Bonetti P, Fontana C, Barausse M, Dambruoso F, Gajofatto F, Santilli V, Smania N (2012) Botulinum toxin type A injection into the gastrocnemius muscle for spastic equinus in adults with stroke: a randomized controlled trial comparing manual needle placement, electrical stimulation and ultrasonography-guided injection techniques. *Am J Phys Med Rehabil* 91:957–964.

Picelli A, Lobba D, Midiri A, Prandi P, Melotti C, Baldessarelli S, Smania N (2014) Botulinum toxin injection into the forearm muscles for wrist and fingers spastic overactivity in adults with chronic stroke: a randomized controlled trial comparing three injection techniques. *Clin Rehabil* 28:232–242.

Schramm A, Bäumer T, Fietzek U, Heitmann S, Walter U, Jost WH (2015) Relevance of sonography for botulinum toxin treatment of cervical dystonia: an expert statement. *J Neural Transm* 122:1457–1463.

Walter U, Dressler D (2014) Ultrasound-guided botulinum toxin injections in neurology: technique, indications and future perspectives. *Expert Rev Neurother* 14:923–936.

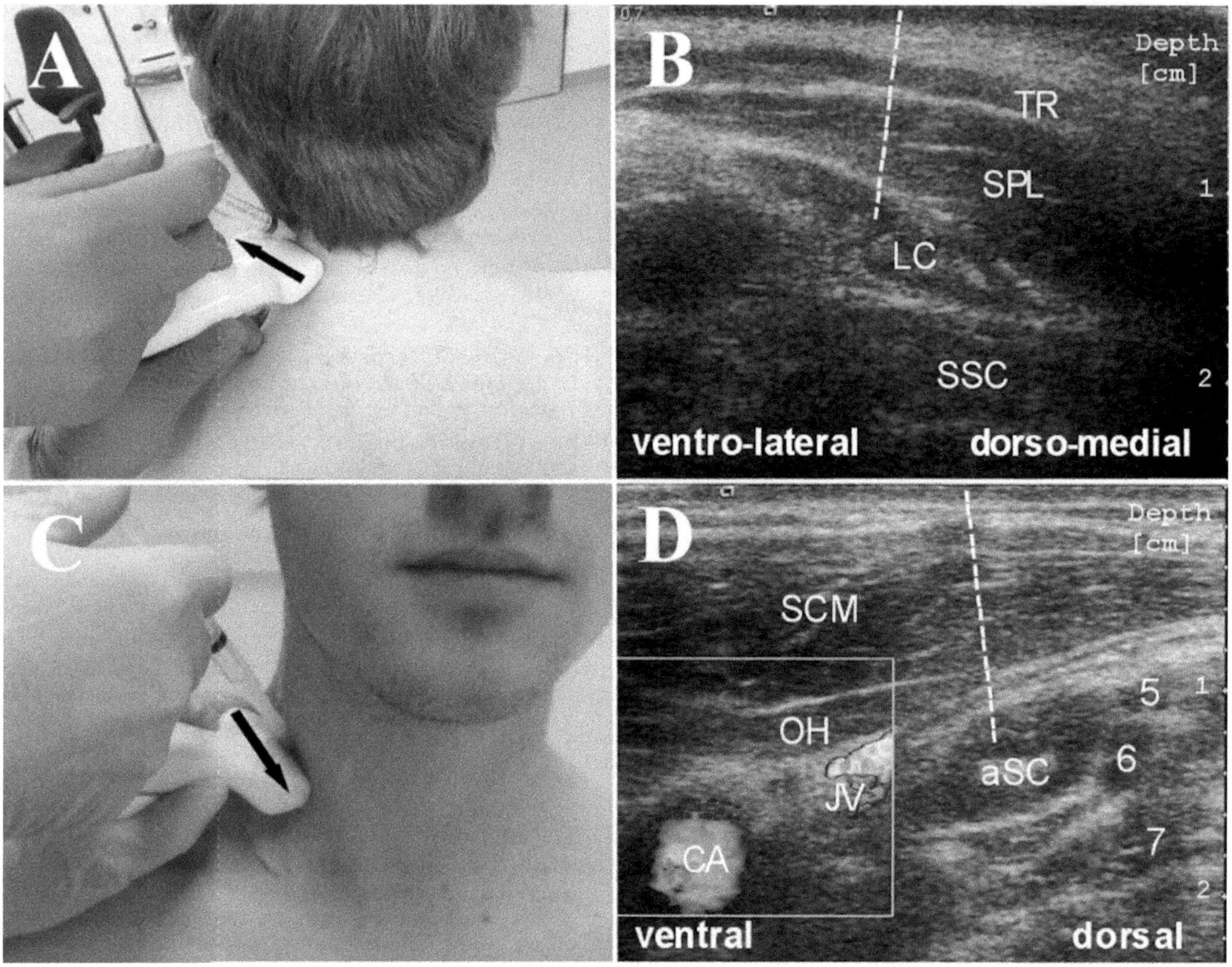

Figure 31.3 Ultrasonography (US) of the lateral neck region for guiding BT injection in patients with cervical dystonia. (a) Position of the US transducer and syringe (off-plane injection technique) for guiding BT injection into the longissimus capitis muscle. The arrow indicates the orientation of the transducer (arrow head corresponding to left side of the US image shown in (b)). (b) US image showing the trapecius (TR), splenius capitis (SPL), longissimus capitis (LC) and semispinalis capitis (SSC) muscles. The dashed line indicates the expected path of the injection needle. (c) Position of the US transducer and syringe (off-plane injection technique) region for guiding BT injection into the anterior scalene muscle. The arrow indicates the orientation of the transducer (arrow head corresponding to left side of US image shown in (d)). (d) US image showing the sternocleidomastoid (SCM), omohyoid (OH) and anterior scalene (aSC) muscles.

CA: common carotid artery; JV: internal jugular vein; 5: fifth cervical nerve root; 6: sixth cervical nerve root; 7: seventh cervical nerve root. The dashed line indicates the expected path of injection.

Table 31.1 Feasibility and necessity of US guidance in various target muscles in dystonia

Necessity for US guidance	Target tissues
Low [1]	Facial mimic muscles [2] Supra- and infrahyoid muscles [2] Pharyngeal muscles [3] Temporalis muscle Masseter muscle Sternocleidomastoid muscle Trapezius muscle Shoulder muscles Proximal arm muscles Intrinsic hand muscles Superficial paravertebral muscles Gluteal muscles Leg adductor muscles Tibialis anterior muscle
Intermediate	Splenius capitis muscle Semispinalis capitis muscle Levator scapulae muscle Abdominal muscles Ischiocrural muscles Gastrocnemius muscle
High	Longus colli muscle [3,4] Longus capitis muscle [3,4] Scalenus anterior muscle [5] Scalenus intermedius muscle [5] Obliquus capitis inferior muscle [5] Longissimus capitis muscle Laryngeal muscles [2] Single forearm muscles [6] Single finger flexors [6] Single finger extensors [6] Psoas muscle (inguinal portion) [5] Gracilis muscle Soleus muscle Tibialis posterior muscle [5] Extensor hallucis longus muscle

[1] Low necessity because of easy manual targeting or low frequency of cases.
[2] Difficult because of small size of target muscles.
[3] Difficult because of depth of target muscles.
[4] Difficult because of neighbouring sensitive structures.
[5] Attention should be paid to correct injection technique.
[6] High necessity in task-related dystonia.

Chapter 32

Treatment Algorithms and Injection Schemes for Botulinum Toxin Therapy of Dystonia

Dirk Dressler

Introduction

Botulinum toxin (BT) therapy of dystonia is based on treatment algorithms describing strategies on how BT therapy is administered and on injection schemes describing target muscles and BT doses used. Both will be outlined in this chapter.

Treatment Algorithms

Treatment algorithms include the intervals between two subsequent injection series (interinjection interval) and the total doses applied. Until recently, there was a general agreement that interinjection intervals should be 12 weeks or more in order to avoid frequent immunologic stimulation increasing the risk for BT antibody formation. Recent studies demonstrated that BT's therapeutic effect often lasts less than 12 weeks, thus identifying an unmet medical need (Dressler et al. 2014). Most recent data show that – when incobotulinumtoxinA is used – reducing interinjection intervals to less than 80 days is immunologically safe (Dressler et al. 2017). In another study it was shown – again, when incobotulinumtoxinA is used – that total BT doses can reach more than 1200 MU (Dressler et al. 2014). This allows improvement of the therapeutic impact in severe cases, extending the duration of action within certain limits and treating more widespread dystonias.

Injection Schemes

The development of an injection scheme for BT therapy requires a skilful analysis of the individual pattern of dystonic posture and dystonic movement. It is based on physiological muscle functioning and its pathological alterations, considering compensatory muscle activity and protective postures and taking into account additional information about pain points and general dose modifiers (Table 32.1). This injection scheme is highly individualised and usually requires several injection series to be optimised.

In selected cases electromyography may be helpful for the development of the injection scheme; imaging techniques are not. Dosing information deriving from registration studies are generally not helpful, either with respect to target muscle selection or with respect to total BT doses.

In the following, injection schemes for the most common forms of dystonia are described. All BT doses are given in mouse units (MU). Doses refer to the use of onabotulinumtoxinA (Botox®, Allergan, Dublin, Ireland) or incobotulinumtoxinA (Xeomin®, Merz Pharmaceuticals, Frankfurt/M, Germany). Doses of abobotulinumtoxinA (Dysport®, Beaufour-Ipsen, Boulogne-Billancourt, France) can be roughly estimated by using 1:2.5 to 1:4 conversion factors. All averages are given as mean ± standard deviation. The injection schemes presented here are derived from patients treated at the Movement Disorders Section of Hannover Medical School. Patient data were randomly collected until preset numbers were reached. These data represent about 40 per cent of all dystonia patients receiving BT therapy in our institution. Usage describes the percentage of patients with a special dystonia diagnosis receiving BT therapy in a particular target muscle. Additional dystonia localisations describe additional dystonia localisations with a severity sufficient to apply additional BT therapy. Additional muscles are infrequently used target muscles.

Cervical Dystonia (Table 32.2)

Cervical dystonia is the most common form of dystonia. In our group of 200 consecutive cervical dystonia patients their age was 58.4 ± 13.5 years and the male/female ratio 38/72 per cent. Of these patients, 23 per cent had additional cranial dystonia, 17 per cent additional oromandibular dystonia, 7 per cent additional axial dystonia, 6 per cent additional arm dystonia and 1 per cent additional leg dystonia. The total BT dose in cervical muscles was 262.6 ± 141.6 MU, with a minimum of 40 MU and a maximum of 860 MU. The number of cervical target muscles was 5.7 ± 1.8, with a

Table 32.1 General dose modifiers

Modifier	Botulinum toxin dose adjustment
Muscle mass	
Old age	↓
Female sex	↓
Iatrogenic atrophy	↓
Athletic training	↑
Comorbidity	
Myasthenia gravis	↓
Lambert–Eaton syndrome	↓
Botulinum toxin antibodies	↑
Increased general botulinum toxin sensitivity	↓

Table 32.2 Cervical dystonia

Age (years)	58.4 ± 13.5	
Males/female (%)	38/72	
Additional dystonia localisations (%)	Cranial dystonia	23
	Oromandibular dystonia	17
	Axial dystonia	7
	Arm dystonia	6
	Leg dystonia	1
Target muscles		
Number (*n*)	5.7 ± 1.8	
Minimum (*n*)	1	
Maximum (*n*)	13	
Total dose		
Mean (MU)	262.6 ± 141.6	
Minimum (MU)	40	
Maximum (MU)	860	

Target muscle	Mean BT dose (MU)	Minimum BT dose (MU)	Maximum BT dose (MU)	Usage (%)
T-PD	44.7 ± 27.5	10	200	78
SC	55.2 ± 33.2	10	300	75
SCM	46.4 ± 21.1	10	120	52
LS	34.2 ± 15.3	10	80	31
SCAL	36.5 ± 14.9	20	80	29
T-PH	46.0 ± 27.4	20	180	20
DNM	32.2 ± 15.4	20	60	3
Additional muscles		Suprahyoidal muscles Platysma		

T-PD. M. trapezius (Pars descends)
SC. M. splenius capitis
SCM. M. sternocleidomastoideus
LS. M. levator scapulae
SCAL. M. scalenii
T-PH. M. trapezius (Pars horizontalis)
DNM. Deep neck muscles

minimum of 1 and a maximum of 13. Most frequently used target muscles were M. trapezius (pars descendens) (78 per cent), M. splenius capitis (75 per cent), M. sternocleidmastoideus (52 per cent), M. levator scapulae (31 per cent), Mm. scalenii (29 per cent), M. trapezius (Pars horizontalis) (20 per cent) and the deep neck muscles (3 per cent). Occasionally, the suprahyoidal muscles and the platysma were target muscles.

The highly visible sternocleidomastoid muscle is not the most frequently involved target muscle. Bilateral BT injections into the M. sternocleidomastoid are possible without major risks of dysphagia. M. trapezius (Pars descendens) describes the nuchal paravertebral muscles, including the M. splenius cervicis and M. semispinalis capitis. The actual M. trapezius (Pars descendens) is a very thin muscle rotating the head into the opposite direction (similar to the M. sternocleidomastoideus) with negligible force. Throughout the literature there is confusion about the anatomical attribution of the nuchal muscles.

Cranial Dystonia (Table 32.3)

Cranial dystonia is the second most frequent form of dystonia. In our group of 100 consecutive cranial dystonia patients, their age was 65.2 ± 13.3 years and the male/female ratio 31/69 per cent. Of these patients, 45 per cent had additional cervical dystonia and 25 per cent additional oromandibular dystonia. The total cranial BT dose was 78.8 ± 31.6 MU with a minimum of 4 MU and a maximum of 220 MU. The number of target muscles was 3.7 ± 1.8 with a minimum of 1 and a maximum of 10. Most frequently used target muscles were M. orbicularis oculi (Pars orbitalis) (91 per cent), M. procerus (32 per cent), M. orbicularis oculi (Pars palpebralis) (26 per cent), M. mentalis (12 per cent), M. frontalis (9 per cent), M. risorius (9 per cent), M. platysma (8 per cent), M. nasolabialis (4 per cent), M. depressor anguli oris (2 per cent) and M. nasalis (2 per cent). Occasionally, the M. orbicularis oris may be a target muscle.

BT injections into perioral muscles are prone to producing paretic adverse effects. The M. frontalis should be used carefully as it is an auxiliary eyelid opening muscle. The M. orbicularis oculi (Pars palpebralis) is used when there is a component of eyelid opening apraxia.

Writer's Cramp (Table 32.4)

Writer's cramp is also a common manifestation of dystonia. It is task-specific, i.e. it only occurs when the specific motor

Table 32.3 Cranial dystonia

Age (years)	65.2 ± 13.3	
Males/female (%)	31/69	
Additional dystonia localisations (%)	Cervical dystonia	45
	Oromandibular dystonia	25
Target muscles		
Number (*n*)	3.7 ± 1.8	
Minimum (*n*)	1	
Maximum (*n*)	10	
Total dose		
Mean (MU)	78.8 ± 31.6	
Minimum (MU)	4	
Maximum (MU)	220	

Target muscle	Mean dose (MU)	Minimum dose (MU)	Maximum dose (MU)	Usage (%)
OOc-PO	32.9 ± 9.9	8	80	91
PROC	6.0 ± 3.5	2	20	32
OOc-PP	12.9 ± 4.8	4	24	26
MENT	6.2 ± 2.6	2	10	12
FRONT	6.2 ± 2.3	4	10	9
RIS	5.3 ± 2.9	2	12	9
PLAT	33.0 ± 21.0	4	80	8
NL	7.0 ± 3.5	4	12	4
DAO	4.8 ± 3.3	4	8	2
NAS	5.0/1.2	4	6	2
Additional muscles		M. orbicularis oris		

OOc-PO. M. orbicularis oculis (Pars orbitalis)
PROC. M. procerus
OOc-PP. M. orbicularis oculi (Pars palpebralis)
MENT. M. mentalis
FRONT. M. frontalis
RIS. M. risorius
PLAT. P. latysma
NL. M. nasolabialis
DAO. M. depressor anguli oris
NAS. M. nasalis

programme of writing is executed. In our group of 50 consecutive writer's cramp patients, their age was 61.6 ± 20.8 years and the male/female ratio 60/40 per cent. Of these patients, 2 per cent had additional cervical dystonia. The total arm BT dose was 70.3 ± 55.3 MU with a minimum of 8 MU and a maximum of 230 MU. The number of target muscles was 2.5 ± 1.5 with a minimum of 1 and a maximum of 6. Most frequently used target muscles were superficial forearm flexors (48 per cent), M. flexor carpi ulnaris (42 per cent), M. extensor carpi ulnaris (34 per cent), M. extensor carpi radialis (30 per cent), profound forearm flexors (30 per cent), M. flexor pollicis longus (28 per cent), M. flexor carpi ulnaris (12 per cent), M. pronator (8 per cent), M. extensor indicis (8 per cent), and M. extensor pollicis (6 per cent). Occasionally, the M. extensor digitorum, M. flexor indicis, M. supinator, M. deltoideus, M. trapezius (Pars descendens) and the M. triceps brachii may be target muscles.

BT application in writer's cramp usually requires guidance either by ultrasound or by electromyography, with or without electrostimulation. BT dosing in writer's cramp is highly individual, including a large number of potential target muscles in a wide range of BT doses.

Oromandibular Dystonia (Table 32.5)

In our group of 40 consecutive oromandibular dystonia patients, their age was 57.9 ± 14.6 years and the male/female ratio 40/60 per cent. Of these patients, 38 per cent had additional cervical dystonia, 30 per cent additional cranial dystonia, 10 per cent additional arm dystonia and 3 per cent additional axial dystonia. The total oromandibular BT dose was 127.5 ± 69.9 MU with a minimum of 40 MU and a maximum of 280 MU. The number of target muscles was 3.68 ± 1.67 with a minimum of 2 and a maximum of 8. Most frequently used target muscles were M. masseter (97 per cent), Mm. pterygoidei (44 per cent), M. temporalis (24 per cent), M. submandibularis (13 per cent) and Platysma (8 per cent). Occasionally, the M. risorius and the M. mentalis may be target muscles. The Mm. pterygoidei can easily be injected through the Incissura mandibulae. Electromyography requiring

Table 32.4 Writer's cramp

Age (years)	61.6 ± 20.8	
Males/female (%)	60/40	
Additional dystonia localisations (%)	Cervical dystonia	2
Target muscles		
Number (*n*)	2.5 ± 1.5	
Minimum(*n*)	1	
Maximum(*n*)	6	
Total dose		
mean (MU)	70.3 ± 55.3	
Minimum (MU)	8	
Maximum (MU)	230	

Target muscle	Mean dose (MU)	Minimum dose (MU)	Maximum dose (MU)	Usage (%)
FF-S	21.8 ± 13.9	8	70	48
FCU	32.7 ± 18.2	10	80	42
ECU	35.4 ± 13.1	10	60	34
ECR	28.0 ± 13.2	10	50	30
FF-P	19.9 ± 10.3	8	40	30
FPL	22.7 ± 13.5	6	60	28
FCR	13.0 ± 5.5	8	20	12
PRON	47.0 ± 39.3	8	100	8
EInd	34.3 ± 43.8	10	100	8
EPol	9.3 ± 1.2	8	10	6
Additional muscles		M. extensor digitorum M. flexor indicis M. supinator M. deltoideus M. trapezius (Pars descendens) M. triceps brachii		

FF-S. Forearm flexors (superficial)
FCU. M. flexor carpi ulnaris
ECU. M. extensor ulnaris
ECR. M. extensor radialis
FF-P. Forearm flexors (profound)
FPL. M. flexor pollicis longus
FCR. M. flexor carpi radialis
PRON. M. pronator
EInd. M. extensor indicis
EPol. M. extensor pollicis

thick combination needles is not necessary since dystonic involvement is usually affecting both the lateral and the medial pterygoid muscles.

Arm Dystonia (Table 32.6)

Non-task-specific arm dystonia is also a less frequent manifestation of dystonia. In our group of ten consecutive arm dystonia patients, their age was 32.7 ± 19.7 years and thus considerably lower than the age of other focal dystonias. The male/female ratio was 40/60 per cent. Of these patients, 80 per cent had additional cervical dystonia, 10 per cent additional oromandibular dystonia. Its isolated occurrence is very rare. Total arm BT dose was 156.0 ± 143.3 MU with a minimum of 40 MU and a maximum of 540 MU. Number of target muscles was 3.8 ± 2.3 with a minimum of 1 and a maximum of 10. Most frequently used target muscles were M. deltoideus (70 per cent), M. flexor carpi ulnaris (70 per cent), M. pectoralis (50 per cent), M. brachioradialis (50 per cent), M. flexor carpi radialis (40 per cent), M. biceps brachii (40 per cent), M. pronator (30 per cent) and M. latissimus dorsi/M. teres major (30 per cent).

Axial Dystonia (Table 32.7)

Axial dystonia is a less frequent manifestation of dystonia. In our group of ten consecutive axial dystonia patients, their age was 61.7 ± 116.0 years and the male/female ratio 30/70 per cent. Axial dystonia usually occurs together with other dystonia manifestations. In 50 per cent of our patients it is cervical dystonia, in 10 per cent cranial dystonia. The total axial BT dose was 318.0 ± 212.2 MU with a minimum of 80 MU and a maximum of 800 MU. The number of segmental levels injected was 3.9 ± 1.4. The dose per segmental level was 40–80 MU.

Table 32.5 Oromandibular dystonia

Age (years)	57.9 ± 14.6	
Males/female (%)	40/60	
Additional dystonia localisations (%)	Cervical dystonia	38
	Cranial dystonia	30
	Arm dystonia	10
	Axial dystonia	3
Target muscles		
Number (*n*)	3.8 ± 2.3	
Minimum (*n*)	1	
Maximum (*n*)	10	
Total dose		
Mean (MU)	127.5 ± 69.9	
Minimum (MU)	40	
Maximum (MU)	280	

Target muscle	Mean dose (MU)	Minimum dose (MU)	Maximum dose (MU)	Usage (%)
M	36.7 ± 14.0	20	60	97
PTER	31.6 ± 13.2	8	60	44
TEMP	42.0 ± 23.9	20	80	24
SUBM	16.0 ± 5.5	10	20	13
PLAT	33.3 ± 11.5	20	40	8

M. M. masseter
PTER. Mm. flexor carpi ulnaris
PECT. M. pterygoidei
TEMP. M. temporalis
PLAT. M. platysma
SUBM. M. submandibularis

Leg Dystonia

Non-task-specific leg dystonia is very rare. It only occurs in widespread dystonia. BT doses are similar to those used in spasticity.

Widespread Dystonia

Widespread dystonia includes all patients with dystonia exceeding two adjacent focal dystonias, i.e. segmental dystonia with more than two localisations, with hemidystonia and with generalised dystonia. BT therapy consists of treatment of the focal dystonic elements. New treatment algorithms allowing high dose application offer improved treatment options.

References

Dressler D, Adib Saberi F (2017) Immunological safety of incobotulinumtoxinA (Xeomin®) therapy with reduced interinjection intervals. *J Neural Transm* 124:437–440.

Dressler D, Tacik P. Adib Saberi F (2014a) Botulinum toxin therapy of cervical dystonia: duration of therapeutic effects. *J Neural Transm* 122:297–300.

Dressler D, Adib Saberi F, Kollewe K, Schrader C (2014b) Safety aspects of incobotulinumtoxinA high dose therapy. *J Neural Transm* 122:327–333.

Table 32.6 Arm dystonia

Age (years)	37.2 ± 19.7	
Males/female (%)	40/60	
Additional dystonia localisations (%)	Cervical dystonia	80
	Oromandibular dystonia	10
Target muscles		
Number (*n*)	3.8 ± 2.3	
Minimum (*n*)	1	
Maximum (*n*)	10	
Total dose		
Mean (MU)	156.0 ± 143.3	
Minimum (MU)	40	
Maximum (MU)	540	

Target muscle	Mean dose (MU)	Minimum dose (MU)	Maximum dose (MU)	Usage (%)
D	40.0 ± 16.3	20	60	70
FCU	40.0 ± 16.3	20	60	70
PECT	40.0 ± 24.5	20	80	50
BR	36.0 ± 16.7	20	60	50
BB	40.0 ± 16.3	20	60	40
FCR	40.0 ± 16.3	20	60	40
PRON	46.7 ± 11.5	40	60	30
LT/TM	53.3 ± 23.1	40	80	30
Additional muscles				

D. M. deltoideus
FCU. M. flexor carpi ulnaris
PECT. M. pectoralis
BR. M. brachioradialis
BB. M. biceps brachii
FCR. M. flexor carpi radialis
PRON. M. pronator
LT/TM. Mm. latissimus dorsi/teres major

Table 32.7 Axial dystonia

Age (years)	61.7 ± 116.0	
Males/female (%)	30/70	
Additional dystonia localisations (%)	Cervical dystonia	50
	Cranial dystonia	10
Number of segmental levels (*n*)	3.9 ± 1.4	
Dose per segmental level (MU)	40–80	
Total dose		
Mean (MU)	318.0 ± 212.2	
Minimum (MU)	80	
Maximum (MU)	800	

Chapter 33

Botulinum Toxin Therapy for Cervical Dystonia

Mary Ann Thenganatt and Joseph Jankovic

Introduction

Cervical dystonia (CD) is the most common form of focal dystonia encountered in movement disorder clinics. More common in women than men, the prevalence estimates of CD in the general population have ranged from 20 to 4100 cases/million, with estimated incidence ranging at 8–12 cases/million person-years (Defazio et al. 2013). Further information on the epidemiology of dystonia can be found in Chapter 5.

Several rating scales used to assess motor and non-motor aspects of CD have been developed and used to assess response to treatment. These include the Tsui Scale, Cervical Dystonia Severity Scale (CDSS), Toronto Western Spasmodic Torticollis Rating Scale (TWSTRS), Craniocervical Dystonia Questionnaire (CDQ-24), Cervical Dystonia Impact Profile-58 (CDIP-58) and the Comprehensive Cervical Dystonia Rating Scale (CCDRS) (Comella et al. 2016). A newly proposed scale called the Dystonia Discomfort Scale (DDS) is a self-assessment scale that reports the temporal profile of BoNT, including information such as the onset, duration, wearing off and reproducibility of botulinum toxin (BoNT) injections (Dressler et al. 2015). This scale has been studied in CD patients and found to correlate with TWSTRS total scores. Further information on rating scales in dystonia can be found in Chapters 15 and 16.

The introduction of BoNT for the treatment of dystonia was a major therapeutic advancement for the field of movement disorders (Jankovic 2017). BoNT was first used in the 1980s for the treatment of blepharospasm and hemifacial spasm; onabotulinumtoxinA (Botox®) was approved by the US Food and Drug Administration (FDA) in 1989 for the treatment of these movement disorders, and along with rimabotulinumtoxinB (MyoBloc®) was approved for CD in 2000. Compared to oral medications, such as trihexyphenidyl (Burke et al. 1986), BoNT is a focal therapy targeted at the muscles involved in dystonia, generally without clinically appreciable widespread side-effects (Thenganatt & Jankovic 2014). While the long-term benefits and safety of BoNT have been well established (Ramirez-Castaneda & Jankovic 2014), there is ongoing research studying different targeting techniques (e.g. electrophysiology, ultrasound), dosing intervals and novel formulations of BoNT. Suboptimal response or secondary non-response can be due to various factors besides the formation of neutralising antibodies, including changes in the pattern or severity of dystonia, the need for dosing adjustments or the presence of contractures. Thus knowledge about the motor (posture and movement) and non-motor (pain and alleviating manoeuvres) (Patel et al. 2014) aspects of CD and experience with BoNT will help a clinician optimise the treatment outcomes.

Formulations of Botulinum Toxin

There are three formulations of BoNT type A (BoNT/A) and one BoNT type B (BoNT/B) formulation that are approved by the FDA for the treatment of CD. The non-proprietary names of the three type A formulations are onabotulinumtoxinA (Botox®), abobotulinumtoxinA (Dysport®) and incobotulinumtoxinA (Xeomin®). The non-proprietary name of the type B formulation is rimabotulinumtoxinB (MyoBloc®). All four of these toxins have been studied in numerous clinical trials and have been shown to be effective for CD (Thenganatt & Fahn 2012; Hallett et al. 2013). IncobotulinumtoxinA is the most recent formulation to be approved by the FDA. Compared to the other type A formulations, this product is free from accessory proteins, suggesting the possibility of lower risk of immunoresistance with this toxin (Jost et al. 2014). The long-term antigenicity of incobotulinumtoxinA compared to the other toxins is yet to be determined. The various formulations of BoNT are not of equal potency labelling and the clinician must be familiar with the specific product when making dosing adjustments. The optimal unit conversion ratio between abobotulinumtoxinA and onabotulinumtoxinA has been debated and a recent study demonstrated that a ratio of 2.5:1 for abobotulinumtoxinA: onabotulinumtoxinA resulted in similar efficacy and side-effects, whereas a higher ratio may result in greater side-effects (Yun et al. 2015). We use this ratio in our practice when converting between abobotulinumtoxinA and onabotulinumtoxinA, 50:1 ratio for rimabotulinumtoxinB:onabotulinumtoxinA conversion and 1:1 for incobotulinumtoxinA: onabotulinumtoxinA.

Further information on pharmacology of BoNT drugs can be found in Chapter 27.

Principles of Treatment

The treatment goal should be to reduce dystonia severity, improve pain and overall quality of life (Albanese et al. 2015; Jankovic et al. 2015). One recent study reported pain related to CD in 88.9 per cent (922/1037) of CD patients with 70.7 per cent (733/1037) reporting their pain as moderate or severe at baseline (Charles et al. 2014). Compared to those with no or mild pain, those with moderate to severe pain were older, had anterocollis, had higher use of analgesics, antianxiety or antidepressant medications and were more likely to be disabled. Those with moderate to severe pain had higher TWSTRS severity (17.7 ± 5.1 vs 16.2 ± 5.6, $p < 0.0001$) and disability (12.7 ± 6.1 vs 7.5 ± 5.6, $p < 0.0001$) scores and received higher doses of onabotulinumtoxinA (177.3 ± 82.9 vs 158.0 ± 67.1 MU, $p = 0.0001$).

When planning treatment of CD with BoNT, the first step is to determine the phenomenology of CD in an individual patient: torticollis (rotation), laterocollis (lateral tilt), retrocollis (backward extension) or anterocollis (forward flexion). This allows one to identify the muscles that are most actively involved in producing the abnormal movement. Of the different forms of CD, anterocollis is most complex in its phenomenology and most challenging to treat, but meaningful improvements can be achieved by experienced and skilled clinicians (Finsterer et al. 2015; Jankovic 2018; Jindal & Jankovic 2017). While muscle hypertrophy or palpable muscle tension may be helpful to identify target muscles, it is important to identify the primary muscles (agonists) responsible for the dystonia vs compensatory muscle contraction (antagonists). A patient's subjective report of localised pain can also be misleading. A classic example is anterocollis (forward flexion), which often results in compensatory contraction of the neck extensors and associated pain in these muscles and in the trapezius muscles. If one were to choose muscles for injection based on these findings, injection of the neck extensors could result in worsening of involuntary neck flexion. Dosing of BoNT should take into consideration the overall size of the patient and the bulk of the muscles being injected. While dosing intervals are often 12–16 weeks based on previous trials, the ideal dosing interval with minimal long-term side-effects is unclear (Evidente et al. 2014). It is not uncommon for patients' symptoms to return before 12 weeks and enquire about more frequent injections with shorter interinjection intervals (Sethi et al. 2012). A post hoc analysis evaluated a flexible dosing schedule with incobotulinumtoxinA for the treatment of CD based on patient request and physician assessment (Evidente et al. 2014). Injection intervals of <12 weeks were performed in 369 of 821 (44.9 per cent) treatment cycles for CD. The most common side-effects were dysphagia and neck pain; however, the frequency of side-effects were similar in the groups injected <12 weeks vs >12 weeks. In a large study on 1289 treatment cycles in 59 patients with CD, 89 per cent of patients had mean durations of their therapeutic effects of less than 12 weeks, 36 per cent of less than 10 weeks, accumulating to 23 per cent of their time being suboptimally treated (Dressler et al. 2015). Further studies confirming these findings and demonstrating the long-term safety without increased risk of immunoresistance are needed.

Efficacy

Since the initial studies in the late 1980s, there have been numerous randomised, placebo-controlled trials demonstrating the benefits and safety of BoNT for CD (Table 33.1). The evidence for BoNT in CD has been summarised in international expert consensus statements and the published evidence supports a Level A recommendation for all four toxins in the treatment of CD (Simpson et al. 2008; Hallett et al. 2013). There have been controlled trials comparing the various toxins, demonstrating similar benefit (Table 33.2).

The long-term benefits and safety of BoNT for CD have also been demonstrated. One of the longest follow-up studies is a retrospective, longitudinal study at a tertiary movement disorder centre (Ramirez-Castaneda & Jankovic 2014). The response to BoNT was evaluated in 89 patients, including 51 with CD, followed for up to 26 years (mean 18.5 years). The majority of patients had sustained long-term benefit with a global response effect of 3.18 (0 = no effect; 4 = marked improvement in severity and function) after the first injection session and 3.57 after the last injection ($p < 0.0001$). Adverse events were reported in 19 per cent of visits, with approximately 10 per cent in CD. The most common adverse events in CD were dysphagia and neck weakness. BoNT has been shown to improve health-related quality of life in CD with one study involving abobotulinumtoxinA demonstrating greater improvement in Physical Functioning, Role Physical, Bodily Pain, General Health and Role Emotional domains of the SF-36 Health Survey compared to placebo ($p \leq 0.03$) (Mordin et al. 2014). According to the American Academy of Neurology practice guidelines, AbobotulinumtoxinA and rimabotulinumtoxinB are established as effective and should be offered (Level A), and onabotulinumtoxinA and incobotulinumtoxinA are probably effective and should be considered (Level B) (Simpson et al. 2016). The Level B recommendation is based on relative lack of published rigorous double-blind controlled trials.

Potential Side-Effects

While BoNT for CD is an effective treatment for focal dystonia, there is the potential for adverse effects that may be mediated via physical spread of toxin, passive diffusion or distant migration, among other factors (Ramirez-Castaneda et al. 2013). The more common side-effects from BoNT for CD include neck weakness, neck pain and dysphagia. When injecting the sternocleidomastoid, injecting into the upper third portion of the muscle may reduce the incidence of dysphagia. Since the effect of BoNT is not permanent, the adverse effects will also wear off with time. A transient flu-like reaction has been reported after injection with BoNT and may be seen in approximately 15 per cent of patients (Baizabal-Carvallo et al. 2011, 2013). Autonomic side-effects, most commonly dry mouth and constipation, can be seen with BoNT, more frequently with type B compared to type A (Lew et al. 1997; Dressler & Benecke 2003).

Suboptimal Response and Secondary Non-Responders

There may be many factors that contribute to a suboptimal or secondary non-response to BoNT (poor response after initial benefit) (Figure 33.1). The presence of contractures may limit the response to BoNT. An international observational

Table 33.1 Randomised, placebo-controlled trials of botulinum toxin

Study	Treatment	# Subjects	Follow-up	Primary outcome
Greene et al. 1990	OnabotulinumtoxinA, varied dose	55	12 weeks	Improvement in functional capacity, pain and results of injections compared to placebo, $p < 0.05$
Lew et al. 1997	RimabotulinumtoxinB 2500, 5000 or 10 000 MU	122	4 weeks	Reduction in TWSTRS 2500 MU (−11.6), 5000 MU (−12.5), 10 000 MU (−16.4) vs placebo (−3.3), $p < 0.05$
Brashear et al. 1999	RimabotulinumtoxinB 5000 or 10 000 MU	109	4 weeks	Reduction in TWSTRS with 5000 MU 9.3, $p = 0.0004$ and 10 000 MU 11.7, $p = 0.0115$ vs placebo 4.3
Brin et al. 1999	RimabotulinumtoxinB 10 000 MU	77	4 weeks	Reduction in TWSTRS toxin vs placebo −11.1 vs −2.0, $p = 0.0001$
Poewe et al. 1998	AbobotulinumtoxinA 250, 500 or 1000 MU	75	4 weeks	Reduction modified Tsui Scale in 500 MU and 1000 MU groups at week 4, $p < 0.05$
Truong et al. 2005	AbobotulinumtoxinA 500 MU	80	4 weeks	Reduction in TWSTRS with toxin vs placebo (9.9 vs 3.8, $p \le 0.013$)
Truong et al. 2010	AbobotulinumtoxinA 500 MU	116	4 weeks	Reduction in TWSTRS (−15.6 ± 2.0) vs placebo (6.7 ± 2.0), $p < 0.001$
Comella et al. 2011	IncobotulinumtoxinA 120 or 240 MU	233	4 weeks	Reduction in TWSTRS with 120 MU (−9.9), 240 MU (−10.9) vs placebo (−2.2), $p < 0.01$
Charles et al. 2012	OnabotulinumtoxinA varied dose maximum 360 MU	88	6 weeks	Greater improvement than placebo on the Cervical Dystonia Severity Scale (−1.81 vs −0.31, $p = 0.012$) and physician Global Assessment Scale (61.7 per cent vs 41.6 per cent improved, $p = 0.022$

TWSTRS = Toronto Western Spasmodic Torticollis Rating Scale.

Table 33.2 Randomised, comparator trials of botulinum toxin

Study	Treatment	# Subjects	Follow-up	Primary Outcome
Odergren et al. 1998	OnabotulinumtoxinA mean 152 MU vs abobotulinumtoxinA mean 477 MU	73	12 weeks	No significant difference in Tsui score at 12 weeks or time to retreatment
Benecke et al. 2005	OnabotulinumtoxinA mean 138.9 MU vs incobotulinumtoxinA mean 140.4 MU	463	4 weeks	IncobotulinumtoxinA non-inferior to onabotulinumtoxinA based on TWSTRS
Comella et al. 2005	OnabotulinumtoxinA vs rimabotulinumtoxinB	139	4 weeks	No difference in improvement in TWSTRS at 4 weeks. Greater frequency of dysphagia and dry mouth with rimabotulinumtoxinB, $p < 0.0001$. Mild longer duration of benefit with onabotulinumtoxinA, $p = 0.033$.
Pappert & Germanson 2008	OnabotulinumtoxinA 150 MU vs rimabotulinumtoxinB 10 000 MU	11	4 weeks	RimabotulinumtoxinB non-inferior to onabotulinumtoxinA based on TWSTRS

TWSTRS = Toronto Western Spasmodic Torticollis Rating Scale.

study found younger age (age <40) and the absence of head tremor to be associated with good response to BoNT in CD (Misra et al. 2012). Change in severity of dystonia and muscles involved, and severity of dystonia may also affect response and require a change in muscle selection and dosing. The involvement of deep cervical muscles that are inaccessible with routine BoNT injections may also contribute to suboptimal response (Bhidayasiri 2011). A study of 35 patients with CD and a reported suboptimal response to BoNT found that most causes were correctible and included inadequate BoNT doses, suboptimal muscle selection, intolerable side-effects, complex movement patterns (head tremor, anterocollis, sagittal shift), incorrect diagnoses and discordant opinions between patient and injector (Jinnah et al. 2016). Only one subject was functionally resistant to BoNT, and 78 per cent of subjects who underwent repeat injections had a satisfactory outcome with a revised treatment plan. Immunoresistance due to the formation of antibodies to BoNT is also a concern with repeated injections. When there is a concern for resistance, a clinical test such as a unilateral brow injection (UBI) into the corrugator or frontalis is a simple test to help determine if there is clinical resistance to BoNT (Hanna & Jankovic 1998). Injection into the corrugator (UBI) over the frontalis is preferable cosmetically. The immunogenicity of onabotulinumtoxinA was studied in 326 patients with CD with a median of nine treatments over a mean of 2.5 years (Brin et al. 2008). Only four out of 326 (1.2

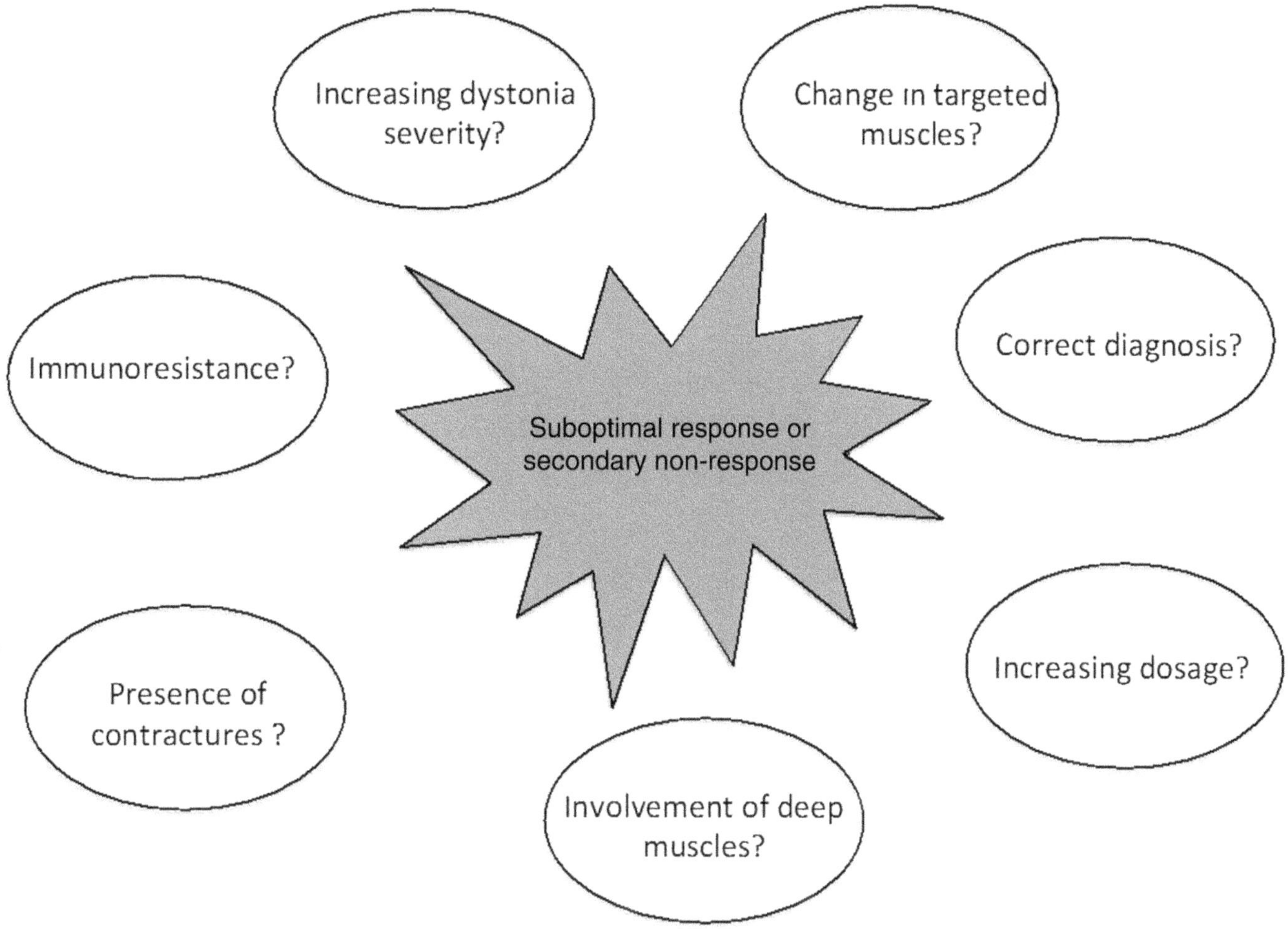

Figure 33.1 Suboptimal response or secondary non-response to botulinum toxin: things to consider.

per cent) subjects tested positive for neutralising antibodies via the mouse protection assay and three of these subjects did not respond clinically. The formation of neutralising antibodies with rimabotulinumtoxinB is higher (Dressler & Bigalke 2004). In one study of 100 CD patients treated with rimabotulinumtoxinB, after 5.1 mean number of treatment visits, one-third of patients developed neutralising antibodies who were negative at baseline (Jankovic et al. 2006). Although immunologically alternate type of BoNT may be effective in patients who develop immunoresistance, because of secondary cross-reactivity, many patients develop blocking antibodies to the new type of BoNT (Sankhla et al. 1998). Further information on the immunogenicity of BoNT therapy can be found in Chapter 28.

When suboptimal response or secondary non-response is encountered, all of these factors listed above should be considered. In some patients that are poor responders to BoNT, deep brain stimulation may be an option.

Future Directions

It is clear that BoNT is a highly effective treatment for CD with long-term safety profile. BoNT not only relieves motor aspects of dystonia (abnormal posture, dystonic tremor), but also ameliorates pain and improves overall quality of life. Furthermore, it may also change the natural history of CD by preventing chronic complications such as contractures. Further optimisation of outcomes can be achieved by better selection and targeting of involved muscles, appropriate dosing and injection intervals and innovations in BoNT formulations. The development of newer toxins with a longer duration of benefit is also desirable. Strategies to minimise adverse effects, the spread of toxin and overcome suboptimal treatment response can always be refined.

The use of electromyography (EMG) as a technique to guide BoNT therapy has been studied in various applications including CD (Dressler 2000; Nijmeijer et al. 2012). While some may find these techniques helpful, they should not replace the clinical evaluation of the patient when selecting the appropriate muscles of injection. A pilot study evaluated the use of multi-channel EMG in nine patients with CD who were non-responders but without blocking antibodies (Kilbane et al. 2012). The investigators inserted 12 EMG recording needles in all major muscles of the neck to identify the most active muscles, prior to BoNT injection. This was followed by a single lead injection 16 weeks later. The mean improvement in TWSTRS was 23.5 per cent using the multi-channel EMG vs

9 per cent using the single channel. Although significant difference was demonstrated between these two techniques, it is unlikely that the use of multi-channel EMG, with its associated problems (e.g. discomfort, time, cost) is justified over administration of BoNT using clinical observation and palpation, which in our experience results in >85 per cent improvement in abnormal movement, posture and pain experienced by most of our patients. One study attempted to compare EMG-guided vs non-EMG-guided injections in 65 patients with CD (Wu et al. 2016). While a small but significant difference in Tsui score was observed between groups 16 weeks after therapy, the EMG-guided group had lower baseline score than the other group, which minimises the observed difference in outcome. Furthermore there was no significant difference in visual analogue scale scores or Clinical and Patient Global Impression of Change (CGIC and PGIC). Although dysphagia was less frequent, there was more injection-site pain with EMG guidance.

The use of ultrasound for BoNT injection has been suggested as a non-invasive method of localising a muscle and improving injection precision in a pre-selected muscle. The use of ultrasound may help avoid side-effects such as dysphagia, injection of blood vessels and may allow for injection into deeper neck muscles that are not easily accessible (Schramm et al. 2015). Future studies using ultrasound in CD may help define its utility in BoNT injections. Although these techniques may possibly improve response to BoNT, the modest gains in outcome measures must be weighed against the increase in time, discomfort and cost. Therefore, well-designed health outcome and cost analyses are needed. Further information on the use of ultrasound BoNT therapy for dystonia is found in Chapter 31.

References

Albanese A, Abbruzzese G, Dressler D, Duzynski W, Khatkova S, Marti MJ, Mir P, Montecucco C, Moro E, Pinter M, Relja M, Roze E, Skogseid IM, Timerbaeva S, Tzoulis C (2015). Practical guidance for CD management involving treatment of botulinum toxin: a consensus statement. *J Neurol* 262:2201–2213.

Baizabal-Carvallo JF, Jankovic J, Pappert E (2011). Flu-like symptoms following botulinum toxin therapy. *Toxicon* 58:1–7.

Baizabal-Carvallo JF, Jankovic J, Feld J (2013). Flu-like symptoms and associated immunological response following therapy with botulinum toxins. *Neurotox Res* 2:298–306.

Benecke R, Jost WH, Kanovsky P, Ruzicka E, Comes G, Grafe S (2005). A new botulinum toxin type A free of complexing proteins for treatment of cervical dystonia. *Neurology* 64:1949–1951.

Bhidayasiri R (2011). Treatment of complex cervical dystonia with botulinum toxin: involvement of deep-cervical muscles may contribute to suboptimal responses. *Parkinsonism Relat Disord* 17 (Suppl. 1):S20–S24.

Brashear A, Lew MF, Dykstra DD, Comella CL, Factor SA, Rodnitzky RL, Trosch R, Singer C, Brin MF, Murray JJ, Wallace JD, Willmer-Hulme A, Koller M (1999). Safety and efficacy of NeuroBloc (botulinum toxin type B) in type A-responsive cervical dystonia. *Neurology* 53:1439–1446.

Brin MF, Lew MF, Adler CH, Comella CL, Factor SA, Jankovic J, O'Brien C, Murray JJ, Wallace JD, Willmer-Hulme A, Koller M (1999). Safety and efficacy of NeuroBloc (botulinum toxin type B) in type A-resistant cervical dystonia. *Neurology* 53:1431–1438.

Brin MF, Comella CL, Jankovic J, Lai F, Naumann M; CD-017 BoNTA Study Group (2008). Long-term treatment with botulinum toxin type A in cervical dystonia has low immunogenicity by mouse protection assay. *Mov Disord* 23:1353–1360.

Burke RE, Fahn S, Marsden CD (1986). Torsion dystonia: a double-blind, prospective trial of high-dosage trihexyphenidyl. *Neurology* 36:160–164.

Charles D, Brashear A, Hauser RA, Li HI, Boo LM, Brin MF; CD 140 Study Group (2012). Efficacy, tolerability, and immunogenicity of onabotulinumtoxinA in a randomized, double-blind, placebo-controlled trial for cervical dystonia. *Clin Neuropharmacol* 35:208–214.

Charles PD, Adler CH, Stacy M, Comella C, Jankovic J, Manack Adams A, Schwartz M, Brin MF (2014). Cervical dystonia and pain: characteristics and treatment patterns from CD PROBE (Cervical Dystonia Patient Registry for Observation of OnabotulinumtoxinA Efficacy). *J Neurol* 261:1309–1319.

Comella CL, Jankovic J, Shannon KM, Tsui J, Swenson M, Leurgans S, Fan W; Dystonia Study Group (2005). Comparison of botulinum toxin serotypes A and B for the treatment of cervical dystonia. *Neurology* 65:1423–1429.

Comella CL, Jankovic J, Truong DD, Hanschmann A, Grafe S; US XEOMIN Cervical Dystonia Study Group (2011). Efficacy and safety of incobotulinumtoxinA (NT 201, XEOMIN(R), botulinum neurotoxin type A, without accessory proteins) in patients with cervical dystonia. *J Neurol Sci* 308:103–109.

Comella CL, Perlmutter JS, Jinnah HA, Waliczek TA, Rosen AR, Galpern WR, Adler CA, Barbano RL, Factor SA, Goetz CG, Jankovic J, Reich SG, Rodriguez RL, Severt WL, Zurowski M, Fox SH, Stebbins GT (2016). Clinimetric testing of the Comprehensive Cervical Dystonia Rating Scale (CCDRS). *Mov Disord* 31:563–569.

Defazio G, Jankovic J, Giel JL, Papapetropoulos S (2013). Descriptive epidemiology of cervical dystonia. *Tremor Other Hyperkinet Mov (NY)* 4:3.

Dressler D (2000). Electromyographic evaluation of cervical dystonia for planning of botulinum toxin therapy. *Eur J Neurol* 7:713–718.

Dressler D, Benecke R (2003). Autonomic side effects of botulinum toxin type B treatment of cervical dystonia and hyperhidrosis. *Eur Neurol* 49:34–38.

Dressler D, Bigalke H (2004). Antibody-induced failure of botulinum toxin type B therapy in de novo patients. *Eur Neurol* 52:132–135.

Dressler D, Tacik P, Saberi FA (2015). Botulinum toxin therapy of cervical dystonia: duration of therapeutic effects. *J Neural Transm* 122:297–300.

Evidente VG, Truong D, Jankovic J (2014). IncobotulinumtoxinA (Xeomin(R)) injected for blepharospasm or cervical dystonia according to patient needs is well tolerated. *J Neurol Sci* 346:116–120.

Finsterer J, Maeztu C, Revuelta G, Reichel G, Truong D (2015). Collum-caput (COL-CAP) concept for conceptual anterocollis, anterocaput, and forward sagittal shift. *J Neurol Sci* 355:37–43.

Greene P, Kang U, Fahn S, Brin M, Moskowitz C, Flaster E. (1990). Double-blind, placebo-controlled trial of botulinum toxin injections for the treatment of spasmodic torticollis. *Neurology* 40:1213–1218.

Hallett M, Albanese A, Dressler D, Segal KR, Simpson DM, Truong D, Jankovic J (2013). Evidence-based review and assessment of botulinum neurotoxin for the treatment of movement disorders. *Toxicon* 67:94–114.

Hanna PA, Jankovic J (1998). Mouse bioassay versus Western blot assay for botulinum toxin antibodies: correlation with clinical response. *Neurology* 50:1624–1629.

Jankovic J (2017). Botulinum toxin: state of the art. *Mov Disod* 32:1131–1138.

Jankovic J (2018). An update on new and unique uses of botulinum toxin in movement disorders. *Toxicon*. Epub ahead of print.

Jankovic J, Hunter C, Dolimbek BZ, Dolimbek GS, Adler CH, Brashear A, Comella CL, Gordon M, Riley DE, Sethi K, Singer C, Stacy M, Tarsy D, Atassi MZ (2006). Clinico-immunologic aspects of botulinum toxin type B treatment of cervical dystonia. *Neurology* 67:2233–2235.

Jankovic J, Adler CH, Charles D, Comella C, Stacy M, Schwartz M, Manack Adams A, Brin MF (2015). Primary results from the cervical dystonia patient registry for observation of onabotulinumtoxinA efficacy (CD PROBE). *J Neurol Sci* 349:84–93.

Jindal P, Jankovic J (2017). Botulinum toxin treatment in Parkinson's disease and atypical parkinsonian disorders. In Bahman Jabbari (ed.) *Botulinum Toxin Treatment*. New York: Springer.

Jinnah HA, Goodmann E, Rosen AR, Evatt M, Freeman A, Factor S (2016). Botulinum toxin treatment failures in cervical dystonia: causes, management, and outcomes. *J Neurol* 263:1188–1194.

Jost WH, Benecke R, Hauschke D, Jankovic J, Kaňovský P, Roggenkämper P, Simpson DM, Comella CL (2014). Clinical and pharmacological properties of incobotulinumtoxinA and its use in neurological disorders. *Drug Des Devel Ther* 9:1913–1926.

Kilbane C, Ostrem J, Galifianakis N, Grace J, Markun L, Glass GA (2012). Multichannel electromyographic mapping to optimize onabotulinumtoxinA efficacy in cervical dystonia. *Tremor Other Hyperkinet Mov (NY)* 2.

Lew MF, Adornato BT, Duane DD, Dykstra DD, Factor SA, Massey JM, Brin MF, Jankovic J, Rodnitzky RL, Singer C, Swenson MR, Tarsy D, Murray JJ, Koller M, Wallace JD (1997). Botulinum toxin type B: a double-blind, placebo-controlled, safety and efficacy study in cervical dystonia. *Neurology* 49:701–707.

Misra VP, Ehler E, Zakine B, Maisonobe P, Simonetta-Moreau M; Interest in CD Group (2012). Factors influencing response to botulinum toxin type A in patients with idiopathic cervical dystonia: results from an international observational study. *BMJ Open* 14(2).

Mordin M, Masaquel C, Abbott C, Copley-Merriman C (2014). Factors affecting the health-related quality of life of patients with cervical dystonia and impact of treatment with abobotulinumtoxinA (Dysport): results from a randomised, double-blind, placebo-controlled study. *BMJ Open* 4:e005150.

Nijmeijer SW, Koelman JH, Kamphuis DJ, Tijssen MA (2012). Muscle selection for treatment of cervical dystonia with botulinum toxin: a systematic review. *Parkinsonism Relat Disord* 18:731–736.

Odergren T, Hjaltason H, Kaakkola S, Solders G, Hanko J, Fehling C, Marttila RJ, Lundh H, Gedin S, Westergren I, Richardson A, Dott C, Cohen H (1998). A double blind, randomised, parallel group study to investigate the dose equivalence of Dysport and Botox in the treatment of cervical dystonia. *J Neurol Neurosurg Psychiatry* 64:6–12.

Pappert EJ, Germanson T; Myobloc/Neurobloc European Cervical Dystonia Study (2008). Botulinum toxin type B vs. type A in toxin-naive patients with cervical dystonia: randomized, double-blind, noninferiority trial. *Mov Disord* 23: 510–517.

Patel N, Hanfelt J, Marsh L, Jankovic J; Members of the Dystonia Coalition (2014). Alleviating manoeuvres (sensory tricks) in cervical dystonia. *J Neurol Neurosurg Psychiatry* 85(8): 882–884.

Poewe W, Deuschl G, Nebe A, Feifel E, Wissel J, Benecke R, Kessler KR, Ceballos-Baumann AO, Ohly A, Oertel W, Künig G; German Dystonia Study Group (1998). What is the optimal dose of botulinum toxin A in the treatment of cervical dystonia? Results of a double blind, placebo controlled, dose ranging study using Dysport. *J Neurol Neurosurg Psychiatry* 64:13–17.

Ramirez-Castaneda J, Jankovic J (2014). Long-term efficacy, safety, and side effect profile of botulinum toxin in dystonia: a 20-year follow-up. *Toxicon* 90:344–348.

Ramirez-Castaneda J, Jankovic J, Comella C, Dashtipour K, Fernandez HH, Mari Z (2013). Diffusion, spread, and migration of botulinum toxin. *Mov Disord* 28:1775–1783.

Sankhla C, Jankovic J, Duane D (1998). Variability of the immunologic and clinical response in dystonic patients immunoresistant to botulinum toxin injections. *Mov Disord* 13:150–154.

Schramm A, Baumer T, Fietzek U, Heitmann S, Walter U, Jost WH (2015). Relevance of sonography for botulinum toxin treatment of cervical dystonia: an expert statement. *J Neural Transm* 122:1457–1463.

Sethi KD, Rodriguez R, Olayinka B (2012). Satisfaction with botulinum toxin treatment: a cross-sectional survey of patients with cervical dystonia. *J Med Econ* 15:419–423.

Simpson DM, Blitzer A, Brashear A, Comella C, Dubinsky R, Hallett M, Jankovic J, Karp B, Ludlow CL, Miyasaki JM, Naumann M, So Y; Therapeutics and Technology Assessment Subcommittee of the American Academy of Neurology (2008). Assessment: botulinum neurotoxin for the treatment of movement disorders (an evidence-based review) – report of the Therapeutics and Technology Assessment Subcommittee of the American Academy of Neurology. *Neurology* 70:1699–1706.

Simpson DM, Hallet M, Ashman, EJ, Cornella CL, Green MW, Gronseth GS, Armstrong MJ, Gloss D, Potrebic S, Jankovic J, Karp BP, Naumann M, So YT, Yablon SA (2016). Practice guideline update summary: botulinum neurotoxin for the treatment of blepharospasm, cervical dystonia, adult spasticity, and headache. Report of the Guidelines Development Subcommittee of the American Academy of Neurology. *Neurology* 86(19): 1818–1826.

Thenganatt MA, Fahn S (2012). Botulinum toxin for the treatment of movement disorders. *Curr Neurol Neurosci Rep* 12:399–409.

Thenganatt MA, Jankovic J (2014). Treatment of dystonia. *Neurotherapeutics* 11: 139–152.

Truong D, Duane DD, Jankovic J, Singer C, Seeberger LC, Comella CL, Lew MF, Rodnitzky RL, Danisi FO, Sutton JP, Charles PD, Hauser RA, Sheean GL (2005). Efficacy and safety of botulinum type A toxin (Dysport) in cervical dystonia: results of the first US randomized, double-blind, placebo-controlled study. *Mov Disord* 20:783–791.

Truong D, Brodsky M, Lew M, Brashear A, Jankovic J, Molho E, Orlova O, Timerbaeva S; Global Dysport Cervical Dystonia Study Group (2010). Long-term efficacy and safety of botulinum toxin type A (Dysport) in cervical dystonia. *Parkinsonism Relat Disord* 16:316–323.

Wu C, Xue F, Chang W, Lian Y, Zheng Y, Xie N, Zhang L, Chen C (2016). Botulinum toxin type A with or without needle electromyographic guidance in patients with cervical dystonia. *Springerplus* 8(5):1292.

Yun JY, Kim JW, Kim HT, Chung SJ, Kim JM, Cho JW, Lee JY, Lee HN, You S, Oh E, Jeong H, Kim YE, Kim HJ, Lee WY, Jeon BS (2015). Dysport and Botox at a ratio of 2.5:1 units in cervical dystonia: a double-blind, randomized study. *Mov Disord* 30:206–213.

Chapter 34

Botulinum Toxin Therapy for Cranial Dystonia

Karoline Wenzel and Carlo Colosimo

Introduction

Blepharospasm (BSP), oromandibular dystonia (OMD) and Meige syndrome (MS) are the most common subtypes of cranial dystonia. Botulinum toxin type A (BT-A) is regarded as the first-line treatment for these conditions. In this chapter the clinical presentation, evidence of treatment efficacy and injection techniques will be discussed.

Blepharospasm and Meige Syndrome

Clinical Presentation

BSP is a focal cranial dystonia characterised by chronic intermittent or persistent involuntary forceful contractions of the orbicularis oculi muscles leading to increased blinking or inappropriate eye closure. The prevalence of BSP is an estimated 5 per 100 000. It usually starts in the fifth to sixth decade and is more prevalent among females (Grandas et al. 1988). The most frequent presentation is an adult-onset idiopathic BSP also called 'essential blepharospasm', but it can also occur as a secondary symptom in neurodegenerative disorders, lesions in the basal ganglia or upper midbrain or as a tardive symptom after intake of neuroleptic drugs (Jankovic & Ford 1983; Grandas et al. 1988). Symptoms appear gradually. At onset patients complain about increased blinking, a feeling of a dry eye or foreign-body sensations and photophobia. The dystonic contractions of the orbicularis oculi muscles can be clonic or rhythmic or tonic and sustained. The latter may lead to functional blindness and thus to a marked reduction of quality of life. The symptoms are increased by stress, emotions, anxiety or by looking into bright light. They can often be relieved by sensory tricks (geste antagoniste) such as slightly touching the skin in the temporal regions or opening the eyelids with the fingers (Kraft & Lang 1988). As the symptoms can show wide variability, a psychiatric origin was often suspected in the past (Jankovic & Ford 1983). In the beginning, BSP can affect one eye only, but almost always it becomes bilateral, contrary to the unilateral hemifacial spasm, which is not considered a form of dystonia. Additional involuntary inhibition of the levator palpebrae superioris muscle, called 'apraxia of eyelid-opening' (ALO) or levator inhibition, is a variant of BSP. It can occur isolated or in combination with BSP. In this condition patients have difficulty initiating the act of lid elevation after lid closure (Goldstein & Cogan 1965). ALO is more common in women and in a variety of neurodegenerative diseases involving the frontal lobes, and its pathophysiology is still unclear. An underlying abnormality in the supranuclear control of voluntary eyelid opening requiring activation of the levator palpebrae superioris and concurrent inhibition of orbicularis oculi activity is assumed (Aramideh et al. 1994).

In 31 per cent of patients with BSP, dystonic movements spread to oromandibular regions, neck muscles or limbs. When the disorder spreads to the lower face it is called 'Meige syndrome' (Meige 1910). Female gender, old age or history of significant cranial trauma are risk factors for spreading. The risk is highest within the first two years after the event, whereas in other dystonic conditions it remains stable (Weiss et al. 2006). An Italian–US study identified genetic factors contributing to the spread of primary BSP. Patients carrying the T-allele of the rs1182 polymorphism of TOR1A were found to carry a higher risk for spreading as compared with the homozygous carriers of the common G-allele (Defazio et al. 2009). DYT6 testing is recommended in patients with generalised dystonia with craniocervical dystonia at onset (Albanese et al. 2011). The underlying pathophysiology of blepharospasm is not entirely clear. Neurophysiological and functional imaging studies suggest a combination of genetic susceptibility, loss of inhibition at various levels of the neuroaxis, abnormal plasticity and defect sensorimotor integration (Colosimo et al. 2010; Hellmann & Torres-Russotto 2015).

Conventional Treatment

BT-A has become the treatment of choice for BSP; however, other management strategies should also be considered. Oral medications include benzodiazepines such as clonazepam or $GABA_B$ drugs (baclofen), anticholinergics (trihexiphenidyl), dopamine depletors (tetrabenazine), clozapine or levodopa in dopamine-responsive dystonias. No Level A recommendation can be given for oral medications. Physical devices are sometimes considered useful: dark or tight glasses, glasses with a palpebral splint, bands across the lower forehead. Myotomy of the orbicularis oculi muscles has more or less been abandoned because of side-effects and recurrence of symptoms. Deep brain stimulation has shown to be effective in severe tardive blepharospasm and in primary generalised dystonias and is under investigation in focal dystonia (Hellmann & Torres-Russotto 2015).

Botulinum Toxin Therapy

In 1981, the American ophthalmologist Alan Scott was the first to use BT-A for treatment of strabismus. His findings were the beginning of clinical research and use in further indications including BSP (Scott et al. 1973). In 1989 BSP was the first indication approved by the US Food and Drug Administration (FDA). A recent literature review by Hallett et al. investigated the efficacy of botulinum toxin in movement disorders for the three botulinum toxin type A drugs onabotulinumtoxinA (Ona, Botox®, Allergan Inc.), abobotulinumtoxinA (Abo, Dysport®, Ipsen Ltd), incobotulinumtoxinA (Inco, Xeomin®, Merz Pharmaceuticals) and the only botulinum toxin type B (BT-B) drug rimabotulinumtoxinB (Rima, Myobloc®/Neurobloc®, US WorldMeds) (Hallett et al. 2013). The available evidence for the treatment of BSP supports a Level A recommendation for Inco based on one class I placebo-controlled trial (Jankovic et al. 2011) and two class I active-comparator trials (Roggenkamper et al. 2006; Wabbels et al. 2011). A Level A recommendation for Ona is given based on two class I active-comparator trials (Jankovic & Orman 1987; Girlanda et al. 1996), two class II placebo-controlled trials (Jankovic & Orman 1987; Girlanda et al. 1996) and one class II active-comparator trial (Nuessgen & Roggenkamper 1997). A Level B recommendation for Abo is based on two class II trials, one placebo-controlled (Truong et al. 2008) and one active-comparator trial (Nuessgens & Roggenkamper 1997). A Level U recommendation is given for Rima due to the lack of controlled studies. A few open-label, retrospective studies showed an effect with shorter duration, but with more spread and side-effects (Colosimo et al. 2003; Hallett et al. 2013). There are no data regarding optimal dosing for BT-A, therefore expert opinion recommendations are used (Brin et al. 2003). Long-term efficacy and safety have been demonstrated in several studies (Colosimo et al. 2012; Ramirez-Castaneda & Jankovic 2013).

All three botulinum toxin type A drugs – Ona, Abo and Inco – are approved by the FDA and European Medicines Agency (EMA) for the treatment of BSP. The botulinum toxin type B drug Rima is not licenced for the treatment of BSP in the United States and European Union. Side-effects are usually mild and transient. The following may occur: ptosis due to spread to the levator palpebrae muscle, a dry eye, eyelid oedema, haematomas, blurred or double vision, lagophthalmus with consecutive keratopathy, entropion and lower eyelid sagging due to injection too close to the lower central eyelid.

Injection Techniques

There is quite a lot of variability in injection techniques among botulinum toxin users concerning dosages, number of injections, sites or dilutions. In general, dose and injection sites should be chosen according to the severity of symptoms and started with a low dose into the orbital part of the orbicularis oculi muscles (Brin et al. 2003). We usually start with four injection sites medial and lateral into the superior palpebral, the lateral canthus and the inferior part of the orbicularis oculi (Figure 34.1). If needed, the injection sites in the orbicularis oculi can be increased to five, and other nearby facial muscles, including the corrugator, procerus, and frontalis, can also be targeted. To prevent ptosis an injection into the median part of the upper orbital part near the levator palpebrae should be avoided. Needle direction should therefore be positioned away from the centre of the eye. Injection of the medial lower lid can produce diplopia due to spread to the inferior oblique or inferior rectus muscle or dysfunction of the lacrimal duct. Low-dose injections of the pretarsal or preseptal part can be additionally helpful, especially in patients with ALO. The treatment should be performed with the patient in a lying position. He should be informed of the procedure and possible side-effects. Patients should document treatment effects and be prepared that symptoms will slowly worsen when the effect wears off. They should be made aware that this will make repeated injections necessary. Symptoms should be evaluated using an objective scale. Consecutive injections should be tailored based on efficacy or side-effects of the previous injection. After the first injection a re-assessment after three to four weeks might be helpful. Usually when the optimal dosage has been found the effects remain remarkably stable. Sterile 27–30 gauge (0.40–0.30 mm) needles should be used to avoid bruises. There are different special recommendations for initial treatment for the different available BT-A formulations:

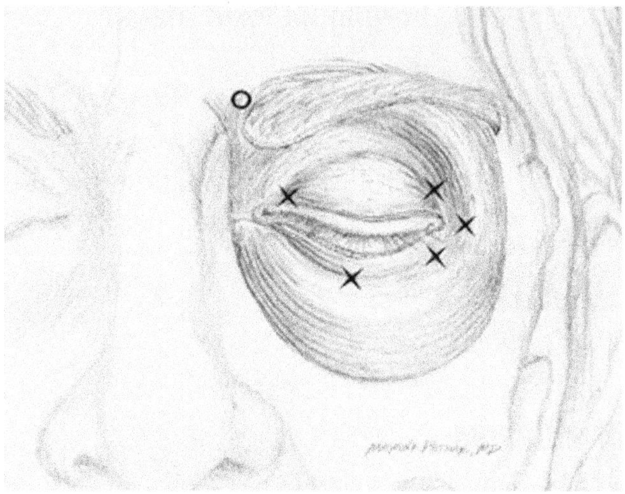

Figure 34.1 Injection points in patient with blepharospasm. X, onabotulinumtoxinA 5 U/abobotulinumtoxinA 20 U; O, onabotulinumtoxinA 2.5 U/abobotulinumtoxinA 10 U.

Ona: The dilution should be 100 MU in 2.0 ml normal saline (5 MU in 0.1 ml). The initial dose should be 1.25–2.5 MU per injection site. The total dose should not be more than 25 MU per eye. A total dose of 100 MU during consecutive injections should not be exceeded.

Abo: The dilution should be 500 MU in 2.5 ml normal saline (20 MU in 0.1 ml). The initial dose should be 40 MU per eye. Higher doses such as 60–80 MU might be necessary for consecutive injections. A total of 120 MU should not be exceeded.

Inco: The dilution should be 100 MU in 2.0 ml normal saline (5 MU in 0.1 ml). The initial dose should be 1.25–2.5 MU per injection site. The total dose should not be more than 25 MU per eye. A total dose of 100 MU during consecutive injections should not be exceeded.

Oromandibular Dystonia

Clinical Presentation

Oromandibular dystonia is characterised by involuntary spasms of the masticatory, lingual and pharyngeal muscles that can be action-induced, tonic or clonic. The spasms can lead to painful jaw-deviation, jaw-opening or jaw-closing, bruxism or temporomandibular joint subluxation, dysphagia, dysarthria or involuntary tongue movements (Thompson et al. 1986; Brin et al. 2003). The quality of life is reduced because of impaired function while eating, swallowing and speaking, as well as social stigma (Colosimo et al. 2010). Symptoms can often, as is typical for all focal dystonias, be alleviated by voluntary actions such as opening of the mouth, singing or yawning (Albanese et al. 2011). Isolated or mainly lingual forms are observed in neurodegenerative diseases such as neuroacanthocythosis, Lesch–Nyhan syndrome or panthothenate kinase-associated neurodegeneration (Schneider et al. 2006). The aetiology is similar to BSP or other focal or segmental dystonia, but tardive cases, which are predominantly confined to the oromandibular region, are relatively common. Differential diagnoses include temporomandibular joint diseases, paroxysmal masticatory spasms occurring in multiple sclerosis or hemifacial atrophy or masticatory pain syndromes (Thompson et al. 1986). Bruxism may be a variant of dystonia or can be caused by several other aetiologies (drugs, Rett's syndrome, cerebellar damage, Whipple's disease and others) (Brin et al. 2003). A recent retrospective study including 27 patients with OMD showed a female preponderance, beginning in the sixth decade, often in association with specific occupations (speaking loudly in public). Occurrence in patients with cerebellar lesions or essential tremor suggests an involvement of cerebellar structures. There are different clinical subtypes: most common are the jaw-opening and jaw-closing variants, followed but markedly less frequent by jaw-deviation or jaw-protrusion dystonias. OMDs responding to sensory tricks are more prone to respond also to dental prosthesis. The jaw-closing type seemed to respond better to botulinum toxin than the jaw-opening type (Gonzalez-Alegre et al. 2014).

Botulinum Toxin Therapy

One class II trial with eight patients supports a Level C recommendation for the treatment of OMD with Ona. Subjective ratings showed an improvement of symptoms severity and pain (Jankovic & Orman 1987). Abo showed significant reduction of bruxism in 12 patients in a placebo-controlled study using nocturnal electromyography of the masseter and temporal muscle (Lee et al. 2010). For Inco or Rima there are no controlled or randomised studies published, resulting in a Level U recommendation (Hallett et al. 2013). These studies showed good clinical efficacy and tolerability, but there is still a lack of larger controlled studies. No data are available for oral medications. Long-term electrical stimulation of the globus pallidus internus has shown an improvement of 72 per cent on dystonia rating scales in six patients with MS. The efficacy in secondary dystonia except in tardive dystonia is less than in primary dystonia (Albanese et al. 2011).

Injection Technique

Sufficient knowledge of the anatomy and function of the masticatory muscles is mandatory and evaluation through a temporomandibular joint specialist might be helpful. Selection of muscles is made according to the clinical pattern. The most common target muscles are the masseter, temporal and internal, and external pterygoid muscles. Also the digastric and rarely the base-of-tongue muscles are options. As muscles are difficult to palpate and accurate needle placement can avoid dysphagia, EMG – and recently also ultrasound – guidance is recommended. The external pterygoid muscles can be injected via a percutaneous or intraoral approach. When using the intraoral approach the full length of the muscle can be reached; percutaneously, in contrast, there is access only to one point perpendicular to the muscle. Injecting too medially can cause dysphagia, rhinolalia, nasal regurgitation and Eustachian tube dysfunction. Other rare side-effects are haematomas and xerostomia. The internal pterygoid muscle can be reached from the mandibular angle, while taking precautions as the injection into lingual muscles should be avoided (Brin et al. 2003; Mendes & Upton 2009). Long-term treatment has been shown to be safe and effective. Side-effects, consisting mostly of dysphagia or dysarthria, are uncommon and particularly rare in the treatment of jaw-closing dystonias (Tan & Jankovic 1999). Initially the most affected muscle should be injected. Treatment should be started with a small dose of BT-A, slowly increasing in subsequent injections when needed. Dilution is usually 100 MU in 2.0 ml normal saline (5 MU in 0.1 ml) for Ona and should be the same for Inco; 500 MU in 2.5 ml normal saline (20 MU in 0.1 ml) for Abo. For the masseter or temporal muscle, 15–50 MU Ona, respectively 60–200 MU Abo divided into four injection sites per muscle is recommended. For the internal pterygoid muscle, 5–40 MU Ona, 20–160 MU Abo in two injection sites; for the external pterygoid 10–20 MU Ona, 40–160 MU Abo in three injection sites; and for the anterior belly of the digastric muscle 2.5–20 MU Ona, 10–30 MU Abo in two sites are used. Tongue thrusting may be associated with jaw-opening and jaw-deviation OMD, mainly resulting from the action of the posterior fibres of the genioglossus muscle. The treatment of lingual dystonia is much debated among experts, but when performed at all then only very cautiously as the amount of BT-A that may be used is limited by the need to preserve functional activity of the patient.

Jaw-Closing Type

In jaw-closing dystonia the best treatment results are seen after bilateral BT injections of the masseter and temporal muscles (Figure 34.2). These injections may easily be performed according to anatomical landmarks. The internal pterygoid muscle might be injected additionally when needed (Figure 34.3).

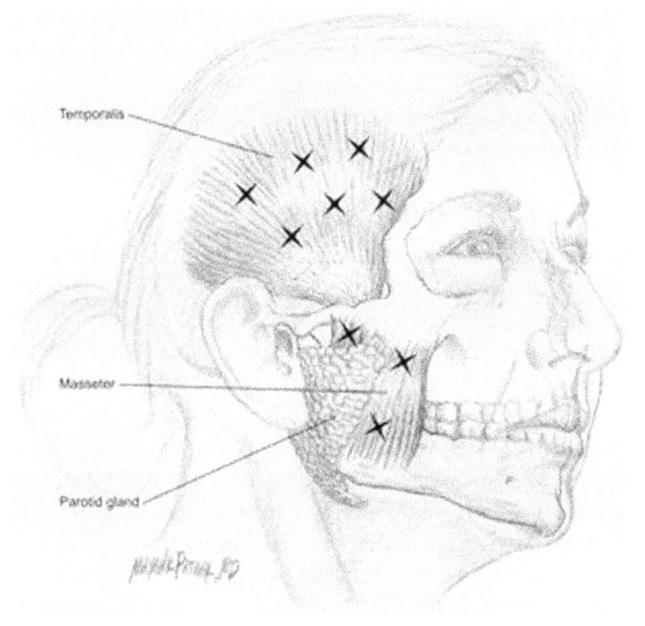

Figure 34.2 The masseter and temporalis muscles.

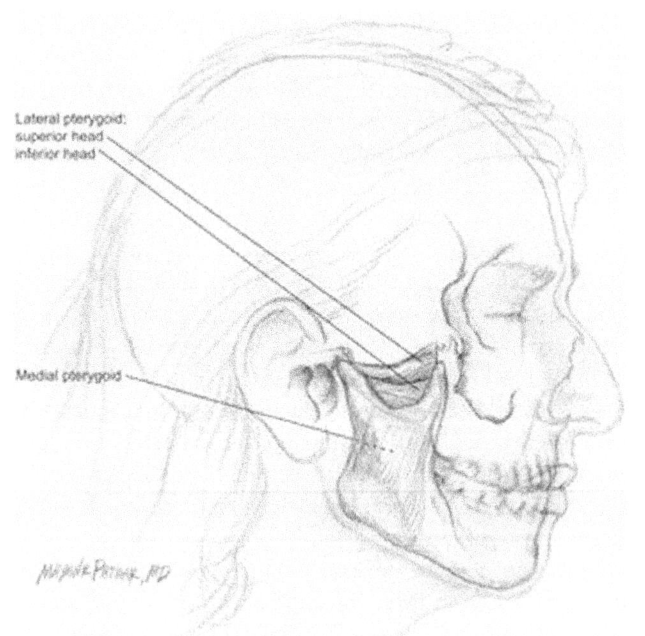

Figure 34.3 The pterygoid muscle.

Jaw-Opening Type

External pterygoid muscles (Figure 34.3) and/or the anterior belly of the digastric muscles can be injected. EMG guidance is recommended for better targeting the respective muscles, thus helping to reduce the dysphagia risk.

Jaw Deviation and Protrusion Type

To treat jaw deviation, the contralateral external pterygoid muscle can be injected. For protrusion, both external pterygoid muscles are targeted. Bilateral injections are also applied in mixed types with an application of a larger dose into the contralateral external pterygoid muscle.

References

Albanese A, Asmus F, Bhatia KP, Elia AE, Elibol B, Filippini G, Gasser T, Krauss JK, Nardocci N, Newton A, Valls-Solé J (2011). EFNS guidelines on diagnosis and treatment of primary dystonias. *Eur J Neurol* 18:5–18.

Aramideh M, Bour LJ, Koelman JH, Speelman JD, Ongerboer de Visser BW (1994). Abnormal eye movements in blepharospasm and involuntary levator palpebrae inhibition: clinical and pathophysiological considerations. *Brain* 117:1457–1474.

Brin M, Danisio F, Blitzer A (2003). Blephaospasm, oromandibular dystonia, Meige's syndrome and hemifacial spasm. In: Moore AP, Naumann M (eds) *Handbook of Botulinum Toxin Treatment*. Oxford: Blackwell Scientific.

Colosimo C, Chianese M, Contarino F, Giovannelli M, Bentivoglio AR (2003). Botulinum toxin type B in blepharospasm and hemifacial spasm. *J Neurol, Neurosurg Psychiatry* 74:687.

Colosimo C, Suppa A, Fabbrini G, Bologna M, Berardelli A (2010). Craniocervical dystonia: clinical and pathophysiological features. *Eur J Neurol* 17 (Suppl. 1):15–21.

Colosimo C, Tiple D, Berardelli A (2012). Efficacy and safety of long-term botulinum toxin treatment in craniocervical dystonia: a systematic review. *Neurotox Res* 22:265–273.

Defazio G, Matarin M, Peckham EL, Peckham EL, Martino D, Valente EM, Singleton A, Crawley A, Aniello MS, Brancati F, Abbruzzese G, Girlanda P, Livrea P, Hallett M, Berardelli A (2009). The TOR1A polymorphism rs1182 and the risk of spread in primary blepharospasm. *Mov Disord* 24(4):613–616.

Girlanda P, Quartarone A, Sinicropi S, Nicolosi C, Messina C (1996). Unilateral injection of botulinum toxin in blepharospasm: single fiber electromyography and blink reflex study. *Mov Disord* 11:27–31.

Goldstein JE, Cogan DG (1965). Apraxia of lid opening. *Arch Ophthalmol* 73:155–159.

Gonzalez-Alegre P, Schneider RL, Hoffman H (2014). Clinical, etiological, and therapeutic features of jaw-opening and jaw-closing oromandibular dystonias: a decade of experience at a single treatment center. *Tremor Other Hyperkinet Mov (NY)* 30(4):231.

Grandas F, Elston J, Quinn N, Marsden CD (1988). Blepharospasm: a review of 264 patients. *J Neurol Neurosurg Psychiatry* 51:767–772.

Hallett M, Albanese A, Dressler D, Segal KR, Simpson DM, Truong D, Jankovic J (2013). Evidence-based review and assessment of botulinum neurotoxin for the treatment of movement disorders. *Toxicon* 67:94–114.

Hellman A, Torres-Russotto D (2015). Botulinum toxin in the management of blepharospasm: current evidence and recent developments. *Ther Adv Neurol Disord* 8(2):82–91.

Jankovic J, Ford J (1983). Blepharospasm and orofacial-cervical dystonia: clinical and pharmacological findings in 100 patients. *Ann Neurol* 13:402–411.

Jankovic J, Orman J (1987). Botulinum A toxin for cranial-cervical dystonia: a double-blind, placebo-controlled study. *Neurology* 37:616–623.

Jankovic J, Comella C, Hanschmann A, Grafe S (2011). Efficacy and safety of incobotulinumtoxinA (NT 201, Xeomin) in the treatment of blepharospasm: a randomized trial. *Mov Disord* 26:1521–1528.

Kraft SP, Lang AE (1988). Cranial dystonia, blepharospasm and hemifacial spasm: clinical features and treatment, including the use of botulinum toxin. *CMAJ* 139:837–844.

Lee SJ, McCall WD Jr, Kim YK (2010). Effect of botulinum toxin injection on nocturnal bruxism: a randomized controlled trial. *Am J Phys Med Rehabil* 89:16–23.

Meige H (1910). Les convulsions de la face: une forme clinique de convulsions faciales, bilaterales et mediane. *Rev Neurol (Paris)* 21:437–443.

Mendes RA, Upton LG (2009). Management of dystonia of the lateral pterygoid muscle with botulinum toxin A. *Br J Oral Maxillofac Surg* 47:481–483.

Nuessgens Z, Roggenkamper P (1997). Comparison of two botulinum-toxin preparations in the treatment of essential blepharospasm. *Graefes Arch Clin Exp Ophthalmo* 235:197–199.

Ramirez-Castaneda J, Jankovic J (2013). Long-term efficacy and safety of botulinum toxin injections in dystonia. *Toxins* 5:249–266.

Roggenkamper P, Jost WH, Bihari K, Comes G, Grafe S; NT 201 Blepharospasm Study Team (2006). Efficacy and safety of a new botulinum toxin type A free of complexing proteins in the treatment of blepharospasm. *J Neural Transm* 113:303–312.

Schneider SA, Aggarwal A, Bhatt M, Dupont E, Tisch S, Limousin P, Lee P, Quinn N, Bhatia KP (2006). Severe tongue protrusion dystonia: clinical syndromes and possible treatment. *Neurology* 26(67):940–943.

Scott AB, Rosenbaum A, Collins CC (1973). Pharmacologic weakening of extraocular muscles. *Invest Ophthalmol Vis Sci* 12:924–927.

Tan EK, Jankovic J (1999). Botulinum toxin A in patients with oromandibular dystonia: long-term follow-up. *Neurology* 53:2102–2107.

Thompson PD, Obeso JA, Delgado G, Gallego J, Marsden CD (1986). Focal dystonia of the jaw and the differential diagnosis of unilateral jaw and masticatory spasm. *J Neurol Neurosurg Psychiatry* 49:651–656.

Truong D, Comella C, Fernandez HH, Ondo WG; Dysport Benign Essential Blepharospasm Study Group (2008). Efficacy and safety of purified botulinum toxin type A (Dysport) for the treatment of benign essential blepharospasm: a randomized, placebo-controlled, phase II trial. *Parkinsonism Relat Disord* 14:407–414.

Wabbels B, Reichel G, Fulford-Smith A, Wright N, Roggenkämper P (2011). Double-blind, randomised, parallel group pilot study comparing two botulinum toxin type A products for the treatment of blepharospasm. *J Neural Transm* 11:233–239.

Weiss EM, Hershey T, Karimi M, Racette B, Tabbal SD, Mink JW, Paniello RC, Perlmutter JS (2006). Relative risk of spread of symptoms among the focal onset primary dystonias. *Mov Disord* 21:1175–1181.

Chapter 35

Botulinum Toxin Therapy for Spasmodic Dysphonia

Christopher Tang and Andrew Blitzer

Introduction

Spasmodic dysphonia (SD) is considered a focal laryngeal dystonia in which a patient experiences inappropriate functionally specific laryngeal muscular contractions, usually during speech. The most common form, adductor spasmodic dysphonia, produces inappropriate muscle contraction causing excessive glottal closure and a strained and strangled speech pattern. Abductor spasmodic dysphonia is less common, and results in a persistently open glottal configuration with breathy breaks or a whispering speaking pattern. Although the task specificity for focal laryngeal dystonia has been observed mostly for speech, there is a low incidence of adductor breathing dystonia that may produce inspiratory stridor, and a variety occurring during singing. The aetiology of laryngeal dystonia falls into the same categories as forms affecting other areas of the body. Drug-induced glottic dystonic reactions have been described as causing acute upper airway obstruction necessitating intubation (Newton-John 1988; Warren & Thompson 1998).

The gold standard of treatment for laryngeal dystonia is EMG-guided botulinum toxin injections into the affected musculature. Medications may also ameliorate symptoms, but rarely have a significant impact. Multiple surgical interventions have been performed, many of which have fallen out of favour as recidivism is seen over time. Selective denervation–reinnervation procedures have shown promising preliminary data, but long-term results are still to be evaluated.

Background

Spasmodic dysphonia was first described by Traube in 1871, within a treatise detailing the effects of typhus on the larynx (Traube 1871). Critchley provided a similar description in 1939: 'there results a peculiarly forced character in the speech, which appears difficult of accomplishment, almost as though the patient were trying to talk whilst being choked' (Critchley 1939). Aronson et al. (1968) reviewed SD and other hyperfunctional voice disorders in detail and proposed this symptom complex could arise from a neurologic aetiology. Dedo (1976) reported a dramatic and immediate normalisation of voice among individuals after transection of the recurrent laryngeal nerve (RLN), further suggesting an organic cause. Abnormalities in autonomic function (Schaefer et al. 1983) and abnormal V-wave latencies from brainstem auditory-evoked potential (BAEP) testing (Finitzo-Hieber et al. 1982; Schaefer 1983; Feldman 1984) implied a central defect, further supported by the lack of consistent abnormalities in histologic studies of the RLN (Ravits et al. 1979; Carlsoo et al. 1987) and intrinsic laryngeal muscles (Chhetri et al. 2003). Functional studies with electromyography (EMG) show that electrical patterns during whispering and non-speech tasks were not different between affected individuals and normal controls (Roark et al. 1995); during speech, if aphonic intervals were excluded, electrical patterns were otherwise normal (Van Pelt et al. 1994). In general, neuroimaging studies have failed to identify consistent anatomic abnormalities among individuals with SD (Schaefer et al. 1985; Aronson & Lagerlund 1991).

In 1980, Jacome and Yanez (Jacome & Yanez 1980) postulated that SD was a disorder of the extrapyramidal system, based on the frequent coexistence with other cranial dystonias and tremor, and the lack of morphometric abnormalities of the RLN in these patients. Marsden and Sheehy noted the frequent coexistence of SD with Meige disease and classified cases of SD as examples of isolated focal laryngeal dystonia (Marsden & Sheehy 1982). Blitzer et al. reviewed EMGs of the laryngeal musculature in focal and generalised dystonia, further supporting SD as a focal dystonia (Blitzer et al. 1985).

Epidemiology

Blitzer et al. (1998) published one of the largest studies of SD in 1998, reviewing a 12-year experience of 901 cases of laryngeal dystonia treated with injections of botulinum toxin. Of these cases, 70 per cent were isolated to laryngeal involvement and the remainder with either segmental cranial or generalised dystonia. The majority (82.5 per cent) were classified as primary dystonia. There was a 63 per cent female preponderance and 12 per cent had a family history of dystonia. In this group, 82 per cent were of the adductor type, 17 per cent of the abductor type and 1 per cent had adductor-breathing dystonia. The average age of onset was 39 years. Of patients with primary laryngeal involvement, 14–16 per cent (Blitzer et al. 1998) had eventual spread to other areas of the body; therefore patients with laryngeal dystonia should be examined on a regular basis.

Diagnosis

The diagnosis of SD relies on clinical history, voice analysis and physical exam, including flexible fibreoptic laryngoscopy. Spasmodic dysphonia is a chronic adult-onset disorder, although some children with generalised dystonia may have laryngeal involvement. Patients often first notice their symptoms after an illness, during a period of increased stress, or during a public-speaking exercise. Some individuals describe a gradual onset, with symptoms noted only during periods of stress or increased speaking demands; others describe a sudden occurrence which may be related to an illness or life event. Individuals usually report that singing, laughing, yelling, crying and falsetto are relatively spared. Coughing and swallowing, along with other vegetative laryngeal tasks, are preserved. Vocal tremor is frequently coexistent (Meyer & Blitzer 2006).

Vocal characteristics vary depending on the type of SD. Patients with adductor SD have a characteristic strained, strangled, effortful speech, often with vocal breaks and frequency shifts. There is often a reduction in loudness and prosody. These individuals have spasmodic hyperadduction during tasks in which the vocal folds are already adducted to create voiced sounds such as vowels. Therefore, instead of creating the appropriate degree of glottic closure to allow controlled airflow past the vocal folds, creating vocal fold vibration and consequently sound, the larynx squeezes shut, completely interrupting the airflow through the glottis and thereby precluding sound formation. These patients will have difficulty with sentences containing a predominance of voiced consonants and vowels such as 'We mow our lawn all year' or counting from 80 to 90 (Meyer & Blitzer 2006).

Patients with abductor SD have a breathy, though still effortful, voice quality with aphonic whispered segments. These are particularly marked when attempting to phonate a vowel after a voiceless consonant such as /p/, /f/, /t/, /s/, /d/, /k/ or /h/. During the voiceless consonant, the cords are held apart so that no vocal cord vibration is created and the sound is thereby formed, not at the glottic level, but rather at the lips (/p/,/f/), tongue/teeth (/t/, /s/, /d/, /k/) or oropharynx (/h/). To experience the difference between voiceless and voiced sounds, try saying a prolonged /f/ and then transitioning to a /v/. The oral cavity, tongue and pharyngeal articulators are held in the same position with the two sounds, but when transitioning from /f/ to /v/, the glottis is engaged to add phonation. The same can be experienced when transitioning from /s/ to /z/. Abductor SD patients have hyper**ab**duction of the vocal folds during the voiceless consonant and then have trouble overcoming this opening spasm to bring the folds together to create a voiced vowel sound. Examples of sentences that these individuals have particular difficulty with are: 'Harry's happy hat', 'The pretty puppy bit the tape', or 'Taxi' (Meyer & Blitzer 2006).

Some individuals with SD exhibit compensatory behaviour in an effort to overcome their spasms. This is most common in adductor SD in which individuals will exhibit compensatory abduction, producing a breathy voice by whispering or incomplete contraction of the vocal folds. Compensatory adduction in abductor dysphonia is rare. These behaviours can create diagnostic confusion with functional voice disorders such as muscle tension dysphonia in which there is no neurologic defect and often responds to speech therapy and psychological counselling (Meyer & Blitzer 2006). In an effort to find better diagnostic markers, Sapienza et al. performed acoustic analysis of ten patients with SD compared to ten patients with muscle tension dysphonia and found voice breaks only in the SD group (Sapienza et al. 2000).

On flexible fibreoptic laryngeal exam the patient should have normal anatomy with no evidence of extreme inflammatory mucosal disease. In general the patient should exhibit a normal glottic aperture and movement with vegetative laryngeal tasks such as sniffing, coughing and swallowing. The patient is then asked to perform eliciting speech tasks as described above. For adductor SD the patients will have excessive glottal closure with false vocal fold approximation. For abductor SD, the patient will have hyperabduction of the vocal folds with the appearance of a delay in closure of the vocal fold or 'hanging' of the arytenoid with speech tasks. Patients with adductor breathing dystonia will have vocal fold adduction with inspiration and with sniffing manoeuvres, but this will not affect speech or swallowing (Meyer & Blitzer 2006).

It is strongly suggested that all patients exhibiting signs and symptoms of spasmodic dystonia be evaluated by both a neurologist and an otolaryngologist with an interest or specialisation in movement disorders to confirm the diagnosis, exclude other body part involvement, examine for additional neurological signs or symptoms, and discover causative disorders (e.g. Wilson's disease, multiple sclerosis, storage diseases) if it exists. Sixty per cent of spasmodic dysphonia is idiopathic (Meyer & Blitzer 2006).

Treatments

Botulinum Toxin

Trans-cutaneous EMG-guided injection of botulinum toxin is the gold standard for the treatment of SD (Figure 35.1). Most individuals will report an excellent effect, and it can temporarily restore the voice to near-normal with both a reduction in voice breaks and effort required for speaking. The specific adductor or abductor muscle groups responsible can be targeted and the dose can be titrated to produce just enough weakness to relieve spasm in target muscles without causing unnecessary weakness in neighbouring muscles, resulting in dysphagia, prolonged breathiness (adductor), or airway compromise (abductor). Rarely is the dose high enough to cause frank paralysis of the targeted muscle group (Meyer & Blitzer 2006).

The thyroarytenoid or lateral cricoarytenoid are usually targeted for adductor SD. If a too-high dose is given, the patient may experience excessive breathiness from an inability to fully adduct the vocal folds, or dysphagia from diffusion of toxin to the pharyngeal constrictors. Our initial dose is 1 unit bilaterally, which can be titrated up or down depending on each individual's response weighed against their side-effect profile. Some patients are remarkably sensitive and we have successfully used doses of less than 0.1 units to achieve spasm amelioration. Some patients do well with a higher dose given unilaterally, alternating the side and decreasing the injection interval. In especially refractory patients, injection of supraglottic musculature, the cricothyroid (Bielamowicz 2002) or the interarytenoideus has shown success (Hillel 2004).

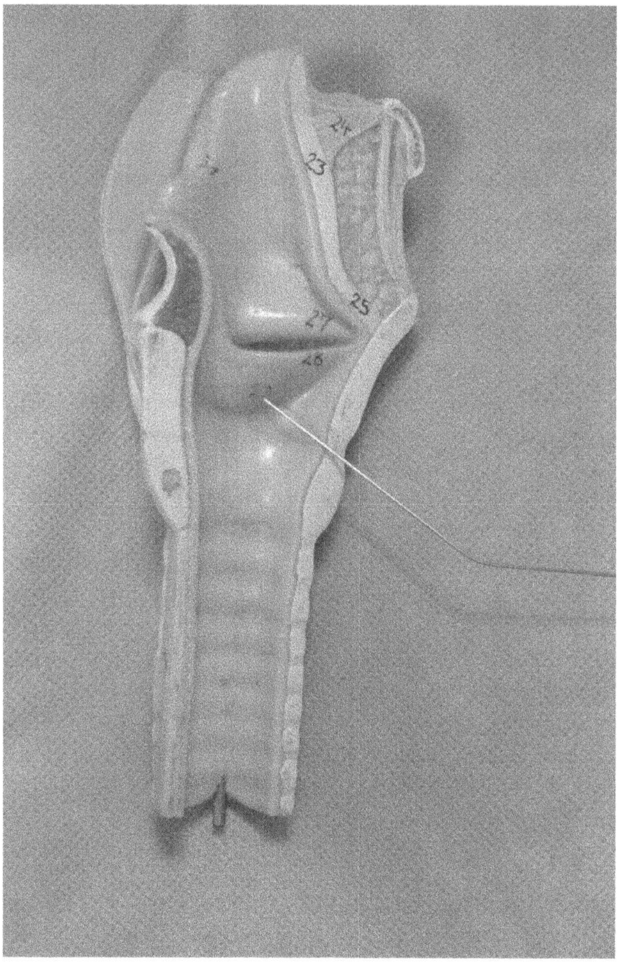

Figure 35.1 Trans-cutaneous laryngeal injection of botulinum toxin. Under EMG guidance to confirm the location of the muscle, a needle is inserted through the cricothyroid membrane into the thyroarytenoid muscle. A positive signal can be detected when the patient adducts the cords to phonate. From sagittal cut of plastic model: 23 – epiglottic cartilage, 24 – thyroepiglottic ligament, 25 – petiole, 27 – false vocal cord, 28 – true vocal cord, 29 – thyroarytenoid muscle.

The posterior cricoarytenoid muscle is targeted for abductor SD. Although there are differences in technique, most authors favour doses only unilaterally during a session since bilateral abductor weakness can lead to stridor and airway obstruction requiring tracheotomy. All patients are evaluated with flexible fibreoptic exam prior to any injection to determine which cord has the strongest abductor spasms and to verify an adequate glottic aperture. The usual starting dose is 3.75 units unilaterally. If abductor spasms are satisfactorily ameliorated the patient can return in two weeks for re-evaluation, at which time a booster can be given to the original side, or a carefully planned dose can be given to the contralateral side. Individuals requiring injection of bilateral posterior cricoarytenoid muscles for speech benefit may be treated in a staggered fashion at two-week intervals, always evaluating the airway endoscopically prior to injection to assure an adequate glottal aperture (Meyer & Blitzer 2006).

Excellent results from adductor SD toxin injections are well accepted. In a series (Blitzer et al. 1998) of 901 patients treated over 12 years evaluating 6280 injection sessions, the average dose was 1 unit bilaterally, producing an effect in 2.4 days and achieving a rate of nearly 90 per cent of normal function (37 per cent average improvement) lasting 15 weeks. Mild breathiness occurred in 35 per cent of patients lasting for less than one week and 15 per cent described mild coughing when drinking fluids (Meyer & Blitzer 2006).

In the same series, abductor SD was successfully treated with staggered injections to the PCA muscle in 80 per cent and unilateral injections in 20 per cent. The average dose was 3.2 units to one side and 0.6–2.5 units to the contralateral side two weeks later. The effect lasted 10.5 weeks and achieved a rate of 70 per cent of normal function (43 per cent average improvement). Because these patients did not achieve the same degree of voice normalisation, 30 per cent received additional systemic agents including clonazepam, trihexiphenidyl or baclofen (Meyer & Blitzer 2006).

Novakovic et al. examined the longitudinal functional effects of botulinum toxin injections with individuated dosing for SD and quality of life using a patient-specific dosing regimen. Out of 133 patients with 1457 patient-specific treatments, there was a mean Voice Handicap Index improvement of 9.6 per cent, which correlated with a mean overall improvement of 30.3 per cent of normal (percentage of normal function scale). With an individuated dosing regimen, 28.5 per cent of treatments (not patients) had an initial functional decline, which was designated as a type 2 curve (see Figure 35.2b), while those that did not have a functional decline were designated as a type 1 curve (see Figure 35.2a). In the 28.5 per cent of treatments that had a functional decline, the period of decline lasted 5.7 per cent of the treatment cycle followed by improvement of voice function to an optimal plateau that lasted 42.5 per cent of the treatment cycle, followed by functional decline back down to baseline (Figure 35.2). According to the paper, 'An individuated dosing regimen helps minimize side effects and maximize functional and quality-of-life outcomes' (Novakovic et al. 2011).

There is some thought that individual patients may develop antibodies to botulinum toxin type A over a period of time. Atassi et al. describe in several articles the binding regions where auto-antibodies bind to the light and heavy chain of the Botox toxin and the mechanism of immunogenicity (Atassi 2009; Atassi et al. 2011). Atassi showed in his studies that immunoresistance to toxin therapy can appear in some patients after a few injections with the toxin (Atassi 2004). Laryngeal secondary non-response is very rare for laryngeal dystonias, perhaps because of the small doses utilised during botulinum toxin injections for treatment. A forehead test can be performed by injecting roughly 10 units into the frontalis and observing for effect within a week.

For this reason, if subjects do not demonstrate good response with botulinum toxin type A, a trial of botulinum toxin type B should be considered (Adler et al. 2004). The relative toxin potencies are a bit different, with dose ratio being approximately 52.3:1 (Myobloc units:Botox units) with a more rapid onset of two days, benefit of ten weeks (compared to 17 with Botox), and a more abrupt end (Blitzer 2005).

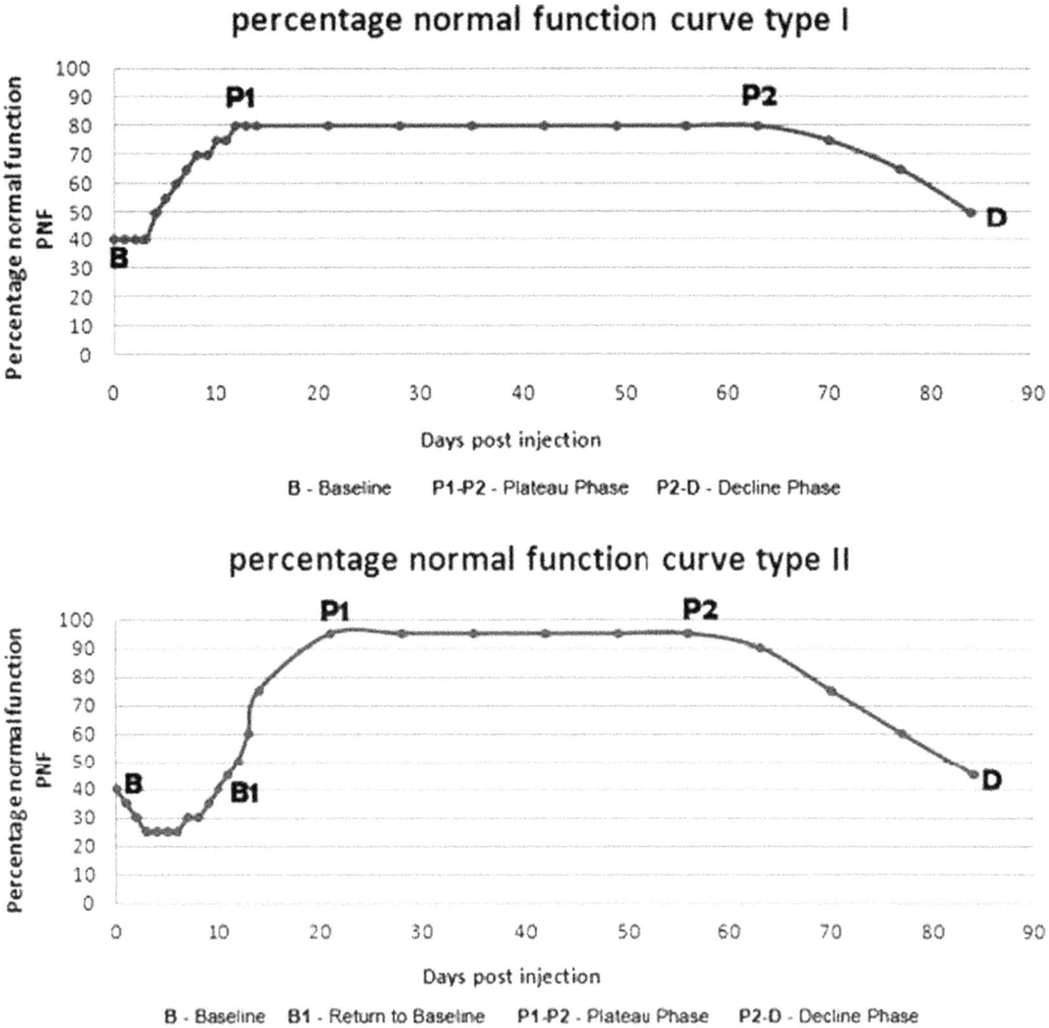

Figure 35.2 Percentage of normal function over time after botulinum toxin injection for spasmodic dysphonia. (a) Percentage of normal function curve type 1: out of all treatments given, 71.5 per cent did not have any functional decline. (b) Percentage of normal function curve type 2: out of all treatments given, 28.5 per cent had a functional decline that lasted on average 5.7 per cent of the treatment cycle.

Source: Novakovic et al. (2011).

Oral Medications and Voice Therapy

Oral medications such as muscle relaxants, anxiolytics, anticholinergic drugs or beta-blockers are usually not effective as primary therapy, but may be useful as an adjunct or agent to prolong the duration of improvement from botulinum toxin injection. Voice therapy is generally unsuccessful as a sole treatment, although may be essential for diagnosis and prevention of unwanted compensatory patterns. Use of breath support strategies and easy onset phonation may prolong the duration of benefit from toxin in patients with adductor SD (Murry & Woodson 1995).

Surgery

The first surgical therapy for adductor SD was the RLN section by Dedo, first reported in 1976 (Dedo 1976). Initially, patients demonstrated a dramatic normalisation of vocalisation, although over time a failure rate of up to 64 per cent was noted (Aronson & De Santo 1983). Overcompensation of the normal cord with central exaggeration of the dystonic symptoms was implicated as the cause of recurrent spasms and thinning of the vocal fold with lasers was used as salvage (Dedo & Izdebski 1984), although with only temporary success. Neural regeneration was discovered during re-exploration (Netterville 1991), but even with subsequent avulsion of a segment of the recurrent nerve, significant recidivism was seen over long-term follow-up (Weed 1996).

Several procedures designed to mechanically relax the vocal folds through alterations in the laryngeal framework have been attempted (Tucker 1989; Isshiki et al. 2004). Although successful in isolated centres, the results are not widely reproducible and have not gained general acceptance.

In 1999, Berke et al. developed a selective adductor denervation–reinnervation surgery which has shown promising preliminary results (Berke et al. 1999). Postoperatively all patients can expect 3–6 months of moderate breathiness, and 10 per cent experience temporary aspiration. Because this procedure creates a permanent alteration in laryngeal function and significant short-term vocal dysfunction, it should only be performed in patients with relatively severe symptoms. Long-term follow-up needs to be evaluated before the true efficacy of these procedures can be determined.

Conclusions

Spasmodic dysphonia is classified as a focal laryngeal dystonia. To date the majority of interventions are targeted at the end organ and provide only symptomatic control. The central nervous system eventually adapts to the change created in the neural inputs by these interventions and returns to sending out an inappropriate signal to the involved muscles. Future developments will hopefully target the central nervous system through medical or surgical means in hope of a durable cure.

References

Adler CH, Bansberg SF, Krein-Jones K, Hentz JG. 2004. Safety and efficacy of botulinum toxin type B (Myobloc) in adductor spasmodic dysphonia. *Mov Disord* 19(9): 1075–1079.

Aronson AE, De Santo LW. 1983. Adductor spastic dysphonia: three years after recurrent laryngeal nerve resection. *Laryngoscope* 93(1): 1–8.

Aronson AE, Lagerlund TD. 1991. Neuroimaging studies do not prove the existence of brain abnormalities in spastic (spasmodic) dysphonia. *J Speech Hear Res* 34(4): 801–811.

Aronson AE, Brown JR, Litin EM, Pearson JS. 1968. Spastic dysphonia: I. Voice, neurologic, and psychiatric aspects. *J Speech Hear Disord* 33(3): 203–218.

Atassi MZ. 2004. Basic immunological aspects of botulinum toxin therapy. *Mov Disord* 19(Suppl. 8): S68–S84.

Atassi MZ. 2009. Immune recognition of BoNTs A and B: how anti-toxin antibodies that bind to the heavy chain obstruct toxin action. *Toxicon* 54(5):600–613.

Atassi MS, Dolimbek BZ, Jankovic J, Steward LE, Aoki KR. 2011. Regions of botulinum neurotoxin A light chain recognized by human anti-toxin antibodies from cervical dystonia patients immunoresistant to toxin treatment: the antigenic structure of the active toxin recognized by human antibodies. *Immunobiology* 216(7):782–792.

Berke GS, Blackwell KE, Gerratt BR, Verneil A, Jackson KS, Sercarz JA. 1999. Selective laryngeal adductor denervation-reinnervation: a new surgical treatment for adductor spasmodic dysphonia. *Ann Otol Rhinol Laryngol* 108(3): 227–231.

Bielamowicz S, Stager SV, Badillo A. Godlewski A. 2002. Unilateral versus bilateral injections of botulinum toxin in patients with adductor spasmodic dysphonia. *J Voice* 16(1): 117–123.

Blitzer A. 2005. Botulinum toxin A and B: a comparative dosing study for spasmodic dysphonia. *Otolaryngol Head Neck Surg* 133(6): 836–838.

Blitzer A, Lovelace RE, Brin MF, Fahn S, Fink ME. 1985. Electromyographic findings in focal laryngeal dystonia (spastic dysphonia). *Ann Otol Rhinol Laryngol* 94(6 Pt 1): 591–594.

Blitzer A, Brin MF, Stewart CF. 1998. Botulinum toxin management of spasmodic dysphonia (laryngeal dystonia): a 12-year experience in more than 900 patients. *Laryngoscope* 108(10): 1435–1441.

Carlsoo B, Izdebski K, Dahlqvist A, Domeij S, Dedo HH. 1987. The recurrent laryngeal nerve in spastic dysphonia: a light and electron microscopic study. *Acta Otolaryngol* 103(1–2): 96–104.

Chhetri DK, Blumin JH, Vinters HV, Berke GS. 2003. Histology of nerves and muscles in adductor spasmodic dysphonia. *Ann Otol Rhinol Laryngol* 112(4): 334–341.

Critchley M. 1939. Spastic dysphonia 'inspiratory speech'. *Brain* 62: 96–103.

Dedo HH. 1976. Recurrent laryngeal nerve section for spastic dysphonia. *Ann Otol Rhinol Laryngol* 85(4 Pt 1): 451–459.

Dedo HH, Izdebski K. 1984. Evaluation and treatment of recurrent spasticity after recurrent laryngeal nerve section: a preliminary report. *Ann Otol Rhinol Laryngol* 93(4 Pt 1): 343–345.

Feldman M, Nixon JV, Finitzo-Hieber T, Freeman FJ. 1984. Abnormal parasympathetic vagal function in patients with spasmodic dysphonia. *Ann Intern Med* 100(4): 491–495.

Finitzo-Hieber T, Freeman FJ, Gerling IJ, Dobson L, Schaefer SD. 1982. Auditory brainstem response abnormalities in adductor spasmodic dysphonia. *Am J Otolaryngol* 3(1): 26–30.

Hillel AD, Maronian NC, Waugh PF, Robinson L, Klotz DA. 2004. Treatment of the interarytenoid muscle with botulinum toxin for laryngeal dystonia. *Ann Otol Rhinol Laryngol* 113(5): 341–348.

Isshiki N, Yamamoto I, Fukagai S. 2004. Type 2 thyroplasty for spasmodic dysphonia: fixation using a titanium bridge. *Acta Otolaryngol* 124(3): 309–312.

Jacome DE, Yanez GF. 1980. Spastic dysphonia and Meigs disease. *Neurology* 30(4): 349.

Marsden CD, Sheehy MP. 1982. Spastic dysphonia, Meige disease, and torsion dystonia. *Neurology* 32(10): 1202–1203.

Meyer T, Blitzer A. 2006. Spasmodic dysphonia. In: Stacy M, ed. *Handbook of Dystonia*. London: CRC Press, pp. 179–188.

Murry T, Woodson GE. 1995. Combined-modality treatment of adductor spasmodic dysphonia with botulinum toxin and voice therapy. *J Voice* 9(4): 460–465.

Netterville JL, Stone RE, Rainey C, Zealear DL, Ossoff RH. 1991. Recurrent laryngeal nerve avulsion for treatment of spastic dysphonia. *Ann Otol Rhinol Laryngol* 100(1): 10–14.

Newton-John H. 1988. Acute upper airway obstruction due to supraglottic dystonia induced by a neuroleptic. *BMJ* 297(6654): 964–965.

N'ovakovic D, Waters HH, D'Elia JB, Blitzer A. 2011. Botulinum toxin treatment of adductor spasmodic dysphonia: longitudinal functional outcomes. *Laryngoscope* 121(3): 606–612.

Ravits JM, Aronson AE, DeSanto LW, Dyck PJ. 1979. No morphometric abnormality recurrent laryngeal nerve in spastic dysphonia. *Neurology* 29(10): 1376–1382.

Roark RM, Dowling EM, DeGroat RD, Watson BC, Schaefer SD. 1995. Time-frequency analyses of thyroarytenoid myoelectric activity in normal and spasmodic dysphonia subjects. *J Speech Hear Res* 38(2): 289–303.

Sapienza CM, Walton S, Murry T. 2000. Adductor spasmodic dysphonia and muscular tension dysphonia: acoustic analysis of sustained phonation and reading. *J Voice* 14(4): 502–520.

Schaefer SD. 1983. Neuropathology of spasmodic dysphonia. *Laryngoscope* 93(9): 1183–1204.

Schaefer S, Freeman F, Finitzo T, Close L, Cannito M, Ross E, Reisch J, Maravilla K. 1985. Magnetic resonance imaging findings and correlations in spasmodic dysphonia patients. *Ann Otol Rhinol Laryngol* 94(6 Pt 1): 595–601.

Schaefer SD, Finitzo-Hieber T, Gerling IJ, Freeman FJ. 1983. Brainstem conduction abnormalities in spasmodic dysphonia. *Ann Otol Rhinol Laryngol* 92(1 Pt 1): 59–64.

Traube L. 1871. *Zur Lehre von den Larynxaffectionen beim Ileotyphus.* Berlin: Verlag Van August Hisschwald, pp. 674–678.

Tucker HM. 1989. Laryngeal framework surgery in the management of spasmodic dysphonia: preliminary report. *Ann Otol Rhinol Laryngol.* 98(1 Pt 1): 52–54.

Van Pelt F, Ludlow CL, Smith PJ. 1994. Comparison of muscle activation patterns in adductor and abductor spasmodic dysphonia. *Ann Otol Rhinol Laryngol* 103(3): 192–200.

Warren J, Thompson P. 1998. Drug-induced supraglottic dystonia and spasmodic dysphonia. *Mov Disord* 13(6): 978–979.

Weed DT, Jewett BS, Rainey C, Zealear DL, Stone RE, Ossoff RH, Netterville JL. 1996. Long-term follow-up of recurrent laryngeal nerve avulsion for the treatment of spastic dysphonia. *Ann Otol Rhinol Laryngol* 105(8): 592–601.

Chapter 36

Botulinum Toxin Therapy for Writer's Cramp and Other Focal Hand Dystonias

Barbara Illowsky Karp

Writer's Cramp and Focal Hand Dystonia

Writer's cramp is a task-specific focal dystonia of the dominant hand during writing (Sheehy & Marsden 1982). The term is sometimes used, however, as a generic term for other focal hand dystonias, both task-specific and non-task-specific. For example, the term may be used for focal hand dystonia elicited by playing a musical instrument (also called 'musician's cramp'), typing, buttoning, knitting, or performing any skilled motor act. In this chapter, the term 'focal hand dystonia' (FHD) will be used to encompass all task-specific and non-specific variants; the term 'writer's cramp' (WC) will be used specifically for dystonia elicited by writing.

The definition of dystonia as a syndrome of 'sustained or intermittent muscle contractions causing abnormal, often repetitive movements, postures or both' applies well to FHD. In FHD, performance of an eliciting task activates upper-limb muscles that should not be activated. Other muscles needed for the task may fail to activate or may show excessive contraction. There may be abnormal co-contraction of agonist/antagonist pairs (Cohen & Hallett 1988). In this way, skilled movement is undermined.

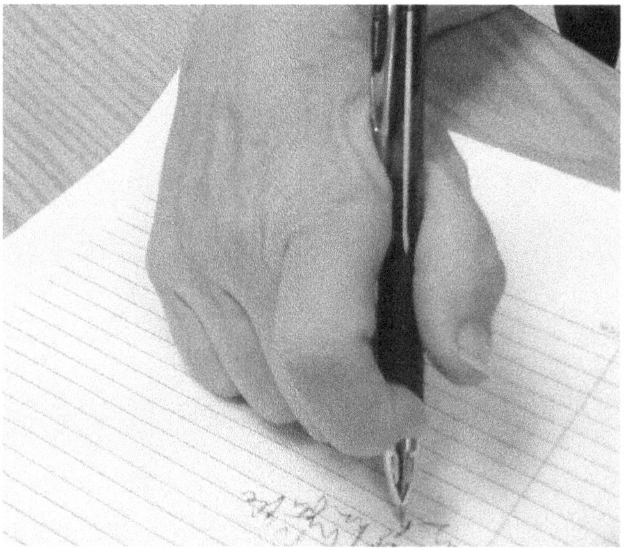

Figure 36.1 Writer's cramp with a flexion pattern.

Symptoms and Natural History

Focal hand dystonia often begins with vague hand discomfort. Within weeks to months, abnormal muscle contraction is noted. When mild, the affected tasks are possible, but may be performed awkwardly (Figure 36.1). When severe, posture is distorted and tasks are exceedingly impaired or impossible.

The combination of muscles affected in FHD is specific to the individual; however, certain patterns are more common than others. In writer's cramp, forearm and hand intrinsic muscles are more commonly affected than proximal arm muscles. The wrist and finger flexor muscles are more frequently affected than the extensors. Pronation is more common than supination. Mixed patterns, however, are also frequent (Figure 36.2). In musician's cramp, the muscles most commonly affected reflect those bearing the highest technical demands specific to the instrument being played.

Aetiology

Focal hand dystonia is usually idiopathic but may be associated with an underlying inherited disease or an acquired lesion, particularly of the basal ganglia. The role of peripheral limb trauma as a cause of focal hand dystonia is controversial (Jankovic & Van der Linden 1988). It is clear, however, from the earliest reports that prolonged repetitive use of small hand muscles contributes to its development.

An increasing number of genes have been associated with focal dystonias, some with hand involvement in their phenotype such as DYT1, DYT7 and DYT13. Genetic dystonias can often be differentiated from idiopathic FHD by the family history as many are autosomal dominant, and by other associated signs and symptoms. A family history of dystonia is present in about 15–20 per cent of patients with FHD. Recently, an increase in rare variants in the arylsulphatase G gene was reported for FHD (Nibbeling et al. 2015).

Epidemiology and Pathophysiology

The prevalence of writer's cramp has been reported at 2.7–14 per million (Nutt et al. 1988; Epidemiological Study of Dystonia in Europe Collaborative Group 2000). The sex predilection differs from that of most other focal dystonias, which are more common in women. WC affects men and women about equally; musician's cramp is more common in men. The typical age of onset is in the fourth decade.

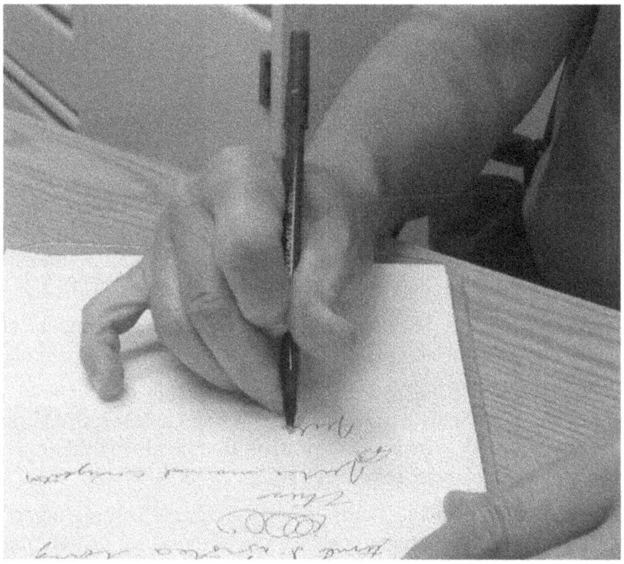

Figure 36.2 Writer's cramp with mixed flexion and extension.

Like other focal dystonias, FHD is characterised by a loss of inhibition at multiple levels within the central nervous system, including reciprocal inhibition, intracortical inhibition, interhemispheric inhibition and surround inhibition, and by changes in connectivity in resting state and sensorimotor networks detected by functional MRI (Karp 2012).

Treatment

Early in its course, many patients do not appreciate that the hand dysfunction is a neurological condition. Before coming to medical attention, some patients try a period of rest. Others try a period of intense practice or to adjust their performance of the affected task. Those with WC try different pens or different grips or switch to writing with the non-dominant hand. Many try splints and seek physical or occupational therapy. These and other functional approaches, such as sensory or motor retraining, have limited success. Oral medications sometimes used for FHD include anticholinergics, benzodiazepines, muscle relaxants, dopamine agonists and dopamine antagonists. These provide little relief in most patients and are often associated with unacceptable side-effects. Stereotactic neurosurgery, including thalamotomy or deep brain stimulation, is increasingly being tried in focal hand dystonia, with some success (Asahi et al. 2014).

Botulinum Toxin Treatment

Botulinum toxin has been used to treat focal hand dystonia since the 1980s and has become the mainstay of treatment (Simpson et al. 2008). One advantage of botulinum toxin for FHD is that it can be safely combined with other approaches, including rehabilitative therapies, surgery and oral medications.

Muscle Selection

For FHD, botulinum toxin is injected into the muscles involved in the dystonia, making proper muscle selection crucial. Because of the number of muscles and complexity of the musculature of the hand and forearm and the many ways it can be distorted by FHD, choosing muscles for injection is particularly challenging. Determining which muscles are involved is further complicated by the adjustments many make to cope with the dystonia. This compensation is often subconscious, so that patients have difficulty reporting what is compensatory and what is dystonic movement.

The selection of muscle begins with talking to the patients about their perception of the dystonia, including where they feel pulling, tightness, deviation or discomfort. Observation by a trained clinician plays an important role. Patients should be examined at rest, while writing, while walking, and during whatever activities elicit the dystonic movement. Viewing activities other than writing or the primary affected activity can help differentiate dystonic from compensatory actions. In some patients there is mirror dystonia, where writing with the non-dominant hand elicits dystonic posturing in the dominant hand. If the involved muscles are not apparent on direct inspection during writing with the affected hand or are possibly masked by compensatory movements, mirror movements can be considered as a guide for which muscles in the dominant hand to inject.

If the pattern of dystonic muscle activation differs between tasks, injection should likely begin using the muscles involved in the primary problematic task identified by the patient. Direct observation and patient report are not always sufficient. In some cases, surface or intramuscular thin wire EMG recorded during activities that elicit the dystonia can help determine whether deep muscles not accessible to direct observation are inappropriately activated.

It is neither necessary nor advisable to inject every dystonic muscle. Many patients have substantial benefit from injection limited to the primarily affected muscles, which also helps to limit weakness from injection.

Approaches to Dose/Toxin Selection

Published clinical trials have not directly compared types or brands of the marketed toxins; however, they do not suggest significant differences in the extent or duration of benefit when used for FHD. There are similarly no studies directly addressing optimal dosing for FHD. Dosing guidelines can be gleaned from various publications, including textbooks and articles (Jost & Valerius 2008; Truong 2014). A typical total dose range for focal hand dystonia is 25–50 units onabotulinumtoxinA and incobotulinumtoxinA, 100–300 units abobotulinumtoxinA and 1000–10 000 units rimabotulinumtoxinB.

Dosing should start at the lower end of the potentially therapeutic range to minimise the risk of weakness from injection. The dose is titrated over time to response, being raised or additional muscles being injected to try to improve the degree of benefit. Correspondingly, the dose should be decreased or redistributed into different muscles if there is impairing weakness.

There is no direct relationship between dose and benefit (Yoshimura et al. 1992). Some patients respond to a low dose, while others require a significantly higher dose into the same muscles. Women tend to require lower doses than men and extensors require lower doses than flexors (Karp et al. 1994). The severity of dystonic spasm also does not appear to predict the dose needed. There is, however, a direct correlation between weakness and dose. Weakness is predictably greater at higher doses. The trade-off between benefit and weakness at a given dose is unique to the individual patient.

Injection Methodology

Accurate injection of the selected muscles should serve to maximise benefit and minimise weakness in unaffected muscles. Use of surface landmarks has been shown to be inaccurate (Molloy et al. 2002). Electromyography, electrical stimulation and ultrasound have been demonstrated to improve the accuracy of injection into the selected muscles in other focal dystonias and in limb spasticity (Grigoriu et al. 2015).

Outcome Assessment

Efficacy of botulinum toxin for FHD can be assessed by patient report of improvement and patient and/or clinician rating on visual analogue scales. Measurement of writing speed and evaluation of the accuracy or neatness of writing are also sometimes used. Rating scales are available for writer's cramp, but are not frequently used in clinical practice (Wissel et al. 1996).

For FHD, about 60–70 per cent of patients have at least moderate benefit, with a decrease in spasm and increased ease in task performance (Yoshimura et al. 1992; Kruisdijk et al. 2007; Lungu et al. 2011). Recent evidence-based reviews of clinical studies comparing botulinum toxin to placebo noted a lack of published gold standard, double-blind placebo-controlled trials, so that it could not be concluded that botulinum toxin is definitely effective for FHD. The recommendations, therefore, were that botulinum toxin is probably effective for FHD (Simpson et al. 2008; Hallett et al. 2013). Efficacy in FHD can be maintained for over 20 years with repeated injections. Patients return for re-injection based on the extent and duration of response (Lungu et al. 2011). Injections are typically given every three months. Originally, loss of response due to neutralising antibodies occurred in about 10 per cent of patients. With current toxins, loss of response due to antibodies is rare and the interval between injection sessions can likely be shortened and adjusted to individual duration of response.

The most common side-effects of injection for FHD are the discomfort from injection and excessive weakness. Long-term follow-up of patients shows no worsening of early adverse effects and no emergent new adverse effects over time (Simpson et al. 2008; Lungu et al. 2011; Hallett et al. 2013).

Conclusions

Botulinum toxin is the current mainstay of treatment for FHD. When used with careful attention to muscle selection, dose and localisation technique, many patients have relief of spasm and improved function. Botulinum toxin injections can safely be combined with oral medications and rehabilitative approaches.

References

Asahi T, Koh M, Kashiwazaki D, Kuroda S. 2014. Stereotactic neurosurgery for writer's cramp: report of two cases with an overview of the literature. *Stereotact Funct Neurosurg* 92:405–411.

Cohen LG, Hallett M. 1988. Hand cramps: clinical features and electromyographic patterns in a focal dystonia. *Neurology* 38:1005–1012.

Epidemiological Study of Dystonia in Europe Collaborative Group. 2000. A prevalence study of primary dystonia in eight European countries. *J Neurol* 247:787–792.

Grigoriu AI, Dinomais M, Remy-Neris O, Brochard S. 2015. Impact of injection-guiding techniques on the effectiveness of botulinum toxin for the treatment of focal spasticity and dystonia: a systematic review. *Arch Phys Med Rehabil* 96:2067–2078.

Hallett M, Albanese A, Dressler D, Segal KR, Simpson DM, Truong D, Jankovic J. 2013. Evidence-based review and assessment of botulinum neurotoxin for the treatment of movement disorders. *Toxicon* 67:94–114.

Jankovic J, Van der Linden C. 1988. Dystonia and tremor induced by peripheral trauma: predisposing factors. *J Neurol Neurosurg Psychiatry* 51:1512–1519.

Jost W, Valerius K-P 2008. *Pictorial Atlas of Botulinum Toxin Injection: Dosage, Localization, Application*. Berlin: KVM.

Karp BI. 2012. Botulinum toxin physiology in focal hand and cranial dystonia. *Toxins* 4:1404–1414.

Karp BI, Cole RA, Cohen LG, Grill S, Lou JS, Hallett M. 1994. Long-term botulinum toxin treatment of focal hand dystonia. *Neurology* 44:70–76.

Kruisdijk JJ, Koelman JH, Ongerboer de Visser BW, de Haan RJ, Speelman JD. 2007. Botulinum toxin for writer's cramp: a randomised, placebo-controlled trial and 1-year follow-up. *J Neurol Neurosurg Psychiatry* 78:264–270.

Lungu C, Karp BI, Alter K, Zolbrod R, Hallett M. 2011. Long-term follow-up of botulinum toxin therapy for focal hand dystonia: outcome at 10 years or more. *Mov Disord* 26:750–753.

Molloy FM, Shill HA, Kaelin-Lang A, Karp BI. 2002. Accuracy of muscle localization without EMG: implications for treatment of limb dystonia. *Neurology* 58:805–807.

Nibbeling E, Schaake S, Tijssen MA, Weissbach A, Groen JL, Altenmüller E, Verbeek DS, Lohmann K. 2015. Accumulation of rare variants in the arylsulfatase G (ARSG) gene in task-specific dystonia. *J Neurol* 262:1340–1343.

Nutt JG, Muenter MD, Melton LJ, 3rd, Aronson A, Kurland LT. 1988. Epidemiology of dystonia in Rochester, Minnesota. *Adv Neurol* 50:361–365.

Sheehy MP, Marsden CD. 1982. Writers' cramp: a focal dystonia. *Brain* 105 (Pt 3):461–480.

Simpson DM, Blitzer A, Brashear A, Comella C, Dubinsky R, Hallett M, Jankovic J, Karp B, Ludlow CL, Miyasaki JM, Naumann M, So Y. 2008. Assessment: botulinum neurotoxin for the treatment of movement disorders (an evidence-based review): report of the

Therapeutics and Technology Assessment Subcommittee of the American Academy of Neurology. *Neurology* 70:1699–1706.

Truong D, Hallett M, Zachary C, Dressler D (Eds). 2014. *Manual of Botulinum Toxin Therapy*, 2nd edn. Cambridge: Cambridge University Press.

Wissel J, Kabus C, Wenzel R, Klepsch S, Schwarz U, Nebe A, Schelosky L, Scholz U, Poewe W. 1996. Botulinum toxin in writer's cramp: objective response evaluation in 31 patients. *J Neurol Neurosurg Psychiatry* 61:172–175.

Yoshimura DM, Aminoff MJ, Olney RK. 1992. Botulinum toxin therapy for limb dystonias. *Neurology* 42:627–630.

Chapter 37

Botulinum Toxin Therapy for Bruxism

Olga Orlova

Bruxism

Bruxism (from the Greek 'brugmos' – gnashing) or sleep bruxism are stereotyped jaw movements during sleep producing teeth grinding and clenching. They may also occur at daytime and are often seen in families. It was suggested that bruxism is a form of dystonia (Frisardi et al. 2013; Gjovreku & Vyshka 2013) as it may occur together with writer's cramp. An association with tics, with a family history of movement disorders and with jaw tremor was also described (Laine et al. 2015).

Most of the patients may not realise that they are suffering from bruxism. Often the spouse or parents will notice the bruxism first. Initial findings include orofacial pain, limitation of mouth opening, periodontal impairment and aesthetic defects with square face, dental abrasion and hypertrophy of masticatory muscles.

The diagnosis of bruxism is based on the patient's history and the symptoms described above. In unclear cases, polysomnography may reveal bruxism episodes on electromyography (EMG). Alternatively, brux-checkers, special thin splints registering jaw movements by abrasion of their coloured surface, may be helpful. They allow confirmation of the presence of bruxism as well as assessment of its intensity (Onodera & Sato 2008).

Botulinum Toxin Therapy of Bruxism

General

Treatment with botulinum toxin type A (BT-A) should be considered as the first choice (as in the case of dystonia). Treatment should be initiated without delay to reduce the risk of dental damage. BT-A therapy of bruxism came from treating oromandibular dystonia. Despite the fact that the first publication on BT-A injections in bruxism appeared in the 1990s, the need and efficacy of BT-A therapy in this indication remains debatable as extended data on safety and efficacy are lacking. Evidence-based reviews (Long et al. 2012; Persaud et al. 2013; Sposito & Teixeira 2014) are based on only three publications (Guarda-Nardini et al. 2008; Lee et al. 2010; Shim et al. 2014). In these studies, BT-A was injected either into each masseter only (Dysort 80 MU (Lee et al. 2010); Botox 25 MU (Shim et al. 2014)) or rarely into each masseter (Botox 30 MU) and each temporalis (Botox 20 MU) muscle (Guarda-Nardini et al. 2008). It was concluded that BT-A therapy is safe and effective for reducing bruxism episode frequency during sleep, teeth clenching intensity and pain, improving mood, but not for inhibiting the occurrence of bruxism episodes. It was emphasised that there are no validated questionnaires to assess bruxism severity. Despite the fact that the review of Persaud (Persaud et al. 2013) suggests level 1 evidence for efficacy of BT-A therapy for bruxism, many publications do not support this view. Negative results may result from injecting the masseter, sometimes the masseter and temporalis muscles, only. There were no studies injecting the lateral pterygoid muscles (LPM), although the LPM are the main horizontal jaw movers and the strongest muscles producing grinding (Murray et al. 2001; Tintner & Jankovic 2002). Thus, for the treatment of classical bruxism the LPM, the temporalis and masseter muscles should be target muscles. The medial pterygoid muscle (MPM) is a direct agonist of the masseter. In severe bruxism it may also be injected. LPM spasm is a typical cause of pain and temporomandibular joint disorder (TMD) (Guarda-Nardini et al. 2008; Ernberg et al. 2011). Therefore, BT-A therapy may have been ineffective in myofascial TMD pain when only the masseter was injected (Ernberg et al. 2011). EMG studies revealed that clenching is terminated only in injected muscles. It is, therefore, necessary to inject all the involved muscles (Shim et al. 2014).

Practical Aspects

The first step towards use of BT-A therapy for bruxism is to diagnose bruxism and to discuss it with the patient. As bruxism is an interdisciplinary disorder, it may be diagnosed by neurologists, dentists or sleep specialists. However, the latter usually do not offer BT-A therapy and the patient will need to be referred to a neurologist. Typically, BT-A therapy is started after complications such as pain, sleep disturbances or dental abrasions occur. The patient should be aware of the potential benefits of BT-A therapy in masticatory muscles as their hyperactivity is the underlying cause of these complications.

After the BT-A injection, it is necessary to ask the patient to chew for 30 minutes to activate the injected muscles. No serious complications have been reported with this protocol in our experience. Some patients may report transient weakness of chewing or enhanced pain, which may be treated with non-steroidal anti-inflammatory drugs. Repeated injections are performed 2–3 times a year or as needed. The duration of muscle relaxation is a good therapeutic 'window' to restore physiological teeth occlusion (Soikher et al. 2010).

BT-A Dosing

We suggest first choosing the total BT-A dose based on bruxism severity and then distributing it across the involved muscles. In severe bruxism with excessive muscle hypertrophy, pain, severe teeth abrasion, teeth grinding at night and disturbed sleep, males should receive 150–200 MU of Botox (Xeomin, Lantox, Relatox and other '100-units' toxins) or 400–500 MU of Dysport. In females total doses should be 100–150 MU or 300–400 MU, respectively. Approximately 50 per cent of the dose is injected into the masseters, 35 per cent into the temporalis muscles and 15 per cent into the LPM. In moderate cases, the total dose for males should be 100–125 MU of Botox or 250–300 MU of Dysport. For females it should be 80–100 MU or 250–300 MU, respectively. For example, in moderate bruxism 100 MU of Botox may be injected as follows: 25 MU into each masseter, 17–18 MU into each temporalis and 7–8 MU into each LPM. In mild forms the total dose may be 40–60 MU of Botox or 100–150 MU of Dysport, with no gender adjustments required; LPM injections may be skipped.

BT-A Injection Into the Temporalis Muscle

The temporalis muscle can be injected with insulin syringes using 12.7 mm length needles. After palpation and identification of painful areas, the patient is asked to clench his teeth to locate the margins of the muscle. Figure 37.1 shows the front margin of the muscle. The needle should be inserted with clenched teeth to feel the anatomy of the muscle better. In moderate cases three injections (Figure 37.1) may be needed. In severe cases with marked muscle hypertrophy (Figure 37.1), 5–6 injections are necessary. EMG guidance is preferred, but is not obligatory.

BT-A Injection Into the Masseter Muscle

The masseter muscle can be injected with insulin syringes, as shown in Figure 37.1, but only in mild cases. In severe bruxism it is better to use EMG guidance with a 37 mm length needle. The masseter may be hypertrophic (Figure 37.1). To improve results it is necessary to inject not only the superficial but also the deeper layers of the muscle, especially in the upper part adjacent to the maxilla. In moderate cases the masseter can be injected in three sites (Figure 37.1). Additional sites may be used in severe bruxism with muscle hypertrophy (Figure 37.1). The patient is asked to clench his teeth to locate the edges of the muscle. The first two injections are performed between the front and rear edges of the muscle, 1.5 cm above the edge of the jaw. The third point is the top of the triangle. Additional points are spread over the entire area of the muscle. The insertion of the needle is usually made with clenched teeth to feel the needle hitting the muscle, while BT-A may be administered with unclenched teeth. The depth of needle insertion is from 12.7 mm to 20–30 mm in the thickest part of this three-layer muscle. Too superficial insertion will not achieve adequate clinical response and may cause facial asymmetry.

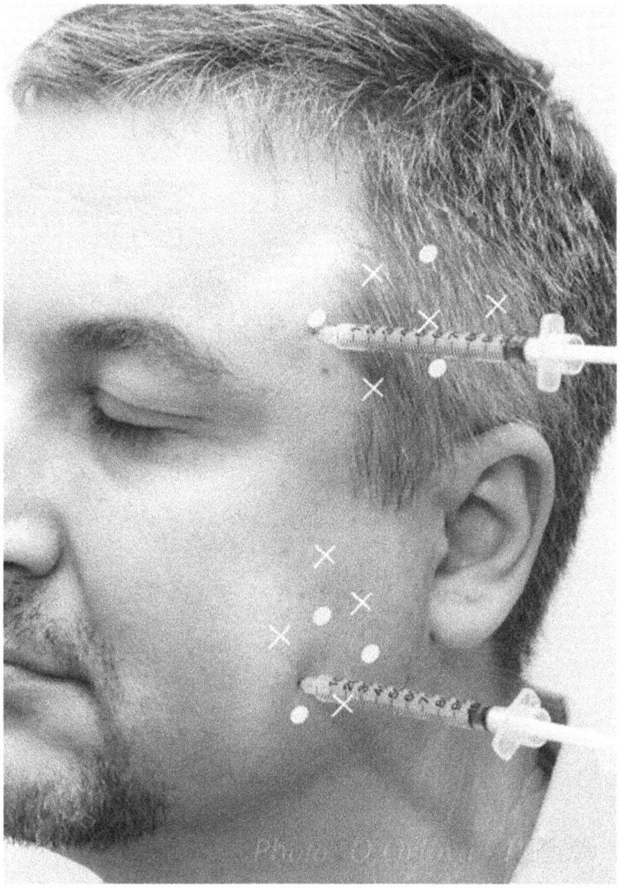

Figure 37.1 Sites of BT-A injection into the temporalis and masseter muscles in moderate and severe bruxism.

BT-A Injection Into the Lateral Pterygoid Muscle

LPM injection is performed with EMG guidance. The muscle can be injected from both the oral cavity (Mor et al. 2015) (this is the way dentists and surgeons work) and from the outside (Carrillo 2011). For the external injection, the recess formed by the maxillary notch (about 3–3.5 cm anterior to the tragus) is palpated and the needle is inserted perpendicularly to the surface and directed slightly anteriorly (5–7°) (Figure 37.2). First, the electrode passes through the deep layer of the masseter and at a depth of 2–2.5 cm a small BT-A dose may be administered. Then, moving the needle, the EMG LPM sound appears. The patient may then be asked to move the jaw to the opposite side, thus intensifying the EMG signal. The total LPM dose is then injected into one site.

BT-A Injection Into the Medial Pterygoid Muscle

The MPM is an agonist of the masseter, with which it forms a 'loop' thrown over the edge of the jaw. It is injected to increase the therapeutic effect in patients with strong jaw clenching. The electrode is inserted under the edge of the mandible around the projection of the middle of the masseter and directed upwards for 1.5–2 cm until the MPM EMG sound appears. The usual dose is the same as for the LPM.

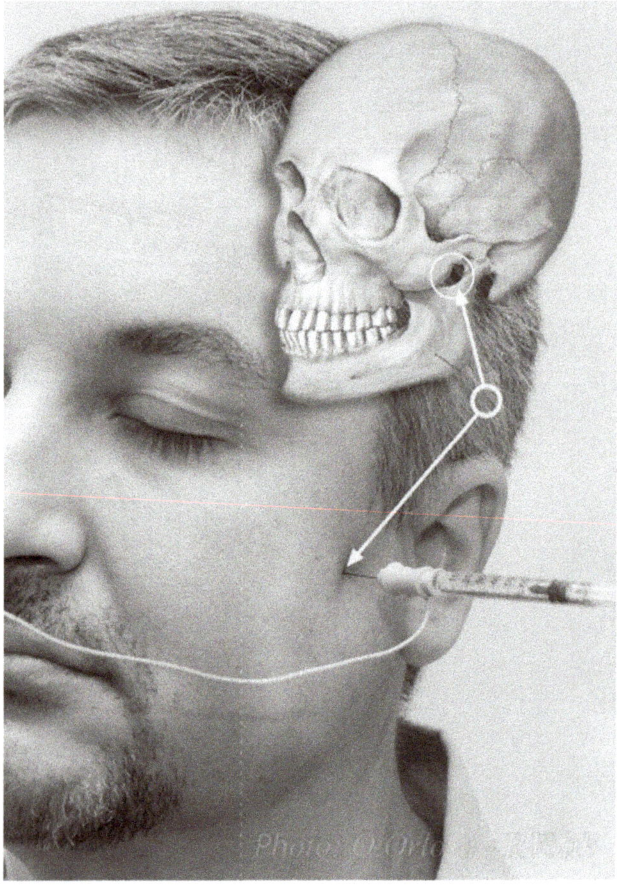

Figure 37.2 Site of lateral pterygoid muscle (LPM) injection in bruxism.

Finally, dentists should be encouraged to pay more attention to masticatory muscles, which are the main structures of the stomatognatic system, and offer BT-A treatment in their practice (Nayyar et al. 2014).

References

Carrillo RJC (2011). Pterygoid botulinum toxin injection. *Philipp J Otolaryngol Head Neck Surg* 26:55–56.

Ernberg M, Hedenberg-Magnusson B, List T, Svensson P (2011). Efficacy of botulinum toxin type A for treatment of persistent myofascial TMD pain: a randomized, controlled, double-blind multicenter study. *Pain* 152:1988–1996.

Frisardi G, Iani C, Sau G, Frisardi F, Leornadis C, Lumbau A, Enrico P, Sirca D, Staderini EM, Chessa G (2013). A relationship between bruxism and orofacial dystonia? A trigeminal electrophysiological approach in a case report of pineal cavernoma. *Behav Brain Funct* 9:41.

Gjovreku E, Vyshka G (2013). Nocturnal bruxism: still a nosological conundrum? *WebmedCentral Dentistry* 4(5):WMC004234.

Guarda-Nardini L, Manfredini D, Salamone M, Salmaso L, Tonello S, Ferronato G (2008). Efficacy of botulinum toxin in treating myofascial pain in bruxers: a controlled placebo pilot study. *Cranio* 26:126–135.

Laine CM, Yavuz ŞU, D'Amico JM, Gorassini MA, Türker KS, Farina D (2015). Jaw tremor as a physiological biomarker of bruxism. *Clin Neurophysiol* 126:1746–1753.

Lee SJ, McCall WD, Kim YK, Chung SC, Chung JW (2010). Effect of botulinum toxin injection on nocturnal bruxism: a randomized controlled trial. *Am J Phys Med Rehabil* 89:16–23.

Long H, Liao Z, Wang Y, Liao L, Lai W (2012). Efficacy of botulinum toxins on bruxism: an evidence-based review. *Int Dent J* 62:1–5.

Mor N, Tang C, Blitzer A (2015). Temporomandibular myofascial pain treated with botulinum toxin injection. *Toxins* 7:2791–2800.

Murray GM, Phanachet I, Uchida S, Whittle T (2001). The role of the human lateral pterygoid muscle in the control of horizontal jaw movements. *J Orofac Pain* 15: 279–292; discussion 292–305.

Nayyar P, Kumar P, Nayyar PV, Singh A (2014). Botox: broadening the horizon of dentistry. *J Clin Diagn Res* 8:ZE25–ZE29.

Onodera K, Sato S (2008). Bruxism evaluating sheet. United States Patent Application: 20080211123. www.freepatentsonline.com/y2008/0211123.html (accessed 11 October 2016).

Orlova O, Soikher MI, Soikher MG, Mingazova L, Kotlyarov V, Slavicek G (2010). Therapeutic application of botulinum toxin A in patients with local muscle dystonia and oral dyskinesia. *J Stomat Occ Med* 3:23–28.

Persaud R, Garas G, Silva S, Stamatoglou C, Chatrath P, Patel K (2013). An evidence-based review of botulinum toxin (Botox) applications in non-cosmetic head and neck conditions. *JRSM Short Rep* 4:10.

Shim YJ, Lee MK, Kato T, Park HU, Heo K, Kim ST (2014). Effects of botulinum toxin on jaw motor events during sleep in sleep bruxism patients: a polysomnographic evaluation. *J Clin Sleep Med* 10: 291–298.

Sposito M, Teixeira S (2014). Botulinum toxin A for bruxism: a systematic review. *Acta Fisiatr* 21:201–204.

Tintner R, Jankovic J (2002). Botulinum toxin type A in the management of oromandibular dystonia and bruxism. In: Brin MF, Hallett M, Jankovic J (Eds). *Scientific and Therapeutic Aspects of Botulinum Toxin.* Lippincott Williams & Wilkins, Philadelphia, PA.

Chapter 38

Treatment of Blepharospasm With Eyelid-Opening Apraxia

Rainer Laskawi and Dirk Dressler

Introduction

Blepharospasm is a neurological condition characterised by forceful involuntary eyelid closures which may be painful and which, in severe cases, may lead to functional blindness. It was the historical achievement of C. David Marsden to recognise blepharospasm as part of the clinical spectrum of focal dystonias (Marsden 1976). In some patients blepharospasm may be accompanied by the inability to activate the levator palpebrae muscle, presenting with the characteristic facial impression of surprise caused by frontalis muscle activation in order to support the function of the levator palpebrae muscle (Figure 38.1). Often patients try to support eyelid-opening by using their index fingers (Figure 38.1). In the absence of paresis or myopathy this symptom was named eyelid-opening apraxia (EOA) (Roggenkämper & Nüssgens 1993) or apraxia of eyelid-opening. Alternatively, the term levator inhibition may be used. Detailed electromyographic (EMG) studies of the orbicularis oculi and the levator palpebrae increased the pathophysiological understanding of EOA (Aramideh et al. 1994). Frequently, blepharospasm with EOA occurs in patients with progressive supranuclear palsy.

Conventional Treatment

Conventional treatment of EOA aims at reducing orbicularis oculi activity. Reduction of orbicularis oculi activity can be achieved by botulinum toxin (BT) therapy (Scott et al. 1985; Kollewe et al. 2015), especially when the pretarsal parts are injected (Aramideh et al. 1995; Boghen et al. 2002; Forget et al. 2002). However, results are limited and EOA is the most common cause of BT therapy failure in blepharospasm. Classic myectomy (Georgescu et al. 2008), myectomy in combination with mechanical devices (Rana & Shah 2012) and denervation operations (Patel & Anderson 1995) have also been suggested, but are problematic because of uncontrollable effects and induction of severe neuralgic pain. Levodopa is reported to have positive effects on EOA (Dewey & Maraganore 1994; Lee et al. 2004; Yamada et al. 2005). Some patients use simple mechanical devices ('eyelid crutches') originally designed to compensate ptosis such as spectacle frames with special springs attached (Moss 1982; Ramasamy et al. 2007); some use their fingers or attach adhesive tapes to their eyelids.

Frontalis Suspension Operation

Frontalis suspension operations were originally used to treat blepharospasm (Putterman & Urist 1972), where they were not effective in overcoming the very forceful orbicularis oculi contractions. In 1993 Peter Roggenkämper introduced a modified frontalis suspension operation (FSO) to treat EOA, as all conventional treatment strategies for EOA were of limited benefit (Roggenkämper & Nüssgens 1993, 1997; Nüssgens & Roggenkämper 1995; Wabbels & Roggenkämper 2007). FSO tries to mechanically restore the impaired function of the levator palpebrae by enhancing the natural function of the

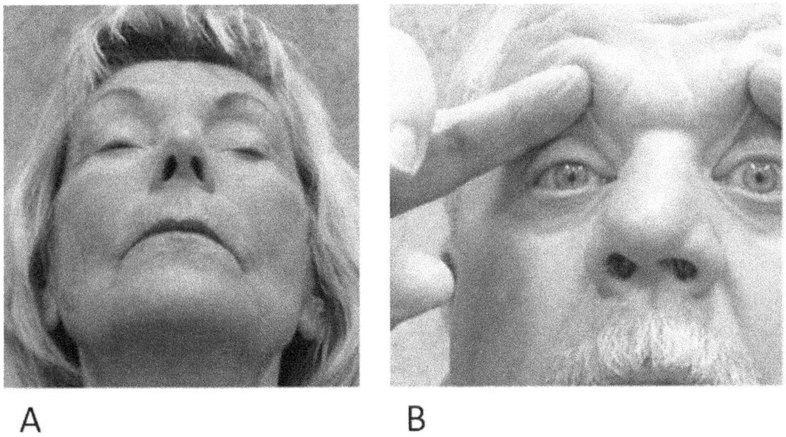

A B

Figure 38.1 Patients with eyelid-opening apraxia. Preoperative state. (a) This patient shows the typical head extension. (b) This patient uses his index fingers to lift the upper eyelids as a compensatory manoeuvre.

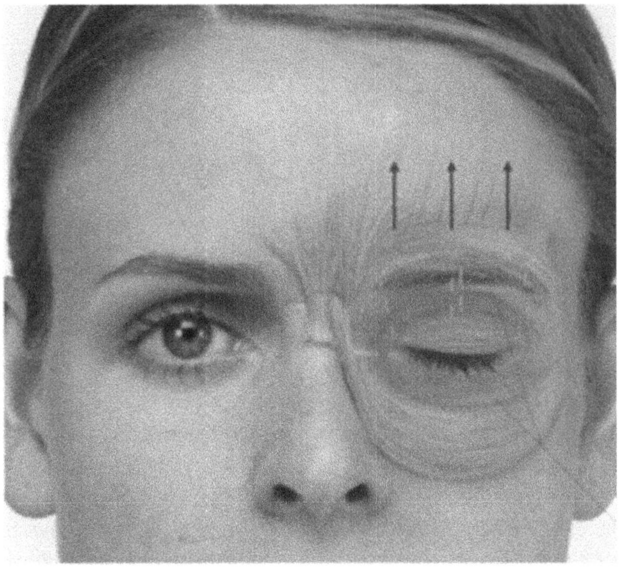

Figure 38.2 Surgical technique of the frontalis suspension operation. The applied polytetrafluoroethylene (PTFE, Gore-Tex®) sutures enable the patients to lift the upper eyelid by innervating the frontalis muscle. The sutures guarantee power transmission from the frontalis muscle to the upper eyelid. *Source*: Picture modified after Jost (2007).

frontalis muscle as an auxillary eyelid opener. This is achieved by connecting the frontalis muscle to the upper eyelid through a non-elastic string. As EOA usually occurs in combination with blepharospasm, FSO is usually complemented by blepharospasm treatment with BT. FSO may also be used to treat ptosis (Takahashi et al. 2010). FSO modifications (Ramasamy et al. 2007; Patil & Foss 2009) have been suggested, but could not gain widespread use. There is an ongoing discussion about the best suited string material (Lemagne & Liu 1991; Wasserman et al. 2001; Ben Simon et al. 2005; Hayashi et al. 2013).

Surgical Technique

We perform the FSO under general anaesthesia, usually in a single session to treat both eyes in the following way (Karapantzou et al. 2014). Three skin incisions are placed above the upper edge of the eyelid and the eyebrow. Polytetrafluoroethylene (PTFE, Gore-Tex®) sutures are used for the suspension (Figure 38.2). Depending on the thickness of the eyelid, a size 3-0 or 4-0 suture is passed through the medial caudal incision in the upper border of the eyelid cephalad to the medial incision just above the eyebrow. On retraction, the needle is used to pull a second subcutaneous PTFE suture caudally through the medial incisions. Starting from the medial incision, two loops (squares) of rectangular shape are then formed with subcutaneous PTFE sutures (medial, lateral; Figure 38.2). Finally, the ends of each suture are brought out through the medial upper incision for the first square and out of the lateral upper incision for the second square and are tied together. The skin incisions, except for the lateral and medial upper incisions above the eyebrow, are then closed. The position of the eyelid is assessed and adjusted to produce a slight overcorrection with a 2–3 mm wide palpebral fissure. The protruding sutures are knotted together and placed subcutaneously. All incisions are then closed with skin sutures. Ointment (Polyspectran®, Alcon Pharma, Freiburg/Breisgau, Germany) is applied to the eyes and the forehead and upper eyelid are covered with sterile dressing.

Efficacy

Fifteen patients of ours with blepharospasm and EOA received bilateral FSO together with BT therapy (Dressler et al. 2017). Overall subjective improvement on a 0–100 per cent self-assessment calendar (0 per cent: lack of any improvement after the operation; 100 per cent: optimal treatment results and resolution of all complaints after the operation) throughout the entire observation period of at least one year was 71.9 ± 25.6 per cent. All 19 items of a self-developed quality of life questionnaire (except for the presence of involuntary eyelid closure) showed postoperative improvement. Daily activities and social life were also improved (Karapantzou 2013). Figure 38.3 shows a patient before and after FSO.

In our patients, the complication rate was 9.1 per cent for suture extrusions, 6.1 per cent for suture granulomas, 5.0 per cent for lacrimation and 7.5 per cent for infections (Karapantzou et al. 2014). If suture extrusion occurs, waiting for some weeks is recommended. Revision surgery with placement of a new PTFE suture is possible and minimally invasive. Suture tension can be corrected under local anaesthesia if the tension between the frontalis muscle and the upper lid decreases. Postoperative BT injections should be performed with sparing the caudal part of the frontalis muscle near the eyebrow in order to protect the elevation force of the frontalis muscle.

In all patients BT therapy had to be continued to treat orbicularis oculi contractions. Our long-term results demonstrate that FSO is a benign procedure producing robust and stable therapeutic effects on EOA in blepharospasm.

Other authors also observed similarly positive effects of FSO (Roggenkämper & Nüssgens 1993, 1997; Grivet et al. 2005; Wabbels & Roggenkämper 2007).

References

Aramideh M, Ongerboer de Visser BW, Devriese PP, Bour LJ, Speelman JD (1994) Electromyographic features of levator palpebrae superioris and orbicularis oculi muscles in blepharospasm. *Brain* 117:27–38.

Aramideh M, Ongerboer de Visser BW, Brans JW, Koelman JH, Speelman JD (1995) Pretarsal application of botulinum toxin for treatment of blepharospasm. *J Neurol Neurosurg Psychiatry* 59:309–311.

Ben Simon GJ, Macedo AA, Schwarcz RM, Wang DY, McCann JD, Goldberg RA (2005) Frontalis suspension for upper eyelid ptosis: evaluation of different surgical designs and suture materials. *Am J Ophthalmol* 140:887–885.

Boghen D, Tozlovanu V, Iancu A, Forget R (2002) Botulinum toxin therapy for apraxia of lid opening. *Ann NY Acad Sci* 956:482–483.

Dewey RB Jr, Maraganore DM (1994) Isolated eyelid opening apraxia: report of a new levodopa-responsive syndrome. *Neurology* 44:1752–1754.

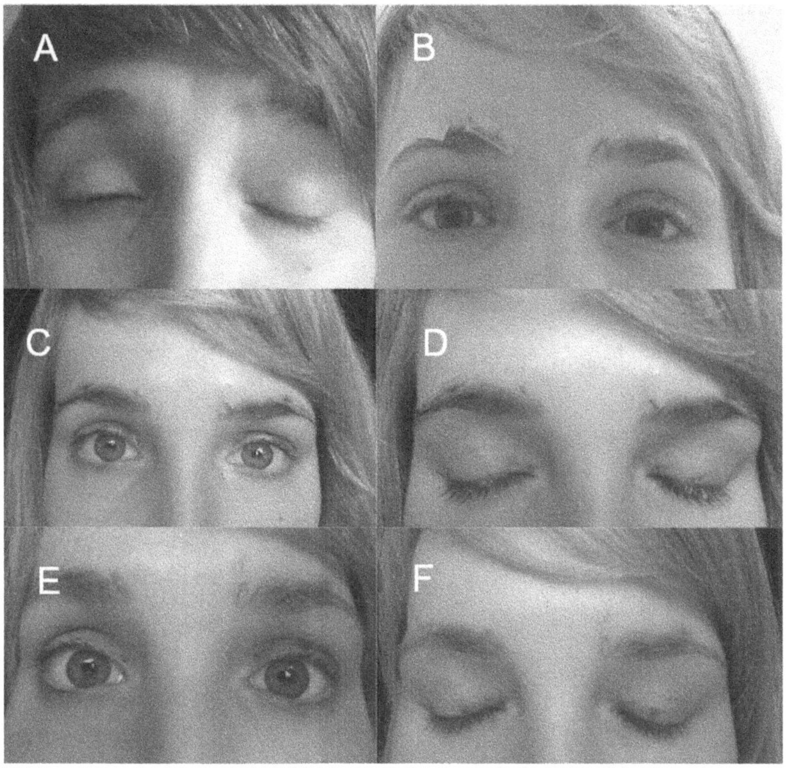

Figure 38.3 Patient with eyelid-opening apraxia, before and after frontalis suspension operation (FSO). Continued botulinum toxin therapy is necessary. (a) Before FSO the patient attempts to open her eyes, but is unable to do so. (b) Immediately after FSO the patient can promptly open her eyes. (c) Two weeks after FSO the patient can promptly open her eyes. (d) Two weeks after FSO the patient can fully close her eyes. (e) Four weeks after FSO the patient can promptly open her eyes. (f) Four weeks after FSO the patient can fully close her eyes.

Dressler D, Karapantzou C, Rohrbach S, Schneider S, Laskawi R (2017) Frontalis suspension surgery to treat patients with blepharospasm and eyelid opening apraxia: long-term results. *J Neural Transm* 124:253–257.

Forget R, Tozlovanu V, Iancu A, Boghen D (2002) Botulinum toxin improves lid opening delays in blepharospasm-associated apraxia of lid opening. *Neurology* 58:1843–1846.

Georgescu D, Vagefi MR, McMullan TFW, McCann JD, Anderson RL (2008) Upper eyelid myectomy in blepharospasm with associated apraxia of lid opening. *Am J Ophthalmol* 145:541–547.

Grivet D, Robert PY, Thuret G, De Feligonde OP, Gain P, Maugery J, Adenis JP (2005) Assessment of blepharospasm surgery using an improved disability scale: study of 138 patients. *Ophthal Plast Reconstr Surg* 21:230–234.

Hayashi K, Katori N, Kasai K, Kamisasanuki T, Kokubo K, Ohno-Matsui K (2013) Comparison of nylon monofilament suture and polytetrafluoroethylene sheet for frontalis suspension surgery in eyes with congenital ptosis. *Am J Ophthalmol* 155:654-663.

Jost W (2007) *Bildatlas der Botulinumtoxin-Injektion: Dosierung, Lokalisation, Anwendung.* Marburg: KVM.

Karapantzou C (2013) Blepharospasmus vom Levator-Inhibitions-Typ – Analyse von Patienten nach Lid-Frontalis-Suspensions Operation und Literaturübersicht. Medical Dissertation, Göttingen.

Karapantzou C, Dressler D, Rohrbach S, Laskawi R (2014) Frontalis suspension surgery to treat patients with essential blepharospasm and apraxia of eyelid opening-technique and results. *Head Face Med* 10:44.

Kollewe K, Mohammadi B, Köhler S, Pickenbrock H, Dengler R, Dressler D (2015) Blepharospasm: long-term treatment with either Botox®, Xeomin® or Dysport®. *J Neural Transm* 122:427–431.

Lee KC, Finley R, Miller B (2004) Apraxia of lid opening: dose-dependent response to carbidopa-levodopa. *Pharmacotherapy* 24:401–403.

Lemagne JM, Liu C (1991) Complications of frontalis suspension using polytetrafluoroethylene (Gore-Tex). *Orbit* 10:29–31.

Marsden CD (1976) Blepharospasm-oromandibular dystonia syndrome (Brueghel's syndrome): a variant of adult-onset torsion dystonia? *J Neurol Neurosurg Psychiatry* 39:1204–1209.

Moss HL (1982) Prothesis for blepharoptosis and blepharospasm. *J Am Optom Assoc* 53:661–667.

Nüssgens Z, Roggenkämper P (1995) Long-term treatment of blepharospasm with botulinum toxin type A. *Ger J Ophthalmol* 4:363–367.

Patel BC, Anderson RL (1995) Blepharospasm and related facial movement disorders. *Curr Opin Ophthalmol* 6:86–99.

Patil B, Foss AJE (2009) Upper lid orbicularis muscle strip and sequential brow suspension with autologous fascia lata is beneficial for selected patients with essential blepharospasm. *Eye* 23:1549–1553.

Putterman AM, Urist M (1972) Treatment of essential blepharospasm with a frontalis sling. *Arch Ophthalmol* 88:278–281.

Ramasamy B, Rowe F, Freeman G, Owen M, Noonan C (2007) Modified Lundie loops improve apraxia of eye lid opening. *J Neuroophthalmol* 27:32–35.

Rana AQ, Shah R (2012) Combination of blepharospasm and apraxia of eye lid opening: a condition resistant to treatment. *Acta Neurol Belg* 112:95–96.

Roggenkämper P, Nüssgens Z (1993) Frontalis suspension in the treatment of essential blepharospasm unresponsive to botulinum toxin therapy: first results. *Ger J Ophthalmol* 2: 426–428.

Roggenkämper P, Nüssgens Z (1997) Frontalis suspension in the treatment of essential blepharospasm unresponsive to botulinum toxin therapy: long-term results. *Graefe's Arch Clin Exp Ophthalmol* 235: 486–489.

Scott AB, Kennedy RA, Stubbs HA (1985) Botulinum A toxin injection as a treatment for blepharospasm. *Arch Ophthalmol* 103:347–350.

Takahashi Y, Leibovitch I, Kakzaki H (2010) Frontalis suspension surgery in upper eyelid blepharoptosis. *Open Ophthamol J* 4:91–97.

Wabbels B, Roggenkämper P (2007) Long-term follow up of patients with frontalis sling operation in the treatment of essential blepharospasm unresponsive to botulinum toxin therapy. *Graefe's Arch Clin Exp Ophthalmol* 245: 45–50.

Wasserman B, Springer DT, Helveston EM (2001) Comparison of materials used in frontalis suspension surgery. *Arch Ophthalmol* 118:687–691.

Yamada S, Matsuo K, Hirayama M, Sobue G (2005) The effects of levodopa on apraxia of lid opening: a case report. *Neurology* 62:830–831.

Chapter 39

Organisation of a Botulinum Toxin Clinic

Austen Peter Moore

Introduction

Botulinum toxin clinics come in many shapes and sizes. They usually begin with a single practitioner dealing with occasional patients with a single disease. Many grow steadily to become large multi-practitioner systems treating a variety of conditions. As the list of disorders treated with botulinum toxin grows, the process of gaining experience and a reputation for treating one condition often generates referrals of patients with other disorders to the local botulinum toxin 'expert', and the skills gained are indeed often transferable. However, the botulinum toxin 'expert' can slip into dealing with patients whose illness is otherwise outside their usual practice, possibly leading to inappropriate use of toxin when other treatments might be preferable. Alternatively, as more specialties develop their own indications, the relevant specialists learn to use botulinum toxin and keep management 'in-house' and potentially use toxin at more appropriate points in treatment pathways. There are many different combinations of these models, depending on the local configuration of medical services and accidents of history.

Perhaps the most common service model began with a neurologist or ophthalmologist treating focal dystonia. Many then expanded to treat spasticity, drooling, hyperhidrosis, headache and other neurologically related disorders, and may now involve or link with medical neurorehabilitationists, ENT and orthopaedic surgeons, urologists, dermatologists, paediatricians and pain specialists. In some countries, clinics deploy paramedical staff such as specialist nurses and physiotherapists to help not just with assessment and post-injection monitoring, but increasingly to give toxin injections, under varying degrees of supervision depending on experience, local custom and regulations.

Increased Complexity

In the early stages of this process it is relatively straightforward to run the small, low-throughput, single-disease clinic, with the disease specialist ensuring an optimal blend of toxin with other treatments and able to decide alone how best to run an effectively isolated clinic. Toxin clinics have a habit of growing, as many patients need regular treatment indefinitely. The isolated clinician must ensure funding and service capacity planning includes growth, leave cover and backup. As complexity increases, cooperation and coordination between teams can increase efficiency, safety and economies of scale.

Building a Clinic

Treating patients in a toxin clinic is more time-efficient than giving occasional treatments in a more general clinic, not least because set-up time can be considerable. The injecting clinician's time is the key resource and limiting factor in most clinics. Clinics must decide whether they are for single or many disorders. Are they for toxin treatment only, with other matters off-limits? How much time will you make for patient or disease assessments in the injection clinic? Remember that from the patient's viewpoint it is preferable to have all their issues dealt with in one visit, and this can create tensions if time is short.

As many sub-tasks as possible should be done by someone else. Protocols can be very helpful in guiding the non-clinicians involved. They include follow-up booking, availability of equipment and supplies, and some parts of the medical procedures. For instance, in some countries nursing staff can prepare the toxin for injection and complete the documentation.

Controlling Clinic Size

As a clinic becomes established it is generally easy to predict how many treatment slots are needed each week. The required clinic frequency depends directly on the cohort size and average desired interval between injection cycles. Two new patients per week will expand the cohort by 80–100 patients per year as there are few dropouts. Remember to allow for staff leave. In the long term it is important to avoid undue pressure on individual staff to treat too many patients, a recipe for mistakes. If there are multiple injectors, it works well for each to establish their own cohort of patients – who much prefer to see the same face each time. Injectors know more clearly what happened last time and get efficient feedback on their decisions.

Some conditions, such as hemifacial spasm, blepharospasm, migraine or other single-area disorders, seem 'simpler', more formulaic and quicker to manage in the toxin clinic than multi-region dystonias or spasticity or conditions requiring ultrasound or EMG-directed treatments. There is evidence that suitably trained nurses can run injection sessions for selected straightforward patients, with results statistically indistinguishable from doctors (Whitaker et al. 2001; Moore & Naumann 2003). In my unit, nurses administer 40–50 per cent of the injections, with ready access to medical support. Some services run separate, lower-throughput clinics deploying more experienced injectors for the more complex patients.

Review Appointments

As toxin treatment for dystonia is largely a symptomatic treatment, within safety constraints such as the customary 10–12 week recommended interval between injections to minimise the risk of toxin resistance, patients ought to receive treatment when their symptoms recur (an aspiration). Some patients like to arrange a date for their next injections before they leave the clinic, others to ring up as soon as they feel the need. Ideally, clinics should be able to accommodate both, but this is not always possible, and many patients do not receive treatment as often or as promptly as they would like (the reality). Patients should be able to postpone their injections if their previous treatment is still working.

Which Toxin Should You Use?

Many clinics use one toxin brand for most of their patients, as this simplifies the clinic, minimises confusion and allows injectors to develop a 'feel' for how best to use it. However, it can be valuable to have other brands available. Patients resistant to type A toxin may respond to type B and vice versa. Patients transferring from elsewhere may be long established on, and unwilling to change from, a particular brand. Converting them (or the clinic as a whole) to another preparation exposes patients to one or more potentially suboptimal injection cycles as the chosen dose conversion may need to be adjusted or the adverse effect profile may change.

There is no universally accepted evidence that one type A toxin is superior overall. Competition on grounds of efficacy is intimately linked to price per unit, hence the long-standing and vigorous commercial arguments over dose equivalence 'ratios'. Other factors include availability, ease of use, perceived risk of adverse effects or toxin resistance, the experience of the injectors, and any legal restrictions on off-licence uses.

Injectors should know enough about their less favoured brands to use them when needed, or to convert patients to their favoured brand. They should have a standard dose-conversion strategy and can choose to use a lower equivalent dose to maximise safety or a higher equivalent dose to maximise efficacy.

Keeping Records

Good records at the first injection session are crucial. Document the diagnosis, other medical problems, pregnancy, allergies and other drugs, especially antithrombotic medication. Give a clear description of the involuntary movements including their severity. List the treatment goals, document discussion of the benefits and risks and record patient consent. For the first and all subsequent cycles you should record enough details of the injections to enable someone else to understand what happened and repeat them. This will allow you to repeat them if they work well and will facilitate appropriate modifications if there are problems. I routinely record

- any difficulties in deciding the injection pattern, reasons for non-standard patterns, and special measures such as use of EMG or ultrasound;
- the brand used (it is surprising how often clinics do not record this);
- dose and number of injection sites/muscle;
- a right/left grid for named muscles, and/or use a diagram, e.g. for face muscles or hyperhidrosis; and
- total dose, and dilution if non-standard.

Measuring Benefit

There are many disease- or situation-specific scales. They may be objective or subjective. Some are prescriptive, such as the Tsui or TWSTRS for cervical dystonia; others are adaptable, such as Goal Attainment Scales (GAS) for spasticity. Many excellent research scales are rather cumbersome for use in a service clinic and it can be confusing to be switching scales repeatedly in a multi-disease clinic. Within a single cycle, isolated measures of effect onset, peak effect and duration of benefit may be misleading as patterns of response vary widely.

Homework

Few clinics can routinely review patients in mid-cycle. Many clinics, including mine, ask patients to document their progress weekly on a homework sheet. This makes it much easier to extract the story of the injection cycle at the next visit, and thus to adapt the injections appropriately. It can be helpful to combine this with a record of the injections given and thus collect all the data on one sheet. The injector can readily compare doses, patterns and responses between cycles and optimise the injection strategy.

The homework sheet uses the same scales for all conditions, supplemented if necessary by separate situation-specific scales. Patients record the following:

- A weekly Visual Analogue Score (VAS) from 0 ('worst possible') to 100 ('no problem') (Dressler et al. 2014) in five-point steps. Any aspect of the illness can be scored, usually by agreement between patient and injector. Different facets of disease (e.g. pain and posture) can be scored separately using distinct symbols or colours. Adverse effects can also be rated weekly, and their timing gives valuable clues to causality.
- Key timings such as effect onset and duration of effect.
- Two supplementary seven-point Likert scores for the cycle as a whole. One scores the peak effect (major deterioration to major benefit). The other compares this cycle with the previous cycle (much worse to much better) for fine-tuning.
- Adverse effects.

A sample sheet is shown in Figure 39.1. The various elements can be cross-referenced to clarify discrepancies. With encouragement, most patients are capable of completing this sheet, if necessary with help from a friend or carer. In practice, it greatly speeds up consultations – sometimes virtually no conversation is required. It provides patient-reported outcome measures (PROMs) and generates audit and research data that can be applied across the whole clinic.

Drug Preparation and Giving Injections

Depending on the preparations available, you may need a refrigerator in the clinic. Always check you are diluting with

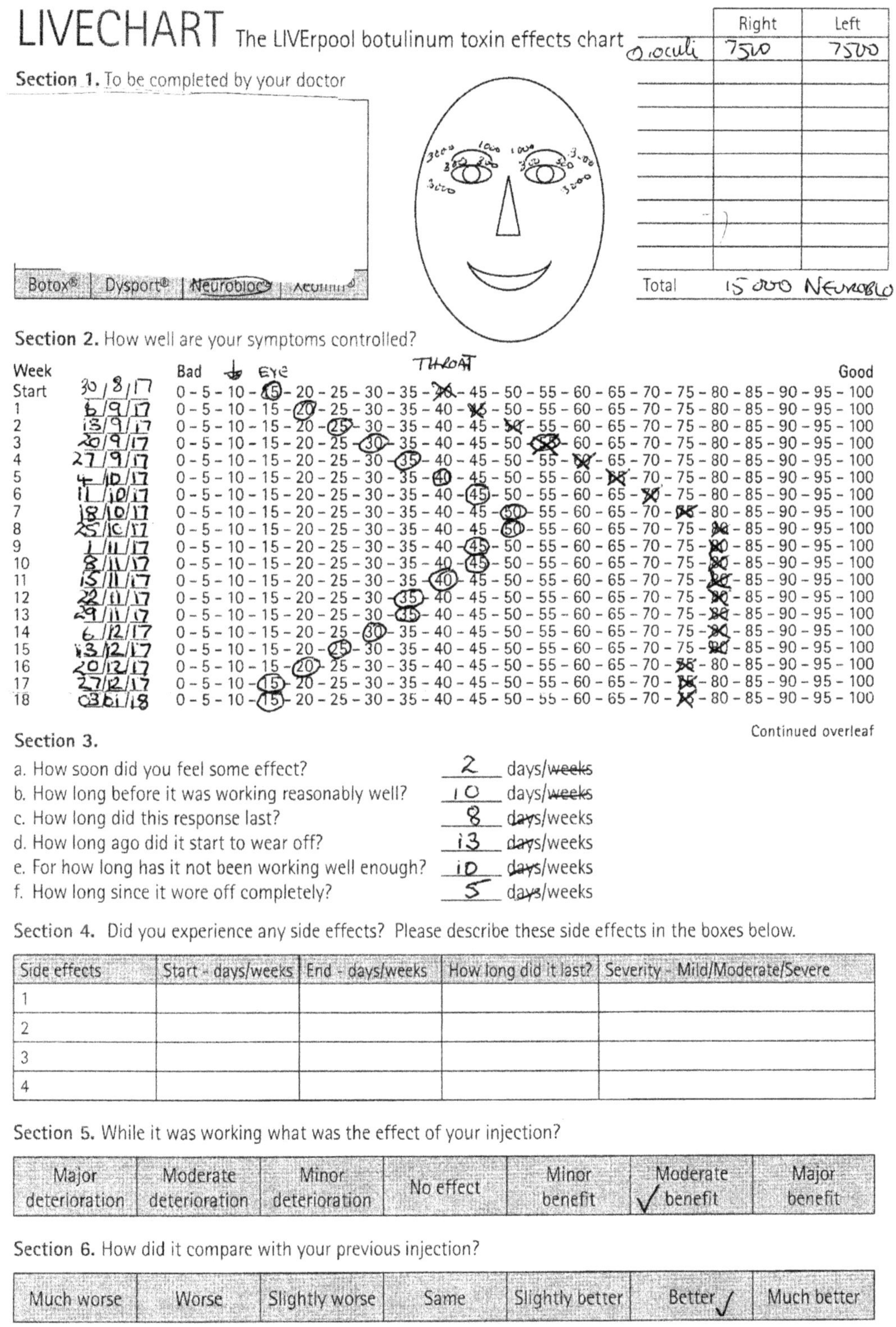

LIVECHART The LIVErpool botulinum toxin effects chart

Section 1. To be completed by your doctor

	Right	Left
O.oculi	7500	7500
Total	15 000 Neurobloc	

Botox® | Dysport® | Neurobloc® | Xeomin®

Section 2. How well are your symptoms controlled?

Week — Bad … Good (EYE / THROAT)

Week	Date	Scale
Start	30/8/17	0 - 5 - 10 - 15 - 20 - 25 - 30 - 35 - 40 - 45 - 50 - 55 - 60 - 65 - 70 - 75 - 80 - 85 - 90 - 95 - 100
1	6/9/17	0 - 5 - 10 - 15 - 20 - 25 - 30 - 35 - 40 - 45 - 50 - 55 - 60 - 65 - 70 - 75 - 80 - 85 - 90 - 95 - 100
2	13/9/17	0 - 5 - 10 - 15 - 20 - 25 - 30 - 35 - 40 - 45 - 50 - 55 - 60 - 65 - 70 - 75 - 80 - 85 - 90 - 95 - 100
3	20/9/17	0 - 5 - 10 - 15 - 20 - 25 - 30 - 35 - 40 - 45 - 50 - 55 - 60 - 65 - 70 - 75 - 80 - 85 - 90 - 95 - 100
4	27/9/17	0 - 5 - 10 - 15 - 20 - 25 - 30 - 35 - 40 - 45 - 50 - 55 - 60 - 65 - 70 - 75 - 80 - 85 - 90 - 95 - 100
5	4/10/17	0 - 5 - 10 - 15 - 20 - 25 - 30 - 35 - 40 - 45 - 50 - 55 - 60 - 65 - 70 - 75 - 80 - 85 - 90 - 95 - 100
6	11/10/17	0 - 5 - 10 - 15 - 20 - 25 - 30 - 35 - 40 - 45 - 50 - 55 - 60 - 65 - 70 - 75 - 80 - 85 - 90 - 95 - 100
7	18/10/17	0 - 5 - 10 - 15 - 20 - 25 - 30 - 35 - 40 - 45 - 50 - 55 - 60 - 65 - 70 - 75 - 80 - 85 - 90 - 95 - 100
8	25/10/17	0 - 5 - 10 - 15 - 20 - 25 - 30 - 35 - 40 - 45 - 50 - 55 - 60 - 65 - 70 - 75 - 80 - 85 - 90 - 95 - 100
9	1/11/17	0 - 5 - 10 - 15 - 20 - 25 - 30 - 35 - 40 - 45 - 50 - 55 - 60 - 65 - 70 - 75 - 80 - 85 - 90 - 95 - 100
10	8/11/17	0 - 5 - 10 - 15 - 20 - 25 - 30 - 35 - 40 - 45 - 50 - 55 - 60 - 65 - 70 - 75 - 80 - 85 - 90 - 95 - 100
11	15/11/17	0 - 5 - 10 - 15 - 20 - 25 - 30 - 35 - 40 - 45 - 50 - 55 - 60 - 65 - 70 - 75 - 80 - 85 - 90 - 95 - 100
12	22/11/17	0 - 5 - 10 - 15 - 20 - 25 - 30 - 35 - 40 - 45 - 50 - 55 - 60 - 65 - 70 - 75 - 80 - 85 - 90 - 95 - 100
13	29/11/17	0 - 5 - 10 - 15 - 20 - 25 - 30 - 35 - 40 - 45 - 50 - 55 - 60 - 65 - 70 - 75 - 80 - 85 - 90 - 95 - 100
14	6/12/17	0 - 5 - 10 - 15 - 20 - 25 - 30 - 35 - 40 - 45 - 50 - 55 - 60 - 65 - 70 - 75 - 80 - 85 - 90 - 95 - 100
15	13/12/17	0 - 5 - 10 - 15 - 20 - 25 - 30 - 35 - 40 - 45 - 50 - 55 - 60 - 65 - 70 - 75 - 80 - 85 - 90 - 95 - 100
16	20/12/17	0 - 5 - 10 - 15 - 20 - 25 - 30 - 35 - 40 - 45 - 50 - 55 - 60 - 65 - 70 - 75 - 80 - 85 - 90 - 95 - 100
17	27/12/17	0 - 5 - 10 - 15 - 20 - 25 - 30 - 35 - 40 - 45 - 50 - 55 - 60 - 65 - 70 - 75 - 80 - 85 - 90 - 95 - 100
18	03/01/18	0 - 5 - 10 - 15 - 20 - 25 - 30 - 35 - 40 - 45 - 50 - 55 - 60 - 65 - 70 - 75 - 80 - 85 - 90 - 95 - 100

Continued overleaf

Section 3.

a. How soon did you feel some effect? 2 days/~~weeks~~
b. How long before it was working reasonably well? 10 days/~~weeks~~
c. How long did this response last? 8 ~~days~~/weeks
d. How long ago did it start to wear off? 13 ~~days~~/weeks
e. For how long has it not been working well enough? 10 ~~days~~/weeks
f. How long since it wore off completely? 5 ~~days~~/weeks

Section 4. Did you experience any side effects? Please describe these side effects in the boxes below.

Side effects	Start - days/weeks	End - days/weeks	How long did it last?	Severity - Mild/Moderate/Severe
1				
2				
3				
4				

Section 5. While it was working what was the effect of your injection?

Major deterioration	Moderate deterioration	Minor deterioration	No effect	Minor benefit	Moderate benefit ✓	Major benefit

Section 6. How did it compare with your previous injection?

Much worse	Worse	Slightly worse	Same	Slightly better	Better ✓	Much better

Figure 39.1 Anonymised homework sheet (LIVEchart ©), showing muscles and doses injected and good response to the area treated. Intriguingly, in previous cycles, this lady had reported parallel improvement in her spasmodic dysphonia, which was never directly treated. I asked her to score this on the LIVEchart © to clarify the timing and perceived degree of benefit. Her throat symptoms deteriorated back to baseline in weeks 20–24 (not shown). Arrow indicates 'worst ever' symptoms. VAS shows weekly scores. Higher scores are better. Onset, peak and wearing off, and relative benefit in each symptom are clearly appreciated. Note that this is an unusually large dose for blepharospasm.

normal saline (water for injection is very painful). Label any vials not used immediately with: the dilution, a use-by time and your name. I operate one Golden Rule: syringes containing normal saline have a green needle, syringes containing toxin solution have a blue or orange needle.

Although many patients can be successfully treated with freehand injections, it is worth having EMG and/or ultrasound available in your service, and needles that are long enough to reach deep muscles. These topics are covered in more detail elsewhere in this book.

Advantages and Disadvantages of Running a Botulinum Toxin Clinic

Clinics can create demand – the 'new motorway' syndrome – and can easily grow too big and require increasing resources. Clinics that are too focused on giving botulinum toxin treatment can inhibit holistic care and there is a temptation to treat everything with toxin. Clinics risk generating the perception that botulinum toxin is an expensive treatment, as all the costs are visible and highlighted, by comparison with oral medication and other therapy costs that are distributed through the region – even though toxin may well be cheaper on analysis of cost per day of successful treatment.

On the plus side, clinics promote efficient use of toxin and scarce medical time. They allow proper short- and long-term planning of staffing, training and facilities. They facilitate links between service professionals. Finally – and these topics are not covered here – they provide a nucleus encouraging publicity and better diagnosis, patient education and support services, and a resource for audit and research.

References

Dressler D, Kupsch A, Seitzinger A, Paus S (2014) The Dystonia Discomfort Scale (DDS): a novel instrument to monitor the temporal profile of botulinum toxin therapy in cervical dystonia. *Eur J Neurol* 21:459–462.

Moore P, Naumann M (2003) General and clinical aspects of treatment with botulinum toxin. In: Moore P, Naumann M (eds) *Handbook of Botulinum Toxin Treatment*, 2nd edition. Blackwell Science, Malden, MA, pp. 68–69.

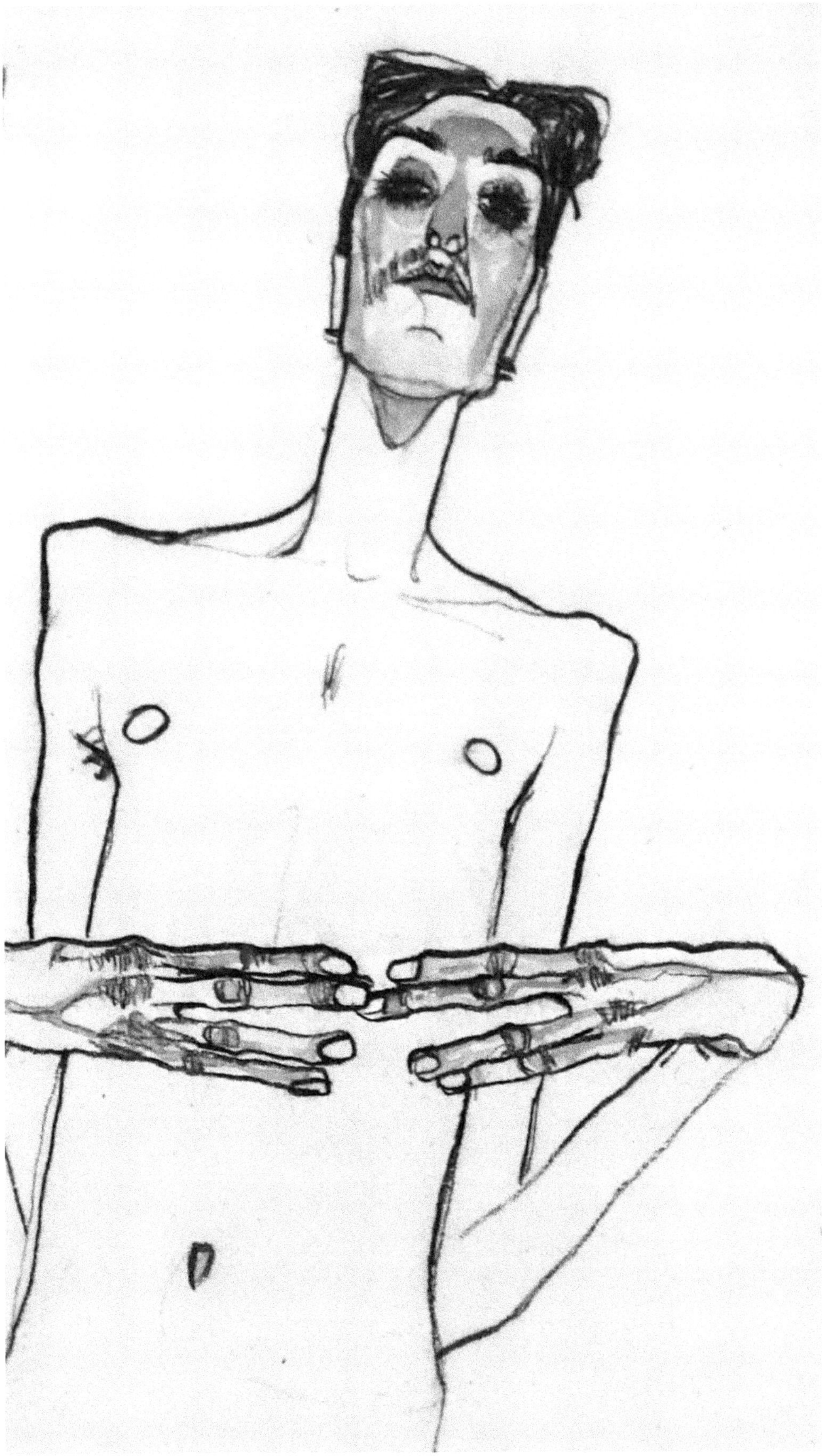

Chapter 40

Phenomenology of Musician's Dystonia

Steven J. Frucht

Framing the Problem

Musician's dystonia (MD) refers to dystonia affecting a part of the body involved in performance of a musical instrument. While dystonia may spread to involve other tasks or even other body regions, MD in its purest form is an exquisite focal task-specific dystonia. MD most commonly affects the arm, and in a sizable minority of patients involves the lower cranial structures (so-called 'embouchure dystonia'). The occurrence of rare patients with singer's dystonia (vocal cord) (Halstead et al. 2015) or even rock-drummer's dystonia of the leg (Lee & Altenmuller 2014) illustrates that any body region can be involved. The incidence and prevalence of MD are unknown, but estimates from the Hannover group's series of over 1000 patients supports a lifetime prevalence as high as 1 in 200 (Altenmuller et al. 2015). For perspective, the prevalence of torticollis (the most common form of focal dystonia) is only 30 per 100 000 (Evatt et al. 2011). MD differs from other forms of focal dystonia in its striking male predominance, at 4:1 (Schmidt et al. 2013), seen in both European and Western series. Genetic factors are also likely important, illustrated by the recent discovery of familial MD and writer's cramp associated with the arylsulphatase A locus (Lohmann et al. 2014).

Symptoms of MD usually begin in the late thirties, and most patients present either a decade before or after this mark. Onset of the disorder before age 18 is almost unheard of. Compared to other forms of focal dystonia, MD occurs at nearly the same age as writer's cramp or torticollis, and earlier than blepharospasm, Meige syndrome, spasmodic dysphonia, leg dystonia and truncal dystonia (Altenmuller et al. 2015). Several factors have been shown to influence the development of MD besides male gender and family history. Onset of musical training after age ten and increasing accumulated practice hours predispose to development of the condition (Altenmuller & Jabusch 2010). Psychological factors such as anxiety and perfectionism are also more common in MD patients (Baur et al. 2011; Enders et al. 2011).

Historical Perspective

Descriptions of MD date back nearly 200 years. Neurologists of the late nineteenth and early twentieth centuries wrote about MD with a beauty and insight that is still unsurpassed today. In 1830 Sir Charles Bell first described writer's cramp, later expanded upon by Samuel Sully in his elegant description of 'scrivener's palsy'. Duchenne, Hammond, Oppenheim and, especially, Gowers devoted significant portions of their neurologic texts to focal task-specific dystonia, including MD (Frucht 2014). These pioneers recognised MD as an organic centrally mediated disorder, allied to other occupational dystonias such as 'writer's paralysis, telegrapher's paralysis, hammer paralysis, and so on'. More than a decade prior to his seminal work coining the term dystonia, Oppenheim wrote:

> Piano-player's cramp consists, as a rule, in abnormal muscular contractions, from which a finger or several remain lifted from the keys or are pressed upon them.... Violinists' cramp may affect the bowing hand or the hand pressing upon the strings, occasionally both.... An occupational neurosis of the labial muscles was seen by me in a horn-blower. As soon as he placed the mouthpiece to his lips a spasm came on in the orbicularis oris, so that the patient was unable to bring out a tune.

In the early part of the twentieth century, neurologists used the term 'geigen-neurosis' (occupational neurosis) to describe focal task-specific dystonia, including MD. Misinterpretation of this moniker led to the view that these disorders were psychiatric in origin, a perversion of the original intent of the word. It was not until David Marsden's seminal observation that blepharospasm, spasmodic dysphonia, torticollis and writer's cramp were related conditions that MD was again viewed as an organic disorder (Marsden 1976).

Several famous musicians have been afflicted with MD, with profound personal and professional impact. Robert Schumann developed MD in his right hand at age 19, ending his career as a public performer and forcing him to concentrate on composition and music criticism (Garcia de Yebenes 1995). Yehudi Menuhin likely developed MD in his bowing arm in his thirties, impairing his confidence and resulting in playing that was unpredictable for the remainder of his career. His later explorations of yoga and meditation may have been an attempt to understand and remedy his condition. Leon Fleisher and Gary Graffman, two of the most celebrated American pianists of the twentieth century, developed nearly identical forms of MD affecting the fourth and fifth fingers of their right hands (Newmark 1999). Both expanded their artistic outlets to master the left-hand repertoire, and to teach and mentor several generations of American pianists.

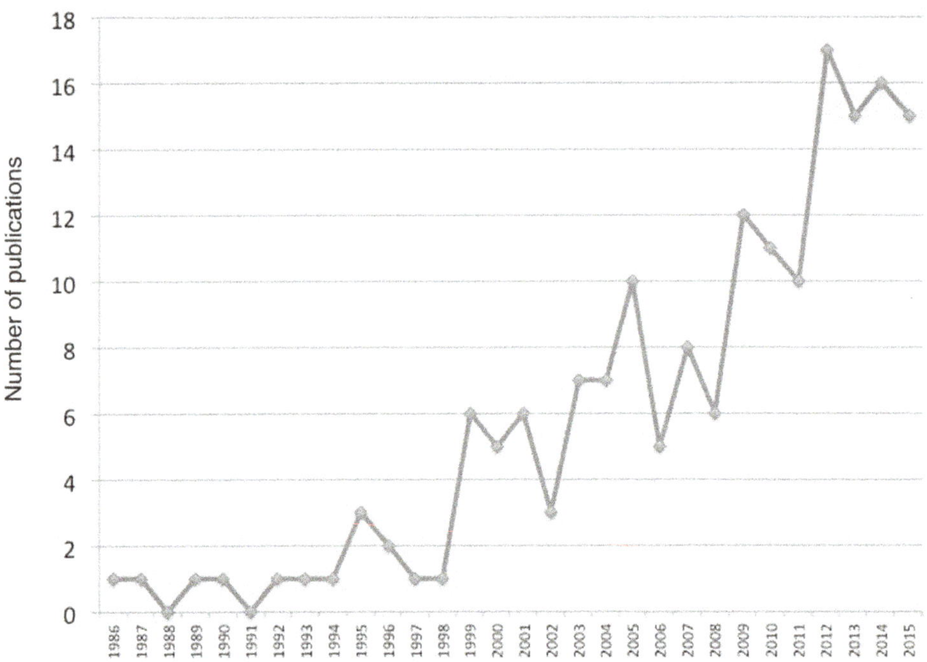

Figure 40.1 The graph demonstrates the growth of PubMed publications involving music and dystonia over the last 30 years.

Modern interest in MD developed in the 1980s and 1990s (Figure 40.1), coincident with the emergence of the field of performing arts medicine. Alice Brandfonbrener and Richard Lederman spearheaded this movement, with important contributions from Richard Wilson, Michael Charness, Fred Hochberg, Mark Hallett, Eckart Altenmuller and Hans-Christian Jabusch. In 2000, Glen Estrin and I formed the organisation *Musicians with Dystonia* under the auspices of the Dystonia Medical Research Foundation (DMRF) to raise awareness and encourage research. In 2004, Leon Fleisher partnered with the DMRF in a public awareness campaign, 'Freedom to Play', coincident with the release of the Academy-award-nominated short film *Two Hands* which documented his 35-year saga with MD. This rise in public awareness has been accompanied by an exponential increase in scientific investigation of MD.

What is Known About Phenomenology?

Current understanding of the phenomenology of MD is robust, thanks to large patient series published by Newmark, Wilson, Hochberg, Charness, Bradnfonbrener, Lederman, Frucht, Jabusch and Altenmuller (Newmark & Hochberg 1987; Hochberg et al. 1990; Wilson et al. 1993; Charness et al.1996; Brandfonbrener & Robson 2004; Schuele & Lederman 2004; Conti et al. 2008; Altenmuller et al. 2014; van Vugt et al. 2014). Cases of task-specific drummer's foot dystonia and singer's dystonia are rare, and do not allow a complete picture of these disorders. In contrast, well over 1000 patients with MD affecting the upper extremity have been reported. MD usually begins insidiously, expressed as a loss of automaticity or as a need to expend greater effort to accomplish musical tasks that were previously automatic. Symptoms often begin with specific techniques – for example, ascending scales in pianists or specific keys in woodwind players. One finger may be involved initially, with spread to other adjacent fingers over time. Office evaluation should always include careful observation of patients playing their instrument; dystonic movements typically begin within seconds of playing. A history of prominent pain, numbness or paresthesias, spontaneous remissions, symptoms present only after sustained playing or difficulty with other arm tasks should alert the examiner that the diagnosis is likely *not* dystonia.

MD has been described with virtually every instrument, including keyboard, strings, plectrum, woodwind, brass and drums. The relative paucity of certain instruments such as double bass or cello and the overrepresentation of piano, violin and guitar suggests the possibility that instruments that demand fine simultaneous finger placement may predispose to the development of dystonia.

The distribution of the hand involved in MD is likely not random. Among pianists and guitarists the right hand is preferentially involved, among violinists the left hand and among woodwind players both hands are involved equally, with the exception of flautists where the left hand is more common (Conti et al. 2014; see Figure 40.2). These trends correlate with differences in the technical demands imposed by each instrument. The virtuoso piano repertoire demands more from the right hand than the left as the right hand must play the inner harmonies while also carrying the treble melodic line with the third, fourth and fifth fingers. On the violin the technical demands of the fingering hand (left) are extreme, requiring sub-millimetre precision for professional-level playing. The right and left hands perform similar roles in woodwind instruments (clarinet, oboe, bassoon), which may explain the relatively equal distribution of hand involvement. The one exception is flute, where the left hand must support the weight of the instrument as well as depress the keys.

The majority of MD patients have been reported with involvement of individual fingers. Flexion dystonia clearly predominates over extension, likely due to the mechanical

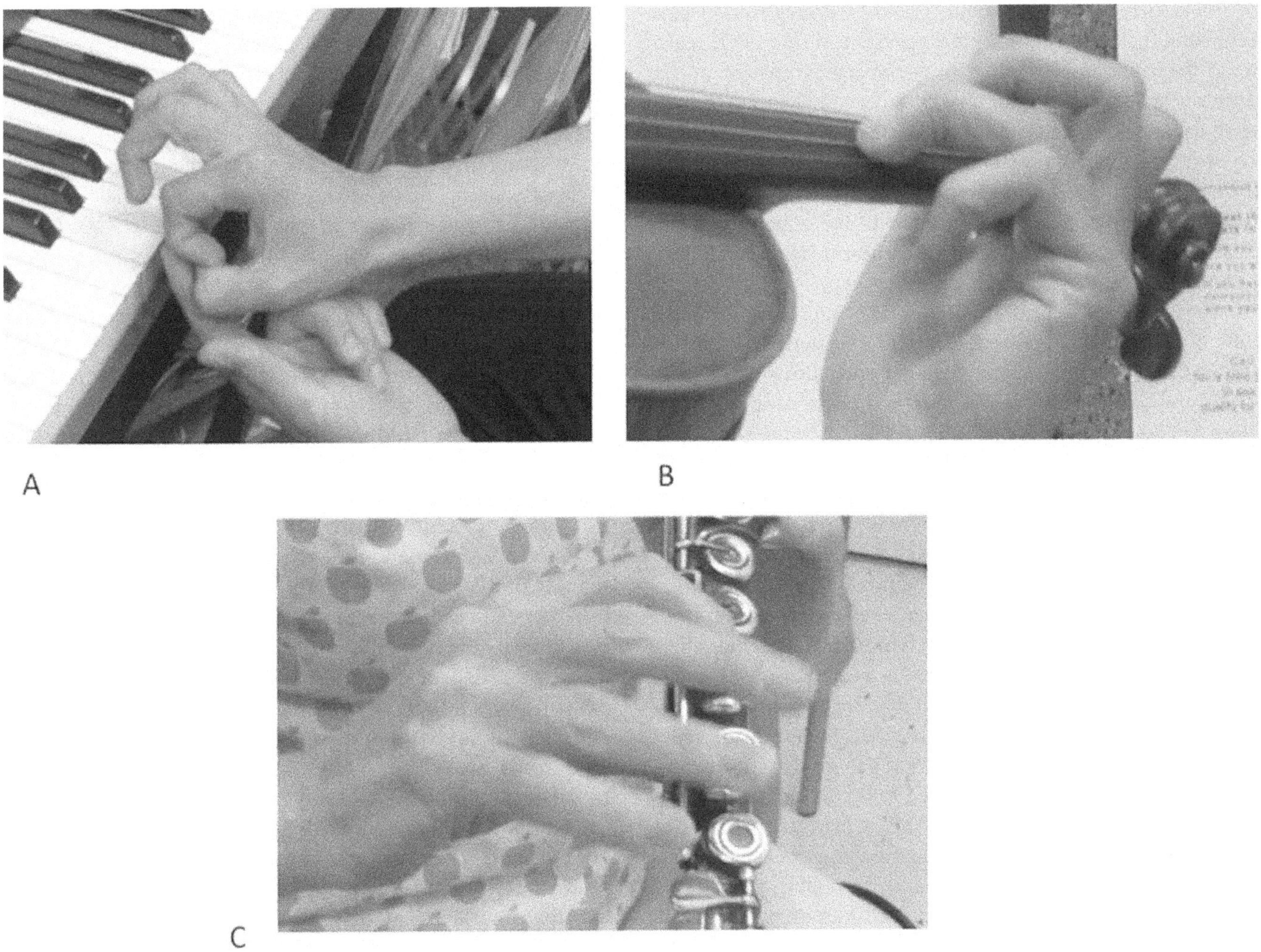

A B C

Figure 40.2 Three still photos taken from video recordings of MD dystonia illustrate classic phenotypes: (a) pianist with flexion of the thumb and index finger; (b) violinist with flexion of the left fifth finger; (c) flautist with extension of the third finger.

demands of pressing a key, covering an open hole or stopping a string. Two patterns emerge in analysing finger involvement. First, most finger patterns involve adjacent fingers – it is quite rare for dystonia to skip a finger. Second, the fourth and fifth fingers are much more commonly involved than the first three fingers (Conti et al. 2014). Finally, early reports drew attention to patterns of dystonic phenotypes in MD, including flexion of the thumb and index finger, extension of the middle finger, and flexion of the fourth and fifth fingers. Thumb and index flexion was common in plectrum instrumentalists (e.g. banjo), extension of the middle finger in woodwind players, and flexion of the fourth and fifth fingers in string players (left hand), and guitarists and pianists (right hand) (Newmark & Hochberg 1987).

In 2001 we reported the first large series of patients with task-specific dystonia of the embouchure, the muscles and structures of the face, lips, jaw, tongue and pharynx used to control the flow of air into the mouthpiece of a brass or woodwind instrument (Frucht et al. 2001). In 2009 we extended these observations to 89 patients, the largest series reported to date (Frucht 2009). The embouchure is a complex motor activation network, and the fine movements of the facial muscles are the only part of the system visible to the examiner. There are four distinct types of embouchures, each with different technical demands. Brass players modulate the tension of their lips to control the diameter of the opening through which air flows. They also must create a 'buzz' by precisely vibrating their lips to control the pitch and tone quality of their sound. Single-reed players such as clarinet and saxophone create this buzz differently, by controlling the pressure applied to the instrument's reed with their lower jaw. Double-reed players (oboe, bassoon) control the vibration of their instruments by exerting pressure with both the upper and lower teeth. Finally, flute and piccolo players must create sound using a fixed opening while stabilising the instrument with their lower jaw and lip.

The typical patient with embouchure dystonia presents similarly to musician's hand dystonia, with an insidious, painless deterioration in their playing, present from the moment they play. Office evaluation should ask brass players to 'free buzz' (vibrate their lips as if they were playing), and also to simulate playing using only their mouthpiece. Patients should be asked to perform passages that are easy, and also passages or techniques that specifically trigger dystonia. The majority of embouchure dystonia patients present with register-specific problems (i.e. dystonic symptoms present in one pitch register of the instrument), and technique-specific impairment (i.e. dystonic symptoms present only with certain techniques, such as sharp attacks or smooth legato playing). Six distinct phenotypes of embouchure dystonia occur: tremor, lip-pulling, lip-lock, jaw, tongue and task-specific Meige. Patients with tremor phenotype show a rapid, 8 Hz tremor of the upper and lower lips that is typically register-specific and noticeable with sustained legato notes. In lip-pulling phenotype, one lip (usually the upper) moves aberrantly to one side, interfering with the flow of air. Lip-lock refers to a peculiar pattern of coactivation of the lips, bringing them together and cutting off the flow of air and sound. Tongue dystonia and jaw dystonia are less common and much more difficult to visualise on exam. Task-specific Meige is exceptionally rare, similar in appearance to ordinary Meige with the exception of its specific trigger.

As in MD affecting the hand, there is not a 1:1 link between instrument and dystonic phenotype – for example, tremor phenotype may occur in trumpeters, tuba players, clarinettists or bassoonists. However, certain patterns do emerge. Tremor and lip-pulling phenotypes are much more common in higher-register brass instruments (trumpet and French horn), while lip-lock is exclusively observed in low-register brass instrumentalists (trombone and tuba). Jaw and tongue phenotypes are much more common in woodwind players than brass players. These tendencies may be related to the technical demands of each instrument. High-register brass instruments such as trumpet and French horn impose significant physical demands on the embouchure, and tremor and lip-pulling phenotypes may be a response to these demands. Lip-lock phenotype's link to low-register brass instruments may relate to the technical demands of these instruments, i.e. these instruments prize performance of separated notes as accompanying lines. Jaw and tongue phenotypes are markedly overrepresented in woodwind players. This may relate to the embouchure mechanics of a single reed, double reed or flute that constrain upper and lower jaw. As many as 50 per cent of patients with jaw or tongue phenotypes experience spread of dystonia to speaking or eating, and these dystonic features can persist even if the patient stops playing. For this reason we recommend that patients with jaw or tongue embouchure dystonia quit playing, even though they may be reluctant to do so.

Phenomenology as a Guide to Investigation of Mechanism

The motor training programme required for a performer to achieve instrumental mastery is intense, requiring study in childhood through early adulthood of at least 10 000 hours. Intuitively, it makes sense that training should play a role in the development of dystonia. For example, the only convincing animal model of focal hand dystonia demonstrated disordered cortical somatotopy in the primate primary sensory and motor cortex, linking over-performance of a motor task with structural brain changes. However, intense acquired motor training is not required to develop task-specific dystonia. Some patients with adductor or abductor spasmodic dysphonia have vocal breaks triggered by specific vowels or consonant combinations, and rare forms of writer's cramp may be triggered by writing specific letters or words. Task-specific speaking dystonia may affect certain dialects or speech patterns, and even task-specific leg dystonia may affect patients with specific walking patterns such as walking up or down stairs. None of these patients trained excessively to learn to speak, to write or to walk. Highly attended, skilled motor training is thus not a requirement for the development of task-specific dystonia.

A striking feature of MD is the variety of different phenotypes, and the stability of these dystonic patterns in a given patient over time. Once a pianist develops dystonic flexion of the fourth and fifth fingers of the right hand, for example, this pattern is invariant and almost always permanent. By analogy, stability of the phenotype is a cardinal feature of blepharospasm and torticollis, and this stability allows patients to enjoy a robust and stable response to botulinum toxin injections. One possible explanation for this phenomenon might involve the role of the striatum in motor subroutine selection and the importance of centre–surround inhibition. Ordinarily a musician enjoys almost unlimited degrees of freedom in selecting muscles needed to perform a task. For whatever reason, an event triggers a marked reduction in the degrees of freedom and constrains motor programme selection. This new constrained circuit becomes stable and entrained, either by facilitation or inhibition of other motor pathways.

Another striking feature of phenomenology seen in MD (and by analogy in dystonia in general) is the idea of spread. A small minority of MD patients relates a history of dystonia affecting one finger at onset, with gradual spread to involve adjacent fingers. A similar story occurs frequently in embouchure dystonia, where patients describe onset of difficulty with one particular note and continuous spread of dystonia to higher and lower pitches over weeks to months. Spread may also occur in the hand from dystonia limited to specific technical passages (i.e. scales in certain keys) to more generalised dystonia while playing. The idea of spread from a task-specific trigger, to any motor activity, to occurrence at rest, dates back more than a century to Gowers' original description (Frucht 2014).

Although involuntary movements are the most obvious feature of MD, detailed histories of MD patients usually reveal another complaint that often precedes the involuntary movements – 'loss of automaticity'. Patients describe this phenomenon as a 'lack of control', 'lack of fine touch', 'having to exert more effort to accomplish the same task' or 'having to think about what was previously automatic'. Loss of automaticity might reflect a change in the performer's relationship to their instrument. In performing artists, the instrument is a complex tool, which becomes integrated into the performer's body and sensorimotor system. Loss of automaticity might be the inciting event in the development of MD. Compensatory mechanisms might be activated to compensate for this loss of automaticity, leading to overactivation and overselection of a motor subroutine. By the time the patient is seen by the neurologist in the office, involuntary movements are usually well

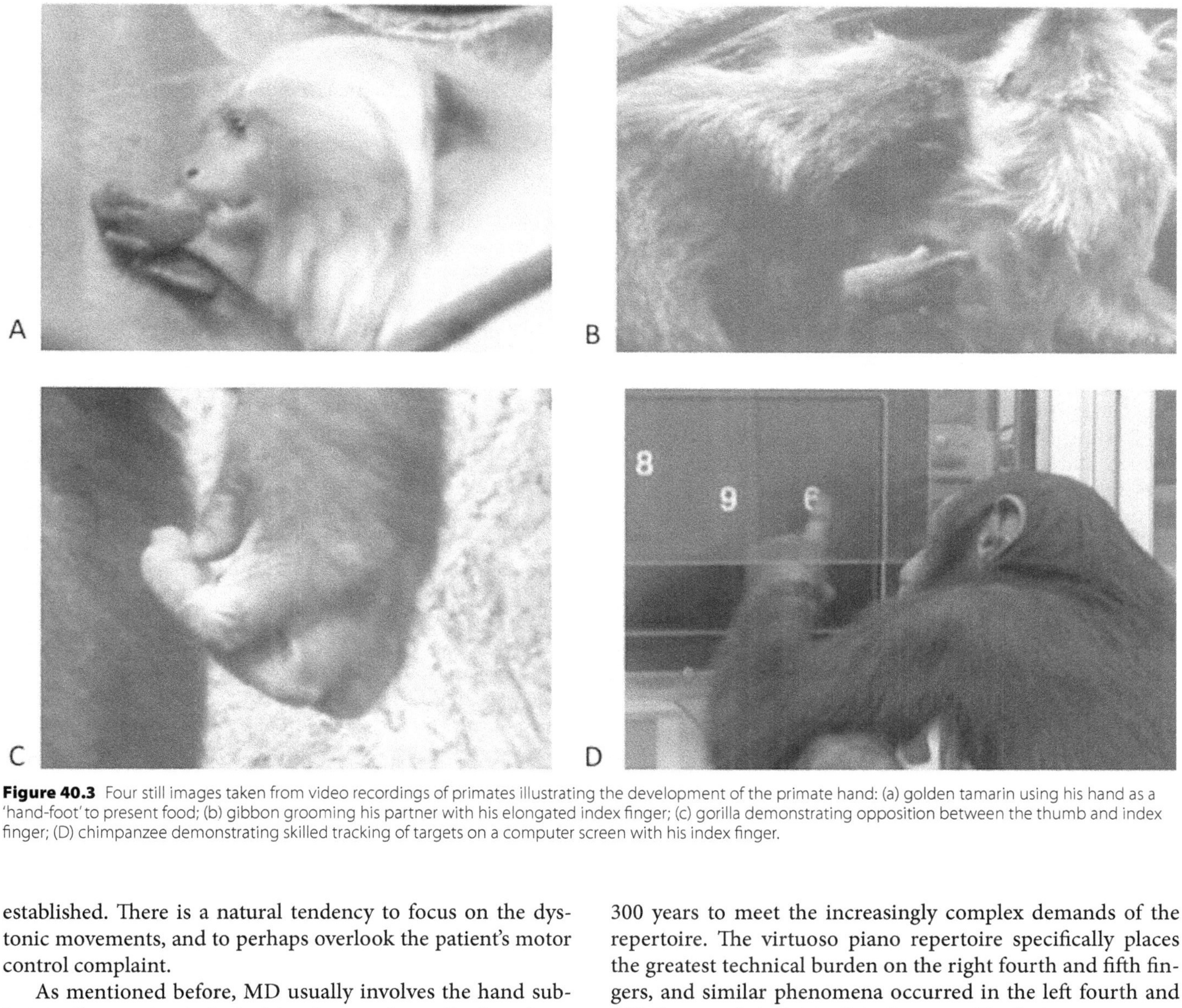

Figure 40.3 Four still images taken from video recordings of primates illustrating the development of the primate hand: (a) golden tamarin using his hand as a 'hand-foot' to present food; (b) gibbon grooming his partner with his elongated index finger; (c) gorilla demonstrating opposition between the thumb and index finger; (D) chimpanzee demonstrating skilled tracking of targets on a computer screen with his index finger.

established. There is a natural tendency to focus on the dystonic movements, and to perhaps overlook the patient's motor control complaint.

As mentioned before, MD usually involves the hand subject to the greater technical burden, and usually the ulnar-innervated hand more than the median-innervated hand. The prevalence of ulnar-innervated involvement could be related to the interplay between the biomechanical demands of the instrument and the evolutionarily derived limitations of the primate hand. Over 60 million years, the primate hand began as a 'hand-foot', grasping food and presenting it to be eaten with crude flexion-extension of all fingers together. Over time individual finger movements developed, especially the index finger (for grooming) and the thumb (for opposition with the index and middle fingers in the great apes) (Figure 40.3). Napier proposed a seminal idea in the mid-twentieth century, separating hand tasks into those performed by the *precision grip* (thumb, index and middle finger) and those performed by the *power grip* (fourth and fifth fingers, transmitting a striking or power impulse from the upper arm) (Napier 1962). Most precision tasks such as writing, using a paintbrush or threading a needle are performed by the precision hand. String and keyboard instruments changed dramatically over the last 300 years to meet the increasingly complex demands of the repertoire. The virtuoso piano repertoire specifically places the greatest technical burden on the right fourth and fifth fingers, and similar phenomena occurred in the left fourth and fifth fingers of violinists. It is then possible that overrepresentation of dystonia in these ulnar-innervated muscles relates to the excessive mechanical demands placed on the power hand, which was not designed by millions of years of evolution to meet requirements that are usually better served by the precision hand.

Phenomenology as a Guide to Treatment

As with any disease, it is worth approaching the idea of treatment of MD from three perspectives: prevention, cure and symptomatic therapy. The idea of preventing MD may seem far-fetched, especially since such factors as male gender, age at onset of training and amount of practice time are out of the control of the neurologist. However, it may be worth considering the possibility that pedagogical factors could enhance or inhibit the development of MD. The following recommendations remain a suggested guide based on the experience of the author with his patients. A focus on efficiency of movement, relaxation and playing that requires a minimum of expended effort seems wise. Avoidance of simultaneous forced activation of adjacent fingers, avoiding rapid shifts in repertoire difficulty and practice time and avoiding peripheral biomechanical injuries (sprain, peripheral neuropathy) that might trigger the onset of dystonia also seems reasonable.

Once symptoms of MD occur they are almost always permanent. Refraining from playing usually does not result in disappearance of symptoms; however, it may be that symptoms are already well established when this is tried. Gowers noted the benefits of complete rest from the offending task in writer's cramp, noting that rest was often employed too late to achieve real benefit (Frucht 2014). Most patients with MD are initially evaluated by their music teachers, and it may be more than a year before an affected patient is evaluated by a neurologist with familiarity with the disorder.

Treatments for MD are considered in other chapters of this volume, and we will confine our comments to the role phenomenology may play in guiding therapy. Distinguishing the primary dystonic movement from compensatory movements is the single most important, and most difficult, part of the evaluation. If muscles that trigger dystonia are injected, the patient will usually improve, while if compensatory muscles are inadvertently injected they will worsen. Injection techniques including e-stim and ultrasound have dramatically improved the accuracy of targeting. Patients may often notice that the period following initial weakness from injections allows them a window to retrain and explore accommodation techniques to adapt to their dystonia. Details of administration of toxin, the role of medications, and the use of physical therapy and sensory modulation techniques are covered in other chapters within this volume.

Acknowledgement/Dedication

I wish to acknowledge the expert and compassionate role that my good friend and patient Glen Estrin has played over the last 15 years, guiding and improving the lives of patients with MD throughout the world. I am grateful for the courage and inspiration of Leon Fleisher in sharing his story, bringing the entity of MD and indeed the word dystonia to more than 200 million people. Finally, this chapter is dedicated to my late friend, Dr Oliver Sacks. Oliver lent his support to our foundation, and also helped to raise awareness of MD by writing so eloquently of his meeting with Leon in his book, *Musicophilia*. A lifelong lover of music and a believer in the power of music to inspire and heal, he was and is an inspiration to me and to other neurologists who believe in the value of careful observation and individualised attention to patients.

References

Altenmuller E, Jabusch HC. 2010. Focal dystonia in musicians: phenomenology, pathophysiology, triggering factors, and treatment. *Med Probl Perform Art* 25:35d.

Altenmuller E, Ioannou CI, Raab M, Lobinger B. 2014. Apollo's curse: causes and cures of motor failure in musicians – a proposal for a new classification. *Adv Exp Med Biol* 826:161–178.

Altenmuller E, Ioannou CI, Lee A. 2015. Apollo's curse: neurological causes of motor impairments in musicians. *Prog Brain Res* 217:89–106.

Baur V, Jabusch HC, Altenmuller E. 2011. Behavioral factors influence the phenotype of musician's dystonia. *Mov Disord* 26:1780–1781.

Brandfonbrener AG, Robson C. 2004. Review of 113 musicians with focal dystonia seen between 1985 and 2002 at a clinic for performing artists. *Adv Neurol* 94:255–256.

Charness ME, Ross MH, Shefner JM. 1996. Ulnar neuropathy and dystonic flexion of the fourth and fifth digits: clinical correlation in musicians. *Muscle Nerve* 19:431–437.

Conti AM, Pullman S, Frucht SJ. 2008. The hand that has forgotten its cunning: lessons from musicians' hand dystonia. *Mov Disord* 23:1398–1406.

Enders L, Spector JT, Altenmuller E, Schmidt A, Klein C, Jabusch HC. 2011. Musician's dystonia and comorbid anxiety: two sides of one coin? *Mov Disord* 26:539–542.

Evatt ML, Freeman A, Factor S. 2011. Adult-onset dystonia. *Handb Clin Neurol* 100:481–511.

Frucht SJ. 2009. Embouchure dystonia: portrait of a task-specific cranial dystonia. *Mov Disord* 24:1752–1762.

Frucht SJ. 2014. Focal task-specific dystonia: from early descriptions to a new, modern formulation. *Tremor Other Hyperkinet Mov* 4:230. doi:10.7916/D8VD6WHP

Frucht SJ, Fahn S, Greene PE, O'Brien C, Gelb M, Truong DD, Welsh J, Factor S, Ford B. 2001. The natural history of embouchure dystonia. *Mov Disord* 16:899–906.

Garcia de Yebenes J. 1995. Did Robert Schumann have dystonia? *Mov Disord* 10:413–417.

Halstead LA, McBroom DM, Bonilha HS. 2015. Task-specific singing dystonia: vocal instability that technique cannot fix. *J Voice* 29:71–78.

Hochberg FH, Harris SU, Blattert TR. 1990. Occupational hand cramps: professional disorders of motor control. *Hand Clin* 6:417–428.

Lee A, Altenmuller E. 2014. Heavy metal curse: a task-specific dystonia in the proximal lower limb of a professional percussionist. *Med Probl Perform Art* 29:174–176.

Lohmann K, Schmidt A, Schillert A Winkler S, Albanese A, Baas F, Bentivoglio AR, Borngräber F, Brüggemann N, Defazio G, Del Sorbo F, Deuschl G, Edwards MJ, Gasser T, Gómez-Garre P, Graf J, Groen JL, Grünewald A, Hagenah J, Hemmelmann C, Jabusch HC, Kaji R, Kasten M, Kawakami H, Kostic VS, Liguori M, Mir P, Münchau A, Ricchiuti F, Schreiber S, Siegesmund K, Svetel M, Tijssen MA, Valente EM, Westenberger A, Zeuner KE, Zittel S, Altenmüller E, Ziegler A, Klein C. 2014. Genome-wide association study in musician's dystonia: a risk variant at the arylsufatase G locus? *Mov Disord* 29:921–927.

Marsden CD. 1976. The problem of adult-onset idiopathic torsion dystonia and other isolated dyskinesias in adult life (including blepharospasm, oromandibular dystonia, dystonic writer's cramp, and torticollis, or axial dystonia). *Adv Neurol* 14:259–276.

Napier J. 1962. The evolution of the hand. *Sci Am* 207:56–62.

Newmark J. 1999. Musicians' dystonia: the case of Gary Graffman. *Semin Neurol* 19S1:41–45.

Newmark J, Hochberg FH. 1987. Isolated painless manual incoordination in 57 musicians. *J Neurol Neurosurg Psychiatry* 50:291–295.

Schmidt A, Jabusch HC, Altenmuller E, Kasten M, Klein C. 2013. Challenges of making music: what causes musician's dystonia? *JAMA Neurol* 70:1456–1459.

Schuele S, Lederman RJ. 2004. Long-term outcome of focal dystonia in string instrumentalists. *Mov Disord* 19:43–48.

van Vugt FT, Boullet L, Jabusch HC, Altenmuller E. 2014. Musician's dystonia in pianists: long-term evaluation of retraining and other therapies. *Parkinsonism Relat Disord* 20:8–12.

Wilson FR, Wagner C, Homberg V. 1993. Biomechanical abnormalities in musicians with occupational cramp/focal dystonia. *J Hand Ther* 6:298–307.

Chapter 41

Aetiological Concepts of Musician's Dystonia

Eckart Altenmüller and Christos I. Ioannou*

Degradation of Motor Control in Musicians

Motor disturbances in musicians are common and include mild forms, such as temporary motor fatigue with short-term reduction of motor skills, painful overuse injuries following prolonged practice, anxiety-related motor failures during performances ('choking under pressure'), as well as more persistent losses of motor control, here termed 'dynamic stereotypes'. Musician's dystonia (MD), which is characterised by the permanent loss of control of highly skilled movements when playing a musical instrument, is the most severe manifestation of dysfunctional motor programmes and is frequently linked to a genetic susceptibility to develop such motor disturbances.

Based on the phenomenology, duration, triggering mechanisms, psychological background, symptomatology, response to the treatments and the genetic predisposition, we propose the following classification of motor disturbances in musicians (Altenmüller et al. 2014, 2015):

Motor Fatigue

Most musicians, at some point, experience a loss of motor control when playing their instrument. Frequently this phenomenon is short term and bound to either lack of practice or overuse. It is accompanied by mental or bodily fatigue and linked to reduced attention and insufficient movement monitoring. Usually these deteriorations of movement coordination are short term: they disappear overnight and do not compromise overall performance. Although these incidents seem to be frequent, there are almost no scientific data available. A recent questionnaire given to German orchestral brass instrumentalists identified temporary crises of embouchure coordination in as many as 30 per cent (Steinmetz et al. 2014). In clinical practice, the symptoms are lack of regularity in scales, trills and other fast, repetitive movements, and loss of sound quality and occasional early fatigue. Pain is not usually reported. There is no information available as to whether any medical intervention other than rest is useful to treat this condition.

Overuse Injury

In contrast to the former condition, overuse should only be diagnosed when pain is a dominating symptom and a history of either prolonged or unaccustomed practice exists. In this case, local inflammation of over-strained tissues, the release of pain-mediators, and spinal reflexes with increased or occasionally lowered muscle tone may lead to a deterioration of motor control, mostly accompanied by relieving movements (Szeto & Lin 2011). This condition may last a couple of days and, if the patient rests, subsides after a few weeks at the latest.

Choking Under Pressure

Another condition leading to a deterioration of motor control is 'choking under pressure' (CuP) (Hill et al. 2010). CuP describes the situation in which the individual perceives a situation to be unmanageable. This is accompanied by fear of failure, anxiety and increased arousal, leading to reduced motor control and worse performance outcome. In musicians, CuP is a relatively frequent experience, especially among performing novices, and is usually subsumed under the term 'performance anxiety'. According to questionnaires, 15–60 per cent of performing musicians occasionally suffer from this condition (Brugués 2011). It may lead to loss of agility, heightened muscular stiffness accompanied by increased co-contraction of antagonist muscles and, as a consequence, reduction of temporo-spatial precision of movements and sound quality. This has been impressively demonstrated in pianists (Yoshie et al. 2009). In brass players, the so-called tongue stopper prior to an important cue is a typical manifestation.

Dynamic Stereotype in Musicians

If motor incoordination and lack of motor control persist for more than four weeks despite the patient resting and careful rehabilitation under the guidance of a therapist or teacher, one can assume that there is a more severe alteration of sensorimotor networks leading to a deterioration of motor programmes in the central nervous system. We have called this condition 'dynamic stereotype', a term borrowed from the eminent Russian physiologist Ivan Pavlov (1951; for a critical review, see Windholz 1996). Originally, this condition can be understood as a reflection of fatal compensation strategies, which become automated. It can, at least in part, be conceptualised

* The work on this short review chapter has been funded by a grant from the Federal Ministry of Education and Research (BMBF) in the framework of the 'Rare-Diseases' Initiative DysTract.

Part of the current text has been previously published in Altenmüller E, Ioannou CI (2016). Music performance: expectations, failures and prevention. In: Raab M et al. (Eds) *Performance Psychology: Perception, Action, Cognition, and Emotion*. New York: Elsevier, pp. 103–119.

as a consequence of long-term CuP when these dysfunctional movements are stored in procedural memory traces, possibly as a consequence of conditioned reactions to previous choking experiences and procedural memory formation under stress (Klämpfl et al. 2013; Lobinger et al. 2014).

In many aspects, the phenomenology of dynamic stereotypes resembles focal, task-specific dystonia (see below). However, in contrast to the latter, it seems to be more modifiable and more fluctuating, especially during stressful performances. Dynamic stereotypes respond occasionally to sensory trick manoeuvres, such as alterations of either tactile input from the body parts affected by dystonia or alterations of auditory input, for example by delaying the produced sound. We were able to demonstrate that the improvement in motor control when the patient plays with a latex glove is related to better outcome of retraining and behavioural therapies (Paulig et al. 2014). It should be mentioned, however, that responses to sensory tricks and objective improvement are rare and highly variable (Cheng et al. 2013). Therefore, we prefer to consider this phenomenon a 'soft-sign' with respect to the classification of motor control problems.

Focal Dystonia in Musicians

The most severe movement disorder among instrumental performers is task-specific MD. Commonly, two major forms are distinguished: focal hand dystonia and embouchure dystonia. This movement disorder is characterised by persistent muscular incoordination or loss of voluntary motor control during task-specific highly trained movements, such as playing a musical instrument (Jankovic & Ashoori 2008). In most cases, pain does not accompany the disorder; occasionally, some muscular strain can occur when patients attempt to compensate for the dystonic movement by over-activating the antagonist muscles. However, lack of pain distinguishes it from the above-mentioned overuse injuries. It is important to make this distinction while bearing in mind that prolonged pain syndromes may lead to symptomatic dystonia. MD frequently terminates professional careers and is highly disabling among musicians (Altenmüller & Jabusch 2010).

Risk Factors for Developing Musician's Dystonia

Demographic data demonstrate a preponderance of male musicians, with a male:female ratio of about 4:1 (Lim & Altenmüller 2003). Hereditary factors play a role in the aetiology of MD, as a family history of dystonia exists in up to 36 per cent of affected musicians (Schmidt et al. 2009). According to epidemiological data, the probability of developing MD depends on the instrument played: guitar players, pianists and brass instrument players have the highest risk of developing dystonia (Altenmüller & Jabusch 2010). Repetitive use, controllability of motor actions, temporo-spatial demands, and extra-instrumental fine motor burdens, such as writing, are triggering factors (Baur et al. 2011; Altenmüller et al. 2012). Furthermore, musicians who start practising after age ten are at a much higher risk of developing MD (Schmidt et al. 2013).

While there is probably a certain overlap between MD and the above-described dynamic stereotypes, each of these disorders is distinct from the other. Generally, focal dystonia is more severe, and the dysfunctional movements are more obvious and more resistant to any attempt to correct them voluntarily. Furthermore, movements are less likely to respond to sensory tricks. Sudden spontaneous improvements are rare exceptions, and psychological stressors do not influence the loss of motor control to a major degree. Furthermore, in contrast to dynamic stereotypes, MD has a tendency to spread from the specific movement when playing the instrument to general, everyday movements (Rosset-Llobet et al. 2007). Moreover, MD and dynamic stereotypes respond to a lesser degree to the above-mentioned sensory tricks. Finally, one out of two musicians with focal dystonia were found to be additionally characterised by psychological traits related to increased levels of stress, anxiety and perfectionism (Ioannou & Altenmüller 2014). Recent studies revealed that those features could contribute significantly to the manifestation of dystonia by accelerating (about 10–15 years) or even promoting the triggering of the symptoms in musicians (Ioannou et al. 2016).

A Heuristic Model of Motor Disturbances in Musicians

Summarising the previous paragraphs, we can classify the five types of motor disorders according to the duration of motor degradation, the accompanying symptoms, the underlying neurophysiological mechanisms and the response to treatment. In Figure 41.1, we depict a heuristic model that goes from a continuous worsening of motor control to temporary subtle awkwardness, then to increasingly unstable motor control, and finally to fully developed focal dystonia. Furthermore, we have added triggering factors, identified in our previous epidemiological studies (Altenmüller 2003; Altenmüller & Jabusch 2010; Altenmüller et al. 2012; Ioannou et al. 2016).

In the beginning, motor fatigue may cause a temporary degradation of motor skills, or, in highly skilled experts, additional/alternative recruitment of muscles contributing to dysfunctional movements. This mechanism has been convincingly demonstrated in skilled table-tennis players (Aune et al. 2008) and most likely also applies to instrumental musicians. For example, in skilled piano players, fatigue of the long flexor muscles in the forearm may be compensated by activation of the intrinsic muscles in the hand, which in turn results in dysfunctional movements in the metacarpophalangeal (MCP) joints, with lack of fine control of touch and degraded sound quality. These changes are accompanied by central nervous adaptations due to short-term plasticity. These changes result in reduced amplitude of movement-related potentials and in an alteration of the topography of motor and premotor cortex activations (Dirnberger et al. 2004). Interestingly, in a study of musicians suffering from dystonia, a fatiguing muscular contraction significantly improved motor performance. In contrast, in healthy musicians, performance consistently worsened following fatigue (Pesenti et al. 2004).

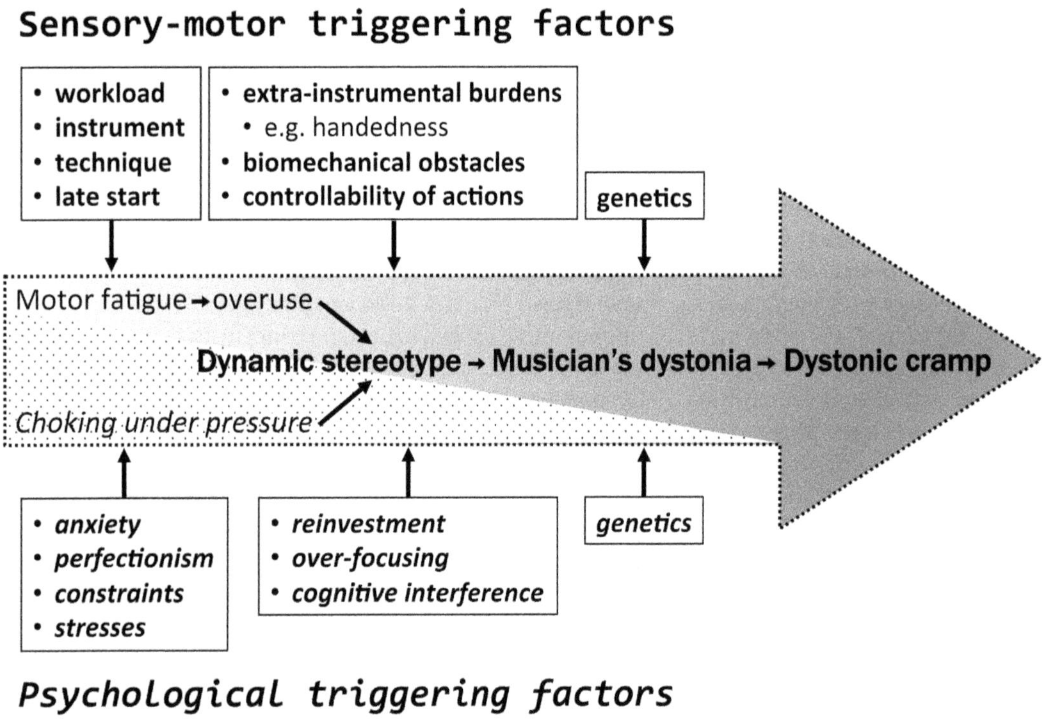

Figure 41.1 Heuristic model demonstrating the proposed interplay of sensorimotor and psychological triggering factors and their contribution to the different motor disturbances. The assumed degree of 'psychological' triggering factors is displayed as the dotted space; the increasing grey shading represents the increasing degree of loss of motor control.

In the overuse condition, dysfunctional CNS plasticity might play an important role in motor degradation (Byl et al. 1996; see also Flor 2012 for a review). Although in most instances the prognosis is good and quick recovery common, under conditions with heightened anxiety and other stressors, such as a high professional workload, these dysfunctional motor patterns may stabilise in procedural memory. Here, psychological stress might induce a cascade of emotionally induced memory consolidation, which has been previously described for different forms of memory and which mainly relies on noradrenergic activation of the basolateral amygdala (McGaugh 2000). The primary motor cortex, which is essentially involved in the storage of motor memories (Karni et al. 1998), receives a basolateral amygdala projection (Sripanidkulchai et al. 1984). Thus, it can be assumed that consolidation of these dys-coordinated movements as dysfunctional motor programmes is a BLA-mediated process in the primary motor cortex (Jabusch & Altenmüller 2004). This may also be the link to conditions we discuss in the following paragraphs, namely CuP and dynamic stereotypes.

Choking under pressure is common in sports and has been investigated in golfers suffering from the yips. This condition is defined as involuntary movements during the execution of putting strokes, resulting in a serious decrease in the success rate in putting. It has been classified by some authors as a task-specific focal dystonia (Adler et al. 2005); however, many authors believe that the yips is instead related to CuP, since it occurs not only in professionally trained golfers but also in golfing beginners (Lobinger et al. 2014).

The term CuP has not been applied in music, but the phenomenon clearly exists. The above-mentioned tongue-stopper felt by brass players, or the short-action bowing tremor of violinists playing soft notes with the tip of the bows are good examples. Here, it is most likely that anxiety-induced 'reinvestment' leads to cognitive interference, resulting in dysfunctional movements due to the attempt to prevent or even correct feared errors.

Dynamic stereotype is characterised by a more permanent reduction of motor control. As outlined above, it differs from focal dystonia only over time, but is more likely linked to psychological triggering factors than to underlying genetic causes (Ioannou & Altenmüller 2014).

Musician's dystonia can be distinguished from the former by the more pronounced worsening of motor control, the lack of sudden, but short-term, improvement, and the tendency to progress to dystonic cramps. We argue that musician's focal dystonia is the product of a hereditary susceptibility, probably related to a general lack of central nervous inhibition and the above-mentioned triggering factors. This leads not only to task-specific functional alterations of CNS-networks – as we predict in patients suffering from a dynamic stereotype – but also to structural alterations found in numerous studies (for a review, see Altenmüller et al. 2015).

Prevention of Musician's Dystonia

Since successful treatment of MD is still a challenge, preventing MD is important. On the basis of the heuristic model outlined in this chapter, we now possess the theoretical means to intervene at an early stage. From the first lesson on, music educators should strive to do the following: create a friendly, supportive atmosphere; introduce reasonable practice schedules; teach energy-efficient techniques; and prevent overuse and pain by including mental practice and varying the movements performed by the student. By avoiding mechanical repetitions, and hence frustration, teachers can help maintain students' motivation. Students should be taught to adopt healthy living habits, which include warm-up and cool-down exercises, regular physical exercise, sufficient breaks, and sleep as the cornerstones of healthy musical practice.

References

Adler CH, Crews D, Hentz JG, Smith AM, Caviness JN (2005). Abnormal co-contraction in yips-affected but not unaffected golfers: evidence for focal dystonia. *Neurology* 64:1813–1814.

Altenmüller E (2003). Focal dystonia: advances in brain imaging and understanding of fine motor control in musicians. *Hand Clin* 19: 1–16.

Altenmüller E, Jabusch HC (2010). Focal dystonia in musicians. *Eur J Neurol* 17(Suppl. 1):31–36.

Altenmüller E, Baur V, Hofmann A, Lim VK, Jabusch HC (2012). Musician's cramp as manifestation of maladaptive brain plasticity: arguments from instrumental differences. *Ann NY Acad Sci* 1252:259–265.

Altenmüller E, Ioannou CI, Raab M, Lobinger B (2014). Apollo's curse: causes and cures of motor failures in musicians – a proposal for a new classification. *Adv Exp Med Biol* 826:161–178.

Altenmüller E, Ioannou CI, Lee A (2015). Apollo's curse: neurological causes of motor impairments in musicians. *Prog Brain Res* 217:89–106.

Aune TK, Ingvaldsen RP, Ettema GJ (2008). Effect of physical fatigue on motor control at different skill levels. *Percept Mot Skills* 106:371–386.

Baur V, Jabusch HC, Altenmüller E (2011). Behavioral factors influence the phenotype of musician's dystonia. *Mov Disord* 26:1780–1781.

Brugués AO (2011). Music performance anxiety: part 1 – a review of its epidemiology. *Med Probl Perform Art* 26(2):102–105.

Byl NN, Merzenich MM, Jenkins WM (1996). A primate genesis model of focal dystonia and repetitive strain injury: I. Learning-induced dedifferentiation of the representation of the hand in the primary somatosensory cortex in adult monkeys. *Neurology* 47(2):508–520.

Cheng FP, Großbach M, Altenmüller E (2013). Altered sensory feedbacks in pianist's dystonia: the altered auditory feedback paradigm and the glove effect. *Front Hum Neurosci* 7:868.

Dirnberger G, Duregger C, Trettler E, Lindinger G, Lang W (2004). Fatigue in a simple repetitive motor task: a combined electrophysiological and neuropsychological study. *Brain Res* 1028:26–30.

Flor H (2012). New developments in the understanding and management of persistent pain. *Curr Opin Psychiatry* 25:109–113.

Hill DM, Hanton S, Matthews N, Fleming S (2010). Choking in sport: a review. *Int Rev Sport Exerc Psychol* 3:24–39.

Ioannou CI, Altenmüller E (2014). Psychological characteristics in musician's dystonia: a new diagnostic classification. *Neuropsychol* 61:80–88.

Ioannou CI, Furuya S, Altenmüller E (2016). The impact of stress on motor performance in skilled musicians suffering from focal dystonia: physiological and psychological characteristics. *Neuropsychol* 85:226–236.

Jabusch HC, Altenmüller E (2004). Anxiety as an aggravating factor during onset of focal dystonia in musicians. *Med Probl Perf Art* 19:75–81.

Jankovic J, Ashoori A (2008). Movement disorders in musicians. *Mov Disord* 23:1957–1965.

Karni A, Meyer G, Rey-Hipolito C, Jezzard P, Adams MM, Turner R, Ungerleider LG (1998). The acquisition of skilled motor performance: fast and slow experience-driven changes in primary motor cortex (M1). *Proc Natl Acad Sci USA* 95(3):861–868.

Klämpfl MK, Lobinger BH, Raab M (2013). How to detect the yips in golf. *Human Mov Sci* 32:1270–1287.

Lim V, Altenmüller E (2003). Musicians' cramp: instrumental and gender differences. *Med Probl Perform Art* 18:21–27.

Lobinger B, Klämpfl M, Altenmüller E (2014). We are able, we intend, we act – but we do not succeed: a theoretical framework for a better understanding of paradoxical performance in sports. *J Clin Sport Psychol* 8(4):357–377.

McGaugh JL (2000). Memory: a century of consolidation. *Science* 287:248–251.

Paulig J, Jabusch HC, Großbach M, Boullet L, Altenmüller E (2014). Sensory trick phenomenon improves motor control in pianists with dystonia: prognostic value of glove-effect. *Front Psychol* 5:1012.

Pavlov IP (1951). Dinamicheskaya stereotipiya vysshego otdela golovnogo mozga [The dynamic stereotype of the higher section of the brain]. In: *I. P Pavlov, polnoe sobraniie sochineniy* (2nd ed., enlarged, vol. 3, pt. 2, pp. 240–244). Moscow: Izdatel'stvo Akademii Nauk SSSR.

Pesenti A, Barbieri S, Priori A (2004). Limb immobilization for occupational dystonia: a possible alternative treatment for selected patients. *Adv Neurol* 94:247–254.

Rosset-Llobet J, Candia V, Fàbregas S, Ray W, Pascual-Leone A (2007). Secondary motor disturbances in 101 patients with musician's dystonia. *J Neurol Neurosurg Psychiatry* 78(9):949–953.

Schmidt A, Jabusch HC, Altenmüller E, Hagenah J, Brüggemann N, Lohmann K, Enders L, Kramer PL, Saunders-Pullman R, Bressman SB, Münchau A, Klein C (2009). Etiology of musician's dystonia: familial or environmental? *Neurology* 72:1248–1254.

Schmidt A, Jabusch HC, Altenmüller E, Kasten M, Klein C (2013). Challenges of making music: what causes musician's dystonia? *JAMA Neurol* 70(11):1456–1459.

Sripanidkulchai K, Sripanidkulchai B, Wyss JM (1984). The cortical projection of the basolateral amygdaloid nucleus in the rat: a retrograde fluorescent dye study. *J Comp Neurol* 229(3):419–431.

Steinmetz A, Stang A, Kornhuber M, Röllinghoff M, Delank. KS, Altenmüller E (2014). From embouchure problems to embouchure dystonia? A survey of self-reported embouchure disorders of 585 professional orchestra brass players. *Int Arch Occup Environ Health* 87(7):783–792.

Szeto GP, Lin JK (2011). A study of forearm muscle activity and wrist kinematics in symptomatic office workers performing mouse-clicking tasks with different precision and speed demands. *J Electromyogr Kinesiol* 21:59–66.

Windholz H (1996). Pavlov's conceptualization of the dynamic stereotype in the theory of higher nervous activity. *Am J Psychol* 109:287–295.

Yoshie M, Kudo K, Murakoshi T, Ohtsuki T (2009). Music performance anxiety in skilled pianists: effects of social-evaluative performance situation on subjective, autonomic, and electromyographic reactions. *Exp Brain Res* 199(2):117–126.

Chapter 42

Treatment of Musician's Dystonia With Botulinum Toxin

Miriam Sklerov and Seth L. Pullman

Introduction

Focal task-specific dystonia of musicians (FTSDm) is an occupational movement disorder in which playing an instrument triggers muscle spasms and abnormal postures that interfere with performance, while other actions in the same limb remain unaffected. Musicians are specially prone to FTSDm due to their extensive training and years of performing complex, repetitive movements. FTSDm affects about 1 per cent of all professional musicians, usually at the fingers or wrist (Altenmüller & Jabusch 2009). Great pianists such as Robert Schumann in the nineteenth century, Leon Fleisher and Gary Graffman today have suffered from FTSDm. Skilled musicians playing any instrument can be affected, and have had to radically alter their performing careers, play without one hand, or stop altogether because there have not been adequate forms of treatment. However, since the 1980s intramuscular injection of botulinum toxin (BoNT) has been found successful in relieving the spasms, unwanted movements and postures in patients with movement disorders, including FTSDm (Pullman et al. 1996; Simpson et al. 2008).

Though it remains unclear why some musicians develop dystonia, the technical demands, years of learned, repetitive motor tasks and stresses of giving performances may contribute to the development of FTSDm (Jabusch et al. 2004a). FTSDm may be due to a combination of reduced inhibition at multiple levels of nervous system, dysfunctional sensory processing and an exaggeration of brain plasticity (Rosenkranz et al. 2000). The postulated basis of task-driven changes in dystonia relates to the dynamic synapse concept of Hebb in which neuronal connectivity is modulated by activation. Plastic reorganisation of the cortex has been demonstrated by augmentation of finger projection areas after repetitive tasks, and with practice (Elbert et al. 1995). While this may improve performance, it arguably may set the stage for dystonia (Tinazzi et al. 2000). These mechanisms also help explain why treatment with BoNT and rehabilitation efforts are effective for FTSDm.

Intramuscular BoNT injection is a first-line treatment for FTSDm. Other therapies include oral medications such as anticholinergics, benzodiazepines and muscle relaxants (Jabusch et al. 2005), rehabilitation efforts such as constraint-induced training and immobilisation techniques, and making ergonomic changes to the musical instrument (Altenmüller & Jabusch 2010). However, these methods are not as effective, well tolerated, or long-lasting as BoNT (which can be effective up to three months), with its high potency at low doses and minimal adverse effects (Schuele & Lederman 2004). Limb muscles in FTSDm are often not superficial or palpable, and need to be targeted with a high degree of accuracy, so intramuscular BoNT injections need to be done under guidance, usually with electromyography (EMG) or ultrasound.

BoNT Mechanisms

BoNT works through presynaptic blockade of acetylcholine on both extrafusal and intrafusal muscle fibres. Blocking alpha motor neurons results in relaxation of skeletal muscle through denervation at the neuromuscular junction. Blocking gamma motor neurons results in altered sensorimotor and proprioceptive input through modulation of spindle Ia and type II afferent activity (Hallett 2000; Rosales & Dressler 2010). These mechanisms may explain how peripherally administered BoNT can affect the central nervous system and brain plasticity. They also may explain how BoNT is effective in treating FTSDm for several months with minimal muscle weakness.

BoNT Formulations

There are two clinically effective BoNT serotypes (A and B), manufactured as different BoNT formulations that are available today. OnabotulinumtoxinA (Botox, Allergan, Inc.), abobotulinumtoxinA (Dysport, Ipsen, Ltd) and incobotulinumtoxinA (Xeomin, Merz Pharmaceuticals) are three type A preparations. RimabotulinumtoxinB (Myobloc, US WorldMeds, LLC) is the available type B preparation. Though each has different labelled indications, there are many 'off-label' uses of BoNT, which include first-line therapies for limb disorders such as FTSDm. Two comprehensive evidence-based reviews and practice guidelines on BoNT for movement disorders have recommended that BoNT be offered as a Level B treatment option for limb dystonia such as FTSDm (Simpson et al. 2008; Hallett et al. 2013).

Patient Characteristics

In our series of 79 musicians treated with BoNT at Columbia University Medical Center over the last 25 years, we have found that there are many factors that lead to the development of FTSDm. The type of music played, such as classical and other rigorously demanding genres, compared to more casual improvisational music, appears to be important in causing dystonia. Anxious 'type A' personalities are also more prone to developing FTSDm (Jabusch et al. 2004a) and there is likely a genetic predisposition as well (Schmidt et al. 2006; Defazio et al. 2007). During patient selection, the only clinical findings are the dystonic movements and postures. No weakness, muscle atrophy, sensory loss, reflex asymmetry or other localising signs should be present.

The majority of musicians in our series play piano or guitar, followed by strings, drums and brass. Limb region affected varies by class of instrument: keyboard (piano, organ, harpsichord and accordion), strummed/plucked string (guitar, banjo), woodwind (clarinet, flute, saxophone), bowed string (violin, viola), percussion (drums, tabla) and brass (trumpet, trombone). Different forms of FTSDm are related to overuse of specific muscles, the technical demands of the instrument and type of music (Conti et al. 2008). For example, higher string instrument players, i.e. violinists and violists, are more likely to develop dystonia than lower string players, explained perhaps by the higher demand for precision and smaller spatial resolution of movements. Similarly, the FTSDm affects the hand that has greater demand for complex fine motor movements. Contiguous digits are typically involved, e.g. the second/third or fourth/fifth, reflecting the exaggerated cortical representation of limb action in FTSDm.

Approach to Treatment

Before injecting BoNT for FTSDm, it is important that the musician understands the specific goals and limitations of this treatment. Involuntary muscle action should be distinguished from compensatory activity to prevent misdirected injections that could make the symptoms worse. Compensatory activity is defined as voluntary or semi-voluntary movement or posture meant to negate the effect of the pathologic spasms, typically involving antagonist muscles. For example, if it is determined that flexor actions are compensatory attempts to overcome extensor dystonia, the extensors are injected. On the first injection visit it is often difficult to determine which of several actions may be compensatory.

BoNT doses vary by muscle size and function. In general, less complex forms of FTSDm, or those requiring fewer injections, are the most effectively treated. Larger, proximal muscles require higher BoNT doses than distal muscles, and flexors and pronators of the forearm and hand also require higher doses than extensors and supinators (Pullman et al. 1996). Extensor dystonia may be more easily treated with lower BoNT doses than flexor dystonia, though with the caveat that unwanted spread and weakness of digits, particularly the third, is more common. The main unwanted effect of BoNT is weakness in targeted or neighbouring muscles. Some patients exhibit complex abduction, adduction, flexion or extension of fingers mediated by small hand muscles that are difficult to isolate. Targeting individual digital fascicles within a muscle is critical but can be problematic as their topographical arrangement is not straightforward in multi-digit muscles (Figure 42.1).

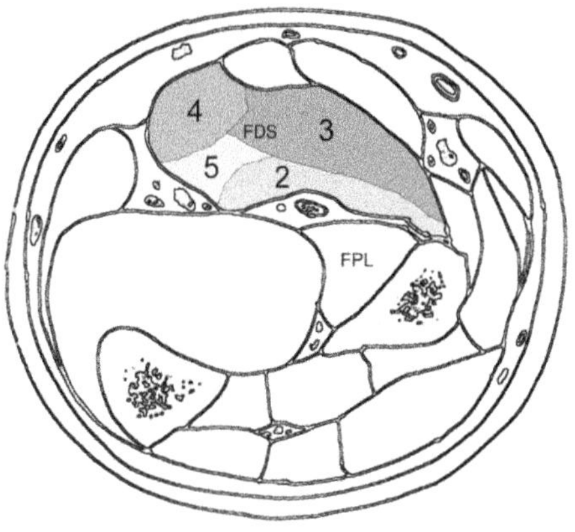

Figure 42.1 Cross-section of the forearm to highlight the topographic arrangement of individual muscle fascicles of the FDS, based on personal (SLP) experience. Note that fibres to the third digit are superficial to the second and next to the fifth digit. It is critical to understanding how to treat specific finger actions.

Source: From Perotto (1994) with permission.

Instrument-Specific Issues

Piano and Other Keyboard Players

Pianists commonly develop FTSDm in the right hand, typically causing abnormal flexion in the proximal interphalangeal joints of the third, fourth, fifth and/or second digits. Less often there is flexion at distal interphalangeal or extension at metacarpal interphalangeal joints, usually the second or third digit. The latter can be problematic in specific instances where finger extension of one hand interferes with crossing over of the other hand, an unusual but remarkably treatable FTSDm (Figure 42.2). Thus, keyboard instrumentalists typically require injection of finger flexors, less commonly finger extensors, supinators and pronators of the wrist, small hand muscles or more proximal arm and shoulder muscles. The flexors that are commonly involved include the flexor digitorum superficialis (FDS), flexor digitorum profundus (FDP) and flexor pollicus longus (FPL). Common extensors include the extensor digitorum communis (EDC), extensor indicis proprius (EIP), extensor carpi ulnaris (ECU) and extensor carpi radialis (ECR).

Strummed/Plucked String Instruments

Most affected are the right wrist and finger flexors, typically the third, fourth and fifth digits. The right fifth digit often extends to compensate. The muscles commonly injected are flexor carpi radialis (FCR), flexor carpi ulnaris (FCU), pronator teres, FDS and FDP. When a finger tends to flex at the metacarpal phalangeal joint, the lumbricals or other intrinsic hand muscles can be treated with low doses of BoNT.

Bowed String Instruments

More often the fingering left hand is involved, but the bowing right hand is subject to FTSDm in many cases. For the

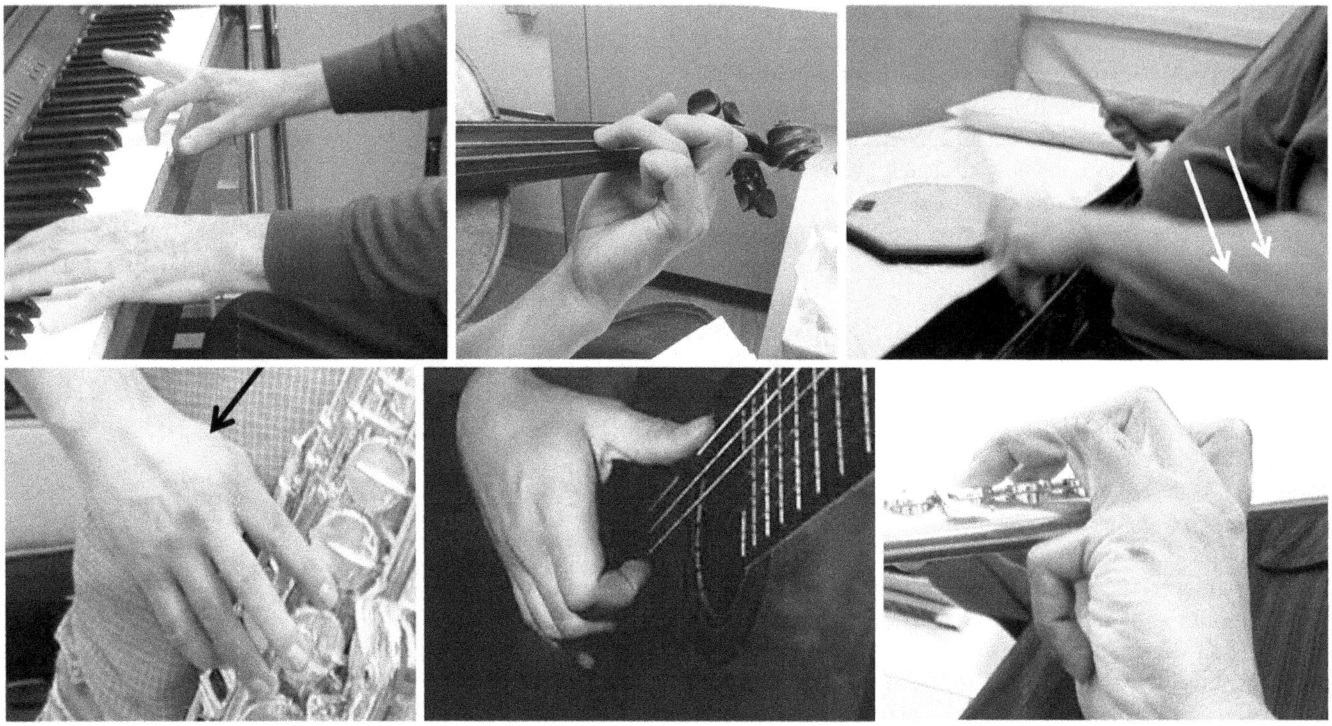

Figure 42.2 Examples of FTSDm that have all done well with BoNT injections. Top panel: pianist extensor dystonia of the right third digit; violinist fingering hand dystonia involving flexion of the proximal and distal interphalangeal joints of the fourth and fifth digits; drummer with wrist and finger extensor spasms (arrows: EDC and ECU spasms). Bottom panel: saxophonist with right second digit abduction dystonia (arrow: FDI spasm); guitar player with flexor spasms of right second, third and fourth digits; flautist with left fifth digit metacarpal phalangeal and proximal interphalangeal flexor dystonia.

left hand, most muscle spasms involve flexion of the proximal and distal interphalangeal joints of the fourth and fifth digits (Figure 42.2) and wrist pronation, so FDS, FDP and pronator teres are injected. Wrist tremors are also frequent, and difficult to treat as often both wrist flexors and extensors need injections. Right-arm bowing dystonia may involve wrist and more proximal elbow and shoulder muscles. The muscles involved will typically be the right pronator teres, biceps, triceps, trapezius, FPL, FCU, FCR, ECU and ECR.

Woodwinds

FTSDm mostly involves the finger flexors where the key pressing and release becomes difficult. Rarely, the second finger abducts away from the others as part of the dystonic spasm in saxophone players (Figure 42.2). Proximal shoulder muscles may be involved as well. The distal muscles often injected are the FDS, EDC and first dorsal interosseus (FDI). The proximal muscles involved are typically the deltoid, teres minor and trapezius.

Brass

Apart from embouchure dystonia, brass players get FTSDm affecting the right-hand finger flexors and extensors, as well as proximal arm rotators and shoulder muscles. Single digits, e.g. the second or third, are involved in isolation. The most common muscles injected are FDS, EIP, pronator teres and trapezius.

Percussion

Depending on the type of grip, drummers may have overactive extensors of the wrist and fingers, and require injections into the ECR, ECU or EDC. Flexors are less commonly affected, in which case the FTSDm will involve the FCU, and rarely the FCR.

Outcomes

There are four possible overall outcomes after BoNT injections (Pullman et al. 1996), each requiring a different approach at follow-up (see Table 42.1). The first is that there is no improvement in muscle spasms, and no evident weakness. In this case, the same muscles are usually re-injected later at higher BoNT doses on the assumption that at least some initial weakness indicates the BoNT is effective. Non-responsiveness can be due to a number of causes, but most commonly the dosage was too low or improperly placed. A second possible outcome is a submaximal or partial response. In this case, the same muscles are usually re-injected at three months with 1.5–2 times the original dose. A third outcome is an unexpected response with overactivity uncovered in non-injected muscles, caused by BoNT injection into uninvolved or compensatory muscles. In this case, the choice of muscles and dose regimen have to be reconsidered. The last possibility is the desired response and improvement in musical performance. When this optimal response is obtained, follow-up injections with the same doses are usually given every 3–4 months.

Table 42.1 BoNT injection algorithm

On the first visit:	Start with low to average BoNT doses, in fewest muscles
For the next visits:	Schedule with respect to musical performances to obtain peak BoNT effect. Try to re-inject every 3–4 months
If there is:	*Then:*
No response	Inject same muscle(s) at higher doses
Submaximal response	Inject same muscle(s) at higher doses, consider additional muscles
Unexpected response	Unwanted clinical pattern emerges, with excessive weakness in injected muscles, overactivity in missed muscles. Re-think strategy – consider antagonists
Good response	Wait for BoNT to wear off, re-inject the same regimen

Results are dependent on the musician's personality and expectations, complexity of dystonia and experience of the injecting physician. Functional improvement is based almost entirely on the musician's subjective assessment. Musicians generally know when they have, or have not, improved. There are no fully objective, quantifiable methods to assess the severity of FTSDm, or reliably measure BoNT treatment effects. Improvement may be measured indirectly by a better orchestra position, expansion of repertoire or increased number of performances. Subjective and objective rating scales with varying degrees of sophistication have been proposed (Jabusch et al. 2004b). Musical instrument digital interface (MIDI)-based analysis stands out as a valid way to objectively rate musician's dystonia (Spector & Brandfonbrener 2007;Peterson et al. 2013). At our centre, we have musicians play the involved passages before and six weeks after injections, and judge the BoNT effects. For objective measures, we use surface EMG, kinematic measurements and MIDI-based analyses.

About 60 per cent of FTSDm patients do well enough to continue playing or teaching, but only 10–15 per cent maintain high professional levels of activity. Some musicians comment that fast 16th-note measures remain difficult, and prefer to play more chordal music, avoiding fast, scalar passages. Nevertheless, BoNT injections administered by an experienced physician can offer hope and continued success for one of the most challenging professions affected by dystonia.

References

Altenmüller E, Jabusch HC. 2009. Focal hand dystonia in musicians: phenomenology, etiology, and psychological trigger factors. *J Hand Ther* 22(2):144–154.

Altenmüller E, Jabusch HC. 2010. Focal dystonia in musicians: phenomenology, pathophysiology, triggering factors, and treatment. *Med Probl Perform Art* 25(1):3–9.

Conti AM, Pullman S, Frucht SJ. 2008. The hand that has forgotten its cunning: lessons from musicians' hand dystonia. *Mov Disord* 23(10):1398–1406.

Defazio G, Berardelli A, Hallett M. 2007. Do primary adult-onset focal dystonias share aetiological factors? *Brain* 130(Pt 5):1183–1193.

Elbert T, Pantev C, Wienbruch C, Rockstroh B, Taub E. 1995. Increased cortical representation of the fingers of the left hand in string players. *Science* 270(5234):305–307.

Hallett M. 2000. How does botulinum toxin work? *Ann Neurol* 48(1):7–8.

Hallett M, Albanese A, Dressler D, Segal KR, Simpson DM, Truong D, Jankovic J. 2013. Evidence-based review and assessment of botulinum neurotoxin for the treatment of movement disorders. *Toxicon* 67:94–114.

Jabusch HC, Muller SV, Altenmüller E. 2004a. Anxiety in musicians with focal dystonia and those with chronic pain. *Mov Disord* 19(10):1169–1175.

Jabusch HC, Vauth H, Altenmüller E. 2004b. Quantification of focal dystonia in pianists using scale analysis. *Mov Disord* 19(2):171–180.

Jabusch HC, Zschucke D, Schmidt A, Schuele S, Altenmüller E 2005. Focal dystonia in musicians: treatment strategies and long-term outcome in 144 patients. *Mov Disord* 20(12):1623–1626.

Perotto A. 1994. *Anatomical Guide for the Electromyographer: The Limbs and Trunk.* 3rd ed. Springfield, IL: Charles C Thomas.

Peterson DA, Berque P, Jabusch HC, Altenmüller E, Frucht SJ. 2013. Rating scales for musician's dystonia: the state of the art. *Neurology* 81(6):589–598.

Pullman SL, Greene P, Fahn S, Pedersen SF. 1996. Approach to the treatment of limb disorders with botulinum toxin A: experience with 187 patients. *Arch Neurol* 53(7):617–624.

Rosales RL, Dressler D. 2010. On muscle spindles, dystonia and botulinum toxin. *Eur J Neurol* 17(Suppl. 1):71–80.

Rosenkranz K, Altenmüller E, Siggelkow S, Dengler R. 2000. Alteration of sensorimotor integration in musician's cramp: impaired focusing of proprioception. *Clin Neurophysiol* 111(11):2040–2045.

Schmidt A, Jabusch HC, Altenmüller E, Hagenah J, Bruggemann N, Hedrich K, Saunders-Pullman R, Bressman SB, Kramer PL, Klein C. 2006. Dominantly transmitted focal dystonia in families of patients with musician's cramp. *Neurology* 67(4):691–693.

Schuele S, Lederman RJ. 2004. Long-term outcome of focal dystonia in string instrumentalists. *Mov Disord* 19(1):43–48.

Simpson DM, Blitzer A, Brashear A, Comella C, Dubinsky R, Hallett M, Jankovic J, Karp B, Ludlow CL, Miyasaki JM, Naumann M, So Y. 2008. Assessment: botulinum neurotoxin for the treatment of movement disorders (an evidence-based review): report of the Therapeutics and Technology Assessment Subcommittee of the American Academy of Neurology. *Neurology* 70(19):1699–1706.

Spector JT, Brandfonbrener AG. 2007. Methods of evaluation of musician's dystonia: critique of measurement tools. *Mov Disord* 22(3):309–312.

Tinazzi M, Priori A, Bertolasi L, Frasson E, Mauguiere F, Fiaschi A. 2000. Abnormal central integration of a dual somatosensory input in dystonia: evidence for sensory overflow. *Brain* 123 (Pt 1):42–50.

Chapter 43

Experimental Occupational and Brain Stimulation Therapies for Musician's Dystonia

Eckart Altenmüller and Shinichi Furuya

Trials with Pedagogical Retraining in Musicians

In the last decade, based on the hypotheses of aberrant learning and maladaptive plasticity, several treatment protocols have been designed, aiming to reverse the central nervous system degradation that accounts for one origin and expression of musician's dystonia. These therapies aim to re-differentiate representations of the disturbed somatotopy of the hand in musician's hand dystonia and lips in embouchure dystonia respectively.

The principles of neuroplasticity are most closely related to constraint-induced training, immobilisation, learning-based sensorimotor training and retraining at the instrument. In a study of 11 musicians with focal hand dystonia, the unaffected fingers of the dystonic hands were constrained with splints (Candia et al. 2002). Patients were trained to use the dystonic fingers on fine motor tasks emphasising instrumental play for 2–3 hours a day over two weeks. When control of the digits most affected by dystonia improved, the splints on the less affected digits were gradually removed and practice at the instrument was increased. Eight out of the eleven musicians showed an improvement in their motor skills. A brain imaging study, demonstrating that patients with focal hand dystonia showed some reorganisation of receptive fields in the somatosensory cortex after treatment, supported this approach (Candia et al. 2003). Combining constraint-induced therapy and motor control retraining in eight musicians suffering from hand dystonia seemed to be even more successful when analysing dystonic postures and abnormal movements before and after the intervention (Berque et al. 2010).

Based on evidence showing that the somatotopic representation of the hand is abnormal in patients with focal hand dystonia, immobilisation of the hand has been proposed as an appropriate treatment at the first signs of dystonia. In individuals without dystonia, limb immobilisation leads to a shrinkage of the cortical representation of the immobilised limb. Thus, the objective of immobilisation in patients with limb dystonia is to place the affected finger, hand, wrist and forearm into a static splint to stop all movement in order to decrease the size of the representational area of the involved hand. In a study by Pesenti et al. (2004), 19 patients wore the splint 24 hours a day for 4–6 weeks. Subsequently, a careful retraining and physiotherapy approach was applied. The outcome of this study was heterogeneous: in 6 out of 19 patients, there was marked improvement, while in the other group no or only minor improvements could be observed. It is probable that retraining effects were the most important component in this approach.

Learning-based sensorimotor training (LBST) is another approach to rehabilitation for patients with focal hand dystonia (Byl & McKenzie 2002). The objective of LBST is to redefine spatial and temporal processing capacities in the sensory and motor cortices in order to restore task-specific skills, like writing. Different exercise strategies address sub-tasks of the target tasks, emphasising different aspects of sensory feedback (i.e. somatosensation, proprioception, kinaesthesia, haptics). Patients begin by making relatively simple distinctions between relatively large stimuli, with task difficulty increasing following mastery of each distinction. One set of tasks includes reading Braille or embossed letters, making roughness estimations and performing grating orientation discriminations. A series of haptic tasks requires subjects to manipulate and identify surface features and shapes of three-dimensional objects held in their hands.

This training protocol has been tested in a series of patients with focal hand dystonia, including patients suffering from musician's dystonia (for a review, see Byl et al. 2009). In the first study that focused on this training protocol, all 12 trained patients showed improvements in performance ability on a variety of tests of sensory discrimination, fine motor accuracy and speed, strength, flexibility and functional independence. Motor control improved, with the resulting control ranging from 70 per cent to 94 per cent of normal performance. All but three patients were able to return to their usual work following treatment.

Pedagogical retraining has been applied to patients with all forms of musician's dystonia. A variety of behavioural approaches have been taken under the supervision of instructors, including elements based on the following principles: (1) movements of affected body parts were limited to a level of tempo and force at which the dystonic movement would not occur; (2) compensatory movements (e.g. of adjacent fingers) were avoided, partially under the application of splints; (3) instant visual feedback with mirrors or monitors helped patients to recognise dystonic and non-dystonic movements; (4) body awareness techniques (e.g. Feldenkrais®) were used to increase patients' perception of non-dystonic movements. Common to all these therapies is the 'long-term' approach. For example, in a large study series of 145 musicians, an average rehabilitation time of 24 months was reported, after which 35 musicians returned to playing in public (Sakai 2006).

We applied pedagogical retraining with an experienced piano pedagogue to 50 pianists suffering from focal hand dystonia (Boullet 2003). Improvements in motor performance were reported by 82 per cent of the subjects, with four patients reporting a complete recovery. Objective gains in task-specific motor performance were documented in 50 per cent of the patients. Subjectively, 80 per cent of subjects reported improvement. It should be mentioned that this treatment requires a long period of training: those patients reporting an improvement had undergone retraining for an average of 28 months (van Vugt et al. 2014).

In embouchure dystonia, several experienced brass pedagogues have expertise in improving the situation considerably, although no controlled clinical trials have been conducted up to now. In many cases, embouchure dystonia is accompanied by a lack of control of tongue movements and dysfunctional muscular activations in the larynx and in the breathing musculature of the trunk (Iltis et al. 2015, 2016). Successful retraining seems to depend mainly on the severity of the embouchure dystonia, and is more common in brass instrumentalists who have only a subtle loss of control and who do not suffer from lip spasms and involuntary clenching of the masseter muscles (Steinmetz et al. 2014). In general, it seems that problems relating to proper air-guidance and relaxed breathing are easier to rehabilitate than involuntary muscular spasms in facial and/or chewing muscles. Training of body awareness, relaxation techniques and general stress management seem to be useful for the retraining process.

Open Questions Concerning Retraining Therapy

Limitations of the above studies are typical of small-scale trials, as these trials lack control groups, blinding and randomisation. As the rehabilitation research in musician's dystonia develops, it will be important to compare the effectiveness of different interventions to understand which approach holds the most promise and which neurophysiological mechanism is affected. Given the nascent stage of rehabilitation research in musician's dystonia, controlled full-scale clinical trials have yet to be conducted. Here, objective assessment of dystonic movements is extremely important (Peterson et al. 2013).

A major challenge of retraining intervention studies in musicians is determining an appropriate control and clearly specifying the interventions to improve reproducibility. The hallmark of retraining is that it involves active participation by the patient and is tailored to each patient's unique needs, which can create problems for reproducibility. For a control to be effective, it must be believable as a true intervention but not contain the key components of the experimental condition. Both blinding and control are essential for future studies, as care from a therapist may impart benefits caused by feeling cared for in addition to a pure placebo effect. Consequently, future investigations in retraining of musician's dystonia need to carefully address this issue by comparing different treatment strategies with similar frequency, duration and interaction between patient and therapist.

Trials with Repetitive Transcranial Magnetic Stimulation

Non-invasive brain stimulation techniques, such as repetitive transcranial magnetic stimulation (rTMS) and transcranial direct current stimulation (tDCS), have been applied to do both basic research into the pathophysiology of hand dystonia and therapeutic trials (for a recent review, see Cho & Hallett 2016). Both methods alter brain excitability in sensorimotor networks, and are also suitable to reduce abnormal hyper-excitation in sensorimotor cortices in patients with musician's dystonia. The precise neurophysiological mechanisms are not fully understood. As a rule of thumb, high-frequency rTMS and anodal tDCS reduce resting potential in cortical pyramidal cells and in this way increase excitability in the upper neuronal layers of the sensorimotor cortices, whereas low-frequency rTMS and cathodal tDCS work in an inhibitory manner (Nitsche & Paulus 2000). However, effects are far more complex and are not limited to the site of the stimulating electrodes, but rather extend to frontal and parietal networks, as well as to basal ganglia and to cerebellar structures (Havrankova et al. 2010; Sehm et al. 2012).

With respect to therapeutic trials, inhibitory slow-frequency rTMS has been applied in several controlled trials, including a few musicians suffering from hand dystonia (for a recent review, see Cho & Hallett 2016). Studies typically included fewer than ten (mostly writer's cramp) subjects and most used a cross-over design, stimulating the contralateral side of the dystonic hand. Siebner et al. (1999) could show that motor cortex (M1) stimulation had some beneficial effects; however, Murase et al. (2005) showed that the premotor cortex (PMC) was a better target when compared with M1 and supplementary motor area (SMA). Subsequently, more studies used PMC as the target and showed promising results, either by physiologic or behavioural measures (e.g. Borich et al. 2009; Huang et al. 2012). In order to investigate sustained effects of 1 Hz rTMS, Kimberley et al. (2015) investigated eight writer's cramp subjects over five consecutive days with stimulation over the left premotor cortex while subjects underwent sensorimotor retraining. However, rTMS, either with or without sensorimotor training, did not substantially improve objective measures, although six of nine participants reported improvement in self-rated function.

In summary, the results of clinical trials with low-frequency rTMS do not currently justify its clinical application.

Trials with Direct Current Stimulation

In recent years, tDCS has gained popularity partly due to its simple applicability and its inexpensive availability, with little risk of adverse effects. In patients with musician's dystonia (professional guitarists), a single session of cathodal tDCS of the affected M1 did not improve the performance of guitar playing (Buttkus et al. 2010). Also in pianists, a single session of cathodal or anodal tDCS of the affected M1 combined with simultaneous retraining consisting of slow, voluntarily controlled movements on the piano did not result in any improvement of dystonia (Buttkus et al. 2011). A similar finding was reported in patients with writer's cramp (Benninger et al. 2011). In contrast, cathodal tDCS of the affected M1 and simultaneous anodal tDCS of the unaffected M1 in dystonic pianists resulted in improvement in the rhythmic accuracy of sequential finger movements with the affected hand, but only if concurrently bimanual mirrored finger movements were performed (Furuya et al. 2014). This improvement was retained four days after the intervention. The reversed montage of electrodes (anodal tDCS of the affected M1, cathodal tDCS of the unaffected M1), unilateral anodal tDCS of the unaffected M1 and sham stimulation all failed to yield any improvement (Furuya et al. 2014). Furthermore, the amount of motor improvement correlated directly with the severity of the symptoms, i.e. the most severely affected patients benefited most from the intervention. These findings suggest a therapeutic potential of behavioural training assisted by bihemispheric and polarity-specific tDCS in restoring fine motor control in musician's dystonia (Furuya et al. 2014). A further single case study determined augmented therapeutic effects through the bihemispheric tDCS with bimanual mirrored retraining over two successive days (Furuya & Altenmüller 2015).

Open Questions Concerning Non-Invasive Brain Stimulation Techniques

The therapeutic application of transcranial brain stimulation in musician's dystonia is based on clear evidence of abnormal (elevated) sensorimotor excitability and maladaptive plasticity in this disorder. However, as it stands, treatment with brain stimulation is still experimental. It seems that rTMS is less promising than a combination of bilateral tDCS and retraining. Long-term effects of repeated stimulations are currently under investigation. Furthermore, larger-scale randomised controlled trials are clearly needed. To make progress, future trials will need to take the following into consideration: (1) the target(s) of stimulation (including novel targets such as the cerebellum, and concomitant stimulation of more than one network; (2) predictive markers for a therapeutic response – e.g. whether musician's cramp is more susceptible for beneficial effects as compared to writer's cramp; (3) dose and duration of the stimulation protocol; and (4) combination with specific motor retraining procedures.

References

Benninger DH, Lomarev M, Lopez G, Pal N, Luckenbaugh DA, Hallett M (2011). Transcranial direct current stimulation for the treatment of focal hand dystonia. *Mov Disord* 26, 1698–1702.

Berque P, Gray H, Harkness C, McFadyen A (2010). A combination of constraint-induced therapy and motor control retraining in the treatment of focal hand dystonia in musicians. *Med Probl Perform Art* 25:149–161.

Borich, M, Arora, S, Kimberley, TJ (2009). Lasting effects of repeated rTMS application in focal hand dystonia. *Restor Neurol Neurosci* 27:55–65.

Boullet L (2003). Treating focal dystonia: a new retraining therapy for pianists. Available from: www.epos.uni-osnabrueck.de/music/books/k/klww003/pdfs/268_Boullet_Abs.pdf

Buttkus F, Weidenmüller M, Schneider S, Jabusch HC, Nitsche MA, Paulus W, Altenmüller E (2010). Failure of cathodal direct current stimulation to improve fine motor control in musician's dystonia. *Mov Disord* 25:389–394.

Buttkus F, Baur V, Jabusch HC, de la Cruz Gomez-Pellin M, Paulus W, Nitsche MA, Altenmüller E (2011). Retraining and transcranial direct current stimulation in musician's dystonia: a case report. *Restor Neurol Neurosci* 29:85–90.

Byl NN, McKenzie A (2002). The effect of sensory discrimination training on structure and function in patients with focal hand dystonia: 3 case series. *Arch Phys Med Rehabil* 84:1505–1514.

Byl NN, Archer ES, McKenzie A (2009). Focal hand dystonia: effectiveness of a home program of fitness and learning-based sensorimotor and memory training. *J Hand Ther* 22:183–197.

Candia V, Schäfer T, Taub E, Rau H, Altenmüller E, Rockstroh B, Elbert T (2002). Sensory motor retuning: a behavioral treatment for focal hand dystonia of pianists and guitarists. *Arch Phys Med Rehabil* 83:1342–1348.

Candia V, Wienbruch C, Elbert T, Rockstroh B, Ray W (2003). Effective behavioral treatment of focal hand dystonia in musicians alters somatosensory cortical organization. *PNAS* 100:7942–7946.

Cho HJ, Hallett, M (2016). Non-invasive brain stimulation for treatment of focal hand dystonia: update and future direction. *J Mov Disord* 9:55–62.

Furuya S, Altenmüller E (2015). Acquisition and reacquisition of motor coordination in musicians. *Ann NY Acad Sci* 1337:118–124.

Furuya S, Nitsche MA, Paulus W, Altenmüller E (2014). Surmounting retraining limits in musicians' dystonia by transcranial stimulation. *Ann Neurol* 75:707.

Havrankova P, Jech R, Walker ND, Operto G, Tauchmanova J, Vymazal J, Dusek P, Hromcik M, Ruzicka E (2010). Repetitive TMS of the somatosensory cortex improves writer's cramp and enhances cortical activity. *Neuro Endocrinol Lett* 31:73–86.

Huang YZ, Lu CS, Rothwell JC, Lo CC, Chuang WL, Weng YH, Lai SC, Chen RS (2012). Modulation of the disturbed motor network in dystonia by multisession suppression of premotor cortex. *PLoS One* 7(10):e47574. doi: 10.1371/journal.pone.0047574

Iltis PW, Frahm J, Voit D, Joseph A, Schoonderwaldt E, Altenmüller E (2015). Divergent oral cavity motor strategies between healthy elite and dystonic horn players. *J Clin Mov Disord* 2:15. doi: 10.1186/s40734-015-0027-2

Iltis PW, Frahm J, Voit D, Joseph A, Burke R, Altenmüller E (2016). Inefficiencies in motor strategies of horn players with embouchure dystonia: comparisons to elite performers. *Med Probl Perform Art* 31:69–77.

Kimberley TJ, Borich MR, Schmidt RL, Carey JR, Gillick B (2015). Focal hand dystonia: individualized intervention with repeated application of repetitive transcranial magnetic stimulation. *Arch Phys Med Rehabil* 96:122–128.

Murase N, Rothwell JC, Kaji R, Urushihara R, Nakamura K, Murayama N, Igasaki T, Sakata-Igasaki M, Mima T, Ikeda A, Shibasaki H (2005). Subthreshold low-frequency repetitive transcranial magnetic stimulation over the premotor cortex modulates writer's cramp. *Brain* 128:104–115.

Nitsche MA, Paulus W (2000). Excitability changes induced in the human motor cortex by weak transcranial direct current stimulation. *J Physiol* 527:633–639.

Pesenti A, Barbieri S, Priori A (2004). Limb immobilization for occupational dystonia: a possible alternative treatment for selected patients. *Adv Neurol* 94:247–254.

Peterson DA, Berque P, Jabusch HC, Altenmüller E, Frucht SJ (2013). Rating scales for musician's dystonia: the state of the art. *Neurology* 81:589–598.

Sakai N (2006). Slow-down exercise for the treatment of focal hand dystonia in pianists. *Med Probl Perform Art* 21:25–28.

Sehm B, Schäfer A, Kipping J, Margulies D, Conde V, Taubert M, Villringer A, Ragert P (2012). Dynamic modulation of intrinsic functional connectivity by transcranial direct current stimulation. *J Neurophysiol* 108:3253–3263.

Siebner HR, Tormos JM, Ceballos-Baumann AO, Auer C, Catala MD, Conrad B, Pascual-Leone A (1999). Low-frequency repetitive transcranial magnetic stimulation of the motor cortex in writer's cramp. *Neurology* 52:529–553.

Steinmetz A, Stang A, Kornhuber M, Röllinghoff M, Delank KS, Altenmüller E (2014). From embouchure problems to embouchure dystonia? A survey of self-reported embouchure disorders of 585 professional orchestra brass players. *Int Arch Occup Envir Health* 87:783–792.

van Vugt FT, Boullet L, Jabusch HC, Altenmüller E (2014). Musician's dystonia in pianists: long-term evaluation of retraining and other therapies. *Parkinsonism Relat Disord* 20:8–12.

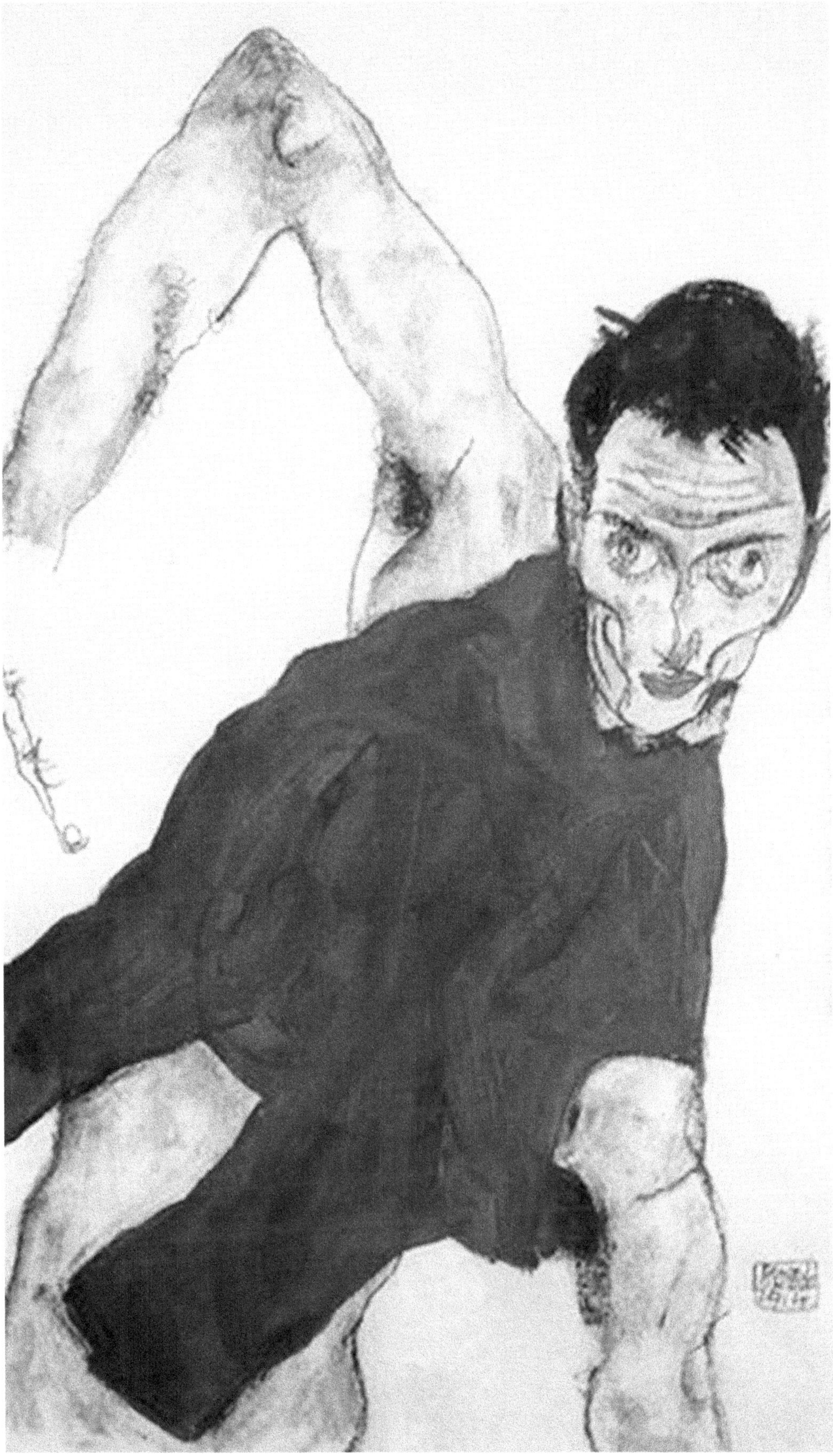

Chapter 44

The Clinical Spectrum of Functional/Psychogenic Dystonia

Thomas D. L. Steeves and Anthony E. Lang

Introduction

The diagnosis of psychogenic or functional dystonia (F/PDys) is a task filled with pitfalls. No reliable biomarkers currently exist to assist in this undertaking, and the spectrum of organic dystonia itself, which forms the basis for any comparison, is both broad and characterised by seemingly improbable clinical features. At the same time, a misdiagnosis in either direction imposes a multiplicity of negative consequences, directing the patient away from appropriate interventions or needlessly imposing invasive and potentially harmful ones. Increasingly, in a consumerist and litigious culture, a clinical misjudgement also imposes upon the physician negative consequences far in excess of any benefits received for the provision of care.

In this brief chapter our limited goals are to provide a concise description of the clinical spectrum of F/PDys and to enumerate the historical and clinical examination features that allow it to be distinguished from its organic counterparts. The investigation, treatment and clinical outcomes of F/PDys are reviewed elsewhere in this book.

The 'Psyche' in Dystonia

Physicians have long been aware of the significance of the psyche in the generation of disease states, and the study of the relationship between the two has a varied and distinguished history in medicine. Speculation over the role of psychological states in the generation of abnormal movements has likewise permeated the conceptualisation of both the organic and psychogenic dystonias over the course of their documented histories.

The conceptualisation of F/PDys has evolved over the last 150 years as the work of Charcot at the Salpetriere Hospital illustrates. Charcot, who was perhaps the dominant figure in the study of psychogenic conditions in the latter half of the nineteenth century, felt throughout much of his career that such conditions, referred to as hysteria, reflected organic mechanisms. He classified hysteria, along with seizures, as '*nevroses*', conditions lacking identifiable neuropathological substrates, but which nonetheless arose from transient functional or structural disturbances which he assumed would be found in due course. In such cases Charcot believed that the manifestation of disease resulted from a combination of a hereditary predisposition and an environmental provocation, usually in the form of a physical or emotional shock.

Many, including Sigmund Freud, who was Charcot's student, and Paul Broca, an academic contemporary in Paris, criticised Charcot's conceptualisation of hysteria, postulating instead purely psychological bases for the manifestation of such disorders, and later in his life Charcot's own approach to the disorder appears to have evolved and conformed to the views of his critics. He is known subsequently to have made passing remarks that hysteria could be 'for the most part a mental illness' (Goetz 2006). However, this evolution in the conceptualisation of psychogenic conditions demonstrates that throughout history the term 'psychogenic' cannot always be considered equal to non-organic.

Ironically, over the last decade the study of functional/psychogenic movement disorders (F/PMDs) has arguably come full circle, as developments in functional imaging have identified a variety of disturbances associated with both organic and psychogenic neurologic presentations that are now contributing to the emergence of a mechanistic view of psychogenic disorders, which may in fact approach Charcot's original conception. Currently, key elements in the generation of F/PDys seem to be an abnormal pattern of attention and an accompanying loss of the sense of agency over movement. Attempts to elucidate the neuroanatomic bases of these specific elements through functional imaging are currently among the most active areas of research in F/PMDs.

What's in a name? Psychogenic Versus Functional

Over the last three decades the term 'psychogenic' has come into widespread use within the field of movement disorders to describe conditions that are not obviously organic or secondary to structural disturbances. However, the term is not without its detractors. It has been criticised for potentially reinforcing an outdated concept of mind–body dualism, in place of a more mechanistic or biological approach to the condition, consistent with our current understanding of many physical syndromes, and also for implying a somewhat nebulous relationship between the condition and psychopathology that has at best been inconsistently demonstrated.

In general the results of studies evaluating the frequency with which psychological disorders can be identified in patients with F/PMDs remain mixed. In patients with psychogenic motor disorders, reported rates of depression have ranged from 26 per cent to 71 per cent, and rates of anxiety from 7 per cent to 38 per cent. Likewise, personality disorders have been reported in 42–67 per cent, with dependent and borderline personality features predominating (Factor et al. 1995; Williams et al. 1995; Crimlisk et al. 1998; Feinstein et al. 2001). However, the results of such studies may also depend significantly on the methodology and instruments used in testing, as at least one case-control study of patients with F/PMDs demonstrated no difference in frequency of DSM-IV diagnoses of psychiatric disorders, disordered personality traits, or histories of physical or sexual abuse compared to healthy controls and patients with organic dystonia, although greater symptoms of anxiety and depression as well as incidence of childhood traumas were noted in patients with F/PMDs (Kranick et al. 2011).

Given the purported inadequacies of the term psychogenic, a number of authors have proposed alternatives to the term which are said, variously, to be more neutral and more able to avoid implying a specific psychiatric causation, including 'non-organic', 'medically unexplained' and 'functional'. Among these alternatives, the term 'functional' in particular has acquired a wider currency among neurologists over the last decade, and in at least one report the term has been shown to be better accepted by patients than 'psychogenic' (Edwards et al. 2014).

In addition to the above terms, the psychiatric literature, summated in the *Diagnostic and Statistical Manual of Psychiatric Disorders 5* (DSM-V), proposes a number of diagnostic terms that are contained within the movement disorders rubric of functional or psychogenic. These are, first, conversion disorder and somatic symptom disorder (previously somatisation disorder in DSM-IV-TR). As defined in DSM-V, conversion disorder (also referred to in DSM-V as functional neurological symptom disorder) is 'one or more symptoms of altered voluntary motor or sensory function' which, importantly, no longer requires as an essential criterion the identification of an acute stressor prior to symptom onset. Somatic symptoms disorder by definition consists of one or more symptoms, of which dystonia may be one, in association with excessive thoughts, feelings or behaviours related to the somatic symptoms.

Factitious disorder and malingering are two other entities listed in the DSM-V that can generate a 'non-organic' dystonia. Although factitious disorder is classified as one of the somatic symptoms disorders, malingering is not a psychiatric condition. Both terms describe conditions in which symptoms are by definition consciously produced, and therefore exist as entities distinct from the more common F/PMD presentations.

Epidemiology

Accurate epidemiological data related to F/PDys are limited and restricted by the usual shortcomings of such studies, including reporting and ascertainment biases.

Functional/psychogenic disorders as a whole have been proposed to account for anywhere from 1 to 9 per cent of all neurological presentations (Lempert et al. 1990). Likewise, the literature suggests that F/PDys accounts for anywhere from 1 to 5 per cent of all patients presenting with dystonia (Fahn & Williams 1988). Conversely, and somewhat paradoxically, given the low incidence of dystonia relative to other organic movement disorders, the condition is reported to be among the more common F/PMDs, accounting for anywhere from 20 to 50 per cent of reported psychogenic cases (Factor et al. 1995; Williams et al. 1995).

Less is known of F/PDys in children and adolescents; however, on the basis of limited descriptions, childhood and adult F/PDys appears similar in relative frequency, phenomenology and additional clinical characteristics. In the reported series the average age of diagnosis ranges from 12.3 to 14 years, and a female predominance seems evident (Schwingenschuh et al. 2008).

The Clinical Assessment of Functional/Psychogenic Dystonia

With the exception of the genetically determined dystonias, which currently comprise only a minority of cases, and some instances of secondary dystonia, no specific biomarkers readily distinguish a functional from an organic dystonia. The diagnosis of F/PDys, therefore, typically reduces to a balance of probabilities related to positive and negative signs and the clinician's reference to an accumulated experience with similar presentations. The room for error is large, as evidenced by the shared experience of tertiary movement disorder centres that have accumulated patients who have undergone surgery for dystonic conditions subsequently shown to be psychogenic (Kobayash et al. 2011).

Historical Features Suggesting the Presence of Functional/Psychogenic Dystonia

Several large case series of F/PMDs published over the last three decades have described the clinical spectrum of F/PDys. Together these studies have identified commonalities in the history, phenomenology of the movements, and findings on examination that can be used to diagnose F/PDys (Table 44.1; Fahn & Williams 1988; Factor et al. 1995; Lang 1995). None of the features outlined in Table 44.1 are specific; many can be seen in either functional or organic dystonia, and the clinician must first weigh and then sum these elements in formulating a diagnosis.

F/PDys is often characterised by a number of positive features on history, a subset of these shared with other F/PMDs. The condition is more likely to occur with an abrupt onset, commonly precipitated by minor injury, and the dystonic movements themselves may remit suddenly or be inconsistent over time. F/PDys not uncommonly affects the lower limb, whereas adult-onset idiopathic dystonia rarely begins in a lower limb. When this occurs it is typically a manifestation of a secondary dystonia, for example that of a neurodegenerative disease in which other neurologic features such as parkinsonism would typically accompany the presentation. Rapid progression of symptoms and spread to remote body parts are more typical of a psychogenic presentation; conversely, most organic dystonias are more likely to have a gradual onset and progress, if at all, slowly over time. Post-lesional dystonia and the dystonia of rapid-onset dystonia-parkinsonism are exceptions that highlight this rule.

Table 44.1 Historical and examination features differentiating psychogenic from organic dystonia

	Typical of functional/psychogenic dystonia	Typical of 'organic' dystonia
Past medical history	Prior somatisations Psychological stressors present No family history	PMHx unremarkable No psychological stressors identified Family history may be present
Time-course	Sudden onset/rapid progression Paroxysmal presentations common Marked fluctuation over time; remissions common	Gradual onset/slow spread Paroxysmal presentations rare Little fluctuation; remissions uncommon
Inciting events	Precipitating event – onset after minor injury common	Onset after injury rare
Distribution	Onset in legs common Pattern changes over time	Onset in legs seen typically in childhood Lower-limb presentation rare in adulthood; exception is neurodegenerative conditions Pattern consistent over time
Associated symptoms	Significant pain Multiple other somatisations Degree of disability inconsistent or in excess of pattern of dystonia	Little pain with exception of cervical dystonia Degree of disability consistent with or even less than expected for pattern of dystonia
Social history	Question of secondary gain, litigation, compensation claim	
Psychiatric assessment	Depression and anxiety may coexist Presence of disordered personality features History of sexual or physical abuse	Depression and anxiety may coexist
Pattern of activation	Often fixed dystonia Variable patterns of activation Increased resistance to passive movements in the dystonic limb	Usually mobile dystonia Action-specific pattern may be seen (including task specificity)
Modifications	Distractible (variable; much less than in other functional movement disorders) May increase with attention Suggestible with stimuli or trigger points Sensory tricks/gestes antagonistes very rare	Rarely modifiable Sensory tricks (gestes antagonistes) improve
Additional features	Other pseudo neurologic signs (e.g. give-way weakness, non-anatomic sensory loss) Organic signs consistent with disuse may be present in severe cases Presence of other functional/psychogenic movement disorders Selective abilities Features of complex regional pain syndrome (usually Type I)	Other organic neurologic findings Other movement disorders may be present in secondary causes Reported abilities in excess of apparent severity of dystonia
Common 'phenotypes'	Fixed limb dystonia: Hand: flexed fingers, thumb and index finger may be spared Foot: curling of toes, arching of foot, inversion and plantarflexion Face: tonic sustained lateral and/or downward protrusion of one side of the lower lip with ipsilateral deviation Head/neck: tonic contraction with head tilt and shoulder elevation (latter can occur in isolation)	See other chapters in this text: action-induced dystonia; task-specific dystonias

Paroxysmal presentations are relatively common for all psychogenic disorders, whereas they are rare in organic ones. When present in organic disease, they point to a relatively narrow range of conditions that are typically genetically determined. A cluster of appropriate features on history, such as brief episodes triggered by movement or onset after exercise or caffeine intake, may increase the index of suspicion for one of the genetically determined paroxysmal movement disorders, and prompt further testing.

The phenomenology of the movements themselves may provide clues to their aetiology. Fixed, often painful dystonia is extremely common in F/PDys. In contrast, organic dystonias typically occur with some reliability during the performance of a specific action and with considerable consistency over the short and medium term. Pain is also much less common, except in patients with cervical dystonia. Over the longer term, the distribution of an organic dystonia may progress slowly, particularly to adjacent body regions; whereas in F/PDys, much greater variability and inconsistency may be observed in the space of a single examination, or within the period of timely follow-up.

Likewise, a more detailed exploration of the medical history may suggest the presence of other neurological symptoms, including movement disorders, or other poorly explained medical conditions that have since resolved or symptoms indicating a broader somatoform illness. Alternatively, the clinician should also be aware that patients with somatoform illnesses often under-report their past evaluations or report histories of prior specific diagnoses whose somatoform nature only becomes apparent when the outcomes of specific investigations are subsequently confirmed to have been negative (Schrag et al. 2004b). Further careful discussions with the patient may reveal more complex illness behaviours such as doctor shopping, or personality features and attitudes that result in the patient 'splitting' opinions relating to the healthcare professionals previously involved in the patient's care.

The Psychiatric History

Acknowledging the mixed results of studies evaluating the frequency with which psychological disorders and life stressors can be identified in patients with F/PMDs, the psychiatric history remains an important element in the evaluation of the patient with any dystonia. Psychiatric diagnoses are seen at increased frequency in a number of organic dystonia syndromes, such as myoclonus-dystonia and idiopathic torsion dystonia. Likewise a variety of neurometabolic conditions, such as Wilson's disease, Huntington's disease, neuroacanthocytosis and Niemann-Pick type C, commonly present initially with psychiatric manifestations before developing movement disorders later in their courses. The interpretation of the significance of any given patient's psychiatric history, therefore, must occur in the context of the broader clinical picture.

A further consideration when interpreting the significance of psychiatric disease is that it is also possible that psychiatric disorders may be relatively more common in patients with organic movement disorders simply because of physical, psychological and social stressors related to physical demands and disability. Conversely, organic movement disorders have likewise been reported at relatively higher frequency in patients with primary psychiatric diagnoses, whether due to medication side-effects or for reasons that reflect underlying basal ganglia pathology (Saint-Cyr et al. 1995).

However, attempting to document a psychiatric history in a patient with a psychogenic movement disorder can prove challenging in its own right. Many such patients report normal mental states and deny histories of psychological trauma and are therefore reluctant to undergo an evaluation with a psychiatrist. A recent study provides a potential explanation for such observations by demonstrating significantly higher levels of alexithymia, an impaired ability to identify and appreciate emotional states, in patients with F/PMDs compared to controls (Demartini et al. 2014).

Examination Findings Supporting a Diagnosis of Functional/Psychogenic Dystonia

Although the physical examination of the patient with a F/PMD can often provide clues to the non-organic nature of the presentation, we would caution the reader that of all F/PMDs, dystonia is the most challenging for the clinician to identify reliably.

Much of the potential difficulty lies is the complexity and the unusual nature of organic dystonia, which serves as the baseline for comparison. The phenomenology of an organic dystonia can evolve with disease progression and can display profound variability in relation to the performance of voluntary actions, compensatory strategies, sensory inputs and psychological states – precisely the features that contributed to the belief predominant throughout much of the early and mid-twentieth century that organic dystonia was a psychogenic condition.

Table 44.1 lists the examination features seen more commonly in F/PDys than in organic dystonia.

The first important feature of the examination is the absence of hard neurological signs. However, patients with isolated (primary) organic dystonia also lack other neurological abnormalities; conversely, psychogenic disorders can overlie and amplify organic ones, and the presence of genuine neurological abnormalities therefore does not rule out the presence of a psychogenic disorder contributing to the presentation.

A second point of caution is that in more severe cases of F/PDys resulting in prolonged immobilisation, physical consequences of immobility, including wasting, trophic changes and osteoporosis, may indeed be present. The examiner should also be wary of confusing pseudo-neurological signs including asymmetry of reflexes induced by voluntarily holding a limb rigid, or a pseudo-Babinski sign, often presenting as a delayed, slowed or prolonged plantar extension following stimulation. Additional physical examination findings suggesting a psychogenic disorder include give-way weakness not attributable to guarding because of pain, and false weakness, sometimes with the presence of a Hoover's sign. The presence of scars from self-inflicted injuries or multiple prior operations may signal underlying psychiatric disease, abnormal illness behaviours or somatisation.

A number of specific positive signs, some of which are common more broadly to psychogenic disorders, may also suggest an underlying diagnosis of F/PDys. These include the appearance of distractibility and, conversely, an increase in the severity of the movements with attention. However, distractibility is less likely to be seen in patients with F/PDys than in other F/PMDs, as a fixed posture is easier to maintain in the face of multiple distractors and skill demanding tasks than are dynamic or rhythmic movements. Conversely, given the fluctuating and variable nature of organic dystonia, the distractibility of abnormal movements must be relatively marked to justify a psychogenic designation. When tremor is an associated feature, the usual examination strategies for the evaluation of psychogenic tremor, with distraction and entrainment, should be attempted. However, organic dystonic tremor may be quite variable in presence, frequency and amplitude.

The presence of other non-organic signs may also act as positive indicators of F/PDys. The patient may dramatise the effort involved in specific examination tasks by grimacing and using the whole body to perform what should otherwise be discrete or simple movements; additional dramatising behaviours include episodes of whole-body shaking and excessive startle responses, as well as extreme or acrobatic responses on postural pull testing. Alternatively, an extreme slowness of movement not associated with a decrement in the amplitude of movement may be present, or the patient may simply fail to complete tasks on examination that would not be precluded by the severity of the dystonia. Likewise the presence of additional, bizarre involuntary movements, including bizarre gait, may provide a clue to the non-organic nature of the presentation, although the examiner will need to be familiar with the sometimes bizarre gaits of organic dystonia. Likewise, a recognition of the influence of sensory tricks in ameliorating organic dystonia is important. The presence of a geste antagoniste should strongly suggest an organic cause, although rarely have these been reported in the presence of confirmed F/PDys (Munhoz & Lang 2004).

A number of non-anatomic sensory signs, such as loss of vibration sense splitting the midline, might be helpful in alerting the examiner to the possibility of a F/PDys, but given the lack of reliability and reproducibility of the sensory exam in organic disease, these have poor specificity and should therefore not weigh heavily in any formulation.

A more useful sign, if present, is the suggestibility of dystonic postures induced by non-physiologic stimuli such as a vibrating tuning fork, passive movements of another limb or body part, or the activation of 'pressure points' as originally emphasised by Charcot. However, the most reliable feature permitting a relatively confident diagnosis is significant improvement with placebo or suggestion, and ultimately psychotherapy. The observed response to such interventions, however, must be marked and sustained for more than a few minutes, since brief (and sometimes even more prolonged) placebo responses can occur in organic movement disorders (Goetz et al. 2002).

Finally, the clinician may note considerable discrepancy between objective signs and reported disability and requirements for supportive care. Conversely, the presence of selective abilities – with the patient inexplicably able to perform some tasks (especially desirable ones) that would otherwise be precluded by a continuous degree of dystonia – should act as a clue to the presence of an F/PDys. This contrasts with the selective pure task-specific nature of some forms of organic dystonia.

Functional/Psychogenic Dystonia Associated with Peripheral Injury

A significant literature has accumulated describing the temporal association between either soft tissue or nerve injury and the emergence of dystonia. Analysis of these cases has demonstrated psychogenic features in a large proportion; however, the degree of overlap of this condition with F/PDys and the extent to which this condition represents a purely psychogenic presentation remain major points of contention in the field. Table 44.2 outlines the clinical features of these cases reported under different terms. When the limbs are affected, additional features of complex regional pain syndrome (CRPS) may be present (almost always 'Type I', without evidence of a peripheral nerve lesion). Although we and others believe that most of these patients suffer from a type of F/PDys, some authors favour an organic origin (van Hilten 2010) and have even championed the use of intrathecal baclofen in its treatment, although videotapes demonstrating this response (van Hilten et al. 2002) to our eyes strongly suggest F/PDys and a probable placebo response.

Diagnostic Accuracy in Functional/Psychogenic Dystonia

The growing awareness of the broad spectrum of organic movement disorders that emerged in the mid-1970s and early 1980s engendered an initial reluctance to consider psychogenic aetiologies for movement disorder presentations. A now much criticised early study suggested that such fears were in fact justified and that a large proportion of patients with organic conditions were typically diagnosed with psychogenic disorders in error (Slater & Glithero 1965). More recent reports, however, suggest that, following detailed neurological assessment and in the era of modern imaging, the percentage of obvious misdiagnosis of F/PMDs is considerably less than 1 per cent of patients (Stone et al. 2009).

Standardised diagnostic criteria for F/PDys may assist the clinician in the task of diagnosis, but they do not guarantee diagnostic accuracy, which still depends on the traditional clinical skills of history taking, a skilled examination technique, and the clinician's powers of close observation, interpreted in the context of knowledge and experience. However, once the clinician has concluded that a presentation is most consistent with an F/PDys, some statement can be made regarding the relative certainty of the diagnosis. Fahn and Williams (1988) first established the diagnostic criteria for F/PDys, and subsequent modifications have been proposed (Williams et al. 1995; Gupta & Lang 2009). In contrast to tremor and myoclonus, where electrophysiological techniques can often assist in making a 'laboratory supported definite' clinical diagnosis (Gupta & Lang 2009), as will be discussed elsewhere in this text, a reliable diagnostic test for F/PDys is sorely needed, particularly as this is the most challenging F/PMD to diagnose.

Conclusion

Neurology, probably more than any other specialty in medicine, relies upon the art of its clinical practice. Successful clinicians develop an intuitive understanding of the presentations that form the basis of their work. Careful history taking and a flexible examination technique form the foundation of this understanding, but the clinician must then interpret the acquired information in the context of accumulated personal experience and a wide knowledge of the field. F/PMDs, notoriously, test this process to its limits, at times to the point of failure. F/PDys represents an even further challenge since its diagnosis calls upon an exhaustive knowledge of an organic counterpart with varied and sometimes bizarre manifestations. All these elements can summate in a successful formulation and accurate diagnosis. But this end is only a beginning. The outcome for most patients with F/PDys remains tenuous and depends in no small measure on acceptance by the patient, empathy from the physician and a respect for the limitations of our current knowledge on the part of both.

References

Bhatia KP, Bhatt MH, Marsden CD. 1993. The causalgia-dystonia syndrome. *Brain* 116:843–851.

Crimlisk H, Bhatia K, Cope H, David A, Marsden C, Ron M. 1998. Slater revisited: 6 year follow-up study of patients with medically unexplained motor symptoms *BMJ* 316(7131):2–6.

Demartini B, Petrochilos P, Ricciardi L, Price G, Edwards M, Joyce E. 2014. The role of alexthymia in the development of functional

Table 44.2 Clinical subtypes of dystonia associated with peripheral injury

	Dystonia associated with peripheral injury	Causalgia –dystonia syndrome	Syndrome of fixed dystonia	Posttraumatic painful torticollis
Representative papers	Marsden et al. 1984 van Rooijen et al. 2011	Bhatia et al. 1993	Schrag et al. 2004b	Sa et al. 2003
Clinical features of dystonia	Fixed posture Sympathetic blockade helpful in some cases	Fixed posture Often lower limb Absence of geste antagoniste Sympathetic blockade sympathectomies unhelpful Poor response to botulinum toxin injections	Fixed posture Limbs in 90 per cent Neck or shoulder region in 6 per cent Spread of dystonia to other body regions in 56 per cent Medical and surgical treatments largely unsuccessful Multidisciplinary treatment, including psychotherapy produced remission in small proportion	Fixed posture Typically shoulder elevation and head tilt Rapid onset following inciting event
Associated historical features	Onset after minor injury common	Female preponderance Acute- or subacute-onset after minimal trauma Litigation or workers' compensation often involved	84 per cent female Minor peripheral trauma, including operations or immobilisation in a plaster cast in 63 per cent of patients	Precipitants always trivial with no serious structural injury identified Injuries often work-related involving neck or shoulder area Litigation or compensation involved in majority of cases
Associated clinical features	Severe pain Tremor, myoclonus Complex regional pain syndrome (with other autonomic phenomena: vasomotor, sudomotor and trophic changes)	Severe pain (accompanied by vasomotor, sudomotor and trophic changes)	Pain 'major component' in 41 per cent of all cases Continuous pain at rest in 38/41 of prospectively followed group Of 41/103 patients prospectively evaluated: 20 per cent fulfilled criteria for CRPS 24 per cent 'documented' psychogenic dystonia 12 per cent clinically established psychogenic dystonia 29 per cent DSM-IV criteria for somatisation disorder 24 per cent criteria for DSM-IV somatisation disorder and clinically established psychogenic dystonia	Pain prominent Frequent additional findings suggesting a psychogenic disorder: 'give way' weakness Non-anatomic sensory loss (typically changed or resolved under Amytal) Distractibility Improvement with sham botulinum toxin injections Surreptitious observation of a symptom-free period in some instances Minnesota Multiphasic Personality inventory suggested presence of a conversion disorder Sodium Amytal interview resulted in improvement of pain and posturing in most

motor symptoms (conversion disorder). *J Neurol Neurosurg Psychiatry* 85(10):1132–1137.

Edwards M, Stone J, Lang A. 2014. From psychogenic movement disorder to functional movement disorder: it's time to change the name. *Mov Disord* 29:849–852.

Factor S, Podskalny G, Molho E. 1995. Psychogenic movement disorders: frequency, clinical profiles and characteristics. *J Neurol Neurosurg Psychiatr* 59(4):406–412.

Fahn S, Williams D. 1988. Psychogenic dystonia. *Adv Neurol* 50:431–455.

Feinstein A, Stergiopoulos V, Fine J, Lang A. 2001. Psychiatric outcome in patients with a psychogenic movement disorder: a prospective study. *Neuropsychiatry Neuropsychol Behav Neurol* 14:169–176.

Goetz C. 2006. Charcot and psychogenic movement disorders. In: Hallet M, Fahn S, Jankovic J, Lang AE, Cloninger CR, Yudofsky SC, editors. *Psychogenic Movement Disorders Neurology and Neuropsychiatry*. Philadelphia, PA: Lippincott Williams & Wilkins; pp. 3–13.

Goetz C, Leurgans S, Raman R. 2002. Placebo associated improvement in motor function: comparison of subjective and objective sections of the UPDRS in early Parkinson's disease. *Mov Disord* 17:283–288.

Gupta A, Lang A. 2009. Psychogenic movement disorders. *Curr Opin Neurol* 22(4):430–436.

Kobayash J, Lang A, Hallett M, Lenz F. 2011. Thalamic neuronal and EMG activity in psychogenic dystonia compared with organic dystonia. *Mov Disord* 26:1348–1352.

Kranick S, Ekanayak V, Martinez V, Ameli R, Hallett M, Voon V. 2011. Psychopathology and psychogenic movement disorders. *Mov Disord* 26:1844–1850.

Lang A. 1995. Psychogenic dystonia: a review of 18 cases. *Can J Neurol Sci* 22:136–143.

Lempert T, Dieterich M, Huppert D, Brandt T. 1990. Psychogenic disorders in neurology: frequency and clinical spectrum. *Acta Neurol Scand* 82:335–340.

Marsden CD, Obeso JA, Traub MM, Rothwell JC, Kranz H, LaCruz F. 1984. Muscle spasms associated with Sudeck's atrophy after injury. *BMJ* 288:173–176.

Munhoz R, Lang A. 2004. Gestes antagonistes in psychogenic dystonia. *Mov Disord* 19(3):331–332.

Sa, DF, Mailis-Gagnon A, Nicholson K, Lang AE. 2003. *Mov Disord* 18(12):1482–1491.

Saint-Cyr J, Taylor A, Nicholson K. 1995. Behavior and the basal ganglia. *Adv Neurol* 65:1–28.

Schrag A, Brown R, Trimble M. 2004a. The reliability of self-reported diagnoses in patients with neurologically unexplained symptoms. *J Neurol Ches Neurosurg Psychiatry* 75:608–611.

Schrag A, Trimble M, Quinn N, Bhatia K. 2004b. The syndrome of fixed dystonia: an evaluation of 103 patients. *Brain* 127:2360–2372.

Schwingenschuh P, Pont-Sunyer C, Surtees R, Edwards M, Bhatia K. 2008. Psychogenic movement disorders in children: a report of 15 cases and a review of the literature *Mov Disord* 23(13):1882–1888.

Slater E, Glithero E. 1965. Follow-up of patients diagnosed as suffering from 'hysteria.' *J Psychosom Res* 9(1):9–13.

Stone J, Carson A, Duncan R, Coleman R, Roberts R, Warlow C, Hibberd C, Murray G, Cull R, Pelosi A, Cavanagh J, Matthews K, Goldbeck R, Smyth R, Walker J, Macmahon AD, Sharpe M. 2009. Symptoms 'unexplained by organic disease' in 1144 new neurology out-patients: how often does the diagnosis change at follow-up. *Brain* 132:2878–2888.

van Hilten J. 2010. Movement disorders in complex regional pain syndrome. *Pain Med* 11(8):1274–1277.

van Hilten J, van de Beek W, Hoff J, Voormolen J, Delhaas E. 2002. Intrathecal baclofen treatment of dystonia in reflex sympathetic dystrophy. *Mov Disord* 17(4):745–746.

van Rooijen DE, Geraedts EJ, Marinus J, Jankovic J, van Hilten JJ. 2011. Peripheral trauma and movement disorders: a systematic review of reported cases. *J Neurol Neurosurg Psychiatry* 82(8):892–898.

Williams D, Ford B, Fahn S. 1995. Phenomenology and psychopathology related to psychogenic movement disorders. *Adv Neurol* 65:231–257.

Chapter 45

Diagnosis of Psychogenic Dystonias

Carine W. Maurer and Mark Hallett*

Historically, dystonia has been one of the movement disorders most commonly misdiagnosed as psychogenic in underlying aetiology (Lesser & Fahn 1978; Munhoz & Lang 2004). Although our understanding of the natural history, phenomenology and physiology of dystonia has improved considerably, the diagnosis of psychogenic dystonia remains a challenge.

Clinical Features of Psychogenic Dystonia

While the diagnosis of psychogenic dystonia can be quite difficult even for the experienced clinician, several clues can be of assistance in distinguishing clinically between psychogenic and organic dystonia (see Box 45.1). As with other types of psychogenic movements, psychogenic dystonia may be distractible and suggestible, and symptoms may be relieved completely with non-physiological interventions (Munhoz & Lang 2004). The clinical course of psychogenic dystonia is often abrupt to subacute, with symptoms reaching their maximum around the time of disease onset, compared to a more protracted course in organic dystonia. The presence of a fixed posture early in the course of the disease is also suggestive of psychogenic dystonia, whereas organic dystonia tends to be action-induced, especially at disease onset (Hallett 2010). In addition to maintenance of a fixed posture, resistance to manipulation is also characteristic of psychogenic dystonia (Espay & Lang 2011). Sensory tricks, common in organic dystonia, are rare in patients with psychogenic dystonia (Schrag et al. 2004; Hawley & Weiner 2011). Pain also commonly accompanies psychogenic dystonia (Hawley & Weiner 2011), and continuous pain at rest has been proposed to be a key feature of patients with this disorder (Schrag et al. 2004).

In a combined retrospective and prospective study examining 103 patients with fixed dystonia, many of whom were thought to have psychogenic dystonia, Schrag and colleagues found fixed dystonia affected predominantly young females, with an average age of onset around 30 years of age. Unlike organic dystonia, which frequently affects the neck and shoulder, patients with fixed dystonia had symptoms predominantly involving the limbs (90 per cent), and only rarely involving the neck (6 per cent). While spread to other body regions occurred in the majority of patients, none of the patients examined exhibited overflow dystonia (Schrag et al. 2004), a phenomenon often seen in organic dystonia and thought to reflect lack of surround inhibition. Schrag and colleagues also found that peripheral injury preceded symptom onset in a large subset of patients with fixed dystonia, an observation that has also been made in a number of additional studies (Tarsy 1998; Sa et al. 2003). Sa and colleagues observed that patients who developed cervical dystonia very quickly after onset of trauma were more likely to exhibit other signs suggestive of psychogenic dystonia, including maximum disability shortly after disease onset, fixed immobile posture, severe pain, absence of sensory tricks, distractibility and improvement with non-physiological interventions (Sa et al. 2003).

Box 45.1 Clinical Clues Suggestive of Psychogenic (Functional) Dystonia

Abrupt onset
Fixed postures present from early stage of disease
Resistance to manipulation
Sensory tricks are rare
Distractibility
Suggestibility
Associated pain is common
Poor response to treatment

Another pattern of dystonia typically psychogenic involves lateral deviation of the mouth, including the lower lip and jaw (Fasano et al. 2012). This form of psychogenic dystonia appears as slow intermittent spasms, and can also involve the eyelid, perinasal region and forehead.

Electrophysiologic Testing in Psychogenic Dystonia

Despite the clinical clues listed above, reliable clinical diagnosis of psychogenic dystonia remains a challenge. Achieving a 'laboratory-supported' level of certainty has been suggested as a means of improving the level of diagnostic certainty for psychogenic movement disorders (Gupta & Lang 2009); electrophysiological testing has in fact proven to be quite useful in assisting the diagnostic process in a variety of psychogenic movement disorders, including psychogenic tremor and psychogenic myoclonus (Brown & Thompson 2001; Hallett 2010).

* Supported by the NINDS Intramural Program.

A handful of studies have explored the electrophysiological findings in patients with psychogenic dystonia, with a minority of these having potential diagnostic utility.

Somewhat surprisingly, a number of studies have detected similar abnormalities in patients with psychogenic and organic dystonia. Intraoperative microelectrode recordings in the globus pallidus interna (Ramos et al. 2015) and the thalamus (Kobayashi et al. 2011) of patients who had been operated on erroneously indicate that simple intraoperative neurophysiology measures, including spontaneous firing rate and bursting, as well as movement-related discharges, are not sufficient to distinguish between patients with psychogenic dystonia and those with organic dystonia. Studies using transcranial magnetic stimulation (TMS) have demonstrated that both psychogenic and organic dystonia patients exhibit impaired measures of cortical inhibition, including reduced short-interval intracortical inhibition (SICI), reduced long-interval intracortical inhibition (LICI) and shortened contralateral silent period (SP) (Espay et al. 2006; Avanzino et al. 2008; Quartarone et al. 2009). Spinal reciprocal inhibition has similarly been demonstrated to be impaired in both psychogenic and organic dystonia (Espay et al. 2006). The impaired cortical inhibition seen in psychogenic dystonia has been interpreted in a number of ways. One possibility is that it is due to secondary brain changes resulting from chronic maintenance of an abnormal posture. It has also been hypothesised to reflect a predisposition to developing dystonia, with additional factors contributing to the further specification of the dystonia as either psychogenic or organic. The presence of bilateral cortical abnormalities in patients with unilateral symptoms (Avanzino et al. 2008) favours the latter hypothesis, although the mechanism for this predisposition remains unclear.

Patients with psychogenic dystonia have also been found to exhibit abnormal tactile temporal discrimination, with the temporal discrimination threshold (TDT) for tactile stimuli comparably elevated in patients with psychogenic dystonia and those with primary torsion dystonia, as compared to controls (Morgante et al. 2011). It has been speculated that this impaired somatosensory processing may be linked to impaired temporal inhibition in the sensory cortex, and may represent a predisposing trait for the development of both psychogenic and organic dystonia.

In addition to being characterised by reduced excitability of inhibitory systems, patients with organic dystonia also exhibit increased plasticity in sensorimotor circuits. One study suggests that this increased plasticity may distinguish patients with organic dystonia from their counterparts with psychogenic dystonia. Using a paired associative stimulation (PAS) protocol in which an electrical stimulus to the median nerve at the wrist is subsequently paired with a TMS pulse to the hand area of the contralateral motor cortex, Quartarone and colleagues found that, while patients with organic dystonia had facilitation of motor-evoked potentials (MEPs) to both median- and ulnar-innervated muscles, patients with psychogenic dystonia and controls only showed facilitation of median-innervated muscles (Quartarone et al. 2009). The authors subsequently suggest that, whereas the development of organic dystonia may require both reduced cortical inhibition as well as enhanced plasticity, impaired cortical inhibition may be sufficient for the predisposition to psychogenic dystonia.

In patients with organic blepharospasm, the blink reflex recovery cycle is characterised by an abnormally enhanced R2 blink reflex recovery cycle, reflecting impaired brainstem interneuron excitability. Schwingenschuh and colleagues demonstrated that, in contrast, patients with presumed psychogenic blepharospasm had blink reflex recovery cycles that did not differ from healthy controls (Schwingenschuh et al. 2011). While the findings need to be confirmed in a larger study with a better characterised group of patients, the high specificity (90 per cent) of the abnormality suggests that it may prove to be a useful diagnostic tool to distinguish between organic and psychogenic dystonia.

Conclusions

In this chapter, we have described some of the challenges inherent to the diagnosis of psychogenic dystonia, and provided some of the clinical clues that can be useful in the diagnostic process. While challenging, proper diagnosis of patients with psychogenic dystonia is critical, as it will prevent unnecessary additional testing and procedures, and help to guide optimal treatment.

References

Avanzino L, Martino D, van de Warrenburg BP, Schneider SA, Abbruzzese G, Defazio G, Schrag A, Bhatia KP, Rothwell JC. 2008. Cortical excitability is abnormal in patients with the 'fixed dystonia' syndrome. *Movement Disorders: Official Journal of the Movement Disorder Society* 23(5):646–652.

Brown P, Thompson PD. 2001. Electrophysiological aids to the diagnosis of psychogenic jerks, spasms, and tremor. *Movement Disorders: Official Journal of the Movement Disorder Society* 16(4):595–599.

Espay AJ, Lang AE. 2011. The psychogenic toe signs. *Neurology* 77(5):508–509.

Espay AJ, Morgante F, Purzner J, Gunraj CA, Lang AE, Chen R. 2006. Cortical and spinal abnormalities in psychogenic dystonia. *Annals of Neurology* 59(5):825–834.

Fasano A, Valadas A, Bhatia KP, Prashanth LK, Lang AE, Munhoz RP, Morgante F, Tarsy D, Duker AP, Girlanda P, Bentivoglio AR, Espay AJ. 2012. Psychogenic facial movement disorders: clinical features and associated conditions. *Movement Disorders: Official Journal of the Movement Disorder Society* 27(12):1544–1551.

Gupta A, Lang AE. 2009. Psychogenic movement disorders. *Current Opinion in Neurology* 22(4):430–436.

Hallett M. 2010. Physiology of psychogenic movement disorders. *Journal of Clinical Neuroscience: Official Journal of the Neurosurgical Society of Australasia* 17(8):959–965.

Hawley JS, Weiner WJ. 2011. Psychogenic dystonia and peripheral trauma. *Neurology* 77(5):496–502.

Kobayashi K, Lang AE, Hallett M, Lenz FA. 2011. Thalamic neuronal and EMG activity in psychogenic dystonia compared with organic dystonia. *Movement Disorders: Official Journal of the Movement Disorder Society* 26(7):1348–1352.

Lesser RP, Fahn S. 1978. Dystonia: a disorder often misdiagnosed as a conversion reaction. *The American Journal of Psychiatry* 135(3):349–352.

Morgante F, Tinazzi M, Squintani G, Martino D, Defazio G, Romito L, Albanese A, Di Matteo A, Quartarone A, Girlanda P, Fiorio M, Berardelli A. 2011. Abnormal tactile temporal discrimination in psychogenic dystonia. *Neurology* 77(12):1191–1197.

Munhoz RP, Lang AE. 2004. Gestes antagonistes in psychogenic dystonia. *Movement Disorders: Official Journal of the Movement Disorder Society* 19(3):331–332.

Quartarone A, Rizzo V, Terranova C, Morgante F, Schneider S, Ibrahim N, Girlanda P, Bhatia KP, Rothwell JC. 2009. Abnormal sensorimotor plasticity in organic but not in psychogenic dystonia. *Brain: A Journal of Neurology* 132(Pt 10):2871–2877.

Ramos VF, Pillai AS, Lungu C, Ostrem J, Starr P, Hallett M. 2015. Intraoperative neurophysiology in deep brain surgery for psychogenic dystonia. *Annals of Clinical and Translational Neurology* 2(6):707–710.

Sa DS, Mailis-Gagnon A, Nicholson K, Lang AE. 2003. Posttraumatic painful torticollis. *Movement Disorders: Official Journal of the Movement Disorder Society* 18(12):1482–1491.

Schrag A, Trimble M, Quinn N, Bhatia K. 2004. The syndrome of fixed dystonia: an evaluation of 103 patients. *Brain: A Journal of Neurology* 127(Pt 10):2360–2372.

Schwingenschuh P, Katschnig P, Edwards MJ, Teo JT, Korlipara LV, Rothwell JC, Bhatia KP. 2011. The blink reflex recovery cycle differs between essential and presumed psychogenic blepharospasm. *Neurology* 76(7):610–614.

Tarsy D. 1998. Comparison of acute- and delayed-onset posttraumatic cervical dystonia. *Movement Disorders: Official Journal of the Movement Disorder Society* 13(3):481–485.

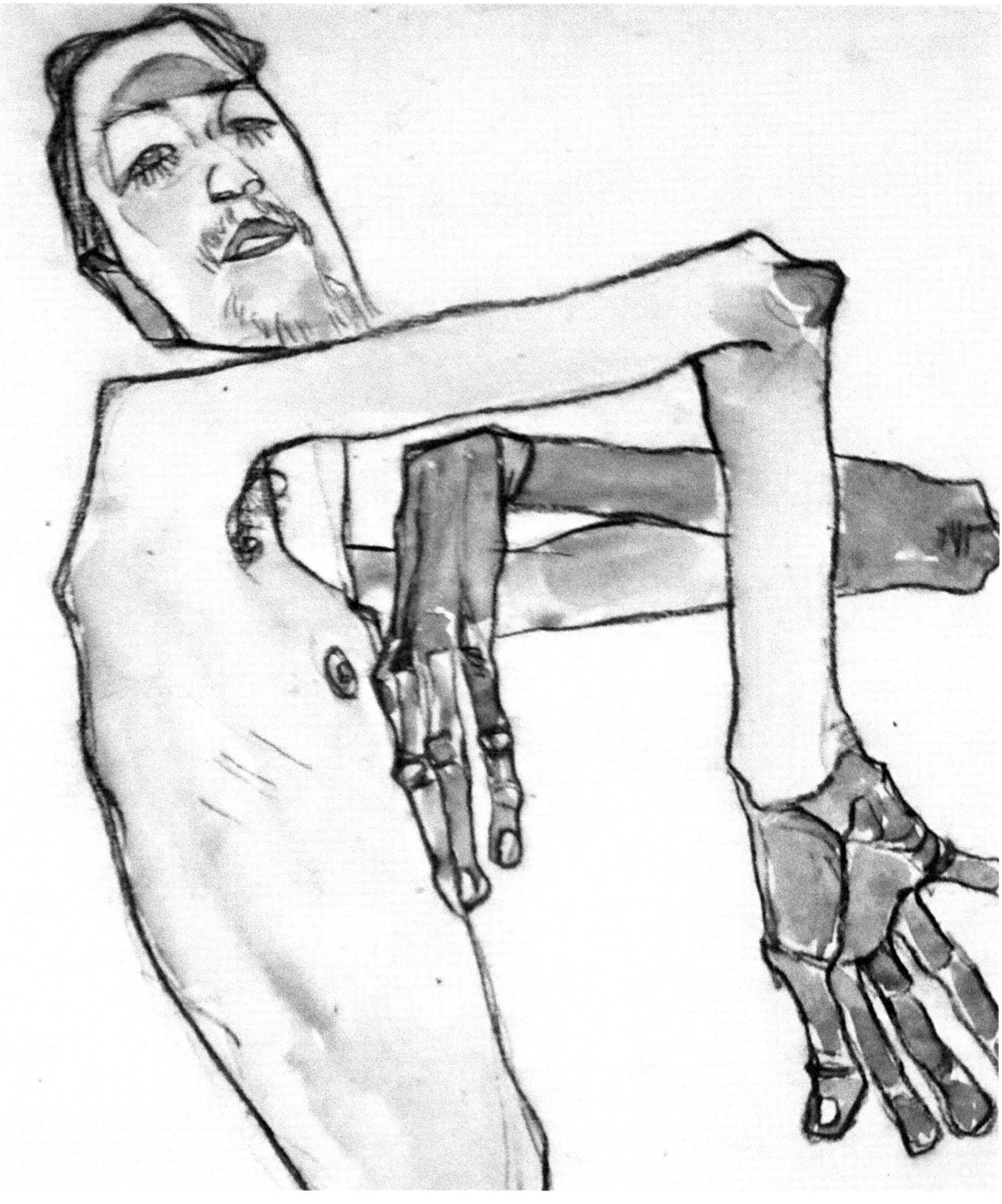

Chapter 46

Intrathecal Baclofen for Dyskinetic Cerebral Palsy

R. Jeroen Vermeulen, Laura A. Bonouvrie, Annemieke I. Buizer, Willem J. R. van Ouwerkerk, Jasper van Aalst, Onno Teernstra, Dan Soudant and Jules G. Becher

Cerebral palsy (CP) is a frequent cause of childhood disability, with an incidence of 1.77 per 1000 live births (Sellier et al. 2016). Most children (80 per cent) suffer from spasticity and approximately 5–16 per cent suffer from dyskinetic CP (Howard et al. 2005; Himmelmann & Uvebrant 2014; Sellier et al. 2016). Children with perinatal events are most likely to develop dyskinetic CP and these children are the most severely affected (Himmelmann et al. 2007). In dyskinetic CP, two types of involuntary movements can be distinguished: slow movements (dystonic) and fast movements (choreathetotic, also described as hyperkinetic).

Aetiology

The cause of dyskinetic CP is mainly asphyxia due to perinatal events, causing damage in the basal nuclei and central cortex (Krageloh-Mann et al. 2002). Another cause of dyskinetic CP is the occurrence of hyperbilirubinaemia in term and premature born children (McDonald 1963; Wu et al. 2015). The dyskinetic movement disorder in these children is associated with accumulation of bilirubin in the globus pallidus (Groenendaal et al. 2004). This aetiology of CP is often accompanied by severe hearing loss. Brain malformations are another cause of dyskinetic CP. These malformations are often associated with abnormal basal ganglia (e.g. fusion of the thalamus) (Krageloh-Mann & Horber 2007).

Dystonia Rating

For primary dystonia the Fahn–Burke–Marsden dystonia rating scale and the Unified dystonia rating scale are used. Both scales are reliable and reproducible (Monbaliu et al. 2010). Another clinical rating scale, the Barry–Albright dystonia rating scale for secondary dystonia, does not take rest or activity during rating into account.

Dyskinesia Scale

Recently, Monbaliu presented a newly developed scale, the dyskinesia impairment scale (DIS), to measure secondary dystonia (Monbaliu et al. 2012). Not only does this instrument have a strict activity/rest protocol, it also has a separate score for choreoathetosis. This scale is reliable for scoring both choreoathetosis and dystonia in dyskinetic CP. In addition, using this score, Monbaliu and coworkers showed that dystonia is correlated with severity of disability. So far, the responsiveness of this scale to treatment-induced changes is unclear.

Functional Severity Rating

Based on the international classification of function from the World Health Organization, effects can be measured at the body function and structure level (e.g. dystonia), at the activity level (e.g. mobility) and at the participation level (Wright et al. 2008).

At the activity level, children with dyskinetic CP are commonly classified for mobility, hand use and communication. For mobility, the Gross Motor Function Classification System (GMFCS) is used. This classification has five levels; a child is classified as level I if he or she can walk on stairs without assistance and as level V if she or he is completely wheelchair-bound and cannot move alone (Palisano et al. 2000). Children with dyskinetic CP are generally rated as more severe at GMFCS IV and V (Himmelmann et al. 2007). A similar classification scale has been developed for hand use when handling objects in daily activities, the Manual Ability Classification System (MACS) (Eliasson et al. 2006). This system classifies the collaborative use of both hands together and the scores range from I (handles objects easily and successfully) to V (requires total assistance). For communication, the Communication Function Classification System (CFCS) has been developed (Hidecker et al. 2011). This system classifies communication from I (sends and receives with familiar and unfamiliar partners effectively and efficiently) to V (seldom effectively sends and receives, even with familiar partners).

Intrathecal Baclofen

Baclofen is a spasmolytic drug. The first studies on intrathecal administration of baclofen (intrathecal baclofen therapy = ITB) in the 1980s showed an effect on spasticity in major neurological diseases, e.g. multiple sclerosis, but also in spastic CP (Hoving et al. 2007; Pin et al. 2011). In an elegant randomised placebo-controlled study with 19 participants with spastic CP, Hoving et al. showed the effectiveness of a bolus ITB on spasticity and daily care (Hoving et al. 2008).

Albright was one of the first investigators to use intrathecal baclofen in dyskinetic CP in several large uncontrolled studies (Albright et al. 1991, 2001). More recently, a small randomised

Table 46.1 Clinical effects of intrathecal baclofen in patients with dyskinetic cerebral palsy

Overview of effects	improved (%)	unchanged (%)	worsened (%)	*n*	reference
Effect on daily activities					
Hygiene	68	32	0	19	Motta et al. 2008
Dressing	95	5	0	19	Motta et al. 2008
Ease of care	86	11	3	86*	Albright et al. 2001
Feeding	53	42	5	19	Motta et al. 2008
Comfort	50	0	50	4	Bonouvrie et al. 2011
Sleeping	53	42	5	19	Motta et al. 2008
Speaking	35	61	4	103*	Albright et al. 2001; Bonouvrie et al. 2011
Swallowing	26	66	8	86*	Bonouvrie et al. 2011
Quality of life					
Quality of life	85	11	4	86*	Albright et al. 2001
Happiness	75	0	25	3	Bonouvrie et al. 2011
Mood	47	53	0	19	Motta et al. 2008
Autonomy	37	63	0	19	Motta et al. 2008
Pain	52	35	13	23	Motta et al. 2008; Bonouvrie et al. 2011
Dystonia and motor function					
Dystonia	96	4	0	23	Motta et al. 2008; Bonouvrie et al. 2011
Control of head	95	5	0	19	Motta et al. 2008
Control of trunk	93	7	0	19	Motta et al. 2008
Sitting	89	11	0	19	Motta et al. 2008
Upper extremity control	49	65	5	119*	Albright et al. 2001; Motta et al. 2008; Bonouvrie et al. 2011
Lower extremity control	36	58	6	86*	Albright et al. 2001
Overall outcome					
GAS	70	30	0	16	Ward et al. 2009

Abbreviations used: *n*, number; GAS, goal attainment scaling; * 70 per cent of the patients in the study of Albright were diagnosed as CP (Albright et al. 2001).

pilot study confirmed the effect of ITB on dyskinetic CP, especially with regard to caregiving (Bonouvrie et al. 2013).

Pharmacological Properties

Baclofen is a $GABA_B$ receptor agonist. This receptor is present at the spinal interneurons and mediates inhibition of the reflex arch. As a result of the $GABA_B$ properties of baclofen, the disturbed pyramidal tract activity is inhibited. In spasticity this is the most likely mode of action. This mode of action is supported by the effect of ITB on the Hoffman (H)-reflex (Macdonell et al. 1989; Hoving et al. 2006). The H-reflex is dose dependently affected by ITB (Hoving et al. 2006; Stokic et al. 2006). Another possible mechanism is baclofen-induced inhibition of atrial natriuretic peptide-mediated cGMP synthesis in laminae I–III as demonstrated in the rat cervical spinal cord (de Louw et al. 2002).

It remains unsolved, however, whether the effect of ITB in patients with dyskinetic CP is also mediated at the spinal level. Since the dyskinetic movements are thought to originate from the basal ganglia, the working mechanism of ITB is also supposed to act though its effect in the basal ganglia.

Chen and coworkers showed that the activity of pallidal neurons is suppressed by activation of the $GABA_B$ receptor by modulating glutamatergic input at a presynaptic site (Chen et al. 2002). Ikeda and coworkers expanded this work and showed that $GABA_B$ receptors in the globus pallidus and substantia nigra pars reticulata are activated depending on motor function (Ikeda et al. 2010). These results suggest a central role for the basal ganglia in the effect of intrathecal baclofen in dyskinesia.

Clinical Effect of Intrathecal Baclofen on Dystonia

Several studies point towards a beneficial effect of ITB on daily activities, daily care and quality of life in dyskinetic CP (Albright et al. 2001; Motta et al. 2008; Bonouvrie et al. 2011). ITB clearly reduces dystonic movements (see Table 46.1). The available studies on dyskinetic CP and ITB differ in outcome measures, though in general caregiving as part of daily activities is improving in most patients.

Intrathecal baclofen seems also to have a good effect on pain, though pain worsened in about 10 per cent of patients. Sitting improved in most patients. Importantly, upper and lower extremity control did improve in about half of the patients.

A larger randomised placebo-controlled study on ITB in dyskinetic CP patients, the IDYS trial, is underway (Bonouvrie et al. 2013). In this study the effect of ITB versus placebo is investigated over a longer period of time (three months).

Catheter Placement

In spasticity (i.e. exaggerated stretch reflex activity) the placement of the tip of the catheter is usually at a low thoracic level (Sanger et al. 2003). In line with the presumed origin of dyskinetic movements, it is advocated that in patients with dyskinetic CP catheter placement should be achieved at a cervical level. It should be noted, however, that the effect of catheter location has not been systematically investigated.

Dose Adaptation of Intrathecal Baclofen

In general during the first months of treatment dosage increases are necessary. For CP the doses range between 50 and 1500 μg/24 h with a mean dose around 500 μg/24 h (Boster et al. 2016). Therefore regular checks should be scheduled in the first months. Some advocate an inpatient setting for ITB dose titration, though this will probably be strongly influenced by geographical characteristics of each country.

Further, it seems that introduction of bolus injection might be a solution when continuous administration is insufficient or when the effect fades away quickly after increasing the dosage (Boster et al. 2016).

Complications of Intrathecal Baclofen Pumps

Reported complications include CSF leak, seroma, infection, skin erosion at the pump site, catheter fracture, catheter disconnection, catheter occlusion, catheter sagging/migration, pump refill problems, baclofen withdrawal, baclofen overdose, truncal hypotonia, neck hyperextension, low-pressure CSF headache, and excessive frequency of refills. As several improved types of spinal catheters are being developed, data about the present rate of catheter dysfunction are not available. Infection is the most serious reported complication (Ward et al. 2009). There is some evidence that the complication rate in patients with dyskinetic CP is higher than in those with spastic CP (complication rate 0.25 vs 0.71) (Ward et al. 2009).

Intrathecal Withdrawal Syndrome

Sudden withdrawal of ITB can cause a very serious life-threatening withdrawal syndrome in spastic CP (Cruikshank & Eunson 2007). This syndrome can present with fever, exaggerated movements, itching, painful muscle spasms, vegetative signs (e.g. heavy sweating) and pulmonary oedema. When pulmonary oedema occurs intensive care treatment, including sedation and artificial ventilation, may be necessary. Especially in the group of severely disabled patients (GMFCS IV and V), recognition of ITB withdrawal syndrome can be difficult and is sometimes mistakenly interpreted as a common (respiratory) infection. Causes of withdrawal can be diverse and include shortage of medication, catheter dislocation, breakage or occlusion, and, in rare cases, mechanical pump failure.

As a first step in suspected withdrawal syndrome the administration of oral baclofen 0.75–2 mg/kg/24h is advised to prevent the development of more severe withdrawal symptoms. In addition, a plan for systematic troubleshooting should be installed (Dvorak et al. 2010; Saulino et al. 2016).

Intrathecal Baclofen Overdose Syndrome

The dosage of baclofen is usually higher in dyskinetic CP than in spastic CP. Signs of overdosing are increased swallowing problems with risk of pneumonia, slurred speech (in the case of a speaking patient), loss of consciousness, decreased heart rate and respiratory depression. There is no antidote to counteract the effect of ITB. One of the few options is to collect cerebrospinal fluid in order to influence pharmacokinetics (usually 20 ml cerebrospinal fluid in a child >25 kg).

Causes of overdosing are using the wrong concentration when refilling a baclofen pump or wrong programming of the daily dosage. Therefore, the filling protocol should be very strict and double-checking of the dose is mandatory in order to prevent a devastating overdose or withdrawal syndrome. It is important to note that intrathecal baclofen concentration can be assessed using high-performance liquid chromatography (HPLC) (Albright et al. 2007).

Conclusions

The evidence for intrathecal baclofen to improve the level of functioning in dyskinetic CP is currently weak. Clear effects are reported at the body function and structure level (e.g. dystonia). Effects at the activity level (e.g. mobility, communication) and participation (e.g. school attendance) are less clear. Randomised controlled trials are necessary in order to support the use of ITB in dyskinetic CP. On the other hand, currently there is a lack of other effective treatment options for these severely affected patients.

References

Albright AL, Cervi A, Singletary J. 1991. Intrathecal baclofen for spasticity in cerebral palsy. *JAMA* 265(11):1418–1422.

Albright AL, Barry MJ, Shafton DH, Ferson SS. 2001. Intrathecal baclofen for generalized dystonia. *Dev Med Child Neurol* 43(10):652–657.

Albright AL, Thompson K, Carlos S, Minnigh MB. 2007. Cerebrospinal fluid baclofen concentrations in patients undergoing continuous intrathecal baclofen therapy. *Dev Med Child Neurol* 49(6):423–425.

Bonouvrie LA, van Schie PE, Becher JG, van Ouwerkerk WJ, Reeuwijk A, Jeroen Vermeulen R. 2011. Effects of intrathecal baclofen on daily care in children with secondary generalized dystonia: a pilot study. *Eur J Paediatr Neurol* 15(6):539–543.

Bonouvrie LA, Becher JG, Vles JS, Boeschoten K, Soudant D, de Groot V, van Ouwerkerk WJ, Strijers R, Foncke E, Geytenbeek J, van de Ven PM, Teernstra O, Vermeulen RJ. 2013. Intrathecal baclofen treatment in dystonic cerebral palsy: a randomized clinical trial – the IDYS trial. *BMC Pediatr* 13:175.

Boster AL, Adair RL, Gooch JL, Nelson ME, Toomer A, Urquidez J, Saulino M. 2016. Best practices for intrathecal baclofen therapy: dosing and long-term management. *Neuromodulation* 19(6):623–631.

Chen L, Chan SC, Yung WH. 2002. Rotational behavior and electrophysiological effects induced by GABA(B) receptor activation in rat globus pallidus. *Neuroscience* 114(2):417–425.

Cruikshank M, Eunson P. 2007. Intravenous diazepam infusion in the management of planned intrathecal baclofen withdrawal. *Dev Med Child Neurol* 49(8):626–628.

de Louw AJ, de Vente J, Steinbusch HP, Steinbusch HW, Troost J, Vles JS. 2002. Baclofen inhibits ANP-mediated cyclic GMP synthesis in the rat cervical spinal cord. *Neurosci Lett* 321(1–2):120–122.

Dvorak EM, McGuire JR, Nelson ME. 2010. Incidence and identification of intrathecal baclofen catheter malfunction. *PM R* 2(8):751–756.

Eliasson AC, Krumlinde-Sundholm L, Rosblad B, Beckung E, Arner M, Ohrvall AM, Rosenbaum P. 2006. The manual ability classification system (MACS) for children with cerebral palsy: scale development and evidence of validity and reliability. *Dev Med Child Neurol* 48(7):549–554.

Groenendaal F, van der Grond J, de Vries LS. 2004. Cerebral metabolism in severe neonatal hyperbilirubinemia. *Pediatrics* 114(1):291–294.

Hidecker MJ, Paneth N, Rosenbaum PL, Kent RD, Lillie J, Eulenberg JB, Chester K Jr, Johnson B, Michalsen L, Evatt M, Taylor K. 2011. Developing and validating the communication function classification system for individuals with cerebral palsy. *Dev Med Child Neurol* 53(8):704–710.

Himmelmann K, Uvebrant P. 2014. The panorama of cerebral palsy in Sweden: XI. Changing patterns in the birth-year period 2003–2006. *Acta Paediatr* 103(6):618–624.

Himmelmann K, Hagberg G, Wiklund LM, Eek MN, Uvebrant P. 2007. Dyskinetic cerebral palsy: a population-based study of children born between 1991 and 1998. *Dev Med Child Neurol* 49(4):246–251.

Hoving MA, van Kranen-Mastenbroek VH, van Raak EP, Spincemaille GH, Hardy EL, Vles JS, Dutch Study Group on Child Spasticity. 2006. Placebo controlled utility and feasibility study of the H-reflex and flexor reflex in spastic children treated with intrathecal baclofen. *Clin Neurophysiol* 117(7):1508–1517.

Hoving MA, van Raak EP, Spincemaille GH, Palmans LJ, Sleypen FA, Vles JS, Dutch Study Group on Child Spasticity. 2007. Intrathecal baclofen in children with spastic cerebral palsy: a double-blind, randomized, placebo-controlled, dose-finding study. *Dev Med Child Neurol* 49(9):654–659.

Hoving MA, Evers SM, Ament AJ, van Raak EP, Vles JS, Dutch Study Group on Child Spasticity. 2008. Intrathecal baclofen therapy in children with intractable spastic cerebral palsy: a cost-effectiveness analysis. *Dev Med Child Neurol* 50(6):450–455.

Howard J, Soo B, Graham HK, Boyd RN, Reid S, Lanigan A, Wolfe R, Reddihough DS. 2005. Cerebral palsy in Victoria: motor types, topography and gross motor function. *J Paediatr Child Health* 41(9–10):479–483.

Ikeda H, Kotani A, Koshikawa N, Cools AR. 2010. Differential role of GABAA and GABAB receptors in two distinct output stations of the rat striatum: studies on the substantia nigra pars reticulata and the globus pallidus. *Neuroscience* 167(1):31–39.

Krageloh-Mann I, Horber V. 2007. The role of magnetic resonance imaging in furthering understanding of the pathogenesis of cerebral palsy. *Dev Med Child Neurol* 49(12):948.

Krageloh-Mann I, Helber A, Mader I, Staudt M, Wolff M, Groenendaal F, DeVries L. 2002. Bilateral lesions of thalamus and basal ganglia: origin and outcome. *Dev Med Child Neurol* 44(7):477–484.

Macdonell RA, Talalla A, Swash M, Grundy D. 1989. Intrathecal baclofen and the H-reflex. *J Neurol Neurosurg Psychiatry* 52(9):1110–1112.

McDonald AD. 1963. Cerebral palsy in children of very low birth weight. *Arch Dis Child* 38:579–588.

Monbaliu E, Ortibus E, Roelens F, Desloovere K, Deklerck J, Prinzie P, de Cock P, Feys H. 2010. Rating scales for dystonia in cerebral palsy: reliability and validity. *Dev Med Child Neurol* 52(6):570–575.

Monbaliu E, Ortibus E, De Cat J, Dan B, Heyrman L, Prinzie P, De Cock P, Feys H. 2012. The dyskinesia impairment scale: a new instrument to measure dystonia and choreoathetosis in dyskinetic cerebral palsy. *Dev Med Child Neurol* 54(3):278–283.

Motta F, Stignani C, Antonello CE. 2008. Effect of intrathecal baclofen on dystonia in children with cerebral palsy and the use of functional scales. *J Pediatr Orthop* 28(2):213–217.

Palisano RJ, Hanna SE, Rosenbaum PL, Russell DJ, Walter SD, Wood EP, Raina PS, Galuppi BE. 2000. Validation of a model of gross motor function for children with cerebral palsy. *Phys Ther* 80(10):974–985.

Pin TW, McCartney L, Lewis J, Waugh MC. 2011. Use of intrathecal baclofen therapy in ambulant children and adolescents with spasticity and dystonia of cerebral origin: a systematic review. *Dev Med Child Neurol* 53(10):885–895.

Sanger TD, Delgado MR, Gaebler-Spira D, Hallett M, Mink JW, Task Force on Childhood Motor Disorders. 2003. Classification and definition of disorders causing hypertonia in childhood. *Pediatrics* 111(1):e89–97.

Saulino M, Anderson DJ, Doble J, Farid R, Gul F, Konrad P, Boster AL. 2016. Best practices for intrathecal baclofen therapy: troubleshooting. *Neuromodulation* 19(6):632–641.

Sellier E, Platt MJ, Andersen GL, Krageloh-Mann I, De La Cruz J, Cans C, Surveillance of Cerebral Palsy Network. 2016. Decreasing prevalence in cerebral palsy: a multi-site European population-based study, 1980 to 2003. *Dev Med Child Neurol* 58(1):85–92.

Stokic DS, Yablon SA, Hayes A, Vesovic-Potic V, Olivier J. 2006. Dose-response relationship between the H-reflex and continuous intrathecal baclofen administration for management of spasticity. *Clin Neurophysiol* 117(6):1283–1289.

Ward A, Hayden S, Dexter M, Scheinberg A. 2009. Continuous intrathecal baclofen for children with spasticity and/or dystonia: goal attainment and complications associated with treatment. *J Paediatr Child Health* 45(12):720–726.

Wright FV, Rosenbaum PL, Goldsmith CH, Law M, Fehlings DL. 2008. How do changes in body functions and structures, activity, and participation relate in children with cerebral palsy? *Dev Med Child Neurol* 50(4):283–289.

Wu YW, Kuzniewicz MW, Wickremasinghe AC, Walsh EM, Wi S, McCulloch CE, Newman TB. 2015. Risk for cerebral palsy in infants with total serum bilirubin levels at or above the exchange transfusion threshold: a population-based study. *JAMA Pediatr* 169(3):239–246.

Chapter 47

Deep Brain Stimulation for the Treatment of Paediatric Dystonia

Laura Cif and Philippe Coubes

Dystonia is the most frequent movement disorder in paediatric populations. According to the recently revised classification, dystonia is classified along two axes: clinical characteristics, including age of onset, body distribution, temporal pattern and associated features; and aetiology, which includes nervous system pathology and inheritance (Albanese et al. 2013). In children, dystonia has many diverse aetiologies; the underlying pathobiology as well as related phenotypes are heterogeneous and complex (Mink 2013). Unlike dystonia in adults, which most frequently remains focal or spreads only to neighbouring muscle groups, childhood-onset dystonia often generalises, progressively involving an increasing number of body parts and highly impacting the evolving functional capacities at various developmental stages; furthermore, it may be combined with associated neurological and systemic signs and symptoms, rendering assessment and prognosis challenging. Several treatment options of childhood dystonia are available and include oral pharmaceutical agents, botulinum toxin injections and deep brain stimulation (DBS) (Mink 2013). DBS in dystonia followed ablative procedures and DBS for Parkinson's disease and essential tremor, and it was initiated in paediatric dystonia in 1999 (Coubes et al. 1999). DBS is a symptomatic therapy addressed to improve a spectrum of symptoms, from moderate to highly impairing muscle spasms or involuntary movements, abnormal postures, associated pain, respiratory distress or swallowing difficulties, as well as additional movement disorders like tremor or myoclonic jerks. Under the assumption that surgery is optimally performed to reach the intended anatomical target, therapeutical response depends on aetiology, the distribution and type of dystonia, associated symptoms, morphological integrity of the motor network and DBS settings, aspects we will discuss in the current chapter.

Current Indications and Patient Selection Criteria

One of the major limitation of DBS addressed for treating dystonia in both children and adults is the lack of validated selection criteria like response to medication as in Parkinson's disease or quantified severity criteria. Reduction in quality of life (QoL) and disability non-responsive to medical treatment were proposed as the main factors guiding the decision to consider DBS, independently of age (Moro et al. 2013). The prevalence of phasic components of dystonia, short disease duration, absence of skeletal deformities, DYT1 gene mutations in isolated dystonia and no associated weakness and spasticity in acquired forms were all regularly reported as being good prognostic indications (Coubes et al. 2004; Alterman & Tagliati 2007; Vasques et al. 2009). The response to treatment seems to decline with the proportion of life lived with dystonia in both primary and secondary paediatric dystonia – one further argument to offer the therapy early (Lumsden et al. 2013a). Therefore, surgery should not be delayed when disability and QoL are impaired to the extent that justifies the surgical risk (Moro et al. 2013).

DBS Management

DBS Target

Several concurrent targets are proposed for DBS administration while treating dystonia, but so far the best evidence-based established DBS target is the sensorimotor posteroventral globus pallidus internus (GPi) (Kupsch et al. 2006). The subthalamic nucleus (STN) and several motor thalamic nuclei are targeted mainly when the GPi is structurally impaired by the disease process (Chakraborti et al. 2013), to avoid side-effects related to GPi DBS (Ostrem et al. 2011), but also to treat associated tremor or myoclonus (Gruber et al. 2010).

DBS Settings

There is no consensus regarding the optimal settings for treating dystonia because systematic evaluations of varying stimulus parameters have not been conducted (Alterman & Tagliati 2007). Evidence-based recommendations and guidelines are not available for therapy initiation and adjustment for the treatment of dystonia in children and settings do not differ from those used in adult dystonia. However, a systematic approach to optimise stimulation parameters is highly recommended (Kupsch et al. 2011). Postoperative programming may begin the day after connection of the electrodes with the implantable pulse generators (IPGs), but also a few weeks later in order to overcome potential improvement related to the lead insertion lesional effect. High-frequency stimulation (frequency >100 Hz) is most frequently reported as efficient; however, lower frequencies (60 Hz) have been reported also to improve dystonic features (Alterman & Tagliati 2007; Marks et al. 2011). A frequency of 130 Hz, monopolar or bipolar stimulation, with various combinations of amplitudes and narrower pulse widths (PWs; 60–210 μsec) have been used more commonly, but wider PWs may provide similar efficacy in treating dystonia (Coubes et al. 2004).

Therapeutical Outcome

Isolated Dystonia

While the application of DBS in adults continues to expand, paediatric indications for DBS have been more limited (DiFrancesco et al. 2012). Although there is now Level A evidence that pallidal DBS is effective in treating adult patients with isolated generalised, segmental and cervical dystonia, prospective, controlled studies reporting on DBS in paediatric isolated and acquired dystonia are not available. Well-documented retrospective studies in paediatric dystonia maintain full interest since they can add valuable information to the currently limited available experience. Cumulative data point towards a lasting efficacy of GPi DBS mainly in isolated dystonia (Cif et al. 2010), frequently more than 50–60 per cent improvement in motor scores in both generalised and segmental dystonias, reaching sometimes up to 80–90 per cent improvement (Coubes et al. 2000). In isolated forms of dystonia, the initial clinical outcome was reported to be slightly superior in children than in adults (Coubes et al. 2004), possibly related to shorter disease duration in the childhood dystonia groups. DBS outcome has been reported to be superior in DYT1 dystonia related to single mutations in the TOR1A gene compared to DYT6 dystonia related to THAP1 gene mutations; however, very few data are available for children. Anecdotal reports indicate that the thalamic ventral lateral anterior nucleus may be a more successful DBS alternative in DYT6 dystonia (Mure et al. 2014). Similar results to that obtained in DYT1 dystonia are reported in myoclonus-dystonia related to *SGCE* gene mutations in both children and adults (Cif et al. 2004; Gruber et al. 2010).

Acquired and Degenerative Dystonia

The response to DBS is highly variable in acquired and degenerative dystonia. Limited responses are often related to associated symptoms (spasticity and weakness, cerebellar symptoms) and impaired motor network (Lumsden et al. 2013a). However, the DBS-related benefit may be underestimated when considering only impairment-level measures such as the motor (M) and disability sections (D) of the Burke–Fahn–Marsden Dystonia Rating Scale (BFMDRS), which will not capture the full amount of clinical changes, especially those related to care, comfort and quality of life. DBS may offer meaningful changes across multiple domains of functioning, disability and health, even in the absence of significant change in dystonia rating scales, as reported by the patients and families in these groups of secondary dystonia (Gimeno et al. 2012). Indeed, several subgroups from the vast group of acquired and degenerative dystonias deserve further attention.

Dyskinetic (Dystonic) Cerebral Palsy (DCP)

Cerebral palsy is arguably the most common cause of dystonia in childhood (Alterman & Tagliati 2007; Marks et al. 2011). Marks and colleagues reported a mean improvement of 37.8 per cent on the M-BFMDRS in a subgroup of DCP aged under 16 with DBS (Marks et al. 2011), comparable to responses reported by Keen and colleagues in paediatric DCP (Keen et al. 2014). These results are superior to outcomes reported by the only controlled DBS trial in adults with DCP (Vidailhet et al. 2009) and by a meta-analysis on DBS in DCP (Koy et al. 2013), but in line with other data in adults with DCP (Cif 2015). The differences in DBS outcome may be related to differences between populations (extent of brain insult and sequellae, functional reorganisation in the motor network, motor phenotype, age at DBS administration), the modality of assessment or therapy characteristics (site of DBS electrode and DBS settings), sample sizes but also the difficulties in capturing subtle clinical changes while using the available tools (Cif 2015).

Neurodegeneration With Brain Iron Accumulation (NBIA)

NBIA encompasses a genetically and phenotypically heterogeneous expanding group of disorders with the common hallmark of brain iron accumulation. DBS was performed mainly for the most common subtype, pantothenate kinase-associated neurodegeneration (PKAN), related to mutations in the PANK2 gene, since it is frequently associated with severe, generalised forms of dystonia. Castelnau et al. reported on the positive effect of GPi DBS at a mean follow-up of 20.6 months in a group of six patients with PKAN-related dystonia, three of them younger than 18 years at DBS administration (Castelnau et al. 2005). A multicentre retrospective study on 23 subjects (age at operation 23 years) confirmed that dystonia in NBIA benefits from bilateral GPi DBS with a mean M-BFMDRS improvement of 25.7 per cent at 9–15 months postoperatively (Timmermann et al. 2010). Of interest, five out of the six patients from the study by Castelnau and colleagues survived with a maintained clinical and functional benefit ten years after the initial report (personal experience of the authors) in this highly disabling progressive disorder. Multicentre, controlled prospective studies are necessary to get large numbers of cases of this heterogeneous condition and thus be able to better predict the outcome from surgery (Timmermann et al. 2010).

The effect of DBS in other acquired and degenerative dystonias (glutaric aciduria, Lesch–Nyhan syndrome, Mohr–Tranebjaerg syndrome) in children was only occasionally reported, with highly variable results. Children with secondary dystonia should continue to be offered DBS, but goals and expectations should expect a less dramatic improvement than in primary dystonia (Lumsden et al. 2013a).

Status Dystonicus

Children with both isolated or acquired dystonia may experience acute deterioration of their condition, termed 'status dystonicus', defined as 'generalized, intense and potentially fatal exacerbation of muscle contractions'. These acute episodes represent the most severe state of worsening dystonia and require prompt medical or surgical care. Early recognition may potentially facilitate intervention and prevent progression (Lumsden et al. 2013b). Several case reports of acquired, degenerative as well as of isolated dystonia, including the very first child treated with GPi DBS for dystonia (Coubes et al. 1999), presented with this condition at the time of DBS surgery (Castelnau et al. 2005). Fasano and colleagues reported on DBS efficiency in reverting the condition in 33.7 per cent of episodes compared to 10.1 per cent for the best medical management in a population of 15 patients with status dystonicus (Fasano et al. 2012).

Other Target Symptoms for DBS in Children With Dystonia

Pain is often concurrent with severe dystonic spasms. It has been reported frequently that DBS, early after initiation, alleviates painful spasms independently of the underlying aetiology of dystonia (Coubes et al. 1999, 2000; Koy et al. 2013). Impaired swallowing can sometimes be improved by GPi DBS with recovery of oral feeding in children with dystonia who had an exclusive percutaneous enteral gastrostomy feeding (Coubes et al. 1999), as opposed to dysphagia worsened or related to STN DBS in adults with Parkinson's disease (PD). Improvement in verbal communication has been reported less frequently (Castelnau et al. 2005; Keen et al. 2014) than improvement of axial (Zorzi et al. 2005) and appendicular dystonia. Tongue protrusion dystonia was anecdotally reported as being improved by GPi DBS in adults. It can occur also in children with PKAN, DCP and other forms of dystonia, and it is a symptom difficult to treat (Zorzi et al. 2005).

Recovery of postural abnormalities and walking impairment can be frequently achieved in isolated primary dystonias (Coubes et al. 1999, 2004; Castelnau et al. 2005; Zorzi et al. 2005) but more rarely in acquired dystonias (Coubes et al. 2000). Comfort related to sitting tolerance and ability to attend school and other leisure activities may be realistic objectives that can be reached, as captured by the Canadian Occupational Performance Measure (COPM) and Goal Attainment Scaling (GAS) (Gimeno et al. 2012). Fixed dystonic postures (Coubes et al. 1999; Zorzi et al. 2005), isolated tonic components involving the limbs, as well as decreased muscle tone will negatively impact DBS outcome.

Staged DBS

Multiple electrodes in the GPi have been proposed to address incomplete therapeutical effects and symptom progression under DBS (likely a manifestation of disease progression, DBS-induced plasticity changes in the basal ganglia-thalamocortical circuits involved in dystonia, or both) in patients with primary dystonia who initially improved with DBS but deteriorated later, and as a rescue therapy (Cif et al. 2010, 2012). These important issues should be clearly discussed with the patient, family and caregivers at the time of initial DBS indication.

Combined DBS to distinct targets, such as GPi and the motor nuclei of the thalamus was used to treat myoclonus features in myoclonus-dystonia (Gruber et al. 2010) and suggested to better address altered motor networks in acquired dystonia (Gonzalez et al. 2015).

Discussion

DBS is now a recognised treatment in childhood primary and secondary dystonias. However, the response to DBS is highly variable and depends on several factors, as previously described. One aspect that deserves to be highlighted is that frequently symptoms targeted by DBS in paediatric dystonia remain progressive and fluctuating, and also during follow-up with DBS therapy, in both primary and secondary dystonia. The phenomenology of dystonic symptoms upon DBS discontinuation varies highly from one patient to another, from no clinical worsening for days or even months, to immediate recurrence or even rebound of severe dystonic symptoms (Cif et al. 2010).

DBS mechanisms of action are not fully understood. However, there are now arguments in favour of alteration of the main physiological parameters underlying dystonia pathophysiology: decreased inhibition and excessive plasticity. The time-course of the different physiological changes is not identical, with intracortical inhibition normalising in parallel with the clinical changes, while excessive plasticity changes faster after DBS initiation, to normalise at the time of the clinical steady state (Ruge et al. 2011b). It has been documented that in the long term, LTP-like plasticity will be further altered by DBS to reach a level, after years of continuous DBS, inferior to that measured in healthy controls (Ruge et al. 2011a). DBS-induced alterations of plasticity seem to be correlated with the level of DBS administered: the higher the levels of energy delivered, the more profoundly the LTP-like plasticity decreases, resembling measures in naïve PD patients. The amount of residual plasticity under DBS was correlated with the degree of clinical worsening at DBS discontinuation (Cif et al. 2013).

It has been reported that pallidal stimulation may induce bradykinetic symptoms or parkinsonism in patients who receive effective stimulation for dystonia (Schrader et al. 2011). This has also been identified in paediatric dystonia under DBS. Consequently, alternative targets such as the STN were proposed for DBS; however, there are scant comparative data on the efficacy of STN DBS in dystonia, especially in the long term. The role of the site of therapy administration as well as the way the therapy is delivered to a given target should be taken into consideration when discussing the side-effects of the therapy. Long-term effects of alternative targets such as STN and thalamic nuclei are not yet sufficiently available. DBS is a lifelong therapy since physiological changes induced by prolonged, continuous DBS seem to be reversible at DBS discontinuation (Ruge et al. 2014).

The most challenging questions remain the following: in whom will the DBS benefit/risk ratio favour in the long term, especially in the secondary static and progressive groups of dystonia? And which would be the best and most physiological way to administer DBS, in order to maintain in the long term the reacquired physiological equilibrium state (Ruge et al. 2014)?

The way the therapy is administered in a given target is critical. Careful management of the therapy with the lowest efficient doses should be proposed since the pathological but also the physiological background could be altered by DBS.

DBS should be considered early in the management of childhood-onset dystonia compared to adult-onset dystonia, given the propensity of early-onset dystonia to worsen within this vulnerable age window, and the lack of comparable efficient medical therapies. While DBS has been considered as the last remedy in the therapeutical arsenal of dystonia, cumulative data point towards a better therapeutical outcome when DBS is addressed early in the management of progressive childhood dystonias.

Remarkably, clinical outcome of DBS in a crossover trial for primary generalised dystonia was greater than the effect of high-dosage trihexyphenidyl, the most efficient treatment of dystonia (Kupsch et al. 2011). Complementary physical and occupational therapies, as well as speech therapy, are useful in optimising motor function and enhancing communication skills.

DBS surgery is well tolerated with limited surgical, hardware and therapy-related adverse events. The most frequent hardware-related complications are infection/skin erosion and extension cable fractures. The size of rechargeable batteries and their prolonged life span and the limited rate of complications (transient recharging problems as the most common complication) render them more suitable for DBS therapy in children (Kaminska et al. 2012).

Conclusions

DBS is a recognised therapy in childhood dystonia, with objectives depending on the type of dystonia to be treated. The response of childhood dystonia to DBS therapy varies according especially to aetiology, phenotype and underlying physiology, but also within the same patient group. DBS efficacy is superior in isolated dystonia when compared to acquired and degenerative dystonias. Delivering DBS therapy to treat dystonia in children requires a multidisciplinary team to select adequate candidates, identify reasonable target symptoms, perform the procedure, optimise DBS administration, support the patients and families over the changing life and cope with complications related to therapy and devices. Treating dystonia earlier with lower, efficient doses in paediatric populations seems to have a better impact on the long-term outcome. Considering the economic burden of complementary therapeutical approaches in childhood dystonia, DBS can represent a reasonable therapeutical approach when candidates are well selected and requirements related to selection criteria are fulfilled.

References

Albanese A, Bhatia K, Bressman SB, Delong MR, Fahn S, Fung VS, Hallett M, Jankovic J, Jinnah HA, Klein C, Lang AE, Mink JW, Teller JK. 2013. Phenomenology and classification of dystonia: a consensus update. *Mov Disord* 28(7):863–873.

Alterman RL, Tagliati M. 2007. Deep brain stimulation for torsion dystonia in children. *Childs Nerv Syst* 23(9):1033–1040.

Castelnau P, Cif L, Valente EM, Vayssiere N, Hemm S, Gannau A, Digiorgio A, Coubes P. 2005. Pallidal stimulation improves pantothenate kinase-associated neurodegeneration. *Ann Neurol* 57(5):738–741.

Chakraborti S, Hasegawa H, Lumsden DE, Ali W, Kaminska M, Lin JP, Ashkan K. 2013. Bilateral subthalamic nucleus deep brain stimulation for refractory total body dystonia secondary to metabolic autopallidotomy in a 4-year-old boy with infantile methylmalonic acidemia: case report. *J Neurosurg Pediatr* 12(4):374–379.

Cif L. 2015. Deep brain stimulation in dystonic cerebral palsy: for whom and for what? *Eur J Neurol* 22(3):423–425.

Cif L, Valente EM, Hemm S, Coubes C, Vayssiere N, Serrat S, Di Giorgio A, Coubes P. 2004. Deep brain stimulation in myoclonus-dystonia syndrome. *Mov Disord* 19(6):724–727.

Cif L, Vasques X, Gonzalez V, Ravel P, Biolsi B, Collod-Beroud G, Tuffery-Giraud S, Elfertit H, Claustres M, Coubes P. 2010. Long-term follow-up of DYT1 dystonia patients treated by deep brain stimulation: an open-label study. *Mov Disord* 25(3):289–299.

Cif L, Gonzalez-Martinez V, Vasques X, Corlobe A, Moura AM, Bonafe A, Coubes P. 2012. Staged implantation of multiple electrodes in the internal globus pallidus in the treatment of primary generalized dystonia. *J Neurosurg* 116(5):1144–1152.

Cif L, Ruge D, Gonzalez V, Limousin P, Vasques X, Hariz MI, Rothwell J, Coubes P. 2013. The influence of deep brain stimulation intensity and duration on symptoms evolution in an OFF stimulation dystonia study. *Brain Stimul* 6(4):500–505.

Coubes P, Echenne B, Roubertie A, Vayssiere N, Tuffery S, Humbertclaude V, Cambonie G, Claustres M, Frerebeau P. 1999. Treatment of early-onset generalized dystonia by chronic bilateral stimulation of the internal globus pallidus: apropos of a case. *Neurochirurgie* 45(2):139–144.

Coubes P, Roubertie A, Vayssiere N, Hemm S, Echenne B. 2000. Treatment of DYT1-generalised dystonia by stimulation of the internal globus pallidus. *Lancet* 355(9222):2220–2221.

Coubes P, Cif L, El Fertit H, Hemm S, Vayssiere N, Serrat S, Picot MC, Tuffery S, Claustres M, Echenne B, Frerebeau P. 2004. Electrical stimulation of the globus pallidus internus in patients with primary generalized dystonia: long-term results. *J Neurosurg* 101(2):189–194.

DiFrancesco MF, Halpern CH, Hurtig HH, Baltuch GH, Heuer GG. 2012. Pediatric indications for deep brain stimulation. *Childs Nerv Syst* 28(10):1701–1714.

Fasano A, Ricciardi L, Bentivoglio AR, Canavese C, Zorzi G, Petrovic I, Kresojevic N, Kostic VS, Svetel M, Kovacs N, Balas I, Roubertie A, Mishra D, Mariotti P, Temudo T, Nardocci N. 2012. Status dystonicus: predictors of outcome and progression patterns of underlying disease. *Mov Disord* 27(6):783–788.

Gimeno H, Tustin K, Selway R, Lin JP. 2012. Beyond the Burke–Fahn–Marsden Dystonia Rating Scale: deep brain stimulation in childhood secondary dystonia. *Eur J Paediatr Neurol* 16(5):501–508.

Gonzalez V, Le Bars E, Cif L, van Dokkum LE, Laffont I, Bonafe A, Menjot de Champfleur N, Zanca M, Coubes P. 2015. The reorganization of motor network in hemidystonia from the perspective of deep brain stimulation. *Brain Imaging Behav* 9(2):223–235.

Gruber D, Kuhn AA, Schoenecker T, Kivi A, Trottenberg T, Hoffmann KT, Gharabaghi A, Kopp UA, Schneider GH, Klein C, Asmus F, Kupsch A. 2010. Pallidal and thalamic deep brain stimulation in myoclonus-dystonia. *Mov Disord* 25(11):1733–1743.

Kaminska M, Lumsden DE, Ashkan K, Malik I, Selway R, Lin JP. 2012. Rechargeable deep brain stimulators in the management of paediatric dystonia: well tolerated with a low complication rate. *Stereotact Funct Neurosurg* 90(4):233–239.

Keen JR, Przekop A, Olaya JE, Zouros A, Hsu FP. 2014. Deep brain stimulation for the treatment of childhood dystonic cerebral palsy. *J Neurosurg Pediatr* 14(6):585–593.

Koy A, Hellmich M, Pauls KA, Marks W, Lin JP, Fricke O, Timmermann L. 2013. Effects of deep brain stimulation in dyskinetic cerebral palsy: a meta-analysis. *Mov Disord* 28(5):647–654.

Kupsch A, Benecke R, Muller J, Trottenberg T, Schneider GH, Poewe W, Eisner W, Wolters A, Muller JU, Deuschl G, Pinsker MO, Skogseid IM, Roeste GK, Vollmer-Haase J, Brentrup A, Krause M, Tronnier V, Schnitzler A, Voges J, Nikkhah G,Vesper J, Naumann M, Volkmann J, Deep-Brain Stimulation for Dystonia Study Group. 2006. Pallidal deep-brain stimulation in primary generalized or segmental dystonia. *N Engl J Med* 355(19):1978–1990.

Kupsch A, Tagliati M, Vidailhet M, Aziz T, Krack P, Moro E, Krauss JK. 2011. Early postoperative management of DBS in dystonia: programming, response to stimulation, adverse events, medication changes, evaluations, and troubleshooting. *Mov Disord* 26(Suppl. 1):S37–S53.

Lumsden DE, Kaminska M, Gimeno H, Tustin K, Baker L, Perides S, Ashkan K, Selway R, Lin JP. 2013a. Proportion of life lived with dystonia inversely correlates with response to pallidal deep brain stimulation in both primary and secondary childhood dystonia. *Dev Med Child Neurol* 55(6):567–574.

Lumsden DE, Lundy C, Fairhurst C, Lin JP. 2013b. Dystonia severity action plan: a simple grading system for medical severity of status dystonicus and life-threatening dystonia. *Dev Med Child Neurol* 55(7):671–672.

Marks WA, Honeycutt J, Acosta F, Jr, Reed M, Bailey L, Pomykal A, Mercer M. 2011. Dystonia due to cerebral palsy responds to deep brain stimulation of the globus pallidus internus. *Mov Disord* 26(9):1748–1751.

Mink JW. 2013. Special concerns in defining, studying, and treating dystonia in children. *Mov Disord* 28(7):921–925.

Moro E, Gross RE, Krauss JK. 2013. What's new in surgical treatment for dystonia? *Mov Disord* 28(7):1013–1020.

Mure H, Morigaki R, Koizumi H, Okita S, Kawarai T, Miyamoto R, Kaji R, Nagahiro S, Goto S. 2014. Deep brain stimulation of the thalamic ventral lateral anterior nucleus for DYT6 dystonia. *Stereotact Funct Neurosurg* 92(6):393–396.

Ostrem JL, Racine CA, Glass GA, Grace JK, Volz MM, Heath SL, Starr PA. 2011. Subthalamic nucleus deep brain stimulation in primary cervical dystonia. *Neurology* 76(10):870–878.

Ruge D, Cif L, Limousin P, Gonzalez V, Vasques X, Hariz MI, Coubes P, Rothwell JC. 2011a. Shaping reversibility? Long-term deep brain stimulation in dystonia – the relationship between effects on electrophysiology and clinical symptoms. *Brain* 134(Pt 7):2106–2115.

Ruge D, Tisch S, Hariz MI, Zrinzo L, Bhatia KP, Quinn NP, Jahanshahi M, Limousin P, Rothwell JC. 2011b. Deep brain stimulation effects in dystonia: time course of electrophysiological changes in early treatment. *Mov Disord* 26(10):1913–1921.

Ruge D, Cif L, Limousin P, Gonzalez V, Vasques X, Coubes P, Rothwell JC. 2014. Long term deep brain stimulation withdrawal: clinical stability despite electrophysiological instability. *J Neurol Sci* 342(1–2):197–199.

Schrader C, Capelle HH, Kinfe TM, Blahak C, Bazner H, Lutjens G, Dressler D, Krauss JK. 2011. GPi-DBS may induce a hypokinetic gait disorder with freezing of gait in patients with dystonia. *Neurology* 77(5):483–488.

Timmermann L, Pauls KA, Wieland K, Jech R, Kurlemann G, Sharma N, Gill SS, Haenggeli CA, Hayflick SJ, Hogarth P, Leenders KL, Limousin P, Malanga CJ, Moro E, Ostrem JL, Revilla FJ, Santens P, Schnitzler A, Tisch S, Valldeoriola F, Vesper J, Volkmann J, Woitalla D, Peker S. 2010. Dystonia in neurodegeneration with brain iron accumulation: outcome of bilateral pallidal stimulation. *Brain* 133(Pt 3):701–712.

Vasques X, Cif L, Gonzalez V, Nicholson C, Coubes P. 2009. Factors predicting improvement in primary generalized dystonia treated by pallidal deep brain stimulation. *Mov Disord* 24(6):846–853.

Vidailhet M, Yelnik J, Lagrange C, Fraix V, Grabli D, Thobois S, Burbaud P, Welter ML, Xie-Brustolin J, Braga MC, Ardouin C, Czernecki V, Klinger H, Chabardes S, Seigneuret E, Mertens P, Cuny E, Navarro S, Cornu P, Benabid AL, Le Bas JF, Dormont D, Hermier M, Dujardin K, Blond S, Krystkowiak P, Destee A, Bardinet E, Agid Y, Krack P, Broussolle E, Pollak P, French SPIDY-2 Study Group. 2009. Bilateral pallidal deep brain stimulation for the treatment of patients with dystonia-choreoathetosis cerebral palsy: a prospective pilot study. *Lancet Neurol* 8(8):709–717.

Zorzi G, Marras C, Nardocci N, Franzini A, Chiapparini L, Maccagnano E, Angelini L, Caldiroli D, Broggi G. 2005. Stimulation of the globus pallidus internus for childhood-onset dystonia. *Mov Disord* 20(9):1194–1200.

Chapter 48

Deep Brain Stimulation for Small Children With Dystonia

Keyoumars Ashkan and Jean-Pierre Lin

Neuromodulation with deep brain stimulation (DBS) for childhood dystonia was introduced in the mid-1990s (Coubes et al. 2000). Diagnostic confusion given neuro-inflammatory and genetic causes of dystonia, particularly 'genetic pleiotropy and phenotypic heterogeneity', have primed the introduction of a 'field guide' to understanding movement disorders in children (Silveira-Moriyama & Lin 2015). Diagnostic difficulties also contribute to late referral of children for DBS 'after all other options have been considered' and the relative lack of experience of DBS in young children. Here, we explore the rationale and advantages for earlier referral for DBS in children and current clinical practice barriers along with the neurosurgical challenges to DBS implantation.

General Considerations of Performing Deep Brain Stimulation in Small Children

The Impact of Dystonia in Childhood

Dystonia severely impairs activity and participation in children. A recent large cross-sectional study of 279 children referred for possible DBS or intrathecal baclofen (ITB) pump implantation painted a pessimistic picture for children living with dystonia today (Lin et al. 2014).

Worsening Dystonia With Age in Children

Dystonia in childhood worsened in almost two-thirds of cases, remained static in a further one-third of cases, and less than 8 per cent experienced amelioration. Causes of dystonia in descending order included dystonic cerebral palsy (CP) in 150/279 (53.7 per cent), acquired brain injury in 51/279 (18.2 per cent), heredodegenerative dystonias, mostly neurodegeneration with brain iron accumulation (NBIA) in 29/279 (10.3 per cent), primary dystonia in 30/279 (10.7 per cent) and primary-plus dystonia in 19/279 (6.8 per cent) (Lin et al. 2014).

Whereas about two-thirds of primary, primary-plus and heredogenerative dystonias experience a period of normal development, only one-fifth of non-progressive, secondary dystonias do so, leaving the remaining 80 per cent never experiencing normal development. A period of normal motor development may be considered 'money in the bank' or 'archived patterns of movement and motor learning' which may be released or become available after neuromodulation of dystonia with DBS.

Risk of Deformity With Dystonia in Children

By the age of five, 50 per cent of children with early-onset secondary dystonia, mostly of CP origin, have musculoskeletal deformities – a figure which rises to 80 per cent by age ten years and to 90 per cent by age 15 years.

Frequency of Adverse Drug Reactions in Children

Adverse drug reactions (ADRs) are common, and by age 15 years most children will have experienced at least one ADR.

Interventional Studies in Childhood Dystonia Fail to Measure What Matters Most

A review of 70 dystonia interventional studies, 46 neurosurgical and 24 pharmacological, by concentrating on impairments, failed to measure what matters most to children: pain, activities of daily living, manual function and sitting (Lumsden et al. 2015b).

How Common is Dystonia in Childhood?

The genetic causes of dystonia are individually rare, though the genetic contribution to causation will inevitably rise with the availability of modern genomic techniques to screen whole exomes. Cerebral palsy is clearly the commonest cause of dystonia in childhood, and it is estimated that 6–14 per cent of children with CP have dystonia.

Abnormal and Normal Imaging in Cerebral Palsy

The finding of normal scans in children with CD may occur in 5–17 per cent of cases and is interesting on two counts. The first challenge is the definition of 'normal scan' and the second challenge is the concept of CP arising as a non-progressive injury to the developing brain. However, the finding of a normal scan highlights the possibility that the underlying motor disorder has a higher likelihood of being dystonic in origin in the 11–17 per cent of CP scans that are normal (Bax et al. 2006).

Spasticity or Dystonia in Children: Role of Tractography and Transcranial Magnetic Stimulation Studies

A common misconception is the automatic assumption that periventricular white matter disorders (PWMD) or periventricular leucomalacia (PVL), so prevalent in CP, must be synonymous with a 'spastic' phenotype. Elegant tractography studies have demonstrated beyond doubt that even severe dilation of the posterior horns of the lateral ventricles can be associated with intact corticospinal tracts viewed with MRI tractography techniques. The same study also demonstrated that the real lesion was not to the 'upper motor neuron' pathways but to the posterior thalamic radiation (Hoon et al. 2002).

Exoneration of the corticospinal tracts as implicated in the motor pathology in CP and many other symptomatic causes of motor dysfunction has been reported using transcranial magnetic stimulation (TMS) to measure central motor conduction times (CMCTs) in children with dystonia being assessed as potential candidates for DBS. The rationale was to exclude cases with absent or prolonged CMCTs from the DBS programme or to allocate these to the ITB pump implantation programme. In the study, 80 per cent of children with abnormal scans had normal CMCTs, including many with severe white matter signal change (McClelland et al. 2011). Conversely, another study directly compared TMS evaluation of CMCT with fractional anisotropy (FA) values in 49 potential candidates for DBS using tract-based spatial statistics (TBSS). This study could find no differences in FA values between children with and without abnormal CMCT, suggesting that neurophysiology techniques of motor assessment are important in detecting functional impairments not currently picked up by detailed imaging (Lumsden et al. 2015c). Dystonia can therefore occur with and without focal or generalised white matter or grey matter lesions. A matter of immediate concern now relates to the true prevalence and incidence of dystonic syndromes, particularly in the CP population, recognition of which would significantly alter management decisions in children.

Registries, Correct Diagnoses, Classifications and Appropriate Referrals

Two issues have hampered the diagnosis of a dystonic motor phenotype in CP: the first is the assumption that dystonia is rare, and the other is that spasticity phenotypes account for over 80 per cent of cases of CP. Until new therapeutic options such as selective dorsal rhizotomy (SDR) or DBS were available, it might have been of only theoretical interest to delineate the motor phenotype. Accordingly, the Surveillance in Cerebral Palsy in Europe registry defines 'dyskinesia' as *dystonia* and/or *choreoathetosis*; however, health professionals classifying cases of CP for the registry were unable to agree between whole-body spasticity and whole-body dyskinesia, indicating the likelihood that cases of dystonia are being overlooked or misclassified (Gainsborough et al. 2008). The advent of the taskforce on the definition and classification of hyperkinetic movements in childhood has added a North American dimension that may confuse the unwary further since 'hypertonus' is defined as either *spasticity*, *dystonia* or *rigidity* (Sanger et al. 2010).

Efficacy of Deep Brain Stimulation in Children

Burke–Fahn–Marsden Dystonia Rating Scale (BFMDRS): Motor Component

Deep brain stimulation may greatly improve the lives of children with primary dystonias, but the percentage change on the BFMDRS motor score are less dramatic in secondary dystonias – approximately 24 per cent in young adults with choreoathetoid CP and children with dystonic CP (Vidailhet et al. 2009; Koy et al. 2012).

Duration of Dystonia, Proportion of Life Lived With Dystonia and Deep Brain Stimulation Efficacy

Duration of dystonia reduces DBS efficacy in primary dystonias (Isaias et al. 2009). A longer duration of dystonia is another plausible explanation for the lower dystonia reduction in secondary dystonia/CP dystonia children as compared with primary dystonias. When duration of dystonia is divided by the age of the child, the *proportion of life lived with dystonia* (PLD) is 0.5 for primary dystonia compared with more than 0.9 for children with CP at the time of DBS implantation (14). These data suggest that DBS should be offered before a child has lived 80 per cent of life with dystonia, necessitating very early referral in children with CP, i.e. between the ages of three and five years.

Globus Pallidus Internus Volume and Deep Brain Stimulation Efficacy

Globus pallidus internus volume correlates with DBS outcome in primary dystonias (Vasques et al. 2009). This may be even more relevant in secondary dystonias in which pallidal volumes may be markedly reduced. Detailed normalised pallidal to whole-brain ratio data are required to fully understand the underlying neuroanatomical markers of success of DBS in children with dystonia.

Improving Activity and Participation With Deep Brain Stimulation in Childhood

Measuring dystonia reduction alone may not reveal the true benefits of DBS in childhood. Other scales are needed to fully evaluate this. The Canadian Occupational Performance Measure (COPM) may reveal functional gains not demonstrated by the BFMDRS-M (Gimeno et al. 2014). This provides a simple scheme for determining functional priorities in childhood dystonias, measuring goal attainment with a *performance* and *satisfaction* score both of which are significantly improved after DBS in children with primary, secondary-static (including CP) and secondary-progressive dystonias: a result maintained two years after DBS surgery (Gimeno et al. 2014). Manual abilities are clearly important functions to assess and may be tracked with the Melbourne Assessment of Upper Limb Function (MAULF) (Gimeno et al. 2013).

Cognitive Function After Deep Brain Stimulation in Children

Cognitive function is maintained or may improve in children with primary dystonias and those with NBIA (Owen et al. 2015).

Technical Considerations of Performing Deep Brain Stimulation in Small Children

Consent

Obtaining informed consent remains an essential issue when operating on paediatric patients. While in most countries, depending on the local laws of consent, parents or the legal guardians of the child are responsible for providing consent, it is important to engage the child where possible. Age-specific literature to explain the rationale, the surgical procedure and what the child can expect after the surgery is an important tool that can help prepare the child for the operation.

Precaution Against Infection

Children, especially those under the age of five years, are more prone to infective complications of surgery. The reasons may include a weaker, less mature immune system and also the increased likelihood of handling the surgical wound. Meticulous surgical technique and reduction in the length of the operative procedure may help in reducing the risks. Presurgical skin disinfection using octenidine hair and body wash the day before surgery may also help here. We also routinely use prophylactic cephalosporins starting at the time of the surgery and continued for a week in all our paediatric DBS patients.

Anaesthetic Considerations

While in adult patients undergoing DBS the opinion is divided over the relative benefits of awake surgery with test stimulation compared to surgery done under general anaesthetic, in paediatric patients the general consensus is in favour of the latter. Compliance and the stress caused to the child precludes awake surgery. Intraoperative physiological monitoring with techniques such as impedance measurement, field potential or micro-electrode recording remain important and are feasible under general anaesthesia (Pinsker et al. 2009). Maintaining the child in the optimal metabolic state while under general anaesthetic may prove challenging, especially in those with inherent disorders of metabolism.

Stereotactic Frame

The majority of DBS centres use a stereotactic frame to help placement of the DBS electrodes. In children between the ages of three and seven, the thickness of the skull must be kept in mind when tightening the screws and hand tightening may prove safer than using a screwdriver. Once the frame is in place particular attention and support need to be given to the child's neck, especially during transfers. In children under the age of three, placement of a stereotactic frame may not be possible and developments in frameless stereotaxy or robotics may ultimately pave the way here.

Shape of the Head

The variation in head shape encountered in children is far greater than that in adults. Plagiocephaly is not uncommon in children and scaphocephaly and brachicephaly are sometimes seen. These may have implications for the placement of the stereotactic frame or positioning of the child's head and warrant careful preoperative planning.

Intracranial Anatomy

Targeting

Given the variation in the head size of the children, indirect surgical targeting based on adult stereotactic atlases is not valid. Direct visualisation of the DBS target is therefore required (Ashkan et al. 2007). In the majority of paediatric patients undergoing DBS, dystonia is the indication and therefore globus pallidus internus (GPi) is the target. Proton density and T2-weighted MRI sequences are particularly useful in defining the internal lamina and therefore distinguishing GPi from the globus pallidus externus. Given the very small size of the target in young children, attention to details during surgery, especially to avoid cerebrospinal fluid (CSF) leak and brain shift, are of utmost importance.

Disease-Related Anatomical Variations

A proportion of paediatric candidates for DBS have dystonias secondary to metabolic conditions that alter brain structure. MRI of the patients with neurodegeneration with brain iron accumulation typically shows the eye-of-the-tiger sign secondary to a signal change in the medial aspect of the GPi. In such patients PET imaging may be useful to identify viable tissue at the site of the target before proceeding to DBS. Further functional imaging, volumetric and tractography correlations are required to determine case-specific prognostic indicators of DBS neuromodulation success in children.

In other patients, such as those with methylmalonic acidaemia, the entire GPi may be destroyed and replaced with CSF. In such patients alternative targets such as the thalamus or the subthalamic nucleus may be used to treat the dystonia (Chakraborti et al. 2013).

Non-Disease-Related Anatomical Variations

Anatomical anomalies such as arachnoid or porencephalic cysts are encountered in paediatric patient groups undergoing DBS. The choice of the trajectory to the target is critical and may have to be inventive to avoid entering such cysts both to circumvent haemorrhagic complications and to prevent CSF leak and brain shift which would then lead to mis-targeting.

Head Growth and Electrode Migration

The child's head continues to grow until at least the age of seven years. Given that the DBS electrode is anchored at the skull, gradual shortening of the electrode with the growth of the head when the operation is done in very young children remains a concern. In practice, however, loss of efficacy of DBS is only seen in a minority of such children and the electrode revision rates are low (Lumsden et al. 2015a). This may partly be due to surgical technique of placing the most distal contact of the DBS electrode at the most ventral part of the GPi. Another explanation may be the development of a CSF-filled tract as the electrode shortens from the target, which then conducts the electricity down the path of least resistance to the target.

Implantable Pulse Generator (IPG) Considerations

Battery Size and Location

In very young children, obtaining sufficient tissue cover for the IPG can be a challenge. Dual-chamber IPGs such as the Kinetra or Activa PC (Medtronic) are often too large to place in an infraclavicular pocket in small children. An abdominal pocket may be more suitable, although in some patients proximity to feeding tubes may increase the risk of infection. Using two single-chamber IPGs such as the Soletra or Activa SC, which are smaller than dual-chamber IPGs, to empower bilateral electrodes and placing each in a separate infraclavicular pocket is an alternative solution. The problem of 'cross talk' when programming the two IPGs located close together may occur, however. The newer generation of smaller IPGs such as the Activa Rechargeable Cell (Medtronic), Brio (Abbott) or Vercise (Boston) are much better suited to the paediatric population and can be placed in an infraclavicular pocket even in very small children (Figure 48.1).

Choice of Rechargeable Versus Non-Rechargeable IPG

Rechargeable IPGs are well tolerated and effective in the paediatric population (Kaminska et al. 2012). They have the advantage of substantially reducing the number of operations required to change the battery throughout the child's life. This is an important consideration both to reduce the risk of infection and also repeated surgery and anaesthetic procedures in often medically challenging patients. The carers are readily able to recharge the battery and in many children it becomes part of their routine and something they can do for themselves as they grow up.

Wound Closure

Meticulous wound closure is critical in reducing the risk of infection. We recommend the use of absorbable sutures, as removing stitches can cause anxiety and discomfort in children. Protective dressing and a head bandage will prevent the child from scratching the wound, which can delay healing and result in infection.

Postoperative Analgesia

Comfort of the child in the postoperative period is critical. A nurse-controlled analgesia system is an efficient means of providing pain control after surgery. Non-steroidal anti-inflammatory drugs are best avoided, given their anti-platelet action.

Lessons from the Early History of Cochlear Implantation in Children

Cochlear implantation for the neuromodulation of deafness, available since 1980 for sensorineural deafness in children, has been shown to relieve disability and improve activity and participation in deaf children. From 1980 to 1995 cochlear implant teams demonstrated that very early implantation under the age of five years and duration of cochlear stimulation of at least

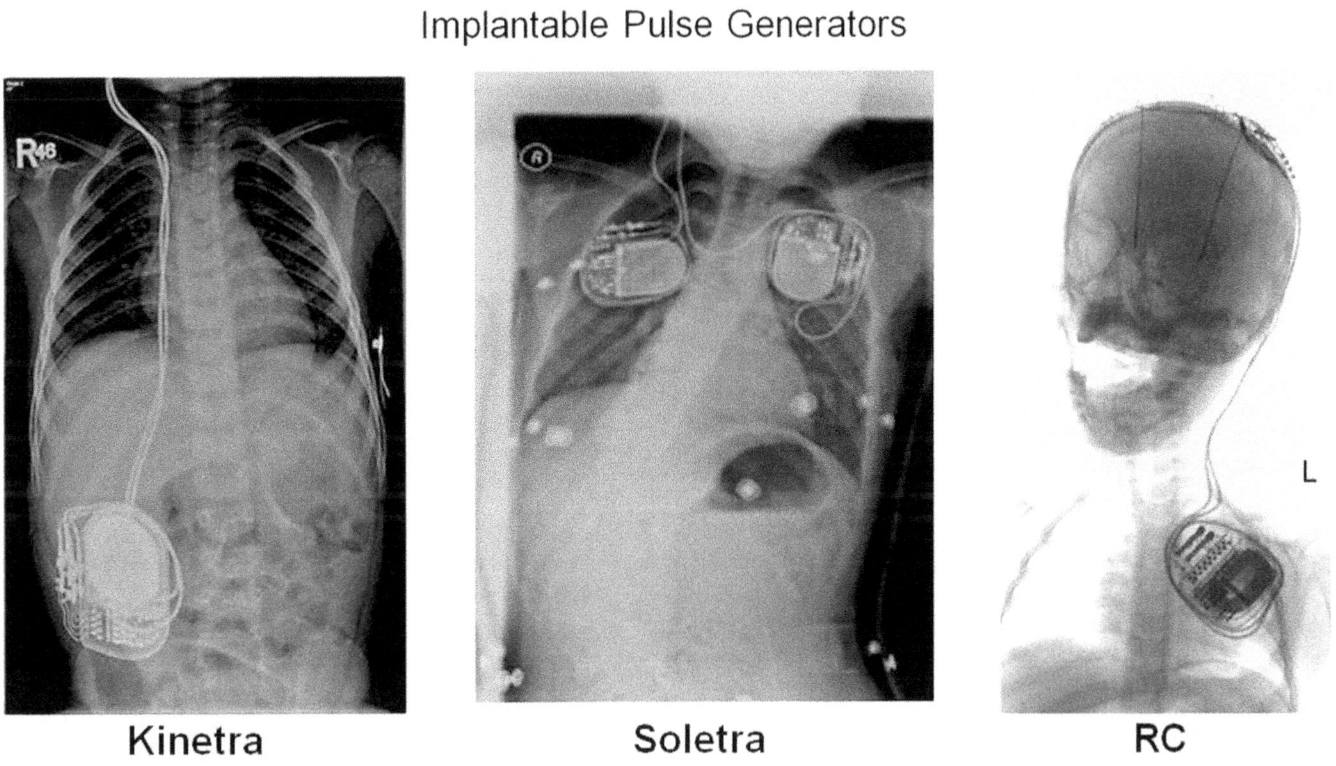

Figure 48.1 Range of implantable pulse generators: (Medtronic) Kinetra dual-channel, Soletra single-channel and the Activa RC rechargeable dual-channel.

four years of neuromodulation produces the best responses, resulting in acquisition of normal language and educational prospects. This is particularly the case in children with congenital or very early-acquired deafness, before language development: i.e. often under one year of age.

The comparison with dystonic CP and other early-acquired dystonias is evident, raising the question of even earlier DBS administration, i.e. by age two years. DBS neuromodulation must confront and explore the same developmental biological questions facing the early cochlear implantation community.

Conclusions

Deep brain stimulation is now recognised as an effective tool for the management of dystonia in small children. More definitive and convincing proof is required to establish the benefits of very early intervention with DBS. This work can only be delivered with experienced multidisciplinary teams using a cross-registration of neurophysiological, neuroimaging and clinical evaluation tools in the context of growth, development and the backdrop of the natural history of the underlying childhood dystonia.

References

Ashkan K, Blomstedt P, Zrinzo L, Tisch S, Yousry T, Limousin-Dowsey P, Hariz MI. 2007. Variability of the subthalamic nucleus: the case for direct MRI guided targeting. *Br J Neurosurg* 21(2):197–200.

Bax M, Tydeman C, Flodmark O. 2006. Clinical and MRI correlates of cerebral palsy: the European Cerebral Palsy Study. *JAMA* 296(13):1602–1608.

Chakraborti S, Hasegawa H, Lumsden DE, Ali W, Kaminska M, Lin JP, Ashkan K. 2013. Bilateral subthalamic nucleus deep brain stimulation for refractory total body dystonia secondary to metabolic autopallidotomy in a 4-year-old boy with infantile methylmalonic acidemia: case report. *J Neurosurg Pediatr* 12(4):374–379.

Coubes P, Roubertie A, Vayssiere N, Hemm S, Echenne B. 2000. Treatment of DYT1-generalised dystonia by stimulation of the internal globus pallidus. *Lancet* 355(9222):2220–2221.

Gainsborough M, Surman G, Maestri G, Colver A, Cans C. 2008. Validity and reliability of the guidelines of the surveillance of cerebral palsy in Europe for the classification of cerebral palsy. *Dev Med Child Neurol* 50(11):828–831.

Gimeno H, Tustin K, Selway R, Lin JP. 2012. Beyond the Burke-Fahn-Marsden Dystonia Rating Scale: deep brain stimulation in childhood secondary dystonia. *Eur J Paediatr Neurol* 16(5):501–508.

Gimeno H, Lumsden D, Gordon A, Tustin K, Ashkan K, Selway R, Lin JP. 2013. Improvement in upper limb function in children with dystonia following deep brain stimulation. *Eur J Paediatr Neurol* 17(4):353–360.

Gimeno H, Tustin K, Lumsden D, Ashkan K, Selway R, Lin JP. 2014. Evaluation of functional goal outcomes using the Canadian Occupational Performance Measure (COPM) following deep brain stimulation (DBS) in childhood dystonia. *Eur J Paediatr Neurol* 18(3):308–316.

Hoon AH, Jr, Lawrie WT, Jr, Melhem ER, Reinhardt EM, Van Zijl PC, Solaiyappan M, Jiang H, Johnston MV, Mori S. 2002. Diffusion tensor imaging of periventricular leukomalacia shows affected sensory cortex white matter pathways. *Neurology* 59(5):752–756.

Isaias IU, Alterman RL, Tagliati M. 2009. Deep brain stimulation for primary generalized dystonia: long-term outcomes. *Arch Neurol* 66(4):465–470.

Kaminska M, Lumsden DE, Ashkan K, Malik I, Selway R, Lin JP. 2012. Rechargeable deep brain stimulators in the management of paediatric dystonia: well tolerated with a low complication rate. *Stereotact Funct Neurosurg* 90(4):233–239.

Koy A, Hellmich M, Pauls KA, Marks W, Lin JP, Fricke O, Timmermann L. 2013. Effects of deep brain stimulation in dyskinetic cerebral palsy: a meta-analysis. *Mov Disord* 28(5):647–654.

Lin JP, Lumsden DE, Gimeno H, Kaminska M. 2014. The impact and prognosis for dystonia in childhood including dystonic cerebral palsy: a clinical and demographic tertiary cohort study. *J Neurol Neurosurg Psychiatry* 85(11):1239–1244.

Lumsden DE, Kaminska M, Gimeno H, Tustin K, Baker L, Perides S, Ashkan K, Selway R, Lin JP. 2013. Proportion of life lived with dystonia inversely correlates with response to pallidal deep brain stimulation in both primary and secondary childhood dystonia. *Dev Med Child Neurol* 55(6):567–574.

Lumsden DE, Ashmore J, Charles-Edwards G, Selway R, Lin JP, Ashkan K. 2015a. Observation and modeling of deep brain stimulation electrode depth in the pallidal target of the developing brain. *World Neurosurg* 83(4):438–446.

Lumsden DE, Gimeno H, Tustin K, Kaminska M, Lin JP. 2015b. Interventional studies in childhood dystonia do not address the concerns of children and their carers. *Eur J Paediatr Neurol* 19(3):327–336.

Lumsden DE, McClelland V, Ashmore J, Charles-Edwards G, Mills K, Lin JP. 2015c. Central motor conduction time and diffusion tensor imaging metrics in children with complex motor disorders. *Clin Neurophysiol* 126(1):140–146.

McClelland V, Mills K, Siddiqui A, Selway R, Lin JP. 2011. Central motor conduction studies and diagnostic magnetic resonance imaging in children with severe primary and secondary dystonia. *Dev Med Child Neurol* 53(8):757–763.

Owen T, Gimeno H, Selway R, Lin JP. 2015. Cognitive function in children with primary dystonia before and after deep brain stimulation. *Eur J Paediatr Neurol* 19(1):48–55.

Pinsker MO, Volkmann J, Falk D, Herzog J, Steigerwald F, Deuschl G, Mehdorn HM. 2009. Deep brain stimulation of the internal globus pallidus in dystonia: target localisation under general anaesthesia. *Acta Neurochir (Wien)* 151(7):751–758.

Sanger TD, Chen D, Fehlings DL, Hallett M, Lang AE, Mink JW, Singer HS, Alter K, Ben-Pazi H, Butler EE, Chen R, Collins A, Dayanidhi S, Forssberg H, Fowler E, Gilbert DL, Gorman SL, Gormley ME, Jr, Jinnah HA, Kornblau B, Krosschell KJ, Lehman RK, MacKinnon C, Malanga CJ, Mesterman R, Michaels MB, Pearson TS, Rose J, Russman BS, Sternad D, Swoboda KJ, Valero-Cuevas F. 2010. Definition and classification of hyperkinetic movements in childhood. *Mov Disord* 25(11):1538–1549.

Silveira-Moriyama L, Lin JP. 2015. A field guide to current advances in paediatric movement disorders. *Curr Opin Neurol* 28(4):437–446.

Vasques X, Cif L, Hess O, Gavarini S, Mennessier G, Coubes P. 2009. Prognostic value of globus pallidus internus volume in primary dystonia treated by deep brain stimulation. *J Neurosurg* 110(2):220–228.

Vidailhet M, Yelnik J, Lagrange C, Fraix V, Grabli D, Thobois S, Burbaud P, Welter ML, Xie-Brustolin J, Braga MC, Ardouin C, Czernecki V, Klinger H, Chabardes S, Seigneuret E, Mertens P, Cuny E, Navarro S, Cornu P, Benabid AL, Le Bas JF, Dormont D, Hermier M, Dujardin K, Blond S, Krystkowiak P, Destee A, Bardinet E, Agid Y, Krack P, Broussolle E, Pollak P, French SPIDY-2 Study Group. 2009. Bilateral pallidal deep brain stimulation for the treatment of patients with dystonia-choreoathetosis cerebral palsy: a prospective pilot study. *Lancet Neurol* 8(8):709–717.

Section VI

Rehabilitation of Dystonia

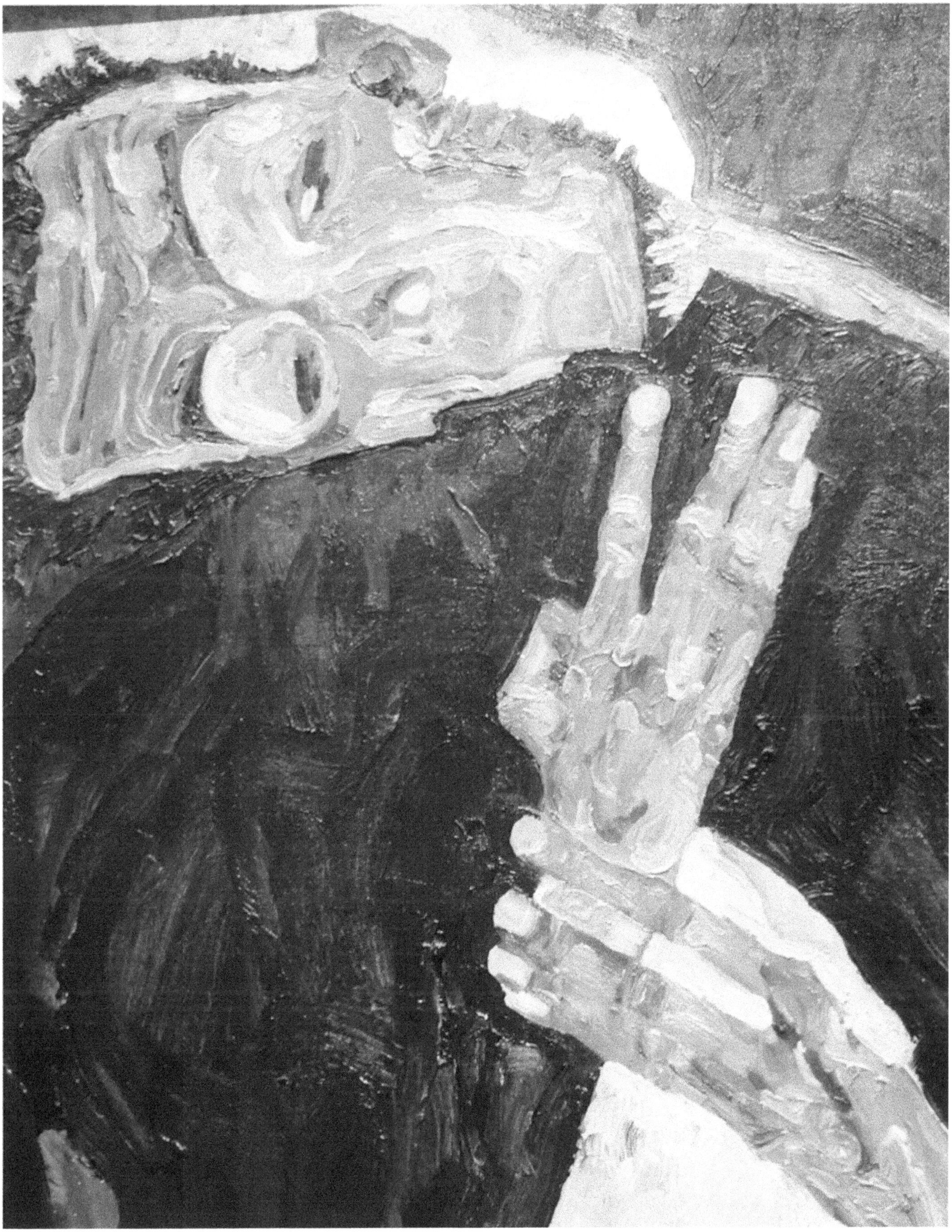

Chapter 49

Treatment Strategies for the Rehabilitation of Dystonia

Teresa Jacobson Kimberley, Heidrun Pickenbrock and Lena Zetterberg

Introduction

For the treatment of dystonia, the current standard of care emphasises the use of botulinum toxin, which is shown to be effective at managing the muscle spasms associated with the disease (Costa et al. 2009; Kalliainen & O'Brien 2014), but patient satisfaction is surprisingly low (Sethi & Olayinka 2012), with small or no changes in overall quality of life (Queiroz et al. 2012).

Clinical experience suggests that physiotherapy (PT) and occupational therapy (OT) are potentially effective in reducing disability and improving quality of life in people with dystonia. The rehabilitation treatment plan must be adapted to the individual patient's resources, problems and needs.

This chapter is based on a 'bio-psycho-social' model that addresses biological, psychological, behavioural, social and environmental factors involved in an overlapping and reciprocal process. This model offers the therapist an understanding of the full consequences of dystonia for each patient, i.e. the sources of the disability. The approach also provides a framework for treatment and the development of symptom self-management.

Clinical Presentation of the Patient With Dystonia

The patient with dystonia often presents to PT/OT with a different diagnosis, such as repetitive strain injury in the hand instead of focal hand dystonia (HD) or neck strain instead of cervical dystonia (CD). Lack of diagnostic tests for dystonia makes diagnosis difficult. The patient with dystonia usually complains of pain and cramping muscles which interfere with activity; symptoms which are also common with orthopaedic injuries. For example, patients with CD present with a twisted neck with spasms, but treatments like stretching or traction have no benefit or may worsen the symptoms. When assessing tone, the therapist often can feel a sustained or intermittent resistance against stretching. This may indicate that the 'neck strain' diagnosis is incorrect.

Two unique features of focal dystonia can assist diagnosis: task specificity and sensory trick. Task specificity means the dystonic movement occurs only during a specific task. For example, someone with HD may have symptoms while writing, but no problem performing other hand tasks that require similar movements, such as typing. Due to this feature, dystonia is also classified according to the specific task that triggers the symptoms (e.g. musician's dystonia, golfer's yip, writer's cramp). An individual with foot dystonia may have symptoms while walking forwards or running, but no problems while walking backwards or riding a bike. The other unique feature is the 'sensory trick', where sensory input will help to temporarily disrupt the dystonic posture. For example, in cervical dystonia the patient can touch a part of his or her face and the head can be briefly held upright.

Bio-Psycho-Social Consequences of Dystonia

There are many factors that influence the patient's experience of disability. In addition to the visually apparent motor symptoms, symptoms that affect psychological wellbeing and social participation must also be addressed in the rehabilitation setting (see Table 49.1).

Biological Factors

The biological factors of dystonia is an active area of investigation particularly related to the genetic risk factors (see Chapter 10). Other hypothesised risk factors for the development of focal dystonia include: highly repetitive work or avocation, poor stress management, hypermobility and poor physical fitness.

Pathophysiology

The pathophysiologic factors associated with dystonia have not been fully elucidated. It is understood that the brain networks responsible for motor control, sensorimotor integration and motor learning are dysfunctional. A combination of these factors may contribute to cortical reorganisation with enlarged and overlapping representation fields (Byl et al. 1996). The dystonic patient presents with a loss of inhibition throughout involved and uninvolved muscles (Samargia et al. 2014). In addition to cortical and basal gangliar impairment, cerebellar dysfunction is also implicated in dystonia, with structural abnormalities in Purkinje cell number (Prudente et al. 2013) and metabolic hyperactivity during symptomatic tasks (Simonyan et al. 2013). This lack of inhibitory tone might explain the difficulties of relearning new movement patterns (Filip et al. 2013) or may cause maladaptive brain plasticity. That is, instead of brain reorganisation with functional benefits, unintended associations are made that reinforce dystonic movements.

Table 49.1 Treatment strategies across the biological, psychological and social perspective adapted individually to the patient's prioritised goal, impairments and context

Disease	Goal	Sensorimotor perspective	Motor learning perspective	Psychological-social perspective	Compensation strategies
General principles for rehabilitation					
Dystonia	Prioritise goals that are challenging, meaningful and achievable that will contribute to improved quality of life	Active exercises in activities and daily life to promote self-management Find exercise the patient can perform and enjoy to promote physical activity in daily life (e.g. dancing, swimming, stationary bike, yoga)	Determine level of activity that challenges but doesn't flare the dystonia Increase of demand Sufficient repetition Use of feedback Concentrate on achieving *one* goal	Motivation, reduce catastrophising thoughts, belief that improvement is possible, identify progress towards the goal, empowerment to manage their condition, help patient learn how to describe their neurologic disorder to others, develop courage to participate in activities	Avoid or reduce triggers of the dystonic postures Self-awareness of stress and fatigue and relaxation strategies
Examples					
Cervical dystonia	Being able to drive the car back and forth to the store for 15 minutes three times/week	Stretching muscles to increase range of motion of the cervical spine and the trunk Exercises to promote strengthening of postoral muscles	Modification of some daily tasks progressively with more left rotation Graded exposure to driving	Belief the patient can drive Gradually progress difficulty so the patient can have success and develop comfort and confidence in all traffic situations Seek support from friends and colleagues	Add another mirror to assist with potential blind spot Determine ideal support and positioning of seat and headrest
Writer's cramp: severe problems in right hand during keyboard use	Being able to stay employed as an administrative assistant	Address secondary proximal muscle issues in forearm and neck, perform sensory retraining	Training in progressive programme in daily practice of sensory retraining	Advocate to employer for adaptive equipment and ability to modify the patient's day to allow for flexible schedule that allows for rest	Training in a voice-to-text typing system Modify mouse

Sensorimotor Impairment

Patients with dystonia have excessive muscle contraction that may be sustained or oscillating. They often suffer from pain. Antagonists may be weak and movement production requires more energy than usual, leading to fatigue. Specific impairments vary according to the location of the dystonia. The patient with dystonia does not generally have sensory loss, but does have other sensory system impairments. For example, patients with CD may suffer from postural orientation problems, whereas patients with HD may present with impaired temporal and spatial tactile discrimination.

Psycho-Social Involvement

Besides the obvious motor problems, patients may suffer from a multitude of non-motor symptoms such as alterations of mood, disturbed sleep patterns, fatigue and loss of self-confidence due to stigma of visible dystonia (Motl et al. 2009; Stamelou et al. 2012). Physical and mental quality of life scores are typically decreased in dystonic patients. Patients with CD state that they have difficulty keeping up with personal and professional demands, feel uneasy in public, are hindered by pain, depressed, annoyed, bitter and feel lonely and isolated (Werle et al. 2014). The patient's rating of self-efficacy in daily activities has been identified as one of the primary non-motor factors for perceived disability in CD (Zetterberg et al. 2012).

HD can be triggered by excessive use of the hand during a task, and for many people the diagnosis has an existential threat. Often the repetitive task is central to the person's profession, such as playing a musical instrument, writing or performing other tasks requiring fine motor control, such as surgery. Due to the loss of motor control, the dystonia can be career-ending. Clearly, this realisation has psychological and social implications for the patient.

Principles of Physical Therapy and Occupational Therapy in the Treatment of Dystonia

Assessment

A primary question to ask patients during the initial evaluation is which activities are most impaired. This helps to identify the patient's main functional goal. The assessment should focus on the bio-psycho-social components that might interfere with the specific goal. For example, biological – passive and active range of motion, pain, strength, endurance; psychological/social – mood, self-esteem, social support, work and hobby implications.

Tests and Measurements

Disease-specific scales (Chapter 15) should be complemented by quality of life, participation and motor performance measures to effectively evaluate the severity of dystonia, with its consequences on activity and participation. Although the following measures are not yet validated for dystonia, we recommend their use to address specific issues. The 'Self-Efficacy Scale' measures the patient's perceived self-efficacy in performing common daily activities. The 'Neck Disability Index' assesses the level of perceived disability in different domains. The 'International Physical Activity Questionnaire' estimates overall physical activity. The 'Goal Attainment Scale' allows the patient and therapist to identify the key tasks that are most impaired and provides an objective measurement to identify progress.

Goal Setting

The overarching goal of rehabilitation in dystonia is the reduction of disability in addition to emphasising health-promoting behaviour. The identification of the patient's prioritised goals should start the sessions. The PT/OT guides the patient in the goal-defining process, but still empowers the patient to list and rank activities that are most important to him or her. The patient identifies important and specific activities that are difficult to perform and the expectation of the treatment. Importantly, goals should be challenging but attainable and prioritised by the patient in order to help the patient stay active over the long term.

The guiding rehabilitation treatment principles addressing the motor impairment is based on developing strategies to inhibit expression of the dystonic posture and practice of non-/less-affected movements to retrain the maladaptive brain patterns. Treatment strategies are incorporated in a goal-oriented treatment tailored to individual patient characteristics and directed towards the key goals.

Treatment Strategies

General/Overarching Principles

There is a strong need for randomised controlled trials of physiotherapy in dystonia. Research has demonstrated that physiotherapy improves head position, pain, cervical range of motion, quality of life and activities of daily living, which is promising, but cautious interpretation of the effectiveness is required as the scientific level of the studies are limited (De Pauw et al. 2014). The treatment strategies provided here are based on clinical experience and small-scale rehabilitation studies (Tassoreli et al. 2006; Queiroz et al. 2012).

We believe that treatment strategies in dystonia must address all aspects of the person. Treatment focused solely on motor impairment rarely results in lasting reduction in disability. The lack of reduction in disability and small or no changes in overall quality of life in patients with CD, despite reduction in motor impairment following botulinum toxin, supports this statement (Sethi & Olayinka 2012). Success is brought about by working multidimensionally towards the prioritised goal. The therapist's task is to determine the key components required to achieve a desired goal. For example, if the goal is to walk long distances, endurance is required; the goal of driving requires rotation of the spine. From the psycho-social perspective, these tasks may be frightening as falls or failure has been previously experienced. The therapist analyses which components are interfering with progress, which helps guide treatment. In some cases adaptive equipment may need to be utilised to help facilitate the goal. For example, in the case of driving, additional mirrors may need to be added. In the case of writer's cramp, voice-activation software may need to be learned to allow for less reliance on hand use.

General motor learning principles should be applied to practice (Mulder & Hochstenbach 2003). Broadly, task practice should begin at a level that is challenging but appropriate for the level of impairment. Practice should be repetitive with feedback, and advanced when a level is achieved. Together with the patient the therapist may determine rewards.

Fatigue can have an aggravating effect on the severity of dystonia. Strategies to reduce fatigue include planning of type and amount of activity, scheduling time for rest and recognising factors, such as stress, that might increase the experience of fatigue. It may be useful to analyse whether a patient's active movements are performed in the most energy-efficient way, especially if the patient is already functioning at the limit of her or his ability.

In general, in the rehabilitation setting it is important to recognise the organic origin of dystonia, but also emphasise the role of psycho-social factors maintaining and exacerbating symptoms and disability.

Modification and Training of the Desired Activity or Participational Task

The treatment should focus on guiding the patient towards the goal, which may require modifying the task. Imagine a woman with CD. Her desired activity is 'collecting mushrooms in the forest'. To be able to walk in the forest she needs an initial goal to increase her walking distance/endurance. Initially, she has difficulty walking 500 metres; thus, the first goal is to increase walking capacity to 2000 metres within 4–6 weeks. Further, 'biological factors' to address in the treatment plan would be physical activity, balance, muscle strength and endurance. Motor relearning exercises will address the position of the head because it hinders her in the activity. If she is afraid to walk alone, a 'psycho-social' treatment strategy is for her to seek social support, such as asking a friend to go along with her in the beginning. A home exercise programme could consist of exercises related to the goal; exercises for the body and neck such as simulated bending, searching and/or picking motions. Progression could be carrying a basket and increased duration of activity, then walking in the forest for 20 minutes, etc. Feedback should be given on performance at each stage. Self-efficacy to the task is essential for improvement, thus the therapist needs to help identify progression towards the components of the task.

Another patient with CD might want to be able to talk in a crowded environment. The treatment plan involves the therapist and the patient working together to determine what causes the avoidance behaviour. Because of his dystonia it is nearly impossible to talk to somebody to his right side. Therefore, the patient avoided meetings and parties and became socially isolated. The treatment plan would involve strategies to modify the environment in order to not require right cervical rotation. Initially, for example, he should plan to sit at the end of a rectangular table. Concurrently, practice tasks are developed that progressively require more right rotation in other daily activities, such as shaving or washing dishes to help progress this ability.

For some individuals the desired task may require assistive technology. In a patient with writer's cramp, voice-activated software may need to be learned to maintain job performance, with careful consideration of vocal cord rest. In this case, the task progression will involve maintaining a relaxed posture while the task is gradually progressed (Byl et al. 2009).

Treatment of Sensory and Motor Impairment

The treatment of the underlying impairments which are interfering with the patient's goals also include addressing motor and sensory impairments. Ideally, this aspect of rehabilitation is combined with the task training to keep practice as relevant as possible.

Motor

Interventions that specifically address the motor impairment, which include botulinum toxin injections into the involved muscles, sometimes accompanied by oral medication, is the current standard care for most focal dystonia (Chapters 32, 33, and 36). For a rehabilitation perspective, muscle shortening and stiffness is a key motor problem. This may be treated with manual therapy such as stretching. As early as possible the patient should learn to practice active stretching independently. Besides the obvious problems in the involved body part, there are often secondary joint problems due to compensatory postural alterations. In all types of dystonia, strengthening exercises have to be put into practice to increase isometric muscle endurance and dynamic strength, especially in the antagonist muscles (Bleton 2010). Many patients benefit from a general fitness programme with exercises to increase physical activity, balance and coordination. This increases overall wellbeing and sets a positive foundation for retraining the brain.

Pain, generally secondary to the involuntary muscle contractions, is also a major concern of many patients. Progressive muscle relaxation might be necessary, especially in the beginning of the treatment, to stop the cycle between tension and pain (Zetterberg et al. 2008).

Sensory and Proprioceptive

Patients may have proprioceptive impairments. For example, a patient with CD may not know how to put the head in an upright position, but the difficulty is not due to the motor impairment, rather a lack of postural orientation. In this case, the therapist could attempt to improve body perception in different positions with manual, verbal and visual guidance.

Patients, particularly those with HD, may benefit from sensory retraining due to possible abnormal finger sensory representation in the primary somatosensory cortex (Zeuner et al. 2002; Candia et al. 2003). Sensory training seeks to discriminate between textures, thumb and fingers and different weights (Byl et al. 2009). Therapeutic putty can be used to train the different fingers individually (Zeuner et al. 2002).

'Psycho-Social' Intervention Strategies

As mentioned above, the psychological and social implications are also within the domain of PT/OT treatment. Key to this is self-efficacy. Self-efficacy is the situation-specific belief in one's capability to successfully perform a particular behaviour. Self-efficacy in daily activities has been identified as one of the primary agents for perceived disability in cervical dystonia (Zetterberg et al. 2012). Psycho-social intervention strategies could include training in how to plan the type and dose of activity or exercise that is tolerated and how to increase it to build capacity. Also, learning when to rest or seek social support. It includes belief in one's ability to participate in the activities they love, learning how to adapt the physical environment as needed, manage stress, and recognise negative thoughts when they occur.

Future Considerations

There is tremendous opportunity for advancement in the area of rehabilitation in the treatment of dystonia. It is essential that solutions are developed and tested regarding behavioural treatment incorporated into PT/OT for reduction of disability in patients with dystonia across the lifespan.

Dystonia is still rarely known and therefore diagnosing is often delayed. From the perspective of brain plasticity and relearning, it is possible that the chance of substantially improving dystonia is greater if the patient has not had long-standing performance of the dystonic movement. Efforts should be directed to educate health providers to be aware of the disease.

To date, several different options have been developed to inhibit undesirable neural pathways. These include transcranial magnetic stimulation or transcranial direct current stimulation (see also Chapter 78). Future research will show whether these methods can improve the outcomes in patients with dystonia.

Summary

The rate of utilisation of PT/OT in the treatment of dystonia is unknown, but anecdotal evidence suggests it is low, but variable, depending on the region. We believe the reason for the low utilisation rate is that many physicians currently treating patients with focal dystonia are unaware of the success that can be associated with rehabilitation. Further, many physiotherapists misunderstand the neurologic basis of the disorder and are unaware of the treatment principles. Current standard of care can help manage some aspects of the disorder, but PT/OT have the potential to make significant impact in patients' quality of life.

References

Bleton J-P. 2010. Physiotherapy of focal dystonia: a physiotherapist's personal experience. *European Journal of Neurology* 17(Suppl. 1):107–112.

Byl NN, Merzenich MM, Jenkins WM. 1996. A primate genesis model of focal dystonia and repetitive strain injury. *Neurology* 47(2):508–520.

Byl NN, Archers ES, McKenzie A. 2009. Focal hand dystonia: effectiveness of a home program of fitness and learning-based sensorimotor and memory training. *Journal of Hand Therapy* 22(2):183–197.

Candia V, Wienbruch C, Elbert T, Rockstroh B, Ray W. 2003. Effective behavioral treatment of focal hand dystonia in musicians alters somatosensory cortical organization. *Proceedings of the National Academy of Science* 100(13):7942–7946.

Costa J, Espírito-Santo CC, Borges AA, Ferreira J, Coelho MM, Moore P, Sampaio C. 2009. Botulinum toxin type B for cervical dystonia. *Cochrane Database of Systematic Reviews* 25:1–93.

De Pauw J, Van der Velden K, Meirte J, Van Daele U, Truijen S, Cras P, Mercelis R, De Hertogh W. 2014. The effectiveness of physiotherapy for cervical dystonia: a systematic literature review. *Journal of Neurology* 261(10):1857–1865.

Filip P, Lungu OV, Bareš M. 2013. Dystonia and the cerebellum: a new field of interest in movement disorders? *Clinical Neurophysiology* 124(7):1269–1276.

Kalliainen LK, O'Brien VH. 2014. Current uses of botulinum toxin A as an adjunct to hand therapy interventions of hand conditions. *Journal of Hand Therapy* 27(2):85–95.

Motl RW, McAuley E, Snook EM, Gliottoni RC. 2009. Physical activity and quality of life in multiple sclerosis: intermediary roles of disability, fatigue, mood, pain, self-efficacy and social support. *Psychological Health Medicine* 14(1):111–124.

Mulder T, Hochstenbach J. 2003. Motor control and learning: implications for neurological rehabilitation. In Greenwood RJ (ed.), *Handbook of Neurological Rehabilitation* (pp. 143–147). Psychology Press, New York.

Prudente CN, Pardo CA, Siyo J, Hanfelt J, Hess EJ, Ledoux MS, Jinnah HA. 2013. Neuropathology of cervical dystonia. *Experimental Neurology* 241:95–104.

Queiroz MAR, Chien HF, Sekeff-Sallem FvA, Barbosa ER. 2012. Physical therapy program for cervical dystonia: a study of 20 cases. *Functional Neurology* 27(3):187–192.

Samargia S, Schmidt R, Kimberley TJ. 2014. Shortened cortical silent period in adductor spasmodic dysphonia: evidence for widespread cortical excitability. *Neuroscience Letters* 560:2–15.

Sethi KD, Rodriguez R, Olayinka B. 2012. Satisfaction with botulinum toxin treatment: a cross-sectional survey of patients with cervical dystonia. *Journal of Medical Economics* 15(3):419–423.

Simonyan K, Berman BD, Herscovitch P, Hallett M. 2013. Abnormal striatal dopaminergic neurotransmission during rest and task production in spasmodic dysphonia. *Journal of Neuroscience* 33(37):14705–14714.

Stamelou M, Edwards MJ, Hallett M, Bhatia KP. 2012. The non-motor syndrome of primary dystonia: clinical and pathophysiological implications. *Brain* 135(6):1668–1681.

Tassoreli C, Mancini F, Balloni L, Pacchetti C, Sandrini G, Nappi G, Martignoni E. 2006. Botulinum toxin and neuromotor rehabilitation: an integrated approach to idiopathic cervical dystonia rehabilitation. *Movement Disorders* 21:2240–2243.

Werle RW, Takeda SY, Zonta MB, Guimarães AT, Teive HA. 2014. The physical, social and emotional aspects are the most affected in the quality of life of the patients with cervical dystonia. *Arquivos de Neuro-Psiquiatria* 72(6):405–410.

Zetterberg L, Halvorsen K, Färnstrand C, Aquilonius SM, Lindmark B. 2008. Physiotherapy in cervical dystonia: six experimental single-case studies. *Physiotherapy Theory and Practice* 24(4):275–290.

Zetterberg L, Lindmark B, Söderlund A, Åsenlöf P. 2012. Self-perceived non-motor aspects of cervical dystonia and their association with disability. *Journal of Rehabilitation Medicine* 44(11):950–954.

Zeuner KE, Bara-Jimenez W, Noguchi PS, Goldstein SR, Dambrosia JM, Hallett M. 2002. Sensory training for patients with focal hand dystonia. *Annals of Neurology* 51(5):593–598.

Chapter 50

Rehabilitation of Cervical Dystonia

Jean-Pierre Bleton

Introduction

Cervical dystonia (CD) is characterised by an intermittent or permanent abnormal head position in relation to the location of involuntary contractions of one or more neck muscles. It occurs or is accentuated during voluntary movements and maintenance of posture. It manifests as functional disability to enable and maintain muscle synergies necessary for the implementation of corrective movements (Häkkinen et al. 2004). CD alters the position of the head during everyday activities. It is responsible for aesthetic, social and relational disorders that are difficult to accept for the patient.

Injections of botulinum neurotoxin (BoNT) are the primary treatment of CD. However, rehabilitation has always played an important role in the treatment of this ailment. Already in the 1950s, Wilson (1955) advised re-educative measures in favour of the muscles, which correct the abnormal posture. Rehabilitation has been recognised as a useful associated treatment with the introduction of the EMG-biofeedback in the 1970s (Brudny et al. 1976), which showed the first tangible effects of the rehabilitation programme (RP) on the CD.

Since the introduction of BoNT for its 'inhibitor' effects on dystonic muscles, activation of the antagonist muscles, which correct the abnormal posture, remains one of the key points of rehabilitation. Nowadays, several strategies prevail, essentially multimodal rehabilitation, which deal with the various clinical features. Active exercises are included in the RP (Delnooz et al. 2009), as well as postural exercises aiming to correct the impaired position of the head.

Cervical Dystonia Assessment

In front of such different clinical features, the initial assessment is an important point base to establish RP. It allows identifying dystonic and inhibited muscles. In addition to this, a precise assessment allows distinguishing the initial deformations due to dystonia from secondary compensations, in order to concentrate RP on dystonia itself.

Schematically, the CD is analysed in the three dimensional planes. It may occur in a single spatial plane or be the result of a combination of deformities in different planes. The cervical spine is divided into two parts: the lower cervical spine (C3 to C7) and upper cervical spine (C0 to C2). These two parts complement each other to achieve pure rotation, pure lateral flexion or pure flexion-extension of the head. Various measurement devices have been used for characterising kinematics of the patient's cervical spine (Salvia et al. 2006), such as the cervical range of motion device or universal inclinometer, goniometer and electrogoniometer, and recently the use of inertial sensors for characterising kinematics.

The tonic spasms occur during neck movements when dystonic muscles are forced to intervene to maintain the balance of the head on the midline (de Beyl & Salvia 2009). Palpation gives a reliable assessment on muscle trophicity and muscle tone. So, the involuntary and intermittent spasms lead to hypertrophy of the involved muscles. If the sternocleidomastoid muscle seems to be the most commonly implicated muscle, this is probably because it is the most superficial anterior and lateral muscle of the neck and the easiest to observe. Other muscles including the muscles of the deepest layers are also affected: trapezius, scalene, splenius capitis, semispinalis capitis, levator scapulae, platysma, suboccipital (such as obliquus capitis inferior muscles). The muscles that cause CD are not always on the same side and we can observe the most singular cross-associations. Following their location, dystonic muscles are involved in the movements of the lower cervical spine or upper cervical spine, or both parts.

The manual examination is performed with the patient lying comfortably on the back. Then, the patient sits up in order to assess the influence of posture and voluntary movements on the severity of the spasms (de Beyl & Salvia 2009). Manual examination also allows discovery of pain spots on some of the overactive muscles.

Strength and endurance of the neck muscles are used as an indicator of neck dysfunction (Strimpakos 2011). Although strength and endurance are separate phenomena, they are interrelated. Strength is defined as the ability of skeletal muscle to develop force for the purpose of providing stability, mobility and muscle endurance (Guide to Physical Therapy Practice 2001) as the ability of muscle to sustain forces repeatedly or to generate forces over a period of time.

For example: the deficit of contraction of the weak sternocleidomastoid muscle appears during the attempts to voluntarily correct CD. Its 'impersistence' of contraction in the case of a rotational torticollis is easy to observe at its muscular body on the lateral face of the neck. The patient cannot manage to

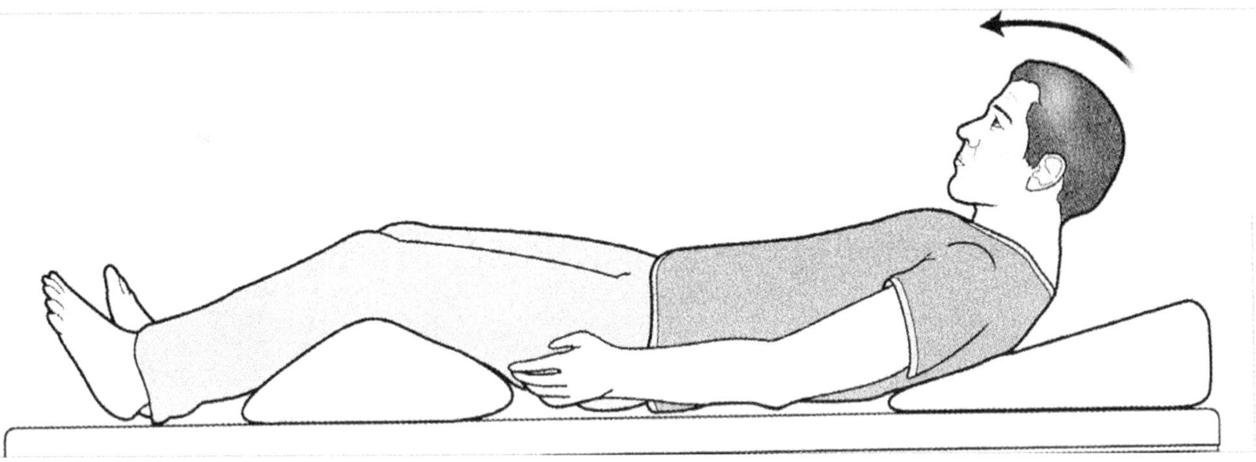

Figure 50.1 Cervical flexion – sternocleidomastoid muscles.
Source: Bleton (2014).

maintain the effort of contraction throughout the duration of the rotation of the head to the corrective side. The assessment of strength and endurance is completed in supine position with maintenance of the cervical flexion position, and against gravity (head lift test; Figure 50.1). The difficulty to lift up or maintain the head above the examining table reveals the muscular deficit. The craniocervical flexion is the primary action of the longus colli muscles. It is tested by feedback pressure, the patient in supine position (craniocervical flexion test) (Jull et al. 2008). The cervical flexion is one of the main actions of the sternocleidomastoid muscles.

Subjective evaluation is based on a clinical interview, taking into account various aspects of the subject's personal experience, such as pain or difficulty in performing certain activities of daily living and their consequences for quality of life. Various scales provide a quantitative score based on standardised clinical examination (Boyce et al. 2012).

The features of CD can change due to its natural evolution or under the effect of BoNT injections. Successive assessments allow rehabilitation to adapt to eventual clinical change. It is preferable to perform the initial assessment out of the periods of BoNT efficiency in order to establish the RP on the primary clinical presentation of the CD, not temporarily modified by BoNT injections.

Rehabilitation Programme Procedures

Although there is no standard RP, we can, however, distinguish a number of strategies for different forms of CD. In the tonic form, the RP focuses on the reinforcement and sustained contraction of the corrective muscles. Conversely, in mobile forms, the objectives are to stop moving the head, to control the head by a low level of contraction of the overactive muscles.

Seeking Immobility

Reducing head movement is the main objective for the mobile forms. The RP tries to achieve muscle relaxation and obtain more or less complete immobility of the head. This therapy is based on the relearning process. The patient learns to recognise his or her muscular spasms. The more the patient knows his or her muscular spasms, the better he or she can control them. Then, the patient strives to maintain immobility during a progressively increasing time period. Once a burst spasm reappears, he or she keeps calm, breathes deeply and relaxes the muscles of the neck region. The control of immobility is repeated several times per day while facing a mirror for self-training. This requires calm attention and a good perception of the muscular contraction.

Positions of 'Lesser Dystonia'

The severity of the CD diminishes thanks to some specific stimuli or situations. Lying on the back abolishes or greatly reduces the spasms in the majority of cases. The contact of the occipital region against the plane of the examination table seems to play the main role. In a few cases of 'clinostatic torticollis', the spasms appear only when the patients are lying on their backs. In these cases, the supine position is not recommended.

The elevation of arms upward, when sitting or standing, also attenuates CD. A classical release position consists of correcting the position of the head with the fingers folded behind the head. It is then easier to control spasm and bring the head to the opposite side of the CD.

Effect of Tactile Stimuli on Motor Behaviour

Antagonist gestures show the influence of sensory inputs on dystonic phenomena. In the same way, gentle strokes applied on the jaw of the contralateral side of CD attract the head towards the correction side.

Orthopaedic correction devices supposed to block the neck generally cause nociceptive stimuli responsible for an increase of the severity of CD.

Eye–Neck Coordination

Eye position plays an important role. The orientation of the gaze to the opposite side of CD reduces spasm and promotes correction of postures. That is why daily activities should be organised in such a way as to rotate the head to the opposite side of CD.

Stretching

The constant head rotation causes a chronic muscle twist. The restoration of the optimal functioning of the body requires untwisting and release of the neck and trunk, to enable the body to return symmetrical. Maintaining gradual tension leads to muscular relaxation. Each specific range of motion can be loosened by gentle stretching exercises. This must not generate pain either during or after the stretching programme.

Relaxation

Relaxation helps to feel and locate tension and muscle contractions for better control. By creating conditions of deep mental and physical relaxation, spasm is reduced. The patient is encouraged to settle comfortably and breathe deeply, calmly and steadily for 2–3 minutes, then release the facial, shoulders and neck muscles. By frequent repetition, it is possible to acquire a sufficient relaxed state that can be extended in the activities of daily life.

Quest for Right Movement

From a rehabilitative standpoint, CD appears as a disorder that can be more or less completely controlled by the patient at the cost of effort. It is important that their pathology be explained to them, and that they are helped to discover the factors that can alleviate or aggravate it.

Reinforcement of the Corrective Muscles

Inhibition of the antagonist dystonic muscles is a part of the dystonic phenomenon. Even though muscular contraction cannot be maintained, this capability to correct CD is developed during RP. The choice of which muscles to strengthen is a fundamental step conditioning the result of the rehabilitation. Corrective muscles are trained in strength and endurance. For this, the head is placed in reverse position (in the exact opposite position to the CD) during periods of time that progressively increase. This posture stimulates the contraction of the corrective muscles and prevents the spread to the muscles that are not involved in the corrective movement.

Particular attention is paid to the muscles of the deepest layers of the nape of the neck, which are frequently deficient. Longus colli and multifidi muscles are the deep muscles most notably involved in head posture (Mayoux- Benhamou 2006). If they properly fulfil their role of head support, they allow superficial muscles to act with less tension. Postural correction consists of an active axial cervical lengthening. The position in mild axial extension is the postural correction reference (Figure 50.2). It serves as the basis for most other corrective exercises.

Exercise Progression

Spasms tend to reappear in the corrective effort to turn the head to the opposite side. At the beginning of the RP, the movements are assisted by the therapist, who partially supports the head. Progressively, the patient is trained to overcome the resistance of the spasms without help. Sustained activity in the corrective muscles is a good prognosis.

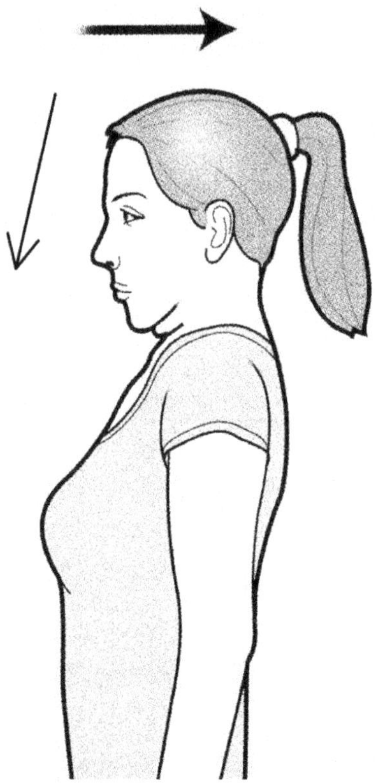

Figure 50.2 Postural correction – longus colli muscles.
Source: Bleton (2014).

The corrective muscles are reinforced in the inner range of movement in order to avoid muscular overflow. The overall control of the entire cervical and craniocervical region is then extended to the shoulder girdle.

The exercises are initially performed in supine position to more easily obtain voluntary contraction of corrective muscles, then when seated, when standing and finally when walking. In each of these positions, the patient is trained to overcome the resistance of increasing intensity. Sudden and uncontrolled efforts are avoided. The period of full effectiveness of BoNT is ideal for this training.

Postural Readjustments Using Proprioception

The consequences of CD are not limited to an imbalance between weak and overactive muscles. Many patients have lost the exact notion of the symmetrical position of their head (Leis et al. 1992). Proprioceptive training consists of: eyes closed, replacing the head on the midline. This jointly develops the ability to stabilise the head and adjust the postural reactions between agonist and antagonist muscles.

Control of Head Movements

The control of head movements is envisaged once the patient is able to control the immobility of his or her head for a long enough time. He or she has to replace involuntary movements with appropriate and controlled movements when turning his or her head to the side of CD and to the opposite side. These head movements are performed slowly, regularly and controlling the occurrence of clonic jerking.

Double-Task Activities

Control of the head when performing double tasks or whole-body activities, such as exercises of the upper limbs while maintaining stability of the head, allows gain of an automatic control of cervical posture. The head posture is also controlled when walking. The patient must repeat the corrective exercises at home (Boyce et al. 2013).

Prospects for Rehabilitation in the BoNT Era

The evolution is capricious and unpredictable. The result is considered acquired when head control is transferred to daily activities. Positive results can sometimes be obtained in a short time, but it is usually necessary to train for 6–12 months to get a steady positive effect (Bleton 2010).

The RP can be started safely immediately after BoNT injections. At the end of the period of effectiveness of the BoNT, when the CD increases or reappears, RP can be continued without changing its content, until the next BoNT injections.

Conclusion

Currently, RP is prescribed to complement the BoNT injections. The two treatments mutually interact in order to reduce abnormal postures and RT increases the time between two series of BoNT injections (Tassorelli et al. 2006).

Although rehabilitation plays an important role, until now no single method or guidelines have been universally accepted. Rather than one single method, there are several strategies which deal with the various clinical features. There is some evidence that an active and multimodal RP (Queiroz et al. 2012) in adjunction to BoNT injections can ameliorate the symptoms of CD, improve head position and decrease pain (De Pauw et al. 2014).

References

Bleton JP. 2010. Physiotherapy of focal dystonia: a physiotherapist's personal experience. *Eur J Neurol* 17 (Suppl. 1):107–112.

Bleton JP. 2014. *Spasmodic torticollis. A Physiotherapy Handbook.* 3rd edn. Paris, Frison-Roche.

Boyce MJ, Canning CG, Mahant N, et al. 2012. The Toronto Western Spasmodic Torticollis Rating Scale: reliability in neurologists and physiotherapists. *Parkinsonism Relat Disord* 18:635–637.

Boyce MJ, Canning CG, Mahant N, et al. 2013. Active exercise for individuals with cervical dystonia: a pilot randomized controlled trial. *Clin Rehabil* 27:226–235.

Brudny J, Korein J, Grynbaum BB, et al. 1976. EMG feedback therapy: review of treatment of 114 patients. *Arch Phys Med Rehabil* 57:55–61.

de Beyl DZ, Salvia P. 2009. Neck movement speed in cervical dystonia. *Mov Disord* 24:2267–2271.

De Pauw J, Van der Velden K, Meirte J, et al. 2014. The effectiveness of physiotherapy for cervical dystonia: a systematic literature review. *J Neurol* 261:1857–1865.

Delnooz CCS, Horstink MWIM, Tijssen MA, et al. 2009. Paramedical treatment in primary dystonia: a systematic review. *Mov Disord* 24: 2187–2198.

Guide to Physical Therapy Practice. 2001 What types of tests and measures do physical therapists use? *Phys Ther* 81: S72–S73.

Häkkinen A, Ylinen J, Rinta-Keturi M, et al. 2004. Decreased neck muscle strength is highly associated with pain in cervical dystonia patients treated with botulinum toxin injections. *Arch Phys Med Rehabil* 85:1684–1688.

Jull GA, O'Leary SP, Falla DL. 2008. Clinical assessment of the deep cervical flexor muscles: the craniocervical flexion test. *J Manipulative Physiol Ther* 31:525–533.

Leis AA, Dimitrijevic MR, Delapasse JS, et al. 1992. Modification of cervical dystonia by selective sensory stimulation. *J Neurol Sci* 110:79–89.

Mayoux- Benhamou A. 2006. Descriptive and functional anatomy of cervical muscles. In: Bouvier G, de Soultrait F, Molina-Negro P, eds, *Spasmodic Torticollis: Clinical Aspects and Treatment.* Paris, Expression Santé, pp. 19–36.

Queiroz MAR, Chien HF, Sekeff-Sallem FA, et al. 2012. Physical therapy program for cervical dystonia: a study of 20 cases. *Funct Neurol* 27:187–192.

Salvia P, Champagne O, Feipel V, et al. 2006. Clinical and goniometric evaluation of patients with spasmodic torticollis. *Clin Biomech* 21:323–329.

Strimpakos N. 2011. The assessment of the cervical spine. Part 2: strength and endurance/fatigue. *J Bodyw Mov Ther* 15:417–430.

Tassorelli C, Mancini F, Balloni L, et al. 2006. Botulinum toxin and neuromotor rehabilitation: an integrated approach to idiopathic cervical dystonia. *Mov Disord* 21:2240–2243.

Wilson K. 1955. *Neurology.* 2nd edn. London, Butterworth.

Chapter 51

Rehabilitation and Plasticity of Task-Specific Focal Hand Dystonia

Jaume Rosset-Llobet and Sílvia Fàbregas-Molas

Historical Overview of Behavioural Methods

When we first encountered a musician with task-specific focal hand dystonia (TSFHD) in 1992, there was not much knowledge available about this disorder. At that time, many health professionals still believed this was a mental disturbance. Consequently, as there was no effective cure for this condition, most affected musicians had to end their professional careers.

Fortunately, in the 1990s, the scientific world became more aware of this field. Researchers demonstrated that the main cause of this disorder was not linked to any major mental problem (Sheehy & Marsden 1982). Because of this, TSFHD moved from psychology and psychiatry to neurology. To treat these patients, neurologists used pharmacological strategies including injections of botulinum toxin into the cramping muscles, as well as anticholinergic drugs. Although these treatments showed some temporary relief and improvement of symptoms, none of them provided a cure for the underlying causal changes (Altenmüller & Jabusch 2008).

Further research showed no brain damage in these patients; instead, patients exhibited organisational and functional changes of neuronal networks, including sensory processing, sensorimotor integration and motor planning on cortical and subcortical levels (Ridding et al. 1995; Bara-Jimenez et al. 1998; Elbert et al. 1998; Pujol et al. 2000; McKenzie et al. 2003; Quartarone et al. 2006; Tamura et al. 2009). It is quite probable that many of these alterations are interrelated. It could be that some alterations are the result of others, but do not cause TSFHD.

Because most of these central nervous system changes are considered to be the result of maladaptive changes to practice and since there is no structural brain damage, it seems logical that retraining, i.e. behavioural methods including instrumental practice and slow-motion exercises, should restore brain organisation and functionality. However, most patients report that any kind of basic relearning or intensive repetition of the affected movement to try to correct undesired responses (on the musical instrument if they have musician's dystonia, or doing calligraphy if they have writer's cramp) does not lead to consistent improvements, and can often exacerbate the problem.

Some researchers believe that focusing specifically on restoring some of the detected nervous system alterations could cure TSFHD symptoms. However, although they were able to improve or normalise some brain changes, and this was linked to clinical improvements, none of these protocols produced a complete, consistent and definitive resolution of the problem (Byl & McKenzie 2000; McKenzie et al. 2009; Rosenkranz et al. 2009). This could be due to several factors: the fact that they were retraining non-crucial changes in the brain; their focus on a symptom of TSFHD, not the cause; or the impact of the protocol not being strong and sustained enough to lead to a rearrangement of the disordered sensorimotor system.

At the same time, other researchers used more general and integrative procedures to treat TSFHD. This seemed to produce better results. In fact, for the first time, complete recovery in musicians having TSFHD was reported. Nevertheless, protocols were complex, required years of training, and the rate of success was low (Brockman et al. 1993; Tubiana & Chamagne 2000).

Background of Our Retraining Approach

One of the most distinct features of TSFHD is the sensory trick. This phenomenon, which refers to sensory stimulation, e.g. wearing a latex glove while playing the instrument, is able to ameliorate or even completely restore motor control (Paulig et al. 2014). This kind of trick emphasises the important role of the sensory system as well as sensory motor integration in the pathophysiology of TSFHD. However, these kinds of tricks are not usually useful for retraining, as they have no lasting effects. Candia found a way around this limitation (Candia et al. 1999). He tested the efficacy of finger splinting as a new sensory input that should act as a more permanent sensory trick. He configured splints to place the fingers in a position different from the normal playing position. Candia also realised that splinting the compensatory fingers (those reacting to the original dystonic movement) is more effective than splinting the dystonic ones (for more information about how to identify dystonic and compensatory fingers, see Rosset-Llobet et al. 2013). Therefore, the first part of the daily retraining routine was to repeat different movement patterns on the musical instrument with the non-splinted fingers while some other fingers were splinted. Then, to avoid habituation effects, he used possibilities involving transfer. Transfer is the capability that allows the nervous system to use what has been learned in a specific context within another context, which has different conditions and task variants (for more details on transfer, see Seidler 2010). The second daily part of the retraining involved the repetition of the same

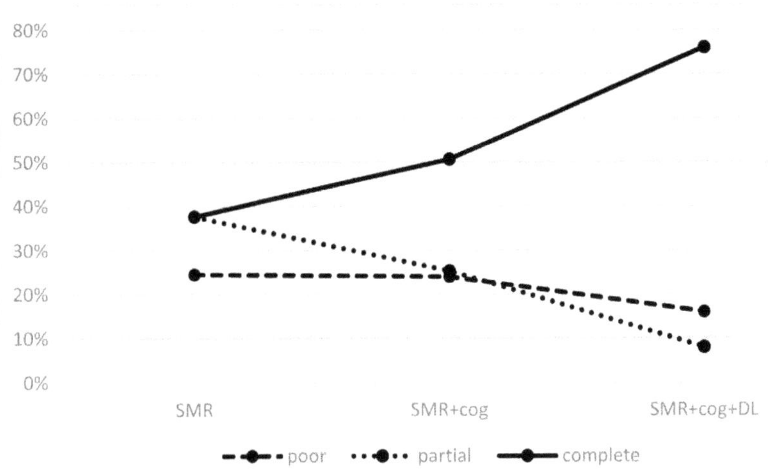

Figure 51.1 Therapy results depending on the strategy used. We have grouped 230 consecutively treated patients into three groups depending on the protocol used: SMR alone, adding cognitive work to SMR, and combining these two strategies with differential learning (DL). Outcomes of patients were classified into three levels: poor, partial and complete recovery (see text for more details). Groups were compared using the *chi square* parametric test to analyse the significance. The confidence level used in all tests was 95 per cent. There were no statistically significant differences between group SMR and SMR + cog ($\chi^2 = 4.084$; $p = 0.130$) nor between SMR + cog and SMR + cog + DL ($\chi^2 = 5.339$; $p = 0.069$). There were statistically significant differences between SMR group and SMR + cog + DL ($\chi^2 = 13.302$; $p = 0.001$).

movement patterns, also on the musical instrument, but now without the splints, in order to transfer the new motor behaviour to the original (unaffected) situation. This procedure was called sensory motor retuning (SMR) and demonstrated a usefulness in reverting symptoms while causing parallel brain reorganisation (Candia et al. 2005). This was the technique that we adopted in 1999 to treat our TSFHD patients.

Results from Our Training Without and With Additional Cognitive Therapy

We consecutively treated 130 musicians using this technique. To analyse the results, we have classified patients into three groups depending on their self-reported functional outcome. These are *complete recovery* (those who returned to instrumental activity with full recovery, with no dystonia symptoms at all), *partial recovery* (those with improvement of dystonia symptoms making a possible return to instrumental activity, but still feeling some functional limitation) and *poor result* (patients who dropped out of treatment or with an improvement not compatible with their musical career). Thirty-two of them (25 per cent) had *poor results*, 49 (38 per cent) *partial recovery*, and 49 (38 per cent) *complete recovery* (see Figure 51.1).

Although these figures constitute an improvement in comparison to other current rehabilitation techniques (Brockman reported 21 per cent successful results but without being clear how many of them had complete recovery), results are still far from acceptable (Brockman et al. 1993).

Patients with TSFHD frequently have certain psychological traits, including proneness to anxiety, perfectionism and obsessive compulsive tendencies. Some of these may be due to dystonia itself, but others probably existed before the onset of dystonia (Jabusch et al. 2004; Ioannou & Altenmüller 2014). We thought that this psychological status could account for the difference between the patients responding well to neurorehabilitation and those not responding to treatment. For this reason, our therapists receive training from a psychologist to be able to use cognitive techniques to improve these psychological factors that can interfere with therapy.

In a second study, we consecutively treated 75 musicians with TSFHD, adding cognitive behavioural therapy to SMR. From this group of patients 18 had *poor results* (24 per cent), 19 *partial recovery* (25 per cent), and 38 *complete recovery* (51 per cent). As can be seen in Figure 51.1, the proportions of patients changed, but the improvement was not statistically significant.

Effects of tDCS on Retraining Results

Bearing in mind that patients with TSFHD exhibit greater activation of the primary sensorimotor cortex, deficits in surrounding inhibition and increased plasticity (Pujol et al. 2000; Hallett 2006), and knowing that transcranial direct current stimulation (tDCS) can safely modulate some of these aspects, we decided to explore the utility of combining this technique with SMR (Rosset-Llobet et al. 2014). As there are no studies demonstrating safety of tDCS if applied over longer periods, we decided to combine SMR and tDCS only during the first two retraining weeks. The results of this pilot study, subsequently confirmed by a larger survey, demonstrate that cathodal biparietal tDCS is a safe technique that enhances the improvement produced by neurorehabilitation on TSFHD and makes retraining easier (Rosset-Llobet et al. 2015). As the retraining protocol for these patients takes many months (average is 15 months), further studies are required to investigate whether two weeks of tDCS will improve not only short-term therapy results but also long-term results. It is also important to examine neurophysiological parameters in cases where brain stimulation is prolonged for more than two weeks. Due to lack of results from basic clinical research concerning the safety of long-term application of tDCS, we decided to stop using the treatment, although previous results have shown promise.

Effects of Differential Training on Rehabilitation of Focal Dystonia

One intriguing characteristic of patients suffering from TSFHD is the stability of the dysfunctional behaviour after inception of dystonic symptoms. It is difficult to understand why, in a group of patients with increased brain plasticity, retraining is so difficult. This question led us to explore approaches that have documented the ability to destabilise brain networks and promote learning. Differential training, also called differential learning (DL) and originally created to improve sports performance, is a technique which, by means of promoting and increasing system fluctuations, has also proven effective in rehabilitation (Schöllhorn et al. 2010). One of the strategies is to introduce noise to the task, constantly changing the way the task is done.

Recently, we have added this new approach to our protocol, introducing noise to SMR exercises. Patients were asked to change, every 3–5 seconds, the way they were performing the exercise, in order to interfere with the activity. For instance, they could change hand, arm or body position, modify the speed or intensity of a part of the movement, or perform it using other biomechanical patterns. We have completed treatment of 25 patients following this strategy (patients in progress are not included in this analysis). From this group, four had *poor results* (16 per cent), two *partial recovery* (8 per cent), and 19 *complete recovery* (76 per cent). These unpublished results are statistically better than those of the SMR group.

Dynamic Systems Theory and Causes and Cures of TSFHD

From our point of view, the above-mentioned experiences open a new perspective to understand how TSFHD emerges and how it can be treated. First, there will not be a single technique useful for every patient, but a tailored combination of procedures, slightly different for each patient. We have seen that when we combine different strategies and adapt these strategies to each patient, results improve. However, we need to go a step further. TFSHD does not seem to have a unique patient profile; in other words, TSFHD patients do not exhibit the same psychological behaviour (Ioannou & Altenmüller 2014). Additionally, they do not exhibit the same behaviour in many other aspects, such as response to sensory tricks, their genetic predisposition, their biomechanical constraints, their gender, and, if they are women, their hormonal status (Rosset-Llobet et al. 2009, 2012; Lohmann et al. 2014; Paulig et al. 2014). In the near future we will need to more precisely identify these profiles and, accordingly, combine and adapt the different available techniques.

The second, and perhaps most challenging, consequence of this analysis is the necessity to see TSFHD from a completely different standpoint, not based on linear systems but rather on dynamic systems theory (Kurz & Stergiou 2004). According to this theory, the human body is an adaptable, complex and dynamic system capable of organising itself, although there is no one single factor inside the system capable of doing this task. Dynamic systems theory states that organisation of movement relies less on sensorimotor representations, and is also less hierarchical when considering how the multitude of interacting parts of the body are integrated into functional, goal-directed movements in dynamic environments. Research from this perspective has illustrated how spontaneous coordination tendencies provide neurobiological systems with the stability and the flexibility needed to adapt to complex, ever-changing environments (Kelso 1995). If a musician, due to his psychological behaviour or his training workload, shapes a very stable but rigid and inflexible nervous system, he or she will not easily be able to adapt to internal or external changes. This can lead to a degradation in the musician's performance or even to dysfunctional coordination when he or she faces challenging new situations or environments.

Interestingly, this way of seeing TSFHD can provide answers to questions that, until now, had no easy explanation. Musician's dystonia characteristically appears in high-level musicians that have practised a certain amount in their lives. Typically, dystonia emerges at a certain point in their careers, when they are under strenuous conditions (e.g. routine changes, physical problems, nerve conduction alterations, psychological stress). However, one of the urgent questions is: why do we occasionally find cases where only some, or even none, of these prerequisites can be identified (Rosset-Llobet et al. 2013)? From the dynamic system point of view, dystonia will appear when there is an imbalance between how able the musician is to adapt to inner or outer environmental changes (how flexible he or she is) and how intense these changes are. If he or she is flexible, the amount of environment changes necessary to produce system breakdown should be high. If he or she is very rigid, breakdown (dystonia, in this case) can occur more easily.

Even the role of genetics can be interpreted under this outlook. We know that 20 per cent of musician's dystonia patients have relatives with either musician's dystonia or writer's cramp (Schmidt et al. 2009). Genome-wide significance with musician's dystonia was observed for an intronic variant in the arylsulphatase G gene (Lohmann et al. 2014). This gene, along with others, could by means of molecular changes make the system more rigid and therefore more likely to suffer a breakdown when facing a destabilising environment. However, the data also suggest that genes are not the only factor causing the system to break under certain situations. TSFHD can be the result of a sum of many factors, genetics being only one of them. Other factors could compensate for the effects of genes, making the system more flexible. Or, conversely, the subject could never be subjected to a situation destabilising enough for the development of dystonia, even if the subject has a genetic predisposition.

Another poorly understood feature of musician's dystonia is the fact that women are less frequently affected (Lim & Altenmüller 2003). There is no evidence that this could be explained by a lower proportion of women playing musical instruments at a high level or by other occupational factors (Rosset-Llobet et al. 2005). We have demonstrated women having a normal menstrual cycle are less prone to suffer from musician's dystonia (Rosset-Llobet et al. 2012). We hypothesised in our paper that the physiological mechanism that protects them could be the hormonal cycle's capability to change cortical excitability and neuronal plasticity (Smith et al. 1999; Fernández et al. 2003), which could produce a protective effect. This hypothesis seems very plausible if viewed from the dynamic systems point of view. Cyclic female hormonal variations can facilitate brain adaptability to changes, promoting system flexibility. When this is reduced (when a woman has a menstrual disorder) or lost (e.g. during menopause or pregnancy), women become more prone to TSFHD due to a reduction of the factors which make them more adaptable to their environment.

Finally, we need to explore in more depth the role that a differential learning and dynamic system approach can have in TSFHD neurorehabilitation and prevention. Both prevention and treatment can probably be done by means of rendering the nervous system more flexible and promoting network plasticity. This will make the nervous system more adaptable and, thus, less prone to dystonia, and also more able to restore its functional organisation. Here, we must develop tools to make rehabilitation possible and test these tools to confirm their impact on this group of patients.

References

Altenmüller E, Jabusch HC (2008). Focal dystonia: diagnostic, therapy, rehabilitation. In: Grunwald M, Srinivasan MA (eds) *Human Haptic Perception: Basics and Applications.* Heidelberg: Birkhäuser. pp. 303–311.

Bara-Jimenez W, Catalan MJ, Hallett M, Gerloff C (1998). Abnormal somatosensory homunculus in dystonia of the hand. *Ann Neurol* 44(5):828–831.

Brockman R, Chamagne P, Tubiana R (1993). The upper extremity in musicians. In: Tubiana R (ed.) *The Hand*, Vol. IV. Philadelphia, PA: WB Saunders. pp. 873–885.

Byl NN, McKenzie A (2000). Treatment effectiveness for patients with a history of repetitive hand use and focal hand dystonia: a planned, prospective follow-up study. *J Hand Ther* 13(4):289–301.

Candia V, Elbert T, Altenmüller E, Rau H, Schäfer T, Taub E (1999). Constraint-induced movement therapy for focal hand dystonia in musicians. *Lancet* 353(9146):42.

Candia V, Rosset-Llobet J, Elbert T, Pascual-Leone A (2005). Changing the brain through therapy for musicians' hand dystonia. *Ann NY Acad Sci* 1060:335–342.

Elbert T, Candia V, Altenmüller E, Rau H, Sterr A, Rockstroh B, Pantev C, Taub E (1998). Alteration of digital representations in somatosensory cortex in focal hand dystonia. *Neuroreport* 9(16):3571–3575.

Fernández G, Weis S, Stoffel-Wagner B, Tendolkar I, Reuber M, Beyenburg S, Klaver P, Fell J, de Greiff A, Ruhlmann J, Reul J, Elger CE (2003). Menstrual cycle-dependent neural plasticity in the adult human brain is hormone, task, and region specific. *J Neurosci* 23:3790–3795.

Hallett M (2006). Pathophysiology of dystonia. *J Neural Transm Suppl* 70:485–488.

Ioannou CI, Altenmüller E (2014). Psychological characteristics in musician's dystonia: a new diagnostic classification. *Neuropsychologia* 61:80–88.

Jabusch HC, Müller SV, Altenmüller E (2004). Anxiety in musicians with focal dystonia and those with chronic pain. *Mov Disord* 19(10):1169–1175.

Kelso JAS (1995). *Dynamic Patterns: The Self-Organization of Brain and Behavior.* Cambridge, MA: MIT.

Kurz MJ, Stergiou N (2004). *Applied Dynamic Systems Theory for the Analysis of Movement. Innovative Analyses of Human Movement.* Champaign, IL: Human Kinetics. pp. 93–120.

Lim VK, Altenmüller E (2003). Musicians' cramp: instrumental and gender differences. *Med Probl Perform Art* 18:21–26.

Lohmann K, Schmidt A, Schillert A, Winkler S, Albanese A, Baas F, Bentivoglio AR, Borngräber F, Brüggemann N, Defazio G, Del Sorbo F, Deuschl G, Edwards MJ, Gasser T, Gómez-Garre P, Graf J, Groen JL, Grünewald A, Hagenah J, Hemmelmann C, Jabusch HC, Kaji R, Kasten M, Kawakami H, Kostic VS, Liguori M, Mir P, Münchau A, Ricchiuti F, Schreiber S, Siegesmund K, Svetel M, Tijssen MA, Valente EM, Westenberger A, Zeuner KE, Zittel S, Altenmüller E, Ziegler A, Klein C (2014). Genome-wide association study in musician's dystonia: a risk variant at the arylsulfatase G locus? *Mov Disord* 29(7):921–927.

McKenzie AL, Nagarajan SS, Roberts TP, Merzenich MM, Byl NN (2003). Somatosensory representation of the digits and clinical performance in patients with focal hand dystonia. *Am J Phys Med Rehabil* 82(10):737–749.

McKenzie AL, Goldman S, Barrango C, Shrime M, Wong T, Byl N (2009). Differences in physical characteristics and response to rehabilitation for patients with hand dystonia: musicians' cramp compared to writers' cramp. *J Hand Ther* 22(2):172–181.

Paulig J, Jabusch HC, Großbach M, Boullet L, Altenmüller E (2014). Sensory trick phenomenon improves motor control in pianists with dystonia: prognostic value of glove-effect. *Front Psychol* 23(5):1012. doi: 10.3389/fpsyg.2014.01012 (accessed 24 July 2015).

Pujol J, Roset-Llobet J, Rosinés-Cubells D, Deus J, Narberhaus B, Valls-Solé J, Capdevila A, Pascual-Leone A (2000). Brain cortical activation during guitar-induced hand dystonia studied by functional MRI. *Neuroimage* 12(3):257–267.

Quartarone A, Siebner HR, Rothwell JC (2006). Task-specific hand dystonia: can too much plasticity be bad for you? *Trends Neurosci* 29(4):192–199.

Ridding MC, Sheean G, Rothwell JC, Inzelberg R, Kujirai T (1995). Changes in the balance between motor cortical excitation and inhibition in focal, task specific dystonia. *J Neurol Neurosurg Psychiatry* 59(5):493–498.

Rosenkranz K, Butler K, Williamon A, Rothwell JC (2009). Regaining motor control in musician's dystonia by restoring sensorimotor organization. *J Neurosci* 29(46):14627–14636.

Rosset-Llobet J, Fàbregas i Molas S, Rosinés i Cubells D, Narberhaus Donner B, Montero i Homs J (2005). Clinical analysis of musicians' focal hand dystonia: review of 86 cases. *Neurologia* 20:108–115.

Rosset-Llobet J, Garcia-Elias M, Montero J, Valls-Solé J, Pascual-Leone A (2009). Linburg's syndrome, can it cause focal dystonia? *Mov Disord* 24(11):1704–1706.

Rosset-Llobet J, Pascual-Leone A, Fàbregas-Molas S (2012). Role of female reproductive hormones in musicians' dystonia. *Med Probl Perform Art* 27(3):156–158.

Rosset-Llobet J, Fàbregas-Molas S, Valls-Solé J (2013). Diagnostic du doigt dystonique et du doight compensatoire. In: Rosset-Llobet J, Fàbregas-Molas S (eds) *La Dystonie du Musicien.* Montauvan: Alexitère editions. pp. 63–83.

Rosset-Llobet J, Fàbregas-Molas S, Pascual-Leone A (2014). Transcranial direct current stimulation improves neurorehabilitation of task-specific dystonia: a pilot study. *Med Probl Perform Art* 29(1):16–18.

Rosset-Llobet J, Fàbregas-Molas S, Pascual-Leone A (2015). The effect of transcranial direct current stimulation on neurorehabilitation of task-specific dystonia: a double blind, randomized clinical trial. *Med Probl Perform Art* 30(3):178–184.

Schmidt A, Jabusch HC, Altenmüller E, Hagenah J, Brüggemann N, Lohmann K, Enders L, Kramer PL, Saunders-Pullman R, Bressman SB, Münchau A, Klein C (2009). Etiology of musician's dystonia: familial or environmental? *Neurology* 72(14):1248–1254.

Schöllhorn WI, Beckmann H, Davids K (2010). Exploiting system fluctuations: differential training in physical prevention and rehabilitation programs for health and exercise. *Medicina (Kaunas)* 46(6):365–373.

Seidler RD (2010). Neural correlates of motor learning, transfer of learning, and learning to learn. *Exerc Sport Sci Rev* 38(1):3–9.

Sheehy MP, Marsden CD (1982). Writers' cramp: a focal dystonia. *Brain* 105(Pt 3):461–480.

Smith MJ, Keel JC, Greenberg BD, Adams LF, Schmidt PJ, Rubinow DA, Wassermann EM (1999). Menstrual cycle effects on cortical excitability. *Neurology* 53:2069–2072.

Tamura Y, Ueki Y, Lin P, Vorbach S, Mima T, Kakigi R, Hallett M (2009). Disordered plasticity in the primary somatosensory cortex in focal hand dystonia. *Brain* 132(Pt 3):749–755.

Tubiana R, Chamagne P (2000). Prolonged rehabilitation treatment of musicians' focal dystonia. In: Tubiana R, Amadio PC (eds) *Medical Problems of the Instrumentalist Musician*. London: Martin Dunitz Ltd.

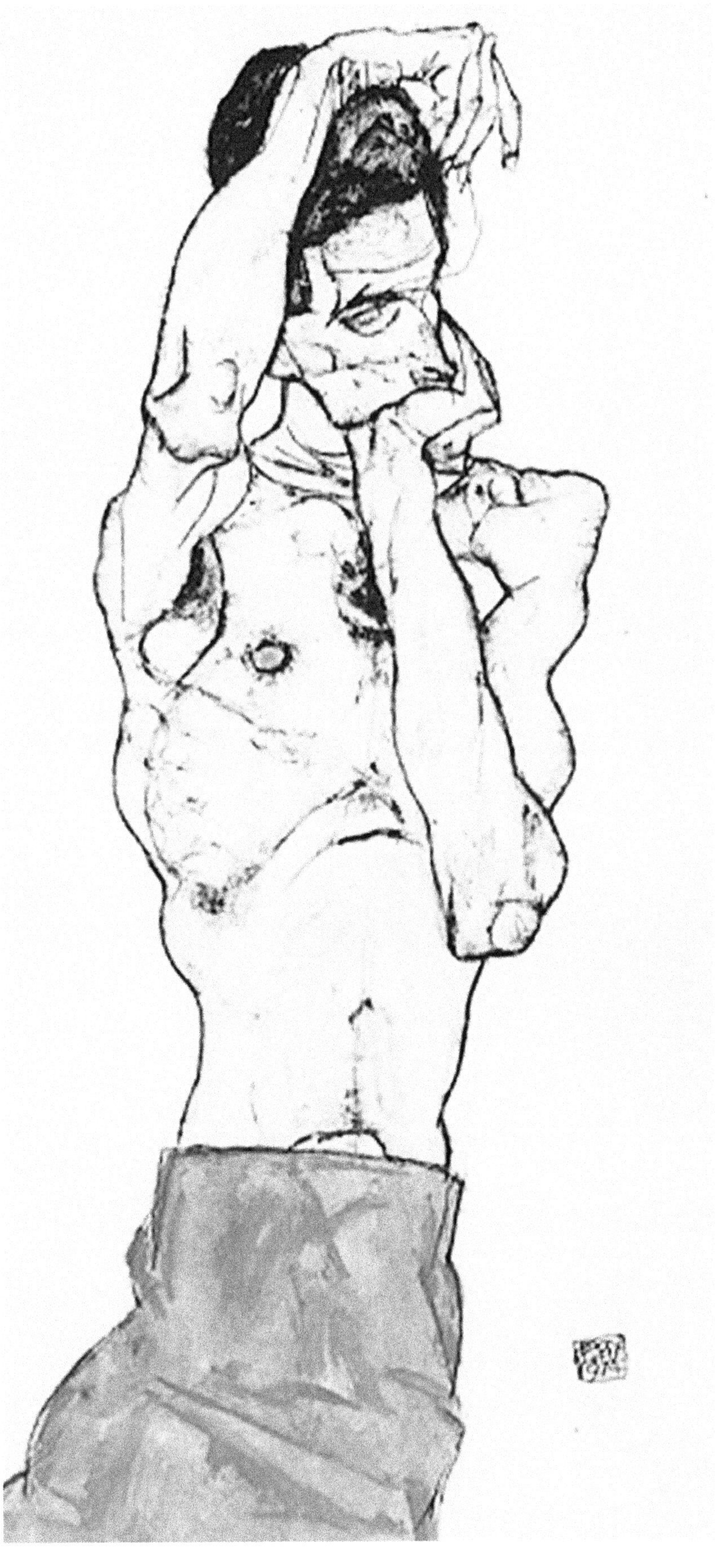

Chapter 52

Pharmacotherapy of Dystonia

An Overview

Vladimir S. Kostić and Zvezdan Pirtošek

Introduction

Before introduction of botulinum toxin (BT) and deep brain stimulation, medical treatment was the cornerstone in symptomatic treatment of dystonia. Its use in dystonia remains extensive, but, unfortunately, efficacious in only a few syndromes and in only selected patients. Many patients do not benefit from drugs, and for many drugs formal proof of efficacy is lacking. Large double-blind placebo-controlled studies are rare and most available data come from anecdotal reports, case series, open and uncontrolled studies. Therefore, medical treatment of dystonia still rests to a large degree on the personal experience of the clinician. Also, as adverse effects of drug treatment may be considerable, many patients with very mild dystonia are better left untreated. For some forms of secondary dystonia, such as Wilson's disease and dopa-responsive dystonia, there are specific causative treatments and therefore their recognition and timely treatment is crucial.

Several systematic reviews on the treatment of dystonia have been published (Balash & Giladi 2004; Albanese et al. 2011; Delnooz & van de Warrenburg 2012; Dressler et al. 2015a). After the initial report of the European Federation of Neurological Societies and Movement Disorders Society-European Section Task Force (EFNS/MDS-ES Task Force) in 2006, five years later the same taskforce pessimistically concluded that 'no new class A or B data are available for oral medications' (Albanese et al. 2011). Still, despite its only modest symptomatic benefit, oral medication is widely used, particularly in generalised dystonia or in focal dystonias when there is an unsatisfactory response to BT therapy.

Anticholinergic Drugs

Anticholinergic drugs considered to be efficacious for all types of dystonia (particularly if applied within five years of disease onset) were largely replaced by BT as a treatment of choice, particularly in focal and segmental dystonia, but did largely retain their role in generalised dystonia (Jankovic 2013). Small class III crossover studies showed that the most widely used, trihexyphenidyl (THP), a muscarinic acetylcholine receptor antagonist, might be superior to placebo for childhood-onset primary or secondary dystonias. It was the only anticholinergic agent that was proved effective by a double-blind, randomised, placebo-controlled trial for the symptomatic treatment of segmental and generalised dystonia (mean dose of 30 mg/d) in young patients (mean age 18.9 years, range 9–32) (Burke et al. 1986). An improvement of up to 72 per cent was registered in 31 patients with primary segmental or generalised dystonia on THP. Benefit continued during follow-up periods of nine months to 2.4 years. Distribution of dystonia, aetiology and gender were not correlated with the treatment effect (Burke et al. 1986). These data support observations obtained in a retrospective analysis of open-label trials of initial treatment with anticholinergic agents on 358 patients with primary focal and generalised dystonia (Greene et al. 1988). A 'good' response (defined as a slight, moderate or marked improvement) was experienced by 40–50 per cent of patients, superior to data obtained in patients receiving clonazepam (21 per cent), baclofen (11 per cent) or benzodiazepines (13 per cent). Mean effective daily doses of THP were 41 mg for children (occasionally they may respond to low doses of even 4 mg/d) and 24 mg for adults (Cloud & Jinnah 2010). Despite a lack of controlled trial of THP in older adults with dystonia, it has been proposed that adults did not exhibit the same benefit as younger patients, probably due to poorer efficacy and/or intolerable adverse effects, as side-effects increase in frequency with age. However, several studies, including double-blind crossover ones, failed to find any consistent benefit from anticholinergics in patients with adult-onset focal dystonia, and concluded that only a minority with cranial dystonia were responsive.

The majority of, but not all, open studies suggest that THP improves motor function in children with dystonic cerebral palsy (primarily upper extremity function and/or oromotor skills in younger children), particularly in absence of spasticity and in those with higher cognitive abilities (Cloud & Jinnah 2010; Jankovic 2013).

Besides THP, some antidystonic effect has also been linked to diphenhydramine, a histamine H_1 antagonist with anticholinergic properties, biperiden, orphenadrine, benztropine, procyclidine and profenamine (Jankovic 2013).

Common, mostly age- and dose-related, adverse effects include dry mouth, blurred vision, constipation, urinary retention, memory loss, drowsiness, confusion, hallucinations and behavioural changes. THP is better tolerated when started low and titrated with small dose increments (1 mg/d, with slow increases by 1 mg every 4–5 days up to 6–10 mg/d and then, if tolerated and particularly in children, by 2 mg increments every 5–7 days up to 80 mg/d or until adverse effects emerge (Jankovic 2013).

Recommendations and good clinical points given by the EFNS/MDS-ES Task Force in 2006, that were not changed in 2011 (Albanese et al. 2011), were: 'The absolute and comparative efficacy and tolerability of anticholinergic agents in dystonia is poorly documented in children and there is no proof of efficacy in adults; therefore, no recommendations can be made to guide prescribing (good practice point).' Further information about the use of anticholinergic drugs for treatment of dystonia can be found in Chapter 53.

GABA-Mimetic Agents

High-dosage oral baclofen (β-parachlorophenyl GABA) (from 40 to 180 mg/d), a presynaptic $GABA_B$ receptor agonist, may be helpful in patients, particularly children, with generalised or segmental dystonia, as well as in those with oromandibular dystonia or in levodopa-related off-dystonia in Parkinson's disease (Jankovic 2013). The mechanism of action is not clear. In a retrospective analysis of open-label trials (Greene et al. 1988; Greene 1992), slight, moderate or marked improvement to baclofen was verified in 20 per cent of the patients: those with blepharospasm responded best (30 per cent), followed by generalised (13 per cent) and cervical dystonia (11 per cent). Predictors of good response were mild-to-moderate severity of dystonia and age <20 years. In patients with DYT1 dystonia, baclofen (>50 mg/d) improved leg dystonia and gait in 42 per cent of children, with stable and prolonged benefit in some of them (Cloud & Jinnah 2010). Unfortunately, the role of baclofen in adult focal dystonia is questionable. While in one series a sustained benefit was registered in 18 per cent of adults with cranial dystonia, other smaller series failed to find significant benefit in adults with focal dystonias (Greene 1992). However, baclofen combined with valproic acid might be useful in a small number of patients with focal dystonias (Cloud & Jinnah 2010). Intrathecal baclofen is an established treatment for spasticity, particularly that of spinal origin. Treatment was tried also in patients with dystonia, with mixed results, with a better outcome in children (Dressler et al. 2015b)

Dose-related adverse effects include lethargy, sedation, dry mouth, dizziness, gastrointestinal complaints and urinary urgency or hesitation. In addition, psychosis and seizures can result from abrupt baclofen withdrawal.

No benzodiazepine, including diazepam, lorazepam and clonazepam, known to potentiate neural inhibitory mechanisms mediated by GABA, has been evaluated in controlled trials, but clinical practice indicates that they might be particularly useful in blepharospasm, cervical dystonia with prominent head tremor and, to some extent, myoclonic dystonia (Cloud & Jinnah 2010), as well as an additional therapy in patients with suboptimal response to anticholinergics. Greene et al. (1988) reported good response to the most frequently used clonazepam in 16 per cent of 115 patients: response rates were best for blepharospasm (23 per cent) and cervical dystonia (21 per cent), respectively, and only 6 per cent for generalised dystonia (these differences were not significant). The authors concluded that anticholinergics were significantly more effective than GABA-mimetics in blepharospasm and cervical dystonia (Greene et al. 1988). Marked relief of dystonic symptoms may be achieved after intravenous application of diazepam (5–10 mg). Adverse effects of benzodiazepines (sedation, confusion, depression, impaired coordination), like with other groups of agents, may limit dose escalation.

Gamma-hydroxybutyric acid, a drug acting on the $GABA_B$ receptors either directly or through conversion to GABA, was effective in patients with ethanol-responsive movement disorders, including two patients with ε-sarcoglycan-linked myoclonus-dystonia. Zolpidem (5–20 mg/d), an imidazopyridine agonist with high affinity for the benzodiazepine receptor α1 subunit site, had promising effects without prominent sedation in blepharospasm, myoclonus-dystonia syndrome, X-linked dystonia-parkinsonism syndrome ('Lubag') and other forms of dystonia (Jankovic 2013).

Dopaminergics

Levodopa was used to treat generalised dystonia, but the results were contradictory, at least partially due to the aetiological heterogeneity of patients recruited in early studies. Lang (1988) reviewed 214 cases; 39 per cent of patients with generalised dystonia showed marked to moderate improvement on levodopa, followed by 27 per cent of patients with cervical dystonia and 6 per cent of patients with cranial dystonia. Levodopa may also be occasionally useful in secondary dystonia. However, there are no evidence-based data to support the use of levodopa or dopamine agonists in other primary dystonias, with the exception of clinically and genetically heterogeneous dopa-responsive dystonia (DRD). In the most frequent autosomal dominant form (DYT5) with heterozygous mutations of GTP-cyclohydrolase 1 (GCH1) and classic phenotype of early-onset lower-limb dystonia causing gait disturbances, levodopa produces an excellent response. Clinical heterogeneity of DRD causes diagnostic uncertainty. A trial with levodopa in every patient with early-onset dystonia without an alternative explanation seems, therefore, mandatory. Most patients exhibit notable and sustained improvement even on small daily doses of levodopa (50–200 mg/d, with a beneficial effect obvious within days or weeks), although some patients need much higher doses (1000–1200 mg/d). The response to low doses of levodopa remains marked and long-lasting. Hallucinations and dyskinesia rarely develop in these patients. If clinical benefit cannot be registered after a month of treatment with adequate doses of levodopa, the diagnosis of DRD is unlikely. Although not based on controlled studies, observations from clinical practice suggest that, besides levodopa, DRD patients might improve on anticholinergics, dopamine agonists and carbamazepine (Jankovic 2006).

Dopamine receptor agonists including bromocriptine, apomorphine and lisuride have also been tried in dystonia, but with inconclusive results and adverse effects in approximately 25 per cent of patients (Balash & Giladi 2004; Albanese et al. 2011). In uncontrolled studies, bromocriptine in doses effective for parkinsonism (50–80 mg/d) improved both generalised and focal dystonia. Contradictory effects of lisuride (2–3 mg/d orally) led to conclusions from 'inconclusive effect' to 'a drug of limited use' in focal dystonias, at best (Nutt et al. 1985).

Although insufficiently explored in generalised and focal dystonia, apomorphine was suggested to have the best effects among dopamine agonists (Lang 1988); an apomorphine test might be useful for the assessment of dopaminergic sensitivity of dystonic symptoms. Adverse effects of dopamine agonists include dyskinesia, sleepiness, orthostatic hypotension, nausea, gastrointestinal symptoms, hallucinations and behavioural changes.

Anti-Dopaminergic Drugs

The possible positive effect of dopamine-blocking agents is paradoxical as they may cause both acute dystonic reactions, mostly in young patients, and tardive dystonia, which together with other adverse effects substantially discouraged their use (Jankovic 2006). However, in small series, symptomatic relief of dystonia, albeit variable, has been reported for phenothiazines, pimozide, perphenazine and haloperidol (Lang 1988).

Open-label studies on atypical antipsychotic clozapine (12.5–300 mg/d), a dibenzodiazepine derivative predominantly blocking the dopamine D4 receptor, failed to improve cervical dystonia after 3–12 weeks of treatment (Thiel et al. 1994).

However, several small, open-label studies on generalised dystonia, Meige syndrome and oromandibular dystonia revealed marked improvement with clozapine. Doses of up to 900 mg/d were required in patients with axial or generalised dystonia (Cloud & Jinnah 2010). Due to a slight risk of granulocytopenia, the usage of the drug requires regular monitoring of haematologic parameters and it should be used with caution in patients with cardiac insufficiency and epilepsy. Clozapine and aripiprazole should be considered in symptomatic patients who developed tardive dystonia while receiving other antipsychotics. Other atypical neuroleptics such as olanzapine, risperidone, quetiapine and tiapride have occasionally demonstrated good to marked improvement in uncontrolled studies. Lin and Chang (2004) reported slow and steady improvement of generalised dystonia by 70 per cent in a patient receiving up to 15 mg of olanzapine in a course of three months. Uncontrolled studies with risperidone (1.5–3 mg/d), however, did not provide sufficient evidence of efficacy, but showed decrease of both duration and amplitude of segmental and generalised dystonia in two uncontrolled studies (Zuddas & Cianchetti 1996; Grassi et al. 2000).

Tetrabenazine

In their review of the literature, Chen and colleagues (2012) identified eight studies on the effectiveness of tetrabenazine (TBZ), an inhibitor of vesicular monoamine transporter 2 and, therefore, a presynaptic catecholamine-depleting agent, in various forms of dystonia. In one prospective, blinded, controlled study TBZ was effective in focal and generalised dystonias, but in another two was ineffective. In four out of five remaining retrospective studies, moderate to marked improvement with TBZ was registered in 45–76 per cent for a variety of dystonias, in particular tardive dystonia (Chen et al. 2012). Also, it was sustainably effective in anecdotal cases with ε-sarcoglycan-related myoclonus-dystonia. TBZ was shown to be beneficial also in a wide range of other dyskinesias. However, the authors proposed that this drug 'should be considered as an alternate treatment option to established therapies', partially due to common adverse effects including drowsiness, parkinsonism, depression, anxiety, akathisia and insomnia which, however, are dose- and age-dependent. Occasionally, TBZ might be combined with lithium or levodopa to augment its effects and to lessen side-effects, enabling usage of smaller doses of TBZ (Jankovic 2013).

Initial doses of 12.5 mg/d should be increased by the same amount in 4–5 day intervals up to a dose of 25–100 mg/d (Cloud & Jinnah 2010). Although it does not induce tardive dyskinesia, rare cases of acute dystonic episodes have been reported (Jankovic 2013).

Various

Antiepileptic Drugs

Although successful in controlling attacks of kinesiogenic paroxysmal dystonia with carbamazepine, antiepileptic drugs including phenytoin, levetiracetam and topiramate are not recommended for routine use in dystonia due to insufficient evidence, mainly based on case reports (Jankovic 2009). Early open trials suggested mild-to-moderate improvement with carbamazepine (400–800 mg/d) in at least a small proportion of patients (19 per cent) (Isgreen 1976). Double-blind randomised crossover studies of oral gamma-vinyl GABA and valproate were considered not representative, due to the small sample size (Cloud & Jinnah 2010; Jankovic 2013). After several case reports on levetiracetam, a pyrrolidine derivate, in segmental and generalised dystonia, open-label trials in patients with cervical dystonia and patients with therapy refractory segmental or generalised dystonia failed to detect any effect in any patients on levetiracetam 3000 mg/d (Jankovic 2009).

Muscle Relaxants

Muscle relaxants (apart from already described benzodiazepines and baclofen) including tizanidine, cyclobenzaprine, metaxalone, carisoprodol, nethocarbamol and chlorzoxazone were supposed to add benefit for patients with unsatisfactory response to anticholinergics (Balash & Giladi 2004; Cloud & Jinnah 2010; Jankovic 2013). In a recent double-blind randomised placebo-controlled crossover study, intramuscular magnesium sulphate (maximal dose 2000 mg/d), that may act as a muscle relaxant, failed to prove superior to placebo for dystonia in complex regional pain syndrome (van der Plus et al. 2013).

Mexiletine

Mexiletine is a derivative oral form of lidocaine, a non-selective voltage-gated sodium channel blocker with a clinical use as an antiarrhythmic drug. A significant improvement in the rating scale for dystonia and in videotape ratings was observed after mexiletine treatment in six patients with dystonia (three with generalised dystonia and three with cervical dystonia) who had failed to respond to previous pharmacotherapy (Lucetti et al. 2000).

Cannabinoids

Early studies of natural and synthetic cannabinoids gave mixed results. In a preliminary open pilot study, cannabidiol, a non-psychoactive cannabinoid of herbal cannabis, was given to five patients with dystonia and a dose-related improvement of 20–50 per cent was observed in all patients (Consroe et al. 1986). Acute administration of nabilone, a psychoactive synthetic 9-trans-ketocannabinoid, failed in a double-blind, randomised placebo-controlled crossover study in reducing dystonia in 15 patients with generalised and segmental primary dystonia (Fox et al. 2002). However, two recent systematic reviews dealing in part with therapeutic potential of cannabinoids in dystonia concluded that, despite some benefit of smoked cannabis or oral cannabinoids suggested by several case reports, this group of agents could not be recommended (Koppel et al. 2014; Kluger et al. 2015).

Combination of Drugs

Based on clinical experience, but without scientific concept, combinations of several drugs were tried in the treatment of adult severe disabling axial dystonia with benzhexol treatment failure. In children with life-threatening generalised dystonia, a triple therapy, named 'Marsden cocktail', consisting of a dopamine antagonist (tetrabenazine), a dopamine-blocking drug (pimozide) and an anticholinergic agent, was used (Marsden et al. 1984).

Others

Anecdotal reports found benefit from various other agents, such as slow release morphine sulphate, oral and intravenous lidocaine, riluzole, topiramate, pregabalin, amantadine and lithium (Balash & Giladi 2004; Cloud & Jinnah 2010; Jankovic 2013).

Summary

This review is unfortunately based on scarce data, with good evidence for only some of the mentioned drugs, lack of sound scientific insight for a majority of them and without enough sufficiently large, randomised controlled trials (Balash & Giladi 2004; Albanese et al. 2011). With these caveats, medical treatment remains an integral part of the modern approach combining drugs, physiotherapy, BT therapy and functional neurosurgery, allowing most patients with dystonia to live independently and enjoy an acceptable quality of life.

References

Albanese A, Asmus F, Bhatia KP, Elia AE, Elibol B, Filippini G, Gasser T, Krauss JK, Nardocci N, Newton A, Valls-Solé J (2011) EFNS guidelines on diagnosis and treatment of primary dystonias. *Eur J Neurol* 18: 5–18.

Balash Y, Giladi N (2004) Efficacy of pharmacological treatment of dystonia: evidence-based review including meta-analysis of the effect of botulinum toxin and other cure options. *Eur J Neurol* 11: 361–370.

Burke RE, Fahn S, Marsden C (1986) Torsion dystonia: a double-blind, prospective trial of high-dosage trihexyphenidyl. *Neurology* 36: 160–164.

Chen JJ, Ondo WG, Dashtipour K, Swope DM (2012) Tetrabenazine for the treatment of hyperkinetic movement disorders: a review of the literature. *Clin Therapeutics* 7: 1487–1504.

Cloud LJ, Jinnah HA (2010) Treatment strategies for dystonia. *Expert Opin Pharmacotherap* 11: 5–15.

Consroe P, Sandyk R, Snider SR (1986) Open label evaluation of cannabidiol in dystonic movement disorders. *Int J Neurosci* 30: 277–282.

Delnooz CCS, van de Warrenburg BPC (2012) Current and future medical treatment in primary dystonia. *Ther Adv Neurol Disord* 5: 221–240.

Dressler D, Altenmueller E, Bhidayasiri R, Boholega S, Chana P, Chung TM, Frucht S, Garcia-Ruiz PJ, Kaelin A, Kaji R, Kanovsky P, Laskawi R, Micheli F, Orlova O, Relja M, Rosales R, Slawek J, Timerbaeva S, Warner TT, Adib Saberi F (2015a) Strategies for treatment of dystonia. *J Neural Transm* 123: 251–258.

Dressler D, Berweck S, Chatzikalfas A, Ebke M, Frank B, Hesse S, Huber M, Krauss JK, Mücke K-H, Nolte A, Oelmann H-D, Schönle PW, Schmutzler M, Pickenbrock H, Van der Ven C, Veelken N, Vogel M, Vogt T, Adib Saberi F (2015b) Intrathecal baclofen therapy in Germany: proceedings of the IAB-Interdisciplinary Working Group for Movement Disorders consensus meeting. *J Neural Transm* 122:1573–1579.

Fox SH, Kellett M, Moore AP, Crossman AR, Brotchie JM (2002) Randomised, double blind, placebo-controlled trial to assess the potential of cannabinoid receptor stimulation in the treatment of dystonia. *Mov Disord* 17:145–149.

Grassi E, Latorraca S, Piacentini S, Marini P, Sorbi S (2000) Risperidone in idiopathic and symptomatic dystonia: preliminary experience. *Neurol Sci* 21:121–123.

Greene P (1992) Baclofen in the treatment of dystonia. *Clin Neuropharmacol* 15: 276–288.

Greene P, Shale H, Fahn S (1988) Analysis of open-label trials in torsion dystonia using high dosages of anticholinergics and other drugs. *Mov Disord* 3: 46–60.

Isgreen WP (1976) Carbamazepine in torsion dystonia. *Adv Neurol* 14: 411–416.

Jankovic J (2006) Treatment of dystonia. *Lancet Neurol* 5: 864–872.

Jankovic J (2009) Treatment of hyperkinetic movement disorders. *Lancet Neurol* 8: 844–855.

Jankovic J (2013) Medical treatment of dystonia. *Mov Disord* 28: 1001–1012.

Kluger B, Triolo P, Jones W, Jankovic J (2015) The therapeutic potential of cannabinoids for movement disorders. *Mov Disord* 30: 313–327.

Koppel BS, Brust JC, Fife T, Bronstein J, Youssof S, Gronseth G, Gloss D (2014) Systematic review: efficacy and safety of medical marijuana in selected neurologic disorders. *Neurology* 82: 1556–1563.

Lang AE (1988) Dopamine agonists and antagonists in treatment of idiopathic dystonia. *Adv Neurol* 50: 561–570.

Lin JJ, Chang DC (2004) Improvement of generalized dystonia by olanzapine treatment. *J Clin Neurosci* 11: 84–86.

Lucetti C, Nuti A, Gambaccini G, Bernardini S, Brotini S, Manca ML, Bonuccelli U (2000) Mexiletine in the treatment of torticollis and generalized dystonia. *Clin Neuropharmacol* 23: 186–189.

Marsden CD, Marion MH, Quinn N (1984) The treatment of severe dystonia in children and adults. *J Neurol Neurosurg Psychiatry* 47: 1166–1173.

Nutt JG, Hammerstad JP, Carter JH, deGarmo PL (1985) Lisuride treatment of focal dystonias. *Neurology* 35: 1242–1243.

Thiel A, Dressler D, Kistel C, Rüther E (1994) Clozapine treatment of spasmodic torticollis. *Neurology* 44: 957–958.

van der Plus AA, Schilder JC, Marinus J, van Hilten JJ (2013) An explanatory study evaluating the muscle relaxant effects of intramuscular magnesium sulphate for dystonia in complex regional pain syndrome. *J Pain* 14: 1341–1348.

Zuddas A, Cianchetti C (1996) Efficacy of risperidone in idiopathic segmental dystonia. *Lancet* 347: 127–128.

Chapter 53

Anticholinergics in the Treatment of Dystonia

Michel Sáenz-Farret and Federico Micheli

Introduction

Anticholinergic drugs have been used to treat dystonia for many years. Most of the studies in the literature have analysed dystonia from the perspectives of mixed aetiologies and distribution patterns. Despite frequent adverse effects in adults, younger patients have benefited more from anticholinergics. With the introduction of botulinum toxin in the treatment of focal and segmental dystonia, this class of drugs is now widely used in the treatment of generalised dystonia. Interestingly, recent studies have focused on the use of anticholinergics for dystonia secondary to cerebral palsy.

Pathophysiology

The exact functional mechanism of anticholinergic drugs for dystonia remains unknown, but evidence from dystonia patients as well as from animal models of dystonia suggest a crucial role for the striatal cholinergic system in the pathophysiology of this disorder. Broad-spectrum muscarinic receptor antagonists, including pirenzepine, trihexyphenidyl, biperiden and orphenadrine, were initially used in the treatment of diverse movement disorders including dystonia.

Both subtypes of acetylcholine receptors (nicotinic and muscarinic) are expressed throughout the striatum on different populations of neurons. Muscarinic acetylcholine receptors (mAChRs) are a family of five G protein-coupled receptors consisting of two major groups: M1-like (M1, M3 and M5) and M2-like receptors (M2 and M4), with the highest levels being the M4 and M1 receptor subtypes, respectively. Nicotinic acetylcholine receptors modulate dopamine release and two subfamilies of subunits have been cloned: an alpha family (α2–α10) and a beta family (β2–β4). The most common type of nicotinic receptor in the striatum is of the α4(non-α6)β2* type, though the α5, α6 and β3 subunits are also expressed at lower levels (Eskow Jaunarajs et al. 2015). The effect of anticholinergic drugs is believed to be mediated through the blockage of muscarinic acetylcholine receptors, thus restoring the imbalance between striatal dopamine and acetylcholine, both involved in the pathophysiology of dystonia (Pisani et al. 2007).

DYT1 dystonia mice models show a significant impairment of corticostriatal synaptic plasticity overexpressing mutant torsinA (Martella et al. 2009). In one study, the novel selective M1 mAChR antagonist VU0255035 rescued striatal synaptic plasticity deficits, providing a potential mechanistic rationale for the development of improved antimuscarinic therapies for this movement disorder (Maltese et al. 2014). Since the M1 muscarinic receptor antagonism has been demonstrated to offset synaptic plasticity deficits in the striatum of mice with the DYT1 dystonia mutation, there is a possible explanation for the development of improved antimuscarinic therapies for this dystonia. Conversely, the non-selective antagonist orphenadrine produces only a partial rescue of synaptic plasticity, whereas biperiden and ethopropazine fail to restore plasticity (Maltese et al. 2014).

Trihexyphenidyl

Fahn was the first to report on the beneficial effect of trihexyphenidyl in children with generalised dystonia. He confirmed this observation afterwards in juvenile and adult dystonia of various aetiologies and distribution patterns (Fahn 1983). Burke et al. conducted a double-blind placebo-controlled crossover trial of a high dosage of trihexyphenidyl for primary torsion dystonia and some forms of secondary dystonia. They included 31 young patients (32 years or younger) with mostly (19/31) generalised dystonia, but also brachial dystonia (8/31), hemidystonia (2/31), focal (1/31) and multifocal (1/31) dystonia. Medication was increased weekly by 5 mg daily until 30 mg per day was reached. The difference in the median Dystonic Movements Scale (DMS) score between the placebo and treatment arms (27 vs 14) was significant at 36 weeks ($p = 0.005$). After a mean follow-up of 2.4 years, 68 per cent of patients continued to take trihexyphenidyl and 42 per cent continued to show a considerable or dramatic benefit (Burke et al. 1986). Possibly, some patients with secondary dystonia showed less benefit. In a further study, none of the nine patients with symptomatic dystonia improved more than mildly and most had no benefit despite the use of high doses (Lang 1986).

Exploring the predictors of treatment success, an analysis of open-label trihexyphenidyl trials for torsion dystonia revealed that benefits from anticholinergics were most likely when treatment began within five years after dystonia onset. In this study, patients with symptomatic dystonia after anoxic birth injury showed more benefit than all other patients, including those with other secondary dystonias (Greene et al. 1988).

Trihexyphenidyl in Dystonia Secondary to Cerebral Palsy

Recent studies have focused on anticholinergics for the treatment of the dyskinetic cerebral palsy, the second most common form of this condition which comprises 15–20 per cent of patients with dystonia (Albright 1996). The rationale for the use of anticholinergics comes from animal models of hypoxic-ischaemic brain injury where the relative preservation of cholinergic neurons in the striatum as compared to surviving dopaminergic neurons creates an imbalance between these neurotransmitters (Kostic et al. 1991). Trihexyphenidyl restores this balance by reducing cholinergic transmission (Sanger et al. 2007).

Trihexyphenidyl also reduces sialorrhoea, affecting 10–58 per cent of children with cerebral palsy (Van der Burg et al. 2006). Thus, Sanger et al. conducted a prospective multicentre pilot trial using high doses of trihexyphenidyl (0.25 mg/kg three times per day) in children aged 4–15 years with cerebral palsy and dystonia affecting function in the dominant upper extremity. All of the 23 children completing the study showed a significant improvement in arm function at 15 weeks ($p = 0.045$), but not at nine weeks ($p = 0.985$). Subsequent post hoc analysis identified a subgroup ($n = 10$) with an excess of involuntary movements who worsened at nine weeks ($p = 0.04$), but returned to baseline following a dose reduction. The authors concluded that the benefit of trihexyphenidyl in this setting remained questionable (Sanger et al. 2007).

A later randomised, double-blind, placebo-controlled, crossover trial evaluated the effect of high doses of trihexyphenidyl (2.5 mg/kg three times per day) in 16 children with cerebral palsy. The mean change for Barry–Albright dystonia score against placebo was 0.9 (−2.2 to 3.9). This pilot study demonstrated that high-dose trihexyphenidyl did not alter the severity of dystonia during the 12 weeks of treatment in a group of children with predominantly severe dystonic cerebral palsy. Even though the results were negative, a higher proportion of participants achieved their individualised goals while taking trihexyphenidyl when compared to placebo (Rice & Waugh 2009).

In contrast to these studies, a subsequent retrospective study found a positive clinical response in children with cerebral palsy and dystonia. The authors found a reduction of dystonia in the upper (59.4 per cent) and lower (37.6 per cent) limbs of participants and concluded that trihexyphenidyl should be started with low doses and gradually increased in a slow stepwise manner over several weeks to increase tolerability and allow for an often delayed beneficial response (Carranza-del Rio et al. 2011).

Because of these conflicting reports regarding the efficacy of trihexyphenidyl for dystonia in cerebral palsy, a retrospective analysis of 31 children (age 8.2 ± 5.8 years) with dystonia receiving high-dose trihexyphenidyl (>0.5 mg/kg per day) was performed. The main goal was to calculate the motor improvements in various affected body areas. Most (21/31) caregivers reported improvements in one or more areas, mainly in arm, hand and oromotor function. Improvement was greater in children without spasticity ($p = 0.02$) and in those with higher cognitive function ($p = 0.02$), indicating that trihexyphenidyl is effective particularly for children with those characteristics (Ben-Pazi 2011).

Other authors have pointed to another subgroup of patients with beneficial response to anticholinergics. In one retrospective study, a statistically significant relationship was found between age at initiation of therapy and selective improvements in upper extremity function as well as language. Earlier therapy produced greater improvement in language (face and jaw dystonia) and upper-limb function (Hoon et al. 2001).

Previously mentioned studies utilised different scales and were not designed for children. Considering that movement disorders in a developmental age are substantially different from those of adults, the MD-Childhood Rating Scale has been proposed as a useful scale for clinical trials in dyskinetic cerebral palsy patients undergoing anticholinergic treatment (Battini et al. 2014). The study introducing this scale found beneficial effects of trihexyphenidyl in this group of patients with dyskinetic cerebral palsy. Nevertheless, the aim of this study was not to test and prove the efficacy of trihexyphenidyl in cerebral palsy (Battini et al. 2014). Overall, it appears that anticholinergics are more likely to be effective in dystonic and other extrapyramidal forms of cerebral palsy (Vidailhet 2013).

Miscellaneous

Case reports have also shown beneficial effects of trihexyphenidyl in young patients with other secondary forms of dystonia, such as bilateral putaminal haemorrhage (Pidcock et al. 1999) and glutaryl-CoA dehydrogenase deficiency (Pidcock et al. 1999). Trihexyphenidyl was reported to be safe during two pregnancies in a patient with early-onset, sporadic, primary generalised dystonia (DYT1 negative) (Robottom & Reich 2011).

Adverse Effects

Anticholinergic adverse effects more frequently occur in adults, including dry mouth, blurred vision, constipation and urinary retention (Thenganatt & Jankovic 2014). Cognitive impairment, such as memory loss and delayed processing, are more likely to occur in older patients (Taylor et al. 1991). In order to avoid adverse effects, a practical recommendation is to start with trihexyphenidyl 1 mg twice daily and to slowly increase the dose over several weeks. Although some patients would probably respond to higher doses, dose-related adverse effects limit the usefulness of this therapy (Jankovic 2013). Usually, doses above 20 mg/d are not tolerated by adults. Adverse effects were more evident in older patients (Taylor et al. 1991).

Biperiden

Evidence for this drug is less than for other anticholinergics. In one study, biperiden was administered to six patients, ages ranging from 15 to 30 years. Five patients had generalised dystonia and one patient had segmental dystonia. All except one (anoxic birth) were of unknown origin. Biperiden was gradually increased to 40 mg/d within a few weeks. All patients had clinically significant responses scales and disability scores after a mean follow-up of 1.9 years. Three patients showed considerable or dramatic benefits. Doses of 40 mg/d were generally well tolerated (Oztekin et al. 1991).

In another study, the acute effects of intravenous injections of biperiden were investigated in 14 patients with various forms of dystonia (two with segmental dystonia, six with generalised dystonia, six with Meige syndrome). The authors reported that 5 mg of intravenous biperiden resulted in improved total and global scores lasting for several hours. The benefit was minor or non-existent in all three patients with secondary generalised dystonia (Povlsen & Pakkenberg 1990).

Diphenhydramine

Diphenhydramine is an antihistaminic with anticholinergic and antidystonic effects. One publication describes five patients with idiopathic truncal dystonia poorly responsive to conventional pharmacotherapies and subsequently benefiting from diphenhydramine 250–400 mg/d (Truong et al. 1995). In another study on five patients with generalised idiopathic torsion dystonia, one with secondary generalised dystonia and one with idiopathic segmental dystonia, all reported benefit (Granana et al. 1999). The role of histamine in dystonia was highlighted by one study showing increased dystonia when histamine was injected in the red nucleus in animal models (van't Groenewout et al. 1995).

Anticholinergics in Hemidystonia

Hemidystonia refers to ipsilateral dystonia of the face, arm and leg, usually contralateral to a structural lesion of the basal ganglia or thalamus (Pettigrew & Jankovic 1985). Chuang et al. analysed 33 cases to determine the most effective treatment strategies. Hemidystonia was due to stroke (ten patients), perinatal injury (nine patients), trauma (eight patients), infection (three patients), congenital lesions (two patients) and tumour (one patient). Anticholinergics were effective in 30 per cent of these patients. They also reviewed 107 cases in the literature and found that only 35 per cent of them improved with medical treatment. Anticholinergics were the most effective drugs with a beneficial response seen in 41 per cent of the cases (Chuang et al. 2002).

Cervical Dystonia

A subanalysis of an open-label trial of patients with cervical dystonia showed a trend towards an improved response in patients with milder disease severity and in those with tonic rather than kinetic forms. This trend, however, did not reach statistical significance (Greene et al. 1988). Older women also seemed to show a better response (Greene et al. 1988). Shorter disease duration and age of onset under 20 were also predictors of benefit (Greene et al. 1988). However, when compared to botulinum toxin in a prospective, randomised, double-blind controlled trial, trihexyphenidyl was significantly less effective in idiopathic cervical dystonia and had more adverse effects (Brans et al. 1996).

Dystonic Tremor

Dystonic tremor is usually defined as a postural and kinetic tremor presenting in a body region affected by dystonia (Deuschl 2003). A recent systematic review failed to find controlled or randomised studies on anticholinergics for this indication. Slight to moderate effects were seen in 16 patients with dystonic tremor of the hand or head (Fasano et al. 2014). However, in three studies of this systematic review, a total of five patients failed to achieve any benefit from anticholinergic treatment. Trihexyphenidyl 4–10 mg/d was the anticholinergic drug most commonly used (Rosenbaum & Jankovic 1988; Hughes et al. 1991; Schneider & Bhatia 2007).

Dystonia in Parkinson's Disease (PD)

Anticholinergic drugs have been reported to alleviate dystonic spasms resulting from chronic levodopa treatment, as in the case of early-morning dystonia in parkinsonian patients (Poewe et al. 1987). In one study, procyclidine was administered to nine PD patients with foot dystonia. In six patients dystonia was abolished and in one ameliorated. In the two remaining patients there was no effect (Poewe et al. 1988).

Conclusions

Trihexyphenidyl is the best studied anticholinergic drug for treatment of dystonia. As young patients tolerate higher doses of anticholinergics they benefit most from this treatment. Improved scales for the assessment of dystonia will further clarify the effects of these compounds.

References

Albright AL (1996) Spasticity and movement disorders in cerebral palsy. *J Child Neurol* 11(Suppl. 1), S1–4.

Battini R, Casarano M, Sgandurra G, Olivieri I, Di Pietro R, Romeo DM, Mercuri E, Cioni G (2014) Responsiveness of the MD-childhood rating scale in dyskinetic cerebral palsy patients undergoing anticholinergic treatment. *Eur J Paediatr Neurol* 18, 698–703.

Ben-Pazi H (2011) Trihexyphenidyl improves motor function in children with dystonic cerebral palsy: a retrospective analysis. *J Child Neurol* 26, 810–816.

Brans JW, Lindeboom R, Snoek JW, Zwarts MJ, van Weerden TW, Brunt ER, van Hilten JJ, van der Kamp W, Prins MH, Speelman JD (1996) Botulinum toxin versus trihexyphenidyl in cervical dystonia: a prospective, randomized, double-blind controlled trial. *Neurology* 46, 1066–1072.

Burke RE, Fahn S, Marsden CD (1986) Torsion dystonia: a double-blind, prospective trial of high-dosage trihexyphenidyl. *Neurology* 36, 160–164.

Carranza-del Rio J, Clegg NJ, Moore A, Delgado MR (2011) Use of trihexyphenidyl in children with cerebral palsy. *Pediatr Neurol* 44, 202–206.

Chuang C, Fahn S, Frucht SJ (2002) The natural history and treatment of acquired hemidystonia: report of 33 cases and review of the literature. *J Neurol Neurosurg Psychiatry* 72, 59–67.

Deuschl G (2003) Dystonic tremor. *Rev Neurol (Paris)* 159, 900–905.

Eskow Jaunarajs KL, Bonsi P, Chesselet MF, Standaert DG, Pisani A (2015) Striatal cholinergic dysfunction as a unifying theme in the pathophysiology of dystonia. *Prog Neurobiol* 127–128C, 91–107.

Fahn S (1983) High dosage anticholinergic therapy in dystonia. *Neurology* 33, 1255–1261.

Fasano A, Bove F, Lang AE (2014) The treatment of dystonic tremor: a systematic review. *J Neurol Neurosurg Psychiatry* 85, 759–769.

Granana N, Ferrea M, Scorticati MC, Diaz S, Arrebola M, Torres L, Micheli F (1999) Beneficial effects of diphenhydramine in dystonia. *Medicina (B Aires)* 59, 38–42.

Greene P, Shale H, Fahn S (1988) Analysis of open-label trials in torsion dystonia using high dosages of anticholinergics and other drugs. *Mov Disord* 3, 46–60.

Hoon AH, Jr, Freese PO, Reinhardt EM, Wilson MA, Lawrie WT, Jr, Harryman SE, Pidcock FS, Johnston MV (2001) Age-dependent effects of trihexyphenidyl in extrapyramidal cerebral palsy. *Pediatr Neurol* 25, 55–58.

Hughes AJ, Lees AJ, Marsden CD (1991) Paroxysmal dystonic head tremor. *Mov Disord* 6, 85–86.

Jankovic J (2013) Medical treatment of dystonia. *Mov Disord* 28, 1001–1012.

Kostic V, Przedborski S, Jackson-Lewis V, Cadet JL, Burke RE (1991) Effect of unilateral perinatal hypoxic-ischemic brain injury in the rat on striatal muscarinic cholinergic receptors and high-affinity choline uptake sites: a quantitative autoradiographic study. *J Neurochem* 57, 1962–1970.

Lang AE (1986) High dose anticholinergic therapy in adult dystonia. *Can J Neurol Sci* 13, 42–46.

Maltese M, Martella G, Madeo G, Fagiolo I, Tassone A, Ponterio G, Sciamanna G, Burbaud P, Conn, PJ, Bonsi P, Pisani A (2014). Anticholinergic drugs rescue synaptic plasticity in DYT1 dystonia: role of M1 muscarinic receptors. *Mov Disord* 29, 1655–1665.

Martella G, Tassone A, Sciamanna G, Platania P, Cuomo D, Viscomi MT, Bonsi P, Cacci E, Biagioni S, Usiello A, Bernardi G, Sharma N, Standaert DG, Pisani A (2009) Impairment of bidirectional synaptic plasticity in the striatum of a mouse model of DYT1 dystonia: role of endogenous acetylcholine. *Brain* 132, 2336–2349.

Oztekin NS, Saygi SS, Dalkara T, Senses I, Zileli T (1991) High dose anticholinergic therapy (biperiden) in dystonia. *Clin Neurol Neurosurg* 93, 35–37.

Pettigrew LC, Jankovic J (1985) Hemidystonia: a report of 22 patients and a review of the literature. *J Neurol Neurosurg Psychiatry* 48, 650–657.

Pidcock FS, Hoon AH, Jr, Johnston MV (1999) Trihexyphenidyl in posthemorrhagic dystonia: motor and language effects. *Pediatr Neurol* 20, 219–222.

Pisani A, Bernardi G, Ding J, Surmeier DJ (2007) Re-emergence of striatal cholinergic interneurons in movement disorders. *Trends Neurosci* 30, 545–553.

Poewe W, Lees AJ, Steiger D, Stern GM (1987) Foot dystonia in Parkinson's disease: clinical phenomenology and neuropharmacology. *Adv Neurol* 45, 357–360.

Poewe WH, Lees AJ, Stern GM (1988) Dystonia in Parkinson's disease: clinical and pharmacological features. *Ann Neurol* 23, 73–78.

Povlsen UJ, Pakkenberg H (1990) Effect of intravenous injection of biperiden and clonazepam in dystonia. *Mov Disord* 5, 27–31.

Rice J, Waugh MC (2009) Pilot study on trihexyphenidyl in the treatment of dystonia in children with cerebral palsy. *J Child Neurol* 24, 176–182.

Robottom BJ, Reich SG (2011) Exposure to high dosage trihexyphenidyl during pregnancy for treatment of generalized dystonia: case report and literature review. *Neurologist* 17, 340–341.

Rosenbaum F, Jankovic J (1988) Focal task-specific tremor and dystonia: categorization of occupational movement disorders. *Neurology* 38, 522–527.

Sanger TD, Bastian A, Brunstrom J, Damiano D, Delgado M, Dure L, Gaebler-Spira D, Hoon A, Mink JW, Sherman-Levine S, Welty LJ, Child Motor Study Group (2007) Prospective open-label clinical trial of trihexyphenidyl in children with secondary dystonia due to cerebral palsy. *J Child Neurol* 22, 530–537.

Schneider SA, Bhatia KP (2007) The entity of jaw tremor and dystonia. *Mov Disord* 22, 1491–1495.

Taylor AE, Lang AE, Saint-Cyr, JA, Riley DE, Ranawaya R (1991) Cognitive processes in idiopathic dystonia treated with high-dose anticholinergic therapy: implications for treatment strategies. *Clin Neuropharmacol* 14, 62–77.

Thenganatt MA, Jankovic J (2014) Treatment of dystonia. *Neurotherapeutics* 11, 139–152.

Truong DD, Sandroni P, van den Noort S, Matsumoto RR (1995). Diphenhydramine is effective in the treatment of idiopathic dystonia. *Arch Neurol* 52, 405–407.

Van der Burg JJ, Jongerius PH, Van Hulst K, Van Limbeek J, Rotteveel JJ (2006) Drooling in children with cerebral palsy: effect of salivary flow reduction on daily life and care. *Dev Med Child Neurol* 48, 103–107.

van't Groenewout JL, Stone MR, Vo VN, Truong DD, Matsumoto RR (1995) Evidence for the involvement of histamine in the antidystonic effects of diphenhydramine. *Exp Neurol* 134, 253–260.

Vidailhet M (2013) Treatment of movement disorders in dystonia-choreoathtosis cerebral palsy. *Handb Clin Neurol* 111, 197–202.

Chapter 54

Tetrabenazine for the Treatment of Dystonia

Christoph Schrader and Saeed A. Bohlega

Introduction

Tetrabenazine (TBZ) is a monoamine-depleting agent mainly acting on dopaminergic terminals within the CNS. It was first introduced in the 1960s as an antipsychotic. Subsequently, it was found to be beneficial in hyperkinetic movement disorders with a better tolerability in terms of extrapyramidal side-effects when compared to neuroleptics. To date, several reports have suggested that TBZ ameliorates hyperkinetic movement disorders; the more phasic the movement, the better the clinical effect. The best data regarding its efficacy are available on chorea in Huntington's disease (HD) (Huntington Study Group 2006; Frank et al. 2008). In fact, it is the only drug that has been shown to be efficacious in suppressing chorea in HD. However, the number of controlled studies for other hyperkinetic movement disorders is very scarce, possibly because the drug is not registered in most countries. This chapter focuses on TBZ and its efficacy in dystonia.

Pharmacology

Tetrabenazine (Ro 1-9569) is a benzoquinoline derivative with the systematic name 3-isobutyl-9,10-dimethoxy-1,3,4,6,7,11b-hexahydro-2H-pyrido[2,1-a]isoquinoline-2-one (Figure 54.1). When given orally, at least 75 per cent of TBZ is rapidly absorbed within one hour. However, the systemic bioavailability of the parent drug is low (5 per cent) due to a high first-pass metabolism by hepatic carbonyl reductase to at least two isomers of dihydrotetrabenazine (DHTBZ), namely a-DHTBZ and b-DHTBZ, of which a-DHTBZ exerts its effect on the striatum. The half-life of a- and b-DHTBZ is individually highly variable and ranges from two to eight hours and two to five hours, respectively (Schrader et al. 2010).

When using clinically typical doses of TBZ between 37.5 and 112.5 mg/d, its kinetics are linear. Meals have no influence on mean plasma concentration or C_{max}. These properties enable the clinician to evaluate its efficacy within 2–3 days. A clinically stable effect is reached after seven days (Schrader et al. 2010).

Mechanism of Action

The monoamines dopamine, norepinephrine and serotonin are synthesised within the neuronal cytoplasm and stored in vesicles (Figure 54.2a). After secretion into the synaptic cleft, the reuptake is mediated by specific monoamine transporters for dopamine (DAT), norepinephrine (NART) and serotonin (SERT). Once in the presynaptic nerve terminal, the monoamines are transported into vesicles again by various vesicular monoamine transporters (VMATs). There are two isoforms of VMAT: VMAT1 is expressed primarily outside the brain, namely in peripheral endocrine and paracrine cells, while VMAT2 is expressed mainly within the brain (Schrader et al. 2010).

TBZ and its active metabolites have two mechanisms of action (Figure 54.2b): first, they bind reversibly to VMAT2 and thereby inhibit competitively the translocation of monoamines into presynaptic vesicles leading to an increased premature degradation of monoamines by cytoplasmatic monoamine oxidases (MAO). Even though TBZ is known as a 'monoamine depletor', it more accurately is a monoamine storage inhibitor (Schrader et al. 2010).

Apart from that, TBZ also blocks postsynaptic D2 receptors. *In vitro* studies found a K_i of approximately 2.1×10^{-6} M. However, its D2 affinity is 1000-fold lower than its VMAT2 affinity. Furthermore, TBZ only weakly inhibits the pharmacologic action of apomorphine, a dopamine agonist. This weak D2 receptor inhibition may be the reason for the practically lacking risk of tardive dyskinesia (TDK). Acute dystonic reactions have been described, but are extremely rare.

Unlike reserpine, TBZ inhibits only VMAT2, but not VMAT1 in the peripheral nervous system, so the typical side-effects of reserpine (i.e. hypotonia, epigastric pain, erectile dysfunction, nasal congestion and diarrhoea) are lacking. Furthermore, TBZ binds to VMAT2 reversibly and has a shorter half-life, making it a safe and a quite easy to handle drug.

Clinical Indications

Two recent double-blind, placebo-controlled studies confirmed the efficacy of TBZ in the treatment of HD chorea (Huntington Study Group 2006; Frank et al. 2008). Acute adverse events (AEs) associated with TBZ are similar to those seen with other neuroleptics, including sedation, parkinsonism, depression and akathisia. However, unlike in neuroleptics, TDK is extremely unlikely: within the last 50 years there is just one reported case (LeWitt 2013). This is a major advantage of TBZ over typical neuroleptics, as up to 25 per cent of those chronically treated with these dopamine receptor-blocking drugs eventually develop TDK. Even the newer 'atypical' neuroleptics have been reported to have a TDK risk (Jankovic 1995), and this may increase with more chronic exposure.

Efficacy in Dystonia

Oral therapy of dystonia is often frustrating: most commonly, anticholinergic agents and muscle relaxants are used. However, frequent and severe adverse effects limit their efficacy in many cases. Nine studies assessed the efficacy of TBZ in various types of dystonia. Two of them have employed a prospective placebo arm, but have included only a small number of patients. The efficacy was equivocal: Asher and colleagues found marked or moderate improvement only in 25 per cent and no change in 50 per cent of treated patients (Asher & Aminoff 1981); Jankovic found TBZ to be more efficacious: 62 per cent improved, while no response or worsening was observed in 16 per cent each (Jankovic 1982). Of all studies on TBZ in dystonia, the latter used the most objective and standardised assessment. Of the retrospective studies, four reported a beneficial effect of TBZ for a variety of dystonias. In a retrospective study, Jankovic and Beach reported results of TBZ therapy in 400 paediatric and adult patients with severe hyperkinetic movement disorders. Within this cohort, 190 patients had various dystonias (idiopathic cranial, cervical and generalised dystonic disorders, tardive dystonias). Clinical response to TBZ was rated on a global response scale (GRS) from 1 to 5 (with 1 meaning 'marked reduction in abnormal movements and excellent improvement in function' and 5 meaning 'worsening of movement disorders, deterioration in function, or both'). Of the patients with idiopathic dystonia (47 with cranial distribution, 41 generalised and 20 cervical), there was no difference in TBZ effectiveness based on affected area of dystonia (p-values not reported). Patients with tardive dystonia showed more of an improvement

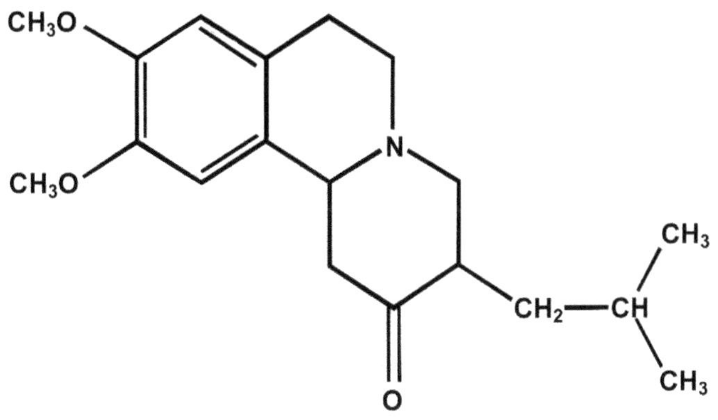

Figure 54.1 Tetrabenazine chemical structure.

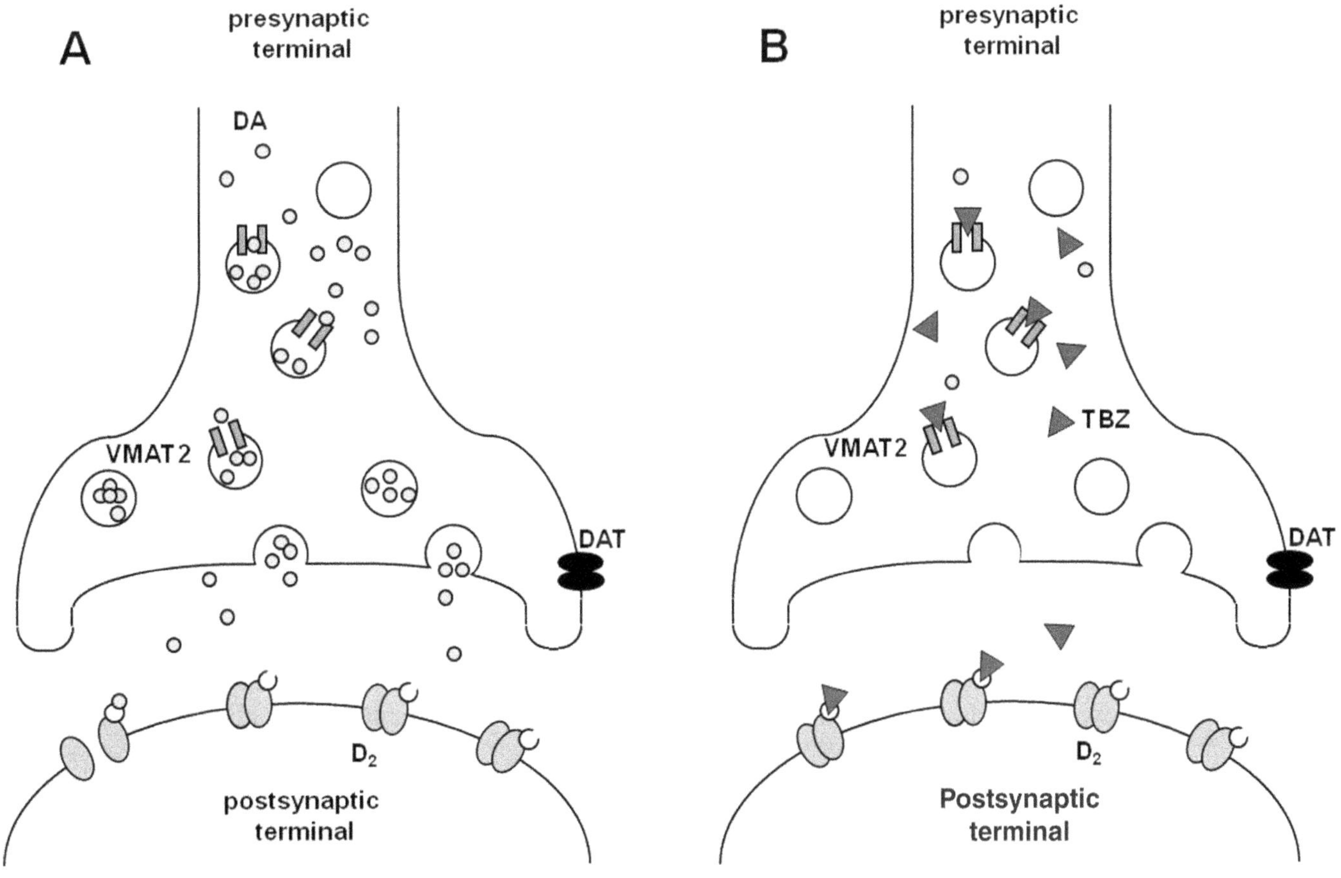

Figure 54.2 Tetrabenazine mechanism of action. (a) DA is stored in vesicles, which merge with the synaptic membrane and thereby excrete DA into the synaptic cleft. After binding to the D2 receptor, DA is re-uptaken into the presynaptic terminal via DAT and then stored in vesicles by VMAT2. (b) TBZ binds reversibly to VMAT2 and thereby inhibits the presynaptic storage of MA, which then are degraded by cytosolic MAO. It thus leads – indirectly – to MA depletion. Furthermore, TBZ inhibits the postsynaptic D2 receptor. D2, dopamine-2 receptor; DA, dopamine; DAT, dopamine transporter; MA, monoamines; MAOs, monoamine oxidases; TBZ, tetrabenazine; VMAT2, vesicular monoamine transporter.

than those with idiopathic dystonia and the antidystonic effect wore off especially in the dystonia group: 45 per cent of dystonia patients had a remarkable response, but 73 per cent of TD patients benefited markedly at last follow-up (Jankovic & Beach 1997). In another retrospective study by the same authors using the same assessment, 31 per cent of patients with dystonia experienced moderate to marked improvement, but 53 per cent of TD patients had a response of at least moderate or better. In this study, the data of patients with dystonia were analysed according to the type of dystonia: patients with generalised dystonia responded better than focal or cranial dystonia, and blepharospasm patients did not have a marked or moderate improvement at all. One important finding was that choreatic movements are more amenable than others (Jankovic & Orman 1988), which was described before (Swash et al. 1972; Asher & Aminoff 1981) and confirmed in later studies (Paleacu et al. 2004; Kenney et al. 2007).

Overall, the evidence from studies on the efficacy of TBZ in dystonia is small and weak, but TBZ seems to have some efficacy for dystonia, being most efficacious for TD (maybe because it often goes along with repetitive phasic movements and least efficacious in very tonic forms of dystonia. On the other hand, as other oral strategies (i.e. anticholinergics, muscle relaxants, whose evidence is no better) are limited by their adverse effects, TBZ could be considered as an alternate treatment option. In one systematic review on dystonic tremor, it is recommended as a second-line therapy despite weak evidence (Fasano et al. 2014). So finally, additional double-blind, placebo-controlled studies are warranted to better characterise TBZ efficacy against other agents as well as to better characterise efficacy in the various types of dystonia (e.g. generalised, segmental, focal).

Efficacy in Tardive Dyskinesia

Tardive dyskinesia is a persistent drug-induced hyperkinetic movement disorder that is most commonly associated with use of central dopamine receptor-blocking agents (e.g. metoclopramide, neuroleptic agents). The term emphasises the delayed ('tardive') onset of choreathetoid, stereotypic movements. Management of TDK is challenging and in a meta-analysis of 45 randomised, placebo-controlled trials, no single agent was identified as a definitive therapy for TDK (Soares-Weiser & Fernandez 2007). Table 54.2 summarises the results of 11 TBZ studies in TDK. Most studies were either retrospective analyses or prospective trials with small numbers of patients. Only two studies report statistics. The biggest disadvantages are that studies employed assessment tools that were not standardised or assessments were done with the bias of subjectivity (Godwin-Austen 1979; Asher & Aminoff 1981; Jankovic & Orman 1988; Watson et al. 1988; Jankovic & Beach 1997; Paleacu et al. 2004; Kenney et al. 2007). However, 9 of these 11 studies reported that TBZ is efficacious in TDK. The largest prospective, single-blind study enrolled 20 patients with a mean age of 65.2 ± 10.8 years and a mean TDK duration 43.7 ± 47.1 months. Patients were videotaped before and after receiving TBZ. Videotapes were blindly assessed in a randomised manner using the Abnormal Involuntary Movement Scale (AIMS). The mean duration of TBZ treatment was 20.3 ± 10.4 weeks and the mean dose was 57.9 ± 22.8 mg/d. The mean score on the AIMS motor subset (questions 1–7) improved by 54.2 per cent from pretreatment ($p = 0.001$) and the subjective scores (questions 8–10) improved by 60.4 per cent ($p = 0.001$). Seventeen patients rated themselves as markedly or moderately improved (assessed by using the GRS). In this study, TBZ provided clinically and statistically significant improvements. In the two largest retrospective studies of patients with various hyperkinetic movement disorders, the effect of TBZ was reported in a subset total of 242 adult patients with TDK. In one study on 149 patients with TDK, TBZ markedly or moderately improved symptoms in 84 per cent of patients. In the other study of 94 adults with TDK, TBZ improved symptoms in approximately 89 per cent of patients. However, the assessment tool (namely the GRS) was somewhat subjective and did not exactly measure the extent of improvement. The results of these and smaller studies are also summarised in Table 54.2.

When compared to other types of dystonia, TDK seems to yield a higher benefit from TBZ. This may be ascribed to the often more phasic and stereotypic nature of the movements in TDK. In fact, TBZ should be deemed an option in TDK, since it is otherwise hard to manage. However, additional randomised, placebo-controlled studies are warranted.

Dosing and Safety Issues

Dosing of TBZ is very individual and needs to be titrated to the lowest tolerable dose that controls symptoms. The considerable inter-individual dose–response variability is possibly due to differences in carbonyl reductase and CYP2D6 metabolic activity. In the studies for dystonia and TDK, TBZ was used with a therapeutic daily dose ranging from 12.5 to 300 mg. The manufacturer recommends a starting dose of 12.5 mg once daily, with weekly titration by 12.5 mg. For doses >37.5 mg, administration should be divided into three doses. The maximum recommended daily dose according to the manufacturer is 100 mg. For patients who require daily doses >50 mg, the manufacturer recommends obtaining CYP2D6 genotyping, even though no published research has been found on the correlation of CYP2D6 genotyping and TBZ dose response.

Overall, TBZ is well tolerated, although fatalities and severe reactions (e.g. hyperthermia, neuroleptic malignant syndrome, severe dysphagia, suicide) have been reported. In clinical studies and in clinical practice, TBZ nowadays is initiated at a subtherapeutic dose and titrated to a dose that provides the best efficacy with tolerable adverse effects. Typical side-effects are listed in Table 54.3. Dose-limiting AEs occur with a likelihood of 10–30 per cent, with the most common being somnolence, insomnia, fatigue, depression, akathisia, anxiety, nausea and parkinsonism. Elderly patients with baseline striatal dopamine deficiency may be at greater risk for experiencing TBZ-induced parkinsonism and patients with a history of depression may be at greater risk of TBZ-induced depression. TBZ can increase the risk of depression and suicidality: in a study of 246 patients with no history of depression, 11.4 per cent developed

Table 54.1 Studies on tetrabenazine in dystonia

Author	Study design	Patients (*n*)	Type of dystonia	Assessment tool	Dose (mg/d)	Outcome	Remarks
Swash et al. 1972	Prospective single observational study	8	3 TC 5 GD	CGIC of seven observers	128 (75–200)	3/8 improved	Choreatic, phasic movements improve better and more quickly, athetoid and tonic movement improve little
Asher & Aminoff 1981	Prospective single-blind randomised placebo-controlled crossover	8	3 TC 2 cranial 3 GD	GCIC of two observers	175 (range not specified)	Marked or moderate improved: TC 1/3; cranial 0/2; GD 1/3 No change: TC + cranial 3/5; GD 1/3	In general more helpful in chorea and very little in dystonic or athetotic states, appendicular symptoms are more responsive than midline symptoms. Only short-term study (three weeks)
Jankovic 1982	Prospective double-blind randomised placebo-controlled crossover	12	6 Meige 1 TC 5 GD	Hyperkinesia Rating Scale	162.5 50–200)	Improved: Meige 4/6; GD 3/5 No change: Meige 1/6; TC 1/1 Worsened: Meige 1/6; GD 1/5	No data on tonic versus phasic movements
Marsden et al. 1984	Retrospective observational	12	9 GD 3 GD (TD)	CGI of seven observers	90 (range not specified)	Dramatically improved: -2/12 Markedly improved: -4/12 Moderately improved: -3/12 Slightly improved: -1/12 No change: -2/12	TBZ in combination with pimozide and trihexyphendyl – no monotherapy!
Jankovic & Orman 1988	Retrospective observational	124	57 cranial 25 focal 19 GD 15 TD 5 BSP 3 hemi-dystonia	GRS	Cranial: 109 (37.5–250) Focal: 119 (75–250) GD: 114.5 (50–200) TD: 155.4 (75–250) BSP: 85 (75–100) Hemidystonia: 150	Markedly or moderately improved: Cranial 17/57; Focal 6/25; GD 10/19; TD 8/15; BSP 0/5; Hemidystonia 0/3 Mild or no response: Cranial 39/57; Focal 18/25; GD 9/19; TD 7/15; BSP 3/5	Choreatic movements are most amenable

(*continued*)

Table 54.1 (*continued*)

Author	Study design	Patients (*n*)	Type of dystonia	Assessment tool	Dose (mg/d)	Outcome	Remarks
Jankovic & Beach 1997	Retrospective observational	190	47 cranial 41 GD 10 TC 82 TD	GRS	Dystonia: 112 (25–400) TD: 97 (25–400)	Markedly improved: Dystonia 49/108; TD 60/82 Moderately improved: Dystonia 15/108; TD 8/82 Mildly improved: Dystonia 18/108; TD 7/82 No change: Dystonia 24/108; TD 7/82 Worsened: Dystonia 2/108	Efficacy slightly wears off especially in idiopathic dystonia
Paleacu et al. 2004	Retrospective observational	41	7 BSP 4 Meige 4 cranial 26 trunkal	CGIC of patients/ spouses	75 (25–175) Not specified for types of dystonia	Markedly or moderately improved: BSP: 2; Meige: 4; Cranial: 3; Trunkal: 9 Mild or no response: BSP: 4; Meige: 1; Cranial: 0; Trunkal: 11 Worsened: BSP: 0; Meige: 0 Cranial: 0; Trunkal: 5	Chorea regardless of which aetiology or facial dyskinesia/dystonia respond best
Kenney et al. 2007	Retrospective observational	132	Not specified	GRS	Not specified (12.5–300)	Markedly or moderately improved: ~ 68 per cent Mild or no response: ~ 27 per cent Worsened: ~ 5 per cent	43.9 per cent remained on TBZ (TD 60.4 per cent, chorea 63.3 per cent) TD and chorea generally respond better than tics, myoclonus or dystonia
Luciano et al. 2014	Prospective observational study	2	2 SGCE (DYT11)	BFMDRS, GDRS, UMRS	75	GDRS: decreased by 86 per cent BFMDRS: decreased by 52 per cent Myoclonus at rest: decreased by 92 per cent	Acute test, no long-term data, small sample size, myoclonus improved best

BFMDRS Burke–Fahn–Marsden Dystonia Rating Scale
BSP blepharospasm
GCIC global clinical impression of change
GD generalised dystonia
GDRS Global Dystonia Rating Scale
SGCE sarcoglycan epsilon
TBZ tetrabenazine
TC torticollis
TD tardive dystonia
UMRS unified myoclonus rating scale

Table 54.2 Studies on tetrabenazine in tardive dyskinesia

Author	Study design	Patients (*n*)	Assessment tool	Treatment daily dose (mg)	Outcome	Remarks
Godwin-Austen 1979	Prospective double-blind placebo-controlled crossover	6	Not exactly noted. 0–4 point scale	100	Complete remission: 3/6 Mildly/moderately improved: 2/6 No change: 1/6	Effective
Kazamatsuri et al. 1972	Prospective single-blind placebo-controlled crossover	24	Abnormal oral movements/min	122.5 (100–150)	Complete remission: 8/24 75–99 per cent less movements: 5/24 50–74 per cent less movements: 1/24 25–49 per cent less movements: 1/24 0–24 per cent less movements: 5/24 Dropouts: 4/24 Overall: reduction from 30 to 10 abnormal movements/min after 6 weeks	Effective
Kazamatsuri et al. 1973	Prospective single-blind placebo-controlled crossover	7	Abnormal oral movements/min	100 12 weeks 200 mg 6 weeks	100 mg: 50–99 per cent less movements: 2/7 0–49 per cent less movements: 5/7 200 mg: Complete remission 2/7 50–99 per cent disappearance 3/7 Dropouts: 2/7	Ineffective
Asher & Aminoff 1981	Prospective single-blind placebo-controlled crossover	10	GCIC of two observers	175 (range not specified)	Markedly/moderately improved: 6/10	Effective
Jankovic 1982	Prospective double-blind placebo-controlled crossover	4	Hyperkinesia Rating Scale	200	4/4 improved	Effective
Jankovic & Orman 1988	Retrospective observational	44	GRS	97.4 (25–200)	Markedly/moderately improved: 31/44, Mild or no response: 12/44	Effective
Watson et al. 1988	Prospective observational	23	CGCI	91.3 [?]	100 per cent improved	Effective
Jankovic & Beach 1997	Retrospective observational	94	GRS	96.9 (25–400)	Markedly/moderately improved: 86/94, Mild or no response: 6/94	Effective
Ondo et al. 1999	Prospective observational	19	AIMS	57.9 (range not specified)	AIMS – 54.2 per cent (17.9 ± 4.4 ≥ 8.2 ± 5.3) Markedly/moderately improved: 17/19 Mildly improved: 2/19	Effective
Paleacu et al. 2004	Retrospective observational	17	CGIC of patients/spouses	Not specified, 75 (25–125 in the whole study)	Markedly/moderately improved: 7/17 Mild or no response: 7/17 Worsening: 1/17 Dropout: 2/17	Ineffective?
Kenney et al. 2007	Retrospective observational	149	GRS	Not specified (12.5–300 in the whole study)	Markedly/moderately improved: ~84 per cent Mild/no response: ~11 per cent Worsening: ~ 5 per cent	Effective

AIMS Abnormal Involuntary Movement Scale
GCIC global clinical impression of change
GD generalised dystonia
GRS global Response Scale

Table 54.3 Side-effects of tetrabenazine in 400 patients with various movement disorders (Jankovic & Beach 1997)

Side-effects	%
Fatigue/somnolence	37
Parkinsonism	30
Depression	15
Insomnia	11
Nervousness/anxiety	10
Akathisia	10
Nausea/emesis	5
Dystonic reactions/oculogyric crisis	3
Tremor	3
Delirium	2
Orthostatic hypotension	3
Zombie-like feeling, sedation	1
Postural instability	1
Dizziness	1
Diarrhoea	<1
Headache	<1
Hallucinations	<1
Paraesthesia	<1
Pharyngeal spasms/pain	<1
Blurred vision	<1
Panic attacks	<1
Dysphagia	<1
Paranoia	<1

depression while taking TBZ. Of the 272 patients with a documented history of depression, 18.4 per cent experienced an exacerbation of depression (Kenney et al. 2006). Being on antidepressants probably prevents a worsening of depressed mood when starting TBZ, so before the initiation of TBZ therapy, patients should be screened and treated for depression when warranted.

Conclusions

TBZ has been studied in paediatric and adult populations. The best data are available for HD. However, for dystonia and TDK, only a small number of studies are randomised and controlled, with the majority of data derived from retrospective studies suggesting a mild to moderate efficacy. In our experience, it is most promising in dystonia displaying predominantly phasic, repetitive movements, while it is not very effective in tonic movements. The common adverse effects of TBZ include somnolence, insomnia, fatigue, depression, akathisia, anxiety, nausea and parkinsonism. Concomitant depression should be treated before initiation of TBZ, and the dose must be titrated properly with monitoring.

References

Asher SW, Aminoff MJ (1981). Tetrabenazine and movement disorders. *Neurology* 31:1051–1054.

Fasano A, Bove F, Lang AE (2014). The treatment of dystonic tremor: a systematic review. *J Neurol Neurosurg Psychiatry* 85:759–769.

Frank S, Ondo W, Fahn S, Hunter C, Oakes D, Plumb S, Marshall F, Shoulson I, Eberly S, Walker F, Factor S, Hunt V, Shinaman A, Jankovic J (2008). A study of chorea after tetrabenazine withdrawal in patients with Huntington disease. *Clin Neuropharmacol* 31:127–133.

Godwin-Austen RB (1979). The treatment of the choreas and athetotic dystonias. *J R Coll Physicians Lond* 13:35–38.

Huntington Study Group (2006). Tetrabenazine as antichorea therapy in Huntington disease: a randomized controlled trial. *Neurology* 66:366–372.

Jankovic J (1982). Treatment of hyperkinetic movement disorders with tetrabenazine: a double-blind crossover study. *Ann Neurol* 11:41–47.

Jankovic J (1995). Tardive syndromes and other drug-induced movement disorders. *Clin Neuropharmacol* 18:197–214.

Jankovic J, Beach J (1997). Long-term effects of tetrabenazine in hyperkinetic movement disorders. *Neurology* 48:358–362.

Jankovic J, Orman J (1988). Tetrabenazine therapy of dystonia, chorea, tics, and other dyskinesias. *Neurology* 38:391–394.

Kazamatsuri H, Chien C, Cole JO (1972). Treatment of tardive dyskinesia. I. Clinical efficacy of a dopamine-depleting agent, tetrabenazine. *Arch Gen Psychiatry* 27:95–99.

Kazamatsuri H, Chien CP, Cole JO (1973). Long-term treatment of tardive dyskinesia with haloperidol and tetrabenazine. *Am J Psychiatry* 130:479–483.

Kenney C, Hunter C, Mejia N, Jankovic J (2006). Is history of depression a contraindication to treatment with tetrabenazine? *Clin Neuropharmacol* 29:259–264.

Kenney C, Hunter C, Jankovic J (2007). Long-term tolerability of tetrabenazine in the treatment of hyperkinetic movement disorders. *Mov Disord* 22:193–197.

LeWitt PA (2013). Tardive dyskinesia caused by tetrabenazine. *Clin Neuropharmacol* 36:92–93.

Luciano AY, Jinnah HA, Pfeiffer RF, Truong DD, Nance MA, LeDoux MS (2014). Treatment of myoclonus-dystonia syndrome with tetrabenazine. *Parkinsonism Relat Disord* 20:1423–1426.

Marsden CD, Marion MH, Quinn N (1984). The treatment of severe dystonia in children and adults. *J Neurol Neurosurg Psychiatry* 47:1166–1173.

Ondo WG, Hanna PA, Jankovic J (1999). Tetrabenazine treatment for tardive dyskinesia: assessment by randomized videotape protocol. *Am J Psychiatry* 156:1279–1281.

Paleacu D, Giladi N, Moore O, Stern A, Honigman S, Badarny S (2004). Tetrabenazine treatment in movement disorders. *Clin Neuropharmacol* 27:230–233.

Schrader C, Dengler R, Dressler D (2010). Tetrabenazin in der Behandlung hyperkinetischer Bewegungsstörungen. *Psychopharmakotherapie* 17:85–90.

Soares-Weiser K, Fernandez HH (2007). Tardive dyskinesia. *Semin Neurol* 27:159–169.

Swash M, Roberts AH, Zakko H, Heathfield KW (1972). Treatment of involuntary movement disorders with tetrabenazine. *J Neurol Neurosurg Psychiatry* 35:186–191.

Watson MW, Skelton D, Jamali F (1988). Treatment of tardive dyskinesia: preliminary report on use of tetrabenazine. *Can J Psychiatry* 33:11–13.

Chapter 55

Treatment of Dopa-Responsive Dystonia

Ryul Kim and Beomseok Jeon

Introduction

As the name implies, there is a remarkable response to low doses of L-dihydroxyphenylalanine (L-dopa) in dopa-responsive dystonia (DRD) (Nygaard et al. 1988; Harwood et al. 1994; Clot et al. 2009). Typically, there are no long-term complications such as motor fluctuations and dyskinesias in DRD, in contrast to Parkinson's disease (PD), where the initial L-dopa response is also excellent (Harwood et al. 1994; Bandmann & Wood 2002; Clot et al. 2009). The autosomal dominant (AD) genetic defect in GTP cyclohydrolase 1 (GCH-1), which is the first rate-limiting step in the biosynthesis of tetrahydrobiopterin (BH_4), is the most classic cause of DRD (Lee et al. 2013). In addition to GCH-1, BH_4 is synthesised from guanosine-5′-triphosphate (GTP) by two additional steps involving pyruvoyltetrahydropterin synthase (PTPS) and sepiapterin reductase (SR), and is recycled by pterin α-carbinolamine dehydratase (PCD) and dihydropteridine reductase (DHPR). BH_4 is an essential cofactor not only for tyrosine hydroxylase (TH) but also for tryptophan hydroxylase (TPH), which is associated with the production of serotonin. TH converts tyrosine to L-dopa, which is then converted to dopamine by aromatic acid decarboxylase (AADC) (Thony et al. 2000; Figure 55.1). Accordingly, it is quite logical that the replacement of L-dopa bypasses and corrects the biochemical defect of GCH-1, thereby showing excellent clinical improvement. However, dyskinesia can be present on initial L-dopa administration, and there are cases in which the L-dopa response is not complete in DRD, described below.

DRD is characterised clinically by childhood onset of dystonia with diurnal fluctuation, which worsens towards evening and improves after sleep. DRD typically presents with lower-limb dystonia which gradually generalises (Segawa et al. 1976). However, there are cases reported as DRD with atypical and much more severe phenotypes (Lee & Jeon 2014). The severe phenotypes have gene defects different from classic DRD, which include the AD GCH-1 defect, and have different L-dopa responses extensively discussed by Jeon et al. (Jeon et al. 1998; Lee & Jeon 2014). In these papers, DRD is proposed to be defined as a syndrome of selective nigrostriatal dopamine deficiency caused by genetic defects in the dopamine synthetic pathway without nigral cell loss. Then, the term 'DRD-plus' is proposed and defined as inherited disorders in dopamine metabolism, which have features of DRD and additional features that are not seen in DRD (Clot et al. 2009), such as an earlier onset (e.g. neonatal onset) than that of DRD (Harwood et al. 1994), more severe motor features such as axial hypotonia, poor sucking and swallowing difficulties (Nygaard et al. 1988), non-motor manifestations such as seizures, psychomotor retardation, mental retardation and autonomic dysfunction (Lee & Jeon 2014). Theoretically, any enzyme defects in the dopamine synthetic pathway including BH_4 biosynthesis could produce DRD and DRD-plus. In general, AD GCH-1 deficiency causes DRD, whereas the autosomal recessive (AR) GCH-1, TH, SR, PTPS, DHPR and AADC deficiencies cause DRD-plus, with rare exceptions. The severity of the phenotype is thought to be related to the severity of the mutation and the biochemical functional defect.

Rationale for Treatment Principles

Deficient neurotransmitters differ depending on the enzyme defect. A decreased level of BH_4 is much more sensitive in the production of dopamine than that of serotonin because TH has a higher K_m value compared to TPH in Michaelis-Menten kinetics (Davis et al. 1992). However, a severe depletion of BH_4 affects the production of both dopamine and serotonin (Lee & Jeon 2014). An AD GCH-1 deficiency has a milder defect than that of other enzyme deficiencies in BH_4 metabolism. Therefore, the AD GCH-1 deficiency induces a greater depletion of dopamine than of serotonin. AR GCH-1, PTPS, SR, DHPR and AADC deficiencies induce a depletion of dopamine, norepinephrine and serotonin (Pons 2009). A TH deficiency induces a depletion of dopamine and norepinephrine, but serotonin is not affected (Figure 55.1). Accordingly, the principle of treatment is aimed at supplementing BH_4 and deficient neurotransmitter precursors. Dopaminergic, serotonergic and norepinephrinergic drugs can be used. Dopaminergic drugs include L-dopa, dopamine agonists, monoamine oxidase (MAO)-B inhibitors, catechol-O-methyl transferase (COMT) inhibitors, anticholinergics and amantadine. Serotonergic drugs include 5-hydroxydryptophan (5-HTP), MAO-A inhibitors, selective serotonin-reuptake inhibitors (SSRIs) and serotonin receptor agonists (Ng et al. 2014). Norepinephrinergic drugs include norepinephrine-reuptake inhibitors, which have been seldom used (Brun et al. 2010).

In general, early treatment is associated with favourable outcomes (Liu et al. 2008; Longo 2009; Niu 2011; Bruggemann et al. 2012; Opladen et al. 2012; Lu et al. 2014). AR GCH-1,

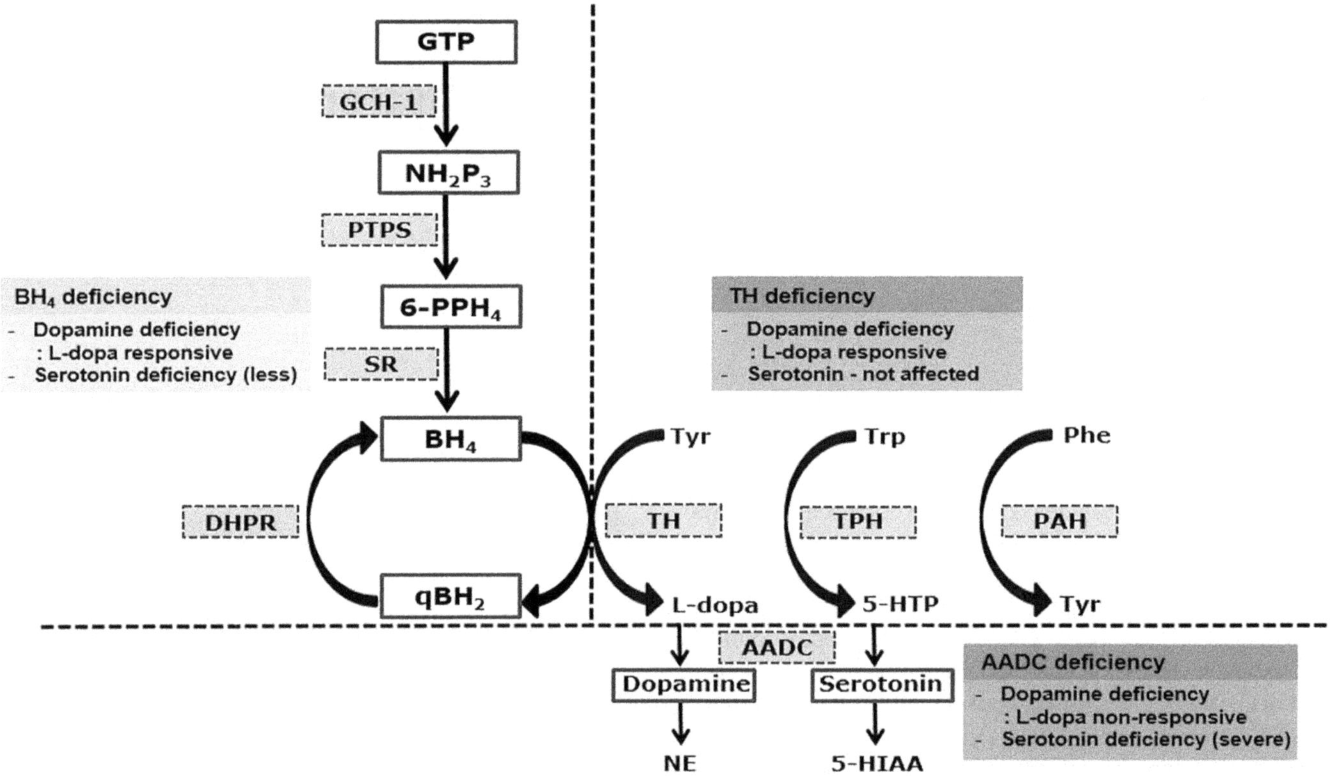

Figure 55.1 Deficient neurotransmitters depending on the enzyme defect. GTP = guanosine triphosphate; NH_2P_3 = dihydroneopterin triphosphate; 6-PPH4 = 6-pyruvoyl-tetrahydropterin; BH_4 = tetrahydrobiopterin; qBH_2 = quinonoid dihydrobiopterin; Tyr = tyrosine; Trp = tryptophan; Phe = phenylalanine; L-dopa = L-dihydroxyphenylalanine; 5-HTP = 5-hydroxydryptophan; NE = norepinephrine; 5-HIAA = 5-hydroxyindolacetic acid; GCH-1 = GTP cyclohydrolase 1; PTPS = 6-pyruvoyltetrahydropterin synthase; SR = sepiaterin reductase; DHPR = dihydropteridine reductase; TH = tyrosine hydroxylase; AADC = aromatic L-amino acid decarboxylase.

PTPS and DHPR deficiencies induce hyperphenylalaninemia (HPA), which can be detected through neonatal screening. This finding makes early intervention possible prior to the onset of clinical manifestations, which showed good clinical outcomes in many cases (Liu et al. 2008; Longo 2009; Niu 2011; Opladen et al. 2012; Lu et al. 2014). In addition, Bruggemann et al. reported a case of AR GCH-1 deficiency with prenatal dopaminergic treatment which resulted in normal motor and mental development without side-effects from the drugs (Bruggemann et al. 2012). Therefore, it is critical to make an early diagnosis and therapeutic intervention.

Classes of drugs

L-dopa

Generally, L-dopa is used with decarboxylase inhibitor (DCI) such as carbidopa or benserazide to prevent conversion to dopamine in the periphery to increase the bioavailability and to reduce the peripheral side-effects. DRD is known to show an excellent and sustained response to small doses of L-dopa without long-term complications such as motor fluctuations and dyskinesias (Nygaard et al. 1988; Harwood et al. 1994; Bandmann & Wood 2002; Clot et al. 2009). The majority of cases have been managed with less than 600 mg/d (Steinberger et al. 2000; Hagenah et al. 2005; Trender-Gerhard et al. 2009; Liu et al. 2010). However, an insufficient response and L-dopa-induced dyskinesias (LIDs) have been described in some cases of DRD. Tassin et al. reported 27 patients from 12 families with DRD due to AD GCH-1 deficiency (Tassin et al. 2000). Thirteen patients showed partial improvement from no response to 90 per cent response to L-dopa. Grimes et al. also reported one patient with DRD who experienced an increase in stiffness during L-dopa treatment and thus did not get any benefits from the treatment (Grimes et al. 2002). Several cases of DRD had intolerable LIDs which made it difficult to increase the doses of L-dopa (de la Fuente-Fernandez 1999; Furukawa et al. 2004; Lopez-Laso et al. 2009; Liu et al. 2010; Wu-Chou et al. 2010). In DRD-plus, L-dopa shows less motor benefit with severe dyskinesias (Lee & Jeon 2014).

LIDs are commonly observed in PD, which has been attributed to neuronal degeneration and denervation superhypersensitivity (Rajput et al. 1997; Pons et al. 2013). In DRD and DRD-plus, neuronal degeneration is absent but depletion of dopamine in the presynaptic nerve terminal may lead to functional denervation and associated supersensitivity (Pons et al. 2013). This functional denervation supersensitivity may explain why LIDs are more common and severe in DRD-plus than in DRD. LIDs are triggered by relatively high starting doses or rapid increments of L-dopa. Inversely, LIDs are improved by reducing the dose of L-dopa or by a gradual escalation to a higher dose, or by increasing the frequency of the dosing, which suggests that LIDs could be regarded as a marker of excessive dosing (Pons et al. 2013). Thus, small doses of L-dopa should be initiated with a gradual dose titration (Pons et al. 2013). If LIDs occur despite the above titration, dopamine agonists, anticholinergics or amantadine are recommended. In addition to LIDs, nausea, vomiting, headache, psychosis, aggravated extrapyramidal symptoms and sleep problems have been reported as side-effects in DRD and DRD-plus (Lipson et al. 1991; Grimes et al. 2002; Ihara et al. 2002; Kaindl et al. 2005; Regula et al. 2007; Sharma et al. 2011; Friedman et al. 2012).

BH_4

The supplementation of BH_4 has been used in order to reduce the phenylalanine levels in the HPA state, which is caused by deficiencies in AR GCH-1, PTPS and DHPR (Ng et al. 2014). BH_4 has been used most frequently in PTPS deficiency. Even though theoretically very appealing, BH_4 is ineffective in correcting neurotransmitter deficiencies because it passes poorly through the blood–brain barrier (Shintaku 2002). Thus, BH_4 is used in combination with L-dopa and 5-HTP rather than as a monotherapy. A trial of BH_4 with neurotransmitter precursors resulted in a marked remission of symptoms in some cases of DRD and DRD-plus; however, BH_4 monotherapy was not generally effective (Furukawa et al. 1996, 1998; Dudesek et al. 2001; Segawa 2011; Ng et al. 2014). Various side-effects such as headaches, throat pain, vomiting, diarrhoea and abdominal pain have been reported in phenylalanine hydroxylase deficiency (Sanford & Keating 2009), but are rarely reported in DRD and DRD-plus (Shintaku & Ohwada 2013; Ye et al. 2013).

Dopamine Agonists

Dopamine agonists have been used mainly in DRD-plus, especially due to AADC deficiency (Brun et al. 2010). Dopamine agonists improve the clinical course in DRD-plus. Two reports by Porta et al. showed that pramipexole in seven patients with DRD-plus due to deficiencies in PTPS and DHPR markedly improved their clinical picture, as well as reduced the L-dopa dose and number of administrations (Porta et al. 2009, 2012). On the other hand, dopamine agonists have only been used as an alternative for L-dopa in DRD (Furukawa et al. 1998; Regula et al. 2007; Sharma et al. 2011; Lopez-Laso et al. 2012). In these cases, L-dopa was changed into dopamine agonists due to side-effects including dyskinesias, headaches and nausea (Furukawa et al. 1998; Regula et al. 2007; Sharma et al. 2011; Lopez-Laso et al. 2012). Pergolide, bromocriptine, pramipexole, ropinirole and rotigotine have been used in DRD and DRD-plus. Pergolide may lead to fibrosis of the heart valves, thus regular monitoring with echocardiography is recommended (Kurian et al. 2011). However, such a complication has not been reported in DRD and DRD-plus (Kurian et al. 2011).

MAO Inhibitors (MAOIs)

MAO breaks down monoamines such as dopamine and serotonin (Allen et al. 2009). There are two isoforms of MAO: MAO-A and MAO-B (Ng et al. 2014). Serotonin and norepinephrine are mainly broken down by MAO-A, whereas dopamine is mainly broken down by MAO-B. Accordingly, MAOIs are used to prevent the degradation of dopamine as well as serotonin and norepinephrine. MAOIs have been used in DRD-plus only, especially due to deficiencies in AADC, PTPS and TH. MAOIs used to treat DRD-plus include tranylcypromine (non-selective MAOI), selegiline (selective MAO-B inhibitor) and moclobemide (selective MAO-A inhibitor). Selective MAO-B inhibitors have been used in most cases of DRD-plus (Schuler et al. 2000; Jaggi et al. 2008; Porta et al. 2009, 2012; Leuzzi et al. 2010; Willemsen et al. 2010; Yosunkaya et al. 2010); however, non-selective MAOIs are the preferred treatment in DRD-plus due to AADC deficiency (Brun et al. 2010). Reported side-effects of MAOIs are dyskinesia, sleep problems, mood swings, aggravated extrapyramidal symptoms and aggressive behaviour (Pons et al. 2004; Manegold et al. 2009; Brun et al. 2010).

COMT Inhibitors

COMT converts L-dopa to the inactive compound 3-O-methyldopa. Blocking the COMT activity results in higher dopamine levels and a longer duration of action. COMT inhibitors have rarely been used in DRD-plus. Entacapone, which is a peripheral COMT inhibitor, has improved the fluctuation of motor symptoms and reduced the L-dopa dose in some cases of PTPS and DHPR deficiencies (Jaggi et al. 2008; Porta et al. 2009).

Anticholinergics

Anticholinergic agents are widely used in patients with generalised dystonia. There have been reports of excellent improvement in some patients with generalised dystonia treated with anticholinergic drugs (Jankovic 2006). Anticholinergic agents including trihexyphenidyl, biperiden and benztropine have been used for the treatment of DRD and DRD-plus, especially due to TH and AADC deficiencies (Jarman et al. 1997; Brun et al. 2010; Liu et al. 2010; Willemsen et al. 2010). DRD showed a favourable response to anticholinergics, even in cases with a partial response to L-dopa (Jarman et al. 1997; Liu et al. 2010). However, response to anticholinergics in DRD-plus is highly variable (Brun et al. 2010; Chi et al. 2012; Friedman et al. 2012). Reported side-effects of anticholinergics are drowsiness, sweating and aggressive behaviour (Pons et al. 2004; Anselm & Darras 2006; Brun et al. 2010).

Amantadine

Amantadine is a partial dopamine agonist and partial N-methyl-D-aspartic acid (NMDA) receptor antagonist that is used to reduce LIDs or improve the condition of a patient in PD. Amantadine is one of the therapeutic options in DRD and DRD-plus if dose adjustment of L-dopa is insufficient to treat LIDs. Furukawa et al. described two cases of DRD showing the beneficial effect of amantadine on LIDs (Furukawa et al. 2004). Pons et al. also reported two patients with DRD-plus due to TH deficiency in which LIDs responded well to amantadine (Pons et al. 2013).

5-HTP

Specific treatment for the serotonin system could be beneficial for DRD-plus with serotonin depletion. Lack of serotonin is likely to cause symptoms such as psychomotor dysfunction, sleep disturbances and gastrointestinal problems. In such cases, 5-HTP, a biosynthetic precursor of serotonin, is used to increase the serotonin level, which results in the improvement of associated symptoms (Friedman et al. 2012). It has been mostly used with L-dopa rather than as a monotherapy. However, 5-HTP has a variety of side-effects such as nausea, vomiting, irritability, abdominal pain, diarrhoea and lethargy that have limited its use in many reports of DRD-plus (Irons et al. 1987; Schmidt et al. 1988; Lipson et al. 1991; Swoboda et al. 1999; Lee et al. 2006; Liu et al. 2008; Brun et al. 2010; Friedman et al. 2012; Mastrangelo et al. 2013).

SSRIs

SSRIs have also been used in DRD-plus with serotonin depletion. Their mechanisms increase the extracellular level of serotonin by blocking its presynaptic reuptake, thus increasing the synaptic serotonin level (Ng et al. 2014). Fluoxetine, sertraline and escitalopram have been used in DRD-plus, especially due to AADC deficiency (Dudesek et al. 2001; Manegold et al. 2009; Leuzzi et al. 2014). However, there have been no reports showing significant clinical improvements from SSRIs.

Therapeutic Approach Based on the Type of Enzyme Defect

BH4 Defects

AD GCH-1 Deficiency

Most cases of AD GCH-1 deficiency show a marked and sustained response to L-dopa (Segawa et al. 2003; Cai et al. 2013; Lee et al. 2013). Reported maintenance doses of L-dopa with DCI have ranged from 25 to 1800 mg/d; however, the majority of cases have been managed with less than 600 mg/d (de la Fuente-Fernandez 1999; Steinberger et al. 2000; Hagenah et al. 2005; Trender Gerhard et al. 2009; Liu et al. 2010; Wu-Chou et al. 2010; Hu et al. 2011; Tachi et al. 2011). In our recent report on 19 cases of AD GCH-1 deficiency, the maintenance doses of L-dopa with DCI ranged from 70 to 250 mg/d (Lee et al. 2013). However, there are cases of AD GCH-1 deficiency showing partial improvement despite L-dopa treatment (Robinson et al. 1999; Tassin et al. 2000; Clot et al. 2009; Trender-Gerhard et al. 2009; Liu et al. 2010, 2014). It could be hypothesised that a prolonged dopamine-deficient state in the basal ganglia results in derangement of the motor circuit associated with dystonia, which leads to partial responsiveness to L-dopa (Lee & Jeon 2014). Thus, other treatments have been used to control residual symptoms. In cases with a partial response to L-dopa, anticholinergics might be successful. In a report on 12 cases of AD GCH-1 deficiency by Liu et al., three patients responded better to trihexyphenidyl than to L-dopa, and two patients were treated with the combination of trihexyphenidyl and L-dopa because their symptoms were not completely controlled with L-dopa monotherapy (Liu et al. 2010). Jarman et al. also reported on two patients showing an excellent response to trihexyphenidyl (Jarman et al. 1997). BH_4 has been used in only a few cases of AD GCH-1 deficiency. Segawa et al. reported that BH_4 with L-dopa led to complete remission of symptoms in some cases that had only a partial response to L-dopa; however, BH_4 monotherapy was not effective (Segawa 2011). Taken together, L-dopa is recommended as a first-line treatment for AD GCH-1 deficiency. If the response to L-dopa is insufficient, anticholinergics might be considered as a second-line treatment.

SR deficiency

SR deficiency may show dopa-responsive movement disorders with diurnal fluctuation as DRD phenotypes (Friedman et al. 2012). However, most cases have additional features such as cognitive impairment, developmental delay, hypotonia and autonomic dysfunction (Friedman et al. 2012). The majority of cases with SR deficiency showed considerable benefits from low doses of L-dopa, especially in motor and sleep symptoms (Friedman et al. 2012). Reported doses of L-dopa have ranged from 0.16 to 20.0 mg/kg per day; however, LIDs were common at initiation or during titration of L-dopa (Dill et al. 2012; Friedman et al. 2012). Despite L-dopa treatment, mild motor and severe cognitive impairment persisted in many cases (Friedman et al. 2006, 2012; Dill et al. 2012; Leuzzi et al. 2013). 5-HTP is recommended for additional benefits in all cases with incomplete resolution of symptoms with L-dopa monotherapy. Friedman et al. reported that some cases of SR deficiency have shown further benefit from the addition of 5-HTP (Friedman et al. 2012). Reported doses of 5-HTP have ranged from 0.75 to 16.0 mg/kg per day (Dill et al. 2012; Friedman et al. 2012). BH_4 is not generally required (Kurian et al. 2011). The reported responses to the dopamine agonists, MAOIs and anticholinergics are limited due to the very small number of cases that have used those drugs (Friedman et al. 2012). Taken together, the combination of L-dopa and 5-HTP is recommended as a first-line treatment for SR deficiency. Unfortunately there is no definite second-line treatment for SR deficiency.

AR GCH-1/PTPS/DHPR Deficiencies

The therapeutic strategies are similar in cases of AR GCH-1, PTPS and DHPR deficiencies. Treatment with BH_4 and neurotransmitter precursors such as L-dopa and 5-HTP should be considered (Kurian et al. 2011). The recommended starting doses of L-dopa and 5-HTP are 1–2 mg/kg per day and titrated up to 10–15 mg/kg per day and 5–10 mg/kg per day, respectively (Niu 2011; Opladen et al. 2012; Ye et al. 2013; Han et al. 2014). It is recommended that the dose of BH_4 is started at 1–2 mg/kg per day and thereafter titrated up to 5–10 mg/kg per day (Opladen et al. 2012; Ye et al. 2013; Han et al. 2014). During the treatment, it is recommended that the BH_4 dose is adjusted to maintain the serum phenylalanine level below 120 umol/L, and the L-dopa dose is titrated based on the serum prolactin level (Spada et al. 1991; Ogawa et al. 2008; Niu 2011; Opladen et al. 2012; Ye et al. 2013; Han et al. 2014). However, neurotransmitter metabolites might not systematically reflect the clinical status (Ponzone et al. 1990; Dudesek et al. 2001). Thus, the dose of L-dopa and BH_4 should be titrated according to the clinical performance and tolerance of side-effects, as well as the level of neurotransmitter metabolites (Lu et al. 2014). Dopamine agonists and MAOIs have been used to improve motor fluctuations and to ameliorate L-dopa-induced side-effects in PTPS and DHPR deficiencies. Porta et al. showed that the concurrent administration of pramipexole with L-dopa is effective in reducing the L-dopa dose and the number of administrations as well as in improving the clinical course (Niu 2011; Porta et al. 2011, 2012). Additionally, several reports have found that selegiline combined with L-dopa showed beneficial effects similar to pramipexole combined with L-dopa (Schuler et al. 1995; Schuler et al. 2000; Ponzone et al. 2004; Niu 2011). Treatment with folic acid is recommended in DHPR deficiency because DHPR has an important role in maintaining the folate levels in its active form (Irons et al. 1987). The recommended dose of folic acid is 15–20 mg/kg per day (Lu et al. 2014). Taken all together, treatment with BH_4 combined with L-dopa and 5-HTP is recommended as a first-line treatment for AR GCH-1, PTPS and DHPR deficiencies. If the response to treatment is unsatisfactory, the addition of MAOIs or dopamine agonists could be considered as a second-line treatment. In DHPR deficiency, additional supplementation of folic acid is recommended.

Non-BH4 Defects

TH Deficiency

L-dopa is the preferred treatment, but the response is highly variable (Schiller et al. 2004). Willemsen et al. divided TH-deficient patients into two main phenotypes: type A with onset of symptoms in the first year presenting as progressive hypokinetic-rigid syndrome, generalised dystonia; and type B with early onset presenting as a more complex encephalopathy associated with hypokinesia, hypotonia, dystonia, myoclonus and eye movement abnormalities (Willemsen et al. 2010). They reported that the response to L-dopa in the type A cases was much better than in those in the type B cases (Willemsen et al. 2010). Most TH-deficient patients meet the criteria of DRD-plus. Only rarely did patients in the type A group fulfil the criteria of DRD. In many cases of TH deficiency, an initial dose of L-dopa at 3 mg/kg per day divided into three doses is acceptable (Willemsen et al. 2010). However, some cases of DRD-plus have showed hypersensitivity to L-dopa. In such cases, a low dose of L-dopa divided into 4–6 doses is recommended, as mentioned above.

Dopamine agonists, anticholinergics and MAO-B inhibitors have been used in TH deficiency (Dionisi-Vici et al. 2000; Haussler et al. 2001; Grattan-Smith et al. 2002; Hoffmann et al. 2003; Willemsen et al. 2010; Yosunkaya et al. 2010; Yeung et al. 2011; Chi et al. 2012). MAO-B inhibitors such as selegiline have been frequently used, which have been effective in many cases with a partial response or side-effects to L-dopa (Dionisi-Vici et al. 2000; Haussler et al. 2001; Grattan-Smith et al. 2002; Hoffmann et al. 2003; Willemsen et al. 2010; Yosunkaya et al. 2010; Yeung et al. 2011; Chi et al. 2012). Dopamine agonists and anticholinergics have rarely been used, which have shown variable responses (Del et al. 2000; Hoffmann et al. 2003; Chi et al. 2012; Stamelou et al. 2012). Taken together, L-dopa is recommended as a first-line treatment for TH deficiency. Nonetheless, if the response to L-dopa is unsuccessful, the addition of MAO-B inhibitors might be considered as a second-line treatment.

AADC Deficiency

The first cases of AADC deficiency were monozygotic twins reported in 1990, who responded well to treatment with MAOI, dopamine agonist and pyridoxine (Hyland & Clayton 1990). This regimen has become a standard treatment for AADC deficiency (Allen et al. 2009; Brun et al. 2010). However, the majority of cases have shown poor responses despite early treatment and various therapeutic trials (Maller et al. 1997; Pons et al. 2004; Abdenur et al. 2006; Brun et al. 2010). Unlike other enzyme defects, L-dopa is seldom used because it might result in the depletion of S-adenosylmethionine, which is enhanced by AADC deficiency and can lead to a deficiency in 5-methyltetrahydrofolate (Surtees & Hyland 1990; Chang et al. 2004; Allen et al. 2009). Although the response with L-dopa has been poor in most cases, some have shown a favourable response with L-dopa (Chang et al. 2004; Manegold et al. 2009; Brun et al. 2010; Mastrangelo et al. 2013). This finding indicates that L-dopa could be tried in AADC deficiency but is generally not recommended. Dopamine agonists are preferred. The dopamine agonists used in AADC deficiency include pergolide, bromocriptine, pramipexole, ropinirole and rotigotine patches, but the response to each drug is variable (Brun et al. 2010). In addition to dopamine agonists, MAOIs, anticholinergics and pyridoxine have been utilised. MAOIs have been frequently used, and have shown favourable responses in some cases of AADC deficiency (Brun et al. 2010). However, selective MAO-B inhibitors are not recommended because they do not block the breakdown of serotonin. Pyridoxine has also been frequently used to boost residual AADC activity through cofactor excess, although patients with AADC deficiency do not have a depletion of pyridoxine 5′-phosphate (Allen et al. 2010; Ng et al. 2014). There have been no reports showing significant clinical improvement with pyridoxine treatment; however, its biochemical response has been reported to have elevated levels of CSF homovalinic acid and plasma serotonin (Hyland et al. 1992; Maller et al. 1997). Anticholinergic medications have been used with dopamine agonists and MAOIs (Brun et al. 2010). Some patients have responded to anticholinergics, although the response has been minimal (Brun et al. 2010). Taken together, dopamine agonists combined with MAOIs are recommended as a first-line treatment for AADC deficiency. Supplementation with folate might be considered. If response to the first-line treatment is unfavourable, the addition of anticholinergics might be considered as a second-line treatment. Therapeutic approach based on the type of enzyme defect is summarised in Table 55.1.

Issues Specific to Women: Pregnancy

The FDA divides drugs into five categories, A, B, C, D and X, based on their safe use during pregnancy. Most drugs used in DRD and DRD-plus fall into category C, while bromocriptine

Table 55.1 Recommended treatment in DRD and DRD-plus patients

Enzyme defect (reference)	First-line treatment	Second-line treatment	Drug	Reported dose (mg/kg per)	Recommended dose (mg/kg per day)	
					Starting	Maintenance
AD GCH-1						
Lee et al. 2013	L-dopa*	Anticholinergics	L-dopa*	25–1800 mg/d	25–50 mg/d	100–300 mg/d
Liu et al. 2010			trihexyphenidyl	2–20 mg/d	2 mg/d	6–10 mg/d
Hagenah et al. 2005						
Steinberger et al. 2000						
Grimes et al. 2002						
Wu-Chou et al. 2010						
Lopez-Laso et al. 2009						
de la Fuente-Fernandez 1999						
Lopez-Laso et al. 2012						
Jarman et al. 1997						
Cai et al. 2013						
Tachi et al. 2011						
Hu et al. 2011						
Karkheiran et al. 2013						
Naiya et al. 2012						
Ling et al. 2011						
Cao et al. 2010						
Zirn et al. 2008						
Wu et al. 2008						
Steinberger et al. 2007						
Theuns et al. 2012						
Uncini et al. 2004						
Saunders-Pullman et al. 2004						
Steinberger et al. 1999						
AR GCH-1[1] / PTPS[2] / DHPR[3]						
[1]Bruggemann et al. 2012	L-dopa* +	MAOIs	L-dopa*	AR-GCH-1~	1–2	10–15
Sato et al. 2014	5-HTP + BH_4	DAs		PTPS~		
Opladen et al. 2011	+ Folic acid			DHPR~		
Horvath et al. 2008	(only DHPR)		5-HTP	AR-GCH~	1–2	5–10
Garavaglia et al. 2004				PTPS~		
Nardocci et al. 2003				DHPR~		
Hwu et al. 1999			BH_4	AR-GCH~	1–2	5–10 (keep the serum Phe
Blau et al. 1995				PTPS		below 120 uM)
Dhondt et al. 1985				DHPR		
[2]Niu 2011			Selegiline	0.088–0.4	0.1	0.2–0.4
Dudesek et al. 2001			Pramipexole	0.02–0.04	n.d.	0.02–0.04
Porta et al. 2009			Folate	2.5–30	5	15–20
Jaggi et al. 2008						
Schuler et al. 2000						
Leuzzi et al. 2010						
Lee et al. 2006						
Gizewska et al. 2009						
Roze et al. 2006						
Demos et al. 2005						
Imamura et al. 1999						
Jardim et al. 1994						
al Aqeel et al. 1991						
[3]Lu et al. 2014						
Lipson et al. 1991						
Porta et al. 2012						
Jaggi et al. 2008						
Schmidt et al. 1988						
Coughlin et al. 2013						
Concolino et al. 2008						
Sedel et al. 2006						
Goldstein et al. 1995						
Leeming et al. 1982						

Enzyme defect (reference)	First-line treatment	Second-line treatment	Drug	Reported dose (mg/kg per)	Recommended dose (mg/kg per day)	
					Starting	Maintenance
SR						
Friedman et al. 2012	L-dopa* +	n.d.	L-dopa*	0.16–20	0.5–1	2–5
Dill et al. 2012	5-HTP		5-HTP	0.75–16	1	2–4
Leuzzi et al. 2013						
Koht et al. 2014						
Thibert et al. 2012						
Arrabal et al. 2011						
Kusmierska et al. 2009						
Verbeek et al. 2008						
Echenne et al. 2006						
Abeling et al. 2006						
Neville et al. 2005						
TH						
Pons et al. 2013	L-dopa*	MAOIs	L-dopa*	0.1–52.1	1	4–10
Chi et al. 2012				(25–)	(25–)	(200–d)
Cai et al. 2013			Selegiline	0.2–0.4	0.1	0.2–0.4
Schiller et al. 2004				(0.5–15 mg/d)	(0.5–)	(5–)
Yeung et al. 2011						
Hoffmann et al. 2003						
Haussler et al. 2001						
Grattan-Smith et al. 2002						
Stamelou et al. 2012						
Del et al. 2000						
Wu et al. 2008						
Sun et al. 2014						
Giovanniello et al. 2012						
Haugarvoll & Bindoff 2011						
Doummar et al. 2009						
Ribases et al. 2007						
Giovanniello et al. 2007						
Chieng et al. 2007						
Moller et al. 2005						
Diepold et al. 2005						
Janssen et al. 2000						
de Rijk-Van Andel et al. 2000						
AADC						
Pons et al. 2004	DAs + MAOIs	Anticholinergics	Rotigotine	6–8 mg/d	1–2 mg/d	6–8 mg/d
Mastrangelo et al. 2013	± Pyridoxine		Bromocriptine	0.5–10 mg/d	1–2 mg/d	5–10 mg/d
Swoboda et al. 1999			Tranylcypromide	5–18 mg/d	5 mg/d	10–15 mg/d
Leuzzi et al. 2014			Pyridoxine	150–1200 mg/d	100 mg/d	200–400 mg/d
Maller et al. 1997			Trihexyphenidyl	n.d.	n.d.	n.d.
Hyland et al. 1992						
Lee et al. 2014						
Fiumara et al. 2002						
Korenke et al. 1997						
Tay et al. 2007						

* L-dopa with decarboxylase inhibitor; n.d. = not determined
GCH-1 = GTP cyclohydrolase 1; AD = autosomal dominant; AR = autosomal recessive; PTPS = 6-Pyruvoyltetrahydropterin synthase; SR = sepiaterin reductase; DHPR = dihydropteridine reductase; TH = tyrosine hydroxylase; AADC = aromatic L-amino acid decarboxylase; 5-HTP = 5-hydroxytryptophan; BH_4 = tetrahydrobiopterin; MAOIs = monoamine oxidase inhibitors; DAs = dopamine agonists

and pergolide fall into category B, and 5-HTP is not classified. In addition, L-dopa with benserazide is contraindicated in pregnant women.

To date, pregnancy has been reported in a few cases of DRD and in only one case of DRD-plus due to PTPS deficiency. In all the cases of DRD, L-dopa with carbidopa or L-dopa alone has only been used during pregnancy (Trender-Gerhard et al. 2009; Watanabe et al. 2009). Rarely have miscarriages been reported in patients with L-dopa combined with carbidopa, described below. In DRD-plus, BH_4, L-dopa with carbidopa and 5-HTP have been used during pregnancy. Gizewska et al. reported the course of two subsequent pregnancies and the follow-up of two offspring in a PTPS-deficient patient (Gizewska et al. 2009). The second child was born normally; however, the first child was born with schizencephaly and the absence of a septum pellucidum. Although the aetiology of congenital brain malformation is unclear, treatment with BH_4, L-dopa with carbidopa, and 5-HTP should be administered with caution.

L-dopa alone rather than L-dopa with carbidopa might be the treatment of choice during pregnancy. Watanabe et al. reviewed nine DRD patients who were pregnant (Watanabe et al. 2009). Six patients with L-dopa alone gave birth to healthy infants; however, miscarriage occurred in one patient out of three patients with L-dopa combined with carbidopa treatment. In the patient with miscarriage, the L-dopa with carbidopa treatment induced spontaneous abortions in two consecutive pregnancies, but L-dopa alone led to full-term normal delivery. It was suggested that the higher concentration of L-dopa in the L-dopa with carbidopa treatment could result in adverse effects on the placenta/embryo.

References

Abdenur JE, Abeling N, Specola N, Jorge L, Schenone AB, van Cruchten AC, et al. 2006. Aromatic l-aminoacid decarboxylase deficiency: unusual neonatal presentation and additional findings in organic acid analysis. *Molecular Genetics and Metabolism* 87(1):48–53.

Abeling NG, Duran M, Bakker HD, Stroomer L, Thony B, Blau N, et al. 2006. Sepiapterin reductase deficiency: an autosomal recessive DOPA-responsive dystonia. *Molecular Genetics and Metabolism* 89(1–2):116–120.

al Aqeel A, Ozand PT, Gascon G, Nester M, al Nasser M, Brismar J, et al. 1991. Biopterin-dependent hyperphenylalaninemia due to deficiency of 6-pyruvoyl tetrahydropterin synthase. *Neurology* 41(5):730–737.

Allen GF, Land JM, Heales SJ. 2009. A new perspective on the treatment of aromatic L-amino acid decarboxylase deficiency. *Molecular Genetics and Metabolism* 97(1):6–14.

Allen GF, Neergheen V, Oppenheim M, Fitzgerald JC, Footitt E, Hyland K, et al. 2010. Pyridoxal 5′-phosphate deficiency causes a loss of aromatic L-amino acid decarboxylase in patients and human neuroblastoma cells, implications for aromatic L-amino acid decarboxylase and vitamin B(6) deficiency states. *Journal of Neurochemistry* 114(1):87–96.

Anselm IA, Darras BT. 2006. Catecholamine toxicity in aromatic L-amino acid decarboxylase deficiency. *Pediatric Neurology* 35(2):142–144.

Arrabal L, Teresa L, Sanchez-Alcudia R, Castro M, Medrano C, Gutierrez-Solana L, et al. 2011. Genotype–phenotype correlations in sepiapterin reductase deficiency: a splicing defect accounts for a new phenotypic variant. *Neurogenetics* 12(3):183–191.

Bandmann O, Wood NW. 2002. Dopa-responsive dystonia: the story so far. *Neuropediatrics* 33(1):1–5.

Blau N, Ichinose H, Nagatsu T, Heizmann CW, Zacchello F, Burlina AB. 1995. A missense mutation in a patient with guanosine triphosphate cyclohydrolase I deficiency missed in the newborn screening program. *The Journal of Pediatrics* 126(3):401–405.

Bruggemann N, Spiegler J, Hellenbroich Y, Opladen T, Schneider SA, Stephani U, et al. 2012. Beneficial prenatal levodopa therapy in autosomal recessive guanosine triphosphate cyclohydrolase 1 deficiency. *Archives of Neurology* 69(8):1071–1075.

Brun L, Ngu LH, Keng WT, Ch'ng GS, Choy YS, Hwu WL, et al. 2010. Clinical and biochemical features of aromatic L-amino acid decarboxylase deficiency. *Neurology* 75(1):64–71.

Cai C, Shi W, Zeng Z, Zhang M, Ling C, Chen L, et al. 2013. GTP cyclohydrolase I and tyrosine hydroxylase gene mutations in familial and sporadic dopa-responsive dystonia patients. *PLoS One* 8(6):e65215.

Cao L, Zheng L, Tang WG, Xiao Q, Zhang T, Tang HD, et al. 2010. Four novel mutations in the GCH1 gene of Chinese patients with dopa-responsive dystonia. *Movement Disorders: Official Journal of the Movement Disorder Society* 25(6):755–760.

Chang YT, Sharma R, Marsh JL, McPherson JD, Bedell JA, Knust A, et al. 2004. Levodopa-responsive aromatic L-amino acid decarboxylase deficiency. *Annals of Neurology* 55(3):435–438.

Chi CS, Lee HF, Tsai CR. 2012. Tyrosine hydroxylase deficiency in Taiwanese infants. *Pediatric Neurology* 46(2):77–82.

Chieng KS, Hussain N, Gosalakkal JA. 2007. Dystonia during feeding as an early sign of dopa-responsive dystonia. *Pediatric Neurology* 37(3):215–217.

Clot F, Grabli D, Cazeneuve C, Roze E, Castelnau P, Chabrol B, et al. 2009. Exhaustive analysis of BH4 and dopamine biosynthesis genes in patients with dopa-responsive dystonia. *Brain: A Journal of Neurology* 132(Pt 7):1753–1763.

Concolino D, Muzzi G, Rapsomaniki M, Moricca MT, Pascale MG, Strisciuglio P. 2008. Serum prolactin as a tool for the follow-up of treated DHPR-deficient patients. *Journal of Inherited Metabolic Disease* 31(Suppl. 2):S193–S197.

Coughlin CR, 2nd, Hyland K, Randall R, Ficicioglu C. 2013. Dihydropteridine reductase deficiency and treatment with tetrahydrobiopterin: a case report. *JIMD Reports* 10:53–56.

Davis MD, Ribeiro P, Tipper J, Kaufman S. 1992. '7-tetrahydrobiopterin', a naturally occurring analogue of tetrahydrobiopterin, is a cofactor for and a potential inhibitor of the aromatic amino acid hydroxylases. *Proceedings of the National Academy of Sciences of the United States of America* 89(21):10109–10113.

de la Fuente-Fernandez R. 1999. Drug-induced motor complications in dopa-responsive dystonia: implications for the pathogenesis of dyskinesias and motor fluctuations. *Clinical Neuropharmacology* 22(4):216–219.

de Rijk-Van Andel JF, Gabreels FJ, Geurtz B, Steenbergen-Spanjers GC, van Den Heuvel LP, Smeitink JA, et al. 2000. L-dopa-responsive infantile hypokinetic rigid parkinsonism due to tyrosine hydroxylase deficiency. *Neurology* 55(12):1926–1928.

Del P, Nassogne MC, van Gennip AH, van Cruchten AC, Billatte de Villemeur T, Cretz M, et al. 2000. Tyrosine hydroxylase deficiency unresponsive to L-dopa treatment with unusual clinical and biochemical presentation. *Journal of Inherited Metabolic Disease* 23(8):819–825.

Demos MK, Waters PJ, Vallance HD, Lillquist Y, Makhseed N, Hyland K, et al. 2005. 6-pyruvoyl-tetrahydropterin synthase deficiency with mild hyperphenylalaninemia. *Annals of Neurology* 58(1):164–167.

Dhondt J-L, Farriaux J-P, Boudha A, Largillière C, Ringel J, Roger M-M, et al. 1985. Neonatal hyperphenylalaninemia presumably caused by guanosine triphosphate-cyclohydrolase deficiency. *The Journal of Pediatrics*. 106(6):954–956.

Diepold K, Schutz B, Rostasy K, Wilken B, Hougaard P, Guttler F, et al. 2005. Levodopa-responsive infantile parkinsonism due to a novel mutation in the tyrosine hydroxylase gene and exacerbation by viral infections. *Movement Disorders: Official Journal of the Movement Disorder Society* 20(6):764–767.

Dill P, Wagner M, Somerville A, Thony B, Blau N, Weber P. 2012. Child neurology: paroxysmal stiffening, upward gaze, and hypotonia – hallmarks of sepiapterin reductase deficiency. *Neurology* 78(5):e29–e32.

Dionisi-Vici C, Hoffmann GF, Leuzzi V, Hoffken H, Brautigam C, Rizzo C, et al. 2000. Tyrosine hydroxylase deficiency with severe clinical course: clinical and biochemical investigations and optimization of therapy. *The Journal of Pediatrics* 136(4):560–562.

Doummar D, Clot F, Vidailhet M, Afenjar A, Durr A, Brice A, et al. 2009. Infantile hypokinetic-hypotonic syndrome due to two novel mutations of the tyrosine hydroxylase gene. *Movement Disorders: Official Journal of the Movement Disorder Society* 24(6):943–945.

Dudesek A, Roschinger W, Muntau AC, Seidel J, Leupold D, Thony B, et al. 2001. Molecular analysis and long-term follow-up of patients with different forms of 6-pyruvoyl-tetrahydropterin synthase deficiency. *European Journal of Pediatrics* 160(5):267–276.

Echenne B, Roubertie A, Assmann B, Lutz T, Penzien JM, Thony B, et al. 2006. Sepiapterin reductase deficiency: clinical presentation and evaluation of long-term therapy. *Pediatric Neurology* 35(5):308–313.

Fiumara A, Brautigam C, Hyland K, Sharma R, Lagae L, Stoltenborg B, et al. 2002. Aromatic L-amino acid decarboxylase deficiency with hyperdopaminuria: clinical and laboratory findings in response to different therapies. *Neuropediatrics* 33(4):203–208.

Friedman J, Hyland K, Blau N, MacCollin M. 2006. Dopa-responsive hypersomnia and mixed movement disorder due to sepiapterin reductase deficiency. *Neurology* 67(11):2032–2035.

Friedman J, Roze E, Abdenur JE, Chang R, Gasperini S, Saletti V, et al. 2012. Sepiapterin reductase deficiency: a treatable mimic of cerebral palsy. *Annals of Neurology* 71(4):520–530.

Furukawa Y, Shimadzu M, Rajput AH, Shimizu Y, Tagawa T, Mori H, et al. 1996. GTP-cyclohydrolase I gene mutations in hereditary progressive and dopa-responsive dystonia. *Annals of Neurology* 39(5):609–617.

Furukawa Y, Kish SJ, Bebin EM, Jacobson RD, Fryburg JS, Wilson WG, et al. 1998. Dystonia with motor delay in compound heterozygotes for GTP-cyclohydrolase I gene mutations. *Annals of Neurology* 44(1):10–16.

Furukawa Y, Filiano JJ, Kish SJ. 2004. Amantadine for levodopa-induced choreic dyskinesia in compound heterozygotes for GCH1 mutations. *Movement Disorders: Official Journal of the Movement Disorder Society* 19(10):1256–1258.

Garavaglia B, Invernizzi F, Carbone ML, Viscardi V, Saracino F, Ghezzi D, et al. 2004. GTP-cyclohydrolase I gene mutations in patients with autosomal dominant and recessive GTP-CH1 deficiency: identification and functional characterization of four novel mutations. *Journal of Inherited Metabolic Disease* 27(4):455–463.

Giovanniello T, Leuzzi V, Carducci C, Carducci C, Sabato ML, Artiola C, et al. 2007. Tyrosine hydroxylase deficiency presenting with a biphasic clinical course. *Neuropediatrics* 38(4):213–215.

Giovanniello T, Claps D, Carducci C, Carducci C, Blau N, Vigevano F, et al. 2012. A new tyrosine hydroxylase genotype associated with early-onset severe encephalopathy. *Journal of Child Neurology* 27(4):523–525.

Gizewska M, Hnatyszyn G, Sagan L, Cyrylowski L, Zekanowski C, Modrzejewska M, et al. 2009. Maternal tetrahydrobiopterin deficiency: the course of two pregnancies and follow-up of two children in a mother with 6-pyruvoyl-tetrahydropterin synthase deficiency. *Journal of Inherited Metabolic Disease* 32(Suppl. 1):S83–S89.

Goldstein DS, Hahn SH, Holmes C, Tifft C, Harvey-White J, Milstien S, et al. 1995. Monoaminergic effects of folinic acid, L-DOPA, and 5-hydroxytryptophan in dihydropteridine reductase deficiency. *Journal of Neurochemistry* 64(6):2810–2813.

Grattan-Smith PJ, Wevers RA, Steenbergen-Spanjers GC, Fung VS, Earl J, Wilcken B. 2002. Tyrosine hydroxylase deficiency: clinical manifestations of catecholamine insufficiency in infancy. *Movement Disorders: Official Journal of the Movement Disorder Society* 17(2):354–359.

Grimes DA, Barclay CL, Duff J, Furukawa Y, Lang AE. 2002. Phenocopies in a large GCH1 mutation positive family with dopa responsive dystonia: confusing the picture? *Journal of Neurology, Neurosurgery, and Psychiatry* 72(6):801–804.

Hagenah J, Saunders-Pullman R, Hedrich K, Kabakci K, Habermann K, Wiegers K, et al. 2005. High mutation rate in dopa-responsive dystonia: detection with comprehensive GCHI screening. *Neurology* 64(5):908–911.

Han B, Zou H, Han B, Zhu W, Cao Z, Liu Y. 2014. Diagnosis, treatment and follow-up of patients with tetrahydrobiopterin deficiency in Shandong province, China. *Brain & Development* 37:592–598.

Harwood G, Hierons R, Fletcher NA, Marsden CD. 1994. Lessons from a remarkable family with dopa-responsive dystonia. *Journal of Neurology, Neurosurgery, and Psychiatry* 57(4):460–463.

Haugarvoll K, Bindoff LA. 2011. A novel compound heterozygous tyrosine hydroxylase mutation (p.R441P) with complex phenotype. *Journal of Parkinson's Disease* 1(1):119–122.

Haussler M, Hoffmann GF, Wevers RA. 2001. L-dopa and selegiline for tyrosine hydroxylase deficiency. *The Journal of Pediatrics* 138(3):451–452.

Hoffmann GF, Assmann B, Brautigam C, Dionisi-Vici C, Haussler M, de Klerk JB, et al. 2003. Tyrosine hydroxylase deficiency causes progressive encephalopathy and dopa-nonresponsive dystonia. *Annals of Neurology* 54(Suppl. 6):S56–S65.

Horvath GA, Stockler-Ipsiroglu SG, Salvarinova-Zivkovic R, Lillquist YP, Connolly M, Hyland K, et al. 2008. Autosomal recessive GTP cyclohydrolase I deficiency without hyperphenylalaninemia: evidence of a phenotypic continuum between dominant and recessive forms. *Molecular Genetics and Metabolism* 94(1):127–131.

Hu FY, Xu YM, Yu LH, Ma MY, He XH, Zhou D. 2011. A novel missense mutation in GTP cyclohydrolase I (GCH1) gene causes dopa-responsive dystonia in Chinese Han population. *European Journal of Neurology: The Official Journal of the European Federation of Neurological Societies* 18(2):362–364.

Hwu WL, Wang PJ, Hsiao KJ, Wang TR, Chiou YW, Lee YM. 1999. Dopa-responsive dystonia induced by a recessive GTP cyclohydrolase I mutation. *Human Genetics* 105(3):226–230.

Hyland K, Clayton PT. 1990. Aromatic amino acid decarboxylase deficiency in twins. *Journal of Inherited Metabolic Disease* 13(3):301–304.

Hyland K, Surtees RA, Rodeck C, Clayton PT. 1992. Aromatic L-amino acid decarboxylase deficiency: clinical features, diagnosis, and treatment of a new inborn error of neurotransmitter amine synthesis. *Neurology* 42(10):1980–1988.

Ihara M, Kohara N, Urano F, Ichinose H, Takao S, Nishida T, et al. 2002. Neuroleptic malignant syndrome with prolonged catatonia in a dopa-responsive dystonia patient. *Neurology* 59(7):1102–1104.

Imamura T, Okano Y, Shintaku H, Hase Y, Isshiki G. 1999. Molecular characterization of 6-pyruvoyl-tetrahydropterin synthase deficiency in Japanese patients. *Journal of Human Genetics* 44(3):163–168.

Irons M, Levy HL, O'Flynn ME, Stack CV, Langlais PJ, Butler IJ, et al. 1987. Folinic acid therapy in treatment of dihydropteridine reductase deficiency. *The Journal of Pediatrics* 110(1):61–67.

Jaggi L, Zurfluh MR, Schuler A, Ponzone A, Porta F, Fiori L, et al. 2008. Outcome and long-term follow-up of 36 patients with tetrahydrobiopterin deficiency. *Molecular Genetics and Metabolism* 93(3):295–305.

Jankovic J. 2006. Treatment of dystonia. *Lancet Neurology* 5(10):864–872.

Janssen RJ, Wevers RA, Haussler M, Luyten JA, Steenbergen-Spanjers GC, Hoffmann GF, et al. 2000. A branch site mutation leading to aberrant splicing of the human tyrosine hydroxylase gene in a child with a severe extrapyramidal movement disorder. *Annals of Human Genetics* 64(Pt 5):375–382.

Jardim LB, Giugliani R, Coelho JC, Dutra-Filho CS, Blau N. 1994. Possible high frequency of tetrahydrobiopterin deficiency in south Brazil. *Journal of Inherited Metabolic Disease* 17(2):223–229.

Jarman PR, Bandmann O, Marsden CD, Wood NW. 1997. GTP cyclohydrolase I mutations in patients with dystonia responsive to anticholinergic drugs. *Journal of Neurology, Neurosurgery, and Psychiatry* 63(3):304–308.

Jeon BS, Jeong JM, Park SS, Kim JM, Chang YS, Song HC, et al. 1998. Dopamine transporter density measured by [123I]beta-CIT single-photon emission computed tomography is normal in dopa-responsive dystonia. *Annals of Neurology* 43(6):792–800.

Kaindl AM, Steinberger D, Heubner G, Müller U, Blau N, Neubert K, et al. 2005. Phenotype of five patients with dopa-responsive dystonia and mutations in GCH1. *Journal of Pediatric Neurology* 3(2):83–87.

Karkheiran S, Hubert B, Moghaddam H, Darvish H, Paisan-Ruiz C. 2013. Phenotypic heterogeneity and full penetrance in a family with dopa-responsive dystonia. *Clinical Genetics* 83(4):392–394.

Koht J, Rengmark A, Opladen T, Bjornara KA, Selberg T, Tallaksen CM, et al. 2014. Clinical and genetic studies in a family with a novel mutation in the sepiapterin reductase gene. *Acta Neurologica Scandinavica Supplementum* 198:7–12.

Korenke GC, Christen HJ, Hyland K, Hunneman DH, Hanefeld F. 1997. Aromatic L-amino acid decarboxylase deficiency: an extrapyramidal movement disorder with oculogyric crises. *European Journal of Paediatric Neurology: Official Journal of the European Paediatric Neurology Society* 1(2–3):67–71.

Kurian MA, Gissen P, Smith M, Heales S, Jr, Clayton PT. 2011. The monoamine neurotransmitter disorders: an expanding range of neurological syndromes. *Lancet Neurology* 10(8):721–733.

Kusmierska K, Jansen EE, Jakobs C, Szymanska K, Malunowicz E, Meilei D, et al. 2009. Sepiapterin reductase deficiency in a 2-year-old girl with incomplete response to treatment during short-term follow-up. *Journal of Inherited Metabolic Disease* 32(Suppl. 1):S5–S10.

Lee JY, Yang HJ, Kim JM, Jeon BS. 2013. Novel GCH-1 mutations and unusual long-lasting dyskinesias in Korean families with dopa-responsive dystonia. *Parkinsonism & Related Disorders* 19(12):1156–1159.

Lee LK, Cheung KM, Cheng WW, Ko CH, Lee HH, Ching CK, et al. 2014. A rare cause of severe diarrhoea diagnosed by urine metabolic screening: aromatic L-amino acid decarboxylase deficiency. *Hong Kong Medical Journal = Xianggang yi xue za zhi/Hong Kong Academy of Medicine* 20(2):161–164.

Lee NC, Cheng LY, Liu TT, Hsiao KJ, Chiu PC, Niu DM. 2006. Long-term follow-up of Chinese patients who received delayed treatment for 6-pyruvoyl-tetrahydropterin synthase deficiency. *Molecular Genetics and Metabolism* 87(2):128–134.

Lee WW, Jeon BS. 2014. Clinical spectrum of dopa-responsive dystonia and related disorders. *Current Neurology and Neuroscience Reports* 14(7):461.

Leeming RJ, Harpey JP, Brown SM, Blair JA. 1982. Tetrahydrofolate and hydroxocobolamin in the management of dihydropteridine reductase deficiency. *Journal of Mental Deficiency Research* 26(Pt 1):21–25.

Leuzzi V, Carducci CA, Carducci CL, Pozzessere S, Burlina A, Cerone R, et al. 2010. Phenotypic variability, neurological outcome and genetics background of 6-pyruvoyl-tetrahydropterin synthase deficiency. *Clinical Genetics* 77(3):249–257.

Leuzzi V, Carducci C, Tolve M, Giannini MT, Angeloni A, Carducci C. 2013. Very early pattern of movement disorders in sepiapterin reductase deficiency. *Neurology* 81(24):2141–2142.

Leuzzi V, Mastrangelo M, Polizzi A, Artiola C, van Kuilenburg AB, Carducci C, et al. 2014. Report of two never treated adult sisters with aromatic L-amino acid decarboxylase deficiency: a portrait of the natural history of the disease or an expanding phenotype? *JIMD Reports* 15:39–45.

Lin Y, Wang DN, Chen WJ, Lin X, Lin MT, Wang N. 2014. Growth hormone deficiency in a dopa-responsive dystonia patient with a novel mutation of guanosine triphosphate cyclohydrolase 1 gene. *Journal of Child Neurology* 30:796–799.

Ling H, Polke JM, Sweeney MG, Haworth A, Sandford CA, Heales SJ, et al. 2011. An intragenic duplication in guanosine triphosphate cyclohydrolase-1 gene in a dopa-responsive dystonia family. *Movement Disorders: Official Journal of the Movement Disorder Society* 26(5):905–909.

Lipson AH, Earl JW, Wilcken B, Yu JS, O'Halloran M, Cotton RG. 1991. Successful treatment of dihydropteridine reductase deficiency, with an interesting effect of 5-hydroxytryptophan deficiency on sleep patterns. *Journal of Inherited Metabolic Disease* 14(1):49–52.

Liu KM, Liu TT, Lee NC, Cheng LY, Hsiao KJ, Niu DM. 2008. Long-term follow-up of Taiwanese Chinese patients treated early for 6-pyruvoyl-tetrahydropterin synthase deficiency. *Archives of Neurology* 65(3):387–392.

Liu X, Zhang SS, Fang DF, Ma MY, Guo XY, Yang Y, et al. 2010. GCH1 mutation and clinical study of Chinese patients with dopa-responsive dystonia. *Movement Disorders: Official Journal of the Movement Disorder Society* 25(4):447–451.

Longo N. 2009. Disorders of biopterin metabolism. *Journal of Inherited Metabolic Disease* 32(3):333–342.

Lopez-Laso E, Ochoa-Sepulveda JJ, Ochoa-Amor JJ, Bescansa-Heredero E, Camino-Leon R, Gascon-Jimenez FJ, et al. 2009. Segawa syndrome due to mutation Q89X in the GCH1 gene: a possible founder effect in Cordoba (southern Spain). *Journal of Neurology* 256(11):1816–1824.

Lopez-Laso E, Beyer K, Opladen T, Artuch R, Saunders-Pullman R. 2012. Dyskinesias as a limiting factor in the treatment of Segawa disease. *Pediatric Neurology* 46(6):404–406.

Lu DY, Ye J, Han LS, Qiu WJ, Zhang HW, Zhou JD, et al. 2014. QDPR gene mutation and clinical follow-up in Chinese patients with dihydropteridine reductase deficiency. *World Journal of Pediatrics* 10(3):219–226.

Maller A, Hyland K, Milstien S, Biaggioni I, Butler IJ. 1997. Aromatic L-amino acid decarboxylase deficiency: clinical features, diagnosis, and treatment of a second family. *Journal of Child Neurology* 12(6):349–354.

Manegold C, Hoffmann GF, Degen I, Ikonomidou H, Knust A, Laass MW, et al. 2009. Aromatic L-amino acid decarboxylase deficiency: clinical features, drug therapy and follow-up. *Journal of Inherited Metabolic Disease* 32(3):371–380.

Mastrangelo M, Caputi C, Galosi S, Giannini MT, Leuzzi V. 2013. Transdermal rotigotine in the treatment of aromatic L-amino acid decarboxylase deficiency. *Movement Disorders: Official Journal of the Movement Disorder Society* 28(4):556–557.

Moller LB, Romstad A, Paulsen M, Hougaard P, Ormazabal A, Pineda M, et al. 2005. Pre- and postnatal diagnosis of tyrosine hydroxylase deficiency. *Prenatal Diagnosis* 25(8):671–675.

Naiya T, Misra AK, Biswas A, Das SK, Ray K, Ray J. 2012. Occurrence of GCH1 gene mutations in a group of Indian dystonia patients. *Journal of Neural Transmission* 119(11):1343–1350.

Nardocci N, Zorzi G, Blau N, Fernandez Alvarez E, Sesta M, Angelini L, et al. 2003. Neonatal dopa-responsive extrapyramidal syndrome in twins with recessive GTPCH deficiency. *Neurology* 60(2):335–337.

Neville BG, Parascandalo R, Farrugia R, Felice A. 2005. Sepiapterin reductase deficiency: a congenital dopa-responsive motor and cognitive disorder. *Brain: A Journal of Neurology* 128(Pt 10):2291–2296.

Ng J, Heales SJ, Kurian MA. 2014. Clinical features and pharmacotherapy of childhood monoamine neurotransmitter disorders. *Paediatric Drugs* 16(4):275–291.

Niu DM. 2011. Disorders of BH4 metabolism and the treatment of patients with 6-pyruvoyl-tetrahydropterin synthase deficiency in Taiwan. *Brain & Development* 33(10):847–855.

Nygaard TG, Marsden CD, Duvoisin RC. 1988. Dopa-responsive dystonia. *Advances in Neurology* 50:377–384.

Ogawa A, Kanazawa M, Takayanagi M, Kitani Y, Shintaku H, Kohno Y. 2008. A case of 6-pyruvoyl-tetrahydropterin synthase deficiency demonstrates a more significant correlation of L-dopa dosage with serum prolactin levels than CSF homovanillic acid levels. *Brain & Development* 30(1):82–85.

Opladen T, Hoffmann G, Horster F, Hinz AB, Neidhardt K, Klein C, et al. 2011. Clinical and biochemical characterization of patients with early infantile onset of autosomal recessive GTP cyclohydrolase I deficiency without hyperphenylalaninemia. *Movement Disorders: Official Journal of the Movement Disorder Society* 26(1):157–161.

Opladen T, Hoffmann GF, Blau N. 2012. An international survey of patients with tetrahydrobiopterin deficiencies presenting with hyperphenylalaninaemia. *Journal of Inherited Metabolic Disease* 35(6):963–973.

Pons R. 2009. The phenotypic spectrum of paediatric neurotransmitter diseases and infantile parkinsonism. *Journal of Inherited Metabolic Disease* 32(3):321–332.

Pons R, Ford B, Chiriboga CA, Clayton PT, Hinton V, Hyland K, et al. 2004. Aromatic L-amino acid decarboxylase deficiency: clinical features, treatment, and prognosis. *Neurology* 62(7):1058–1065.

Pons R, Syrengelas D, Youroukos S, Orfanou I, Dinopoulos A, Cormand B, et al. 2013. Levodopa-induced dyskinesias in tyrosine hydroxylase deficiency. *Movement Disorders: Official Journal of the Movement Disorder Society* 28(8):1058–1063.

Ponzone A, Blau N, Guardamagna O, Ferrero GB, Dianzani I, Endres W. 1990. Progression of 6-pyruvoyl-tetrahydropterin synthase deficiency from a peripheral into a central phenotype. *Journal of Inherited Metabolic Disease* 13(3):298–300.

Ponzone A, Spada M, Ferraris S, Dianzani I, de Sanctis L. 2004. Dihydropteridine reductase deficiency in man: from biology to treatment. *Medicinal Research Reviews* 24(2):127–150.

Porta F, Mussa A, Concolino D, Spada M, Ponzone A. 2009. Dopamine agonists in 6-pyruvoyl tetrahydropterin synthase deficiency. *Neurology* 73(8):633–637.

Porta F, Spada M, Garelli D, Mussa A, Ponzone A. 2011. Tetrahydrobiopterin and phenylketonuria. *The Journal of Pediatrics* 158(5):864.

Porta F, Mussa A, Concolino D, Spada M, Ponzone A. 2012. Dopamine agonists in dihydropteridine reductase deficiency. *Molecular Genetics and Metabolism* 105(4):582–584.

Rajput AH, Fenton M, Birdi S, Macaulay R. 1997. Is levodopa toxic to human substantia nigra? *Movement Disorders: Official Journal of the Movement Disorder Society* 12(5):634–638.

Regula JU, Thoden U, Meinck HM. 2007. Adult-onset dystonia: atypical manifestation of Segawa disease. *Movement Disorders: Official Journal of the Movement Disorder Society* 22(9):1335–1337.

Ribases M, Serrano M, Fernandez-Alvarez E, Pahisa S, Ormazabal A, Garcia-Cazorla A, et al. 2007. A homozygous tyrosine hydroxylase gene promoter mutation in a patient with dopa-responsive encephalopathy: clinical, biochemical and genetic analysis. *Molecular Genetics and Metabolism* 92(3):274–277.

Robinson R, McCarthy GT, Bandmann O, Dobbie M, Surtees R, Wood NW. 1999. GTP cyclohydrolase deficiency: intrafamilial variation in clinical phenotype, including levodopa responsiveness. *Journal of Neurology, Neurosurgery, and Psychiatry* 66(1):86–89.

Roze E, Vidailhet M, Blau N, Moller LB, Doummar D, de Villemeur TB, et al. 2006. Long-term follow-up and adult outcome of 6-pyruvoyl-tetrahydropterin synthase deficiency. *Movement Disorders: Official Journal of the Movement Disorder Society* 21(2):263–266.

Sanford M, Keating GM. 2009. Sapropterin: a review of its use in the treatment of primary hyperphenylalaninaemia. *Drugs* 69(4):461–476.

Sato H, Uematsu M, Endo W, Nakayama T, Kobayashi T, Hino-Fukuyo N, et al. 2014. Early replacement therapy in a first Japanese case with autosomal recessive guanosine triphosphate cyclohydrolase I deficiency with a novel point mutation. *Brain & Development* 36(3):268–271.

Saunders-Pullman R, Blau N, Hyland K, Zschocke J, Nygaard T, Raymond D, et al. 2004. Phenylalanine loading as a diagnostic test for DRD: interpreting the utility of the test. *Molecular Genetics and Metabolism* 83(3):207–212.

Schiller A, Wevers RA, Steenbergen GC, Blau N, Jung HH. 2004. Long-term course of L-dopa-responsive dystonia caused by tyrosine hydroxylase deficiency. *Neurology* 63(8):1524–1526.

Schmidt H, Ullrich K, Korinthenberg R, Peters PE. 1988. Basal ganglion calcification in hyperphenylalaninemia due to deficiency of dihydropteridine reductase. *Pediatric Radiology* 19(1):54–56.

Schuler A, Blau N, Ponzone A. 1995. Monoamine oxidase inhibitors in tetrahydrobiopterin deficiency. *European Journal of Pediatrics* 154(12):997.

Schuler A, Kalmanchey R, Barsi P, Somogyi CS, Toros I, Varadi I, et al. 2000. Deprenyl in the treatment of patients with tetrahydrobiopterin deficiencies. *Journal of Inherited Metabolic Disease* 23(4):329–332.

Sedel F, Ribeiro MJ, Remy P, Blau N, Saudubray JM, Agid Y. 2006. Dihydropteridine reductase deficiency: levodopa's long-term effectiveness without dyskinesia. *Neurology* 67(12): 2243–2245.

Segawa M. 2011. Hereditary progressive dystonia with marked diurnal fluctuation. *Brain & development* 33(3):195–201.

Segawa M, Hosaka A, Miyagawa F, Nomura Y, Imai H. 1976. Hereditary progressive dystonia with marked diurnal fluctuation. *Advances in Neurology* 14:215–233.

Segawa M, Nomura Y, Nishiyama N. 2003. Autosomal dominant guanosine triphosphate cyclohydrolase I deficiency (Segawa disease). *Annals of Neurology* 54(Suppl. 6):S32–S45.

Sharma N, Armata IA, Multhaupt-Buell TJ, Ozelius LJ, Xin W, Sims KB. 2011. Mutation in 5′ upstream region of GCHI gene causes familial dopa-responsive dystonia. *Movement Disorders: Official Journal of the Movement Disorder Society* 26(11):2140–2141.

Shintaku H. 2002. Disorders of tetrahydrobiopterin metabolism and their treatment. *Current Drug Metabolism* 3(2):123–131.

Shintaku H, Ohwada M. 2013. Long-term follow-up of tetrahydrobiopterin therapy in patients with tetrahydrobiopterin deficiency in Japan. *Brain & Development* 35(5):406–410.

Spada M, Parrella T, Ponzone R, Ferraris S, Guardamagna O, Ponzone A, et al. 1991. Monitoring treatment in tetrahydrobiopterin deficiency. *Pteridines*. doi: https://doi.org/10.1515/pteridines.1991.3.12.13.

Stamelou M, Mencacci NE, Cordivari C, Batla A, Wood NW, Houlden H, et al. 2012. Myoclonus-dystonia syndrome due to tyrosine hydroxylase deficiency. *Neurology* 79(5):435–441.

Steinberger D, Topka H, Fischer D, Muller U. 1999. GCH1 mutation in a patient with adult-onset oromandibular dystonia. *Neurology* 52(4):877–879.

Steinberger D, Korinthenberg R, Topka H, Berghauser M, Wedde R, Muller U, German Dystonia Study Group. 2000. Dopa-responsive dystonia: mutation analysis of GCH1 and analysis of therapeutic doses of L-dopa. *Neurology* 55(11):1735–1737.

Steinberger D, Trubenbach J, Zirn B, Leube B, Wildhardt G, Muller U. 2007. Utility of MLPA in deletion analysis of GCH1 in dopa-responsive dystonia. *Neurogenetics* 8(1):51–55.

Sun ZF, Zhang YH, Guo JF, Sun QY, Mei JP, Zhou HL, et al. 2014. Genetic diagnosis of two dopa-responsive dystonia families by exome sequencing. *PLoS One* 9(9):e106388.

Surtees R, Hyland K. 1990. L-3,4-dihydroxyphenylalanine (levodopa) lowers central nervous system S-adenosylmethionine concentrations in humans. *Journal of Neurology, Neurosurgery, and Psychiatry* 53(7):569–572.

Swoboda KJ, Hyland K, Goldstein DS, Kuban KC, Arnold LA, Holmes CS, et al. 1999. Clinical and therapeutic observations in aromatic L-amino acid decarboxylase deficiency. *Neurology* 53(6):1205–1211.

Tachi N, Takahashi S, Jo M, Shinoda M. 2011. A new mutation of GCH1 in triplets family with dopa-responsive dystonia. *European Journal of Neurology: The Official Journal of the European Federation of Neurological Societies* 18(9):1191–1193.

Tassin J, Durr A, Bonnet AM, Gil R, Vidailhet M, Lucking CB, et al. 2000. Levodopa-responsive dystonia: GTP cyclohydrolase I or parkin mutations? *Brain: A Journal of Neurology* 123 (Pt 6):1112–1121.

Tay SK, Poh KS, Hyland K, Pang YW, Ong HT, Low PS, et al. 2007. Unusually mild phenotype of AADC deficiency in 2 siblings. *Molecular Genetics and Metabolism* 91(4):374–378.

Theuns J, Crosiers D, Debaene L, Nuytemans K, Meeus B, Sleegers K, et al. 2012. Guanosine triphosphate cyclohydrolase 1 promoter deletion causes dopa-responsive dystonia. *Movement Disorders: Official Journal of the Movement Disorder Society* 27(11):1451–1456.

Thibert R, Hyland K, Chiles J, Steinberg S, Eichler F. 2012. Levodopa response reveals sepiapterin reductase deficiency in a female heterozygote with adrenoleukodystrophy. *JIMD Reports* 3:79–82.

Thony B, Auerbach G, Blau N. 2000. Tetrahydrobiopterin biosynthesis, regeneration and functions. *The Biochemical Journal* 347(Pt 1):1–16.

Trender-Gerhard I, Sweeney MG, Schwingenschuh P, Mir P, Edwards MJ, Gerhard A, et al. 2009. Autosomal-dominant GTPCH1-deficient DRD: clinical characteristics and long-term outcome of 34 patients. *Journal of Neurology, Neurosurgery, and Psychiatry* 80(8):839–845.

Uncini A, De Angelis MV, Di Fulvio P, Ragno M, Annesi G, Filla A, et al. 2004. Wide expressivity variation and high but no gender-related penetrance in two dopa-responsive dystonia families with a novel GCH-I mutation. *Movement Disorders: Official Journal of the Movement Disorder Society* 19(10):1139–1145.

Verbeek MM, Willemsen MA, Wevers RA, Lagerwerf AJ, Abeling NG, Blau N, et al. 2008. Two Greek siblings with sepiapterin reductase deficiency. *Molecular Genetics and Metabolism* 94(4):403–409.

Watanabe T, Matsubara S, Baba Y, Tanaka H, Suzuki T, Suzuki M. 2009. Successful management of pregnancy in a patient with Segawa disease: case report and literature review. *The Journal of Obstetrics and Gynaecology Research* 35(3):562–564.

Willemsen MA, Verbeek MM, Kamsteeg EJ, de Rijk-van Andel JF, Aeby A, Blau N, et al. 2010. Tyrosine hydroxylase deficiency: a treatable disorder of brain catecholamine biosynthesis. *Brain: A Journal of Neurology* 133(Pt 6):1810–1822.

Wu ZY, Lin Y, Chen WJ, Zhao GX, Xie H, Murong SX, et al. 2008. Molecular analyses of GCH-1, TH and parkin genes in Chinese dopa-responsive dystonia families. *Clinical Genetics* 74(6):513–521.

Wu-Chou YH, Yeh TH, Wang CY, Lin JJ, Huang CC, Chang HC, et al. 2010. High frequency of multiexonic deletion of the GCH1 gene in a Taiwanese cohort of dopa-response dystonia. *American Journal of Medical Genetics Part B, Neuropsychiatric Genetics: The Official Publication of the International Society of Psychiatric Genetics* 153B(4):903–908.

Ye J, Yang Y, Yu W, Zou H, Jiang J, Yang R, et al. 2013. Demographics, diagnosis and treatment of 256 patients with tetrahydrobiopterin deficiency in mainland China: results of a retrospective, multicentre study. *Journal of Inherited Metabolic Disease* 36(5):893–901.

Yeung WL, Wong VC, Chan KY, Hui J, Fung CW, Yau E, et al. 2011. Expanding phenotype and clinical analysis of tyrosine hydroxylase deficiency. *Journal of Child Neurology* 26(2):179–187.

Yosunkaya E, Karaca E, Basaran S, Seven M, Yuksel A. 2010. Marked improvement in Segawa syndrome after L-dopa and selegiline treatment. *Pediatric Neurology* 42(5):348–350.

Zirn B, Steinberger D, Troidl C, Brockmann K, von der Hagen M, Feiner C, et al. 2008. Frequency of GCH1 deletions in dopa-responsive dystonia. *Journal of Neurology, Neurosurgery, and Psychiatry* 79(2):183–186.

Chapter 56

Treatment of Paroxysmal Dystonia

Roberto Erro, Bettina Balint and Kailash P. Bhatia

Introduction

Paroxysmal movement disorders are defined as abnormal involuntary movements that recur intermittently, with abrupt onset, variable duration and without loss of consciousness (Erro et al. 2014a). From the phenomenology point of view, the involuntary movements may be dystonia, chorea, ballismus, or a complex mixture of these, therefore referred to as *paroxysmal dyskinesias* (PxD). Traditionally, the classification of PxD has been based on their clinical characteristics, e.g. trigger(s) and duration of the attacks, but a great advance in our understanding on the aetiology and pathophysiology of these conditions has recently come from the elucidation of the genetic forms of PxD (see Chapter 10). Accordingly, we will discuss the treatment of PxD based on the underlying causative genes (e.g. PPRT2, MR-1, GLUT1). This choice is owing to the evidence that patients with similar clinical features tend to respond differently to treatment according to whether they carry a particular genetic defect or not (Bruno et al. 2007; Li et al. 2013). Treatment in patients who do not carry such genetic mutations, as well as in symptomatic cases, should be pursued on an empirical basis, since there is no robust evidence to guide therapeutic choices. One exception, however, is represented by the clinical syndrome of paroxysmal exercise-induced dystonia (PED) that, beyond GLUT1 deficiency syndrome, has been consistently reported to be associated with some treatable conditions. Hence, PED associated with other conditions will be discussed separately. Furthermore, we will also briefly cover other conditions not classically classified into the PxD that, however, can encompass paroxysmal dystonia in their phenotype, with treatment implications.

Treatment of Paroxysmal Dyskinesias

PRRT2-Related Paroxysmal Dyskinesias

Heterozygous mutations in PRRT2, a gene encoding the proline-rich transmembrane protein 2, have been discovered to be the major cause of the clinical syndrome of paroxysmal kinesigenic dyskinesia (PKD) (see Chapter 10). Nonetheless, recent reports have highlighted that patients with PRRT2 mutations can be clinically heterogeneous (e.g. manifest with other types of PxD), and also that treatment efficacy differs between patients with PKD carrying or not PRRT2 mutations (Li et al. 2013). The identification of PRRT2 mutations has therefore crucial implications in terms of treatment and prognosis.

The first-line option for PRRT2-related dyskinesias is represented by carbamazepine (CBZ). Low dosages of CBZ, usually between 50 and 200 mg daily, are most effective in most PPRT2 patients. The reason why CBZ is the most effective antiepileptic drug to treat this condition is unknown since the biological function of PRRT2 has not been entirely clarified. One recent line of evidence would support a role for the mutant PRRT2 in affecting glutamate signalling, likely through its weakened interaction with SNAP-25, a presynaptic Q-SNARE protein involved in the fusion of neurotransmitter vesicles to the cellular membrane, and the glutamate receptor GRIA1, eventually leading to the increase of glutamate release and subsequent neuronal hyperexcitability (Li et al. 2015). One of the mechanisms of action of CBZ at clinically relevant concentrations is indeed through its ability to enhance the affinity of the postsynaptic glutamate transporter type 3 (EAAT3), hence allowing the glutamate to be pumped out from the synaptic cleft without binding its receptor and activate a postsynaptic potential (Lee et al. 2005).

On the other hand, SNAP-25 seems also able to modulate the kinetics of voltage-gated Ca^{2+} channels such as the Cav2.1 calcium channel (Yokoyama et al. 2005) and the abnormal interaction between the mutant PRRT2 and SNAP-25 might result in an alteration of Cav2.1 properties, leading to neuronal hyperexcitability. On this basis, some authors suggest that any voltage-gated sodium channel blockers, including CBZ, oxcarbazepine, phenytoin and lacosamide, all used at low dosages (Table 56.1), could be chosen according to their side-effect profile and patient comorbidities. However, it should be noted that all these recommendations are based on a class IV level of evidence (e.g. observational studies without controls) and other single papers have also reported on the efficacy of different antiepileptic drugs, including topiramate, valproate and lamotrigine (Erro et al. 2014a). The latter group of drugs can be therefore used in selected patients in whom voltage-gated sodium channel blockers caused cross-hypersensitivity and allergic reactions.

MR-1-Related Paroxysmal Dyskinesias

The MR-1 gene on chromosome 2q35 encodes for a protein with three isoforms with different cellular distribution and presumably distinct biological functions. Mutations in this gene have been discovered to be the major cause of the clinical

Table 56.1 Treatment of PRRT2-related paroxysmal dyskinesias

Drug	Daily dosage	Possible side-effects	Reference
Carbamazepine	50–200 mg	Skin rash (particularly in people of Asian descent), aplastic anaemia, agranulocytosis, dizziness, drowsiness, nausea, vomiting, dry mouth, oedema, loss of balance or coordination	(Bruno et al. 2004)
Oxcarbazepine	75–300 mg	As for carbamazepine	(Yang et al. 2012)
Phenytoin	100–200 mg	Headache, nausea and vomiting, constipation, dizziness, drowsiness, slurred speech, loss of balance or coordination, insomnia, cardiac arrhythmias, skin reactions	(Bruno et al. 2004)
Lacosamide	50–100 mg	Dizziness, spinning sensation, loss of balance or coordination, blurred vision, nausea and vomiting, drowsiness, tiredness, headache, skin reactions	(Mathew et al. 2012)

syndrome of paroxysmal non-kinesigenic dyskinesias (PNKD; see Chapter 10). In PNKD, attacks are mainly precipitated by coffee and alcohol, although other triggers have been reported including stress and sleep deprivation. The biological function of MR-1 is not entirely known. Yet, MR-1 is a homolog of the *hydroxyacylglutathione hydrolase* gene that is implicated in the pathway to detoxify methylglyoxal, a compound present in coffee and alcoholic drinks and also produced as a byproduct of oxidative stress, thereby suggesting a possible mechanism whereby alcohol, coffee and stress can trigger attacks in MR-1-positive patients (Erro et al. 2014a). On the other hand, recent evidence would suggest that MR-1 is a synaptic protein with a regulatory role in calcium-dependent neurotransmitter release (Shen et al. 2015). It is interesting to note that caffeine acts as a ryanodine receptor agonist and can stimulate calcium efflux from the endoplasmic reticulum and the speculation would be that, in MR-1 patients, neurons are more vulnerable to elevated calcium levels and might hence develop hyperexcitability when challenged with coffee, alcohol or stress (Shen et al. 2015).

On this basis, lifestyle modifications and diet (by avoiding triggers) can greatly reduce or almost abolish attacks in up to one-third of patients with MR-1 mutations. In patients who require pharmacological treatment, benzodiazepines are the first-line options and can be used both as prophylactic and rescue drugs. Clonazepam and diazepam have been most commonly used (class IV level of evidence) and have been reported to reduce both the frequency and severity of the attacks in up to 97 per cent of patients (Bruno et al. 2007), but other benzodiazepines can be beneficial, including lorazepam and alternate-day oxazepam. Low dosages are somewhat effective, but the total amount of drug needs to be tailored to single patients. A partial benefit has also been reported in individual cases with a number of different drugs including haloperidol, levetiracetam, valproate or anticholinergics, whereas carbamazepine is ineffective in the majority of patients (Mink 2015).

As for PRRT2-positive patients, also in patients carrying MR-1 mutations the attacks tend to decrease or remit during adulthood, regardless of any treatments.

GLUT1-Related Paroxysmal Dyskinesias

GLUT1 (also named SLC2A1) encodes the glucose transporter type 1 that facilitates the transport of glucose across the blood–brain barrier. Mutations in the GLUT1 gene can cause a broad variety of neurological disorders, ranging from severe encephalopathies with learning disability and epilepsy to pure paroxysmal exercise-induced dyskinesias (PED). The different phenotypes seem, at least partially, to be due to the specific type of genetic mutation, with splice site, nonsense, insertions and deletions (i.e. loss of function mutations) being associated with a more severe clinical phenotype of GLUT1 deficiency syndrome compared with missense mutations that more commonly present with PED (Erro et al. 2014a). Regardless of the phenotype, in patients carrying GLUT1 mutations therapeutic approaches should be attempted to treat the underlying neuroglycopenia. In this regard, good outcomes have been reported with early dietary treatment by means of ketogenic diet (Ramm-Pettersen et al. 2013), even though PED might occasionally worsen with this type of diet (Suls et al. 2008). However, compliance with this type of diet is rather poor and the modified Atkins diet, which has a less strict fat-to-non-fat ratio as well as no restriction of food or fluid intake and is therefore better tolerated by patients, has been proposed as an alternative, with good results on PED and other paroxysmal disorders (Leen et al. 2013). As stated above, one of these diets should be pursued to treat the underlying neuroglycopenia, regardless of the specific outcome on the PED. A single reported case showed some benefit with acetazolamide (Guimaraes & Vale Santos 2000) or L-dopa (Baschieri et al. 2014), but generally PED due to GLUT1 mutations tends to respond less well to pharmacological treatments (Mink 2015), while lifestyle modifications by avoiding sustained exercise might be very important in preventing attacks.

PED and Other Neurological Disorders

Only about 25 per cent of patients with PED carry GLUT1 mutations, implying that other conditions might be responsible for this clinical syndrome. One recent case series has showed that the underlying aetiology of PED is quite heterogeneous, further suggesting that prompt recognition of the cause of PED is crucial, since most of these disorders are treatable, and misdiagnosis can possibly lead to inappropriate management of these patients (Erro et al. 2014b). Beyond GLUT1 deficiency syndrome, which has been discussed above, two other conditions should be kept in mind when faced with a patient with PED: dopa-responsive dystonia due to mutations in the GTP cyclohydrolase 1 gene and young-onset Parkinson disease, possibly due to parkin mutations. In both cases, dopaminergic drugs represent the first-choice treatment, even though anticholinergic drugs or botulinum toxin injections can also be beneficial.

Other Genetic Disorders Encompassing Paroxysmal Dystonia

With the advent of next-generation sequencing techniques, different conditions that can encompass paroxysmal dystonia in their phenotype have been identified. We will here briefly describe three of these disorders, with treatment implications.

Monocarboxylate transporter type 8 (MCT8) deficiency, formerly known as Allan–Herndon–Dudley syndrome, is a rare disorder due to SLC16A2 mutations that are inherited in a X-linked fashion. Typically, affected males present with proximal hypotonia generalised muscular hypotrophy, microcephaly, marked developmental delay, spasticity and ataxia. A number of patients also present with brief paroxysmal attacks, which are dystonic in nature and are induced by passive movements such as changing of their clothes or nappies or by lifting the children from one place to another (Brockmann et al. 2005). The attacks can be further triggered by excitement, happiness or crying. Unfortunately, treatment approaches are disappointing. However, a trial with diiodothyropropionic acid (1–2 mg/kg per day) has been recently published with good short-term outcomes (Verge et al. 2012). Nonetheless, the effects of earlier therapy and long-term outcomes remain to be determined.

Alternating hemiplegia of childhood (AHC) is a rare disorder due to mutations in the ATP1A3 gene (compare Chapter 10) that, despite its name, almost invariably features frequent episodes of either hemidystonia or hemiplegia manifesting together with other paroxysmal symptoms such as nystagmus, anarthria, dysphagia, hypersalivation and seizures. Such attacks can be as long as several days and are typically induced by emotional stressors, but also by hypo- or hyperthermia, respiratory tract infections and bright light. As far as the attacks are concerned, the medical treatment of AHC should focus on episode prophylaxis by avoiding triggers and chronic therapy, and on the acute management of attacks. Despite there being no controlled trials, the actual mainstay for attacks prophylaxis is represented by flunarizine (5–20 mg/day), which has been reported to reduce frequency, duration and severity of the attacks (Neville & Ninan 2007). Because of the consistent relief of symptoms by sleep, early induction of sleep by oral melatonin or, in cases where this is ineffective, sedation by buccal midazolam or rectal diazepam are advocated as soon as an attack starts (Neville & Ninan 2007).

Finally, ADCY5 mutations have been recently described as a novel entity with a heterogeneous clinical presentation that can also feature paroxysmal episodes of choreo-dystonia (Mencacci et al. 2015). Treatment outcomes have only been reported in single families and are generally disappointing, despite a partial benefit being reported with tetrabenazine (Mencacci et al. 2015).

References

Baschieri F, Batla A, Erro R, Ganos C, Cordivari C, Bhatia KP. 2014. Paroxysmal exercise-induced dystonia due to GLUT1 mutation can be responsive to levodopa: a case report. *Journal of Neurology* 261(3):615–616.

Brockmann K, Dumitrescu AM, Best TT, Hanefeld F, Refetoff S. 2005. X-linked paroxysmal dyskinesia and severe global retardation caused by defective MCT8 gene. *Journal of Neurology* 252(6):663–666.

Bruno MK, Hallett M, Gwinn-Hardy K, Sorensen B, Considine E, Tucker S, et al. 2004. Clinical evaluation of idiopathic paroxysmal kinesigenic dyskinesia: new diagnostic criteria. *Neurology* 63(12):2280–2287.

Bruno MK, Lee HY, Auburger GW, Friedman A, Nielsen JE, Lang AE, et al. 2007. Genotype–phenotype correlation of paroxysmal nonkinesigenic dyskinesia. *Neurology* 68(21):1782–1789.

Erro R, Sheerin UM, Bhatia KP. 2014a. Paroxysmal dyskinesias revisited: a review of 500 genetically proven cases and a new classification. *Movement Disorders: Official Journal of the Movement Disorder Society* 29(9):1108–1116.

Erro R, Stamelou M, Ganos C, Skorvanek M, Han V, Batla A, et al. 2014b. The clinical syndrome of paroxysmal exercise-induced dystonia: diagnostic outcomes and an algorithm. *Movement Disorders: Clinical Practice* 1(1):57–61.

Guimaraes J, Vale Santos J. 2000. Paroxysmal dystonia induced by exercise and acetazolamide. *European Journal of Neurology: The Official Journal of the European Federation of Neurological Societies* 7(2):237–240.

Lee G, Huang Y, Washington JM, Briggs NW, Zuo Z. 2005. Carbamazepine enhances the activity of glutamate transporter type 3 via phosphatidylinositol 3-kinase. *Epilepsy Research* 66(1–3):145–153.

Leen WG, Mewasingh L, Verbeek MM, Kamsteeg EJ, van de Warrenburg BP, Willemsen MA. 2013. Movement disorders in GLUT1 deficiency syndrome respond to the modified Atkins diet. *Movement Disorders: Official Journal of the Movement Disorder Society* 28(10):1439–1442.

Li HF, Chen WJ, Ni W, Wang KY, Liu GL, Wang N, et al. 2013. PRRT2 mutation correlated with phenotype of paroxysmal kinesigenic dyskinesia and drug response. *Neurology* 80(16):1534–1535.

Li M, Niu F, Zhu X, Wu X, Shen N, Peng X, et al. 2015. PRRT2 mutant leads to dysfunction of glutamate signaling. *International Journal of Molecular Sciences* 16(5):9134–9151.

Mathew T, Aroor S, Nadig R, Sarma GR. 2012. Lacosamide in paroxysmal kinesigenic dyskinesia. *Movement Disorders: Official Journal of the Movement Disorder Society* 27(6):801–802.

Mencacci NE, Erro R, Wiethoff S, Hersheson J, Ryten M, Balint B, et al. 2015. ADCY5 mutations are another cause of benign hereditary chorea. *Neurology* 85(1):80–88.

Mink JW. 2015. Treatment of paroxysmal dyskinesias in children. *Current Treatment Options in Neurology* 17(6):350.

Neville BG, Ninan M. 2007. The treatment and management of alternating hemiplegia of childhood. *Developmental Medicine and Child Neurology* 49(10):777–780.

Ramm-Pettersen A, Nakken KO, Skogseid IM, Randby H, Skei EB, Bindoff LA, et al. 2013. Good outcome in patients with early dietary treatment of GLUT-1 deficiency syndrome: results from a retrospective Norwegian study. *Developmental Medicine and Child Neurology* 55(5):440–447.

Shen Y, Ge WP, Li Y, Hirano A, Lee HY, Rohlmann A, et al. 2015. Protein mutated in paroxysmal dyskinesia interacts with the active zone protein RIM and suppresses synaptic vesicle exocytosis. *Proceedings of the National Academy of Sciences of the United States of America* 112(10):2935–2941.

Suls A, Dedeken P, Goffin K, Van Esch H, Dupont P, Cassiman D, et al. 2008. Paroxysmal exercise-induced dyskinesia and epilepsy is due to mutations in SLC2A1, encoding the glucose transporter GLUT1. *Brain: A Journal of Neurology* 131(Pt 7):1831–1844.

Verge CF, Konrad D, Cohen M, Di Cosmo C, Dumitrescu AM, Marcinkowski T, et al. 2012. Diiodothyropropionic acid (DITPA) in the treatment of MCT8 deficiency. *The Journal of Clinical Endocrinology and Metabolism* 97(12):4515–4523.

Yang Y, Su Y, Guo Y, Ding Y, Xu S, Jiang Y, et al. 2012. Oxcarbazepine versus carbamazepine in the treatment of paroxysmal kinesigenic dyskinesia. *The International Journal of Neuroscience* 122(12):719–722.

Yokoyama CT, Myers SJ, Fu J, Mockus SM, Scheuer T, Catterall WA. 2005. Mechanism of SNARE protein binding and regulation of Cav2 channels by phosphorylation of the synaptic protein interaction site. *Molecular and Cellular Neurosciences* 28(1):1–17.

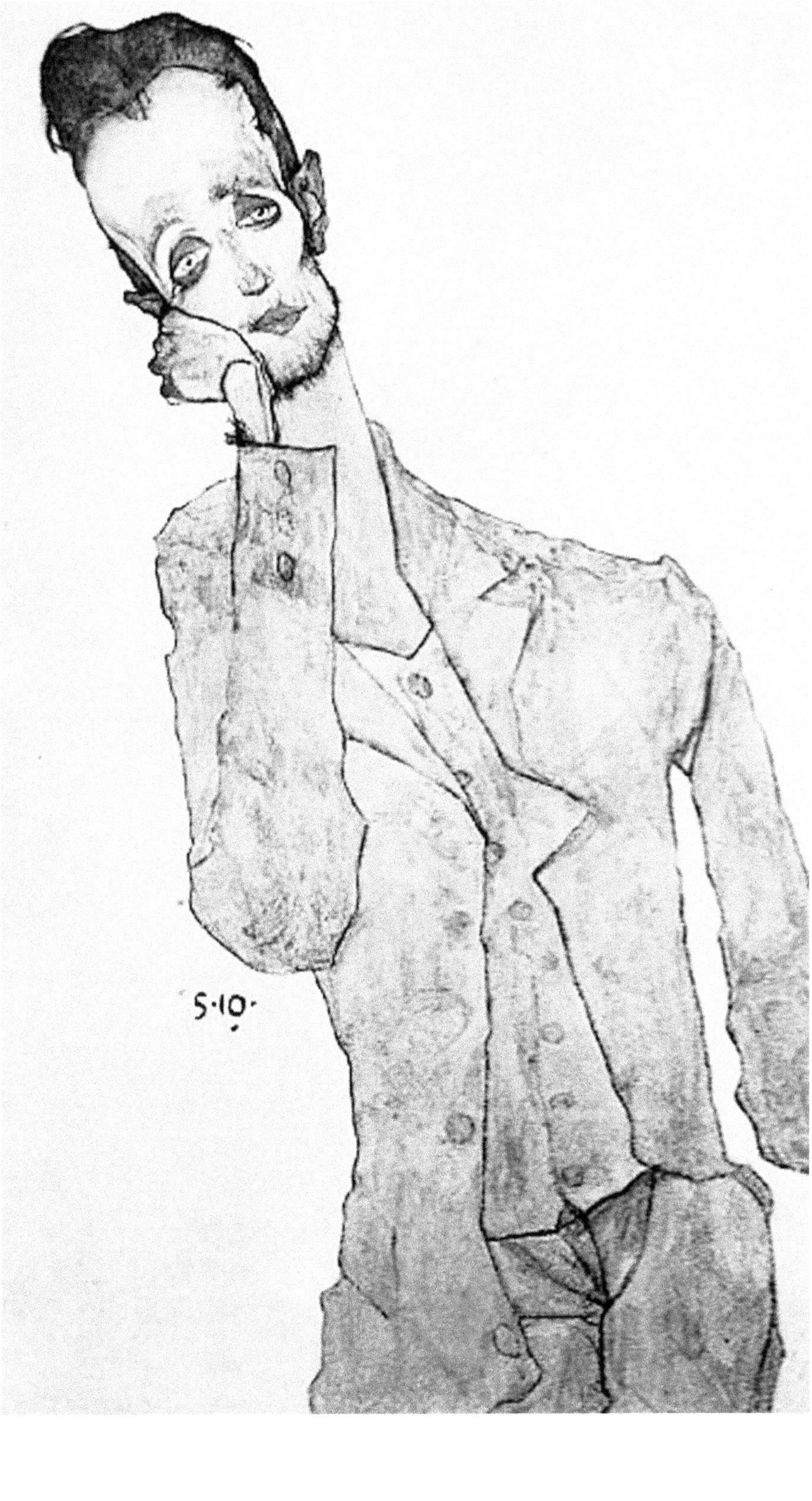
S·10·

Chapter 57

History of Surgical Treatments for Dystonia

Joachim K. Krauss

Surgical treatment of dystonia has a long and convoluted history, with the first procedures having been performed long before the concept of dystonia as a clinical entity had been introduced. Here, a brief overview of the history of surgical treatment of dystonia will be given, with an emphasis on procedures that are not included in the armamentarium of contemporary surgery. For details on the more commonly performed procedures, the reader is being referred to the corresponding chapters in this book.

In the past decades several paradigmatic shifts occurred which resulted in an increased return of interest in surgical treatment options in dystonia. While some methods were abandoned because they were replaced by other techniques with a lower profile of side-effects (e.g. intradural upper cervical anterior rhizotomy was supplanted by selective peripheral denervation using ramisectomy), others were renounced because of lack of proven efficacy (such as microvascular decompression or spinal cord stimulation for cervical dystonia). The most pivotal factor, however, was the introduction of pallidal deep brain stimulation (DBS) as a bilateral procedure to treat all types of dystonia in the 1990s (Krauss et al. 1999b; Coubes et al. 2000). While DBS is now widely available, surgical expertise to perform ablative basal ganglia surgery and selective peripheral denervation has become much more limited (Valadas et al. 2016).

Early Surgical Treatment for Dystonia

It has been said that the first operations to treat cervical dystonia were performed in Ancient Greece (Iskandar & Nashold 1995). It was in 1641 that the German surgeon Minnius sectioned the sternocleidomastoid muscle in a patient with cervical dystonia (Finney & Hughson 1925). Bujalski has been credited with performing the first denervation of cervical muscles for treatment of cervical dystonia in 1834, and de Morgan for sectioning the spinal accessory nerve in 1866 (Finney & Hughson 1925; Vogel et al. 2010).

Surgery for cervical dystonia became more popular in the late nineteenth and early twentieth centuries (Rossitch et al. 1991). Keen introduced sectioning and partial denervation of the posterior neck muscles in cervical dystonia in 1891 (Keen 1891), and de Quervain combined anterior and posterior myotomies several years later (Iskandar & Nashold 1995). Soon thereafter, Taylor introduced posterior rhizotomy of the upper cervical nerve roots, though with limited success (Taylor 1915). Subsequently, attention shifted to the anterior cervical roots.

McKenzie developed unilateral intradural sectioning of the anterior upper cervical nerve roots combined with partial sectioning of the intradural spinal accessory nerve in the 1920s (McKenzie 1954). The procedure was then further refined by Dandy (Dandy 1930) and by Hamby & Schiffer (1969, 1970), who demonstrated the clinical efficacy of bilateral upper cervical anterior rhizotomy. It became the most frequently performed standard procedure for cervical dystonia for many decades.

Intradural Rhizotomy and the Rise of Selective Peripheral Denervation

Several variations of this procedure were developed in different centres worldwide (Ondo & Krauss 2004). The 'standard' procedure included intradural sectioning of the C1–C3 anterior roots and those rootlets of the spinal accessory nerves supplying the sternocleidomastoid muscles. The approach included a small suboccipital craniotomy with widening of the posterior rim of the foramen magnum and laminectomies of the three upper cervical vertebrae. After opening the dura, the upper spinal cord, the medulla oblongata, the cerebellar tonsils, the upper cranial nerve roots, the spinal accessory nerves and the blood vessels at the cervicomedullary junction and the upper cervical medulla were visualised. The anterior roots were identified and then divided, sparing arterial blood vessels which accompany the nerve roots. Denervation with this approach was limited downward to the anterior root of C3 if performed bilaterally. Unilateral rhizotomy of the C4 root was applied by some surgeons, although this manoeuvre was known to endanger functioning of the diaphragm.

It is obvious that this intradural approach could not control dystonic activity mediated via the C4–C6 roots. Since the 'standard' approach was rather non-selective and resulted occasionally in severe complications, modified techniques were developed aiming to denervate the dystonic muscles and to preserve normal activity (Krauss et al. 1997). Thus, for example in a patient with prominent rotational cervical dystonia, unilateral anterior rhizotomy would be combined with contralateral spinal accessory nerve section.

Outcome and complication rates were highly variable in different series (Arseni & Maretsis 1971; Colbassani & Wood

1986; Friedman et al. 1993). Many studies claimed postoperative improvement in 60–90 per cent of their patients. Little data have become available, however, on improvement of functional disability, in particular with regard to the relatively high number of side-effects. In the series of Friedman et al., the head was described to return to a neutral position in 59 per cent of patients postoperatively (Friedman et al. 1993). In this series, the likelihood of the head returning to a normal position postoperatively was inversely related to the duration of CD. Some studies have reported only very modest results after anterior intradural rhizotomy. Hernesniemi and Keränen, for example, reported no patient with an outcome considered as good based on their patients' self-assessments of the surgical result, disability and working capacity (Hernesniemi & Keränen 1990).

Complications of the standard bilateral intradural approach were frequent and sometimes persistent and disabling. Mortality with the standard procedure ranged between 0 and 1 per cent, in general, but was as high as 12 per cent in some series (Arseni & Maretsis 1971). Side-effects included dysphagia, weakness of the neck, cerebrospinal fluid fistulas and infection. Weak or unstable neck has been estimated to occur in about 40 per cent of patients after bilateral anterior rhizotomy, and transient dysphagia in about 30 per cent of patients (Colbassani & Wood 1986). Radiologic swallowing abnormalities were described in as many as 95 per cent of patients postoperatively; sometimes, however, this was thought to represent aggravation of pre-existing pharyngeal dysfunction (Horner et al. 1992). Rarely, bilateral infarctions of the medulla oblongata with Wallenberg syndrome or ischaemia of the upper spinal cord with tetraparesis were reported (Sweet 1975; Scoville 1978). The procedure was much safer and accompanied by far less morbidity with selective approaches.

In the 1970s, Bertrand developed extradural extraspinal approaches for denervation of dystonic muscles, including posterior ramisectomy and peripheral nerve sectioning, which was much less invasive than intradural rhizotomy (Bertrand et al. 1978; Bertrand 1993, 1995). Bertrand emphasised the more selective nature of these procedures and the lower frequency of side-effects. Over the next few years, in many centres worldwide extradural denervations replaced intradural sectioning, which nowadays has been almost aborted and become obsolete, at least in the form of the previously used standard procedure.

Myotomy and Myectomy

Myotomy and myectomy of dystonic muscles have been considered mainly for two indications: cervical dystonia and blepharospasm. While these procedures were and are still being used mainly as an adjunct to denervation procedures in cervical dystonia, they were more popular as a 'curative procedure' before the advent of botulinum toxin for treatment of blepharospasm.

Cervical Dystonia

There are limited data available on the long-term benefits of myotomy and myectomy for cervical dystonia. In only a few series have patients been operated on exclusively by myectomy (Chen 1981; Hernesniemi & Keränen 1990; Chen et al. 1991). Some reviews have concluded that pure myectomies would offer little benefit; and in the past few years exclusive myectomies were widely abandoned. It is evident that patients with complex cervical dystonia would not achieve any benefit from unilateral sectioning of single muscles. The posterior neck muscles are usually adequately denervated by posterior ramisectomies, but dystonic activity in the scalene, levator scapulae and omohyoid muscles is difficult to control by selective denervation. In such patients, selective myotomies or myectomies can still be useful (Krauss et al. 1999a).

The simplest choice is sectioning of the sternocleidomastoid muscle on the side that is opposite to the direction of the chin rotation. Sectioning of the sternocleidomastoid is only appropriate for a few, well-selected patients; namely, those with torticollis who present with marked dystonic activity in the sternocleidomastoid and minimal dystonia in the contralateral posterior neck muscles. This procedure is usually combined with selective denervation of the peripheral branches of the spinal accessory nerve to the sternocleidomastoid muscle. Denervation procedures are not performed in patients who present with painful dystonic activity of the trapezius muscle resulting in elevation and anteversion of the shoulder or ipsilateral head tilt, as this would prohibit the ability to elevate the arm above the horizontal plain. These patients may benefit from partial myotomy/myectomy of the upper portion of the trapezius muscle, using an asleep–awake–asleep operative technique (Krauss et al. 1999a).

Chen published the largest series on myotomies/myectomies for treatment of cervical dystonia (Chen 1981). The procedure was combined occasionally with selective peripheral denervation in certain dystonic patterns. Improvement was described as excellent or marked in 83 per cent of the 60 patients in this series without complications. In another series of 15 patients with retrocollis, bilateral partial resections of the upper part of the trapezius, splenius, semispinalis capitis and semispinalis cervicis muscles were performed (Chen et al. 1991). Outcomes were reported as excellent or markedly improved in 87 per cent of patients at follow-up between three and ten years after surgery without persistent side-effects. Long-term results of nonselective sternocleidomastoid sectioning in another series of 11 patients were less favourable (Hernesniemi & Keränen 1990). At a mean follow-up of four years, outcome was reported as good or fair in 45 per cent of patients.

When used as an adjunct to other surgeries, it is difficult to appreciate the contribution of selective myotomy/myectomy. Nevertheless, additional improvement was achieved in some of the author's patients who underwent selective sectioning of specific muscles as described above. All three patients who underwent partial myectomies of the trapezius muscle benefited (Krauss et al. 1999a). They experienced local pain relief and improvement of the dystonic posture of the shoulder.

Blepharospasm

Since local injection of botulinum toxin has become the preferred treatment option for blepharospasm, the use of orbital myotomies and myectomies for treatment of blepharospasm has decreased markedly. Neurectomies and selective facial nerve avulsions directed at denervation of the contracting muscles in blepharospasm have been abandoned because of their relatively high recurrence rates and frequent side-effects (Bates et al. 1991). Selective myectomy procedures were introduced by Anderson and colleagues in the late 1970s (Anderson et al. 1998), and thereafter became the approaches of choice (Hwang et al. 2001; Patel 2005).

The extended limited myectomy procedure has been suggested as the first step when considering myectomy operations (Hwang et al. 2001). Myectomy is performed through an eyelid crease incision, and involves removal of the pretarsal orbicularis muscle, the preseptal orbicularis muscle, part of the orbital orbicularis muscle and part of the corrugator superficialis muscle. In patients with apraxia of eyelid-opening, the levator aponeurosis can be tightened to correct upper eyelid position, and also the lateral canthal tendon which results in improvement of function and cosmesis while reducing squeezing in the upper eyelid. A few patients may also require frontalis suspension as a second procedure if the eyelids do not open well enough. Extended limited myectomy has been described to result in less lymphoedema, ecchymosis and supraorbital hyperesthesia, with faster recovery as compared to full myectomy procedures. Also, corneal surface exposure problems and dry eyes were reported to be reduced. It has been noted that patients in whom botulinum toxin injections had failed preoperatively responded to residual blepharospasm after extended limited myectomy. Full myectomy is performed through a brow incision above and a blepharoplasty incision in the lower eyelid. The orbicularis oculi muscles, and the procerus and corrugator muscles are removed, and the lateral canthal tendon is tightened. Upper eyelid lymphoedema has been a concern since it may last for weeks, months and even years. The occurrence of chronic lymphoedema has been reported to be rarer with the use of newer techniques. Other potential complications of the myectomy procedures included infection, haematoma, brow hair loss, eyelid retraction, trichiasis and canthal deformity.

In a study from the Mayo Clinic, 94 per cent of patients thought that myectomy procedures had provided both short-term and long-term benefits (Chapman et al. 1999). The long-term need for botulinum toxin injections was decreased in about 50 per cent of patients, and increased efficacy or longer-lasting effects were noted postoperatively. Patients with severe disability from blepharospasm benefited more from myectomies than did patients with relatively mild symptoms.

An alternative procedure, the so-called frontal sling operation, consists of frontalis suspension, which has been used earlier for treatment of ptosis (Wabbels & Roggenkämper 2007). In a series of 132 patients, improvement after surgery was achieved in 73 per cent. No serious corneal complications were observed. The beneficial effect of surgery, in general, remained stable over the years. Most patients continued to have additional botulinum toxin injections. Frontalis suspension may be considered less invasive surgery that is reversible upon removal of the silk or Gore-Tex sutures used in this procedure.

Spinal Cord Stimulation

Spinal cord stimulation (SCS) attracted some attention in the 1980s as a treatment option for cervical dystonia (Gildenberg 1978; Waltz 1998). It was based on the concept that altered sensory input could have an influence on the function of the motor system. The underlying rationales were based mainly on a modified concept of the gate control theory in analogy to the mechanisms thought to be involved in the efficacy of SCS in neuropathic pain. Quadripolar electrodes were placed longitudinally in the epidural space at C2–C4. Usually, stimulation frequencies in the range 500–700 Hz were applied.

SCS was reported to be effective in a few clinical studies (Gildenberg 1978; Waltz 1998). Waltz reported moderate to marked improvement in 69 of 90 patients (76 per cent) with cervical dystonia (Waltz 1998). On the other hand, Fahn noted almost complete lack of benefit in 25 patients on follow-up: while four patients had experienced transient mild benefit, long-lasting improvement was noted in only one instance (Fahn 1985). Subsequently, Goetz and colleagues found no objective improvement in a double-blind study of a series of ten patients with cervical dystonia (Goetz et al. 1988).

Over the next few years, chronic epidural cervical spine SCS for the treatment of cervical dystonia was abandoned – although it might have been an interesting approach from a contemporary perspective.

Microvascular Decompression

Microvascular decompression (MVD) was used for a limited period of time in the 1980s and 1990s for treatment of cervical dystonia (Pagni et al. 1985; Jho & Jannetta 1995). In analogy to other cranial neuropathies such as hemifacial spasm and trigeminal neuralgia, it was based on the (erroneous) concept that in some patients cervical dystonia would be caused by a neurovascular conflict of the spinal accessory nerve. Proponents of MVD suggested the existence of two pathogenetically different types of cervical dystonia: cervical dystonia of 'central origin' and 'spasmodic torticollis of 11th nerve origin' (Pagni et al. 1985). It was always difficult to understand how MVD of the spinal accessory nerve should work, in particular with regard to the fact that cervical dystonia almost never can be attributed only to muscles innervated by the spinal accessory nerve.

In addition to MVD, in many studies also other measures were performed such as sectioning the rootlets of the spinal accessory nerve, the spinal accessory nerve proper, anastomoses between the accessory nerve roots and the posterior C1 and C2 roots, lysis of 'cross-sectional adhesions' and 'hypertrophied dentate ligaments', and division of the posterior C1 and C2 roots (Freckmann et al. 1981; Aksik 1993; Shima et al. 1996). The offending arteries most often were described as loops of the posterior inferior cerebellar artery or the vertebral artery, and, in rare patients, the posterior spinal arteries (Shima et al. 1988, 1996; Alafaci et al. 2000). In a report on a series of 33 patients, the authors concluded that postoperative improvement was not related to vascular decompression per se but rather to lysis from anastomoses and 'adhesions' of the spinal accessory nerve related to 'pathogenic factors in the afferent part of head control' (Freckmann et al. 1981, 1986). In another series of 22 patients who underwent 'microneural decompression' of the spinal accessory nerve, a compressive vessel was thought to be responsible for cervical dystonia in only six patients (Aksik 1993).

Overall, reliable outcome data of MVD for treatment of patients with cervical dystonia were limited. In the series of Freckmann and colleagues, 5 of 33 patients (15 per cent) were reported with 'excellent' results, 10 (30 per cent) with 'good' results, and 12 (36 per cent) with less improvement (Freckmann et al. 1986). Reported side-effects included postoperative death caused by 'medullary symptoms with severe respiratory insufficiency', cerebrospinal fluid leaks, meningitis and stroke. In one series, the frequency of complications was as high as 27 per cent. At long-term follow-up between five and ten years, Jho and Jannetta claimed a cure for cervical dystonia in 65 per cent of their patients (13/20 patients), substantial improvement in four (20 per cent), moderate improvement in one (5 per cent), and minimal improvement in two (10 per cent) (Jho & Jannetta 1995). The majority of these patients were said to have gradual improvement over two years.

MVD for treatment of cervical dystonia has now been completely abandoned. In particular with regard to contemporary concepts of the pathophysiology of cervical dystonia, there are no arguments to support this procedure any longer.

Intrathecal Baclofen Delivery

While intrathecal baclofen was used for treatment of spasticity earlier on, it was first reported to be useful also in dystonia by Narayan and colleagues in 1991 (Narayan et al. 1991). Since then, with the rise of DBS, it has been thought to be indicated mainly in the treatment of patients both with severe generalised dystonia and spasticity, predominantly in those with secondary dystonia (Albright et al. 2001). Concerning the contemporary perspective, the reader is referred to Chapter 46.

Ablative Surgery in the Central Nervous System

Meyers, a true but underappreciated pioneer in neurosurgery, was most likely the first to target the basal ganglia directly via a transventricular approach for the treatment of dystonia (Meyers 1951; Abel et al. 2016). With the advent of the stereotactic technique only a few years later, however, functional stereotactic procedures were introduced also as a therapeutic option in dystonia (Mundinger & Riechert 1961; Cooper 1962, 1964). Initially, functional surgery was mainly used in generalised dystonia, and only later in focal or segmental dystonia (Loher et al. 2004). Remarkably, the main target for cervical dystonia was the thalamus, but there was little agreement on the optimal target within the thalamus (Krauss et al. 1992; Loher et al. 2004). For a detailed account on the development of thalamotomy and pallidotomy, the reader is referred to the chapter on current strategies of lesioning techniques in dystonia.

The Rise of Deep Brain Stimulation

Deep brain stimulation as we know it today was introduced in the late 1980s by the Grenoble group, initially for treatment of tremor in patients who had previously had a thalamotomy on the other side (Benabid et al. 1987; Hariz 2012). It only became more widely known, however, after Benabid and colleagues published a follow-up study on a larger group of patients with tremor including also bilateral implantation of electrodes (Benabid et al. 1991). The discovery that DBS of the subthalamic nucleus (STN) could alleviate all symptoms of Parkinson's disease sparked great enthusiasm and soon, by the mid-1990s, STN DBS became more popular and finally became the preferred surgical treatment over pallidotomy for treatment of advanced Parkinson's disease (Limousin et al. 1995, 1998; Hariz 2012). In parallel, DBS of the globus pallidus internus was introduced in the mid-1990s as a treatment option for dystonia (Krauss et al. 1999b; Coubes et al. 2000), and it became well accepted when larger well-designed confirmatory studies were published about a decade later (Vidailhet et al. 2005; Kupsch et al. 2006).

As outlined by Hariz and colleagues, there was experience with neurostimulation of deep brain targets before 'DBS' became popular as a therapy as we know it today (Blomstedt & Hariz 2010; Hariz et al. 2010). In the early 1970s, Mundinger introduced thalamic stimulation for treatment of cervical dystonia encouraged by his promising results for chronic pain (Mundinger 1977). At that time he had already a large experience with thalamic radiofrequency lesioning for treatment of cervical dystonia which was summarised later in a doctoral thesis submitted in 1990 to the Medical Faculty of the University of Freiburg, but which was never published in detail (Loher et al. 2004). In his publication in 1977, he reported on the effects of intermittent thalamic stimulation of electrodes implanted in the ventralis oralis anterior and the ventralis oralis internus nuclei of the thalamus and the subthalamic region, unilaterally in six patients and bilaterally in one patient (Mundinger 1977). Stimulation was applied via radiofrequency coupling since fully implantable pacemakers were not yet available at that time. Intermittent stimulation with either low frequencies (about 5 Hz) or higher frequencies (25–150 Hz) for 30–40 minutes resulted in improvement of dystonia lasting for 4–7 hours. The results were never published in the English-language literature and the study was almost completely ignored. Several years later, Andy reported improvement of cervical dystonia with chronic unilateral thalamic stimulation (Andy 1983). While the benefit of parkinsonian tremor with thalamic stimulation, which was also published in this manuscript, achieved limited attention, the report on amelioration of dystonia went unnoticed.

When 'modern' DBS became popular for treatment of tremor and Parkinson's disease, thalamic DBS was attempted in the 1990s in several instances of dystonia, mainly in patients with acquired dystonia (see Ondo & Krauss 2004; Krauss & Loher 2007). While Sellal and colleagues published their case report on thalamic stimulation for hemidystonia in 1993, most of the other manuscripts appeared in the early 2000s

(Sellal et al. 1993; Loher et al. 2001; Trottenberg et al. 2001; Vercueil et al. 2001; Ghika et al. 2002). Similar to thalamotomy, there was marked variability in the choice of the thalamic target, and it was debated whether the ventralis oralis anterior, the ventralis oralis posterior or the ventralis intermedius nucleus of the thalamus (according to the terminology of Hassler) would be the target of choice. Thalamic DBS resulted in variable improvement and it remained unclear whether this was related to the patient or to target selection within the thalamus (Ondo & Krauss 2004). With the upcoming success of pallidal DBS, thalamic DBS was never fully explored as an option in dystonia and it became almost abandoned over the next two decades. It is only now, after the bradykinetic side-effects of pallidal DBS have become recognised more commonly, that there is a return of interest in alternative targets such as the STN and the thalamus.

Several factors paved the way for the introduction of DBS of the posteroventral lateral globus pallidus internus as a target for dystonia in the mid-1990s (Krauss 2002): acceptance of the concept of dystonia being a 'basal ganglia disorder'; enhanced knowledge about basal ganglia physiology and the development of pathophysiological models in dystonia; evidence for improvement of dyskinesias and dystonia in Parkinson's disease after pallidotomy; understanding of the need for a bilateral approach to the basal ganglia in dystonia; fear of speech dysfunction with bilateral pallidotomy; the option to perform bilateral DBS in one operative session; the opportunity to adjust stimulation over time; acknowledgement of the limited effects of medication in dystonia, in general; recognition of the limitations of botulinum toxin injections; understanding the failures or the limited efficacy of 'peripheral' surgical treatment options for dystonia; and finally the development of new technology for DBS, among others.

Pallidal DBS for the treatment of dystonia was developed by neurosurgeons almost in parallel in several places worldwide, including Philippe Coubes in Montpellier, Tipu Aziz in Oxford, Andres Lozano in Toronto, and Joachim K. Krauss in Berne. When the author of this chapter was employed at Baylor College of Medicine in Houston in 1995, collaborating with Drs Robert Grossman and Joseph Jankovic performing pallidotomies in patients with advanced Parkinson's disease, he suggested performing pallidal DBS instead of pallidotomy in patients with dystonia. The DBS surgeries, however, at that time could not be realised mainly because of reimbursement issues. In the same year, Dr Hasdemir implanted a DBS electrode unilaterally for chronic DBS in the globus pallidus internus in Berne, Switzerland, in a patient with hemidystonia who had had transient relief after thalamotomy six years earlier (Loher et al. 2000). Chronic stimulation in this probably first instance of pallidal DBS resulted in sustained improvement of dystonia, pain and functional gain at four-year follow-up. The first publications on the beneficial use of pallidal DBS in dystonia came out in 1999 (Coubes et al. 1999; Islekel et al. 1999; Krauss et al. 1999a; Kumar et al. 1999). When Salar convened the *International Congress on Dystonia and Spasticity Treatment: State of the Art and Perspectives for the Third Millennium* in the summer of 1999 in Padova, Italy, it was the first event at which neurosurgeons, neurologists and neuroscientists from different countries came together to realise the potential of the new therapeutic concept.

Systematic studies on pallidal DBS were pioneered in both patients with primary cervical (Krauss et al. 1999a) and primary generalised dystonia (Coubes et al. 1999, 2000) in the late 1990s. While these studies including small numbers of patients were met with some scepticism initially, the results could soon thereafter be replicated in larger multicentre studies applying blinded and randomised designs (Vidailhet et al. 2005; Kupsch et al. 2006). When the first DBS surgeries were performed in Europe, the status of reimbursement varied remarkably. For example, in Switzerland DBS for dystonia was fully reimbursed even at the time when it was considered experimental. However, reimbursement was no longer granted in the mid-2000s for a period of time. In 2002 Drs Aziz, Coubes and Krauss met with the Medtronic administration in Paris to discuss the state of the art, and to gauge the chances for more global reimbursement. As a result of this meeting, documents were prepared to achieve CE certification in Europe in 2003, and FDA approval as a humanitarian device exemption in the same year.

Over the next few years DBS for dystonia became common practice and hundreds of studies were published on its use in several manifestations of dystonia and in different age groups. Several guidelines were produced and a supplement of the *Movement Disorders* journal in 2011 was devoted exclusively to DBS for dystonia (Moro et al. 2011). Pallidal DBS for dystonia nowadays is routine worldwide after a 20-year period of development, and it will probably continue to be the most important surgical technique for dystonia in the near future. The reader is referred to the numerous chapters in this volume to learn more about the various aspects of DBS for dystonia which still remains to be an enigmatic disease, with many aspects also regarding surgical therapy still unresolved.

References

Abel TJ, Walch T, Howard MA 3rd: 2016. Russell Meyers (1905–1999): pioneer of functional and ultrasonic neurosurgery. *J Neurosurg* 125:1589–1595.

Aksik I: 1993. Microneural decompression operations in the treatment of some forms of cranial rhizopathy. *Acta Neurochir* 125:64–74.

Alafaci C, Salpietro FM, Montemagno G, Grasso G, Tomasello F: 2000. Spasmodic torticollis due to neurovascular compression of the spinal accessory nerve by the anteroinferior cerebellar artery: case report. *Neurosurgery* 47:768–771.

Albright AL, Barry MJ, Shafton DH, Ferson SS: 2001. Intrathecal baclofen for generalized dystonia. *Dev Med Child Neurol* 43:652–657.

Anderson RL, Patel BC, Holds JB, Jordan DR: 1998. Blepharospasm: past, present and future. *Ophthal Plast Reconstr Surg* 14:305–317.

Andy OJ: 1983. Thalamic stimulation for control of movement disorders. *Appl Neurophysiol* 46:107–111.

Arseni C, Maretsis M: 1971. The surgical treatment of spasmodic torticollis. *Neurochirurgia* 4:177–180.

Bates AK, Halliday BL, Bailey CS, Collin JR, Bird AC: 1991. Surgical management of essential blepharospasm. *Br J Ophthalmol* 75:487–490.

Benabid AL, Pollak P, Louveau A, Henry S, de Rougemont J: 1987. Combined (thalamotomy and stimulation) stereotactic surgery of the VIM thalamic nucleus for bilateral Parkinson disease. *Appl Neurophysiol* 50:344–346.

Benabid AL, Pollak P, Gervason C, Hoffmann D, Gao DM, Hommel M, Perret JE, de Rougemont J: 1991. Long-term suppression of tremor by chronic stimulation of the ventral intermediate thalamic nucleus. *Lancet* 337(8738):403–406.

Bertrand CM: 1993. Selective peripheral denervation for spasmodic torticollis: surgical technique, results, and observations in 260 cases. *Surg Neurol* 40:96–103.

Bertrand CM: 1995. Surgical management of spasmodic torticollis and adult-onset dystonia. In: Schmidek HH, Sweet WH, eds, *Operative Neurosurgical Techniques*, 3rd ed. Philadelphia, PA: Saunders; 1649–1659.

Bertrand C, Molina-Negro P, Martinez SN: 1978. Combined stereotactic and peripheral surgical approach for spasmodic torticollis. *Appl Neurophysiol* 41:122–133.

Blomstedt P, Hariz MI: 2010. Deep brain stimulation for movement disorders before DBS for movement disorders. *Parkinsonism Relat Disord* 16:429–433.

Chapman KL, Bartley GB, Waller RR, Hodge DO: 1999. Follow-up of patients with essential blepharospasm who underwent eyelid protractor myectomy at the Mayo Clinic from 1980 through 1995. *Ophthal Plast Reconstr Surg* 15:106–110.

Chen X: 1981. Selective resection and denervation of cervical muscles in the treatment of spasmodic torticollis: results in 60 cases. *Neurosurgery* 8:680–688.

Chen XK, Ji SX, Zhu H, Ma AB: 1991. Operative treatment of bilateral retrocollis. *Acta Neurochir* 113:180–183.

Colbassani HJ Jr, Wood JH: 1986. Management of spasmodic torticollis. *Surg Neurol* 25:153–158.

Cooper IS: 1962. Dystonia reversed by operation on basal ganglia. *Arch Neurol* 7:132–145.

Cooper IS: 1964. Effect of thalamic lesions upon torticollis. *N Engl J Med* 270:967–972.

Coubes P, Echenne B, Roubertie A, Vayssière N, Tuffery S, Humbertclaude V, Cambonie G, Claustres M, Frerebeau P: 1999. Treatment of early-onset generalized dystonia by chronic bilateral stimulation of the internal globus pallidus: apropos of a case. *Neurochirurgie* 45:139–144.

Coubes P, Roubertie A, Vayssiere N, Hemm S, Echenne B: 2000. Treatment or DYT1-generalised dystonia by stimulation of the internal globus pallidus. *Lancet* 355: 2220–2221.

Dandy W: 1930. An operation for the treatment of spasmodic torticollis. *Arch Surg* 20:1021–1032.

Fahn S: 1985. Lack of benefit from cervical cord stimulation for dystonia. *N Engl J Med* 313:1229.

Finney JM, Hughson W: 1925. Spasmodic torticollis. *Ann Surg* 81:225–269.

Freckmann N, Hagenah R, Herrmann HD, Müller D: 1981. Treatment of neurogenic torticollis by microvascular lysis of the accessory nerve roots: indication, technique, and first results. *Acta Neurochir* 59:167–175.

Freckmann N, Hagenah R, Herrmann HD, Müller D: 1986. Bilateral microsurgical lysis of the spinal accessory nerve roots for treatment of spasmodic torticollis: follow up of 33 cases. *Acta Neurochir* 83:47–53.

Friedman AH, Nashold BS Jr, Sharp R, Caputi F, Arruda J: 1993. Treatment of spasmodic torticollis with intradural selective rhizotomies. *J Neurosurg* 78:46–53.

Ghika J, Villemure JG, Miklossy J, Temperli P, Pralong E, Christen-Zaech S, Pollo C, Maeder P, Bogousslavsky J, Vingerhoets F: 2002. Postanoxic generalized dystonia improved by bilateral Voa thalamic deep brain stimulation. *Neurology* 58:311–313.

Gildenberg PL: 1978. Treatment of spasmodic torticollis by dorsal column stimulation. *Appl Neurophysiol* 41:113–121.

Goetz CG, Penn RD, Tanner CM: 1988. Efficacy of spinal cord stimulation in dystonia. *Adv Neurol* 50:645–649.

Hamby WB, Schiffer S. 1969. Spasmodic torticollis: results after surgical rhizotomy in 50 cases. *J Neurosurg* 31:323–326.

Hamby WB, Schiffer S. 1970. Spasmodic torticollis: results after cervical rhizotomy in 80 cases. *Clin Neurosurg* 17:28–37.

Hariz M: 2012. Twenty-five years of deep brain stimulation: celebrations and apprehensions. *Mov Disord* 27:930–933.

Hariz MI, Blomstedt P, Zrinzo L: 2010. Deep brain stimulation between 1947 and 1987: the untold story. *Neurosurg Focus* 29:E1.

Hernesniemi J, Keränen T: 1990. Long-term outcome after surgery for spasmodic torticollis. *Acta Neurochir* 103:128–130.

Horner J, Riski JE, Ovelmen-Levitt J, Nashold BS Jr: 1992. Swallowing in torticollis before and after rhizotomy. *Dysphagia* 7:117–125.

Hwang IP, Anderson RL, Jordan DR: 2001. Surgical treatment of blepharospasm. In: Krauss JK, Jankovic J, Grossman RG, eds, *Surgery for Parkinson's Disease and Movement Disorders*. Philadelphia, PA: Lippincott Wiliams and Wilkins; 382–392.

Iskandar BJ, Nashold BS Jr: 1995. History of functional neurosurgery. *Neurosurg Clin North Am* 6:1–25.

Işlekel S, Zileli M, Zileli B: 1999. Unilateral pallidal stimulation in cervical dystonia. *Stereotact Funct Neurosurg* 72:248–252.

Jho HD, Jannetta PJ: 1995. Microvascular decompression for spasmodic torticollis. *Acta Neurochir* 134:21–26.

Keen WW: 1891. III. A new operation for spasmodic wry-neck. *Ann Surg* 13:44–47.

Krauss JK: 2002. Deep brain stimulation for dystonia in adults: overview and developments. *Stereotact Funct Neurosurg* 78:168–182.

Krauss JK, Loher TJ: 2007. Surgery for dystonia. In: Warner TT, Bressman S, eds, *Clinical Diagnosis and Management of Dystonia*. London: Informa Healthcare; 209–222.

Krauss JK, Mohadjer M, Braus DF, Wakhloo AK, Nobbe F, Mundinger F: 1992. Dystonia following head trauma: a report of nine patients and review of the literature. *Mov Disord* 7:263–272.

Krauss JK, Toups EG, Jankovic J, Grossman RG: 1997. Symptomatic and functional outcome of surgical treatment of cervical dystonia. *J Neurol Neurosurg Psychiat* 63:642–648.

Krauss JK, Koller R, Burgunder JM: 1999a. Partial myotomy/myectomy of the trapezius muscle with an asleep–awake–asleep anesthetic technique for treatment of cervical dystonia. *J Neurosurg* 91:889–991.

Krauss JK, Pohle T, Weber S, Ozdoba C, Burgunder JM: 1999b. Bilateral stimulation of globus pallidus internus for treatment of cervical dystonia. *Lancet* 354:837–838.

Kumar R, Dagher A, Hutchison WD, Lang AE, Lozano AM: 1999. Globus pallidus deep brain stimulation for generalized dystonia: clinical and PET investigation. *Neurology* 11(53):871–874.

Kupsch A, Benecke R, Müller J, Trottenberg T, Schneider GH, Poewe W, Eisner W, Wolters A, Müller JU, Deuschl G, Pinsker MO, Skogseid IM, Roeste GK, Vollmer-Haase J, Brentrup A, Krause M, Tronnier V, Schnitzler A, Voges J, Nikkhah G, Vesper J, Naumann M, Volkmann J, Deep-Brain Stimulation for Dystonia Study Group: 2006. Pallidal deep-brain stimulation in primary generalized or segmental dystonia. *N Engl J Med* 355:1978–1990.

Limousin P, Pollak P, Benazzouz A, Hoffmann D, Le Bas JF, Broussolle E, Perret JE, Benabid AL: 1995. Effect of parkinsonian signs and symptoms of bilateral subthalamic nucleus stimulation. *Lancet* 14(345):91–95.

Limousin P, Krack P, Pollak P, Benazzouz A, Ardouin C, Hoffmann D, Benabid AL: 1998. Electrical stimulation of the subthalamic nucleus in advanced Parkinson's disease. *N Engl J Med* 15(339):1105–1111.

Loher TJ, Hasdemir MG, Burgunder JM, Krauss JK: 2000. Long-term follow-up study of chronic globus pallidus internus stimulation for posttraumatic hemidystonia. *J Neurosurg* 92:457–460.

Loher TJ, Krauss JK, Burgunder JM, Taub E, Siegfried J: 2001. Chronic stimulation of the ventrointermediate thalamus is effective for treatment of dystonic paroxysmal nonkinesigenic dyskinesia. *Neurology* 56:268–270.

Loher TJ, Pohle T, Krauss JK: 2004. Functional stereotactic neurosurgery for treatment of cervical dystonia: review of the experience from the lesional era. *Stereo Funct Neurosurgery* 82:1–13.

McKenzie KG: 1954. The surgical treatment of spasmodic torticollis. *Clin Neurosurg* 2:37–43.

Meyers R: 1951. Surgical experiments in the therapy of certain extrapyramidal diseases: a current evaluation. *Acta Psychiatr Neurol* 67:7–42.

Moro E, Albanese A, Krauss JK, Metman LV, Vidailhet M, Hariz MI: 2011. Guest editors' introduction. *Mov Disord* 26(Suppl. 1):S1–S2.

Mundinger F: 1977. New stereotactic treatment of spasmodic torticollis with a brain stimulation system (author's transl.). *Med Klin* 18(72):1982–1986.

Mundinger F, Riechert T: 1961. Long-term results of stereotactic treatment of extrapyramidal movement disorders (in German). *Dtsch Z Nervenheilkd* 182:542–576.

Narayan RK, Loubser PG, Jankovic J, Donovan WH, Bontke CF: 1991. Intrathecal baclofen for intractable axial dystonia. *Neurology* 41:1141–1142.

Ondo WG, Krauss JK: 2004. Surgical therapies for dystonia. In: Brin MF, Comella C, Jankovic J, eds, *Dystonia: Etiology, Clinical Features and Treatment*. Philadelphia, PA: Lippincott, Williams & Wilkins; 125–147.

Pagni CA, Naddeo M, Faccani G: 1985. Spasmodic torticollis due to neurovascular compression of the 11th nerve. *J Neurosurg* 63:789–791.

Patel BC: 2005. Surgical management of essential blepharospasm. *Otolaryngol Clin North Am* 38:1075–1098.

Rossitch E Jr, Khoshbin S, Black PM, Moore MR, Tyler HR: 1991. Kenneth McKenzie, Harvey Cushing, and the early neurosurgical treatment of spasmodic torticollis. *Neurosurgery* 28:278–282.

Scoville WB: 1978. Motor tics of the head and neck: surgical approaches and their complications. *Acta Neurochir* 45:338.

Sellal F, Hirsch E, Barth P, Blond S, Marescaux C: 1993. A case of symptomatic hemidystonia improved by ventroposterolateral thalamic electrostimulation. *Mov Disord* 8:515–518.

Shima F, Fukui M, Kitamura K, Kuromatsu C, Okamura T: 1988. Diagnosis and surgical treatment of spasmodic torticollis of 11th nerve. *Neurosurgery* 22:358–363.

Shima F, Fukui M, Matsubara T, Kitamura K: 1996. Spasmodic torticollis caused by vascular compression of the spinal accessory root. *Surg Neurol* 26:431–434.

Sweet WH: 1975. What should the neurosurgeon do when faced with a malpractice suit? *Clin Neurosurg* 23:112–124.

Taylor AS: 1915. Operation for relief of spasmodic torticollis. In: Johnson AB, ed., *Operative Therapeutics*, New York: Appleton Century Crofts 525–612.

Trottenberg T, Paul G, Meissner W, Maier-Hauff K, Taschner C, Kupsch A: 2001. Pallidal and thalamic neurostimulation in severe tardive dystonia. *J Neurol Neurosurg Psychiatry* 70:557–559.

Valadas A, Contarino MF, Albanese A, Bhatia KP, Falup-Pecurariu C, Forsgren L, Friedman A, Giladi N, Hutchison M, Kostic VS, Krauss JK, Lokkegaard A, Marti MJ, Milanov M, Pirtosek Z, Relja M, Skorvanek M, Stamelou M, Stepens A, Tamas G, Taravari A, Tzoulis C, Vandenberghe W, Vidailhet M, Ferreira JJ, Tijssen MAJ: 2016. Management of dystonia in Europe: a survey of the European network for the study of the dystonia syndromes. *Eur J Neurol* 23:772–779.

Vercueil L, Pollak P, Fraix V, Caputo E, Moro E, Benazzouz A, Xie J, Koudsie A, Benabid AL: 2001. Deep brain stimulaüon in the treatment of severe dystonia. *J Neurol* 248:695–700.

Vidailhet M, Vercueil L, Houeto JL, Krystkowiak P, Benabid AL, Cornu P, Lagrange C, Tézenas du Montcel S, Dormont D, Grand S, Blond S, Detante O, Pillon B, Ardouin C, Agid Y, Destée A, Pollak P: 2005. French Stimulation du Pallidum Interne dans la Dystonie (SPIDY) Study Group: bilateral deep-brain stimulation of the globus pallidus in primary generalized dystonia. *N Engl J Med* 352:459–467.

Vogel TD, Pendleton C, Quinoñes-Hinojosa A, Cohen-Gadol AA: 2010. Surgery for cervical dystonia: the emergence of denervation and myotomy techniques and the contributions of early surgeons at the Johns Hopkins Hospital. *J Neurosurg Spine* 12:280–285.

Wabbels B, Roggenkämper P: 2007. Long-term follow-up of patients with frontalis sling operation in the treatment of essential blepharospasm unresponsive to botulinum toxin therapy. *Graefes Arch Clin Exp Ophthalmol* 245:45–50.

Waltz JM: 1998. Chronic stimulation for motor disorders. In: Gildenberg PL., Tasker RR, eds, *Textbook of Stereotactic and Functional Neurosurgery*. New York: McGraw-Hill; 1087–1099.

Chapter 58

Selective Neurotomy for the Treatment of Dystonia

Takaomi Taira, Shiro Horisawa, Nobuhiko Takeda and Tomoko Hanada

Selective peripheral neurotomy is generally indicated for certain types of cervical dystonia (CD) as described in another chapter of this book. The basic and well-established procedure is the 'Bertrand operation' in which the extradural C1–C6 posterior branches of the spinal nerves are denervated to control the abnormal contractions of posterior neck muscles (Molina-Negro 1988; Bertrand & Bouvier 1991; Bertrand 1993). Denervation of the neck muscles for CD is not a curative treatment but merely a symptomatic suppression of abnormal contractions of the neck muscles. Selective peripheral denervation (SPD) for CD, as described by Bertrand, is a safe and effective surgical option (Braun & Richter 1991; Bertrand 1993; Cohen-Gadol et al. 2003). However, this technique does not provide a proper approach to the levator scapulae muscle (LS) in laterocollic CD (Taira et al. 2003), and for some patients seems to be responsible for a certain discomfort in the occipital area.

Thus, in this chapter we describe two new approaches for surgical neurotomy of CD: an anterior approach for denervation of the LS (Taira et al. 2003); and intradural denervation to avoid sensory loss in the cutaneous area innervated by the greater occipital nerve (Taira 2009; Taira et al. 2002).

We also describe some forms of other dystonias, though not very common, that may be treated with peripheral neurotomy.

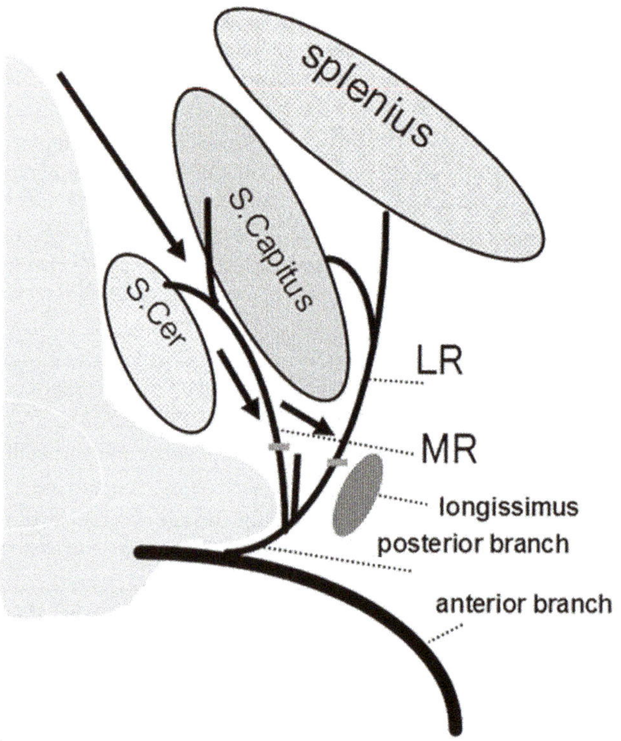

Figure 58.1 Surgical approach to the posterior branches of the cervical nerves. Note that the semispinalis capitus muscle has double innervation from the lateral ramus (LR) and the medial ramus (MR) of the posterior branch. The splenius muscle is innervated from the lateral branching of LR. S.Capitus: semispinalis capitus muscle; S.Cer: semispinalis cervicalis muscle.

3D Anatomy of the Posterior Branches

Reappearance of abnormal contraction of the 'denervated' muscle may be seen even after seemingly complete denervation with the Bertrand operation. This is because of the complex anatomy of the posterior branches of the cervical nerves. The semispinalis capitus (SSCap) receives innervation from both the medial and lateral surfaces. The SSCap separates the posterior branch into medial and lateral rami. The splenius muscle (SPL) is innervated from the lateral branch of the lateral rami, while the semispinalis cervicis (SSCer) receives nerve supply from the medial branch of the medial rami. The SSCap has double innervation from both the medial branch of the lateral rami and the medial branch of the lateral rami. This anatomical relation is complex and difficult; this is very important when performing the Bertrand operation, as shown in Figure 58.1. In most cases of recurrence, we had dissected the plane between the semispinalis capitus and cervicalis muscles where only the medial rami of the posterior branch were exposed. For complete denervation of SPL, the lateral rami of the posterior branch should be cut. The lateral rami of the posterior branch run in the anterolateral aspects of SSCap, and we have to cut the insertions of SSCap to the vertebral body to expose these rami. After cutting the insertions of SSCap, we can observe another muscle of which fibres run parallel to the rostro-caudal direction. This muscle is distinct from SSCap, of which fibres are oblique to the vertebral column; it is the longissimus muscle. The lateral rami are found on the dorsal aspect of the longissimus muscle, and they run perpendicular to the vertebral column. We believe understanding this anatomy is key for a successful operation. After realising the detailed anatomy of the spinal posterior nerves, the incidence of reoperation dramatically decreased in our series. Bogduk (1982) reported an excellent review on the posterior branches of the cervical nerves. Layer-by-layer anatomy of the cervical muscles and posterior branches is helpful for our understanding of the 3D anatomy.

Anterior Approach to the Levator Scapulae Muscle

The LS elevates the shoulder and produces lateral tilting of the neck, responsible for laterocollis. This muscle is innervated by the anterior branches of the C2–C5 nerves. The contribution of nerve supply is reported to be 5.5 per cent from C2, 100 per cent from C3 and C4, and 19 per cent from C5 anterior branches (Kato & Sato 1984; Frank et al. 1997). The innervation arises from the ventrolateral surface of the muscle. Palpation in the deep cervical area between the posterior border of SCM and the anterior border of the trapezius in various postures confirms its abnormal contraction. One hundred and twenty patients were referred for surgical treatment of their dystonia; eight showed major involvement of LS. Patients with laterocollis related to abnormal contraction of the posterior muscles of the neck and/or SCM should be excluded.

Because the nerve supply to LS comes from the ventrolateral surface of the muscle and because of its anatomy, the denervation procedure is not difficult in the anterior approach. An average of approximately two nerves from the cervical plexus emerges from beneath the posterior border of SCM in a cephalad to caudal progression to enter the posterior triangle of the neck on their way to innervating LS.

Patients are operated on under general anaesthesia in the supine position, with the head rotated towards the opposite side of the surgical field. Muscle relaxants are not used except at the induction of anaesthesia to monitor intraoperative neurostimulation. We use an operative microscope from the skin incision which is about 8 cm long on the posterior border of SCM. The greater auricular nerve, the branches of the external jugular vein, and the accessory nerve are carefully identified and preserved. The greater auricular nerve is followed along the posterior surface of SCM to the LS. At the anterior border of the LS, the high cervical nerve plexus is identified. With electrical stimulation (5 Hz or 50 Hz, 1 msec pulse width, 0.2–1 V), the nerve branches to LS are identified and cut (Figure 58.2). The distal part of the nerve is pulled out from the muscle to prevent reinnervation. The C5 nerve is identified with electrically induced contractions of the deltoid muscle. If there is a branch from the C5 nerve to LS, it is also cut. The phrenic nerve is identified with neurostimulation, which induces contraction of the diaphragm and is carefully preserved (Taira et al. 2003).

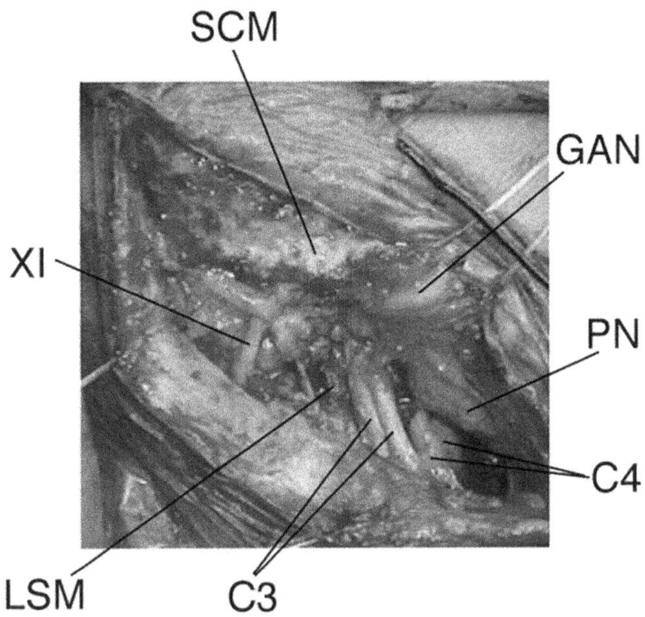

Figure 58.2 Intraoperative view for denervation of the levator scapulae muscle. SCM: sternocleidomastoid muscle; GAN: great auricular nerve; LSM: levator scapulae muscle; XI: accessory nerve.

Intradural Denervation

After the Bertrand procedure some patients complain about numbness in the occipital area, and rarely about deafferentation pain. This is because the sensory components of the C2 nerve are sacrificed. A sensory deficit in the C2 region may not be very troublesome for daily life, but some patients in our series had an uneasy feeling upon C2 sensory loss which made them emotionally unstable. We considered that this could be improved by performing intradural innervation limited to C1 and C2.

To decrease venous bleeding, to preserve occipital sensory function and to decrease total invasiveness, we modified the technique of denervation. This method consists of the sectioning of intradural ventral roots of C1 and C2 through a limited C1 hemilaminectomy. We complete this denervation with the section of the posterior rami from C3 to C6 and the SCM denervation as described in the original Bertrand procedure (Figure 58.3). This procedure can be regarded as a combination of Foerster-Dandy's anterior rhizotomy and Bertrand's ramisectomy. Thus it is no longer a pure peripheral technique. The anterior branches of C1 and C2 have important functions in swallowing, and bilateral sectioning of these branches results in swallowing difficulties. With the traditional Bertrand procedure, we can identify the anterior and posterior branches and selectively cut the nerve to avoid complications. However, in the intradural approach, we cannot make a distinction of the rootlets supplying the anterior or posterior nerves. Therefore, our new intradural approach is only indicated for unilateral denervation. In case of retrocollis that requires bilateral denervation, we still use an entirely extradural approach.

We perform the operation in the prone position. Under general anaesthesia, the head is fixed in a slightly flexed position with a Mayfield clamp. The upper half of the body is elevated about 30 degrees. Muscle relaxants are not used except at the induction of anaesthesia. We use a short, straight skin incision from the inion to the C4 level. The midline nuchal ligament is cut and the inferior oblique muscle and the posterior arch of C1 are exposed. The suboccipital rectus muscles are cut unilaterally at their insertions, but we always preserve the

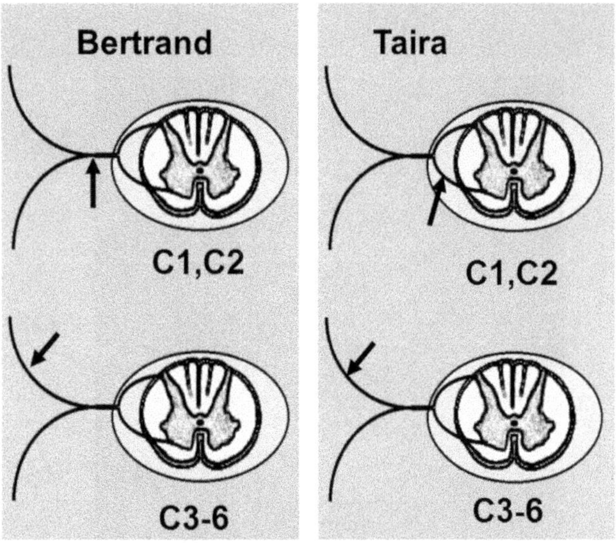

Figure 58.3 Cross-sectional scheme of Bertrand's and Taira's procedure. Arrows indicate the location of cutting the nerves.

inferior oblique muscle. A C1 hemilaminectomy is performed and the dura is opened for a length of 1.5 cm. We them identify the C1 and C2 roots, and the intradural vertebral artery through the small dural incision. We do not drill the occipital bone. After dissection of the arachnoid membrane and the dentate ligament, the C1 and C2 ventral rootlets are exposed and sectioned. The small vessels running with the rootlets must be preserved. For the intradural procedure, very fine microsurgical instruments are required. After dural closure with a 5-0 nylon continuous suture, the space between SSCap and the SSCer is dissected to expose the posterior rami from C3 to C6. These branches are cut completely and we confirm complete denervation with strong monopolar electrical stimulation. By tilting the microscope we perform the procedure through a much smaller opening than in the traditional Bertrand procedure. At closure, the space surrounded by the bilateral SSCap muscles and the inferior oblique muscle is closed in a watertight fashion to prevent cerebrospinal fluid (CSF) leakage. No drainage is used.

For denervation of SCM, we make a straight skin incision of 3 cm along the posterior border of SCM. We always use a microscope for the skin incision to avoid damage to the great auricular nerve. After identification of the main trunk of the accessory nerve, we follow the nerve in both distal and proximal directions and all the branches to SCM are cut and coagulated. We do not cut the SCM itself. The disadvantages of this method are that it requires a C1 hemilaminectomy and dural opening. Theoretically these may increase the risk of instability of the vertebral column, CSF leakage and meningitis. Because the C1 laminectomy is limited to one side and the suboccipital rectal muscles opposite to the side after operation are preserved, the procedure is minimally invasive and we consider that the laminectomy does not cause serious problems (Taira et al. 2002). We have not experienced postoperative CSF leakage or subcutaneous CSF accumulation.

Other Indications for Neurotomy in the Management of Dystonia

Peripheral neurotomy other than for cervical dystonia is most often used as a surgical treatment for intractable focal spasticity such as spastic equinus fort or inversion of the foot (Sindou & Mertens 1988; Decq et al. 2000). Similar focal abnormalities of posture may persist in dystonia, even if generalised dystonia is controlled with deep brain stimulation. Selective peripheral neurotomy of the tibial nerve is a useful treatment of such focal foot dystonia. Similarly, denervation of the pectoralis major muscle might be considered (Decq et al. 1997).

Conclusions

Peripheral neurotomy needs detailed knowledge about microsurgical anatomy and physiology of the peripheral nerves and related muscles. Sophisticated microsurgical techniques are necessary. Neurosurgeons, in general, are not familiar with this technique. These are the hurdles in management of dystonia with peripheral nerve surgery. However, if properly performed, peripheral neurotomy is very effective and useful for selected patients with dystonia. Neurosurgeons involved in the management of dystonia should be aware of the importance of peripheral neurotomy in management of dystonias.

References

Bertrand C, Bouvier G. 1991. Selective peripheral denervation in patients with spasmodic torticollis. V. Braun and H. P. Richter. *Stereotact Funct Neurosurg* 57(4):228–229.

Bertrand CM, Molina-Negro P. 1988. Selective peripheral denervation in 111 cases of spasmodic torticollis: rationale and results. *Adv Neurol* 50:637–643.

Bertrand CM. 1993. Selective peripheral denervation for spasmodic torticollis: surgical technique, results, and observations in 260 cases. *Surg Neurol* 40(2):96–103.

Bogduk N. 1982. The clinical anatomy of the cervical dorsal rami. *Spine (Phila Pa 1976)* 7(4):319–330.

Braun V, Richter HP. 1991. Selective peripheral denervation in patients with spasmodic torticollis. *Stereotact Funct Neurosurg* 57(3):113–122.

Cohen-Gadol AA, Ahlskog JE, Matsumoto JY, Swenson MA, McClelland RL, Davis DH. 2003. Selective peripheral denervation for the treatment of intractable spasmodic torticollis: experience with 168 patients at the Mayo Clinic. *J Neurosurg* 98(6):1247–1254.

Decq P, Filipetti P, Feve A, Djindjian M, Saraoui A, Keravel Y. 1997. Peripheral selective neurotomy of the brachial plexus collateral branches for treatment of the spastic shoulder: anatomical study and clinical results in five patients. *J Neurosurg* 86(4):648–653.

Decq P, Filipetti P, Cubillos A, Slavov V, Lefaucheur JP, Nguyen JP. 2000. Soleus neurotomy for treatment of the spastic equinus foot. groupe d'evaluation et de traitement de la spasticite et de la dystonie. *Neurosurgery* 47(5):1154–1160.

Frank DK, Wenk E, Stern JC, Gottlieb RD, Moscatello AL. 1997. A cadaveric study of the motor nerves to the levator scapulae muscle. *Otolaryngol Head Neck Surg* 117(6):671–680.

Kato K, Sato T. 1984. Innervation of the levator scapulae, the serratus anterior, and the rhomboideus in crab-eating macaques and its morphological significance. *Anat Anz* 157(1):43–55.

Sindou M, Mertens P. 1988. Selective neurotomy of the tibial nerve for treatment of the spastic foot. *Neurosurgery* 23(6):738–744.

Taira T. 2009. Peripheral procedures for cervical dystonia. In: *Textbook of Stereotactic and Functional Neurosurgery*. Lozano AM, Gildenberg PL,Tasker RR, editors. Berlin, Heidelberg: Springer; 1885–1909.

Taira T, Kobayashi T, Takahashi K, Hori T. 2002. A new denervation procedure for idiopathic cervical dystonia. *J Neurosurg* 97(Suppl. 2):201–206.

Taira T, Kobayashi T, Hori T. 2003. Selective peripheral denervation of the levator scapulae muscle for laterocollic cervical dystonia. *J Clin Neurosci* 10(4):449–452.

Chapter 59

Selective Peripheral Denervation for the Treatment of Cervical Dystonia

James Palmer

With a clear understanding of the anatomy of the neck, the combination of muscles that produce dystonic postures can be established through clinical examination supported by electromyography (EMG). The aim of selective peripheral denervation is to permanently paralyse those muscles responsible for the posture by removing their nerve supply. Dividing muscles surgically fails to deliver a lasting clinical outcome, but denervation produces a functionally relevant benefit and improves the range of neck movements.

Anatomy

Anterolateral Muscles

Two muscles play a core role in cervical dystonic posture. The *sternocleidomastoid* connects the back of the skull (along the superior nuchal line) to the sternum and clavicle. The clavicular part of the muscle is a lateral flexor, the tendinous part is a strong rotator. The *levator scapulae* runs from the transverse processes of C1 to C4, passing obliquely to the scapula and is pulling the head towards the shoulder provided the shoulder is fixed, or the shoulder to the head if the neck is fixed.

Superficial Posterior Muscles

The most relevant posterior muscles are the *semispinalis capitis* and *semispinalis cervicis*, both of which extend the head and neck respectively. They are long and strong muscles extending into the upper thoracic spine posteriorly. To the lateral side of the semispinalis on the back of the skull the *splenius capitis* then curves around the side of the neck to insert into the spinous processes of the lower four cervical and upper three thoracic vertebrae. The splenius is the most commonly involved muscle in cervical dystonia; it is a broad and strong muscle.

Deep Posterior Muscles

Deep to the muscle layer of semispinalis capitis and splenius lies the occipital muscles running from the skull onto the C1 and C2 vertebrae. These short muscles can deliver substantial leverage moment and are involved in dystonic postures. *Rectus capitis posterior major* is the main extensor muscle and *obliquus capitis superior* is a lateral flexor. Where rotation of the head is a key component the *obliquus capitis inferior* muscle plays a substantial role. It connects the spine of C2 to the lateral mass of C1, and as the centre of rotation is placed anteriorly the moment of force is strong. This muscle becomes hypertrophied in dystonia, a feature that can be seen on the MRI of the neck. The involvement of these short muscles can lead to accelerated degenerative changes in the atlantoaxial and C1/C2 joints, restricting the range of movement and leading to pain in the upper part of the neck and onto the back of the head (through C2 radicular pain).

Dystonic Postures

The positions of the head and neck are the result of a lead muscle contraction (primary agonist), further muscle contraction recruited in the movement (synergists) and those muscles that would normally be contracting to oppose the movement (antagonists) which do not deliver significant counter contraction as they are paradoxically inhibited by the dystonia.

Rotation

The most common phenotype is rotation (torticollis), seen in 63 per cent. A twist to the right involves the sternal head of the left sternocleidomastoid, the right splenius capitis and the right inferior oblique. A sensory geste is most common in rotation; this usually involves raising the hand towards the side of the chin. Quite often the sensory geste relieves the rotation before the skin is touched, or only a very light touch on the skin is required. Where the sternocleidomastoid is the primary agonist, substantial muscle hypertrophy can be present; where the splenius is primary, there is often associated posterior cervical pain. Clinical examination is best conducted standing behind the patient with the thumbs on each splenius and the fingers across the sternocleidomastoid.

Lateral Flexion

Tilt of the head (laterocollis) can be present without rotation, but can be an additional component with a torticollis in 27 per cent. Tilt to the right results from combined contraction of the clavicular head of the right *sternocleidomastoid* and the right *splenius capitis*. The tilt can be extreme, with the ear forced onto the tip of the shoulder. *Levator scapulae* is often involved and it is usually possible to palpate the tendinous heads of the contracting muscle. Posttraumatic postures are most commonly a laterocollis. Functional presentation is more common as a laterocollis; if this is suspected a general anaesthetic wake-up test can be helpful. The sensory geste appears less effective for laterocollis; lying flat may resolve the posture.

Extension

Extension (retrocollis) can be the most disabling posture in 10 per cent. In the severe form, minimal forward vision is possible, with pain a significant part. The muscles involved include the *semispinalis capitis* and *cervicis*, both *splenius capitis*, *rectus capitis* and the *superior oblique*. The sensory geste of preference is commonly a scarf or similar that provides sensory input to the back of the head. Clinical examination is usually unable to determine which are the lead dystonic muscles.

Flexion

A flexed position of the neck (antecollis) is less common. The muscles involved include both sternomastoid muscles, but commonly the platysma and anterior strap muscles of the neck are involved. As these muscles are innervated by the ventral rami, denervation surgery is contraindicated.

Innervation

The ventral and dorsal nerve roots join to form the ganglion, lying just within the exit foramen. The anterior and posterior rami of C3 to C6 emerge from the ganglion. The posterior rami run close to the lateral mass of the vertebra, emerging in an anatomical plane that lies between the semispinalis capitis and semispinalis cervicis. These posterior rami supply the posterior muscle groups. Additionally, there is innervation supplied by the suboccipital nerve (C1) and the greater occipital nerve (C2).

The sternocleidomastoid innervation comes from the accessory nerve and from the C1/C2 plexus. After emerging from the jugular foramen close to the styloid process, the nerve passes through the sternocleidomastoid muscle and emerges into the posterior triangle of the neck to pass down obliquely to enter the trapezius muscle. Within the early course of the nerve there are 2–4 separate branches of the nerve that pass into and innervate the sternocleidomastoid muscle.

Table 59.1 provides a summary.

Table 59.1 Innervation of the most commonly involved muscles in cervical dystonia

Muscle	Innervation
Semispinalis capitis	Posterior rami C1–8
Semispinalis cervicis	Posterior rami C1–8
Splenius capitis	Posterior rami C1–5
Rectus capitis posterior major	Posterior rami C1–2
Obliquus capitis superior	Posterior rami C1–2
Obliquus capitis inferior	Posterior rami C1–2
Levator scapulae	Anterior rami C1–4
Sternocleidomastoid	Accessory nerve (ventral rami C2–3)
Trapezius	Accessory nerve (ventral rami C3–4)

Electromyography

Electromyography is used to provide supportive analysis of the primary agonist muscles. It is most helpful in trying to establish the contribution of the levator scapulae in a laterocollis. A video EMG method (Munchau et al. 2001a) was developed to provide simultaneous multi-channel EMG.

History

Early surgery for cervical dystonia included sternocleidomastoid muscle section by Isaac Minnius in 1641. In 1867 Mr Campbell de Morgan reported that he removed a section of the accessory nerve before the branches to the sternocleidomastoid. W.W. Keen in 1891 divided the first three cervical nerves at laminectomy along with a section of the spinal accessory nerve (Vogel et al. 2010).

By 1924 Cushing and McKenzie were using an intradural section of the anterior C1–4 roots (rhizotomy). They achieved good outcomes but with significant morbidity, with limitation of neck movements, neck instability, pain and dysphagia. Along with a 4 per cent mortality the surgery developed a poor reputation.

In 1925 Finney undertook most of the surgery for torticollis with Cushing and described the first approach to the posterior rami as an extraspinal operation (ramisectomy). McKenzie identified that the trapezius muscle was not involved in the dystonic postures and hence the selective denervation of sternocleidomastoid was developed.

Claude Bertrand in Montreal started to combine thalamotomy with ramisectomy, eventually dropping the former in 1982 and using EMG assessment to deliver a selective denervation.

Patient Selection

Patients should only be selected for surgery if they have tried botulinum toxin and it has failed (primary failures) or have subsequently reduced benefit of botulinum (secondary failures). Surgery can also be considered if repeated three-monthly botulinum toxin injections are difficult to organise. The pattern of dystonia should be stable for at least two years.

Surgical Technique

The surgical procedure is somewhat technically daunting, since the anatomical relationships are not seen in other operations and dissection is required around the vertebral artery to expose the C1 nerve. Surgery is not for the occasional surgeon.

A CT scan of the upper cervical spine can be helpful; some patients have been wrongly diagnosed as cervical dystonia – for example in atlantoaxial subluxation. Many patients are referred to surgery very late in the course of their dystonia management and the CT scans show extensive degenerative change, which is a common cause for the associated spinal pain.

MRI is not helpful in the preoperative work-up. There are usually degenerative disc changes at multiple levels. Even if there is radicular pain, a corrected posture by selective denervation often significantly improves the symptoms.

General clinical examination should include auscultation of the heart to exclude a murmur when the preferred surgical position is sitting. The risk of air embolism is very low for this technique, but a patent foramen ovale should be excluded using a trans-oesophageal echocardiogram.

Selective Accessory Denervation

A skin incision is made from just anterior to the tip of the mastoid towards the tip of the shoulder. The greater auricular nerve is found and dissected free up to the top of the incision anterior to the mastoid tip. The nerve is then followed posteriorly as it curves around the posterior margin of the sternocleidomastoid. Just superior to this point separating the tissues in the same direction as the expected trajectory of the accessory nerve, the nerve is found by direct stimulation and observing the muscular twitch of the trapezius.

One technique consists of following the accessory nerve through the sternocleidomastoid by dividing the muscle fibres over the nerve using an operating microscope. This dissection is continued until the nerve emerges anterior to the sternocleidomastoid high in the wound deep to the mastoid tip. The palpating finger should be able to feel the styloid process; it is important to reach the most anterior part of the nerve.

The branches of the accessory nerve to sternocleidomastoid are identified using nerve stimulation. There are usually three branches, sometimes two, and rarely four that are found. These nerves are divided close to the trunk of the accessory nerve. Once the nerves are divided, the accessory nerve is mobilised free from the deep part of the sternocleidomastoid and the muscle fully divided. The accessory nerve is followed inferiorly to the insertion into the trapezius. Further careful nerve stimulation checks the bed of the sternocleidomastoid as there may be other small motor rootlets, sometimes from cervical ventral rami that innervate the lower part of the muscle; each should be divided.

In order to prevent the accessory nerve being in contact with residual muscle, the upper part is resected and then the lower part is pulled upwards using a Duval clamp, and as much of the remaining muscle removed using bipolar scissors.

Posterior Ramisectomy

A midline incision is made and extended well above the external occipital protuberance and down to just below the C7 spinous process. Bertrand used an incision extending laterally towards the mastoid process; a linear incision heals well with less wound pain. The top end of the wound is exposed to the occipital bone and the attachments of the semispinalis capitis and splenius capitis are dissected off the superior nuchal line as far laterally as possible. The dissection is deepened in the midline and the suboccipital muscle (rectus capitis) is preserved in its position attached to the inferior nuchal line at this stage.

Dissection inferiorly identifies the tip of the C2 spinous process and the inferior oblique muscle lateral to it. The muscle is left attached to the spinous process (unlike a standard cervical approach) and the plane is found between the semispinalis cervicis and capitis. There is loose connective tissue in this plane and occasional insignificant blood vessels. Retraction is careful without too much tension to avoid neuropraxia of the nerves so they maintain the ability to be stimulated.

The branches of the C3 and C4 posterior rami come into view lying attached to the elevated semispinalis capitis and under microsurgical dissection they are followed to the lateral masses of the vertebra and a vessel loop placed around the nerve. The posterior rami of C5 and C6 can be found on the medial aspect in the fascia of the semispinalis cervicis using nerve stimulation and using the previously identified nerves as a reference.

The inferior oblique is often very hypertrophied, after exposing its lateral surface as much as possible the muscle is divided fully and beneath it the C2 posterior ramus is exposed. The bone of the most lateral part of C1 is exposed and the C1 posterior ramus position is identified with stimulation. It emerges under the vertebral artery where it can be isolated and divided, up to a 1 cm length of nerve can be removed and the stumps are diathermied.

Sequentially the C2 to C5 (or C6) posterior rami are divided and long sections of the nerves (2–4 cm) are removed. The attachment of the splenius capitis to the lateral mass of the vertebra is divided until the inferolaterally directed fibres of levator scapulae are seen. Further branches of C2/C3 and sometimes C4 can be found in this plane, which need to be divided and diathermied. Finally lateral mass are exposed, with cutting diathermy removing all innervation (particularly if pain is a key feature).

Postoperative inpatient stay is usually 2–3 days, there is very little wound pain (in part due to the denervation). Numbness is inevitable over the back of the head supplied by C2 and patients need to be warned not to scratch this area. If a bilateral posterior ramisectomy has been carried out care should be taken introducing fluids and feed. Patients stay in accommodation up to a week after the surgery to learn a series of exercises to encourage a range of movements and to induce activity in the paradoxically inhibited muscles.

Results

Prior to introduction of deep brain stimulation for cervical dystonia, selective peripheral denervation was the most common procedure for its treatment (Krauss 2011). While deep brain stimulation initially was introduced for patients with 'complex' cervical dystonia who were not suitable candidates for selective peripheral denervation (Krauss et al. 1999), it was subsequently used also for less 'complex' cases, and gradually almost replaced selective peripheral denervation over the past few years (Volkmann et al. 2014). Injection with botulinum toxin only works if the paralysis is achieved in the main muscles producing the dystonia. Well-placed injections are the mainstay of treatment of cervical dystonia. Selective peripheral denervation follows the same therapeutic strategy delivering permanent paralysis of specifically targeted muscles.

The manual skills of the surgeon are key to the success of the treatment. Treatment failure is mostly through reinnervation. Since simple nerve section is not sufficient, nerve segments

(a) (b)

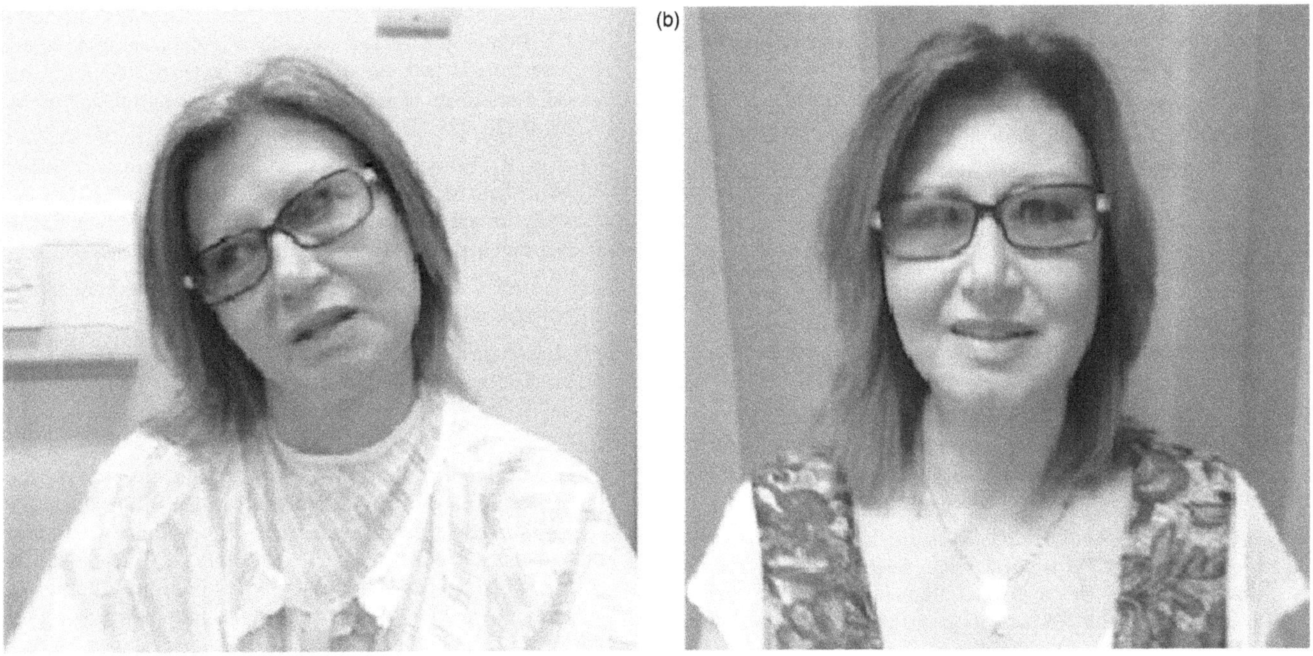

Figure 59.1 Selective peripheral denervation is a treatment of choice for 'simple' cervical dystonia where the agonist muscles can be easily identified, such as laterocollis or torticollis with 'pure' rotation.

should be removed, the nerve stumps cauterised and nearby muscle excised. Rough handling of tissues leads to neuropraxia so that smaller branches cannot be found. Much of the reported reinnervation is failure to achieve adequate denervation.

The experience gained by Claude Bertrand and subsequently Guy Bouvier in Montreal was pivotal. In 1993, 260 cases were reported with total or marked relief of symptoms with preservation of normal or near-normal neck movements in 88 per cent. Forty per cent had no detectable abnormal movements, 48 per cent had slight residual movements, 10 per cent had an appreciable amount of residual movement, and 1 per cent had no improvement or worse (Bertrand 1993).

More recently, Wang has reported the largest series of 648 patients, the mean preoperative TWSTRS score was 54.7 ± 18.3 points (range, 39–67 points), which decreased to 31.1 ± 11.6 points postoperatively (range, 1–67 points) (Wang et al. 2015).

In the first of my two series (the first 37 operated on) functionally relevant improvement was achieved in 68 per cent with a 30 per cent mean reduction of TWSTRS score (Munchau et al. 2001b). In the second cohort of 27 patients, functionally relevant improvement was achieved in more than 80 per cent with a 52 per cent mean reduction of TWSTRS score (Ashida & Palmer 2011). An example of the functionally relevant response is shown in Figure 59.1. Other surgeons have replicated similar results in substantial series sizes (Braun & Richter 1994, 2002; Krauss et al. 1997; Ford et al. 1998; Taira et al. 2002; Cohen-Gadol et al. 2003; Taira & Hori 2003; Chen 2007; Bergenheim et al. 2015).

The morbidity of SPD is limited to fewer than 10 per cent of patents: wound infection; mild dysphagia; neuralgia; and haematoma. There is skin numbness on the back of the head from C2 denervation, which is well tolerated. Postoperative hospital stay is usually two days.

In the search to answer the question of whether surgery is best by DBS or SPD, only one small study has compared DBS with SPD. Twenty-four patients with CD underwent operations: either SPD (16) or DBS (8). All patients showed gradual improvement after SPD and DBS. No statistically significant differences were seen between the SPD group and the DBS group, with limited follow-up. However, there was a trend towards greater pain reduction in the DBS group ($p = 0.094$) (Huh et al. 2010).

Conclusions

With two effective treatments for cervical dystonia refractory to botulinum toxin therapy available, DBS and SPD, we need to continue to refine the former and manage succession planning of expert surgeons to prevent the latter from being lost from our toolbox. A recent survey on the availability of surgical treatment options for dystonia in European countries identified that SPD was still offered only in a few places (Valadas et al. 2016). For those offering botulinum injections, do not delay consideration of surgery if the results are limited or resistance is developing, since severe degenerative changes of the cervical spine follow and surgical outcome worsens (Chawda et al. 2000).

Importantly, SPD may also be combined with DBS in selected patients. The experience with such combined surgical treatment, however, is quite limited and needs further study.

References

Ashida R, Palmer JD. 2011. Cohort 2: selection for and outcome of selective peripheral denervation for cervical dystonia. *Acta Neurochir* 153:1833–1905.

Bergenheim AT, Nordh E, Larsson E, Hariz MI. 2015. Selective peripheral denervation for cervical dystonia: long-term follow-up. *J Neurol Neurosurg Psychiatry* 86(12):1307–1313.

Bertrand CM. 1993. Selective peripheral denervation for spasmodic torticollis: surgical technique, results, and observations in 260 cases. *Surg Neurol* 40(2):96–103.

Braun V, Richter HP. 1994. Selective peripheral denervation for the treatment of spasmodic torticollis. *Neurosurgery* 35(1):58–62.

Braun V, Richter HP. 2002. Selective peripheral denervation for spasmodic torticollis: 13-year experience with 155 patients. *J Neurosurg* 97(Suppl. 2):207–212.

Chawda SJ, Munchau A, Johnson D, Bhatia K, Quinn NP, Stevens J, Lees AJ, Palmer JD. 2000. Pattern of premature degenerative changes of the cervical spine in patients with spasmodic torticollis and the impact on the outcome of selective peripheral denervation. *J Neurol Neurosurg Psychiatry* 68(4):465–471.

Chen X, Ma A, Liang J, Ji S, Pei S. 2000. Selective denervation and resection of cervical muscles in the treatment of spasmodic torticollis: long-term follow-up results in 207 cases. *Stereotact Funct Neurosurg* 75(2–3):96–102.

Cohen-Gadol AA, Ahlskog JE, Matsumoto JY, Swenson MA, McClelland RL, Davis DH. 2003. Selective peripheral denervation for the treatment of intractable spasmodic torticollis: experience with 168 patients at the Mayo Clinic. *J Neurosurg* 98(6):1247–1254.

Ford B, Louis ED, Greene P, Fahn S. 1998. Outcome of selective ramisectomy for botulinum toxin resistant torticollis. *J Neurol Neurosurg Psychiatry* 65(4):472–478.

Huh R, Han IB, Chung M, Chung S. 2010. Comparison of treatment results between selective peripheral denervation and deep brain stimulation in patients with cervical dystonia. *Stereotact Funct Neurosurg* 88(4):234–238.

Krauss JK. 2011. Selective peripheral denervation for cervical dystonia. In: *Youmans Textbook Neurological Surgery*, 6th edn, Winn HR, ed. Elsevier, Amsterdam: 996–1000.

Krauss JK, Toups EG, Jankovic J, Grossman RG. 1997. Symptomatic and functional outcome of surgical treatment of cervical dystonia. *J Neurol Neurosurg Psychiatry* 63(5):642–648.

Krauss JK, Pohle T, Weber S, Ozdoba C, Burgunder JM. 1999. Bilateral stimulation of globus pallidus internus for treatment of cervical dystonia. *Lancet* 354(9181):837–838.

Munchau A, Bahlke G, Allen PJ, Quinn NP, Lees AJ, Rothwell JC, Palmer JD, Bhatia KP. 2001a. Polymyography combined with time-locked video recording (video EMG) for presurgical assessment of patients with cervical dystonia. *Eur Neurol* 45(4):222–228.

Munchau A, Palmer JD, Dressler D, O'Sullivan JD, Tsang KL, Jahanshahi M, Quinn NP, Lees AJ, Bhatia KP. 2001b. Prospective study of selective peripheral denervation for botulinum-toxin resistant patients with cervical dystonia. *Brain* 124(Pt 4):769–783.

Taira T, Hori T. 2003. A novel denervation procedure for idiopathic cervical dystonia. *Stereotact Funct Neurosurg* 80(1–4):92–95.

Taira T, Kobayashi T, Takahashi K, Hori T. 2002. A new denervation procedure for idiopathic cervical dystonia. *J Neurosurg* 97(Suppl. 2):201–206.

Valadas A, Contarino MF, Albanese A, Bhatia KP, Falup-Pecurariu C, Forsgren L, Friedman A, Giladi N, Hutchinson M, Kostic VS, Krauss JK, Lokkegaard A, Marti MJ, Milanov I, Pirtosek Z, Relja M, Skorvanek M, Stamelou M, Stepens A, Tamas G, Taravari A, Tzoulis C, Vandenberghe W, Vidailhet M, Ferreira JJ, Tijssen MA. 2016. Management of dystonia in Europe: a survey of the European network for the study of the dystonia syndromes. *Eur J Neurol* 23(4):772–779.

Vogel TD, Pendleton C, Quinones-Hinojosa A, Cohen-Gadol AA. 2010. Surgery for cervical dystonia: the emergence of denervation and myotomy techniques and the contributions of early surgeons at the Johns Hopkins Hospital. *J Neurosurg Spine* 12(3):280–285.

Volkmann J, Mueller J, Deuschl G, Kuhn AA, Krauss JK, Poewe W, Timmermann L, Falk D, Kupsch A, Kivi A, Schneider GH, Schnitzler A, Sudmeyer M, Voges J, Wolters A, Wittstock M, Muller JU, Hering S, Eisner W, Vesper J, Prokop T, Pinsker M, Schrader C, Kloss M, Kiening K, Boetzel K, Mehrkens J, Skogseid IM, Ramm-Pettersen J, Kemmler G, Bhatia KP, Vitek JL, Benecke R, DBS Study Group for Dystonia. 2014. Pallidal neurostimulation in patients with medication-refractory cervical dystonia: a randomised, sham-controlled trial. *Lancet Neurol* 13(9):875–884.

Wang J, Li J, Han L, Guo S, Wang L, Xiong Z, Ma J, Liang J, Wang L. 2015. Selective peripheral denervation for the treatment of spasmodic torticollis: long-term follow-up results from 648 patients. *Acta Neurochir (Wien)* 157(3):427–433.

Chapter 60

Stereotactic Lesioning for the Treatment of Dystonia

Robert E. Gross and Matthew A. Stern

Whereas focal dystonias often are successfully treated locally with botulinum toxin and dopa-responsive dystonia can be treated with dopaminergic medication, generalised dystonia often cannot be pharmacologically managed effectively, regardless of whether it is primary or secondary in origin (Krack & Vercueil 2001). Surgical treatments, particularly lesions or neuromodulation through deep brain stimulation (DBS) have been shown to be an effective option for patients suffering from dystonia. Ablative procedures including thalamotomy and pallidotomy have been utilised for dystonia treatment for over 60 years to great success. Furthermore, in the last 30 years, with greater understanding of cortical–subcortical physiology and with the significant advances in imaging technology and stereotactic equipment, these neurosurgical procedures have become more effective, accurate and safe, providing patients with years of relief and an improved quality of life.

Historical Background

Surgical interventions to address the symptoms of movement disorders were first undertaken prior to the turn of the twentieth century with the 1890 publication of an article describing the treatment of choreoathetosis by resection of the premotor area (Horsley 1890). The first half of the twentieth century saw surgeries mostly performed to alleviate the symptoms of Huntington's disease and Parkinson's disease (PD). At first the targets selected were varied, including lesions in the cerebral cortex and corticospinal system (Bucy & Buchanan 1932; Bucy & Case 1939; Klemme 1940), the pyramidal motor system (e.g. medullary pyramids and cerebral peduncles) (Putnam 1940; Oliver 1949; Walker 1952), in non-motor nervous system (e.g. sympathetcomy) (Royle 1931; Rees 1933; Gardner & Williams 1949), and in extraneural targets (e.g. thyroid) (Myerson & Berlin 1934). In the mid-1920s, Spatz described the 'extrapyramidal motor system' (EPS) through investigations into the caudate nucleus for Huntington's disease (Hallervorden & Spatz 1922; Spatz 1927), providing a new collection of potential targets for neurosurgical intervention. Putnam was the first to perform surgery on the EPS to treat dystonia, sectioning the extrapyramidal motor tracts in the cervical spinal cord in the 1930s with mixed results (Putnam 1933, 1938). In the 1940s, Meyers began to perform extrapyramidal lesions to address movement disorder symptoms, including the caudate nucleus (Meyers 1940) and the globus pallidus internus (GPi) (Meyers 1942; Meyers & Fields 1958). Furthermore, Spiegel and Wycis ushered in the era of stereotactic neurosurgery in 1947 when they published on their use of a stereotactic apparatus for neurosurgical procedures (Spiegel et al. 1947), notably pallidotomy (Spiegel & Wycis 1954, 1958; Spiegel 1966), which provided a more precise and safer approach to the procedures. With Hassler's work on thalamotomy of the ventrolateral (VL) nucleus (Hassler 1955; Hassler et al. 1960) and Cooper and Bravo's work in chemothalamotomies (Cooper & Bravo 1958; Bravo & Cooper 1959; Cooper 1959a, 1959b, 1965), the thalamus soon became an additional target of choice for these procedures.

It was soon noticed that lesions in the EPS could also relieve dystonic symptoms in PD patients and it was at this point that surgeons began to perform similar ablative procedures to treat the symptoms of generalised dystonia. The work began in the 1950s with many nuclei being attempted, although the majority of the studies chiefly targeted the VL thalamus, particularly the ventralis oralis anterior (Voa), the ventralis oralis posterior (Vop) and the ventralis intermedius (Vim) (Hassler & Riechert 1954; Cooper 1959a, 1959b, 1969; Markham & Rand 1961; Riechert 1962; Hassler & Dieckmann 1970a, 1970b; Mundinger et al. 1970; Hassler 1972; Krayenbühl & Siegfried 1972; Andrew et al. 1974, 1983; Gros et al. 1976; Bertrand et al. 1979; Marsden 1981; Tasker et al. 1988; Speelman & Vanmanen 1989; Yamashiro & Tasker 1993; Cardoso et al. 1995; Sungurov et al. 1998; Tasker 1998a, 1998b). These regions of the VL thalamus were able to be determined through the use of microelectrode recording beginning in the 1960s (Albe-Fessard et al. 1961; Guiot et al. 1962). The largest series of patients was reported by Cooper and colleagues, who performed thalamotomies on over 200 patients for generalised dystonia (Cooper 1976). Around 70 per cent of these patients received at least moderate relief that continued through long-term follow-up for an average of eight years. Cooper's initial target was the VL thalamus, particularly Vim and the ventrocaudalis internus and externus (Vci/e) nucleus, and the centromedian nucleus (CM). If the patient failed to receive desired relief, additional surgeries were performed targeting next the pallidothalamic and cerebellothalamic afferents and, as a last resort, the pulvinar nucleus. The patients often had multiple lesions, requiring multiple surgeries to place them all. Thalamotomies were also used to treat cervical dystonias with mixed results (Loher et al. 2004).

The results from the other contemporary series tended to be a bit more modest, with 25–50 per cent of patients receiving significant relief following thalamotomy. Unlike with ablative procedures in PD, where patients saw immediate benefit following lesioning, the benefits for dystonia were more gradual, with a progression of up to six months postoperatively to receive significant relief (Cooper 1976). The most noticeable complications were speech disturbances, which occurred in roughly 15 per cent of cases. Hemiparesis was also of note, but was transient, resolving within a few weeks (Andrew et al. 1983). Also, the corticobulbar tract being in close proximity to the Vim leads to a risk for pseudobulbar palsy. Finally, the complications rates were significantly higher in bilateral procedures compared with unilateral (Bertrand et al. 1979; Andrew et al. 1983).

Concurrent to the exploration into thalamotomy for dystonia, pallidotomy of the GPi was also examined as a therapy to treat generalised dystonia, beginning in the 1950s, albeit to a lesser extent (Guiot & Brion 1952; Hassler & Riechert 1954; Spiegel et al. 1958; Cooper 1959a, 1959b, 1969 Hassler et al. 1960; Mundinger et al. 1972; Bertrand et al. 1978; Burzaco 1985). Although thalamotomy was regarded as the procedure of choice historically, some believed pallidotomy was the better procedure, as it had a lower rate of complications, most notably with regard to speech (Bertrand et al. 1979; Hariz & De Salles 1997; Hariz 2000). Then, after a renewed interest in pallidotomy for PD begun by Laitinen and coworkers reintroducing Leksell's pallidotomy (Laitinen et al. 1992a, 1992b; Laitinen 1995), advances in brain imaging (CT, MRI) (Kelly et al. 1987), intraoperative electrophysiologic techniques (Lenz et al. 1988) and a greater physiological and anatomical understanding of the EPS circuitry (Delong et al. 1985; Alexander et al. 1986; Miller & Delong 1988; Albin et al. 1989; Bergman et al. 1990; Delong 1990; Filion & Tremblay 1991) (Figure 60.1a), there too was a renewed interest in pallidotomy as a treatment for dystonia (Iacono et al. 1996; Lozano et al. 1997). This interest also stemmed from positive results seen in the relief of hyperkinetic and dystonic symptoms in PD patients who received unilateral posteroventral pallidotomy or pallidoansotomy (Laitinen et al. 1992a, 1994, 1995a, 1995b). Thus began the modern era in stereotactic surgery for dystonia (Krack & Vercueil 2001; Gross 2008). The resurgence of interest in pallidotomy, however, coincided with the introduction of the new DBS procedure in the late 1980s and early 1990s by Benabid and Siegfried and their colleagues. Stimulation of the subthalamic nucleus (STN), GPi and thalamus rapidly became the standard surgical procedure for PD, supplanting lesioning, given its equivalent efficacy, reversibility and improved safety profile (Benabid et al. 1987, 1996, 2006; Siegfried & Lippitz 1994, 1995; Limousin et al. 1995; Schuurman et al. 2000; Krack & Vercueil 2001; Krack et al. 2003; Esselink et al. 2004, 2006; Deuschl et al. 2006; Jiménez et al. 2006; Kleiner-Fisman et al. 2006; Contarino et al. 2007; Gross 2008; Schuurman et al. 2008; Fasano et al. 2012). It soon supplanted ablative procedures for dystonia as well (Krauss et al. 1999; Kumar et al. 1999; Coubes et al. 2004; Vidailhet et al. 2005; Kupsch et al. 2006; Gross 2008). However, the implanted hardware of DBS poses drawbacks in the context of dystonia, as the patients tend to be younger and require higher voltage for DBS, which results in more frequent battery changes being necessary, and the very nature of dystonia might pose an increased risk for lead fracture or dislodgement (Gross 2008). Thus, given these drawbacks of DBS, as well as the decreased need for follow-up, the lower risk of infection and the better affordability of stereotactic ablative procedures, pallidotomy and thalamotomy remain viable options for dystonia treatment (Beric et al. 2001; Oh et al. 2002; Blomstedt & Hariz 2005; Paluzzi et al. 2006; Gross 2008; Hooper et al. 2008; Sillay et al. 2008; Falowski et al. 2012).

Physiologic Basis for Ablation Procedures for Parkinson's Disease as an Analogue for Dystonia

Pallidotomy

Much of the current understanding of dystonia pathophysiology stems from research performed for PD. In PD, the loss of dopaminergic neurons in the substantia nigra pars compacta (SNc) leads to increased inhibitory (GABAergic) output from GPi and the substantia nigra pars reticulata (SNr). This GPi hyperactivity excessively inhibiting the thalamus, coupled with irregular GPi output, leads to the decreased and dysregulated thalamic excitatory drive of the downstream cortical motor systems and brainstem motor areas, which are significantly inhibited and dysregulated (Delong et al. 1985; Alexander et al. 1986; Miller & Delong 1987, 1988; Albin et al. 1989; Bankiewicz et al. 1990; Bergman et al. 1990; Delong 1990; Filion & Tremblay 1991; Obeso et al. 1997; Blanchet et al. 1998). The thalamocortical output controls distal appendicular musculature via the corticospinal and corticobulbar tracts. The GPi also directly projects via the ansa lenticularis' pallidal tegmental bundle to brainstem motor areas such as the pedunculopontine nucleus and mescencephalic tegmental field, which control axial and proximal appendicular musculature via the descending reticulospinal tract (Jackson & Crossman 1983; Garcia-Rill 1986; Iacono et al. 1995b, 1998). With the thalamus and brainstem now being less able to regulate movement, the ability to initiate movement becomes excessively impaired, leading to the classic PD clinical symptoms of disrupted and impoverished movements (Hashimoto et al. 2003). In pallidotomy, the sensorimotor region of GPi is selectively lesioned, decreasing its inhibitory output and thereby normalising downstream thalamocortical activity and brainstem motor area function. The sensorimotor portion of GPi is defined by a population of movement-responsive neurons in the posteroventral region, that project to the ventroanterior (VA) and VL thalamus via the ansa lenticularis and lenticular fasciculus, merging as the thalamic fasciculus. Collaterals are given off to the CM nucleus (Ford 2004). The limbic and associative territories of GPi and the adjacent globus pallidus externus (GPe), optic tract and internal capsule are avoided.

Whereas PD is a hypokinetic disorder, dystonia is hyperkinetic, provoking the question as to why performing the

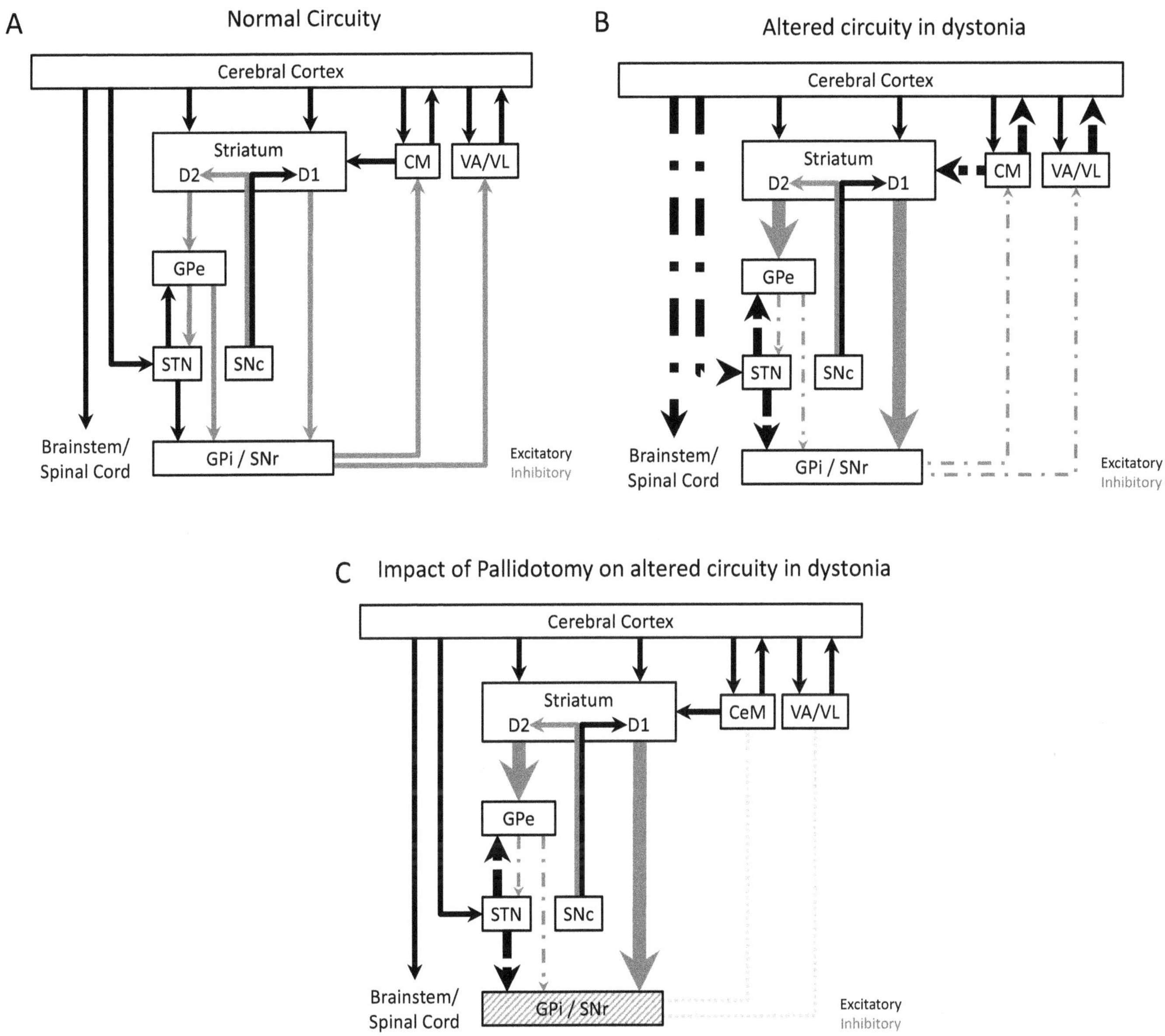

Figure 60.1 Basal ganglia circuitry relevant to dystonia and the impact of ablative surgery. (a) Simplified normal circuit diagram. Grey denotes inhibitory efferent projections; black denotes excitatory efferent projections. Other relevant nuclei are omitted for simplicity (e.g. reticular nucleus of thalamus, pedunculopontine nucleus). (b) Diagram depicting changes in the basal ganglia circuitry in the context of dystonia. Increased line weight denotes increased efferent activity with an increased firing rate; decreased line weight denotes decreased firing rate and efferent output. Irregularly dashed lines indicate pathologically irregular firing patterns, which contribute to the symptomatic features of the disease. Note the increase in inhibition of the GPi via the direct pathway leading to diminished and irregular inhibitory output to the thalamus, hence the overactivity and irregularity of the excitatory thalamocortical pathways. (c) Alteration in the pathological activity of the basal ganglia following pallidotomy. Grey diagonal shading indicates lesion and grey dotted line indicates inactive pathway.

Abbreviations: SNc, substantia nigra compacta; SNr, substantia nigra reticulata; GPe, globus pallidus externa; GPi, globus pallidus interna; STN, subthalamic nucleus; D1, striatopallidal neurons with excitatory postsynaptic D1 dopamine receptors; D2, striatopallidal neurons with inhibitory D2 receptors; CM, centromedian nucleus of the thalamus; VA/VL, ventroanterior/ventrolateral thalamus.

same surgery would correct two seemingly opposite diseases. It has been shown in dystonia that there is decreased GPi activity, which leads to disinhibition of the thalamus, and hence overactivity of the downstream thalamocortical projections and brainstem motor areas (Vitek et al. 1998b; Delong 1990; Hamada & Delong 1992a, 1992b; Lozano et al. 1997; Ford 2004) (Figure 60.1b). As decreased firing rates are also seen in the GPe, it is believed that the indirect pathway is not responsible for the decreased GPi signalling (Lenz et al. 1998). The increased activity downstream of GPi is supported by functional imaging studies with fluorodeoxyglucose (FDG) positron emission tomography (PET), which shows elevated glucose metabolism in the thalamus, lentiform nucleus, cerebellum and supplementary motor cortex (Ceballos-Baumann et al. 1995; Eidelberg et al. 1998).

In addition to being decreased, the GPi firing rate is irregular, leading to changes in the spatial temporal pattern of cortical input, increasing noise and subsequently decreasing the signal to noise ratio (Figure 60.2). Thus it is believed that there is an increased chance for errors in transmission (Vitek et al.

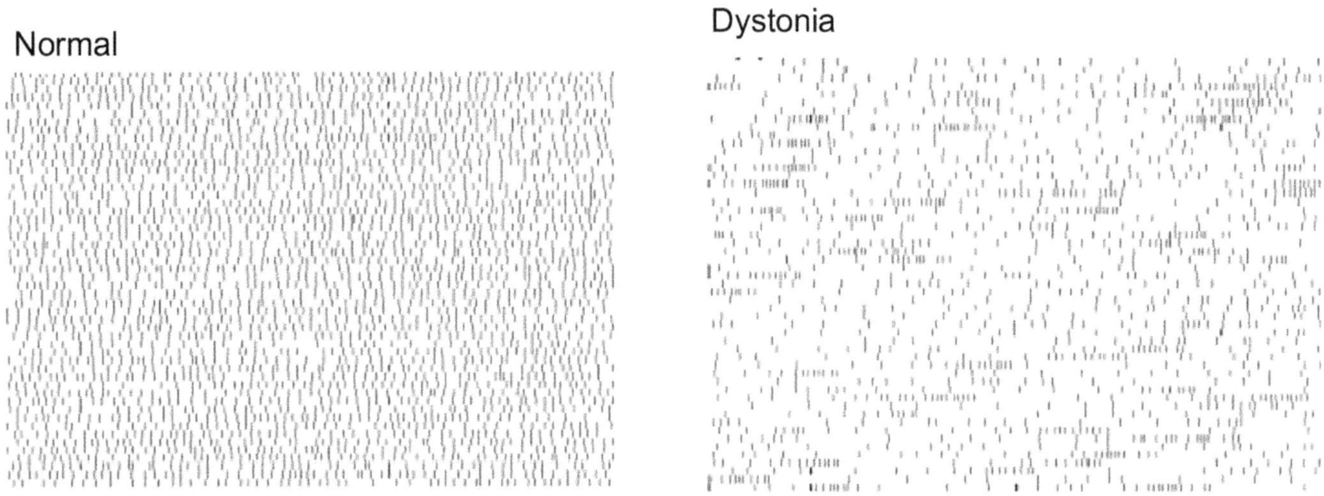

Figure 60.2 Comparison of the globus pallidus internus discharge pattern in dystonia with normal.

Depicted are the digitised rasters of single units recorded from the globus pallidus internus (GPi) during microelectrode mapping in a normal non-human primate (left) and in a patient with primary dystonia undergoing surgery (right) (courtesy of M. DeLong, Emory University). The pattern in dystonia is much more irregular, manifesting increased burstiness and pauses between firing, which is uncharacteristic of normal firing and firing pattern in Parkinson's disease.

1998b). Under the aforementioned basal ganglia circuitry model, one could suspect that lesioning the GPi would further decrease the inhibitory signal to the thalamus, exacerbating the dystonia. However, in as much as pallidotomy causes dystonia relief, it is surmised that dystonic features stem in part from the irregularity of inhibitory signals and not just disinhibition: the disruption of irregular inhibitory signals reaching the thalamus restores its normal function, at least in part (Figure 60.1c).

Thalamotomy

The typical target for thalamotomy today is the Vim nucleus, with some involvement of the Vop nucleus. The Vim thalamus sends projections ipsilaterally to the primary motor cortex, premotor and supplementary motor cortical areas, while predominantly receiving contralateral cerebellar inputs. The Vop thalamus receives both cerebellar and GPi afferents and projects fibres to predominantly the supplementary motor area and premotor cortex (Ohye 2000). Under decreased inhibition from the GPi the downstream activity of these nuclei is overactive and irregular. However, the exact impact of the thalamus, particularly the nuclei of the VL thalamus, on the pathophysiology of dystonia is less understood. Consequently, the use of thalamomtomy for treatment of dystonia is still largely based upon empirical observations that cells which evoke dystonic activity are present within the Vim/Vop and that Vim/Vop thalamotomies provide relief of dystonic symptoms to patients. Specifically, 'dystonia cells' will evoke simultaneous contraction of muscles in the contralateral upper extremity upon microampere stimulation (Bertrand & Lenz 1995). Stimulation can also induce paraesthesia or a sense of muscle contraction (Tasker et al. 1982, 1988). Additionally it has been shown that electromyographic activity can be recorded from the extremities exhibiting dystonic symptoms upon stimulation of such cells (Zirh et al. 1998; Lenz et al. 1999). Furthermore, these cells exhibit characteristic firing patterns in dystonia (Lenz et al. 1990b).

Presurgical Screening and Contraindications

In general, stereotactic lesion surgery is best performed with the patient awake during the procedure such that they can be clinically examined during the ablation to anticipate the efficacy of the treatment, and also possible adverse effects. Hence general anaesthesia is rarely used and patients therefore must be healthy enough to undergo an awake procedure. Consequently, a variety of medical conditions can contraindicate the surgery. Moreover, if a fixed stereotactic frame is to be used the patient must be able to be fixated without sustaining injury or dislodging the frame. In patients with prominent cervical and/or thoracic axial dystonic features this may be contraindicated. However, if the dystonia is so severe that the patient cannot be operated on while awake, partial general anaesthesia has been used (Lozano et al. 1997; Ondo et al. 1998); performing surgery under these conditions is more suited for DBS than lesion surgery, where the consequences of targeting failure are fewer and reversible.

Neuropsychological assessment, such as through the Folstein Mini-Mental Status Examination (Folstein et al. 1975) or the Mattis Dementia Rating Scale (Vitek et al. 2003), is recommended to screen for patients with cognitive decline. The patients must undergo evaluation via a neurological clinical assessment including a dystonia rating scale both pre- and postoperatively to allow for assessment of surgical outcome. These scales include the Burke–Fahn–Marsden Dystonia Rating Scale (BFMDRS) (Burke et al. 1985), the newer Global Dystonia Rating Scale (GDS) or the Unified Dystonia Rating Scale (UDRS) (Comella et al. 2003) and the Toronto Western Spasmodic Torticollis Rating Scale (TWSTRS) (Consky et al. 1990).

The main complication of any stereotactic surgery is intracranial haemorrhage (Terao et al. 2003) and as such the patient must be haematologically stable. Conditions such as bleeding tendency, coagulopathy and uncontrolled hypertension could preclude a patient from being a candidate for these procedures.

All antiplatelet regimens must be discontinued for at least a week prior to surgery and clearance with a cardiac stress test for patients with a history of cardiovascular disease is suggested.

Image screening should also be performed, preferably by MRI, but CT is acceptable if MRI is contraindicated for the patient. It is important to note any significant cerebral atrophy as this may predispose the patient to increased risk for a subdural haematoma from traction injury to bridging veins during microelectrode insertion. It may preclude the patient from being a candidate for stereotactic lesion surgery.

Indications and Outcomes

The patients who receive the most benefit from pallidotomy typically present with primary generalised dystonia (Iacono et al. 1996, 1997, 1998; Shima et al. 1997; Lenz et al. 1998; Ondo et al. 1998; Vitek et al. 1998b, 1999; Lai et al. 1999; Teive et al. 2001; Yoshor et al. 2001; Eltahawy et al. 2004; Ford 2004; Imer et al. 2005; Szolna et al. 2006; Cersosimo et al. 2008), while the benefits are diminished for those presenting with secondary dystonia (Wang et al. 1997; Weetman et al. 1997; Iacono et al. 1998; Lin et al. 1998, 1999a, 1999b, 2001; Ondo et al. 1998; Vitek et al. 1998b; Justesen et al. 1999; Cubo et al. 2000; Teive et al. 2001, 2005; Yoshor et al. 2001; Choi et al. 2003; Eltahawy et al. 2004; Ford 2004; Kyriagis et al. 2004; Rakocevic et al. 2004; Imer et al. 2005; Lenders et al. 2005; Alkhani & Bohlega 2006). Patients experience slowly progressive improvements, in contrast to the more immediate benefits seen with pallidotomy in PD patients. The published reports, most of which look at 12 months postoperatively or less, predominantly include patients who had received bilateral pallidotomy (Iacono et al. 1996, 1997, 1998; Weetman et al. 1997; Lin et al. 1998, 1999a, 1999b, 2001; Ondo et al. 1998; Lai et al. 1999; Cubo et al. 2000; Teive et al. 2001; Yoshor et al. 2001; Eltahawy et al. 2004; Ford 2004; Kyriagis et al. 2004; Rakocevic et al. 2004; Imer et al. 2005; Teive et al. 2005; Cersosimo et al. 2008), although there are still a number of reports on patients who underwent a unilateral pallidotomy (Wang et al. 1997; Iacono et al. 1998; Lenz et al. 1998; Ondo et al. 1998; Vitek et al. 1998b, 1999; Justesen et al. 1999; Yoshor et al. 2001; Choi et al. 2003; Eltahawy et al. 2004; Ford 2004; Imer et al. 2005; Lenders et al. 2005; Alkhani & Bohlega 2006). A review of recent publications revealed 15 patients with average age 22.3 years with primary dystonia who underwent pallidotomy, with follow-up ranging approximately 3–14 months with outcomes reported via BFMDRS (two patients' ages at time of surgery were not reported (Ondo et al. 1998), four patients' follow-up times were only reported as an average for the study (Ondo et al. 1998) and two patients with follow-up of 96 months were not included (Cersosimo et al. 2008)). The mean preoperative BFMDRS was 51.0 (95 per cent CI 42.6–59.4; median 50) improving to a mean of 19.2 (95 per cent CI 13.2–25.2; median 17), a mean improvement of 61.1 per cent (95 per cent CI 49.3–72.9 per cent; median 66 per cent) (Table 60.1; Figure 60.3).

The secondary aetiologies that have shown dystonic symptom improvement after pallidotomy have included cerebral palsy (Iacono et al. 1998; Lin et al. 1998, 1999a, 2001; Imer et al. 2005; Teive et al. 2005), trauma (Ondo et al. 1998; Teive et al. 2001; Imer et al. 2005), Huntington's disease (Cubo et al. 2000), Hallervorden-Spatz disease (one case was a pallidothalamotomy) (Justesen et al. 1999; Kyriagis et al. 2004; Balas et al. 2006), hypoxia (Ondo et al. 1998; Lin et al. 1999a, 2001), encephalitis (Lin et al. 1999a, 2001; Eltahawy et al. 2004), postinfectious encephalopathy (Lin et al. 1999a, 2001), carbon monoxide intoxication (Lin et al. 1999a, 2001), stroke (Choi et al. 2003; Eltahawy et al. 2004), glutaric aciduria (Eltahawy et al. 2004; Rakocevic et al. 2004) and tardive dystonia (Wang et al. 1997; Weetman et al. 1997; Vitek et al. 1998b, 1999; Hashimoto et al. 2003; Ford 2004; Lenders et al. 2005). There have also been benefits seen with paroxysmal dystonia (Bhatia et al. 1998) and status dystonicus (Kyriagis et al. 2004; Teive et al. 2005; Elkay et al. 2009; Marras et al. 2014). The majority of patients have been adolescents, especially for primary dystonia, although adults who were also treated saw comparable benefit (Gross 2008). Publications contain reports of 13 individual patients with secondary dystonia treated by pallidotomy, with a mean age of 27 at the time of surgery and with follow-up ranging approximately 3–12 months reported via BFMDRS. The mean preoperative BFMDRS was 52.1 (95 per cent CI 36.7–67.5; median 51) improving to a mean of 32.7 (95 per cent CI 17.8–47.7; median 15), a mean improvement of 37.5 per cent (95 per cent CI 18.6–56.5 per cent; median 34 per cent) (Table 60.2; Figure 60.3). Lin et al. (Lin et al. 1999a, 2001) published a series of 18 patients with various aetiologies of secondary dystonia that had undergone bilateral pallidotomies (including two patients from the analysis above (Lin et al. 1998, 1999b)). Average age was 26 years old. Preoperative BFMDRS was 58.0 ± 20.9, improving to 50.5 ± 17.6 at 12 months postoperatively; mean reduction was 13 per cent. Thus Lin et al. is consistent with other smaller series, both showing decreased benefits as compared to primary dystonia after pallidotomy. Long-term outcome series for both primary and secondary dystonia following pallidotomy are lacking.

Complications specific to pallidotomy for dystonia treatment have included speech disturbances (Yoshor et al. 2001; Eltahawy et al. 2004; Cersosimo et al. 2008), lethargy/somnolence/stupor (Lin et al. 1999a; Cubo et al. 2000; Teive et al. 2001; Yoshor et al. 2001) and hemiparesis (Lin et al. 1999a; Teive et al. 2001), although the rates of occurrence are low. It has also been reported that pallidotomy has no significant neuropsychological complications, although the published data available are significantly limited (Gryz et al. 2006; Szolna et al. 2006).

Although bilateral pallidotomies in PD have been associated with increased risk of impairment to speech, swallowing, cognition and gait (Ghika et al. 1999; Higuchi & Iacono 2003), bilateral pallidotomies for dystonia have not shown the same risk of complications (Ford 2004). As such, given the two-sided benefit of bilateral procedures, particularly the improvement in axial symptoms (Vitek et al. 1999; Vitek & Giroux 2000; Abosch & Lozano 2003), they are preferred to unilateral procedures for generalised dystonia. Nevertheless, should the patient be presenting asymmetrically, then unilateral pallidotomy has been implemented (Ondo et al. 1998).

Table 60.1 Outcomes of pallidotomy for primary dystonia

Study	Surgery (yr)		Follow-up (mo)	BFMDRS (M)		
	Age (yr)	Side		Pre	Post	Decrease (%)
Lozano et al. 1997						
Dyt1–	9	b/l	3	75	16	79
Ondo et al. 1998						
Idiopathic	51	b/l	3*	57	9	84
Dyt1+	9	b/l	3*	26	13	50
Dyt1+	14	b/l	3*	50	17	66
Dyt1+	13	b/l	3*	48	17	65
Vitek et al. 1998; Vitek et al. 1999						
Idiopathic	54	u/l	14	34	7	79
Idiopathic	24	u/l	7	41	31	24
Teive et al. 2001						
Dyt1–	35	b/l	6	60	18	70
Idiopathic	?	b/l	6	50	28	44
Idiopathic	28	b/l	6	48	4	92
Idiopathic	?	b/l	6	28	12	57
Eltahawy et al. 2004						
Dyt1+	10	b/l	6	75	25	67
Dyt1+	12	b/l	6	71	38	46
Dyt1+	15	b/l	6	53	13	75
Dyt1–	16	b/l	6	49	40	18
Cersosimo et al. 2008 **						
Dyt1+	19	b/l	96	108	21	81
Dyt1+	14	b/l	96	42	50	–19

* Only mean follow-up time was reported
** Excluded from descriptive statistics given 96-month outcome

The patients who have received the most benefit from thalamotomy have had non-progressive generalised dystonia with extremity involvement, but little or no trunk or neck involvement. Although relief is seen in both primary and secondary dystonia, most research has shown more benefit in the context of secondary dystonia (Andrew et al. 1983; Tasker et al. 1988; Bertrand & Lenz 1995; Cardoso et al. 1995; Szolna et al. 2006). However, one modern series, although it too found secondary dystonia to show more benefit from thalamotomy than primary dystonia, found this difference not to be statistically significant (Yoshor et al. 2001). The relief of dystonic symptoms following thalamotomy has been shown to slightly diminish over time (Yoshor et al. 2001). Patients with the DYT1 mutation have also been shown to have strong response to pallidotomy and thalamotomy (Krack & Vercueil 2001; Ford 2004). Cooper originally showed that his Ashkenazi Jewish patients often had some of the best responses to these lesion procedures (Cooper 1969, 1976), of which lineage the DYT1 mutation is linked (Kramer et al. 1990).

Complication rates for thalamotomy have been varied throughout its history as a procedure, but for more recent unilateral procedures, the complication rates are lower. Complications continue to include speech disturbances, contralateral weakness and pseudobulbar palsy (Yoshor et al. 2001). Significant neuropsychological complications for thalamotomy have not been reported, although the published data available are sparse (Szolna et al. 2006).

Bilateral thalamotomies have been shown to have an increased risk of dysarthria (Andrew et al. 1983; Ford 2004). Cooper would not perform simultaneous bilateral surgeries because of the increased incidence of speech disturbances in his series (Cooper 1976); Bertrand would only perform unilateral surgeries given the risk for speech disturbances (Bertrand et al. 1979); and Andrew saw hemidystonia as a better indication for thalamotomy as a unilateral procedure would be sufficient and he could better avoid the complications associated with bilateral procedures (Andrew et al. 1983; Krack & Vercueil 2001).

In the case of focal dystonia where botulinum toxin injections have failed or have been contraindicated stereotactic ablative procedures have also been used. Thalamotomy in particular has been the procedure of choice. There has been considerable benefit seen with ventralis oralis thalamotomy in patients with focal hand dystonia (Siegfried et al. 1969; Andrew et al. 1983; Mempel et al. 1986; Goto et al. 1997; Iacono et al. 1998; Taira et al. 2003; Zhuang et al. 2004; Shibata et al. 2005; Taira et al. 2006; Taira 2007; Kim et al. 2008; Horisawa et al. 2013; Asahi et al. 2014; Taira & Horisawa 2016), such as writer's cramp and musician's cramp, with low rates of recurrence,

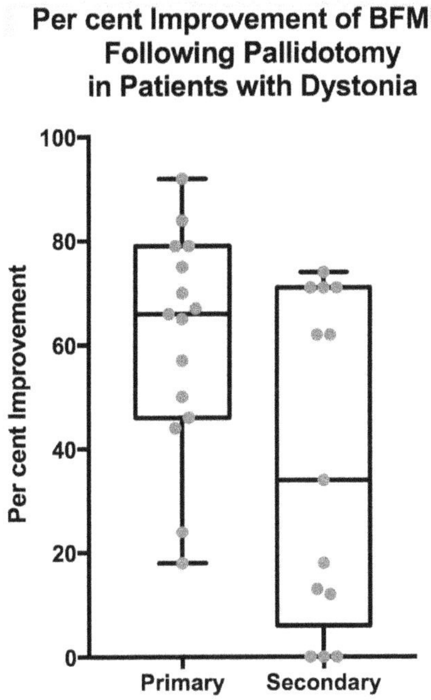

Figure 60.3 Improvement of BMFDRS following pallidotomy for primary and secondary dystonia. Descriptive statistics were run on the percentage improvement in BMFRDS of the patients summarised in Tables 60.1 and 60.2 (excluding those denoted as such in the tables). Box plots are presented in black with each patient represented as a dot. Primary dystonia: range 18–92, interquartile range 46–79, median 66; secondary dystonia: range 0–74, interquartile range 6–71, median 34.

low complication rates and sustained relief seen as far out as 15 years, as well as with Vim thalamotomy (Ohye et al. 1982), although it has been far less studied. Additionally, benefit has been seen in cases where patients experience focal dystonia as the result of a lesion or infarction in the basal ganglia (Andrew et al. 1982; Imer et al. 2005; Alvarez et al. 2014). The use of pallidotomy for focal dystonia has been reported far less, although unilateral lesions for Meige syndrome (Valalik et al. 2011) and focal hand dystonia (Horisawa et al. 2016a) have shown some benefit.

These ablative procedures have also been useful in treating cervical dystonia (Loher et al. 2004). Also known as spasmodic torticollis, cervical dystonia was first treated through stereotactic lesions of the EPS, including the thalamus and GPi, beginning in the 1960s with Mundinger, Riechert (Mundinger & Riechert 1961) and Cooper (Cooper 1964), among others (Handa et al. 1962; Yasargil 1962; Laitinen 1963; Mazars et al. 1968). Then in the 1970s, beginning with Hassler and Dieckmann's work (Hassler & Dieckman 1970a, 1970b), and continuing into the 1980s, the thalamus was the primary target (Meares 1971; Caracalos 1972; Mundinger et al. 1972; Andrew et al. 1974, 1983; Cooper 1977; Goldhahn & Goldhahn 1977; Hernesniemi & Laitinen 1977; Bertrand et al. 1978; von Essen et al. 1980; Stejskal et al. 1981; Hassler & Dieckmann 1982; Burzaco 1985). From the 1990s onwards only a few reports have included thalamotomy (Krauss et al. 1992; Iacono et al. 1998; Imer et al. 2005). It has been shown that while bilateral surgeries are associated with better outcomes than unilateral, they are associated with an elevated risk of complications including dysarthria, dysphagia, ataxia and cognitive impairments (Meares 1971; Andrew et al. 1974, 1983; Cooper 1977; Hernesniemi & Laitinen 1977; Bertrand et al. 1978; Iacono et al. 1998; Lang 1998; Loher et al. 2004; Imer et al. 2005). Pallidotomy has been the focus of more recent ablative treatments for cervical dystonia. The majority of these studies showing benefit with pallidotomy for cervical dystonia have been focused on treating patients with primary generalised dystonia (Lozano et al. 1997; Ondo et al. 1998; Lin et al. 1999b; Teive et al. 2001; Teive et al. 2001), although there have been a few reports on patients specifically with cervical dystonia (Iacono et al. 1998; Horisawa et al. 2016b). While both unilateral (Iacono et al. 1998) and bilateral pallidotomies (Lozano et al. 1997; Ondo et al. 1998; Lin et al. 1999b; Teive et al. 2001; Horisawa et al. 2016b) have provided relief for cervical dystonia, as axial symptoms are best treated with bilateral procedures, it is not surprising that the best outcomes have been with bilateral pallidotomy, although, as mentioned previously, the risk of complications and adverse outcomes is higher for bilateral procedures (Adler & Kumar 2000).

In a few series, pallidotomy has shown better outcomes than thalamotomy for treatment of primary dystonia, although this may be related to performing bilateral procedures for pallidotomy (Yoshor et al. 2001; Szolna et al. 2006). Nevertheless, both pallidotomy and thalamotomy provide significant relief for dystonia and the decision to choose one over another or instead choose a non-destructive procedure, such as DBS, should be made on an individual basis, weighing each of the aforementioned factors accordingly.

Surgical Techniques

The basic stereotactic lesioning procedures for pallidotomy and thalamotomy are quite similar so they are described here together (Tasker 1990; Hutchison et al. 1994; Lozano et al. 1995, 1996; Tasker et al. 1997; Vilela & da Silva 2002; Coban et al. 2009). The procedure used for dystonia is the same as is used with PD (Bertrand & Lenz 1995; Lozano et al. 1997; Ohye 2000). In the following we will give an overview on our techniques.

Imaging and Planning

Although pallidotomy and thalamotomy can be performed today using more advanced frameless techniques or with newer frame technology such as customised frames (e.g. microTargeting™ platform, FHC) or image-guidance frames (e.g. Nexframe', Medtronic), the published lesions were all performed using a classic type stereotactic frame. As such, this is the procedure detailed here. It begins with 3D image acquisition with the patient in a stereotactic frame, either a contrast-enhanced MRI, or, if a previous MRI has been obtained without a frame, a volumetric CT scan, with the two image sets subsequently being co-registered. If MRI acquisition is contraindicated for the patient, such as due to implanted MRI-incompatible hardware, a stereotactic CT scan alone will suffice. If the patient's dystonia is severe such that it precludes

Table 60.2 Outcomes of pallidotomy for secondary dystonia

Study aetiology	Surgery (yr)		Follow-up (mo)	BFMDRS (M)		
	Age (yr)	Side		Pre	Post	Decrease (%)
Weetman et al. 1997						
Tardive dystonia	31	b/l	8	76	21	71
Ondo et al. 1998						
Traumatic	56	u/l	3*	34	13	62
Traumatic	18	b/l	3*	56	46	18
Hypoxic	16	b/l	3*	59	17	71
Peripheral trauma	20	u/l	3*	23	6	74
Vitek et al. 1998; Vitek et al. 1999)						
Tardive dystonia	30	u/l	11	31	9	71
Lin et al. 1998						
Hypoxic	36	b/l	9	74	28	62
Lin et al. 1999b						
Cerebral palsy	29	b/l	12	51	33.5	34
Cubo et al. 2000						
Huntington's disease	13	b/l	3	56	49	13
Lin et al. 1999a; Lin et al. 2001**	26	b/l	12	58	50	13
Teive et al. 2001						
Traumatic	40	b/l	6	51	51	0
Eltahawy et al. 2004						
Postencephalitis	22	u/l	6	28	28	0
Poststroke	30	u/l	6	25	25	0
Glutaric aciduria	10	b/l	6	113	99	12

* Only mean follow-up time was reported

** Only average values of 18 patients reported (8 cerebral palsy, 6 hypoxic, 2 carbon monoxide, 1 postinfectious, 1 postencephalitis) and therefore this cohort is excluded from the descriptive statistical analysis, except the patients from Lin et al. (Lin et al. 1998, 1999b), which were included in this cohort but were reported individually previously

getting an adequate image set, the patient may be imaged under general anaesthesia.

The imaging set(s) are imported into a neuronavigation computer workstation with software that allows for stereotactic targeting. GPi or Vim targeting can be done using consensus indirect targeting coordinates in stereotactic space, i.e. with respect to the intercommisural line between the anterior and posterior commissures. Given the advancements in imaging parameters and MRI field strength, the GPi can be directly targeted although the Vim cannot, as it is not directly observable in clinical strength magnets. Atlases may also be used to assist in target identification. Additionally, some centres may have access to software that implements patient-specific atlas conformation or probabilistic atlases based on large previous data sets. One such package, One Track©, developed by the Georgia Institute of Technology and Emory University, allows for the adjustment of the contours of the basal ganglia and thalamus from an interpolated digital version of the Schaltenbrand and Wahren atlas to the boundaries visible on standard 1.5T T1 weighted image sets. This is then further utilised to plan the best trajectory to approach the target.

The original GPi target coordinates proposed by Laitinen (Laitinen et al. 1992a) are more or less still used today, 2–3 mm anterior to the midcommissural point, 3–6 mm below the intercommissural (IC) line and 20–21 mm lateral to the midline. The thalamic target is usually 25 per cent of the AC–PC length posterior to midcommissural point on the IC plane and 11.5 mm lateral to the ventricle (Machado et al. 2006) (Figure 60.4).

Neurophysiologic Mapping

To begin, a burr hole or twist drill craniostomy is made at a precoronal entry that avoids venous, sulcal or ventricular penetration. The dura and pia/arachnoid are opened so that traction from insertion of the electrodes does not induce a subdural haematoma. If possible, sharp penetration of the dura is recommended, following careful stereotactic planning, as this will minimise egress of cerebrospinal fluid and ingress of air, thus minimising resultant pneumocephalus and brain shift (Khan et al. 2008). Here macroelectrodes or cannulas for guiding the microelectrode may be introduced, for macroelectrode stimulation mapping or microelectrode recording/stimulation respectively (Gross et al. 2006). Macroelectrode stimulation mapping generates a map of responses to stimulation and although it is the faster and less intricate method, the map provides a lower

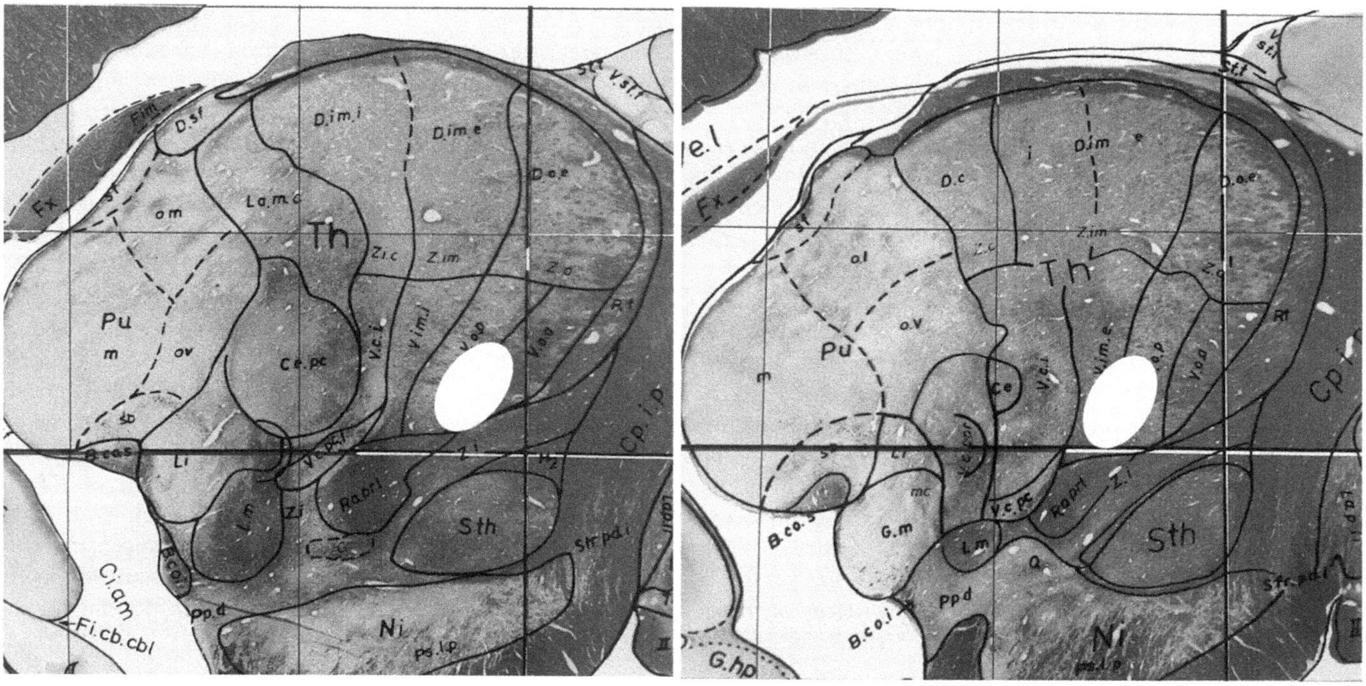

Figure 60.4 Stereotactic targets of thalamotomy. The typical location and size of a Vim thalamotomy is depicted on the 14.5 mm lateral sagittal plane of the Schaltenbrand and Wahren human stereotaxic atlas (left); a typical Voa/Vop lesion is depicted on the 12 mm lateral map.

Source: Modified with permission from Schaltenbrand & Wahren (1977).

resolution of the target anatomy. Microelectrode recording/stimulation records individual neuronal activity, and although it is the more time-consuming method and requires both more expertise and intricate equipment, it yields a more detailed resolution of the basal ganglia and thalamic nuclei receptive fields. These neurophysiologic recordings are then used to further refine the structural contours models used to direct the final trajectory. A microdrive platform used to drive the electrodes and probes into the target structures is mounted to the frame arc. C-arm fluoroscopy or 3D imaging with intraoperative CT scan or MRI is then used to confirm the stereotactic position of the electrode (Lokuketagoda et al. 2011).

During mapping of the GPi for posteroventral pallidotomy, the optic tract, internal capsule and sensorimotor region are determined so as to ensure the proper and safe placement of GPi lesions within the sensorimotor region. There is naturally a slight variance between patients with regards to locations of specific neurons within a given structure and, as such, it is useful to determine the physiological boundaries of these populations. Thus to ensure correct laterality, in addition to recording sensorimotor activity, mapping of the lateral border of the GPi is recommended, with adjustment of the target to lie 2.5 mm medial to the lateral border (Vitek et al. 1998a). Hence the lesion can be localised within the motor portion of GPi, avoiding the more anteromedial cognitive-associative regions, where less benefit and more potential for detrimental effects on cognition would be observed.

For proper placement of a Vim/Vop thalamotomy, lesions are positioned relative to the Vci/e, anterior to the border of this tactile sensory relay thalamic nucleus (Lenz et al. 1995). The neurons here are responsive to innocuous mechanical cutaneous stimulation, whereas the neurons in the Vim and Vop are much less responsive to cutaneous stimulation, so it serves as a good landmark for neurophysiological mapping (Lenz et al. 1988; Bertrand & Lenz 1995). The Vim and the Vop have deep sensory cells, which respond to active and passive movements of the limbs (Lenz et al. 1990a). However, some reports suggest the Vop does not have deep sensory cells and only responds to contralateral extremity muscle contraction (Ohye 2000). In dystonia patients, it has been shown that there is a higher density of neurons which respond to joint, muscle and ligament movement present in the Vim (Lenz et al. 1999). Once the boundaries of the Vim and Vop are defined, the population of dystonia-related cells is determined through stimulation. The lesion is generated in this region. An additional track can be made 2–3 mm lateral ensuring the internal capsule will be avoided (Bertrand & Lenz 1995).

Lesion Generation

Often, several recording and/or stimulation tracks may be necessary to refine the targeting, before lesion generation can be performed. For the radiofrequency lesion generation procedure, a radiofrequency generator that heats a 1.1 mm diameter probe with a 2 or 3 mm exposed tip is used to thermocoagulate the surrounding tissue. The lesioning electrode insertion location is dependent on the previously determined physiological map. If necessitated, the lesion electrode can be repositioned during the procedure. Before permanent lesioning, as a safety measure to prevent adverse effects, a test lesion is performed at the subablative temperature of 42 °C for 60 seconds, where neuronal activity is impaired, but no neuronal damage occurs. Continuous clinical testing is performed concurrently to observe for any changes in sensorimotor and speech functions and – in the case of GPi – visual changes. Lesioning is then performed, each for 60 seconds, beginning at 60 °C and increasing up to 85 °C incrementally. Symptomatic changes and adverse effects should be noted with each lesion. Lesions can continue to be placed so long as adverse effects are not noted so as to maximise lesion size. Ultimately, the lesions must be large enough to produce a long-standing clinical benefit, but small enough to avoid unwanted side-effects or complications. It is important to note that temperature has been shown to be the parameter best correlated with lesion volume (Hirabayashi et al. 2012). Some may also choose to make the lesions based on somatotopic findings and the patient's intraoperative clinical presentation (Gross et al. 1999). However, there has yet to be any conclusive evidence as to the superiority of any of these techniques over the others. Pallidotomy lesions should be oblate spheroidal, measuring approximately 6 mm in height and 4 mm in diameter (Lozano et al. 1996; Vitek et al. 1998a) (Figure 60.5). The lesions in the Vim/Vop are typically cylindrical, measuring 3 mm in diameter and 5 mm in length (Bertrand & Lenz 1995).

Following the procedure, the patients must undergo a neurological exam and be monitored overnight. An MRI scan should be acquired the next day.

Alternate Ablative Options

Radiofrequency Ablation Through *In Situ* DBS Leads

Dystonia patients who have been treated through DBS occasionally require hardware explantation for reasons such as hardware malfunction, hardware erosion or recurring infection (Sillay et al. 2008; Falowski et al. 2012). The typical course of action is for these patients to undergo reimplantation, but this could be contraindicated in the context of advanced disease or comorbid medical conditions. These patients may elect to receive radiofrequency ablation, but again they will be undergoing a subsequent surgery after explantation, which comes with the risks of a second stereotactic surgery, and the possibility that the site of this lesion will not be the same as the original effective DBS lead site. Furthermore, whether these patients undergo reimplantation or radiofrequency ablation, they will have to endure a period without symptomatic treatment between explantation and subsequent surgery. To circumvent these drawbacks, a recent approach has been undertaken in which radiofrequency lesions are generated at the stimulated target site through the implanted DBS leads immediately before explantation, in which the DBS lead is connected to a lesion generator where a potential of 15–40 V is generated for a period of up to 60 seconds. Either monopolar or bipolar fields between lead contacts are employed depending on the target. Although DBS leads lack thermistors or thermocouples, preventing temperature monitoring through the lesion, these parameters have been shown to produce adequate lesions through coagulation and tissue studies (Raoul et al. 2007; Strickland et al. 2013). Thus far there is one report of using this approach for treating a patient with primary generalised dystonia. Two unilateral lesions were produced in GPi using bipolar fields with a potential of 40 V for 30 seconds. This patient saw comparable relief to that seen prior with DBS (Marras et al. 2009). An additional study exists in which DBS electrodes were used in lieu of radiofrequency exposed tip electrodes to produce a lesion in GPi for a patient with secondary dystonia as the first line of surgical treatment (i.e. the DBS electrodes were implanted specifically to be used for lesioning) where the patient also saw symptom relief (Franzini et al. 2015). This technique has also been reported for the treatment of PD and essential tremor with favourable results (Oh et al. 2001; Raoul et al. 2003; Deligny et al. 2009). Although this approach is not approved by the US Food and Drug Administration, it is potentially a viable technique in the context of the aforementioned extenuating circumstances.

Magnetic Resonance-Guided Stereotactic Laser Ablation

In addition to radiofrequency ablation, lasers have more recently been employed for laser interstitial thermal therapy using diode lasers to produce a thermocoagulative lesion under MR guidance. A cooling cannula is stereotactically inserted through which is introduced a fibreoptic with a diffusing tip to distribute the laser energy. Lasers provide highly controlled heating, where the heating properties are dependent upon source wavelength, and as such allow for selection of a laser source specific for the target (Wyman et al. 1997; Atsumi et al. 2001). With intracranial tissue, rapid and localised heating with sharp boundaries at a relatively lower power is preferable, so 980 nm wavelength light is chosen (McNichols et al. 2004). It has also been shown that the thermal energy supplied by the laser tends to conform to anatomical boundaries, where cerebrospinal fluid filled spaces function as heat sinks, preventing transmission of thermal energy, thus allowing for better prevention of off-target damage in neighbouring tissue (Curry et al. 2012; Willie et al. 2014). Even with all of this control, the impact of tissue perfusion and the properties of the delivery element cannot be fully predicted (Wyman et al. 1992; Kahn et al. 1994; Schwarzmaier et al. 1998). As such, real-time thermometry and anatomical monitoring of the target and surrounding tissue via proton magnetic resonance spectroscopy is employed, known as magnetic resonance thermal imaging (MRTI) (Jolesz et al. 1988; Le Behin et al. 1989; Tracz et al. 1992; Corbett et al. 1995, 1997; De Poorter et al. 1995; Kahn et al. 1998; Vogl et al. 1998; Busse et al. 1999; Peters et al. 2000; Fiedler et al. 2001; McNichols et al. 2001; Stroszczynski et al. 2001). This monitoring also allows for a feedback mechanism to regulate the ablation where user-defined thermal thresholds (45 °C) are employed at the target and surrounding tissue such that the laser delivery will be automatically terminated should

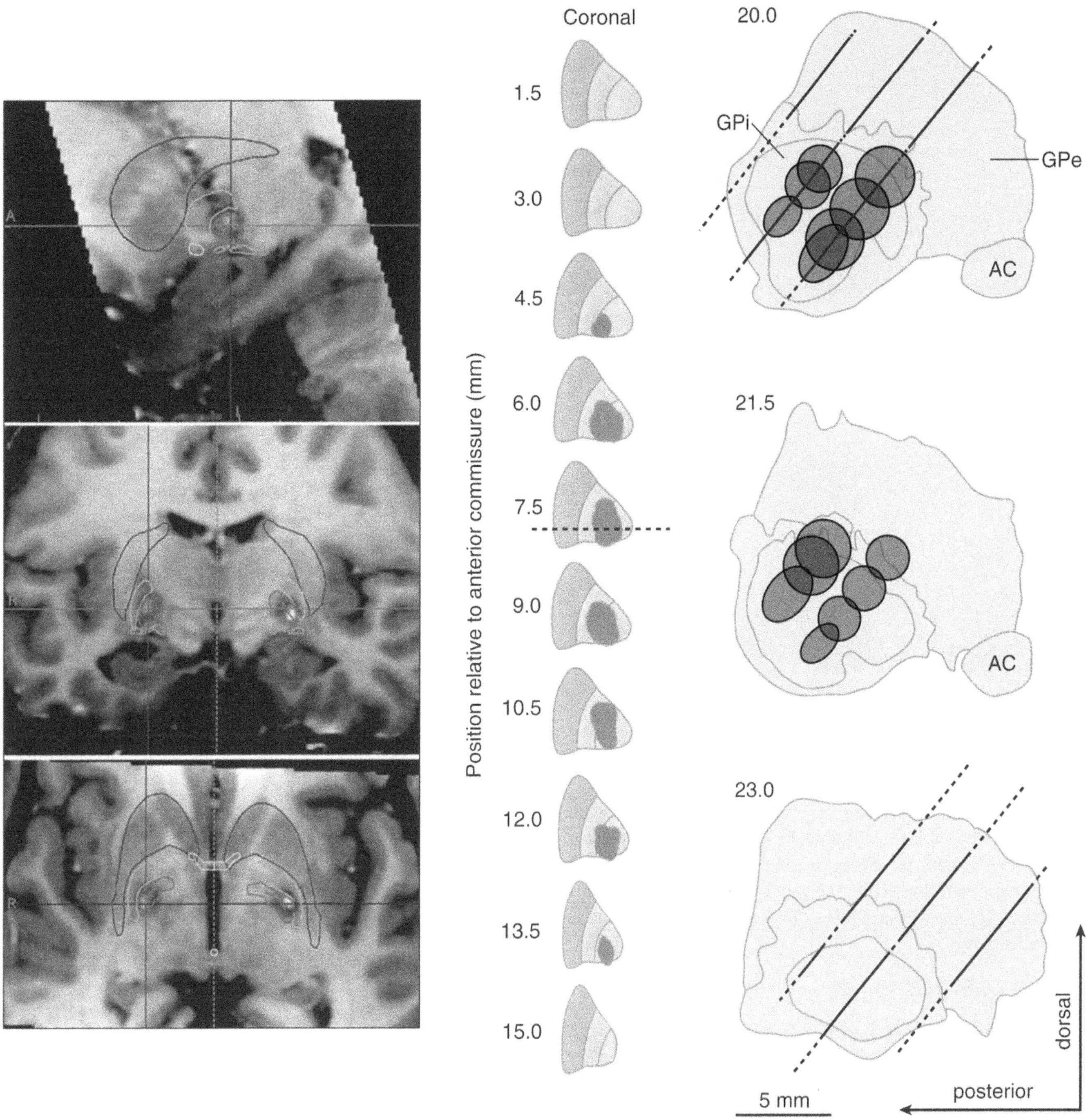

Figure 60.5 Postoperative imaging and reconstruction following pallidotomy. Left MER-guided radiofrequency pallidotomy is shown in sagittal (left, top), coronal (left, centre) and axial (left, bottom) planes. The lesions were performed with overlapping lesions as shown on the right in coronal series and in sagittal reconstructions. Microelectrode tracks were performed at 20 and 23 mm lateral, and the lesions were made at 20 and 21.5 mm lateral.

Source: illustrations redrawn from Vitek et al. (1998a); MRI images from Lokuketagoda & Gross (2011).

a threshold be excited at one of the selected sites (Kangasniemi et al. 2004; McNichols et al. 2004). This ensures not only that the ablation is limited to the desired target, but also can be used to ensure that the acute coagulative necrosis induced during this process does not occur too rapidly, which could lead to tissue vaporisation and damage of the optical fibre. Ultimately this allows for tighter control and better safety for lesion generation. We have performed MR-guided laser interstitial thermal therapy (MRg-LITT) pallidotomy on two patients. One was a 30-year-old male with a history of generalised idiopathic dystonia diagnosed age nine (although his MRI showed right parietal and occipital cystic encephalomalacia first noted in 2013). He underwent right laser pallidotomy under general anaesthesia without complication (Figure 60.6). His BFMDRS decreased from 23 to 12.5 after one year, and TWSTRS declined from 26 to 15, with sustained benefits at two years. The second patient

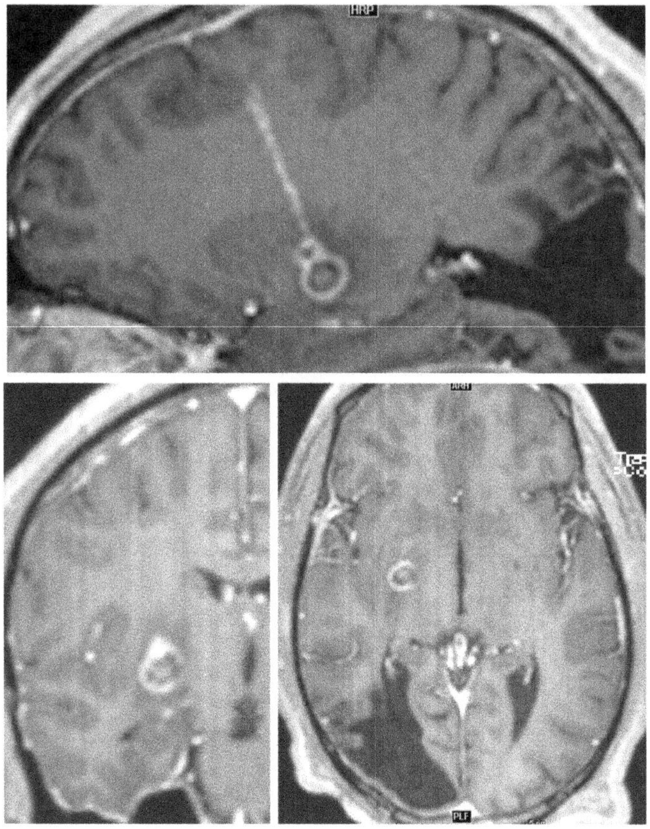

Figure 60.6 Pallidotomy performed with MR-guided laser interstitial thermal therapy. Immediate postoperative contrast enhanced MRI in three planes following MRg-LITT pallidotomy performed on the right for patient with generalised dystonia. Top, sagittal; bottom left, coronal; bottom right, axial.

was an 11-year-old boy with DYT1+ primary dystonia who underwent bilateral laser pallidotomy. His BFMDRS improved from 94 to 56, with no change in his disability score (26 to 28) after nine months. While the benefit was sustained on one side, they have progressed on the other and further ablation is being considered.

Gamma Knife Radiosurgery

Gamma knife radiosurgery, where a lesion is generated through the focusing of ionising radiation, has also been employed for the treatment of dystonia, particularly in patients where invasive surgery was contraindicated. Mainly gamma knife thalamotomies have been performed for dystonia, including two cases of torsional hemidystonia (Pan et al. 2000), two cases of cervical dystonia (Ohye et al. 2005; Yen et al. 2012) and one case of generalised dystonia (Ohye et al. 2002). Of these cases only two reports indicated the laterality of the surgery, both unilateral, and the outcomes (Pan et al. 2000; Yen et al. 2012). Gamma knife thalamotomy has shown considerable benefit for dystonic symptoms as far out as 18 months postoperatively, and a reduction in medications. There have been two reports of using unilateral gamma knife pallidotomy for dystonia, both secondary focal dystonias (Kwon & Whang 1995; Stancanello et al. 2009). While it shows promising results with a decrease in dystonic symptoms and a substantial reduction in medications, the quality of life measures did not show significant improvement and one patient developed homonymous hemianopsia. It is important to note that gamma knife often requires more intense monitoring as well as medical and surgical management due to the potential complications associated with radiation necrosis (Okun et al. 2001).

Magnetic Resonance (Imaging)-Guided Focused Ultrasound

Another non-invasive approach to lesion generation is MRI-guided focused ultrasound (MRgFUS). A thousand ultrasound transducers are positioned around the patient's head to create a sonication at the lesion target site. The temperature of the tissue at the sonication point rises by a few degrees per second, leading to a thermal ablation, while the tissue the beams are travelling through to the target remains unaffected. MRTI is used concurrently to generate a thermal map of the target and surrounding tissue to monitor the process. The tissue is heated to a subablative temperature such as 43 °C, where neuronal activity is impaired without tissue damage, which allows for optimisation of the target and of symptom relief in the conscious patient, similar to using a 'temporary' lesion during radiofrequency ablation. After these adjustments the thermocoagulative lesion is performed at a temperature of 60 °C. Each sonication lasts 10–20 second and generates a lesion 1–2 mm in diameter. Typically 10–30 sonications are performed to ablate the target (Martin et al. 2009; Jeanmonod et al. 2012; Elias et al. 2013a; Lipsman et al. 2013, 2014). While the risks of invasive surgery are circumvented, as are the complications associated with the ionising radiation of gamma knife, it is important to note that intracranial haemorrhage is still a possibility, as vasculature can still be damaged at the lesion site. The risk is theoretically diminished without the insertion of a lesioning probe or microelectrodes. While MRg-FUS has yet to be reported for treatment of dystonia, there are currently several clinical trials evaluating its efficacy for thalamotomy in treating essential tremor (Elias et al. 2013a, 2013b; Lipsman et al. 2013; Chang et al. 2015) and neuropathic pain (Martin et al. 2009; Jeanmonod et al. 2012). These have thus far shown substantial and significant improvement in tremor, disability and quality of life. Pallidotomies, thalamotomies and subthalamotomies have also begun to be evaluated in PD (Lipsman et al. 2014; Na et al. 2015; Shah et al. 2015). Thus MRgFUS has the promise of being a viable treatment option for dystonia in the future.

Conclusions

Stereotactic ablative surgeries remain a safe, effective and established therapeutic strategy in patients with generalised dystonia. Pallidotomy has provided substantial relief, especially in the context of primary dystonia and when performed bilaterally. Thalamotomy has also provided relief, especially in the context of secondary dystonia. Even with the success of DBS to treat generalised dystonia, having equal efficacy and potentially improved safety profile, these ablative procedures should not be abandoned. There are significant advantages to ablations including circumventing the drawbacks of implanted DBS hardware such as malfunctions, infection risk, need for maintenance and battery replacement and lead damage or dislodgment in the context of dystonia. Ablative procedures are typically more cost-effective and require minimal follow-up. Furthermore with the advent of new non-invasive ablative techniques (Martin et al. 2009), lesion surgery may become a preferred option for many who cannot or do not want to undergo an invasive or minimally invasive procedure. However, comparative effectiveness and cost–benefit analysis of pallidotomy/thalamotomy vs pallidal/thalamic DBS has never been performed for dystonia, nor likely will ever be in a sufficiently sized trial to draw inferences. It is also important to note that should an ablative procedure not provide adequate symptom relief, this does not preclude a patient from receiving subsequent DBS, provided some of the target remains unablated or an alternate target is selected for DBS than the nucleus that underwent ablation. Several reports have demonstrated this to be an effective option for patients in these circumstances (Muta et al. 2001; Novak et al. 2008; Kim et al. 2011; Fonoff et al. 2012; Waln et al. 2013; Dec et al. 2014). Ultimately, the decision to perform ablative surgery or DBS will rely on the clinical judgement and experience of movement disorder neurologists and neurosurgeons, and by patient preference.

References

Abosch A, Lozano A. 2003. Stereotactic neurosurgery for movement disorders. *Can J Neurol Sci* 30 (Suppl. 1):S72–S82.

Adler C, Kumar R. 2000. Pharmacological and surgical options for the treatment of cervical dystonia. *Neurology* 55(12):S9–S14.

Albe-Fessard D, Arfel G, Guiot G, Hardy J, Vourc'h G, Hertzog E, Aleonard P. 1961. Identification et delimitation precise de certaines structures sous-corticales de l'homme par l'electrophysiologie: son interet dans la chirurgie stereotaxique des dyskinesies. *C R Hebd Seances Acad Sci, Ser D, Sci Nat* 253(21):2412–2414.

Albin RL, Young AB, Penney JB. 1989. The functional anatomy of basal ganglia disorders. *Trends Neurosci* 12(10):366–375.

Alexander G, Delong M, Strick PL. 1986. Parallel organization of functionally segregated circuits linking basal ganglia and cortex. *Annu Rev Neurosci* 9:357–381.

Alkhani A, Bohlega S. 2006. Unilateral pallidotomy for hemidystonia. *Mov Disord* 21(6):852–855.

Alvarez M, Quintanal N, Diaz A, Prince J, Garcia I, Carballo M, Rodriguez R, Maragoto C, Pedroso I, Macias R. 2014. Dystonia and tremor secondary to thalamic infarction successfully treated with thalamotomy of the ventralis intermedius nucleus. *Mov Disord* 29(9):1188–1190.

Andrew J, Edwards JMR, Rudolf N. 1974. The placement of stereotaxic lesions for involuntary movements other than in Parkinson's disease. *Acta Neurochir* 34(1):29–47.

Andrew J, Fowler C, Harrison M. 1982. Hemi-dystonia due to focal basal ganglia lesion after head-injury and improved by stereotaxic thalamotomy. *J Neurol Neurosurg Psychiatr* 45(3):276.

Andrew J, Fowler C, Harrison M. 1983. Stereotaxic thalamotomy in 55 cases of dystonia. *Brain* 106(4):981–1000.

Asahi T, Koh M, Kashiwazaki D, Kuroda S. 2014. Stereotactic neurosurgery for writer's cramp: report of two cases with an overview of the literature. *Stereotact Funct Neurosurg* 92(6):405–411.

Atsumi H, Matsumae M, Kaneda M, Muro I, Mamata Y, Komiya T, Tsugu A, Tsugane R. 2001. Novel laser system and laser irradiation method reduced the risk of carbonization during laser interstitial thermotherapy: assessed by MR temperature measurement. *Lasers Surg Med* 29(2):108–117.

Balas I, Kovacs N, Hollody K. 2006. Staged bilateral stereotactic pallidothalamotomy for life-threatening dystonia in a child with Hallervorden–Spatz disease. *Mov Disord* 21(1):82–85.

Bankiewicz KS, Plunkett RJ, Jacobowitz DM, Porrino L, di Porzio U, London WT, Kopin IJ, Oldfield EH. 1990. The effect of fetal mesencephalon implants on primate MPTP-induced parkinsonism. histochemical and behavioral studies. *J Neurosurg* 72(2):231–244.

Benabid A, Pollak P, Louveau A, Henry S, Derougemont J. 1987. Combined (thalamotomy and stimulation) stereotactic surgery of the Vim thalamic nucleus for bilateral Parkinson disease. *Appl Neurophysiol* 50(1):344–346.

Benabid A, Pollak P, Gao D, Hoffmann D, Limousin P, Gay E, Payen I, Benazzouz A. 1996. Chronic electrical stimulation of the ventralis intermedius nucleus of the thalamus as a treatment of movement disorders. *J Neurosurg* 84(2):203–214.

Benabid A, Deuschl G, Lang A, Lyons K, Rezai AR. 2006. Deep brain stimulation for Parkinson's disease: introduction. *Mov Disord* 21:S168–S170.

Bergman H, Wichmann T, Delong MR. 1990. Reversal of experimental parkinsonism by lesions of the subthalamic nucleus. *Science* 249(4975):1436–1438.

Beric A, Kelly PJ, Rezai A, Sterio D, Mogilner A, Zonenshayn M, Kopell B. 2001. Complications of deep brain stimulation surgery. *Stereotact Funct Neurosurg* 77(1-4):73–78.

Bertrand CM, Lenz FA. 1995 Surgical treatment of dystonia. In: Tsui JKC, Calne DB, editors, *Handbook of Dystonia*. New York: Marcel Dekker, pp 329–345.

Bertrand C, Molina NP, Martinez SN. 1978. Combined stereotactic and peripheral surgical approach for spasmodic torticollis. *Appl Neurophysiol* 41(1):122–133.

Bertrand C, Molina NP, Martinez SN. 1979. Stereotaxic targets for dystonias and dyskinesias: relationship to corticobulbar fibers and other adjoining structures. In: Poirier LJ, Sourkes TL, Bedard PJ, editors. *Advances in Neurology*. Vol 24. New York: Raven Press. 395–399.

Bhatia K, Marsden C, Thomas D. 1998. Posteroventral pallidotomy can ameliorate attacks of paroxysmal dystonia induced by exercise. *J Neurol Neurosurg Psychiatr* 65(4):604–605.

Blanchet PJ, Konitsiotis S, Hyland K, Arnold LA, Pettigrew KD, Chase TN. 1998. Chronic exposure to MPTP as a primate model of progressive parkinsonism: a pilot study with a free radical scavenger. *Exp Neurol* 153(2):214–222.

Blomstedt P, Hariz MI. 2005. Hardware-related complications of deep brain stimulation: a ten year experience. *Acta Neurochir* 147(10):1061–1064.

Bravo G, Cooper IS. 1959. A clinical and radiological correlation of the lesions produced by chemopallidectomy and thalamectomy. *J Neurol Neurosurg Psychiatr* 22(1):1–10.

Bucy P, Buchanan DN. 1932. Athetosis. *Brain* 55:479–492.

Bucy P, Case TJ. 1939. Tremor: physiologic mechanism and abolition by surgical means. *Arch Neurol Psychiatry* 41(4):721–746.

Burke R, Fahn S, Marsden C, Bressman S, Moskowitz C, Friedman J. 1985. Validity and reliability of a rating-scale for the primary torsion dystonias. *Neurology* 35(1):73–77.

Burzaco J. 1985. Stereotaxic pallidotomy in extrapyramidal disorders. *Appl Neurophysiol* 48(1):283–287.

Busse H, Rassek M, Grust A, Kahn T, Schwarzmaier HJ. 1999. Improved quantitative MR thermometry using a 1.5-T scanner to monitor cooled applicator systems during laser-induced interstitial thermotherapy (LITT). In: Ryan TP, editor, Society of Photo-Optical Instrumentation-SPIE. Bellingham/wash, Proceedings. 24–25 January 1999, San Jose, CA.

Caracalos A. 1972. Results of 103 cryosurgical procedures in involuntary movement disorders. *Confin Neurol* 34(1):74–83.

Cardoso F, Jankovic J, Grossman R, Hamilton WJ. 1995. Outcome after stereotaxic thalamotomy for dystonia and hemiballismus. *Neurosurgery* 36(3):501–507.

Ceballos-Baumann A, Passingham R, Warner T, Playford E, Marsden C, Brooks DJ. 1995. Overactive prefrontal and underactive motor cortical areas in idiopathic dystonia. *Ann Neurol* 37(3):363–372.

Cersosimo M, Raina G, Piedimonte F, Antico J, Graff P, Micheli FE. 2008. Pallidal surgery for the treatment of primary generalized dystonia: long-term follow-up. *Clin Neurol Neurosurg* 110(2):145–150.

Chang W, Jung H, Kweon E, Zadicario E, Rachmilevitch I, Chang JW. 2015. Unilateral magnetic resonance guided focused ultrasound thalamotomy for essential tremor practices and clinicoradiological outcomes. *J Neurol Neurosurg Psychiatr* 86(3):257–264.

Choi SJ, Lee SW, Kim MC, Kwon JY, Park CK, Sung JH, Hong JT, Woo HK. 2003. Posteroventral pallidotomy in medically intractable post-apoplectic monochorea: case report. *Surg Neurol* 59(6):486–490.

Coban A, Hanagasi H, Karamursel S, Barlas O. 2009. Comparison of unilateral pallidotomy and subthalamotomy findings in advanced idiopathic Parkinson's disease. *Br J Neurosurg* 23(1):23–29.

Comella C, Leurgans S, Wuu J, Stebbins G, Chmura T. 2003. Rating scales for dystonia: a multicenter assessment. *Mov Disord* 18(3):303–312.

Consky E, Basinski A, Belle L, Ranawaya R, Lang AE. 1990. The Toronto Western Spasmodic Torticollis Rating Scale (TWSTRS) assessment of validity and inter-rater reliability. *Neurology* 40(4):445–445.

Contarino M, Daniele A, Sibilia A, Romito L, Bentivoglio A, Gainotti G, Albanese A. 2007. Cognitive outcome 5 years after bilateral chronic stimulation of subthalamic nucleus in patients with Parkinson's disease. *J Neurol Neurosurg Psychiatr* 78(3):248–252.

Cooper IS. 1959a. Chemopallidectomy and chemothalamectomy for parkinsonism and dystonia. *Proc Roy Soc Med* 52: 47–60.

Cooper IS. 1959b. Dystonia musculorum deformans alleviated by chemopallidectomy and chemopallidothalamectomy. *Arch Neurol Psychiatry* 81(1):5–19.

Cooper IS. 1964. Effect of thalamic lesions upon torticollis. *N Engl J Med* 270(19):967–972.

Cooper IS. 1965. Surgical treatment of parkinsonism. *Annu Rev Med* 16:309–330.

Cooper IS. 1969. Dystonia musculorum deformans: natural history and neurosurgical alleviation. *J Pediatr* 74(4):585–592.

Cooper IS. 1976. 20-year follow-up study of the neurosurgical treatment of dystonia musculorum deformans. In: Eldridge R, Fahn S, editors. *Advances in Neurology*. Vol 14. New York: Raven Press, pp. 423–452.

Cooper IS. 1977. Neurosurgical treatment of the dyskinesias. *Clin Neurosurg* 24:367–390.

Cooper I, Bravo G. 1958. Chemopallidectomy and chemothalamectomy. *J Neurosurg* 15(3):244–250.

Corbett R, Laptook A, Tollefsbol G, Kim R. 1995. Validation of a noninvasive method to measure brain temperature in-vivo using H-1-NMR spectroscopy. *J Neurochem* 64(3):1224–1230.

Corbett R, Laptook A, Weatherall P. 1997. Noninvasive measurements of human brain temperature using volume-localized proton magnetic resonance spectroscopy. *J Cereb Blood Flow Metab* 17(4):363–369.

Coubes P, Cif L, El Fertit H, Hemm S, Vayssiere N, Serrat S, Picot MC, Tuffery S, Claustres M, Echenne B, Frerebeau P. 2004. Electrical stimulation of the globus pallidus internus in patients with primary generalized dystonia: long-term results. *J Neurosurg* 101(2):189–194.

Cubo E, Shannon K, Penn R, Kroin JS. 2000. Internal globus pallidotomy in dystonia secondary to Huntington's disease. *Mov Disord* 15(6):1248–1251.

Curry D, Gowda A, McNichols R, Wilfong AA. 2012. MR-guided stereotactic laser ablation of epileptogenic foci in children. *Epilepsy Behav* 24(4):408–414.

De Poorter J, De Wagter C, De Deene Y, Thomsen C, Stahlberg F, Achten E. 1995. Noninvasive MRI thermometry with the proton-resonance frequency (PRF) method: in-vivo results in human muscle. *Magn Reson Med* 33(1):74–81.

Dec M, Tutaj M, Rudzinska M, Szczudlik A, Koziara H, Bonicki W, Nauman P, Mandat T. 2014. Subthalamic nucleus deep brain stimulation after bilateral pallidotomy in the treatment of generalized dystonia. *Parkinsonism Relat Disord* 20(1):131–133.

Deligny C, Drapier S, Verin M, Lajat Y, Raoul S, Damier P. 2009. Bilateral subthalamotomy through DBS electrodes: a rescue option for device-related infection. *Neurology* 73(15):1243–1244.

Delong MR. 1990. Primate models of movement-disorders of basal ganglia origin. *Trends Neurosci* 13(7):281–285.

Delong M, Crutcher M, Georgopoulos AP. 1985. Primate globus pallidus and subthalamic nucleus: functional-organization. *J Neurophysiol* 53(2):530–543.

Deuschl G, Schade-Brittinger C, Krack P, Volkmann J, Schäfer H, Bötzel K, Daniels C, Deutschländer A, Dillmann U, Eisner W, Gruber D, Hamel W, Herzog J, Hilker R, Klebe S, Kloss M, Koy J, Krause M, Kupsch A, Lorenz D, Lorenzl S, Mehdorn HM, Moringlane J, Oertel W, Pinsker M, Reichmann H, Reuss A, Schneider G, Schnitzler A, Steude U, Sturm V, Timmermann L, Tronnier V, Trottenberg T, Wojtecki L, Wolf E, Poewe W, Voges J, Group German Parkinson Study, Section Neurostimulation. 2006. A randomized trial of deep-brain stimulation for Parkinson's disease. *N Engl J Med* 355(9):896–908.

Eidelberg D, Moeller J, Antonini A, Kazumata K, Nakamura T, Dhawan V, Spetsieris P, de Leon D, Bressman S, Fahn S. 1998. Functional brain networks in DYT1 dystonia. *Ann Neurol* 44(3):303–312.

Elias WJ, Huss D, Voss T, Loomba J, Khaled M, Zadicario E, Frysinger RC, Sperling SA, Wylie S, Monteith SJ, Druzgal J, Shah BB, Harrison M, Wintermark M. 2013a. A pilot study of focused ultrasound thalamotomy for essential tremor. *N Engl J Med* 369(7):640–648.

Elias WJ, Huss D, Voss T, Loomba J, Khaled M, Zadicario E, Frysinger RC, Sperling SA, Wylie S, Monteith SJ, Druzgal J, Shah BB, Harrison M, Wintermark M. 2013b. A pilot study of focused ultrasound thalamotomy for essential tremor. *G Pub Health* 8(5):640–648.

Elkay M, Silver K, Penn R, Dalvi A. 2009. Dystonic storm due to Batten's disease treated with pallidotomy and deep brain stimulation. *Mov Disord* 24(7):1048–1053.

Eltahawy H, Saint-Cyr J, Giladi N, Lang A, Lozano AM. 2004. Primary dystonia is more responsive than secondary dystonia to pallidal interventions: outcome after pallidotomy or pallidal deep brain stimulation. *Neurosurgery* 54(3):613–619.

Esselink RA, de Bie RM, de Haan RJ, Lenders MW, Nijssen PC, Staal MJ, Smeding HM, Schuurman PR, Bosch DA, Speelman JD. 2004. Unilateral pallidotomy versus bilateral subthalamic nucleus stimulation in PD: a randomized trial. *Neurology* 62(2):201–207.

Esselink RA, de Bie RM, de Haan RJ, Steur ENHJ, Beute GN, Portman AT, Schuurman PR, Bosch DA, Speelman JD. 2006. Unilateral pallidotomy versus bilateral subthalamic nucleus stimulation in Parkinson's disease: one year follow-up of a randomised observer-blind multi centre trial. *Acta Neurochir* 148(12):1247–1255.

Esselink RA, de Bie RM, de Haan RJ, Lenders M, Nijssen P, van Laar T, Schuurman P, Bosch D, Speelman JD. 2009. Long-term superiority of subthalamic nucleus stimulation over pallidotomy in Parkinson disease. *Neurology* 73(2):151–153.

Falowski S, Ooi Y, Smith A, Metman L, Bakay R. 2012. An evaluation of hardware and surgical complications with deep brain stimulation based on diagnosis and lead location. *Stereotact Funct Neurosurg* 90(3):173–180.

Fasano A, Daniele A, Albanese A. 2012. Treatment of motor and non-motor features of Parkinson's disease with deep brain stimulation. *Lancet Neurol* 11(5):429–442.

Fiedler VU, Schwarzmaier HJ, Eickmeyer F, Muller FP, Schoepp C, Verreet PR. 2001. Laser-induced interstitial thermotherapy of liver metastases in an interventional 0.5 tesla MRI system: technique and first clinical experiences. *J Magn Reson Imaging* 13(5):729–737.

Filion M, Tremblay L. 1991. Abnormal spontaneous activity of globus pallidus neurons in monkeys with MPTP-induced parkinsonism. *Brain Res* 547(1):142–151.

Folstein M, Folstein S, McHugh PR. 1975. Mini-mental state: practical method for grading cognitive state of patients for clinician. *J Psychiatr Res* 12(3):189–198.

Fonoff E, Campos W, Mandel M, Lopes Alho EJ, Teixeira MJ. 2012. Bilateral subthalamic nucleus stimulation for generalized dystonia after bilateral pallidotomy. *Mov Disord* 27(12):1559–1563.

Ford B. 2004. Pallidotomy for generalized dystonia. *Adv Neurol* 94:287–299.

Franzini A, Cordella R, Penner F, Rosa M, Messina G, Rizzi M, Nardocci N, Priori A. 2015. Posteroventrolateral pallidotomy through implanted DBS electrodes monitored by recording local field potentials. *Br J Neurosurg* 29(6):888–890.

Garcia-Rill E. 1986. The basal ganglia and locomotor regions. *Brain Res Rev* 396(1):47–63.

Gardner W, Williams GH. 1949. Interruption of the sympathetic nerve supply to the brain-effect on Parkinson's syndrome. *Arch Neurol Psychiatry* 61(4):413–421.

Ghika J, Ghika-Schmid F, Fankhauser H, Assal G, Vingerhoets F, Albanese A, Bogousslavsky J, Favre J. 1999. Bilateral contemporaneous posteroventral pallidotomy for the treatment of Parkinson's disease: neuropsychological and neurological side effects. Report of four cases and review of the literature. *J Neurosurg* 91(2):313–321.

Goldhahn G, Goldhahn WE. 1977. Experience with stereotaxic brain surgery for spasmodic torticollis. *Zentralbl Neurochir* 38(1):87–96.

Goto S, Tsuiki H, Soyama N, Okamura A, Yamada K, Yoshikawa M, Hashimoto Y, Ushio Y. 1997. Stereotactic selective vo-complex thalamotomy in a patient with dystonic writer's cramp. *Neurology* 49(4):1173–1174.

Gros C, Frerebeau P, Perezdominguez E, Bazin M, Privat J, Gillingham FJ. 1976. Long-term results of stereotaxic surgery for infantile dystonia and dyskinesia. *Neurochirurgia* 19(4):171–178.

Gross RE. 2008. What happened to prosteroventral pallidotomy for Parkinson's disease and dystonia? *Neurotheraputics* 5(2):281–293.

Gross RE, Lombardi WJ, Lang AE, Duff J, Hutchison WD, Saint-Cyr J, Tasker RR, Lozano AM. 1999. Relationship of lesion location to clinical outcome following microelectrode-guided pallidotomy for Parkinson's disease. *Brain* 122 (Pt 3):405–416.

Gross RE, Krack P, Rodriguez-Oroz M, Rezai A, Benabid AL. 2006. Electrophysiological mapping for the implantation of deep brain stimulators for Parkinson's disease and tremor. *Mov Disord* 21 (Suppl. 14):S259–S283.

Gryz J, Szolna A, Harat M, Olzak M, Gorzelanczyk EJ. 2006. Early postoperative assessment of cognitive functions after stereotactic pallidotomy in patients with primary dystonia: preliminary results. *Neurol Neurochir Pol* 40(6):493–500.

Guiot G, Brion S. 1952. Traitement neurochirurgical de syndromes choreo-athetosique et parkinsonien. *Sem Hop* 28:2095–2099.

Guiot G, Hardy J, Albefessard D. 1962. Delimitation precise des structures sous-corticales et identification de noyaux thalamiques chez lhomme par lelectrophysiologie stereotaxique. *Neurochirurgia* 5(1):1–18.

Hallervorden J, Spatz H. 1922. Eigenartige Erkankung im extrapyramidalen System mit besonderer Beteiligung des globus pallidus und der substantia nigra. Ein Beitrag zu den Beziehungen zwischen diesen beiden Zentren. *Arch Psychiatr Nervenkr Z Gesamte Neurol Psychiatr* 79:254–302.

Hamada I, Delong MR. 1992a. Excitotoxic acid lesions of the primate subthalamic nucleus result in transient dyskinesias of the contralateral limbs. *J Neurophysiol* 68(5):1850–1858.

Hamada I, Delong MR. 1992b. Excitotoxic acid lesions of the primate subthalamic nucleus result in reduced pallidal neuronal-activity during active holding. *J Neurophysiol* 68(5):1859–1866.

Handa H, Ito M, Araki C, Mizawa I, Mori K. 1962. Spasmodic torticollis treated by chemothalamotomy and chemopallidotomy. *Confin Neurol* 22(3):393–396.

Hariz MI. 2000. Complications of movement disorder surgery and how to avoid them. In: Lozano A, editor, *Movement Disorder Surgery*. Basel: Karger, pp. 246–265.

Hariz MI, De Salles A. 1997. The side-effects and complications of posteroventral pallidotomy. *Acta Neurochir Suppl* 68:42–48.

Hashimoto T, Elder C, Okun M, Patrick S, Vitek JL. 2003. Stimulation of the subthalamic nucleus changes the firing pattern of pallidal neurons. *J Neurosci* 23(5):1916–1923.

Hashimoto T, Naito K, Kitazawa K, Imai S, Goto T. 2010. Pallidotomy for severe tardive jaw-opening dystonia. *Stereotact Funct Neurosurg* 88(2):105–108.

Hassler R. 1955. *The Pathological and Pathophysiological Basis of Tremor and Parkinsonism*. London: Excerpta Medical Foundation.

Hassler R. 1972. Sagittal thalamotomy for relief of motor disorders in cases of double athetosis and cerebral-palsy. *Confin Neurol* 34(1):18–28.

Hassler R, Dieckman G. 1970a. Stereotactic treatment of different kinds of spasmodic torticollis. *Confin Neurol* 32(2):135–143.

Hassler R, Dieckmann G. 1970b. Die stereotaktische Behandlung des Torticollis aufgrund tierexperimenteller Erfahrungen über die richtungsbestimmenden Bewegungen. *Nervenarzt* 41(10):437–487.

Hassler R, Dieckmann G. 1982. Stereotaxic treatment for spasmodic torticollis. In: Schaltenbrand G, Walker AE, editors, *Stereotaxy of the Human Brain*. Stuttgart: Thieme pp. 525–531.

Hassler R, Riechert T. 1954. Indikationen und Lokalisationsmethode der gezielten Hirnoperationen. *Nervenarzt* 25(11):441–447.

Hassler R, Riechert T, Mundinger F, Umbach W, Ganglberger JA. 1960. Physiological observations in stereotaxic operations in extrapyramidal motor disturbances. *Brain* 83:337–350.

Hernesniemi J, Laitinen L. 1977. Long-term results of surgery for spasmodic torticollis. *Neurochirurgie* 23(2):123–131.

Higuchi Y, Iacono RP. 2003. Surgical complications in patients with Parkinson's disease after posteroventral pallidotomy. *Neurosurgery* 52(3):558–571.

Hirabayashi H, Hariz M, Wardell K, Blomstedt P. 2012. Impact of parameters of radiofrequency coagulation on volume of stereotactic lesion in pallidotomy and thalamotomy. *Stereotact Funct Neurosurg* 90(5):307–315.

Hooper AK, Okun MS, Foote KD, Fernandez HH, Jacobson C, Zeilman P, Romrell J, Rodriguez RL. 2008. Clinical cases where lesion therapy was chosen over deep brain stimulation. *Stereotact Funct Neurosurg* 86(3):147–152.

Horisawa S, Taira T, Goto S, Ochiai T, Nakajima T. 2013. Long-term improvement of musician's dystonia after stereotactic ventro-oral thalamotomy. *Ann Neurol* 74(5):648–654.

Horisawa S, Goto S, Takeda N, Takano Y, Kawamata T, Taira T. 2016a. Pallidotomy for writer's cramp after failed thalamotomy. *Stereotact Funct Neurosurg* 94(3):129–133.

Horisawa S, Goto S, Takeda N, Terashima H, Kawamata T, Taira T. 2016b. Bilateral pallidotomy for cervical dystonia after failed selective peripheral denervation. *World Neurosurg* 89(728):1–4.

Horsley V. 1890. Remarks on the surgery of the central nervous system. *Br Med J* 2(1562):1286–1292.

Hutchison W, Lozano A, Davis K, Saintcyr J, Lang A, Dostrovsky JO. 1994. Differential neuronal-activity in segments of globus-pallidus in Parkinson's disease patients. *Neuroreport* 21(5):1533–1537.

Iacono R, Lonser R, Mandybur G, Morenski J, Yamada S, Shima F. 1994. Stereotaxic pallidotomy results for Parkinson's exceed those of fetal graft. *Am Surg* 60(10):777–782.

Iacono RP, Lonser RR, Ulloth JE, Shima F. 1995a. Postero-ventral pallidotomy in Parkinson's disease. *J Clin Neurosci* 2(2):140–145.

Iacono R, Shima F, Lonser R, Kuniyoshi S, Maeda G, Yamada S. 1995b. The results, indications, and physiology of posteroventral pallidotomy for patients with Parkinson's disease. *Neurosurgery* 36(6):1118–1127.

Iacono RP, Kuniyoshi SM, Lonser RR, Maeda G, Inae AM, Ashwal S. 1996. Simultaneous bilateral pallidoansotomy for idiopathic dystonia musculorum deformans. *Pediatr Neurol* 14(2):145–148.

Iacono RP, Kuniyoshi SM, Schoonenberg T. 1998. Experience with stereotactics for dystonia: case examples. In: Fahn S, Marsden CD, DeLong MR, editors. *Advances in Neurology*. Philadelphia, PA: Lippincott-Raven, pp. 221–226.

Imer M, Ozeren B, Karadereler S, Yapici Z, Omay B, Hanagasi H, Eraksoy M. 2005. Destructive stereotactic surgery for treatment of dystonia. *Surg Neurol* 64 (Suppl. 2):S89–S94.

Jackson A, Crossman AR. 1983. Nucleus tegmenti pedunculopontinus: efferent connections with special reference to the basal ganglia studied in the rat by anterograde and retrograde transport of horseradish peroxidase. *Neuroscience* 10(3):725–765.

Jeanmonod D, Werner B, Morel A, Michels L, Zadicario E, Schiff G, Martin E. 2012. Transcranial magnetic resonance imaging-guided focused ultrasound: noninvasive central lateral thalamotomy for chronic neuropathic pain. *Neurosurg Focus* 32(1):E1.

Jiménez F, Velasco F, Carrillo-Ruiz J, García L, Madrigal A, Velasco A, Márquez I. 2006. Comparative evaluation of the effects of unilateral lesion versus electrical stimulation of the globus pallidus internus in advanced Parkinson's disease. *Stereotact Funct Neurosurg* 84(2):64–71.

Jolesz F, Bleier A, Jakab P, Ruenzel P, Huttl K, Jako GJ. 1988. MR imaging of laser-tissue interactions. *Radiology* 168(1):249–253.

Justesen C, Penn R, Kroin J, Egel RT. 1999. Stereotactic pallidotomy in a child with Hallervorden-Spatz disease: case report. *J Neurosurg* 90(3):551–554.

Kahn T, Bettag M, Ulrich F, Schwarzmaier HJ, Schober R, Furst G, Modder U. 1994. MRI-guided laser-induced interstitial thermotherapy of cerebral neoplasms. *J Comput Assist Tomogr* 18(4):519–532.

Kahn T, Harth T, Kiwit J, Schwarzmaier H, Wald C, Modder U. 1998. Preliminary experience during MRI-guided laser-induced interstitial thermotherapy of brain tumors. *J Magn Reson Imaging* 8(1):160–164.

Kangasniemi M, McNichols R, Bankson J, Gowda A, Price R, Hazle JD. 2004. Thermal therapy of canine cerebral tumors using a 980 nm diode laser with MR temperature-sensitive imaging feedback. *Lasers Surg Med* 35(1):41–50.

Kelly PJ, Ahlskog JE, Goerss SJ, Daube JR, Duffy JR, Kall BA. 1987. Computer-assisted stereotaxic ventralis lateralis thalamotomy with microelectrode recording control in patients with Parkinson's disease. *Mayo Clin Proc* 62(8):655–664.

Khan M, Mewes K, Gross R, Skrinjar O. 2008. Assessment of brain shift related to deep brain stimulation surgery. *Stereotact Funct Neurosurg* 86(1):44–53.

Kim J, Chang W, Park Y, Chang JW. 2011. Bilateral globus pallidus internus deep brain stimulation for DYT1+ generalized dystonia with previously received bilateral thalamotomy and unilateral pallidotomy. *Stereotact Funct Neurosurg* 89(4):205–209.

Kim M, Jeon S, Yoo H, Kim G, Lee M, Chung SJ. 2008. Effect of thalamotomy on focal hand dystonia in a family with DYT1 mutation. *Mov Disord* 23(15):2251–2255.

Kleiner-Fisman G, Herzog J, Fisman DN, Tamma F, Lyons K, Pahwa R, Lang A, Deuschl G. 2006. Subthalamic nucleus deep brain stimulation: summary and meta-analysis of outcomes. *Mov Disord* 21:S290–S304.

Klemme RM. 1940. Surgical treatment of dystonia paralysis agitans and athetosis. *Acta Neurol Psychiatry* 44:926.

Krack P, Vercueil L. 2001. Review of the functional surgical treatment of dystonia. *Eur J Neurol* 8(5):389–399.

Krack P, Batir A, Van Blercom N, Chabardes S, Fraix V, Ardouin C, Koudsie A, Limousin P, Benazzouz A, LeBas J, Benabid A, Pollak P. 2003. Five-year follow-up of bilateral stimulation of the subthalamic nucleus in advanced Parkinson's disease. *N Engl J Med* 349(20):1925–1934.

Kramer PL, de Leon D, Ozelius L, Risch N, Bressman SB, Brin MF, Schuback DE, Burke RE, Kwiatkowski DJ, Shale H. 1990. Dystonia gene in Ashkenazi Jewish population is located on chromosome 9q32-34. *Ann Neurol* 27(2):114–120.

Krauss J, Mohadjer M, Braus D, Wakhloo A, Nobbe F, Mundinger F. 1992. Dystonia following head trauma: a report of 9 patients and a review of the literature. *Mov Disord* 7(3):263–272.

Krauss J, Pohle T, Weber S, Ozdoba C, Burgunder JM. 1999. Bilateral stimulation of globus pallidus internus for treatment of cervical dystonia. *Lancet* 354(9181):837–838.

Krayenbühl H, Siegfried J. 1972. Dentatectomy or thalamectomy in treatment of hyperkinesia. *Confin Neurol* 34(1):29–33.

Kumar R, Dagher A, Hutchison W, Lang A, Lozano AM. 1999. Globus pallidus deep brain stimulation for generalized dystonia: clinical and PET investigation. *Neurology* 53(4):871–874.

Kupsch A, Benecke R, Muller J, Trottenberg T, Schneider GH, Poewe W, Eisner W, Wolters A, Muller JU, Deuschl G, Pinsker MO, Skogseid IM, Roeste GK, Vollmer-Haase J, Brentrup A, Krause M, Tronnier V, Schnitzler A, Voges J, Nikkhah G, Vesper J, Naumann M, Volkmann J, Deep-Brain Stimulation for DS. 2006. Pallidal deep-brain stimulation in primary generalized or segmental dystonia. *N Engl J Med* 355(19):1978–1990.

Kwon Y, Whang CJ. 1995. Stereotaxic gamma knife radiosurgery for the treatment of dystonia. *Stereotact Funct Neurosurg* 64 (Suppl. 1):222–227.

Kyriagis M, Grattan-Smith P, Scheinberg A, Teo C, Nakaji N, Waugh M. 2004. Status dystonicus and Hallervorden-Spatz disease: treatment with intrathecal baclofen and pallidotomy. *J Paediatr Child Health* 40(5):322–325.

Lai T, Lai J, Grossman RG. 1999. Functional recovery after bilateral pallidotomy for the treatment of early-onset primary generalized dystonia. *Arch Phys Med Rehabil* 80(10):1340–1342.

Laitinen LV. 1963. Stereotaxic treatment of spasmodic torticollis. *Acta Neurol Scand* 39:231–236.

Laitinen LV. 1995. Pallidotomy for Parkinson's disease. *Neurosurg Clin N Am* 6(1):105–112.

Laitinen LV, Bergenheim A, Hariz MI. 1992a. Leksells posteroventral pallidotomy in the treatment of Parkinson's disease. *J Neurosurg* 76(1):53–61.

Laitinen LV, Bergenheim A, Hariz MI. 1992b. Ventroposterolateral pallidotomy can abolish all parkinsonian symptoms. *Stereotact Funct Neurosurg* 58(1):14–21.

Lang AE. 1998. Surgical treatment of dystonia. In: Fahn S, Marsden CD editors. *Advances in Neurology; Dystonia*. Philadelphia, PA: Lippincott-Raven, pp. 185–198.

Le Behin D, Delannoy J, Levin RL. 1989. Temperature mapping with MR imaging of molecular-diffusion: application to hyperthermia. *Radiology* 171(3):853–857.

Lenders M, Buschman H, Vergouwen M, Steur E, Kolling P, Hariz M. 2005. Long term results of unilateral posteroventral pallidotomy for antipsychotic drug induced tardive dyskinesia. *J Neurol Neurosurg Psychiatr* 76(7):1039.

Lenz FA, Dostrovsky J, Kwan H, Tasker R, Yamashiro K, Murphy JT. 1988. Methods for microstimulation and recording of single neurons and evoked-potentials in the human central nervous-system. *J Neurosurg* 68(4):630–634.

Lenz FA, Kwan H, Dostrovsky J, Tasker R, Murphy J, Lenz YE. 1990a. Single unit analysis of the human ventral thalamic nuclear group: activity correlated with movement. *Brain* 113:1795–1821.

Lenz FA, Martin R, Kwan H, Tasker R, Dostrovsky JO. 1990b. Thalamic single-unit activity occurring in patients with hemidystonia. *Stereotact Funct Neurosurg* 54–55:159–162.

Lenz FA, Normand SL, Kwan HC, Andrews D, Rowland LH, Jones MW, Seike M, Lin YC, Tasker RR, Dostrovsky JO. 1995. Statistical prediction of the optimal site for thalamotomy in parkinsonian tremor. *Mov Disord* 10(3):318–328.

Lenz FA, Suarez JI, Metman LV, Reich SG, Karp BI, Hallett M, Rowland LH, Dougherty PM. 1998. Pallidal activity during dystonia: somatosensory reorganisation and changes with severity. *J Neurol Neurosurg Psychiatr* 65(5):767–770.

Lenz FA, Jaeger CJ, Seike MS, Lin YC, Reich SG, DeLong MR, Vitek JL. 1999. Thalamic single neuron activity in patients with dystonia: dystonia-related activity and somatic sensory reorganization. *J Neurophysiol* 82(5):2372–2392.

Limousin P, Pollak P, Benazzouz A, Hoffmann D, Le Bas JF, Broussolle E, Perret JE, Benabid AL. 1995. Effect of parkinsonian signs and symptoms of bilateral subthalamic nucleus stimulation. *Lancet* 345(8942):91–95.

Lin J, Lin S, Lin G, Chang D, Lee CC. 1998. Application of bilateral sequential pallidotomy to treat a patient with generalized dystonia. *Eur Neurol* 40(2):108–110.

Lin J, Lin S, Chang DC. 1999a. Pallidotomy and generalized dystonia. *Mov Disord* 14(6):1057–1059.

Lin J, Lin G, Shih C, Lin S, Chang D, Lee CC. 1999b. Benefit of bilateral pallidotomy in the treatment of generalized dystonia: case report. *J Neurosurg* 90(5):974–976.

Lin J, Lin S, Lin G, Chang D, Lee CC. 2001. Treatment of intractable generalized dystonia by bilateral posteroventral pallidotomy: one-year results. *Zhonghua Yi Xue Za Zhi (Taipei)* 64(4):231–238.

Lipsman N, Schwartz ML, Huang Y, Lee L, Sankar T, Chapman M, Hynynen K, Lozano AM. 2013. MR-guided focused ultrasound thalamotomy for essential tremor: a proof-of-concept study. *Lancet Neurol* 12(5):462–468.

Lipsman N, Mainprize T, Schwartz M, Hynynen K, Lozano AM. 2014. Intracranial applications of magnetic resonance-guided focused ultrasound. *Neurotherapeutics* 11(3):593–605.

Loher T, Pohle T, Krauss JK. 2004. Functional stereotactic surgery for treatment of cervical dystonia: review of the experience from the lesional era. *Stereotact Funct Neurosurg* 82(1):1–13.

Lokuketagoda J, Gross R, Jandial R. 2011. Pallidotomy and thalamotomy. In: Jandial R, editor. *Core Techniques in Operative Neurosurgery*. Philadelphia, PA: Saunders Elsevier, pp. 290–300.

Lozano A, Hutchison W, Dostrovsky JO. 1995. Microelectrode monitoring of cortical and subcortical structures during stereotactic surgery. *Acta Neurochir Suppl* 64:30–34.

Lozano A, Hutchison W, Kiss Z, Tasker R, Davis K, Dostrovsky J. 1996. Methods for microelectrode-guided posteroventral pallidotomy. *J Neurosurg* 84(2):194–202.

Lozano A, Kumar R, Gross R, Giladi N, Hutchison W, Dostrovsky J, Lang AE. 1997. Globus pallidus internus pallidotomy for generalized dystonia. *Mov Disord* 12(6):865–870.

Machado A, Rezai A, Kopell B, Gross R, Sharan A, Benabid AL. 2006. Deep brain stimulation for Parkinson's disease: surgical technique and perioperative management. *Mov Disord* 21 (Suppl. 14.):S247–S258.

Markham C, Rand RW. 1961. Physiological and anatomical influences in dystonia. *Trans Am Neurol Assoc* 86:135–137.

Marras C, Zorzi G, Lenardi C, Rizzi M, Messina G, Alimehmeti R, Nardocci N, Franzini A. 2009. Deep brain stimulation electrode used for radiofrequency lesion of the globus pallidus internus in dystonia. *Stereotact Funct Neurosurg* 87(6):348–352.

Marras CE, Rizzi M, Cantonetti L, Rebessi E, De Benedictis A, Portaluri F, Randi F, Savioli A, Castelli E, Vigevano F. 2014. Pallidotomy for medically refractory status dystonicus in childhood. *Dev Med Child Neurol* 56(7):649–656.

Marsden CD. 1981. Treatment of torsion dystonia. In: Barbeau A, editor. *Disorders of Movement.* Philadelphia, PA: Lippincott, pp. 81–104.

Martin E, Jeanmonod D, Morel A, Zadicario E, Werner B. 2009. High-intensity focused ultrasound for noninvasive functional neurosurgery. *Ann Neurol* 66(6):858–861.

Mazars G, Merienne L, Chodkiew JP. 1968. Surgery of cephalic orientation dyskinesia (surgery of dyskinetic disorders of head orientation). *Neurochirurgie* 14(6):745–752.

McNichols RJ, Gowda A, Wright SM. 2001. Closed-loop feedback control of laser therapy using magnetic resonance imaging. *BiOS 2001 the International Symposium on Biomedical Optics* 4247:158–165.

McNichols R, Gowda A, Kangasniemi M, Bankson J, Price R, Hazle JD. 2004. MR thermometry-based feedback control of laser interstitial thermal therapy at 980 nm. *Lasers Surg Med* 34(1):48–55.

Meares R. 1971. Natural history of spasmodic torticollis and effect of surgery. *Lancet* 2(7716):149–150.

Mempel E, Kucinski L, Witkiewicz B. 1986. Writer's cramp syndrome treated successfully by thalamotomy. *Neurol Neurochir Pol* 20(5):475–480.

Meyers R. 1940. Surgical procedure for postencephalitic tremor with notes on the physiology of the premotor fibres. *Arch Neurol Psychiatry* 44:455–459.

Meyers R. 1942. The modification of alternating tremors rigidity and festination by surgery of the basal ganglia. *Res Publ Assoc Res Nerv Ment Dis* 21(6):02665.

Meyers R, Fields W. 1958. Pathogenesis and treatment of parkinsonism. *Sixth Annual Scientific Meeting of the Houston Neurological Society.* Houston, TX: Springfield.

Miller W, DeLong M. 1987. Altered tonic activity of neurons in the globus pallidus and subthalamic nucleus in the primate MPTP model of parkinsonism. In: Carpenter M, editor. New York: Plenum Press.

Miller W, Delong MR. 1988. Parkinsonian symptomatology: an anatomical and physiological analysis. *Ann NY Acad Sci* 515:287–302.

Mundinger F, Riechert T. 1961. Results of stereotactic brain operations in extrapyramidal movement disorders on the basis of postoperative and long-term studies. *Dtsch Z Nervenheilkd* 182:542–576.

Mundinger F, Riechert T, Disselhoff J. 1970. Long term results of stereotaxic operations on extrapyramidal hyperkinesia (excluding parkinsonism). *Confin Neurol* 32(2):71–78.

Mundinger F, Riechert T, Disselhoff J. 1972. Long-term results of stereotactic treatment of spasmodic torticollis. *Confin Neurol* 34(1):41–50.

Muta D, Goto S, Nishikawa S, Hamasaki T, Ushio Y, Inoue N, Mita S. 2001. Bilateral pallidal stimulation for idiopathic segmental axial dystonia advanced from Meige syndrome refractory to bilateral thalamotomy. *Mov Disord* 16(4):774–777.

Myerson A, Berlin DD. 1934. A case of postencephalitic Parkinson's disease treated by total thyroidectomy. *N Engl J Med* 210:1205–1206.

Na Y, Chang W, Jung H, Kweon E, Chang JW. 2015. Unilateral magnetic resonance-guided focused ultrasound pallidotomy for Parkinson disease. *Neurology* 85(6):549–551.

Novak K, Nenonene E, Bernstein L, Vergenz S, Cozzens J, Rezak M. 2008. Successful bilateral subthalamic nucleus stimulation for segmental dystonia after unilateral pallidotomy. *Stereotact Funct Neurosurg* 86(2):80–86.

Obeso J, Rodriguez M, DeLong MR. 1997. Basal ganglia pathophysiology: a critical review. *Adv Neurol* 74:3–18.

Oh M, Hodaie M, Kim S, Alkhani A, Lang A, Lozano AM. 2001. Deep brain stimulator electrodes used for lesioning: proof of principle. *Neurosurgery* 49(2):363–367.

Oh M, Abosch A, Kim S, Lang A, Lozano AM. 2002. Long-term hardware-related complications of deep brain stimulation. *Neurosurgery* 50(6):1268–1274.

Ohye C, Miyazaki M, Hirai T, Shibazaki T, Nakajima H, Nagaseki Y. 1982. Primary writing tremor treated by stereotactic selective thalamotomy. *J Neurol Neurosurg Psychiatr* 45(11):988–997.

Ohye C. 2000. Use of selective thalamotomy for various kinds of movement disorder based on basic studies. *Stereotact Funct Neurosurg* 75(2):54–65.

Ohye C, Shibazaki T, Zhang J, Andou Y. 2002. Thalamic lesions produced by gamma thalamotomy for movement disorders. *J Neurosurg* 97(5):600–606.

Ohye C, Shibazaki T, Sato S. 2005. Gamma knife thalamotomy for movement disorders: evaluation of the thalamic lesion and clinical results. *J Neurosurg* 102 (Suppl.):234–240.

Okun MS, Stover NP, Subramanian T, Gearing M, Wainer BH, Holder CA, Watts RL, Juncos JL, Freeman A, Evatt ML, Schuele SU, Vitek JL, DeLong MR. 2001. Complications of gamma knife surgery for Parkinson disease. *Arch Neurol* 58(12):1995–2002.

Oliver LC. 1949. Surgery in Parkinson's disease: division of lateral pyramidal tract for tremor – report on 48 operations. *Lancet* 253(6561):910–913.

Ondo W, Desaloms J, Jankovic J, Grossman RG. 1998. Pallidotomy for generalized dystonia. *Mov Disord* 13(4):693–698.

Paluzzi A, Belli A, Bain P, Liu X, Aziz TM. 2006. Operative and hardware complications of deep brain stimulation for movement disorders. *Br J Neurosurg* 20(5):290–295.

Pan L, Zhang N, Dai J, Wang EM. 2000. Gamma knife radiosurgery for torsion spasm: report of two cases. *J Neurosurg* 93 (Suppl. 3):189–190.

Peters RD, Chan E, Trachtenberg J, Jothy S, Kapusta L, Kucharczyk W, Henkelman RM. 2000. Magnetic resonance thermometry for predicting thermal damage: an application of interstitial laser coagulation in an in vivo canine prostate model. *Magn Reson Med* 44(6):873–883.

Putnam TJ. 1933. Treatment of athetosis and dystonia by section of extrapyramidal motor tracts. *Arch Neurol Psychiatry* 29(3):504–521.

Putnam TJ. 1938. Results of treatment of athetosis by section of extrapyramidal tracts in the spinal cord. *Arch Neurol Psychiatry* 39(2):258–275.

Putnam TJ. 1940. Treatment of unilateral paralysis agitans by section of the lateral pyramidal trace. *Arch Neurol Psychiatry* 44(5):950–976.

Rakocevic G, Lyons K, Wilkinson S, Overman J, Pahwa R. 2004. Bilateral pallidotomy for severe dystonia in an 18-month-old child with glutaric aciduria. *Stereotact Funct Neurosurg* 82(2):80–83.

Raoul S, Faighel M, Rivier I, Verin M, Lajat Y, Damier P. 2003. Staged lesions through implanted deep brain stimulating electrodes: a new surgical procedure for treating tremor or dyskinesias. *Mov Disord* 18(8):933–938.

Raoul S, Leduc D, Vegas T, Sauleau P, Lozano AM, Verin M, Damier P, Lajat Y. 2007. Deep brain stimulation electrodes used for staged lesion within the basal ganglia: experimental studies for parameter validation – laboratory investigation. *J Neurosurg* 107(5):1027–1035.

Rees C. 1933. Observations following sympathetic ganglionectomy in cases of post-enchepalitic parkinsonian syndrome. *Am J Surg* 21(3):411–415.

Riechert T. 1962. Long term follow-up of results of stereotaxic treatment in extrapyramidal disorders. *Confin Neurol* 22:356–363.

Royle ND. 1931. The clinical results following the operation of sympathetic ramisection. *Can Med Assoc J* 24:229–234.

Schaltenbrand G, Wahren W. 1977. *Atlas for Stereotaxy of the Human Brain*. Stuttgart: Thieme.

Schuurman P, Bosch D, Bossuyt P, Bonsel G, van Someren E, de Bie R, Merkus M, Speelman JD. 2000. A comparison of continuous thalamic stimulation and thalamotomy for suppression of severe tremor. *N Engl J Med* 342(7):461–468.

Schuurman P, Bosch D, Merkus M, Speelman JD. 2008. Long-term follow-up of thalamic stimulation versus thalamotomy for tremor suppression. *Mov Disord* 23(8):1146–1153.

Schwarzmaier H, Yaroslavsky I, Yaroslavsky A, Fiedler V, Ulrich F, Kahn T. 1998. Treatment planning for MRI-guided laser-induced interstitial thermotherapy of brain tumors: the role of blood perfusion. *J Magn Reson Imaging* 8(1):121–127.

Shah B, Huss D, Harrison M, Wooten G, Sperling S, Elias WJ. 2015. New frontiers in focused ultrasound treatment in Parkinson's disease: a potential paradigm for staged lesioning of the subthalamic nucleus. *Mov Disord* 30:S239.

Shibata T, Hirashima Y, Ikeda H, Asahi T, Hayashi N, Endo S. 2005. Stereotactic Voa–Vop complex thalamotomy for writer's cramp. *Eur Neurol* 53(1):38–39.

Shima F, Ishido K, Kato M. 1997. Roles of the basal ganglia outputs in movement disorders: a viewpoint based on experiences of stereotactic surgery for idiopathic dystonia. *No to Hattatsu* 29(3):206–212.

Siegfried J, Lippitz B. 1994. Bilateral chronic electrostimulation of ventroposterolateral pallidum: a new therapeutic approach for alleviating all parkinsonian symptoms. *Neurosurgery* 35(6):1126–1129.

Siegfried J, Lippitz B. 1995. Chronic electrical stimulation of the VL–VPL complex and of the pallidum in the treatment of movement disorders: personal experience since 1982. *Stereotact Funct Neurosurg* 62(1):71–75.

Siegfried J, Crowell R, Perret E. 1969. Cure of tremulous writer's cramp by stereotaxic thalamotomy: case report. *J Neurosurg* 30(2):182–185.

Sillay K, Larson P, Starr PA. 2008. Deep brain stimulator hardware-related infections. incidence and management in a large series. *Neurosurgery* 62(2):360–366.

Spatz M. 1927. *Spezielle Physiologie des Zentralnervensystems der Wirbeltiere*. Vol. 10. Berlin: Springer.

Speelman J, Vanmanen J. 1989. Cerebral palsy and stereotactic neurosurgery long term results. *J Neurol Neurosurg Psychiatr* 52(1):23–30.

Spiegel EA. 1966. Development of stereoencephalotomy for extrapyramidal diseases. *J Neurosurg* 24(1):433–439.

Spiegel E, Wycis HT. 1954. Ansotomy in paralysis agitans. *AMA Arch Neurol Psychiatry* 71(5):598–614.

Spiegel E, Wycis HT. 1958. Pallido-ansotomy: anatomic-physiological foundation and histopathologic control. In: Field WS, editor. *Pathogenesis and Treatment of Parkinsonisms*. Springfield, IL: Charles C Thomas.

Spiegel E, Wycis H, Marks M, Lee AJ. 1947. Stereotaxic apparatus for operations on the human brain. *Science* 106(2754):349–350.

Spiegel E, Wycis H, Baird HW. 1958. Long-range effects of electropallidoansotomy in extrapyramidal and convulsive disorders. *Neurology* 8(10):734–740.

Stancanello J, Romanelli P, Pantelis E, Sebastiano F, Modugno N. 2009. Atlas-based functional radiosurgery: early results. *Med Phys* 36(2):457–463.

Stejskal L, Vladyka V, Tomanek Z. 1981. Surgical possibilities for alleviation of axial dyskinesias: comparison with forced movements of the head and eyes. *Appl Neurophysiol* 44(5):320–329.

Strickland B, Jimenez-Shahed J, Jankovic J, Viswanathan A. 2013. Radiofrequency lesioning through deep brain stimulation electrodes: a pilot study of lesion geometry and temperature characteristics. *J Clin Neurosci* 20(12):1709–1712.

Stroszczynski C, Hosten N, Puls R, Nagel S, Scholman HJ, Wlodarczyk W, Oettle H, Moesta KT, Schlag PM, Felix R. 2001. Histopathological correlation to MRI findings during and after laser-induced thermotherapy in a pig pancreas model. *Invest Radiol* 36(7):413–421.

Sungurov E, Peresedov V, Markova E, Ivanova-Smolenskaia I, Rebrova O, Tiurnikov VM. 1998. The surgical results in patients with different forms of torsion dystonia. *Zh Vopr Neirokhir Im N N Burdenko* (4):21–23.

Szolna A, Harat M, Gryz J. 2006. Stereotactic pallidotomy and thalamotomy in the treatment of primary dystonia. *Neurol Neurochir Pol* 40(3):186–193.

Taira T. 2007. Stereotactic ventrooral thalamotomy for task-specific focal hand dystonia (writer's or musician's cramp). *Neurosurgery* 61(1):213–214.

Taira T, Hori T. 2003. Stereotactic ventrooralis thalamotomy for task-specific focal hand dystonia (writer's cramp). *Stereotact Funct Neurosurg* 80(1):88–91.

Taira T, Horisawa S. 2016. Long-term improvement of musician's and writer's focal dystonia after ventro-oral thalamotomy. *Mov Disord* 31:S71.

Taira T, Harashima S, Hori T. 2003. Neurosurgical treatment for writer's cramp. *Acta Neurochir Suppl* 87:129–131.

Taira T, Ochiai T, Goto S, Hori T. 2006. Multimodal neurosurgical strategies for the management of dystonias. *Acta Neurochir Suppl* 99:29–31.

Tasker RR. 1990. Thalamotomy. *Neurosurg Clin N Am* 1(4):841–864.

Tasker RR. 1998a. Ablative procedures for dystonia. In: German IM, editor. *Neurosurgical Treatment of Movement Disorders*. Park Ridge: The American Association of Neurological Surgeons, pp. 255–266.

Tasker RR. 1998b. Surgical treatment of the dystonias. In: Gildenberg PL, Tasker RR, editors. *Textbook of Stereotactic and Functional Neurosurgery*. New York: McGraw-Hill, pp. 1015–1032.

Tasker RR, Organ LW, Hawrylyshyn P. 1982. *The Thalamus and Midbrain of Man: A Physiological Atlas Using Electrical Stimulation*. Springfield, IL: Charles C Thomas.

Tasker RR, Doorly T, Yamashiro K. 1988. Thalamotomy in generalized dystonia. In: Fahn S, Marsden CD, Calne DB, editors. *Advances in Neurology, Dystonia 2*. Vol. 50. New York: Raven Press, pp. 615–632.

Tasker RR, Lang A, Lozano AM. 1997. Pallidal and thalamic surgery for Parkinson's disease. *Exp Neurol* 144(1):35–40.

Teive HA, Sa DS, Grande CV, Antoniuk A, Werneck LC. 2001. Bilateral pallidotomy for generalized dystonia. *Arq Neuropsiquiatr* 59(2):353–357.

Teive HA, Munhoz RP, Souza MM, Antoniuk SA, Santos ML, Teixeira MJ, Barbosa ER, Carvalho RC, Scaff M, Werneck LC. 2005. Status dystonicus: study of five cases. *Arq Neuropsiquiatr* 63(1):26–29.

Terao T, Takahashi H, Yokochi F, Taniguchi M, Okiyama R, Hamada I. 2003. Hemorrhagic complication of stereotactic surgery in patients with movement disorders. *J Neurosurg* 98(6):1241–1246.

Tracz RA, Wyman DR, Little PB, Towner RA, Stewart WA, Schatz SW, Pennock PW, Wilson BC. 1992. Magnetic resonance imaging of interstitial laser photocoagulation in brain lasers. *Surg Med* 12(2):165–173.

Valalik I, Jobbagy A, Bognar L, Csokay A. 2011. Effectiveness of unilateral pallidotomy for Meige syndrome confirmed by motion analysis. *Stereotact Funct Neurosurg* 89(3):157–161.

Vidailhet M, Vercueil L, Houeto JL, Krystkowiak P, Benabid AL, Cornu P, Lagrange C, Tezenas DM, Dormont D, Grand S, Blond S, Detante O, Pillon B, Ardouin C, Agid Y, Destee A, Pollak P, French Stimulation du Pallidum Interne dans la Dystonie Study. 2005. Bilateral deep-brain stimulation of the globus pallidus in primary generalized dystonia. *N Engl J Med* 352(5):459–467.

Vilela O, da Silva DJ. 2002. Unilateral subthalamic nucleus lesioning: a safe and effective treatment for Parkinson's disease. *Arq Neuropsiquiatr* 60(4):935–948.

Vitek J, Giroux M. 2000. Physiology of hypokinetic and hyperkinetic movement disorders: model for dyskinesia. *Ann Neurol* 47(4):S131-S140.

Vitek JL, Bakay RA, Hashimoto T, Kaneoke Y, Mewes K, Zhang JY, Rye D, Starr P, Baron M, Turner R, DeLong MR. 1998a. Microelectrode-guided pallidotomy: technical approach and its application in medically intractable Parkinson's disease. *J Neurosurg* 88(6):1027–1043.

Vitek JL, Zhang J, Evatt M. 1998b. GPi pallidotomy for dystonia: clinical outcome and neuronal activity. In: Fahn S, Marsden CD, DeLong MR, editors. *Advances in Neurology; Dystonia*. New York: Raven Press, pp. 211–219.

Vitek JL, Chockkan V, Zhang JY, Kaneoke Y, Evatt M, DeLong MR, Triche S, Mewes K, Hashimoto T, Bakay RA. 1999. Neuronal activity in the basal ganglia in patients with generalized dystonia and hemiballismus. *Ann Neurol* 46(1):22–35.

Vitek JL, Bakay RA, Freeman A, Evatt M, Green J, McDonald W, Haber M, Barnhart H, Wahlay N, Triche S, Mewes K, Chockkan V, Zhang JY, DeLong MR. 2003. Randomized trial of pallidotomy versus medical therapy for Parkinson's disease. *Ann Neurol* 53(5):558–569.

Vogl T, Mack M, Roggan A, Straub R, Eichler K, Müller P, Knappe V, Felix R. 1998. Internally cooled power laser for MR-guided interstitial laser-induced thermotherapy of liver lesions: initial clinical results. *Radiology* 209(2):381–385.

von Essen C, Augustinsson L, Lindqvist G. 1980. Voi thalamotomy in spasmodic torticollis. *Appl Neurophysiol* 43(3):159–163.

Walker AE. 1952. Cerebral pedunculotomy for the relief of involuntary movements. *J Nerv Ment Dis* 116(6):766–775.

Waln O, Jankovic J. 2013. Bilateral globus pallidus internus deep brain stimulation after bilateral pallidotomy in a patient with generalized early-onset primary dystonia. *Mov Disord* 28(8):1162–1163.

Wang Y, Turnbull I, Calne S, Stoessl A, Calne DB. 1997. Pallidotomy for tardive dyskinesia. *Lancet* 349(9054):777–778.

Weetman J, Anderson I, Gregory RP. 1997. Bilateral posteroventral pallidotomy for severe antipsychotic induced tardive dyskinesia and dystonia. *J Neurol Neurosurg Psychiatr* 63(4):554–556.

Willie J, Laxpati N, Drane D, Gowda A, Appin C, Hao C, Brat D, Helmers S, Saindane A, Nour S, Gross RE. 2014. Real-time magnetic resonance-guided stereotactic laser amygdalohippocampotomy for mesial temporal lobe epilepsy. *Neurosurgery* 74(6):569–584.

Wyman DR, Wilson BC, Malone DE. 1992. Medical imaging-systems for feedback: control of interstitial laser photocoagulation. *Proceedings of the IEEE* 80(6):890–902.

Wyman D, Schatz S, Maguire J. 1997. Comparison of 810 nm and 1064 nm wavelengths for interstitial laser photocoagulation in rabbit brain. *Lasers Surg Med* 21(1):50–58.

Yamashiro K, Tasker RR. 1993. Stereotactic thalamotomy for dystonic patients. *Stereotact Funct Neurosurg* 60(1–3):81–85.

Yasargil MG. 1962. Die Ergebnisse der stereotaktischen Operationen bei Hyperkinesien. *Schweiz Med Wochenschr* 92(48):1550–1566.

Yen C, Sheehan J, Pan H. 2012. Successful treatment of cervical dystonia induced by basal ganglion venous angioma with gamma knife thalamotomy. *J Clin Neurosci* 19(3):470–471.

Yoshor D, Hamilton W, Ondo W, Jankovic J, Grossman RG. 2001. Comparison of thalamotomy and pallidotomy for the treatment of dystonia. *Neurosurgery* 48(4):818–824.

Zhuang P, Li Y, Hallett M. 2004. Neuronal activity in the basal ganglia and thalamus in patients with dystonia. *Clin Neurophysiol* 115(11):2542–2557.

Zirh TA, Reich SG, Perry V, Lenz FA. 1998. Thalamic single neuron and electromyographic activities in patients with dystonia. In: Fahn S, Marsden CD, DeLong MR, editors. *Advances in Neurology; Dystonia*, New York: Raven Publishers, pp. 27–32.

Chapter 61

Direct Cortical Stimulation for the Treatment of Dystonia

Giuseppe Messina, Giovanni Broggi, Roberto Cordella and Angelo Franzini

Several forms of dystonia respond poorly to conservative treatments. The main surgical option that is offered to these patients is deep brain stimulation (DBS). There is limited experience with direct cortical stimulation (DCS), which aims at stimulating the premotor cortex (PMC) or the primary motor cortex (MC). In this chapter, we will focus on the results obtained by DCS.

Cortical Stimulation

Surgery for DCS consists of implantation of a paddle-shaped electrode on the dura mater overlying the lateral portion of the MC. Subdural implementation of the electrode, even in the medial surface of the MC, has been advocated by some authors (Saitoh & Yoshimine 2007) because of a presumed more direct effect of DCS and of the possibility covering the cortical representation of the contralateral inferior limb.

This procedure has initially been introduced for the treatment of drug-resistant chronic neuropathic pain (Tsubokawa et al. 1991). There is evidence also for a role of motor cortex stimulation (MCS) for the treatment of movement disorders. It has been well known that removal of the MC abolishes parkinsonian tremor (Bucy 1949), and more recent observations show the efficacy of DCS for treatment of Parkinson's disease (Bentivoglio et al. 2012) and a breakdown of intracortical inhibition caused by dopamine depletion (Lindebach & Bishop 2013). The potential role of transcranial magnetic stimulation (TMS) (Quartarone et al. 2005, 2009; Edwards et al. 2008) in the treatment of aberrant cortical plasticity frequently found in dystonia has also to be taken into account.

Furthermore, several lines of evidence point to the role of MCS for the treatment of fixed forms of dystonia. In fact, more tonic forms seem to respond poorly to DBS (Romito et al. 2007; Vidailhet et al. 2007; Lalli et al. 2012), whereas improvement has been observed in patients with thalamic hand syndrome and in post-stroke fixed postures (Katayama et al. 2002; Franzini et al. 2003).

The theoretical basis for application of DCS in dystonia is the modulatory role of the PMC or MC on the sensorimotor cortical-striatal-pallido-thalamic circuits. Published data are sparse and sometimes contradictory on this specific subject, though useful for future applications.

Surgical Procedure

The surgical procedure varies among different centres. A subdural or epidural (the most frequent) location may be chosen for implementation of the stimulating electrode. Some surgeons prefer to perform a craniotomy and others a single burr-hole. Other important variables comprise the use of single- or multiple-paddle electrodes, as well as its position (parallel or perpendicular to the precentral gyrus). The localisation of the MC can be determined by preoperative functional magnetic resonance imaging (MRI), which we recommend because of the frequent variants due to abnormal intracortical plasticity which might affect the actual position and size of MC. In any case, MRI images are loaded into a dedicated neuronavigation system for anatomical visualisation.

Another useful tool is the preoperative (and intraoperative) use of somatosensory-evoked potentials (SSEP), obtained by contralateral median nerve stimulation. Intraoperatively, these can help in individualising the electrode contacts located anterior or posterior to the central sulcus, through the phase reversal of N20 and P20 potentials.

Surgery can be performed with general or local anaesthesia, and in either case, patient's discomfort versus the advantage of immediate perception of paraesthesias or subthreshold muscular tonic contractions must be considered, and the patient informed about the specific advantages or disadvantages.

The skin incision is planned according to the above-mentioned techniques, and a burr hole (or craniotomy) is performed. If a burr hole is used, the single-plate electrode is inserted between the calvarial bone and dura mater in the appropriate direction. In either case, after epidural positioning of the electrodes, intraoperative electromyography is used by delivering electrical current from various combinations of the epidural contacts, to ascertain which (or which combination) of them is capable to evoke motor potentials in the affected part of the body. Delivered current is gradually increased until motor potentials are recorded; partial or generalised seizures are not an uncommon occurrence, and they can be abolished either by local administration of cold saline or by intravenous diazepam. The anaesthesiologist is of course warned immediately before stimulation. The electrode can eventually be moved from its initial position until satisfying responses are obtained.

At the end of this procedure, the electrode can be secured to the burr hole with a titanium miniplate; in the case of a craniotomy, the electrode(s) can also be directly sutured to underlying dura mater. Surgery is then completed by subcutaneously tunnelling the connection cable (through the lateral cervical region) to an infraclavicular pocket, where the implantable pulse generator (IPG) is positioned.

Premotor Cortex Stimulation

Paddle leads can be positioned over the PMC or over the MC. Lalli et al. (2012) reported an overall improvement in seven patients submitted to PMC stimulation affected by primary focal dystonia (six with cervical dystonia and one with upper-limb dystonia), as assessed by the Burke–Fahn–Mardsen scale (BMFS) and the Toronto Western Spasmodic Torticollis Rating Scale (TWSTRS). The improvement was observed after a 12-month follow-up period.

The rationale for choosing PMC was previous observation of amelioration in writing performance in patients with upper-limb dystonia (Murase et al. 2005) and the partial restoration of defective reciprocal inhibition, following low-frequency TMS applied over the PMC (Huang et al. 2004). In all patients, the electrodes were positioned along the anterior–posterior axis of the hemisphere, after electrophysiological localisation of the central sulcus (N20–P20 phase reversal). It is interesting to note that the patients who benefited less from this procedure were those with prevalent fixed attitude. This study also reported the finding of a baseline (preoperative) and bilateral increased metabolism in the sensorimotor cortex of patients, as compared to controls, as assessed in a ^{18}F-fluoro-deoxy-glucose positron emission tomography (FDG PET) study. After surgery, such metabolic increase was reduced at 12-month follow-up, suggesting a modulatory or rebalancing role of epidural stimulation on hyperactive sensorimotor cortex.

Motor Cortex Stimulation

For MCS the stimulating electrodes are positioned along (or perpendicular to) the central sulcus, thus covering the dura overlying the motor strip. Messina et al. (2012) reported a case series of ten patients affected by secondary fixed dystonic (FD) postures of the upper limb. For this chapter the series has been updated with inclusion of another patient affected by ischaemic thalamic stroke, for a total of 11 cases. Patients were refractory to conventional and non-invasive treatments (benzodiazepines, baclofen, motor rehabilitation and botulinum toxin injections). None of the patients satisfied the criteria for psychogenic dystonia according to the Fahn and Williams' criteria (Fahn & Williams 1988). Patients presented with major disability; we supposed that a certain degree of improvement was still possible if partial restoration of hand function could be obtained; this assumption was based on a previous observation of suboptimal response to GPi DBS treated with the latter modality (Romito et al. 2007). The theoretical rationale for MCS was the hypothesis that an abnormal cortical representation of the affected body segment could follow deep brain lesions (Opavsky et al. 2006).

In five patients, fixed postures were secondary to cortical or subcortical ischaemic stroke; in one patient, to birth anoxia; in two patients, to iatrogenic postsurgical syndromes; in one patient, to postencephalitic syndrome; in one patient, to long-term neuroleptic treatment (tardive dystonia); and in the last patient, secondary to brain injury (Table 61.1).

A movement disorder neurologist evaluated all of the patients both preoperatively and postoperatively. These evaluations confirmed the phenotypic characteristics of unilateral upper-limb fixed dystonia, involving, in various degrees of severity, shoulder, arm, forearm and hand. Electromyographic examinations showed tonic continuous activity in the affected muscles at rest in all patients. Extensive psychiatric examination excluded the diagnosis of psychogenic dystonia (Fahn & Williams 1988), and no clinical feature of complex regional pain syndrome (CRPS) was found in any patient. The latter diseases may in fact often accompany fixed dystonia (Schrag et al. 2004).

In all patients the surgical procedure consisted of positioning a unilateral quadripolar paddle electrode (Resume II, Medtronic, Minneapolis, Minnesota) on the dural surface corresponding to the 'hand-knob' area of the motor cortex of the side contralateral to the affected upper limb. Surgery was performed under general anaesthesia in all patients without curarisation and with assistance of the Stealth Station Software (Medtronic, Minneapolis, MA, USA) and intraoperative electromyography (EMG) for localisation of the hand-knob area.

A 3 cm skin incision was made 4 cm behind the coronal suture and 3 cm lateral from the midline. A burr hole was performed to expose the dura mater overlying the posteromedial portion of the central gyrus. After dissection of the dura from the calvarial bone, the quadripolar electrode was placed parallel to the motor cortex and along its main axis (as indicated by the navigation system); when it was not possible to evoke a motor response, the orientation of the paddle electrode was changed until recording of the appropriate upper limb's EMG responses (abductor pollicis brevis muscle) was obtained.

Muscular sites monitored intraoperatively with EMG were the orbicularis oris, brachioradialis, abductor pollicis brevis, rectus femoris, tibialis anterior and extensor digitorum brevis. After the initial positioning of the electrode, a set of stimulation trials was delivered to evoke EMG responses in the affected muscles, specifically in the abductor pollicis brevis. In all cases, electric stimulation through the epidural quadripolar electrode (60 Hz, 1 ms pulse width) evoked selective motor responses and EMG activation of the hand and upper-limb muscles with 4–7 mA (Figure 61.1).

Every procedure was completed with the subcutaneous implantation of a single-channel IPG and its connection cable to the epidural electrode.

Patients were evaluated with the Disability of Arm, Shoulder and Hand (DASH) scale (Hudak et al. 1996), and the Short Form-36 Physical Activity subscale. In the DASH scale, higher scores indicate greater disability. We chose this scale because it focuses on the whole functionality of the affected segment of the body better than the more traditional scales employed for classical predominant 'mobile' dystonia. Seven out of 11 patients had a >30 per cent improvement in the first scale, and an overall 70 per cent increase in the second.

Postoperative brain computerised tomography examination was merged with the preoperative brain 3D MRI, and the correct positioning of the epidural electrode was confirmed in all patients (Figure 61.2).

Table 61.1 Motor cortex stimulation in patients affected by secondary fixed dystonic postures of the upper limb

Patient	Age at surgery	Origin	Clinical signs	Follow-up, mo
1	56	Striatal stroke	Flexion of right carpal joint and metacarpophalangeal joints	48
2	62	Parieto-temporal stroke	Elevation of the shoulder, adduction of right arm	60
3	67	Temporo-occipital and thalamic stroke	Flexion of the right first three metacarpophalangeal joints	36
4	42	Viral meningo-encephalitis	Flexion of left carpal joint and metacarpophalangeal joints	36
5	61	Bulbopontine cavernous hemangioma	Flexion of right forearm and of carpal joint	36
6	26	Perinatal hypoxia	Elevation of the shoulder, abduction of the right arm, flexion of the right forearm, flexion of right carpal and metacarpophalangeal joints	36
7	38	Neuroleptic-induced dystonia	Flexion of both forearms	36
8	44	Thalamic oligoastrocytoma	Flexion of left forearm and of left carpal and metacarpophalangeal joints	36
9	74	Thalamic stroke	Flexion of the right carpal joint and adduction of all fingers of the right hand	132
10	33	Posttraumatic bilateral putaminal stroke	Adduction of left arm, flexion of left forearm and of left carpal joints	16
11	51	Thalamic stroke	Flexion of left forearm and of left carpal joints	12

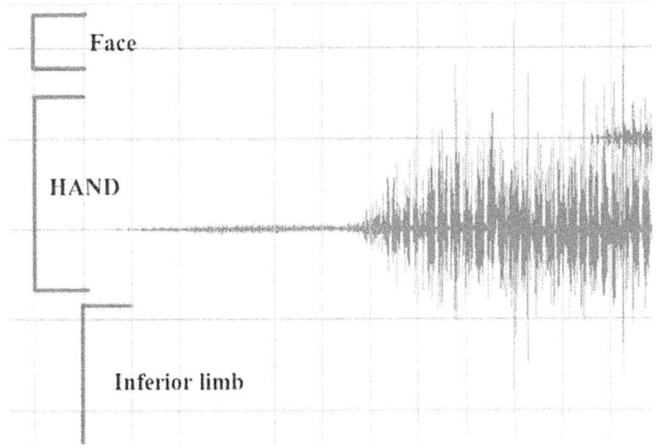

Figure 61.1 Intraoperative EMG showing activation of hand muscles after stimulation with epidural paddle electrode.

The postoperative course was uneventful in all but one patient, who required surgical evacuation for acute epidural haematoma; after six months the whole system was reimplanted.

The day after surgery, the IPG was activated in all patients, and subsequent modifications of stimulation parameters were adapted to the threshold for the elicitation of side-effects (such as paraesthesias) and to the clinical effects observed during follow-up. No patient experienced seizures during programming.

The final stimulation parameters were set at the six-month follow-up examination in all patients and the configuration was quadruple monopolar (case as anode, contacts 0, 1, 2, 3 as cathodes); stimulation parameters are presented in Table 61.2.

The follow-up ranged from 12 to 132 months. Re-evaluations were performed monthly for the first six months and then on a six-monthly basis. The overall degree of disability of patients was high and this, together with their fixed postures being refractory to conservative treatment, led us to consider an improvement of 30 per cent in their DASH scores as indicating a positive result (Figure 61.3). The overall improvement on the SF-36 scale may indicate the high degree of interference resulting from this pathological condition in the overall sense of wellbeing.

Although differences between pre- and postoperative DASH scores found in this series do not seem impressive if only numerical data are taken into account, nevertheless, even small changes in DASH score reflect a significantly higher quality-of-life score (Table 61.3).

Rieu et al. reported a double-blind, crossover, multicentre study involving five patients affected by dystonia secondary to focal post-ischaemic basal ganglia (BG) lesions, who were submitted to cortical stimulation (Rieu et al. 2014). All their patients suffered from left hemidystonia. For every patient, two parallel quadripolar electrodes were positioned in the epidural space overlying both the MC and the PMC, parallel to the central sulcus, with the assistance of a neuronavigation system. Within the MC, the anode was positioned over the motor representation of the most affected limb.

At the level of PMC, the electrodes were positioned over the superior and the middle frontal gyrus. In all patients, postoperative CT scans demonstrated optimal positioning of the electrodes.

In this case series, several scales were used for assessments, including the BFMS, Ashworth scale for spasticity, a visual analogue scale (VAS) for pain and the SF-36 for quality of life for pre- and postoperative evaluations. After one

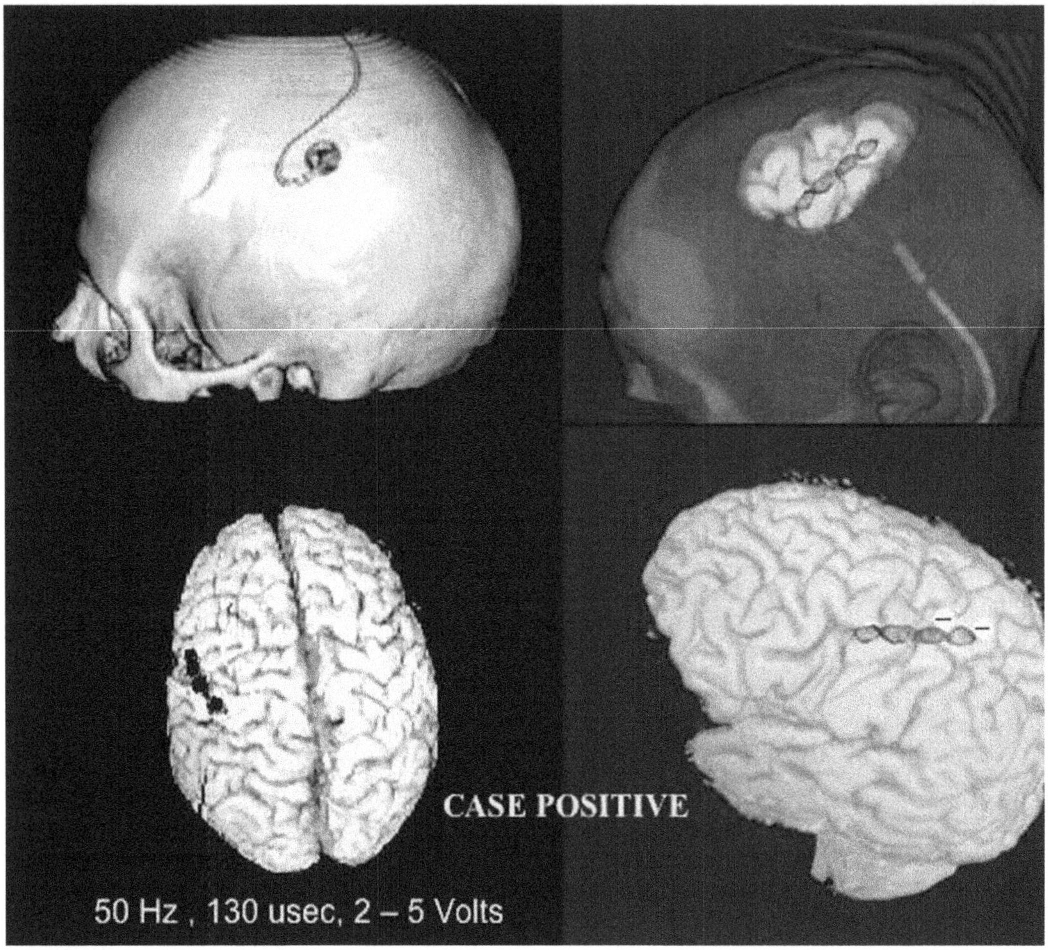

Figure 61.2 Three-dimensional postoperative reconstruction showing the placement of the chronic leads over the motor cortex.

Table 61.2 Stimulation parameters and results

Patient	Before (DASH)	After (DASH)	Stim. parameters	Improvement (%)
1	86	57	120 mcs, 30 Hz, 2.5 V	34
2	90.5	77.6	90 mcs, 50 Hz, 3.5 V	15.1
3	92	49.1	120 mcs, 50 Hz, 3.0 V	47
4	72.4	64.2	120 mcs, 30 Hz, 3.1 V	12.4
5	32.5	18.1	90 mcs, 30 Hz, 3.0 V	44.4
6	48.3	30.8	120 mcs 50 Hz, 3.0 V	36
7	87.1	28.4	90 mcs, 50 Hz, 3.3 V	67
8	66.4	44.8	120 mcs, 50 Hz, 3.5 V	32
9	75	28.4	120 mcs, 30 Hz, 2.8 V	62
10	84	66	150 mcs, 30 Hz, 4.0 V	22.3
11	80	74	150 mcs, 40 Hz, 4.0 V	7.5

month from implantation, patients were randomly assigned to two groups: stimulation-on and stimulation-off groups. Such condition was maintained for three months; after a washout period of one month, a clinical evaluation was performed and the on–off condition was reversed; again, this was maintained for another three months and, then, a second follow-up was carried out. Scores of the above-mentioned scales were not significantly modified at any evaluation time, thus no patient benefited from the procedure. Given the study design and the negative results obtained, the authors concluded that class I evidence would exist that epidural MCS failed to improve dystonia secondary to BG lesions.

Discussion

There is great heterogeneity with regard to the aetiology of abnormal fixed dystonic postures in several body segments;

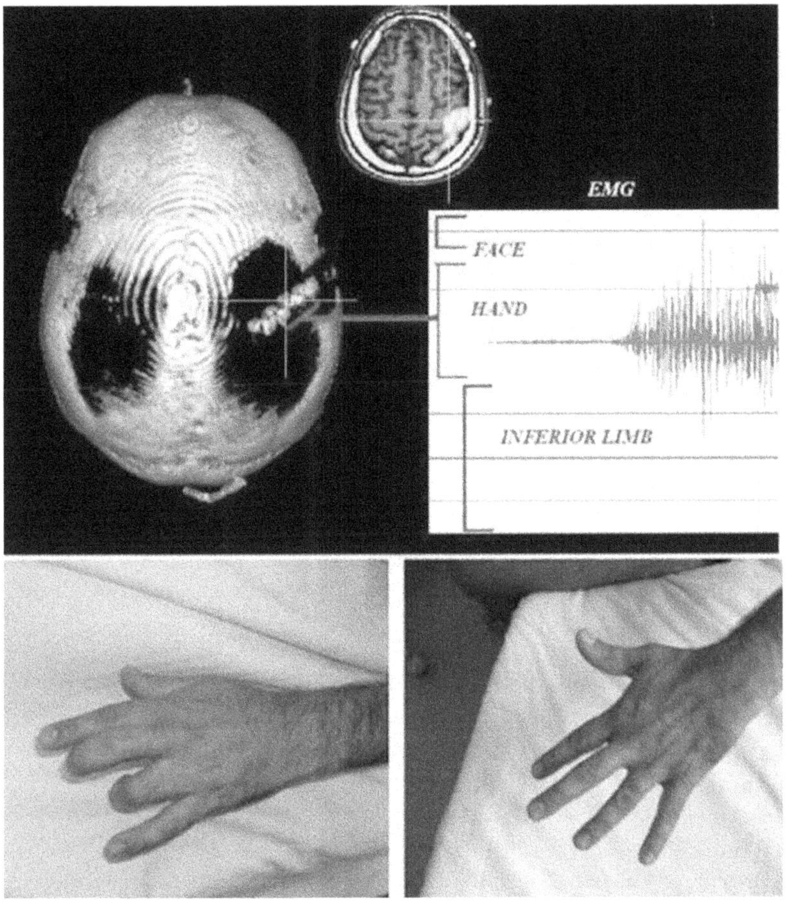

Figure 61.3 *Top*: three-dimensional reconstruction of the postoperative CT showing the contacts of the paddle electrode which allowed stimulation of contralateral hand muscle; above, functional MRI shows aberrant activation of hand motor cortex for the affected contralateral hand. *Bottom*: the affected hand of the patient before (left) and after four months (right) of MCS.

Table 61.3 Pre- and post-treatment comparisons of DASH scores, physical activity and mental state

Patient	DASH before	DASH after	SF-36 Physical Activity Subscale before	SF-36 Physical Activity Subscale after	SF-36 Mental State Subscale before	SF-36 Mental State Subscale after
1	86	57	0	85	64	88
2	90.5	77.6	0	40	24	72
3	92	49.1	30	85	28	48
4	72.4	64.2	10	75	36	60
5	32.5	18.1	20	65	36	44
6	48.3	30.8	75	100	40	52
7	87.1	28.4	0	95	4	100
8	66.4	44.8	20	75	28	60
9	75	28.4	60	80	44	76
10	84	66	40	40	56	60
11	80	74	40	40	50	64

they may in fact develop following a focal brain lesion, be defined as 'psychogenic' or occur in the context of a fixed dystonia syndrome (mainly idiopathic in nature) (Schrag et al. 2004). The hallmark of the disease is permanently fixed abnormal posture of some body segment which never reverts to the normal position, and, as such, it is important to differentiate it from 'typical' forms of mobile dystonia and from segmental spasticity. FD is more frequently focal and less frequently segmental; moreover, Ibrahim reported on a poor prognosis of this condition as far as its natural history is concerned (Ibrahim et al. 2009). In fact, in their study, only 6 per cent of patients reached remission, 25 per cent improved and 33 per cent continued worsening.

The fact that the motor cortex could play a role and influence the subcortical circuitry, thus being a potential target in 'extrapyramidal disorders' can be extrapolated by the historical work of Bucy (Bucy 1949) and Woolsey (Woolsey et al. 1979). Furthermore, several lines of evidence suggest that modulation of the motor cortex could also induce nigrostriatal dopamine release (Brown 2003; Strafella et al. 2003). The therapeutic mechanisms of MCS in the treatment of movement disorders are not known, although some hypotheses suggest activation of inhibitory GABAergic neurons within the motor cortex or a role of the 'hyperdirect' corticosubthalamic nucleus pathway within the basal ganglia circuitry (Dinner et al. 2002). Involvement of cerebellar pathways should also be considered (Franzini et al. 2000, 2003, 2009; Romito et al. 2007).

MCS was originally proposed by Tsubokawa for the treatment of refractory central neuropathic pain and, subsequently, of movement disorders secondary to stroke (Tsubokawa et al. 1991; Katayama et al. 2002, 2003; Canavero & Bonicalzi 2007).

Fixed dystonia typically lacks action specificity and an effect of sensory tricks. It can be idiopathic and can develop as a sign of corticobasal degeneration or within a primary dystonia syndrome in its advanced stages (Marsden 1976). CRPS may also present with abnormal fixed postures (Bhatia et al. 1993). It can be accompanied by severe psychiatric disorders and thus criteria established by Fahn and Williams for psychogenic dystonia (Fahn & Williams 1988).

A causative factor for FD could be an increased thalamocortical drive resulting in hyperexcitability of the sensorimotor cortex. The overactivation of glutamatergic input to the cortex could be caused by an imbalance between the direct and indirect striatopallidal pathways, although why this would result in fixed postures rather than typical (i.e. mobile and twisting) dystonic movements remains unexplained. In fact, according to current concepts, lesions localised in the motor portion of the thalamus (such as those found in three of our patients) would be more likely to cause suppression of movement instead of increasing thalamocortical drive.

Moreover, not all patients affected by acquired basal ganglia lesions present such FD (Micheli et al. 1998; Rivest 2003).

A relevant concept is the increased plasticity of the cerebral cortex as suggested by Quartarone and coworkers (Quartarone et al. 2009). These authors showed that the 'homeostatic' cortical plasticity is disrupted in patients with writer's cramp (Quartarone et al. 2005). Specifically, homeostatic suppression of practice-dependent plasticity is lacking in this pathology (Kang et al. 2011). It is thus possible that the same maladaptive cerebral plasticity might occur in patients with secondary fixed dystonia.

In one of our patients, FD developed after surgery for a right bulbopontine cavernous hemangioma. The role of brainstem lesions in the pathophysiology of dystonia has not been elucidated, but several reports point to a role of dysfunction of ascending and descending pontomesencephalic pathways such as central tegmental tract and dentatothalamic pathway, as well as of the pedunculopontine nucleus and the nucleus interstitialis of Cajal (Malouin & Bedard 1982; Loher & Krauss 2009).

No mutation of the DYT1 gene was detected in the reported series, and none of the patients presented complex regional pain syndrome or psychogenic dystonia at psychiatric examination. The term 'secondary' fixed dystonia might be most appropriate to mark the difference with genetic and secondary mobile dystonia, and also the difference with psychogenic and idiopathic fixed dystonia syndromes. Our series in fact includes patients with acquired brain lesions or with prolonged use of neuroleptic agents.

The patients in this series who did not respond to neuromodulation remain a clinical and conceptual challenge, given that psychological comorbidities were ruled out preoperatively. We can hypothesise that a maladaptive plasticity in some patients affected by a fixed dystonic posture also can occur beyond anatomic sites potentially controlled by cortical stimulation.

References

Bentivoglio AR, Fasano A, Piano C, Soleti F, Daniele A, Zinno M, Piccininni C, De Simone C, Policicchio D, Tufo T, Meglio M, Cioni B. 2012. Unilateral extradural motor cortex stimulation is safe and improves Parkinson disease at 1 year. *Neurosurgery* 71(4):815–825.

Bhatia KP, Bhatt MH, Marsden CD. 1993. The causalgia-dystonia syndrome. *Brain* 116(Pt 4):843–851.

Brown P. 2003. Oscillatory nature of human basal ganglia activity: relationship to the pathophysiology of Parkinson's disease. *Mov Disord* 18(4):357–363.

Bucy PC. 1949. Extirpation in man. In: Bucy PC, ed. *The Precentral Motor Cortex*. Urbana, IL: University of Illinois Press; 355–393.

Canavero S, Bonicalzi V. 2007. Extradural cortical stimulation for movement disorders. *Acta Neurochir Suppl* 97(Pt 2):223–232.

Dinner DS, Neme S, Nair D, Montgomery EB, Jr, Baker KB, Rezai A, Luders HO. 2002. EEG and evoked potential recording from the subthalamic nucleus for deep brain stimulation of intractable epilepsy. *Clin Neurophysiol* 113(9):1391–1402.

Edwards MJ, Talelli P, Rothwell JC. 2008. Clinical applications of transcranial magnetic stimulation in patients with movement disorders. *Lancet Neurol* 7(9):827–840.

Fahn S, Williams DT. 1988. Psychogenic dystonia. *Adv Neurol* 50:431–455.

Franzini A, Ferroli P, Servello D, Broggi G. 2000. Reversal of thalamic hand syndrome by long-term motor cortex stimulation. *J Neurosurg* 93(5):873–875.

Franzini A, Ferroli P, Dones I, Marras C, Broggi G. 2003. Chronic motor cortex stimulation for movement disorders: a promising perspective. *Neurol Res* 25(2):123–126.

Franzini A, Messina G, Marras C, Molteni F, Cordella R, Soliveri P, Broggi G. 2009. Poststroke fixed dystonia of the foot relieved by chronic stimulation of the posterior limb of the internal capsule. *J Neurosurg* 111(6):1216–1219.

Huang YZ, Edwards MJ, Bhatia KP, Rothwell JC. 2004. One-Hz repetitive transcranial magnetic stimulation of the premotor cortex alters reciprocal inhibition in DYT1 dystonia. *Mov Disord* 19(1):54–59.

Hudak PL, Amadio PC, Bombardier C. 1996. Development of an upper extremity outcome measure: the DASH (disabilities of the arm, shoulder and hand) [corrected]: the upper extremity collaborative group (UECG). *Am J Ind Med* 29(6):602–608.

Ibrahim NM, Martino D, van de Warrenburg BP, Quinn NP, Bhatia KP, Brown RJ, Trimble M, Schrag A. 2009. The prognosis of fixed dystonia: a follow-up study. *Parkinsonism Relat Disord* 15(8):592–597.

Kang JS, Terranova C, Hilker R, Quartarone A, Ziemann U. 2011. Deficient homeostatic regulation of practice-dependent plasticity in writer's cramp. *Cereb Cortex* 21(5):1203–1212.

Katayama Y, Oshima H, Fukaya C, Kawamata T, Yamamaoto T. 2002. Control of post-stroke movement disorders using chronic motor cortex stimulation. *Acta Neurochir Suppl* 79:89–92.

Katayama Y, Yamamoto T, Kobayashi K, Oshima H, Fukaya C. 2003. Deep brain and motor cortex stimulation for post-stroke movement disorders and post-stroke pain. *Acta Neurochir Suppl* 87:121–123.

Lalli S, Piacentini S, Franzini A, Panzacchi A, Cerami C, Messina G, Ferre F, Perani D, Albanese A. 2012. Epidural premotor cortical stimulation in primary focal dystonia: clinical and 18F-fluoro deoxyglucose positron emission tomography open study. *Mov Disord* 27(4):533–538.

Lindenbach D, Bishop C. 2013. Critical involvement of the motor cortex in the pathophysiology and treatment of Parkinson's disease. *Neurosci Biobehav Rev* 37(10 Pt 2):2737–2750.

Loher TJ, Krauss JK. 2009. Dystonia associated with pontomesencephalic lesions. *Mov Disord* 24(2):157–167.

Malouin F, Bedard PJ. 1982. Frontal torticollis (head tilt) induced by electrolytic lesion and kainic acid injection in monkeys and cats. *Exp Neurol* 78(3):551–560.

Marsden CD. 1976. Dystonia: the spectrum of the disease. *Res Publ Assoc Res Nerv Ment Dis* 55:351–367.

Messina G, Cordella R, Dones I, Tringali G, Franzini A. 2012. Improvement of secondary fixed dystonia of the upper limb after chronic extradural motor cortex stimulation in 10 patients: first reported series. *Neurosurgery* 70(5):1169–1175.

Micheli F, Cersosimo G, Palacios C, Scorticati MC, Tenembaum S, Tipoli J. 1998. Dystonia and tremor secondary to a pediatric thalamic stroke. *Parkinsonism Relat Disord* 4(3):119–122.

Murase N, Rothwell JC, Kaji R, Urushihara R, Nakamura K, Murayama N, Igasaki T, Sakata-Igasaki M, Mima T, Ikeda A, Shibasaki H. 2005. Subthreshold low-frequency repetitive transcranial magnetic stimulation over the premotor cortex modulates writer's cramp. *Brain* 128(Pt 1):104–115.

Opavsky R, Hlustik P, Kanovsky P. 2006. Cortical plasticity and its implications for focal hand dystonia. *Biomed Pap Med Fac Univ Palacky Olomouc Czech Repub* 150(2):223–226.

Quartarone A, Rizzo V, Bagnato S, Morgante F, Sant'Angelo A, Romano M, Crupi D, Girlanda P, Rothwell JC, Siebner HR. 2005. Homeostatic-like plasticity of the primary motor hand area is impaired in focal hand dystonia. *Brain* 128(Pt 8):1943–1950.

Quartarone A, Rizzo V, Terranova C, Morgante F, Schneider S, Ibrahim N, Girlanda P, Bhatia KP, Rothwell JC. 2009. Abnormal sensorimotor plasticity in organic but not in psychogenic dystonia. *Brain* 132(Pt 10):2871–2877.

Rieu I, Aya Kombo M, Thobois S, Derost P, Pollak P, Xie J, Pereira B, Vidailhet M, Burbaud P, Lefaucheur JP, Lemaire JJ, Mertens P, Chabardes S, Broussolle E, Durif F. 2014. Motor cortex stimulation does not improve dystonia secondary to a focal basal ganglia lesion. *Neurology* 82(2):156–162.

Rivest J. 2003. Myoclonus. *Can J Neurol Sci* 30 (Suppl. 1):S53–S58.

Romito LM, Franzini A, Perani D, Carella F, Marras C, Capus L, Garibotto V, Broggi G, Albanese A. 2007. Fixed dystonia unresponsive to pallidal stimulation improved by motor cortex stimulation. *Neurology* 68(11):875–876.

Saitoh Y, Yoshimine T. 2007. Stimulation of primary motor cortex for intractable deafferentation pain. *Acta Neurochir Suppl* 97(Pt 2):51–56.

Schrag A, Trimble M, Quinn N, Bhatia K. 2004. The syndrome of fixed dystonia: an evaluation of 103 patients. *Brain* 127(Pt 10):2360–2372.

Strafella AP, Paus T, Fraraccio M, Dagher A. 2003. Striatal dopamine release induced by repetitive transcranial magnetic stimulation of the human motor cortex. *Brain* 126(Pt 12):2609–2615.

Tsubokawa T, Katayama Y, Yamamoto T, Hirayama T, Koyama S. 1991. Treatment of thalamic pain by chronic motor cortex stimulation. *Pacing Clin Electrophysiol* 14(1):131–134.

Vidailhet M, Vercueil L, Houeto JL, Krystkowiak P, Lagrange C, Yelnik J, Bardinet E, Benabid AL, Navarro S, Dormont D, Grand S, Blond S, Ardouin C, Pillon B, Dujardin K, Hahn-Barma V, Agid Y, Destee A, Pollak P, French SPIDY Study Group. 2007. Bilateral, pallidal, deep-brain stimulation in primary generalised dystonia: a prospective 3 year follow-up study. *Lancet Neurol* 6(3):223–229.

Woolsey CN, Erickson TC, Gilson WE. 1979. Localization in somatic sensory and motor areas of human cerebral cortex as determined by direct recording of evoked potentials and electrical stimulation. *J Neurosurg* 51(4):476–506.

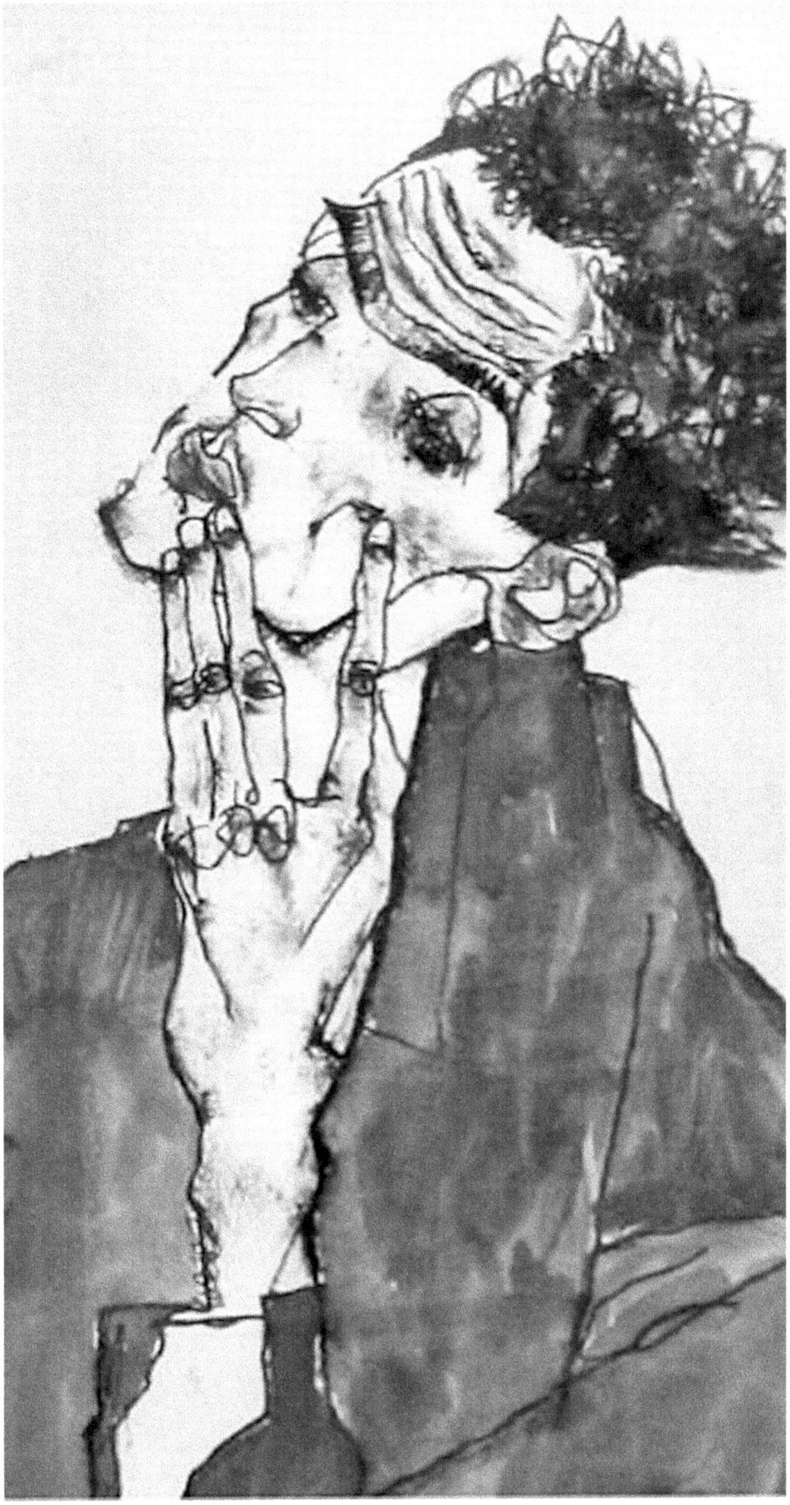

Chapter 62

Functional Mechanisms of Deep Brain Stimulation in Dystonia

Andrea A. Kühn and Angelo Quartarone

Bilateral globus pallidus internus deep brain stimulation (GPi DBS) is a reliable, safe and long-term effective treatment for many forms of medically refractory dystonia (Volkmann et al. 2012; Vidailhet et al. 2013, 2014). The efficacy and safety of GPi DBS have been well established for patients with generalised (Vidailhet et al. 2005) or segmental (Kupsch et al. 2006) isolated dystonia in large, well-designed multicentre trials. In addition to these idiopathic or genetic forms of isolated dystonia, GPi DBS has recently been demonstrated to be markedly effective in myoclonus-dystonia (Gruber et al. 2010) and tardive dystonia (Gruber et al. 2009; Capelle et al. 2010; Welter et al. 2010), but the benefit of GPi DBS for other dystonia-plus syndromes (such as dystonia-choreoathetosis cerebral palsy or inherited metabolic disorders) is variable and still subject to debate (Vidailhet et al. 2009).

Despite the relatively large amount of clinical data available to date, the mechanism by which DBS interacts with the basal ganglia in alleviating and improving dystonic postures is poorly understood. This poor understanding of the DBS mechanisms of action is also paralleled by a largely unclear knowledge of dystonia pathophysiology. Several neural structures, including the motor cortex, cerebellum and the basal ganglia have been identified as part of the structural and functional dystonia network. An intriguing point in DBS in dystonia is that in contrast to the almost immediate effects of DBS on the majority of symptoms in Parkinson's disease, it may take sometimes several weeks or months to achieve maximum clinical benefit in patients with dystonia (Coubes et al. 2000). This delayed improvement suggests that a process of progressive plasticity and neural reorganisation accompanies the long-term effects of GPi DBS in dystonia (Quartarone & Hallett 2013). In the present chapter we will explore the functional mechanisms and network effects underlying motor recovery after pallidal DBS in dystonia.

Insights into Basal Ganglia Pathophysiology of Dystonia from Intracranial Recordings

The basal ganglia have been notoriously difficult to characterise electrophysiologically because of their anatomical distance to the scalp. In recent years, DBS has, beside its highly beneficial therapeutic effects, enabled the unique opportunity to explore basal ganglia pathophysiology by direct recordings of neuronal activity in those patients undergoing functional neurosurgery. Here, two major approaches exist: (1) intraoperative recording of multi-unit activity (MUA) via microelectrodes used for target verification during surgery, and (2) local field potential (LFP) recordings, i.e. population activity that still can be recorded several days after electrode implantation via the implanted macroelectrodes before they are connected to the pulse generator. Insights from direct recordings of neuronal cortical and subcortical activity patterns have shaped our knowledge of the pathophysiology of dystonia that is now seen as a network disorder.

Basal Ganglia Multi-Unit Activity in Dystonia

Microelectrode recording (MER) in dystonia is more challenging as compared to analysis of MUA patterns observed, for example, in the subthalamic nucleus of Parkinson's disease (PD) patients because available data are rare and heterogeneous. The inconsistency of results, however, mirrors the underlying pathophysiological changes in firing pattern of neurons in dystonia. Consistent with the rate model of basal ganglia motor circuits, merely reduced pallidal discharge rate was found in dystonia patients (Lenz et al. 1998; Lenz & Byl 1999; Alam et al. 2016) and was associated with dyskinesia in the MPTP monkey model (Papa et al. 1999) as well as during apomorphine challenge in PD patients undergoing functional neurosurgery (Hutchinson et al. 1997; Merello et al. 1999). However, the reduced discharge rates cannot unambiguously be related to the severity of dystonia (Hutchison et al. 2003; Steigerwald et al. 2005) because the influence of anaesthesia needs to be considered. Propofol anaesthesia may enhance GABAergic inhibition leading to reduced firing rates. Moreover, MUA discharge rates do not differentiate between GPe and GPi, with similar reduced rates between 40 and 70 Hz, which contrasts to findings in PD patients with significantly higher rates for the internal pallidum (Starr et al. 2006). A striking additional feature is the abnormal pattern of neuronal discharge that is encountered in the external and internal pallidum: a change from a regular tonic pattern to irregular grouped discharges with intermittent pauses and high-frequency burst-like discharges in dystonia (Yoshida et al. 1991; Vitek et al. 1999; Hutchison et al. 2003; Merello et al. 2004; Starr et al. 2006; Alam et al. 2016). Moreover, MUA is characterised by an increased degree of synchronisation of pallidal neurons. Thus, a paradigm shift over the last decade has emphasised the abnormal pattern of neuronal activity leading to abnormal pallidal output in dystonia as a pathophysiological hallmark rather than the pallidal discharge rate per se.

Modulation of firing rate during active and passive movement and sensory stimulation is consistently found in pallidal recordings in dystonia. However, it is characterised by widened and less specific receptive fields, i.e. overlapping fields for agonist and antagonist muscles, distorted single-joint movement-related activity changes and enlarged receptive fields (Hutchison et al. 2003). Vitek and colleagues describe that responses are often obtained from more than one joint, more than one body area with single neurons that responded to movement of multiple limb segments or multiple limbs (Vitek et al. 1999), suggesting a significant abnormality in processing sensory input at the level of the basal ganglia.

These altered sensory and motor responses in the basal ganglia may contribute to co-contraction of muscle pairs and inappropriate activation patterns with overflow phenomena in the patients. Again, an abnormal firing pattern with breakdown of focal selection and loss of specificity within the pallidum leads to altered sensorimotor information processing in the cortex–basal ganglia circuit in dystonia. Abnormal basal ganglia activity may thus contribute to the loss in functional selectivity and abnormal scaling of movement in dystonia.

Disease-Specific Oscillatory Basal Ganglia Activity

Physiological markers of particular brain states in patients with movement disorders have emerged from research using the implanted DBS electrodes to record local field potentials (LFP) via externalised leads (Brown 2003) as well as from subdural electrodes to record cortical activity (ECoG) (Crowell et al. 2012). Several studies have demonstrated distinct patterns of oscillatory activity recorded from the basal ganglia of PD patients withdrawn from dopaminergic medication and patients with dystonia (Silberstein et al. 2003). Best characterised are LFP recordings from the subthalamic nucleus in PD patients that show enhanced beta band activity (~20 Hz) that has been associated with bradykinesia and rigidity (Neumann et al. 2016; van Wijk et al. 2016), as beta band activity is decreased with dopaminergic treatment (Priori et al. 2002; Silberstein et al. 2003) and its reduction correlates with clinical improvement in motor symptoms induced by levodopa (Kuhn et al. 2006) and DBS (Kuhn et al. 2008b; Eusebio et al. 2009). In contrast, in dystonia patients basal ganglia activity is characterised by increased low-frequency (5–12 Hz, theta-alpha) activity (Silberstein et al. 2003; Liu et al. 2008; Wang et al. 2016) irrespective of the target area of DBS (Neumann et al. 2012). Pallidal low-frequency activity correlates and is coherent to dystonic EMG activity driving especially phasic EMG bursts (Chen et al. 2006a, 2006b). Recently, a significant correlation of pallidal theta (4–12 Hz) peak amplitude and interhemispheric theta oscillatory activity with preoperative symptom severity has been shown in patients with cervical dystonia (Neumann & Kuhn 2016). Both theta and beta (13–35 Hz) peaks were consistently present across all patients. However, significant associations with dystonic symptoms were only obtained for the theta band. It is of note that beta band activity has been recorded from the subthalamic nucleus in dystonia patients (Wang et al. 2016); however, it was not found related to dystonic movements; and pallidal beta band activity was increased in the subgroup of patients on antidopaminergic drugs (Kuhn et al. 2012). Other hyperkinetic movements such as levodopa-induced dyskinesia, myoclonus, motor tics and hyperkinesia in Huntington's disease patients have been associated with enhanced theta-alpha activity in the BG (Alonso-Frech et al. 2006; Foncke et al. 2007a, 2007b; Groiss et al. 2011) and/or thalamus (Marceglia et al. 2010; Kuhn et al. 2011), supporting a link between mobile hyperkinesias and enhanced theta-alpha activity.

Interestingly, a combined magnetoencephalography-pallidal LFP study in dystonia patients showed that the internal pallidum is interconnected with the cerebral cortex in three spatially and spectrally distinct functional oscillatory networks. Theta band coherence was identified with the temporal cortex, alpha band coherence with a central cerebellar source and the beta band coherence with motor and premotor cortical regions. Importantly, pallidal-cerebellar coherence in the alpha frequency activity was inversely correlated with the severity of motor symptoms (Neumann et al. 2015; Neumann & Kuhn 2016), underlining the importance of cerebellar input for clinical implications of altered network activity. A possible direct connection between the cortex and the pallidum has been proposed by Milardi and coworkers (Milardi et al. 2015). Moreover, an inverse correlation was also found between cerebellar alpha band power (7–13 Hz) and motor cortical beta band power in the dystonia motor network (Neumann & Kuhn 2016).

In sum, these recent data suggest that pallidal low-frequency oscillatory activity could play a key role in the pathophysiology of dystonia and may be a useful biomarker for dystonic symptom severity and monitoring for adaptive DBS strategies.

Modulation of Pallidal Activity by Deep Brain Stimulation

One hypothesis posits that DBS suppresses or overrides pathological oscillatory network activity within the cortex-basal ganglia loop (Hammond et al. 2007; Brown & Eusebio 2008; McIntyre & Hahn 2010; Ruge et al. 2011; Vitek et al. 2012). If pallidal theta activity is considered as a potential pathophysiological hallmark of dystonia, its reduction could offer a feasible mechanism of action of DBS in dystonic symptom alleviation. Support for this comes from the observation of reduced pallidal low-frequency activity observed during a geste manoeuvre along with the alleviation of dystonic posturing in two patients with cervical dystonia (Tang et al. 2007). Monitoring of parallel clinical and neurophysiological DBS effects in dystonia prove difficult, as for the aforementioned delayed stimulation effect in patients with dystonia. However, patients with predominant phasic involuntary movements seem to respond more quickly to pallidal DBS as compared to patients with severe tonic posturing (Krauss 2002; Volkmann & Benecke 2002; Coubes et al. 2004; Krauss et al. 2004; Vidailhet et al. 2005, 2009; Wang et al. 2006; Yianni et al. 2006; Hung et al. 2007; Johnson et al. 2008). Indeed, the immediate effect of DBS on pallidal LFPs in patients with dystonia are limited to those patients with predominant phasic dystonic movements. Here, DBS suppressed pallidal low-frequency activity and this effect was propagated along the cortico-basal ganglia network with DBS-induced reduction of low-frequency coherence between pallidum and motor cortex as well as dystonic EMG activity (Barow et al. 2014). Thus, the reduction in pallidal 4–12 Hz activity may be propagated along the different nuclei of the basal ganglia and to the cerebral cortex, so that DBS influences neuronal activity both locally at the site of stimulation and also over other functionally connected elements of the cortex–basal ganglia network, inducing long-term plastic changes at cortical level that may allow for compensatory strategies to re-establish normal movements. The new generation of bidirectional devices with sensing function (PC+S, Medtronic) allow monitoring of the neuronal signal in chronically implanted patients that will provide important insights of the relation between changes in the pattern of synchronised oscillatory activity and clinical improvement and thus probe low-frequency activity as a reliable biomarker for dystonia to be used for adaptive DBS.

DBS-Related Changes in Cortical Activity as Evaluated by Transcranial Magnetic Stimulation and Electrophysiological Studies

The pathophysiology of dystonia appears to be associated with abnormal plasticity and reduced inhibition at cortical, brainstem and spinal cord levels (Quartarone et al. 2006; Peterson et al. 2010). Indeed, an impaired synaptic function leading to abnormal plasticity has been reported in animal (Martella et al. 2009; Napolitano et al. 2010) and human studies (Chen & Udupa 2009; Quartarone & Hallett 2013).

Abnormalities of Neuronal Inhibition

TMS studies have demonstrated an abnormal short-latency intracortical inhibition (SICI) in the motor cortex (Ridding et al. 1995) and increased cortical excitability during voluntary movement (Ikoma et al. 1996). At brainstem level there is a hyperexcitability as indexed by the abnormal recovery cycle of blink reflex either in patients with cranial dystonia (Berardelli et al. 1985) or in patients with segmental and generalised dystonia. Finally, at spinal cord level several studies have reported an abnormal reciprocal inhibition of forearm H-reflex in patients with focal dystonia and generalised dystonia (Nakashima et al. 1989; Panizza et al. 1989). It is likely that this widespread disinhibition from cortex down to spinal cord could contribute to dystonia by interfering with normal motor selection and suppression of unwanted movements (Quartarone & Hallett 2013).

Abnormal Plasticity

Several lines of evidence point out that an abnormal sensorimotor plasticity plays a pivotal role in the pathophysiology of dystonia (Quartarone et al. 2006; Quartarone & Hallett 2013). More direct evidence for abnormal plasticity in dystonia has come from TMS studies using paired associative stimulation (PAS) or theta-burst repetitive TMS protocols to test motor cortex plasticity.

More in detail, several studies have shown an abnormal plasticity in focal hand dystonia (FHD) patients with greater increases in motor cortex after conditioning with TMS-PAS than healthy subjects (Quartarone et al. 2003; Weise et al. 2006). Similarly, cortical plasticity is increased following theta-burst stimulation in patients with DYT1 dystonia and sporadic cervical dystonia, but reduced in non-manifesting carriers of the DYT1 gene (Edwards et al. 2006). An abnormal response to PAS protocol, similar to FHD, has been reported in patients prior to surgery as compared with healthy individuals (Ruge et al. 2011).

Effect of Deep Brain Stimulation on Cortical Plasticity and Abnormal Neuronal Inhibition

Immediate Effects

Kühn and coworkers evaluated the effects of GPi DBS on several measures of cortical excitability as indexed by TMS and spinal excitability, as determined by forearm H-reflex in patients with severe primary dystonia (Kuhn et al. 2003). Patients were studied three months after implantation in two different conditions: on-stimulation and off-stimulation. In the on-stimulation condition motor threshold was reduced and the slope of the MEP recruitment curve became steeper, while these effects were rapidly reversible when GPi stimulation was turned off (Kuhn et al. 2003). These data suggest that GPi DBS can increase cortical excitability in a rapid and reversible manner. On the contrary, GPi stimulation did not affect short intra-cortical inhibition (SICI), intracortical facilitation (ICF), cortical silent period and forearm H-reflex (Kuhn et al. 2003).

It is likely that increase of cortical excitability is due to a re-modulation of pallidal output to thalamus and cortex. This paradoxical effect of DBS can be solved considering that it is just an acute effect that is different from the long-term effects exerted by chronic DBS stimulation.

Long-Term Effects

Following GPi DBS there is a progressive normalisation of reciprocal inhibition, which correlates with clinical dystonia scores over the time course (Tisch et al. 2006a, 2006b).

This normalisation of spinal cord excitability is probably due again to a re-modulation of the descending inputs controlling the spinal cord circuits of reciprocal inhibition. In another similar study, Tisch and coworkers examined the longitudinal effects of GPi DBS on the blink (trigemino-facial) reflex excitability in patients with primary generalised dystonia (Tisch et al. 2006a, 2006b). In line with previous studies, they found that blink reflex excitability was pathologically increased in dystonia patients compared to healthy subjects (Nakashima et al. 1990). Following DBS, there was a progressive decrease in blink reflex excitability towards normal values which correlated with clinical improvement in dystonia (Tisch et al. 2006a, 2006b). The progressive effect of DBS on spinal cord and brainstem excitability, in parallel with clinical improvement is consistent with the notion that a massive brain reorganisation may play a role.

Chronic Effects of Deep Brain Stimulation on Sensorimotor Plasticity

Motor cortex plasticity following repetitive TMS is increased in patients with DYT1 dystonia and sporadic cervical dystonia, but reduced in non-manifesting carriers of the DYT1 gene (Edwards et al. 2006). This finding has been also reported for focal hand dystonia, where the response of the sensorimotor cortex to paired associative stimulation (PAS) is increased (Quartarone et al. 2003; Weise et al. 2006). These studies are in keeping with the notion that excessive plasticity within the motor cortex may be one factor that contributes to and maintains dystonia. It is likely that convergence of abnormal excitability of inhibitory motor circuits, mis-processing of sensory input and increased cortical synaptic plasticity may result in abnormal neural reorganisation and ultimately clinical dystonia (Tisch et al. 2006a, 2006b; Quartarone & Hallett 2013).

DBS has a long-term effect in reducing this excessive plasticity, which occurs relatively quickly: enhanced preoperative plasticity is absent one month later, and only approaches healthy control levels over the next months. It is worth noting that the effect is observed in ADM and FDI as well as APB, suggesting that the pathological spread to heterotopic ulnar nerve-innervated muscles is not normalised by DBS (Ruge et al. 2011).

The reduction of plasticity induced by DBS is similar to that seen in untreated Parkinson's disease and may explain the parkinsonian symptoms that have sometimes been observed in dystonic patients treated with DBS.

The time-course of the DBS effects on the LTP – like PAS after-effects (an early maximum reduction followed by gradual re-increase towards normal) – differ from the monotonic time-course of its effects on SICI/clinical symptoms. In addition, the reduction of plasticity does not correlate with changes in clinical scores. This apparent paradox can be solved considering that the excess of plasticity promotes an abnormal motor learning that ultimately leads to abnormal involuntary movements. On the other hand, even if the excess of plasticity is normalised by DBS, this has no immediate effects on dystonic movement since the abnormal connections have already been 'learned' and take time to be wiped out (Ruge et al. 2011; Quartarone & Hallett 2013). Interestingly, the larger the response to the PAS protocol the more likely were patients able to maintain the clinical improvement obtained after long-term DBS.

This apparently contradictory effect could be explained considering that patients who have the 'highest plasticity' can better restore a normal motor repertoire after long-term DBS. This paradoxical effect might also explain why patients with the most stable 'memories' (and the highest PAS response after years of DBS) are the ones who experience the least decline in clinical symptoms when turning off DBS.

Interestingly, the amount of PAS-induced plasticity after several years of DBS has been found to be related to current drain (which depends on the parameters of stimulation) in one study (Ruge et al. 2011). The current drain can be calculated from the combination of stimulation parameters (pulse height, duration and frequency) used for DBS and the impedance (Kuncel & Grill 2004). A good response to PAS has been found to be associated with low levels of DBS current drain. If this link is causal, then it might be possible to adjust stimulation parameters during chronic stimulation to maximise long-term clinical effects.

Putative Mechanisms of Action of Deep Brain Stimulation

It is now well established that the beneficial effects of DBS in dystonia are not psychogenic (Kupsch et al. 2006; Volkmann et al. 2014). Certainly, the clinical effects of DBS cannot be simply attributed to normalisation of firing rates. Most likely, they are also mediated by a 'silencing' of pathological electrical activity within the basal ganglia network. In this perspective DBS may act by creating a functional lesion within the basal ganglia network while at the same time establishing a new network that upholds normal function.

Several lines of evidence suggest that DBS may exert local and distant effects. Locally DBS causes a blockade of abnormal firing, creating antidromic spikes close to the somata which collide with orthodromic ones. At the same time, orthodromic spikes travel through axons and activate postsynaptic neurons that alter the overall neuronal activity at the target site. In addition, DBS may have distant effects in that coincident antidromic spikes from axonal collaterals affect distant neurons, leading to a long-term synaptic remodelling.

Such synaptic remodelling may explain why the clinical effects of DBS in dystonia are late, taking weeks to months for the full beneficial effect to become evident. Indeed, clinical evidence suggests that there is a biphasic response to stimulation where the phasic component of dystonia tends to improve more rapidly, whereas the tonic or fixed components have a delayed and sometimes more variable response (Krauss 2002).

It is likely that the early improvement of the mobile aspect of dystonia may reflect the direct, local suppression of the abnormal, i.e. 'noisy signal', within the GPi and the associated basal ganglia-thalamo-cortical loop, whereas late improvement may correspond to the synaptic remodelling at cortical and subcortical levels which will normalise function over several weeks (Barow et al. 2014). Therefore the time needed for the tonic symptoms to subside may correspond to the time needed for the 'new' network to be established.

Interestingly, although the clinical effects of DBS may take months to reach a maximum effect after implantation, symptoms reappear only shortly after DBS is switched off during the first years of DBS (Grips et al. 2007), with the mobile components of dystonia reoccurring first. It is likely that when DBS is started, synaptic remodelling improves dystonic postures; however, when DBS is stopped, dystonia reappears because the new functional network 'producing' the beneficial effects is still dependent on the local effect produced by DBS. In this case, when DBS is turned on again symptoms improve rapidly because this functional network can be functionally restarted by the induced local DBS effects (Quartarone & Hallett 2013).

On the other hand, there are cases of sustained relief after long-term DBS discontinuation that may reflect the capacity of DBS to induce distant effects over time, producing structural synaptic effects that lessen or obviate the need for further treatment in susceptible patients (Quartarone & Hallett 2013).

Future research should combine chronic LFP recordings, non-invasive brain stimulation methods and imaging methods to monitor the evolvement of direct and distant effects of DBS in dystonia.

References

Alam M, Sanghera MK, Schwabe K, Lutjens G, Jin X, Song J, von Wrangel C, Stewart RM, Jankovic J, Grossman RG, Darbin O, Krauss JK. 2016. Globus pallidus internus neuronal activity: a comparative study of linear and non-linear features in patients with dystonia or Parkinson's disease. *J Neural Transm (Vienna)* 123(3):231–240.

Alonso-Frech F, Zamarbide I, Alegre M, Rodriguez-Oroz MC, Guridi J, Manrique M, Valencia M, Artieda J, Obeso JA. 2006. Slow oscillatory activity and levodopa-induced dyskinesias in Parkinson's disease. *Brain* 129(Pt 7):1748–1757.

Barow E, Neumann WJ, Brucke C, Huebl J, Horn A, Brown P, Krauss JK, Schneider GH, Kuhn AA. 2014. Deep brain stimulation suppresses pallidal low frequency activity in patients with phasic dystonic movements. *Brain* 137(Pt 11):3012–3024.

Berardelli A, Rothwell JC, Day BL, Marsden CD. 1985. Pathophysiology of blepharospasm and oromandibular dystonia. *Brain* 108(Pt 3):593–608.

Brown P. 2003. Oscillatory nature of human basal ganglia activity: relationship to the pathophysiology of Parkinson's disease. *Mov Disord* 18(4):357–363.

Brown P, Eusebio A. 2008. Paradoxes of functional neurosurgery: clues from basal ganglia recordings. *Mov Disord* 23(1):12–20.

Capelle HH, Blahak C, Schrader C, Baezner H, Kinfe TM, Herzog J, Dengler R, Krauss JK. 2010. Chronic deep brain stimulation in patients with tardive dystonia without a history of major psychosis. *Mov Disord* 25(10):1477–1481.

Chen CC, Kuhn AA, Trottenberg T, Kupsch A, Schneider GH, Brown P. 2006a. Neuronal activity in globus pallidus interna can be synchronized to local field potential activity over 3–12 Hz in patients with dystonia. *Exp Neurol* 202(2):480–486.

Chen CC, Kuhn AA, Hoffmann KT, Kupsch A, Schneider GH, Trottenberg T, Krauss JK, Wohrle JC, Bardinet E, Yelnik J, Brown P. 2006b. Oscillatory pallidal local field potential activity correlates with involuntary EMG in dystonia. *Neurology* 66(3):418–420.

Chen R, Udupa K. 2009. Measurement and modulation of plasticity of the motor system in humans using transcranial magnetic stimulation. *Motor Control* 13(4):442–453.

Coubes P, Roubertie A, Vayssiere N, Hemm S, Echenne B. 2000. Treatment of DYT1-generalised dystonia by stimulation of the internal globus pallidus. *Lancet* 355(9222):2220–2221.

Coubes P, Cif L, El Fertit H, Hemm S, Vayssiere N, Serrat S, Picot MC, Tuffery S, Claustres M, Echenne B, Frerebeau P. 2004. Electrical stimulation of the globus pallidus internus in patients with primary generalized dystonia: long-term results. *J Neurosurg* 101(2):189–194.

Crowell AL, Ryapolova-Webb ES, Ostrem JL, Galifianakis NB, Shimamoto S, Lim DA, Starr PA. 2012. Oscillations in sensorimotor cortex in movement disorders: an electrocorticography study. *Brain* 135(Pt 2):615–630.

Edwards MJ, Huang YZ, Mir P, Rothwell JC, Bhatia KP. 2006. Abnormalities in motor cortical plasticity differentiate manifesting and nonmanifesting DYT1 carriers. *Mov Disord* 21(12):2181–2186.

Eusebio A, Pogosyan A, Wang S, Averbeck B, Gaynor LD, Cantiniaux S, Witjas T, Limousin P, Azulay JP, Brown P. 2009. Resonance in subthalamo-cortical circuits in Parkinson's disease. *Brain* 132(Pt 8):2139–2150.

Foncke EM, Bour LJ, Speelman JD, Koelman JH, Tijssen MA. 2007a. Local field potentials and oscillatory activity of the internal globus pallidus in myoclonus-dystonia. *Mov Disord* 22(3):369–376.

Foncke EM, Bour LJ, van der Meer JN, Koelman JH, Tijssen MA. 2007b. Abnormal low frequency drive in myoclonus-dystonia patients correlates with presence of dystonia. *Mov Disord* 22(9):1299–1307.

Grips E, Blahak C, Capelle HH, Bazner H, Weigel R, Sedlaczek O, Krauss JK, Wohrle JC. 2007. Patterns of reoccurrence of segmental dystonia after discontinuation of deep brain stimulation. *J Neurol Neurosurg Psychiatry* 78(3):318–320.

Groiss SJ, Elben S, Reck C, Voges J, Wojtecki L, Schnitzler A. 2011. Local field potential oscillations of the globus pallidus in Huntington's disease. *Mov Disord* 26(14):2577–2578.

Gruber D, Trottenberg T, Kivi A, Schoenecker T, Kopp UA, Hoffmann KT, Schneider GH, Kuhn AA, Kupsch A. 2009. Long-term effects of pallidal deep brain stimulation in tardive dystonia. *Neurology* 73(1):53–58.

Gruber D, Kuhn AA, Schoenecker T, Kivi A, Trottenberg T, Hoffmann KT, Gharabaghi A, Kopp UA, Schneider GH, Klein C, Asmus F, Kupsch A. 2010. Pallidal and thalamic deep brain stimulation in myoclonus-dystonia. *Mov Disord* 25(11):1733–1743.

Hammond C, Bergman H, Brown P. 2007. Pathological synchronization in Parkinson's disease: networks, models and treatments. *Trends Neurosci* 30(7):357–364.

Hung SW, Hamani C, Lozano AM, Poon YY, Piboolnurak P, Miyasaki JM, Lang AE, Dostrovsky JO, Hutchison WD, Moro E. 2007. Long-term outcome of bilateral pallidal deep brain stimulation for primary cervical dystonia. *Neurology* 68(6):457–459.

Hutchinson WD, Levy R, Dostrovsky JO, Lozano AM, Lang AE. 1997. Effects of apomorphine on globus pallidus neurons in parkinsonian patients. *Ann Neurol* 42(5):767–775.

Hutchison WD, Lang AE, Dostrovsky JO, Lozano AM. 2003. Pallidal neuronal activity: implications for models of dystonia. *Ann Neurol* 53(4):480–488.

Ikoma K, Samii A, Mercuri B, Wassermann EM, Hallett M. 1996. Abnormal cortical motor excitability in dystonia. *Neurology* 46(5):1371–1376.

Johnson MD, Miocinovic S, McIntyre CC, Vitek JL. 2008. Mechanisms and targets of deep brain stimulation in movement disorders. *Neurotherapeutics* 5(2):294–308.

Krauss JK. 2002. Deep brain stimulation for dystonia in adults: overview and developments. *Stereotact Funct Neurosurg* 78(3–4):168–182.

Krauss JK, Yianni J, Loher TJ, Aziz TZ. 2004. Deep brain stimulation for dystonia. *J Clin Neurophysiol* 21(1):18–30.

Kuhn AA, Meyer BU, Trottenberg T, Brandt SA, Schneider GH, Kupsch A. 2003. Modulation of motor cortex excitability by pallidal stimulation in patients with severe dystonia. *Neurology* 60(5):768–774.

Kuhn AA, Kupsch A, Schneider GH, Brown P. 2006. Reduction in subthalamic 8–35 Hz oscillatory activity correlates with clinical improvement in Parkinson's disease. *Eur J Neurosci* 23(7):1956–1960.

Kuhn AA, Brucke C, Schneider GH, Trottenberg T, Kivi A, Kupsch A, Capelle HH, Krauss JK, Brown P. 2008a. Increased beta activity in dystonia patients after drug-induced dopamine deficiency. *Exp Neurol* 214(1):140–143.

Kuhn AA, Kempf F, Brucke C, Gaynor Doyle L, Martinez-Torres I, Pogosyan A, Trottenberg T, Kupsch A, Schneider GH, Hariz MI, Vandenberghe W, Nuttin B, Brown P. 2008b. High-frequency stimulation of the subthalamic nucleus suppresses oscillatory beta activity in patients with Parkinson's disease in parallel with improvement in motor performance. *J Neurosci* 28(24):6165–6173.

Kuncel AM, Grill WM. 2004. Selection of stimulus parameters for deep brain stimulation. *Clin Neurophysiol* 115(11):2431–2441.

Kupsch A, Benecke R, Muller J, Trottenberg T, Schneider GH, Poewe W, Eisner W, Wolters A, Muller JU, Deuschl G, Pinsker MO, Skogseid IM, Roeste GK, Vollmer-Haase J, Brentrup A, Krause M, Tronnier V, Schnitzler A, Voges J, Nikkhah G, Vesper J, Naumann M, Volkmann J, Deep-Brain Stimulation for Dystonia Study Group. 2006. Pallidal deep-brain stimulation in primary generalized or segmental dystonia. *N Engl J Med* 355(19):1978–1990.

Lenz FA, Byl NN. 1999. Reorganization in the cutaneous core of the human thalamic principal somatic sensory nucleus (ventral caudal) in patients with dystonia. *J Neurophysiol* 82(6):3204–3212.

Lenz FA, Suarez JI, Metman LV, Reich SG, Karp BI, Hallett M, Rowland LH, Dougherty PM. 1998. Pallidal activity during dystonia: somatosensory reorganisation and changes with severity. *J Neurol Neurosurg Psychiatry* 65(5):767–770.

Liu X, Wang S, Yianni J, Nandi D, Bain PG, Gregory R, Stein JF, Aziz TZ. 2008. The sensory and motor representation of synchronized oscillations in the globus pallidus in patients with primary dystonia. *Brain* 131(Pt 6):1562–1573.

Marceglia S, Servello D, Foffani G, Porta M, Sassi M, Mrakic-Sposta S, Rosa M, Barbieri S, Priori A. 2010. Thalamic single-unit and local field potential activity in tourette syndrome. *Mov Disord* 25(3):300–308.

Martella G, Tassone A, Sciamanna G, Platania P, Cuomo D, Viscomi MT, Bonsi P, Cacci E, Biagioni S, Usiello A, Bernardi G, Sharma N, Standaert DG, Pisani A. 2009. Impairment of bidirectional synaptic plasticity in the striatum of a mouse model of DYT1 dystonia: role of endogenous acetylcholine. *Brain* 132(Pt 9):2336–2349.

McIntyre CC, Hahn PJ. 2010. Network perspectives on the mechanisms of deep brain stimulation. *Neurobiol Dis* 38(3):329–337.

Merello M, Balej J, Delfino M, Cammarota A, Betti O, Leiguarda R. 1999. Apomorphine induces changes in GPi spontaneous outflow in patients with Parkinson's disease. *Mov Disord* 14(1):45–49.

Merello M, Cerquetti D, Cammarota A, Tenca E, Artes C, Antico J, Leiguarda R. 2004. Neuronal globus pallidus activity in patients with generalised dystonia. *Mov Disord* 19(5):548–554.

Milardi D, Gaeta M, Marino S, Arrigo A, Vaccarino G, Mormina E, Rizzo G, Milazzo C, Finocchio G, Baglieri A, Anastasi G, Quartarone A. 2015. Basal ganglia network by constrained spherical deconvolution: a possible cortico-pallidal pathway? *Mov Disord* 30(3):342–349.

Nakashima K, Rothwell JC, Day BL, Thompson PD, Shannon K, Marsden CD. 1989. Reciprocal inhibition between forearm muscles in patients with writer's cramp and other occupational cramps, symptomatic hemidystonia and hemiparesis due to stroke. *Brain* 112 (Pt 3):681–697.

Nakashima K, Rothwell JC, Thompson PD, Day BL, Berardelli A, Agostino R, Artieda J, Papas SM, Obeso JA, Marsden CD. 1990. The blink reflex in patients with idiopathic torsion dystonia. *Arch Neurol* 47(4):413–416.

Napolitano F, Pasqualetti M, Usiello A, Santini E, Pacini G, Sciamanna G, Errico F, Tassone A, Di Dato V, Martella G, Cuomo D, Fisone G, Bernardi G, Mandolesi G, Mercuri NB, Standaert DG, Pisani A. 2010. Dopamine D2 receptor dysfunction is rescued by adenosine A2A receptor antagonism in a model of DYT1 dystonia. *Neurobiol Dis* 38(3):434–445.

Neumann WJ, Kuhn AA. 2016. Reply: role of cortico-pallidal connectivity in the pathophysiology of dystonia. *Brain* 139(Pt 9):e49.

Neumann WJ, Huebl J, Brucke C, Ruiz MH, Kupsch A, Schneider GH, Kuhn AA. 2012. Enhanced low-frequency oscillatory activity of the subthalamic nucleus in a patient with dystonia. *Mov Disord* 27(8):1063–1066.

Neumann WJ, Jha A, Bock A, Huebl J, Horn A, Schneider GH, Sander TH, Litvak V, Kuhn AA. 2015. Cortico-pallidal oscillatory connectivity in patients with dystonia. *Brain* 138(Pt 7):1894–1906.

Neumann WJ, Degen K, Schneider GH, Brucke C, Huebl J, Brown P, Kuhn AA. 2016. Subthalamic synchronized oscillatory activity correlates with motor impairment in patients with Parkinson's disease. *Mov Disord* 31(11):1748–1751.

Panizza ME, Hallett M, Nilsson J. 1989. Reciprocal inhibition in patients with hand cramps. *Neurology* 39(1):85–89.

Papa SM, Desimone R, Fiorani M, Oldfield EH. 1999. Internal globus pallidus discharge is nearly suppressed during levodopa-induced dyskinesias. *Ann Neurol* 46(5):732–738.

Peterson DA, Sejnowski TJ, Poizner H. 2010. Convergent evidence for abnormal striatal synaptic plasticity in dystonia. *Neurobiol Dis* 37(3):558–573.

Priori A, Foffani G, Pesenti A, Bianchi A, Chiesa V, Baselli G, Caputo E, Tamma F, Rampini P, Egidi M, Locatelli M, Barbieri S, Scarlato G. 2002. Movement-related modulation of neural activity in human basal ganglia and its L-DOPA dependency: recordings from deep brain stimulation electrodes in patients with Parkinson's disease. *Neurol Sci* 23 (Suppl. 2):S101–S102.

Quartarone A, Hallett M. 2013. Emerging concepts in the physiological basis of dystonia. *Mov Disord* 28(7):958–967.

Quartarone A, Bagnato S, Rizzo V, Siebner HR, Dattola V, Scalfari A, Morgante F, Battaglia F, Romano M, Girlanda P. 2003. Abnormal associative plasticity of the human motor cortex in writer's cramp. *Brain* 126(Pt 12):2586–2596.

Quartarone A, Siebner HR, Rothwell JC. 2006. Task-specific hand dystonia: can too much plasticity be bad for you? *Trends Neurosci* 29(4):192–199.

Ridding MC, Sheean G, Rothwell JC, Inzelberg R, Kujirai T. 1995. Changes in the balance between motor cortical excitation and inhibition in focal, task specific dystonia. *J Neurol Neurosurg Psychiatry* 59(5):493–498.

Ruge D, Cif L, Limousin P, Gonzalez V, Vasques X, Hariz MI, Coubes P, Rothwell JC. 2011. Shaping reversibility? Long-term deep brain stimulation in dystonia. The relationship between effects on electrophysiology and clinical symptoms. *Brain* 134(Pt 7):2106–2115.

Silberstein P, Kuhn AA, Kupsch A, Trottenberg T, Krauss JK, Wohrle JC, Mazzone P, Insola A, Di Lazzaro V, Oliviero A, Aziz T, Brown P. 2003. Patterning of globus pallidus local field potentials differs between Parkinson's disease and dystonia. *Brain* 126(Pt 12):2597–2608.

Starr PA, Turner RS, Rau G, Lindsey N, Heath S, Volz M, Ostrem JL, Marks WJ. 2006. Microelectrode-guided implantation of deep brain stimulators into the globus pallidus internus for dystonia: techniques, electrode locations, and outcomes. *J Neurosurg* 104(4):488–501.

Steigerwald F, Hinz L, Pinsker MO, Herzog J, Stiller RU, Kopper F, Mehdorn HM, Deuschl G, Volkmann J. 2005. Effect of propofol anesthesia on pallidal neuronal discharges in generalized dystonia. *Neurosci Lett* 386(3):156–159.

Tang JK, Moro E, Mahant N, Hutchison WD, Lang AE, Lozano AM, Dostrovsky JO. 2007. Neuronal firing rates and patterns in the globus pallidus internus of patients with cervical dystonia differ from those with Parkinson's disease. *J Neurophysiol* 98(2):720–729.

Tisch S, Limousin P, Rothwell JC, Asselman P, Quinn N, Jahanshahi M, Bhatia KP, Hariz M. 2006a. Changes in blink reflex excitability after globus pallidus internus stimulation for dystonia. *Mov Disord* 21(10):1650–1655.

Tisch S, Limousin P, Rothwell JC, Asselman P, Zrinzo L, Jahanshahi M, Bhatia KP, Hariz MI. 2006b. Changes in forearm reciprocal inhibition following pallidal stimulation for dystonia. *Neurology* 66(7):1091–1093.

van Wijk BC, Beudel M, Jha A, Oswal A, Foltynie T, Hariz MI, Limousin P, Zrinzo L, Aziz TZ, Green AL, Brown P, Litvak V. 2016. Subthalamic nucleus phase-amplitude coupling correlates with motor impairment in Parkinson's disease. *Clin Neurophysiol* 127(4):2010–2019.

Vidailhet M, Vercueil L, Houeto JL, Krystkowiak P, Benabid AL, Cornu P, Lagrange C, Tezenas du Montcel S, Dormont D, Grand S, Blond S, Detante O, Pillon B, Ardouin C, Agid Y, Destee A, Pollak P, French Stimulation du Pallidum Interne dans la Dystonie (SPIDY) Study Group. 2005. Bilateral deep-brain stimulation of the globus pallidus in primary generalized dystonia. *N Engl J Med* 352(5):459–467.

Vidailhet M, Yelnik J, Lagrange C, Fraix V, Grabli D, Thobois S, Burbaud P, Welter ML, Xie-Brustolin J, Braga MC, Ardouin C, Czernecki V, Klinger H, Chabardes S, Seigneuret E, Mertens P, Cuny E, Navarro S, Cornu P, Benabid AL, Le Bas JF, Dormont D, Hermier M, Dujardin K, Blond S, Krystkowiak P, Destee A, Bardinet E, Agid Y, Krack P, Broussolle E, Pollak P, French SPIDY-2 Study Group. 2009. Bilateral pallidal deep brain stimulation for the treatment of patients with dystonia-choreoathetosis cerebral palsy: a prospective pilot study. *Lancet Neurol* 8(8):709–717.

Vidailhet M, Jutras MF, Grabli D, Roze E. 2013. Deep brain stimulation for dystonia. *J Neurol Neurosurg Psychiatry* 84(9):1029–1042.

Vitek JL, Chockkan V, Zhang JY, Kaneoke Y, Evatt M, DeLong MR, Triche S, Mewes K, Hashimoto T, Bakay RA. 1999. Neuronal activity in the basal ganglia in patients with generalized dystonia and hemiballismus. *Ann Neurol* 46(1):22–35.

Vitek JL, Zhang J, Hashimoto T, Russo GS, Baker KB. 2012. External pallidal stimulation improves parkinsonian motor signs and modulates neuronal activity throughout the basal ganglia thalamic network. *Exp Neurol* 233(1):581–586.

Volkmann J, Benecke R. 2002. Deep brain stimulation for dystonia: patient selection and evaluation. *Mov Disord* 17 (Suppl. 3):S112–S115.

Volkmann J, Wolters A, Kupsch A, Muller J, Kuhn AA, Schneider GH, Poewe W, Hering S, Eisner W, Muller JU, Deuschl G, Pinsker MO, Skogseid IM, Roeste GK, Krause M, Tronnier V, Schnitzler A, Voges J, Nikkhah G, Vesper J, Classen J, Naumann M, Benecke R, DBS Study Group for Dystonia. 2012. Pallidal deep brain stimulation in patients with primary generalised or segmental dystonia: 5-year follow-up of a randomised trial. *Lancet Neurol* 11(12):1029–1038.

Volkmann J, Mueller J, Deuschl G, Kuhn AA, Krauss JK, Poewe W, Timmermann L, Falk D, Kupsch A, Kivi A, Schneider GH, Schnitzler A, Sudmeyer M, Voges J, Wolters A, Wittstock M, Muller JU, Hering S, Eisner W, Vesper J, Prokop T, Pinsker M, Schrader C, Kloss M, Kiening K, Boetzel K, Mehrkens J, Skogseid IM, Ramm-Pettersen J, Kemmler G, Bhatia KP, Vitek JL, Benecke R, DBS Study Group for Dystonia. 2014. Pallidal neurostimulation in patients with medication-refractory cervical dystonia: a randomised, sham-controlled trial. *Lancet Neurol* 13(9):875–884.

Wang DD, de Hemptinne C, Miocinovic S, Qasim SE, Miller AM, Ostrem JL, Galifianakis NB, San Luciano M, Starr PA. 2016. Subthalamic local field potentials in Parkinson's disease and isolated dystonia: an evaluation of potential biomarkers. *Neurobiol Dis* 89:213–222.

Wang S, Liu X, Yianni J, Green AL, Joint C, Stein JF, Bain PG, Gregory R, Aziz TZ. 2006. Use of surface electromyography to assess and select patients with idiopathic dystonia for bilateral pallidal stimulation. *J Neurosurg* 105(1):21–25.

Weise D, Schramm A, Stefan K, Wolters A, Reiners K, Naumann M, Classen J. 2006. The two sides of associative plasticity in writer's cramp. *Brain* 129(Pt 10):2709–2721.

Welter ML, Grabli D, Vidailhet M. 2010. Deep brain stimulation for hyperkinetics disorders: dystonia, tardive dyskinesia, and tics. *Curr Opin Neurol* 23(4):420–425.

Yianni J, Wang SY, Liu X, Bain PG, Nandi D, Gregory R, Joint C, Stein JF, Aziz TZ. 2006. A dominant bursting electromyograph pattern in dystonic conditions predicts an early response to pallidal stimulation. *J Clin Neurosci* 13(7):738–746.

Yoshida M, Nagatsuka Y, Muramatsu S, Niijima K. 1991. Differential roles of the caudate nucleus and putamen in motor behavior of the cat as investigated by local injection of GABA antagonists. *Neurosci Res* 10(1):34–51.

Chapter 63

Deep Brain Stimulation for Isolated Generalised Dystonia

Binit B. Shah and Elena Moro

Deep brain stimulation has markedly altered the treatment landscape for patients with dystonia. DBS systems have achieved CE mark for dystonia and the therapy is approved for use by the FDA under a humanitarian device exemption. However, a number of key variables necessary to optimise DBS in dystonia have only recently been defined.

Isolated generalised dystonia (IGD) can be a severe disabling syndrome. As discussed earlier in this volume, pharmacologic treatment, chemodenervation and other tools are available for managing symptoms of dystonia. When more conservative measures are not tolerated or fail to provide adequate benefit, DBS is an effective and relatively safe treatment.

In this chapter, we will review the characteristics of IGD, candidacy and timing factors in DBS for IGD, as well as targets, response and durability of response for DBS. Additionally, we will briefly review adverse effects associated with DBS surgery and stimulation, though this will be discussed in more detail in another chapter. A caveat to this discussion is that class I evidence is scant when discussing DBS in IDG and further prospective studies are necessary to corroborate the current evidence.

Background

As reviewed in earlier chapters, dystonia is a syndrome of sustained or intermittent muscle contractions causing abnormal, often repetitive, movements, postures or both (Albanese et al. 2013). Generalised dystonia refers to the distribution of dystonia involving the trunk and two other sites in the body. Isolated dystonia is dystonia that is either idiopathic or due to a defined monogenetic mutation (e.g. the DYT syndromes). A meta-analysis by Steeves et al. estimated the prevalence of isolated dystonia (generalised and non-generalised) to be 0.44 per 100 000, though this likely is an underestimate of the true figure (Steeves et al. 2012).

Circuit Pathology and DBS

The exact mechanism by which DBS influences dystonia is unknown. Dystonia is thought to involve abnormal network physiology in the direct and indirect basal ganglia pathways. In a recent report, Neumann and colleagues (2015) demonstrated three distinct cortico-pallidal circuits in patients who were undergoing DBS for dystonia. Each of these circuits had distinctive oscillatory patterns and the authors posit that DBS may interfere with these networks and modulate abnormal motor circuit signalling. The globus pallidus internus (GPi) is the main output nucleus of the based ganglia to the thalamus and modulation of this target can therefore affect abnormal pathway signalling. The posteroventral lateral portion of the GPi has become the preferred target for IDG.

Candidacy Factors

A number of factors come into play when considering DBS for IGD. Perhaps most important are the requirements that dystonia is disabling and medical therapy has failed to provide satisfactory improvement in symptoms. Disability secondary to dystonia can be defined as limitation in activities of daily living (ADLs), quality of life and pain; although the latter is not commonly seen in PGD to the degree it can be seen in cervical dystonia.

Age and Symptom Duration

Age and duration of symptoms are two variables that are important to consider. There are no clear minimum or maximum age barriers defined for DBS in IGD. Younger patients usually have a shorter duration of symptoms, and this can correlate with less skeletal deformity development secondary to dystonia. Thus, earlier intervention after symptom onset, and relatedly at an earlier age in IGD, may meet with more improvement. Several studies have shown benefit, mostly as defined by improvement in the Burke–Fahn–Marsden rating scale (BFMDRS) movement score, in younger patients with shorter symptom duration with bilateral GPi DBS at one year compared to older patients and those with longer duration of symptoms. Additional studies have shown correlation between shorter duration of symptoms and improvement, though not with age at time of DBS and improvement, suggesting that the more important factor is duration of symptoms (Holloway et al. 2006; Bronte-Stewart et al. 2011). However, other studies have found that age at time of DBS is better correlated with benefit than duration of symptoms (Valldeoriola et al. 2010). Relatedly, Lumsden and colleagues found that proportion of life lived with dystonia was inversely correlated with benefit in primary and secondary childhood dystonia (Lumsden et al. 2013). As noted above, no class I evidence exists to prove benefit with earlier intervention in terms of age or duration of symptoms.

Genetic Factors

Genetic status of patients with IGD is also a key factor in considering DBS. Several studies have shown consistently more marked benefit in patients with DYT1-positive dystonia with bilateral pallidal DBS (Bronte-Stewart et al. 2011; Moro et al. 2013; Vidailhet et al. 2013). As to whether this benefit is more relevant, however, in DYT1-negative dystonia is not entirely clear, though it may be a better predictor of benefit in children and adolescents (Borggraefe et al. 2010).

A recent large, retrospective study by Bruggemann and colleagues reported long-term results of bilateral GPi DBS in patients with DYT6, DYT1 and isolated dystonia without identified monogenic cause (Bruggemann et al. 2015). Follow-up between 1 and 16 months showed marked improvement in nine subjects with a DYT1 mutation (60 per cent improvement from baseline) and in 38 without identified monogenic dystonia (52 per cent improvement), whereas eight patients with DYT6 showed significant reduction in dystonia (32 per cent improvement), but to a lesser degree. Additionally, the rate of responders was lower in the DYT6 group (57 per cent vs >90 per cent in the other two groups). Long-term follow-up between 22 and 92 months of stimulation, however, showed no difference between groups in dystonia reduction: 42 per cent in the DYT6 group, 44 per cent in the DYT1 group and 61 per cent in the idiopathic group. These results suggest that while there may be differences in shorter-term DBS outcomes, longer-term outcomes are comparable between groups. Of note, the authors reported that regardless of group, subjects with earlier DBS after symptom onset had better outcomes, whereas age at onset and preoperative baseline BFMDRS movement scores did not correlate with a beneficial response to DBS. Further prospective study is warranted in identifying the role of genetics on DBS response.

Cognition and Mood

No consensus criteria exist in terms of cognitive or mood factors when considering DBS in IGD. Certainly, mood disorders such as depression and anxiety should be managed appropriately prior to DBS placement. However, a history of presurgical depression or anxiety does not preclude the use of DBS (Meoni et al. 2015). There have been rare reports of suicide after pallidal DBS in dystonia, and the rate of psychiatric disease might be higher in dystonia patients than in the general population. There is no evidence, though, that pallidal DBS is associated with a higher risk of suicidality. Additionally, cognitive abnormalities are an important factor to consider as it pertains to the ability of patients to participate in programming and monitoring of the DBS system. Nevertheless, no evidence exists for a difference in DBS outcome for patients with diminished cognitive function as compared to unimpaired patients.

Brain Imaging

Typically structural imaging of the brain in IGD is unremarkable. That said, imaging may be helpful to exclude secondary causes of dystonia which may be less amenable to benefit from DBS (Bronte-Stewart et al. 2011).

Deep Brain Stimulation Targets and Outcomes

While the pathophysiology of dystonia has not been fully elucidated, it has been shown that network pathology involves bilateral basal ganglia dysfunction in isolated dystonia. As such, bilateral stimulation is almost invariably used for IGD. Initially, due to success with tremor management, thalamic DBS was attempted for dystonia, with mixed results. The thalamic target is not typically used for IGD currently.

Pallidal Stimulation

Bilateral pallidal DBS has the best evidence for benefit in IGD. A class I study and several other studies have demonstrated efficacy of bilateral pallidal stimulation, giving it level B evidence. Kupsch et al. reported on 40 subjects with bilateral pallidal electrodes who were prospectively randomised to active vs sham stimulation for three months. They found a reduction in the BFMDRS movement score of 15.8 points with pallidal stimulation compared to 1.4 points in the sham stimulation group (Kupsch et al. 2006). Blinded assessments at six months after open-label active treatment for all subjects yielded a mean score reduction of 16.7 points. Other studies have shown a similar magnitude of benefit of 60–90 per cent by BFMDRS with bilateral pallidal DBS. Vidailhet and colleagues performed a prospective trial of bilateral pallidal stimulation in 22 subjects with IGD. Mean reduction in BFMDRS movement score was 25.3 points ($p < 0.001$) at three months. The BFMDRS disability score improved by 5.1 points ($p < 0.001$) at 12 months (Vidailhet et al. 2005).

Subthalamic Nucleus Stimulation

More recently bilateral subthalamic nucleus (STN) DBS has been investigated for primary dystonia. For the most part, this has been isolated cervical dystonia; however, reports in IGD exist. A head-to-head blinded crossover study of 13 subjects – of which six had PGD – involving bilateral STN and GPi DBS showed significant improvement via the BFMDRS movement score and quality of life via the SF-36 physical score for either target compared to preoperative baseline (Schjerling et al. 2013). No difference between baseline and either target stimulation was seen with BFMDRS disability score or SF-36 mental score after six months. Comparison between the targets showed no significant difference in either measure or in adverse effects. Three of these subjects had simultaneous stimulation of bilateral STN and GPI in an open-label fashion and showed an additional benefit in quality of life that was not statistically significant. This was a small study with a heterogeneous dystonia population and further study is necessary to determine the efficacy of bilateral STN DBS in IGD.

Other Outcomes and Duration of Benefit

Owing to the relatively young age of IGD patients undergoing DBS, cognitive deficits are relatively uncommon presurgically. No clear evidence of cognitive decline secondary to bilateral

GPi DBS exists. Rather the opposite – cognitive improvement, post-GPi DBS, has been reported, though this may be confounded by reduction in medications postoperatively, particularly anticholinergic medications which can impair memory (Meoni et al. 2015). A limitation of many reports of DBS in IGD is that cognitive testing is not routinely done prior to or after DBS.

Meoni and colleagues reported a prospectively followed cohort of 57 dystonia patients who underwent DBS for dystonia. Of these, 26 had primary generalised or segmental dystonia (Meoni et al. 2015). Thirteen patients had an axis I diagnosis and, after a mean follow-up of 21 months after bilateral GPi DBS, nine had an axis I diagnosis, a non-significant difference between time points. Only one subject had a new onset axis I diagnosis after DBS placement.

Bilateral GPi has shown long-term benefit according to numerous reports, though these often involved small numbers of patients (Cersosimo et al. 2008; Loher et al. 2008; Tagliati et al. 2011). Volkmann et al. followed 38 subjects for five years (initially randomised between sham and active stimulation, but then all treated in an open-label fashion after three months) (Volkmann et al. 2012). They reported durable and significant benefit in the movement score of the BFMDRS at each year of follow-up, with 47.9 per cent improvement at six months, 61.1 per cent improvement at three years and 57.8 per cent improvement at five years. Indeed they found significant improvement between the three- and five-year assessments compared to the six-month assessment, suggesting better effect in the long-term than short-term follow-up. Another study reported a cohort of 14 children with DYT1 mutations and sustained benefit at a mean follow-up of 32 months and with four subjects followed for over 45 months (Markun et al. 2012).

Cif et al. reported a series of 16 subjects, eight with DYT1 mutations, after bilateral GPi DBS placement (Cif et al. 2012). They found sustained benefit with bilateral GPi DBS, but with either suboptimal benefit or some degree of decay of effect despite optimal programming. At a mean stimulation duration of five years they implanted an additional electrode in each GPi. This led to additional benefit over the original surgery as determined by the BFMDRS movement score, with a mean follow-up after additional lead placement of 4.2 years.

Adverse Effects of DBS in IGD

Stimulation-induced adverse effects are related both to the target itself and adjacent structures. The deeper pallidal contact typically lies near the optic tract and stimulation may induce visual phosphenes in the contralateral visual field at low amplitudes of stimulation.

More recently published reports have demonstrated stimulation-induced bradykinesia, freezing of gait, and other parkinsonian features in bilateral pallidal stimulation. This contrasts with improvement of bradykinesia in pallidal DBS in Parkinson's disease. The mechanism by which this effect is seen is unclear, but it is associated with higher frequency (>100 Hz) stimulation (Moro et al. 2013). A more detailed discussion of this aspect is provided in another chapter.

Another potential adverse effect is the development of status dystonicus associated with IPG depletion. This can be seen in patients who have no prior history of status dystonicus, and it is an important reason to monitor the charge of IPGs regularly (Sobstyl et al. 2014). With the newer generation of IPGs, predicting battery depletion is more accurate, but forgetting to charge rechargeable IPG systems or lead fracture and other disruptions in the circuit could also lead to a similar syndrome and vigilance on an ongoing basis is necessary.

Other Considerations

As outlined in this chapter, patients with IGD often undergo DBS placement at an early age. With relatively high current drain and stimulation that is anticipated for decades, battery replacements are an important consideration. There is some evidence to consider rechargeable pulse generators based on patient preference, diminished frequency of surgical IPG replacements and smaller IPG size (Timmermann et al. 2013).

While it is important to optimise medical therapy in IGD prior to considering DBS, after surgery many patients have substantial reduction in dystonia and as such medication weaning is another consideration. Children tend to tolerate anticholinergic agents with less cognitive adverse effects than adults, but they may also suffer from side-effects. A careful, conservative weaning of anti-dystonia medications post-DBS is prudent, with only the minimal effective medication regimen required in the long term. Indeed, many patients are able to wean off all anti-dystonia medications entirely after bilateral pallidal DBS.

Placement of the IPG also is a unique consideration given the young age of many patients with IGD. For younger children placement in the abdominal wall may be better suited.

Conclusions

Bilateral GPi DBS has level A evidence for benefit in IGD based on the American Academy of Neurology classification of evidence. This benefit is sustained and is seen in motor as well as in quality of life scales in IGD. Younger age at time of surgery, shorter duration of symptoms, dearth of fixed posturing and DYT1 mutation status may be positive predictors of benefit with DBS. It is a generally well-tolerated therapy, though stimulation-induced adverse effects including bradykinesia are possible. Additionally, while DBS is not associated with increased psychiatric morbidity, managing depression and anxiety are of importance prior to referring patients for surgery.

References

Albanese A, Bhatia K, Bressman SB, Delong MR, Fahn S, Fung VS, Hallett M, Jankovic J, Jinnah HA, Klein C, Lang AE, Mink JW, Teller JK. 2013. Phenomenology and classification of dystonia: a consensus update. *Mov Disord* 28(7):863–873.

Borggraefe I, Mehrkens JH, Telegravciska M, Berweck S, Botzel K, Heinen F. 2010. Bilateral pallidal stimulation in children and adolescents with primary generalized dystonia: report of six patients and literature-based analysis of predictive outcomes variables. *Brain Dev* 32(3):223–228.

Bronte-Stewart H, Taira T, Valldeoriola F, Merello M, Marks WJ, Jr, Albanese A, Bressman S, Moro E. 2011. Inclusion and exclusion criteria for DBS in dystonia. *Mov Disord* 26(Suppl. 1):S5–S16.

Bruggemann N, Kuhn A, Schneider SA, Kamm C, Wolters A, Krause P, Moro E, Steigerwald F, Wittstock M, Tronnier V, Lozano AM, Hamani C, Poon YY, Zittel S, Wachter T, Deuschl G, Kruger R, Kupsch A, Munchau A, Lohmann K, Volkmann J, Klein C. 2015. Short- and long-term outcome of chronic pallidal neurostimulation in monogenic isolated dystonia. *Neurology* 84(9):895–903.

Cersosimo MG, Raina GB, Piedimonte F, Antico J, Graff P, Micheli FE. 2008. Pallidal surgery for the treatment of primary generalized dystonia: long-term follow-up. *Clin Neurol Neurosurg* 110(2):145–150.

Cif L, Gonzalez-Martinez V, Vasques X, Corlobe A, Moura AM, Bonafe A, Coubes P. 2012. Staged implantation of multiple electrodes in the internal globus pallidus in the treatment of primary generalized dystonia. *J Neurosurg* 116(5):1144–1152.

Holloway KL, Baron MS, Brown R, Cifu DX, Carne W, Ramakrishnan V. 2006. Deep brain stimulation for dystonia: a meta-analysis. *Neuromodulation* 9(4):253–261.

Kupsch A, Benecke R, Muller J, Trottenberg T, Schneider GH, Poewe W, Eisner W, Wolters A, Muller JU, Deuschl G, Pinsker MO, Skogseid IM, Roeste GK, Vollmer-Haase J, Brentrup A, Krause M, Tronnier V, Schnitzler A, Voges J, Nikkhah G, Vesper J, Naumann M, Volkmann J, Deep-Brain Stimulation for Dystonia Study Group. 2006. Pallidal deep-brain stimulation in primary generalized or segmental dystonia. *N Engl J Med* 355(19):1978–1990.

Loher TJ, Capelle HH, Kaelin-Lang A, Weber S, Weigel R, Burgunder JM, Krauss JK. 2008. Deep brain stimulation for dystonia: outcome at long-term follow-up. *J Neurol* 255(6):881–884.

Lumsden DE, Kaminska M, Gimeno H, Tustin K, Baker L, Perides S, Ashkan K, Selway R, Lin JP. 2013. Proportion of life lived with dystonia inversely correlates with response to pallidal deep brain stimulation in both primary and secondary childhood dystonia. *Dev Med Child Neurol* 55(6):567–574.

Markun LC, Starr PA, Air EL, Marks WJ, Jr, Volz MM, Ostrem JL. 2012. Shorter disease duration correlates with improved long-term deep brain stimulation outcomes in young-onset DYT1 dystonia. *Neurosurgery* 71(2):325–330.

Meoni S, Zurowski M, Lozano AM, Hodaie M, Poon YY, Fallis M, Voon V, Moro E. 2015. Long-term neuropsychiatric outcomes after pallidal stimulation in primary and secondary dystonia. *Neurology* 85(5):433–440.

Moro E, Gross RE, Krauss JK. 2013. What's new in surgical treatment for dystonia? *Mov Disord* 28(7):1013–1020.

Neumann WJ, Jha A, Bock A, Huebl J, Horn A, Schneider GH, Sander TH, Litvak V, Kuhn AA. 2015. Cortico-pallidal oscillatory connectivity in patients with dystonia. *Brain* 138(Pt 7):1894–1906.

Schjerling L, Hjermind LE, Jespersen B, Madsen FF, Brennum J, Jensen SR, Lokkegaard A, Karlsborg M. 2013. A randomized double-blind crossover trial comparing subthalamic and pallidal deep brain stimulation for dystonia. *J Neurosurg* 119(6):1537–1545.

Sobstyl M, Zabek M, Kmiec T, Slawek J, Budohoski KP. 2014. Status dystonicus due to internal pulse generator depletion in a patient with primary generalized dystonia. *Mov Disord* 29(2):188–189.

Steeves TD, Day L, Dykeman J, Jette N, Pringsheim T. 2012. The prevalence of primary dystonia: a systematic review and meta-analysis. *Mov Disord* 27(14):1789–1796.

Tagliati M, Krack P, Volkmann J, Aziz T, Krauss JK, Kupsch A, Vidailhet AM. 2011. Long-term management of DBS in dystonia: response to stimulation, adverse events, battery changes, and special considerations. *Mov Disord* 26(Suppl. 1):S54–S62.

Timmermann L, Schupbach M, Hertel F, Wolf E, Eleopra R, Franzini A, Servello D, Skogseid IM, Rumia J, Aliaga AS, Barbe MT, Pauls KA, Lin JP, Moro E, Lloyd A, Maarouf M. 2013. A new rechargeable device for deep brain stimulation: a prospective patient satisfaction survey. *Eur Neurol* 69(4):193–199.

Valldeoriola F, Regidor I, Minguez-Castellanos A, Lezcano E, Garcia-Ruiz P, Rojo A, Salvador A, Castro A, Grandas F, Kulisevsky J, Marti MJ, Martinez-Martin P, Relova L, Rumia J, Camara A, Burguera JA, Linazasoro G, de Val JL, Obeso J, Rodriguez-Oroz MC, Tolosa E, Grupo ESpanol para el EStudio de la EStimulacion PALidal en la DIStonia. 2010. Efficacy and safety of pallidal stimulation in primary dystonia: results of the Spanish multicentric study. *J Neurol Neurosurg Psychiatry* 81(1):65–69.

Vidailhet M, Vercueil L, Houeto JL, Krystkowiak P, Benabid AL, Cornu P, Lagrange C, Tezenas du Montcel S, Dormont D, Grand S, Blond S, Detante O, Pillon B, Ardouin C, Agid Y, Destee A, Pollak P, French Stimulation du Pallidum Interne dans la Dystonie (SPIDY) Study Group. 2005. Bilateral deep-brain stimulation of the globus pallidus in primary generalized dystonia. *N Engl J Med* 352(5):459–467.

Vidailhet M, Jutras MF, Grabli D, Roze E. 2013. Deep brain stimulation for dystonia. *J Neurol Neurosurg Psychiatry* 84(9):1029–1042.

Volkmann J, Wolters A, Kupsch A, Muller J, Kuhn AA, Schneider GH, Poewe W, Hering S, Eisner W, Muller JU, Deuschl G, Pinsker MO, Skogseid IM, Roeste GK, Krause M, Tronnier V, Schnitzler A, Voges J, Nikkhah G, Vesper J, Classen J, Naumann M, Benecke R, DBS Study Group for Dystonia. 2012. Pallidal deep brain stimulation in patients with primary generalised or segmental dystonia: 5-year follow-up of a randomised trial. *Lancet Neurol* 11(12):1029–1038.

Chapter 64

Deep Brain Stimulation for Isolated Focal and Segmental Dystonia

René Reese and Jens Volkmann

Adult-onset focal dystonias are the most prevalent forms of isolated dystonia. The aetiopathogenesis is usually idiopathic in contrast to young-onset dystonias, which frequently have a monogenetic cause. The clinical picture is typically dominated by an involvement of axial muscles including the face, neck or upper spine, with the exception of task-specific dystonias such as writer's cramp or musician's dystonia. The first-line treatment of focal dystonia is the selective denervation of affected muscles by repeated botulinum toxin injections. Botulinum toxin (BTX) therapy has proven to be more effective than systemic drug therapy with anticholinergics. However, it is not without therapeutic failures despite offering substantial symptomatic relief for the majority of patients. Secondary failure of BTX may result from the development of neutralising antibodies, which previously has been estimated to occur in approximately 5 per cent of patients with prolonged treatment (Kessler et al. 1999), but is of less importance with modern BTX formulations. More relevant are those failures associated with complex dystonic movements involving many or difficult-to-inject muscles.

Deep Brain Stimulation for Isolated Focal (Cervical) Dystonia

Because there are very limited pharmacological treatment alternatives for such patients, surgical treatment alternatives have been used for decades, including rhizotomy and posterior ramisectomy. Since the pattern of dystonia might preclude patients from these procedures, deep brain stimulation (DBS) surgery has been considered an option in selected cases. Krauss was the first to describe excellent outcome of pallidal neurostimulation in three patients with refractory cervical dystonia (CD) in 1999 (Krauss et al. 1999). In 2001, Parkin et al. published another three patients (Parkin et al. 2001) and in 2002, Krauss et al. described the clinical outcome in five patients with CD in a prospective study (Krauss et al. 1999). Both studies could demonstrate relevant reduction of dystonic symptoms with pallidal DBS. In the latter, severity of dystonic symptoms, functional disability and pain were improved by 38 per cent, 54 per cent and about 50 per cent, respectively, in the Toronto Western Spasmodic Torticollis Rating Scale (TWSTRS) at three months after surgery. Symptoms were further improved at six months, twelve months and at last follow-up (mean twenty months). The largest change was apparent between preoperative measures and three months follow-up in all items and between three months and six months in the severity score, indicating a rather rapid response to DBS. Of note, hardware problems initially were more frequent in contrast to what had been observed in Parkinson's disease, such as cable fractures in three instances at the connection between lead and extension cable. This may be a general problem in mobile dystonia probably owing to the higher mechanical stress on the implanted system, and it led to reconsideration of where to place the connection (Volkmann et al. 2014).

So far, three subsequent prospective clinical trials have evaluated the safety and efficacy of pallidal neurostimulation for the treatment of CD, and provide class I evidence in favour of this surgical therapy. The Canadian prospective multicentre observer-blinded study of DBS in CD included ten patients with CD who were followed for 12 months after pallidal DBS (Kiss et al. 2007). Motor improvement was 28 per cent at six months and 43 per cent at twelve months (TWSTRS). Pain and disability scores were also improved by 66 per cent and 64 per cent, as well as mood (Beck's Depression Inventory (BDI)) and quality of life (SF-36), by 58 per cent and 24 per cent, respectively. In another prospective, single-centre study using masked outcome assessment, eight patients with cervical dystonia were followed for up to 48 months (mean: 30 months, range: 12–48 months) (Skogseid et al. 2012). This study reports a median reduction in the TWSTRS motor score of 73 per cent at the last follow-up, which was further improved compared to 50 per cent at six months. In the TWSTRS non-motor symptoms scores 'disability' and 'pain', a median improvement of more than 90 per cent was reported at last follow-up, as well as significant improvements in SF-36.

The German prospective, randomised, sham-controlled multicentre trial for bilateral GPi DBS in CD included 62 patients with a total follow-up of six months (Volkmann et al. 2014). All patients were implanted with a neurostimulation system and randomly assigned to a period of three months with either active or sham stimulation. The blinding of the patients was achieved by setting neurostimulation output to either 0.5 V below the threshold for stimulation-induced adverse effects or to 0 V (sham) after a standardised monopolar review of stimulation effects. After three months, the severity of dystonic symptoms was reduced by 26 per cent in the treatment group as measured by the TWSTRS severity score (primary endpoint of the study) compared to 6 per cent in the sham group. There was a significant 3.8 point difference between both groups. The TWSTRS disability score and the Bain tremor score were also significantly improved in the neurostimulation group, whereas the TWSTRS pain score and quality of life (Craniocervical Dystonia Questionnaire 24-score) were not different. At the three-month visit, all patients received programmed stimulation and a second review of the therapeutic efficacy was done after six months of active stimulation in all patients. There was only a minor incremental effect on dystonia severity, with an additional three months of DBS suggesting that most clinical improvement may be seen within the first three months of stimulation. However, long-term follow-up data are still pending. After six months of active stimulation, significant improvements compared to the presurgical baseline were documented in TWSTRS severity score (28 per cent), disability score (46 per cent) and pain (51 per cent), Tsui score (57 per cent), Bain tremor score (66 per cent), and global clinical impression rated by patients (49 per cent) or physicians (53 per cent). The BDI was reduced by 20 per cent, the Cranio-Cervical Dystonia questionnaire-24 showed a 28 per cent improvement. Cognitive function (as measured by the Mattis dementia rating scale) was unaltered. The latter is corroborated by an additional study on 13 of these patients who underwent more elaborate neuropsychological testing prior to surgery and 12 months after continuous GPi DBS (Dinkelbach et al. 2015). In this study, only verbal fluency exhibited a minor decline. Hardware-related complications comprised device infection (n = 3), misplacement/dislocation of electrodes (n = 3) or of the pacemaker (n = 1), stroke/haemorrhage (n = 1) and seizure (n = 1). Four patients reported pain at the extension cable. The most frequent stimulation-induced side-effect was dysarthria (seven patients), which was directly related to stimulation intensity but could be completely resolved by reprogramming in only one patient. In the others, programming had to find a compromise between symptom control and mild speech impairment.

So far, few studies have ascertained a sustained benefit of pallidal stimulation on cervical dystonia during long-term follow-up. However, such data are urgently needed, because patients are expected to require lifelong therapy. An open-label study presented long-term data of patients with CD beyond five years of continuous bilateral GPi DBS (Walsh et al. 2013). Therapeutic efficacy was retrospectively assessed using video ratings done by two experts blinded to patients and treatment at a presurgical baseline exam, and after 7.7 ± 1.9 (Kiss et al. 2007; Skogseid et al. 2012; Walsh et al. 2013; Asahi et al. 2014; Volkmann et al. 2014; Dinkelbach et al. 2015) years after surgery. This study reports an improvement of 48 per cent in the TWSTRS motor score. In two patients, leads had to be explanted unilaterally due to an infection during follow-up. Of note, both patients had a significant benefit also of unilateral stimulation (one ipsi- and one contralateral to the affected sternocleidomastoid muscle). One patient opted for continuous unilateral stimulation without reimplantation of the other electrode. Two patients claimed difficulties in handwriting and fine motor skills as an adverse effect of DBS. One patient complained about slight rigidity of one arm. Dysarthria was transiently observed in two patients and resolved after reprogramming.

Apart from CD, DBS has been tried in selected cases of writer's cramp (Asahi et al. 2014), Meige syndrome and dystonic camptocormia (Reese et al. 2014), with overall beneficial results.

Recommendation

Pallidal neurostimulation is effective and relatively safe in isolated CD (Volkmann et al. 2014). However, little is known about long-term follow-up and a head-to-head comparison of GPi DBS and BTX therapy has not been undertaken yet. The clinical efficacy of GPi DBS in CD might be underestimated by some unfortunate metric properties of the TWSTRS motor scale, which has mostly been used in the studies to determine therapy effects. The TWSTRS scale adds to the severity of the postural abnormality of the head a duration factor, which leads to an overrating of residual mild but permanent head deviations.

DBS surgery in an experienced centre can be recommended for cases of severe CD, if patients have failed on qualified BTX treatment. For other primary focal dystonia, there is no general recommendation, but patients with relevant symptoms impairing daily or professional activities should be sent to a surgical movement disorder centre as well for further consideration and counselling.

Deep Brain Stimulation for Isolated Segmental Dystonia

Dystonia is classified as 'segmental' when two adjacent segments of the body are affected, such as face, neck, upper extremities, lower extremities or trunk. The typical age at onset for segmental dystonia is around 30 years, mostly combining CD with an involvement of the face (Meige syndrome), an upper extremity or the trunk.

A multicentre randomised trial for GPi DBS in 40 patients with primary segmental or generalised dystonia was published in 2006 (Kupsch et al. 2006). This trial included masked outcome assessment through patient videos and a three-month randomised phase comparing sham to verum stimulation in order to control for a possible placebo effect of GPi DBS. The change from baseline on the BFMDRS was significantly greater in the neurostimulation group (−15.8 ± 14.1 points) than in the sham-stimulation group (−1.4 ± 3.8 points, $p < 0.001$) at three months. Thereafter, all patients continued on effective neurostimulation. Six months of continuous neurostimulation led to a 48 per cent reduction of motor symptoms compared to baseline in both groups. Dystonic movements responded often within hours to GPi DBS, while fixed dystonic postures required weeks or months to improve. Remarkably, there was a great variability in motor outcome among patients from less than 25 per cent to more than 75 per cent, with most patients ranging from 25 per cent to 50 per cent. No predictive factor for favourable outcome could be identified. Neither the distribution of dystonia (segmental vs generalised) nor the genotype (DYT1-positive or -negative) had a bearing on the outcome of DBS. The procedure was found to be cognitively safe, led to a reduction of preoperative depressive symptoms and improved quality of life.

Thirty-two of the patients in the parent trial could be followed for up to five years (Volkmann et al. 2012). Motor improvement (BFMDRS) was 61 per cent at three years of stimulation and 58 per cent at five years compared to baseline. The improvement from six months to three years was significant. These long-term data suggest continuing improvement after surgery for up to three years and sustained benefit thereafter. A progressive improvement was limited to the patients with generalised dystonia and may relate to the greater prevalence of fixed dystonic deformities in this group. Non-motor scores remained basically stable throughout the five-year interval. Adverse events were overall rare and serious adverse events requiring hospitalisation were more frequent in generalised dystonia. Most importantly, lead dislodgement, breakage and wiring problems were reported, probably related to the physical stress upon the implanted material caused by the dystonic movements. The most frequent stimulation-related adverse event was dysarthria followed by worsening of dystonia, which could be managed by reprogramming of stimulation.

The findings of these randomised controlled trials are corroborated by two cohort studies using masked-outcome assessment demonstrating 50–60 per cent motor improvement after 12–36 months and by various uncontrolled, open-label cohort studies (Sensi et al. 2009; Valldeoriola et al. 2010).

Recommendation

There is level I evidence in favour of GPi DBS for the treatment of severe, isolated segmental dystonia from two randomised controlled trials. Because pharmacotherapy is usually ineffective in these cases, the surgical options should be discussed early with affected individuals. Surgery should not be delayed within the course of disease to minimise the impact of dystonia on social life (e.g. professional activities or school education) and to avoid secondary orthopaedic complications.

General Remarks

Shorter disease duration seems to be a predictor of good outcome of GPi DBS. Age seems to be less critical, and a retrospective analysis found that older patients had a longer delay to achieve maximum benefit, but did not differ in the magnitude of symptomatic benefit from younger patients at the final follow-up (Isaias et al. 2008, 2011). A careful clinical analysis of treatment failures in the German multicentre study for GPi DBS in segmental and generalised dystonia did not reveal any consistent predictors of poor outcome (Volkmann et al. 2012). It rather suggested that a primary or secondary non-response to DBS is likely the result of an individual combination of multiple possible factors, which may include suboptimal lead placement, programming issues or disease heterogeneity. Therefore, when informing patients about DBS, physicians should not only discuss the average motor improvement obtained in clinical studies. More importantly, patients should be informed about the variability of outcomes in dystonia and the risk of a treatment failure (as defined by less than 25 per cent motor benefit), which can be up to 25 per cent for primary generalised or segmental dystonia even in experienced centres (Volkmann et al. 2012).

Clinical efficacy of GPi DBS in dystonia is critically dependent on electrode location, but the most effective target point within the posteroventral lateral GPi remains elusive. Data from a small cohort study confirm the posteroventral lateral portion ('motor part') as most effective (Tisch et al. 2007). The 'motor' GPi is bordered laterally and posteriorly by the internal capsule containing corticospinal and corticobulbar fibres. Ventrally the optic tract is forming the boundary. Current spread may stimulate these structures, leading to immediate and non-habituating side-effects limiting higher stimulation intensities.

Improvement of dystonic movements by GPi DBS is delayed by several minutes to hours after stimulation onset, and occasionally it may take months until the full benefit is seen. Clinical outcome and electrode location within the motor portion of the GPi seem to bear no correlation (Hamani et al. 2008), such that the adverse event threshold should guide the implantation procedure of the electrodes to increase the therapeutic window. As a rule of thumb, intraoperative thresholds for tonic muscle contraction should lie between 3 and 6 mA (90 μs, 130 Hz). Lower intraoperative thresholds may imply that clinically relevant stimulation intensities to control dystonic movements may not be achieved in postoperative programming sessions. Thresholds above 6 mA may suggest a target outside the motor GPi (e.g. the electrode being too far lateral or anterior).

There have been several reports of clinically relevant bradykinesia due to GPi DBS in dystonia (Ostrem et al. 2007; Berman et al. 2009; Zauber et al. 2009; Schrader et al. 2010; Blahak et al. 2011; Walsh et al. 2013; Volkmann et al. 2014; Reese et al. 2015). Symptoms may range from difficulties in fine hand skills to relevant hypokinetic gait disturbances and full-blown parkinsonism unresponsive to levodopa. Underlying pathomechanisms and risk factors are not known. The severity of a bradykinetic gait disorder and parkinsonian signs are mostly paralleled by a good control of dystonic symptoms by GPi DBS. In these cases, stimulation parameters must be titrated to a compromise between dystonia relief and bradykinesia. The subthalamic nucleus has already been suggested as an alternative target for the treatment of dystonia, with encouraging clinical results and without bradykinetic side-effects (Kleiner-Fisman et al. 2007; Ostrem et al. 2011), but stimulation caused transient dyskinesia in almost all patients. The small number of patients treated so far with STN DBS, the lack of a controlled trial and the lack of long-term data does not justify a change in clinical practice so far.

References

Asahi T, Koh M, Kashiwazaki D, Kuroda S. 2014. Stereotactic neurosurgery for writer's cramp: report of two cases with an overview of the literature. *Stereotact Funct Neurosurg* 92(6):405–411.

Berman BD, Starr PA, Marks WJ, Ostrem JL. 2009. Induction of bradykinesia with pallidal deep brain stimulation in patients with cranial-cervical dystonia. *Stereotact Funct Neurosurg* 87(1):37–44.

Blahak C, Capelle HH, Baezner H, Kinfe TM, Hennerici MG, Krauss JK. 2011. Micrographia induced by pallidal DBS for segmental dystonia: a subtle sign of hypokinesia? *J Neural Transm* 118(4):549–553.

Dinkelbach L, Mueller J, Poewe W, Delazer M, Elben S, Wolters A, Karner E, Wittstock M, Benecke R, Schnitzler A, Volkmann J, Sudmeyer M. 2015. Cognitive outcome of pallidal deep brain stimulation for primary cervical dystonia: one year follow up results of a prospective multicenter trial. *Parkinsonism Relat Disord* 21(8):976–980.

Hamani C, Moro E, Zadikoff C, Poon YY, Lozano AM. 2008. Location of active contacts in patients with primary dystonia treated with globus pallidus deep brain stimulation. *Neurosurgery* 62(3 Suppl. 1):217–223.

Isaias IU, Alterman RL, Tagliati M. 2008. Outcome predictors of pallidal stimulation in patients with primary dystonia: the role of disease duration. *Brain* 131(Pt 7):1895–1902.

Isaias IU, Volkmann J, Kupsch A, Burgunder JM, Ostrem JL, Alterman RL, Mehdorn HM, Schonecker T, Krauss JK, Starr P, Reese R, Kuhn AA, Schupbach WM, Tagliati M. 2011. Factors predicting protracted improvement after pallidal DBS for primary dystonia: the role of age and disease duration. *J Neurol* 258(8):1469–1476.

Kessler KR, Skutta M, Benecke R, German Dystonia Study Group. 1999. Long-term treatment of cervical dystonia with botulinum toxin A: efficacy, safety, and antibody frequency. *J Neurol* 246(4):265–274.

Kiss ZH, Doig-Beyaert K, Eliasziw M, Tsui J, Haffenden A, Suchowersky O, Functional and Stereotactic Section of the Canadian Neurosurgical Society, Canadian Movement Disorders Group. 2007. The Canadian multicentre study of deep brain stimulation for cervical dystonia. *Brain* 130(Pt 11):2879–2886.

Kleiner-Fisman G, Liang GS, Moberg PJ, Ruocco AC, Hurtig HI, Baltuch GH, Jaggi JL, Stern MB. 2007. Subthalamic nucleus deep brain stimulation for severe idiopathic dystonia: impact on severity, neuropsychological status, and quality of life. *J Neurosurg* 107(1):29–36.

Krauss JK, Pohle T, Weber S, Ozdoba C, Burgunder JM. 1999. Bilateral stimulation of globus pallidus internus for treatment of cervical dystonia. *Lancet* 354(9181):837–838.

Krauss JK, Loher TJ, Pohle T, Weber S, Taub E, Barlocher CB, Burgunder JM. 2002. Pallidal deep brain stimulation in patients with cervical dystonia and severe cervical dyskinesias with cervical myelopathy. *J Neurol Neurosurg Psychiatry* 72(2):249–256.

Kupsch A, Benecke R, Muller J, Trottenberg T, Schneider GH, Poewe W, Eisner W, Wolters A, Muller JU, Deuschl G, Pinsker MO, Skogseid IM, Roeste GK, Vollmer-Haase J, Brentrup A, Krause M, Tronnier V, Schnitzler A, Voges J, Nikkhah G, Vesper J, Naumann M, Volkmann J, Deep-Brain Stimulation for Dystonia Study Group. 2006. Pallidal deep-brain stimulation in primary generalized or segmental dystonia. *N Engl J Med* 355(19):1978–1990.

Ostrem JL, Marks WJ, Volz MM, Heath SL, Starr PA. 2007. Pallidal deep brain stimulation in patients with cranial-cervical dystonia (Meige syndrome). *Mov Disord* 22(13):1885–1891.

Ostrem JL, Racine CA, Glass GA, Grace JK, Volz MM, Heath SL, Starr PA. 2011. Subthalamic nucleus deep brain stimulation in primary cervical dystonia. *Neurology* 76(10):870–878.

Parkin S, Aziz T, Gregory R, Bain P. 2001. Bilateral internal globus pallidus stimulation for the treatment of spasmodic torticollis. *Mov Disord* 16(3):489–493.

Reese R, Knudsen K, Falk D, Mehdorn HM, Deuschl G, Volkmann J. 2014. Motor outcome of dystonic camptocormia treated with pallidal neurostimulation. *Parkinsonism Relat Disord* 20(2):176–179.

Reese R, Fasano A, Knudsen K, Herzog J, Falk D, Mehdorn HM, Deuschl G, Volkmann J. 2015. Full parkinsonian triad induced by pallidal high-frequency stimulation in cervical dystonia. *Mov Disord Clin Pract* 2(1):99–101.

Schrader C, Capelle HH, Luetjens G, Kinfe TM, Dressler D, Krauss JK. 2010. Pallidal deep brain stimulation may induce freezing of gait in patients with focal and segmental dystonia. *Mov Disord* 25(Suppl. 1): S466–S467.

Sensi M, Cavallo MA, Quatrale R, Sarubbo S, Biguzzi S, Lettieri C, Capone JG, Tugnoli V, Tola MR, Eleopra R. 2009. Pallidal stimulation for segmental dystonia: long term follow up of 11 consecutive patients. *Mov Disord* 24(12):1829–1835.

Skogseid IM, Ramm-Pettersen J, Volkmann J, Kerty E, Dietrichs E, Roste GK. 2012. Good long-term efficacy of pallidal stimulation in cervical dystonia: a prospective, observer-blinded study. *Eur J Neurol* 19(4):610–615.

Tisch S, Zrinzo L, Limousin P, Bhatia KP, Quinn N, Ashkan K, Hariz M. 2007. Effect of electrode contact location on clinical efficacy of pallidal deep brain stimulation in primary generalised dystonia. *J Neurol Neurosurg Psychiatry* 78(12):1314–1319.

Valldeoriola F, Regidor I, Minguez-Castellanos A, Lezcano E, Garcia-Ruiz P, Rojo A, Salvador A, Castro A, Grandas F, Kulisevsky J, Marti MJ, Martinez-Martin P, Relova L, Rumia J, Camara A, Burguera JA, Linazasoro G, de Val JL, Obeso J, Rodriguez-Oroz MC, Tolosa E, Grupo ESpanol para el EStudio de la EStimulacion PALidal en la DIStonia. 2010. Efficacy and safety of pallidal stimulation in primary dystonia: results of the Spanish multicentric study. *J Neurol Neurosurg Psychiatry* 81(1):65–69.

Volkmann J, Wolters A, Kupsch A, Muller J, Kuhn AA, Schneider GH, Poewe W, Hering S, Eisner W, Muller JU, Deuschl G, Pinsker MO, Skogseid IM, Roeste GK, Krause M, Tronnier V, Schnitzler A, Voges J, Nikkhah G, Vesper J, Classen J, Naumann M, Benecke R, DBS Study Group for Dystonia. 2012. Pallidal deep brain stimulation in patients with primary generalised or segmental dystonia: 5-year follow-up of a randomised trial. *Lancet Neurol* 11(12):1029–1038.

Volkmann J, Mueller J, Deuschl G, Kuhn AA, Krauss JK, Poewe W, Timmermann L, Falk D, Kupsch A, Kivi A, Schneider GH, Schnitzler A, Sudmeyer M, Voges J, Wolters A, Wittstock M, Muller JU, Hering S, Eisner W, Vesper J, Prokop T, Pinsker M, Schrader C, Kloss M, Kiening K, Boetzel K, Mehrkens J, Skogseid IM, Ramm-Pettersen J, Kemmler G, Bhatia KP, Vitek JL, Benecke R, DBS Study Group for Dystonia. 2014. Pallidal neurostimulation in patients with medication-refractory cervical dystonia: a randomised, sham-controlled trial. *Lancet Neurol* 13(9):875–884.

Walsh RA, Sidiropoulos C, Lozano AM, Hodaie M, Poon YY, Fallis M, Moro E. 2013. Bilateral pallidal stimulation in cervical dystonia: blinded evidence of benefit beyond 5 years. *Brain* 136(Pt 3):761–769.

Zauber SE, Watson N, Comella CL, Bakay RA, Metman LV. 2009. Stimulation-induced parkinsonism after posteroventral deep brain stimulation of the globus pallidus internus for craniocervical dystonia. *J Neurosurg* 110(2):229–233.

Chapter 65

Deep Brain Stimulation for Meige Syndrome

Joachim K. Krauss

Meige syndrome is a unique form of segmental dystonia characterised by blepharospasm combined with oromandibular dystonia which may be associated also with cervical dystonia (Tolosa & Klawans 1979; Jankovic & Ford 1983; Tolosa & Marti 1988). Both primary and secondary manifestations have been described (Jankovic & Ford 1983; Ananth et al. 1988). Most frequently, Meige syndrome starts in the fifth or sixth decade of life with a 3:1 female preponderance (Jankovic & Ford 1983). Blepharospasm may result in functional blindness, and quality of life may be severely compromised in patients with refractory Meige syndrome (Tolosa & Marti 1988).

Treatment Options and Indications for Deep Brain Stimulation

Treatment options for Meige syndrome primarily consist of medication and local injection of botulinum toxin. Medical treatment including tetrabenazine, benzodiazepines and anticholinergics has only limited efficacy, and it is often burdened by side-effects (Jankovic & Ford 1983). Local botulinum toxin injections may be helpful in particular for blepharospasm, but its effect on oromandibular dystonia has been more limited (Jankovic & Orman 1987).

When pallidal deep brain stimulation (DBS) was introduced in the late 1990s, its primary indications were generalised dystonia and complex cervical dystonia (Krauss et al. 1999; Coubes et al. 2000). There were few reports which indicated that both blepharospasm and oromandibular dystonia improved as well in these patients, yet with rather inconsistent results (Muta et al. 2001; Vercueil et al. 2001; Bereznai et al. 2002). Successful pallidal DBS for isolated Meige syndrome was first reported in 2003 (Capelle et al. 2003). Since then several case reports and case series have been published (Ostrem et al. 2007; Blomstedt et al. 2008; Ghang et al. 2010; Limotai et al. 2011; Sako et al. 2011; Sobstyl et al. 2014). Although the efficacy of pallidal DBS for Meige syndrome still needs to be ascertained by a prospective randomised study, it is thought to be indicated nowadays primarily in patients who have been poor responders to botulinum toxin injections.

Outcome of Deep Brain Stimulation

Since the introduction of bilateral pallidal DBS for treatment of isolated Meige syndrome, it has become evident that the quantification of improvement poses particular difficulties because of the lack of appropriate rating scales both with regard to ceiling and bottoming effects and the limited experience with determination of quality of life in these patients. In general, studies have confirmed a beneficial effect for improvement of both blepharospasm and oromandibular dystonia with a lesser effect, however, on speech and swallowing (Reese et al. 2011; Wang et al. 2016). The posteroventral globus pallidus internus (GPi) was targeted bilaterally with only few exceptions. Improvement may be observed rarely directly postoperatively, but more frequently a protracted course with delayed benefit over several weeks or months has been reported (Ostrem et al. 2014).

In a multicentre retrospective study design including video assessment by an independent rater, Reese and colleagues reported long-term outcome for 12 patients with Meige syndrome followed for up to 78 months after bilateral pallidal DBS in 2011 (Reese et al. 2011). Patients' mean age at the time of surgery was 64.5 years with a mean history of dystonia of 8.3 years. The Burke–Fahn–Marsden Dystonia Rating Scale (BFMDRS) motor score was improved by 45 per cent at early follow-up (mean 4.4 months), and by 53 per cent at long-term follow-up (38.8 months). There were significant improvements both for the subscores for eyes (38 per cent at short term, 47 per cent at long term) and mouth (50 per cent at short term, 56 per cent at long term). Speech and swallowing improved by 44 per cent and by 64 per cent, at short term versus long term. Evaluation with the Blepharospasm Movement Scale indicated mean improvement of 25 per cent and 38 per cent, respectively. According to the Abnormal Involuntary Movement Scale, mean improvement was rated as 44 per cent and 49 per cent. Clinically relevant benefit (defined as a change of 25 per cent or more on the BFMDRS motor score) was achieved in all patients. In that regard the clinical benefit obtained was similar to that of patients with generalised dystonia or other forms of segmental dystonia.

More heterogeneous results were reported in a study published by Limotai et al., also in 2011 (Limotai et al. 2011). In that study the BFMDRS motor score in six patients who underwent pallidal DBS improved by 45 per cent at six months and by 64 per cent at twelve months, which was paralleled by a similar benefit as assessed by the Unified Dystonia Rating Scale. Two patients had less than 20 per cent benefit. Remarkably, both had severe speech and swallowing problems. In two patients unilateral DBS was applied initially, but contralateral stimulation was supplemented in the further cause.

Patients' data from different centres with pallidal DBS for Meige syndrome were summarised and collectively analysed in two manuscripts. According to the meta-analysis of Andrews et al., the mean improvement in 17 published patients was 64 per cent on the BFMDRS motor score (Andrews et al. 2010). The more recent review of Wang and colleagues (2016) identified a total of 75 patients with Meige syndrome (some of them were counted twice apparently) who underwent pallidal DBS or (subthalamic nucleus) STN DBS (six patients). Analysis of the pooled data showed a mean improvement of 67 per cent in the BFMDRS motor score, and a mean improvement of 56 per cent in the BFMDRS disability score.

The GPi Target for Meige Syndrome and Postoperative Programming

It is unclear whether patients with Meige syndrome would benefit from targeting a specific area within the posteroventral lateral GPi. Thus far, the somatotopy of the GPi has not been fully clarified and it has been shown that there is a considerable overlap of arm, leg and trunk sensorimotor areas (Vayssiere et al. 2004).

It appears that most centres apply similar algorithms for programming of DBS in patients with Meige syndrome than for other manifestations of dystonia. Usually, a monopolar review is performed first to check system integrity and to gauge thresholds for side-effects. Initial settings may apply either monopolar stimulation of a lower pallidal contact or bipolar stimulation. Stimulation settings in the German multicentre study were within the following ranges: 130–210 Hz, pulse width 60–210 μsec, and amplitude between 2.5 and 5 V (Reese et al. 2011).

Low-frequency stimulation has been used only exceptionally and there is no rigorous study on its use in Meige syndrome (Limotai et al. 2011). Stimulation in cycling mode with stimulation turned off at night has been reported to provide similar relief as continuous stimulation in a single patient after two years of chronic pallidal DBS (Tai et al. 2011).

Side-Effects

Surgical complications and side-effects related to technology are similar in patients with Meige syndrome to other patients with dystonia undergoing DBS. These patients, however, may be more prone to develop bradykinetic side-effects, although systematic studies on this subject are lacking (Ostrem et al. 2007; Berman et al. 2009; Blahak et al. 2011; Limotai et al. 2011; Schrader et al. 2011). Remarkably, in the study of Ostrem and colleagues on pallidal DBS, four out of six patients developed bradykinesia despite good control of dystonia (Ostrem et al. 2007). Bradykinesia was generally mild, but was described to limit overall clinical benefit.

Long-Term Outcome

Outcome beyond a period of three years has only rarely been reported. We have published seven-year follow-up in our pilot patient in 2008 (Loher et al. 2008). At that time there was stable improvement with a slight increase of stimulation amplitude. We still follow this patient, who has sustained benefit after 15 years of chronic DBS.

Long-term follow-up at ten years after pallidal DBS has been published in a patient with acquired segmental dystonia advanced from Meige syndrome after treatment with neuroleptics. The patient previously had undergone bilateral thalamotomy which, however, did not yield sustained relief. Bilateral pallidal DBS provided stable relief both in the BFMDRS motor and disability scores with no worsening in the long term (Inoue et al. 2010).

Sako and colleagues noted sustained and long-lasting improvement in a cohort of five patients with Meige syndrome after bilateral pallidal DBS (Sako et al. 2011). At a mean follow-up of 49 months, the BFMDRS motor score was improved by a mean of 84 per cent and the disability score by a mean 89%. Both higher preoperative BFMDRS motor and disability scores seemed to indicate greater postoperative benefit.

Other Targets

There is little experience with other targets than the GPi for DBS in patients with Meige syndrome. The STN has been chosen in a few instances in two centres with the primary rationale to avoid the possible bradykinetic side-effects associated occasionally with GPi DBS (Ostrem et al. 2014; Wang et al. 2016). Decline of the initial benefit at one year after STN DBS was reported to occur in one patient in the series of Wang and colleagues (Wang et al. 2016). Overall, only three of the six patients with STN DBS had improvement in the BFMDRS motor score exceeding 60 per cent at the last reported follow-up.

Future Prospects

There is ample evidence now that pallidal DBS is a feasible therapeutic strategy in patients with otherwise refractory Meige syndrome with relatively few side-effects. It would be useful to plan a study with a prospective randomised design with sham stimulation and blinded assessment similar to those that have been performed in generalised and cervical dystonia (Kupsch et al. 2006; Volkmann et al. 2014). Because of the rarity of Meige syndrome such a study might be conducted, however, only on a more global geographical level. Another intriguing question is whether or not pallidal DBS should be offered also to patients with blepharospasm only. Proof of principle comes from a recent case report that indicated an 88 per cent improvement in the BFMDRS motor score at 15 months postoperatively (Yamada et al. 2016). Further study on this subject certainly is required.

References

Ananth J, Edelmuth E, Dargan B: 1988. Meige's syndrome associated with neuroleptic treatment. *Am J Psychiatry* 145:513–515.

Andrews C, Aviles-Olmos I, Hariz M, Foltynie T: 2010. Which patients with dystonia benefit from deep brain stimulation? A metaregession of individual patient outcomes. *J Neurol Neurosurg Psychiatry* 81:1383–1389.

Bereznai B, Steude U, Seelos K, Botzel K: 2002. Chronic high-frequency globus pallidus internus stimulation in different types of dystonia: a clinical, video, and MRI report of six patients presenting with segmental, cervical, and generalized dystonia. *Mov Disord* 17:138–144.

Berman BD, Starr PA, Marks WJ, Jr, Ostrem JL: 2009. Induction of bradykinesia with pallidal deep brain stimulation in patients with cranial-cervical dystonia. *Stereotact Funct Neurosurg* 87:37–44.

Blahak C, Capelle HH, Baezner H, Kinfe TM, Hennerici MG, Krauss JK: 2011. Micrographia induced by pallidal DBS for segmental dystonia: a subtle sign of hypokinesia? *J Neural Transm* 118:549–553.

Blomstedt P, Tisch S, Hariz MI: 2008. Pallidal deep brain stimulation in the treatment of Meige syndrome. *Acta Neurol Scand* 118:198–202.

Capelle HH, Weigel R, Krauss JK: 2003. Bilateral stimulation of the globus pallidus for treatment of blepharospasm-oromandibular dystonia (Meige syndrome). *Neurology* 60:2017–2018.

Coubes P, Roubertie A, Vayssiere N, Hemm S, Echenne B: 2000. Treatment of DYT1-generalised dystonia by stimulation of the internal globus pallidus. *Lancet* 355:2220–2221.

Ghang JY, Lee MK, Jun SM, Ghang CG: 2010. Outcome of pallidal deep brain stimulation in Meige syndrome.*J Korean Neurosurg Soc* 48:134–138.

Inoue N, Nagahiro S, Kaji R, Goto S: 2010. Long-term suppression of Meige syndrome after pallidal stimulation: a 10-year follow-up study. *Mov Disord* 25:1756–1758.

Jankovic J, Ford J: 1983. Blepharospasm and orofacial-cervical dystonia: clinical and pharmacological findings in 100 patients. *Ann Neurol* 13:402–411.

Jankovic J, Orman J: 1987. Botulinum A toxin for cranial-cervical dystonia: a double-blind, placebo-controlled study. *Neurology* 37:616–623.

Krauss JK, Pohle T, Weber S, Ozdoba C, Burgunder JM: 1999. Bilateral deep brain stimulation of the globus pallidus internus for treatment of cervical dystonia. *Lancet* 354:837–838.

Kupsch A, Benecke R, Müller J, Trottenberg T, Schneider GH, Poewe W, Eisner W, Wolters A, Müller JU, Deuschl G, Pinsker MO, Skogseid IM, Roeste GK, Vollmer-Haase J, Brentrup A, Krause M, Tronnier V, Schnitzler A, Voges J, Nikkhah G, Vesper J, Naumann M, Volkmann J; Deep-Brain Stimulation for Dystonia Study Group: 2006. Pallidal deep brain stimulation in primary generalized or segmental dystonia. *N Engl J Med* 355:1978–1990.

Limotai N, Go C, Oyama G, Hwynn N, Zesiewicz T, Foote K, Bhidayasiri R, Malaty I, Zeilman P, Rodriguez R, Okun MS: 2011. Mixed results for GPi-DBS in the treatment of cranio-facial and cranio-cervical dystonia symptoms. *J Neurol* 258:2069–2074.

Loher TJ, Capelle HH, Kaelin-Lang A, Weber S, Burgunder JM, Krauss JK: 2008. Deep brain stimulation for dystonia: outcome at long-term follow-up (3 years or longer). *J Neurol* 255:881–884.

Muta D, Goto S, Nishikawa S, Hamasaki T, Ushio Y, Inoue N, Mita S: 2001. Bilateral pallidal stimulation for idiopathic segmental axial dystonia advanced from Meige syndrome refractory to bilateral thalamotomy. *Mov Disord* 16:774–777.

Ostrem JL, Marks WJ Jr, Volz MM, Heath SL, Starr PA: 2007. Pallidal deep brain stimulation in patients with cranial-cervical dystonia (Meige syndrome). *Mov Disord* 22:1885–1891.

Ostrem JL, Markun LC, Glass GA, Racine CA, Volz MM, Heath SL, de Hemptinne C, Starr PA: 2014. Effect of frequency on subthalamic nucleus deep brain stimulation in primary dystonia. *Parkinsonism Relat Disord* 20:432–438.

Reese R, Gruber D, Schoenecker T, Baezner HJ, Blahak C, Capelle HH, Falk D, Herzog J, Pinsker MO, Schneider GH, Schrader C, Deuschl G, Mehdorn HM, Kupsch A, Volkmann J, Krauss JK: 2011. Long-term clinical outcome in Meige syndrome treated with internal pallidum deep brain stimulation. *Mov Disord* 26:691–698.

Sako W, Morigaki R, Mizobuchi Y, Tsuzuki T, Ima H, Ushio Y, Nagahiro S, Kaji R, Goto S: 2011. Meige syndrome: bilateral pallidal deep brain stimulation in primary Meige syndrome. *Parkinsonism Rel Disord* 17:123–125.

Schrader C, Capelle HH, Kinfe TM, Blahak C, Baezner HJ, Lütjens G, Dressler D, Krauss JK: 2011. GPi DBS may induce a hypokinetic gait disorder with freezing of gait in patients with dystonia. *Neurology* 77:483–488.

Sobstyl M, Zabek M, Mossakowski Z, Zaczynski A: 2014. Pallidal deep brain stimulation in the treatment of Meige syndrome. *Neurol Neurochir Pol* 48:196–199.

Tai CH, Wu RM, Liu HM, Tsai CW, Tseng SH: 2011. Meige syndrome relieved by bilateral pallidal stimulation with cycling mode: case report. *Neurosurgery* 69:E1333–E1337.

Tolosa E, Klawans HL: 1979. Meige disease: a clinical form of facial convulsion, bilateral and medial. *Arch Neurol* 36:635–637.

Tolosa E, Marti MJ: 1988. Blepharospasm-oromandibular dystonia syndrome (Meige's syndrome): clinical aspects. *Adv Neurol* 49:73–84.

Vayssiere N, van der Gaag N, Cif L, Hemm S, Verdier R, Frerebeau P, Coubes P: 2004. Deep brain stimulation for dystonia confirming a somatotopic organization in the globus pallidus internus. *J Neurosurg* 101:181–188.

Vercueil L, Pollak P, Fraix V, Caputo E, Moro E, Benazzouz E, Xie J, Koudsie A, Benabid AL: 2001. Deep brain stimulation in the treatment of severe dystonia. *J Neurol* 248:695–700.

Volkmann J, Mueller J, Deuschl G, Kühn AA, Krauss JK, Poewe W, Timmermann L, Falk D, Kupsch A, Kivi A, Schneider GH, Schnitzler A, Südmeyer M, Voges J, Wolters A, Wittstock M, Müller JU, Hering S, Eisner W, Vesper J, Prokop T, Pinsker M, Schrader C, Kloss M, Kiening K, Boetzel K, Mehrkens J, Skogseid IM, Ramm-Pettersen J, Kemmler G, Bhatia KP, Vitek JL, Benecke R; DBS Study Group for Dystonia: 2014. Pallidal neurostimulation in patients with medication-refractory cervical dystonia: a randomised, sham-controlled trial. *Lancet Neurol* 13:875–884.

Wang X, Zhang C, Wang Y, Liu C, Zhao B, Zhang J, Hu W, Shao X, Zhang K: 2016. Deep brain stimulation for craniocervical dystonia (Meige syndrome): a report of four patients and a literature-based analysis of its treatment effects. *Neuromodulation* 19:818–823.

Yamada K, Shinojima N, Hamasaki T, Kuratsu J: 2016. Pallidal stimulation for medically intractable blepharospasm. *BJM Case Rep* doi: 10.1136/bcr-2015-214241.

Chapter 66

Contemporary Thalamotomy for Dystonia

Takaomi Taira, Shiro Horisawa, Nobuhiko Takeda and Tomoko Hanada

Dystonia is not a uniform disorder; it is heterogeneous in symptomatology and there are many different clinical manifestations ranging from focal to generalised forms. Stereotactic functional neurosurgery is an important method for the treatment of dystonias, and used generally for management of severe generalised or segmental dystonias. Patients with focal hand dystonia (FHD), such as writer's cramp and musician's dystonia, though its incidence is much higher, are not considered as surgical candidates in general. Treatment of task-specific FHD (TSFHD) is extremely difficult. Many patients are not satisfied with the existing medical treatment, including botulinum toxin injections, especially when the symptoms disturb their professional activities. Although the incidence of TSFHD is much higher than generalised dystonia, neurosurgical treatment of TSFHD has been rarely performed, probably because the symptoms seem to be too minor for surgeons to select an interventional approach. However, it should be remembered that even if the symptoms of TSFHD may be minor to physicians, they are very serious problems for the patients, as described by Poore many years ago (Poore 1887).

The authors have been treating TSFHD with stereotactic ablation of the ventro-oralis nucleus of the thalamus (Vo thalamotomy). The effect is immediate during the operation and is sustained for a long time. Although this is an invasive treatment that requires highly sophisticated techniques and may carry surgical risks, long-term improvement of TSFHD is possible with such an approach.

History

There have been few reports on neurosurgical treatment of FHD until the 2000s. Siegfried et al. reported a case of cure of tremulous writer's cramp by stereotaxic thalamotomy in 1969 (Siegfried et al. 1969). Mempel et al. reported successful results of cryo-thalamotomy for writer's cramp in 1986 in Polish (Mempel et al. 1986). Dr Sobstyl in Poland, a pupil of Mempel, recently translated it to English (unpublished). They treated three patients with not only FHD but with some other forms of dystonia in other parts of the body, including the face. The target covered a large area of the ventrolateral nucleus of the thalamus, and the final lesion size was 6 × 6 × 8 mm. They reported that writer's cramp symptoms completely disappeared in all patients. Goto et al. reported excellent results of stereotactic selective Vo-complex thalamotomy in a patient with dystonic writer's cramp in 1997 (Goto et al. 1997). Furthermore, Taira and Hitchcock had studied the effect of thalamotomy on dystonias in the late 1980s, and reported that 'immediate improvement occurred in patients with focal limb dystonia', 'improvement was sustained in patients with focal limb dystonia' and 'focal limb dystonia can be greatly improved by thalamotomy without any motor, sensory or intellectual disturbance' (Taira & Hitchcock 1990). These findings are completely consistent with our recent experience of Vo thalamotomy.

In a few patients with TSFHD, the symptom becomes so severe that task specificity is lost and the symptom persists all the time. Very few patients may develop dystonic symptoms in other parts of the body. Especially when the onset of FHD is at a young age (younger than 20 years) (Gasser et al. 1996; Lee et al. 2012), DYT1 dystonia should be suspected. Family history is exceptional in writer's cramp. Some TSFHD may have tremor which is also task-specific but irregular and not rhythmic. When a patient has both dystonia and dystonic tremor of the hand, stereotactic ablation of both Vo and Vim nuclei of the thalamus can control both symptoms. Thus FHD shows symptoms of various combinations of degrees of task specificity, dystonic symptoms and tremor, as shown in Figure 66.1.

Indication for Surgery

The indication for Vo thalamotomy for FHD should not be determined only by the severity of the symptom. Even if the symptom seems minimal to the clinician, the patient may have tremendous difficulty in pursuing his or her profession. Even if the patient has very severe writer's cramp and is unable to hold a pen, he or she may not mind at all because there is no need for handwriting in daily life. Surgical indication should be determined by the degree of the patient's suffering. Very minimal involuntary extension of the little finger may become a serious issue for a professional classic solo-guitarist, while a similar symptom in a violinist in an amateur orchestra may not be that serious.

Our experience shows that the duration of symptoms before surgery does not affect the surgical outcome. Those who suffered for 30–40 years showed similar improvement as 1–2-year sufferers. We do not ask patients to try every possible conservative medical or physical therapy before operating, because permanent improvement of FHD with conservative therapy may take a long time. Most professional musicians cannot wait

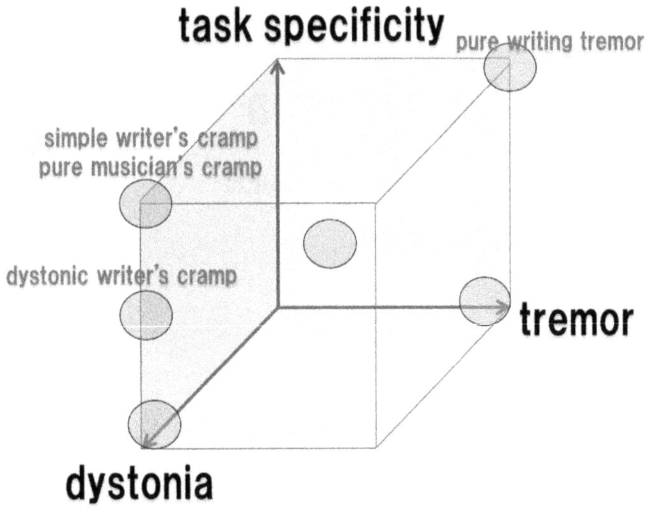

Figure 66.1 Concept of three axes in focal hand dystonia. In focal hand dystonia, three components (task specificity, dystonia and tremor) are present to various degrees. With progression of the disease, task specificity may become less prominent. Some patients may have both dystonia and tremor.

several years to return to their professional performance, even if FHD may improve with an extensive long-term rehabilitation programme. Of course, we would not recommend against conservative therapy, if the patient wants to try. Timing of surgery is appropriate when the patient is convinced about the limitation of the conservative therapy and has made up his or her mind to undergo surgery. We usually avoid operating on patients older than 60 years of age because of the higher risk for surgical complications. The youngest patient (writer's cramp) we operated on was 15 years old.

Some patients may develop FHD in the contralateral hand. This may occur spontaneously, and even after treatment with unilateral thalamotomy. Such patients may ask us to operate on the contralateral side of the thalamus as the second surgery. However, we usually advise against further surgery since bilateral operations are exceptional and more dangerous. Bilateral simultaneous thalamotomy is regarded as contraindicated, in particular because of the high risk of complications such as speech problems and cognitive deterioration. Sequential bilateral thalamotomy may be an option only if the lesion size is minimal. In our series, we performed four bilateral Vo thalamotomies, two for writer's cramp, one in a clarinet musician and one in a pianist. The second surgery was performed 1–3 years after the initial operation, and there were no major subjective or objective side-effects.

Surgical Technique

A Leksell stereotactic frame is fixed onto the skull of the patient under local anaesthesia with 2 per cent lidocaine. Magnetic resonance (1 mm slice) and computer tomographic scan (1 mm slice) images are used to determine the tentative target 2 mm posterior to the midpoint of the anterior commissure (AC) – posterior commissure (PC) line, 1 mm dorsal to the AC–PC line, and 15 mm lateral to the midline (Figure 66.2). In the beginning of our series, we used to take 13.5 mm lateral from the midline. However, because there were about 20 per cent recurrences, we moved the target to 15 mm lateral. This point corresponds to the junction between the ventro-oral anterior (Voa) and posterior (Vop) nuclei of the thalamus according to the stereotactic atlas of Schaltenbrand and Wahren (1998) (Figure 66.2). The operation is performed with the patient under local anaesthesia (1 per cent lidocaine with norepinephrine) without sedation. This is important to check symptoms during surgery. We do not shave off the hair, but clip a small amount along the incision line. After opening a frontal burr hole, we ask the patient to write or play their musical instrument and to report changes in symptoms (Figure 66.3). A monopolar radiofrequency probe (1 mm diameter tip with a 2 mm or 4 mm uninsulated length) is inserted through the burr hole. Electrical stimulation (130–160 Hz, 100-μsec pulse width, up to 15 mA) is applied to identify the optimal position for the lesion. At this target, we have not observed marked changes of symptoms even with the strongest stimulation. Therefore, the Vo target is regarded as an electrically non-responsive silent region. This is interesting, because we generally believe that high-frequency stimulation should improve symptoms, if coagulation works. We do not use microelectrode recording. We carefully check the symptoms and side-effects with a trial lesion created at 45 °C. If the dystonic symptoms improve, we create a permanent lesion by performing thermocoagulation at up to 70–75 °C for 30 seconds. The electrode is then withdrawn in 2 mm increments to increase the lesion size. We do not inform patients regarding the timing of macrostimulation and thermocoagulation in order to avoid a placebo effect. To minimise operative complications, we strictly monitor and control blood pressure. The burr hole is covered with a small ceramic cap for cosmetic purposes and the scalp is closed in two layers. The operation takes less than one hour from skin incision to closure. After operation, the patient is kept flat in bed overnight.

Results

We reported our results in several manuscripts (Taira & Hori 2003; Taira et al. 2003; Horisawa et al. 2013). We have operated on more than 150 patients. The effect of Vo thalamotomy is always immediate during the operation. If there is no improvement during surgery, we cannot expect a delayed response. There are some recurrences; about 10 per cent of patients experience recurrence of the symptoms within three months. Recurrence after three months is very rare. Most patients who have a recurrence ask for another operation, because the improvement of symptoms was substantial immediately after surgery. We plan the location of the target for the second surgery based on the findings of postoperative MR images.

In our series of Vo thalamotomy for writer's cramp, preoperative WCRS was 15.1 ± 4.9 and it improved to 2.2 ± 2.0 (n = 20) after the operation. Such an improvement of the WCRS is extraordinary, as it was reported that a pretreatment score of 9.1 ± 4.5 dropped to 6.6 ± 4.1 (n = 31) in a

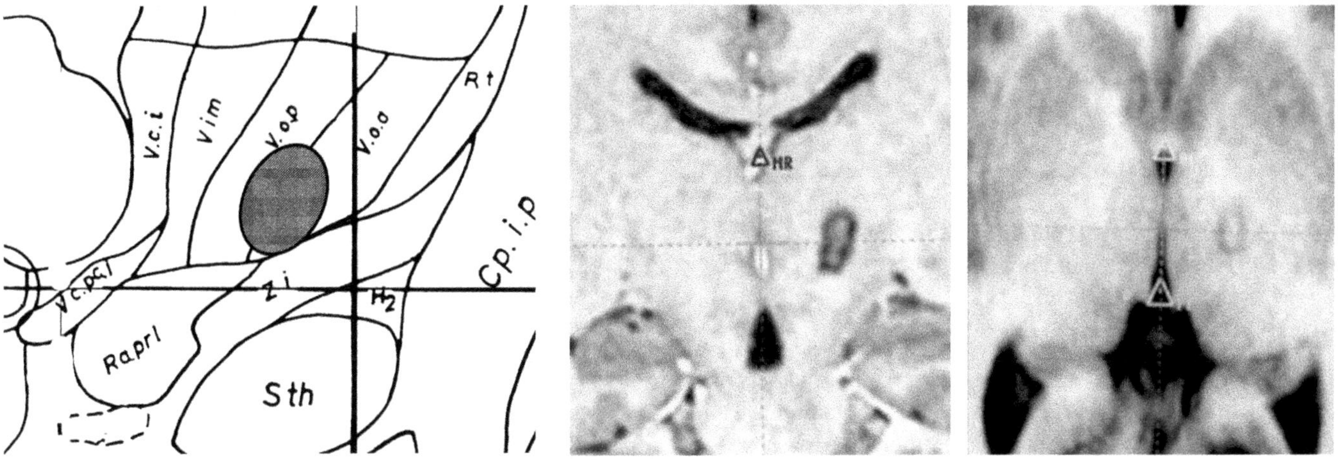

Figure 66.2 Location of the ventro-oral nucleus of the thalamus. Sagittal section from the Schaltenbrand–Wahren atlas 13 mm from the midline. AC: anterior commissure; PC: posterior commissure (left). Postoperative coronal (middle) and axial (right) magnetic resonance images of Vo lesion.

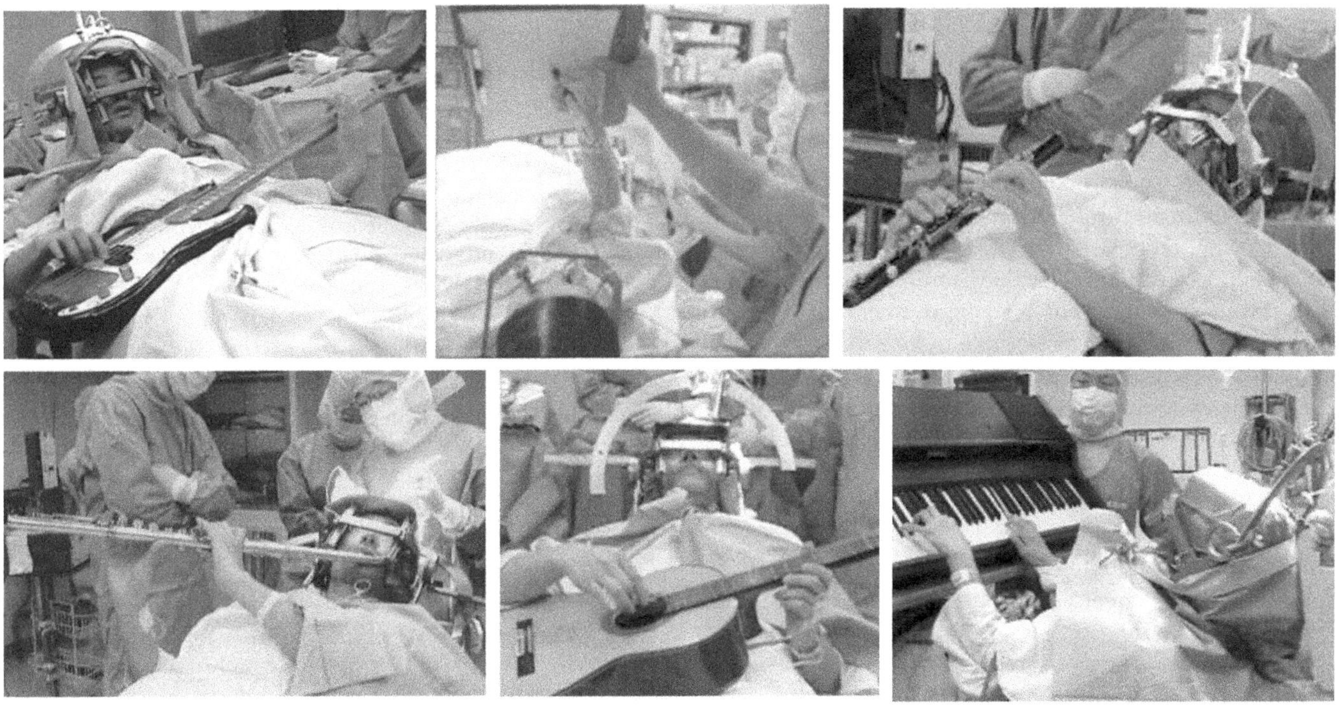

Figure 66.3 Intraoperative set-up in Vo thalamotomy for task-specific focal hand dystonia. Patients are asked to perform activities that induce focal hand dystonia during surgery to check improvement with stereotactic ablation of the Vo nucleus.

study on botulinum toxin therapy for writer's cramp (Wissel et al. 1996). In a study on the long-term effect on musician's FHD (Horisawa et al. 2013), 15 patients were followed up for 4–108 months (mean 30.8 months) after Vo thalamotomy. Fourteen (93 per cent) patients experienced improvement of dystonic symptoms which was sustained without recurrence or deterioration during the follow-up period. The mean preoperative Tubiana scale score was 2.7 (range 1–4). The mean immediate and one-week postoperative scores were both 4.6 (range 2–5). The mean final score was 4.6 (range 2–5). The patient with the longest duration of symptoms (29 years) obtained the best amelioration.

There were two problematic cases in whom we performed thalamotomy twice without sufficient improvement of symptoms. These two patients did not have hand dystonia but abnormal dystonic contractions of the muscles around the shoulder. In our experience, Vo thalamotomy is effective only for symptoms in the distal part of the limb and does not work for symptoms affecting the proximal limb. The latter should be managed with GPi pallidotomy rather than thalamotomy.

Complications

There were no permanent severe complications in our series. There were no postoperative intracerebral haemorrhages or intracranial infections. This is probably because patients are relatively young (20–40 years). The most common transient complication is mild dysarthria and contralateral weakness, which appears 2–3 days after surgery and lasts for 2–3 weeks. About 10 per cent of patients experience such transient episodes. The underlying cause probably is oedema formation around the thermocoagulation lesion. In our experience patients do not lose any acquired skills or abilities to learn new techniques after Vo thalamotomy.

Further Considerations

In the era of DBS, many neurosurgeons and neurologists may consider that lesioning procedures such as thalamotomy and pallidotomy are too risky and old-fashioned. However, the fact is that 63 per cent of functional neurosurgeons are using ablative techniques worldwide even today, not only restricted to lower-/middle-income countries (Jourdain & Schechtmann 2014). The general belief, correct or not, that DBS is more effective and safer than ablative surgery dates back to the 1990s, when ventriculography was still used for identification of stereotactic targets. Modern imaging techniques and computer software for surgical planning became widely available only in the late 1990s, which made stereotactic operations much quicker and safer. DBS gained popularity because of its adjustability and reversibility in the 2000s. DBS is effective, but hardware-related complications may occur even after very long-term follow-up. Because patients with dystonia are younger, in general, and have more favourable long-term effects than those with Parkinson's disease or essential tremor, dystonia patients may have to live with DBS devices for longer than 50–60 years. Even if the dystonic symptoms are well controlled with DBS, they will suffer further emotional and social issues (Hariz et al. 2011). The 'new life' after DBS is stressful, including concern about being dependent on the stimulator as well as having to deal with interfering side-effects. In this sense, DBS does not cure the disease. Lesioning procedures are not inferior to DBS in terms of acute complications in movement disorder surgery (Rughani et al. 2013).

Notably, there are only few reports on DBS for FHD (Fukaya et al. 2007; Cho et al. 2009) and task-specific tremor in a musician (Whitney et al. 2013). Fukaya et al. implanted two DBS electrodes, one in the Vo nucleus of the thalamus and another in the GPi, to treat patients with writer's cramp. They reported that thalamic stimulation was significantly better for writer's cramp (Fukaya et al. 2007).

Our first patient with writer's cramp treated with Vo thalamotomy has not shown any signs of recurrence of the symptoms for 14 years. She is very active as a professional cartoonist even today. The question is 'Can we call it a cure of FHD?' In many textbooks, it is written that there is no cure for dystonia. The term 'remission' is often used when the symptoms of dystonia improve for a certain period of time, which is not rare in cervical dystonia. However, there is no clear definition of both 'remission' and 'cure' in dystonia. It should be discussed how long is long enough to say a cure has occurred in dystonia. We hope that we can provide a 'cure' ultimately for FHD with Vo thalamotomy.

Conclusions

Unilateral Vo thalamotomy is safe and effective as a treatment of FHD when applying modern stereotactic techniques, if the technique of the surgical team is sophisticated enough and if the indication is appropriate. The effect of Vo thalamotomy is immediate and is sustained in the long term. Every effort has to be made to minimise complications for such an invasive treatment to be justified.

References

Cho CB, Park HK, Lee KJ, Rha HK. 2009. Thalamic deep brain stimulation for writer's cramp. *J Korean Neurosurg Soc* 46(1):52–55.

Fukaya C, Katayama Y, Kano T, Nagaoka T, Kobayashi K, Oshima H, Yamamoto T. 2007. Thalamic deep brain stimulation for writer's cramp. *J Neurosurg* 107(5):977–982.

Gasser T, Bove CM, Ozelius LJ, Hallett M, Charness ME, Hochberg FH, Breakefield XO. 1996. Haplotype analysis at the DYT1 locus in Ashkenazi Jewish patients with occupational hand dystonia. *Mov Disord* 11(2):163–166.

Goto S, Tsuiki H, Soyama N, Okamura A, Yamada K, Yoshikawa M, Hashimoto Y, Ushio Y. 1997. Stereotactic selective Vo-complex thalamotomy in a patient with dystonic writer's cramp. *Neurology* 49(4):1173–1174.

Hariz GM, Limousin P, Tisch S, Jahanshahi M, Fjellman-Wiklund A. 2011. Patients' perceptions of life shift after deep brain stimulation for primary dystonia: a qualitative study. *Mov Disord* 26(11):2101–2106.

Horisawa S, Taira T, Goto S, Ochiai T, Nakajima T. 2013. Long-term improvement of musician's dystonia after stereotactic ventro-oral thalamotomy *Ann Neurol* 74(5):648–654.

Jourdain VA, Schechtmann G. 2014. Health economics and surgical treatment for Parkinson's disease in a world perspective: results from an international survey. *Stereotact Funct Neurosurg* 92(2):71–79.

Lee WW, Ahn TB, Chung SJ, Jeon BS. 2012. Phenotypic differences in DYT1 between ethnic groups. *Curr Neurol Neurosci Rep* 12(4):341–347.

Mempel E, Kucinski L, Witkiewicz B. 1986. Writer's cramp syndrome treated successfully by thalamotomy. *Neurol Neurochir Pol* 20(5):475–480.

Poore GV. 1887. Clinical lecture on certain conditions of the hand and arm which interfere with the performance of professional acts, especially piano-playing. *Br Med J* 1(1365):441–444.

Rughani AI, Hodaie M, Lozano AM. 2013. Acute complications of movement disorders surgery: effects of age and comorbidities. *Mov Disord* 28(12):1661–1667.

Schaltenbrand G, Wahren W. 1998. *Atlas for Stereotaxy of the Human Brain,* Thieme Publishing Group, Stuttgart.

Siegfried J, Crowell R, Perret E. 1969. Cure of tremulous writer's cramp by stereotaxic thalamotomy: case report. *J Neurosurg* 30(2):182–185.

Taira T, Hitchcock T. 1990. Stereotactic thalamotomy for patients with dystonia. *Stereotact Funct Neurosurg* 54–55:212–223.

Taira T, Hori T. 2003. Stereotactic ventrooralis thalamotomy for task-specific focal hand dystonia (writer's cramp). *Stereotact Funct Neurosurg* 80(1):88–91.

Taira T, Harashima S, Hori T. 2003. Neurosurgical treatment for writer's cramp. *Acta Neurochir Suppl* 87:129–131.

Whitney N, Kareus S, Cetas JS, Chung K, Brodsky M. 2013. Bilateral deep brain stimulation targeting ventralis intermedius nucleus to treat a professional musician's task-specific tremor. *Mov Disord* 28(13):1896–1897.

Wissel J, Kabus C, Wenzel R, Klepsch S, Schwarz U, Nebe A, Schelosky L, Scholz U, Poewe W. 1996. Botulinum toxin in writer's cramp: objective response evaluation in 31 patients. *J Neurol Neurosurg Psychiatry* 61(2):172–175.

Chapter 67

Deep Brain Stimulation for Myoclonus-Dystonia

Ausaf A. Bari and Andres M. Lozano

Deep brain stimulation (DBS) is an established treatment for movement disorders such as Parkinson's disease and essential tremor. DBS of the globus pallidus has also been shown to be effective in the treatment of primary generalised and cervical dystonia. However, its role in other forms of dystonia such as secondary dystonia and dystonia-plus syndromes is less established. Here we review the role of DBS in the treatment of a dystonia-plus disorder known as myoclonus-dystonia syndrome (MDS).

Myoclonus-dystonia syndrome is a relatively rare and potentially disabling movement disorder characterised by a combination of 'lightning-like' myoclonic jerks and dystonia (Kinugawa et al. 2009). It is designated as DYT11 in the classification scheme for monogenic dystonias. MDS is inherited in an autosomal dominant fashion with maternal imprinting and approximately 50 per cent of cases are associated with mutations in the epsilon-sarcoglycan gene (SGCE) at chromosomal locus 7q21 (Grunewald et al. 2008). However, the disorder displays genetic heterogeneity and can result from mutations at other loci as well (Nygaard et al. 1999; Klein et al. 2000; Vidailhet et al. 2001; Breakefield et al. 2008).

MDS typically presents with bilateral, alcohol-responsive myoclonus with onset typically in childhood and early adolescence (Cif et al. 2004). Myoclonus is usually the initial symptom and most prominent in the head, neck, upper limbs and occasionally the lower limbs (Cif et al. 2004). Myoclonic jerks are often exacerbated by motor tasks and stress. More than half of MDS patients develop dystonia which can present as torticollis or writer's cramp that often coexists with myoclonus, but is occasionally the only manifestation (Cif et al. 2004). MDS is also associated with psychiatric symptoms such as panic attacks and obsessive-compulsive behaviour (Cif et al. 2004).

Pharmacologic treatment for MDS includes levodopa, anticholinergics, benzodiazepines and baclofen, but these generally provide only modest symptomatic relief and are often not well tolerated due to significant side-effects (Sidiropoulos et al. 2014). Thus, in patients with severe symptoms refractory to medical management, DBS may play a significant role. DBS has already been established as a safe and effective treatment for other movement disorders. Large prospective trials have previously shown DBS to be effective for primary generalised dystonia, leading to its approval under a humanitarian device exemption by the US Food and Drug Administration in 2003 (Volkmann et al. 2014; Smith & Spindler 2015). DBS has subsequently been investigated in patients with other forms of dystonia including secondary and combined dystonias such as MDS.

Clinical Evidence Supporting DBS for MDS

To date, 22 publications have described the use of DBS in a total of 49 patients (Smith & Spindler 2015). Based on early case reports, two candidate structures have emerged as efficacious DBS targets for MDS. These are the globus pallidus pars internus (GPi) and the ventral intermediate nucleus of the thalamus (VIM). Our centre previously reported a meta-analysis of 17 publications involving 40 patients as of 2012 (Rughani & Lozano 2013). There were two key findings from this study. First, while DBS resulted in improvement in both myoclonus and dystonia, there was a greater and more consistent improvement in myoclonus (72.6 vs 52.6 per cent) (Rughani & Lozano 2013). Second, while both the GPi and VIM DBS improved myoclonus to a similar degree, stimulation of the GPi was more effective than the VIM in improving dystonia. Given these findings, the meta-analysis concluded that the GPi may be the more efficacious and sufficient target for the treatment of typical MDS (Rughani & Lozano 2013). However, the small number of subjects and lack of randomised trials precluded any definitive recommendation for one target over the other.

Since the publication of this previous meta-analysis, seven additional patients have undergone DBS for MDS, bringing the total number of MDS patients implanted to date to 49 (Smith & Spindler 2015). Clinical results from these additional patients corroborate that bilateral DBS of the GPi significantly improves both myoclonus and dystonia, but with a more consistent and greater improvement in myoclonus (Ghosh & Indulkar 2013; Kim et al. 2014; Papuc et al. 2014; Sidiropoulos et al. 2014; Uruha et al. 2014). Across all cases published to date, the GPi was the most common target, with only nine patients receiving VIM electrodes. One advantage of the GPi over the VIM is the decreased incidence of speech problems such as dysarthria seen after bilateral VIM DBS, a side-effect known from the previous experience of using the VIM as a target for tremor. There is some evidence to suggest that simultaneous targeting of both structures may be synergistic. To date, a single study has evaluated concurrent bilateral GPi and VIM DBS (Gruber et al. 2010). In this cohort, six out of eight patients with bilateral concurrent GPi and VIM DBS had greater efficacy than either target alone (Gruber et al. 2010). As there have been no prospective, randomised controlled trials to date, further studies are necessary to determine the superiority, if any, of one target over the other.

In addition to the characteristic motor symptoms, MDS has a distinct psychiatric component. The efficacy of DBS for these comorbid psychiatric symptoms in MDS patients is not established. While one series reported worsening of psychiatric symptoms following bilateral GPi DBS, others have shown possible improvement (Uruha et al. 2014). It is still unclear whether the psychiatric symptoms in MDS are secondary to the disease burden or whether common basal ganglia networks are involved and potentially amenable to DBS.

Mechanism of DBS in MDS

The initial rationale for choosing the GPi and VIM as DBS targets for MDS was based on the use of these targets for other movement disorders with shared symptomatology, i.e. the GPi for primary dystonia and VIM for hereditary myoclonus (Schaefer & Wieser 1964; Volkmann et al. 2014). Although the selection of these targets was empirically corroborated by their successful use in pilot cases of MDS, the neurophysiologic mechanisms of MDS and the role of these structures are still unclear. Several theories have been postulated, including hyperactivity of the cortico-striato-pallido-thalamo-cortical pathway, abnormal sensorimotor integration and involvement of the cerebello-thalamo-cortical pathway (van der Meer et al. 2012). Although cortical changes are found in patients with MDS, these may be secondary as overwhelming neurophysiological evidence suggests a subcortical origin for the disorder (Popa et al. 2014). For example, neuronal recordings obtained from patients undergoing GPi DBS for MDS show a correlation between myoclonus and bursting activity within the GPi (Liu et al. 2002; Welter et al. 2015). In addition to the basal ganglia, there is also evidence that the cerebellum may play a role. Cerebellar involvement is supported by the fact that the VIM receives primarily cerebellar afferents. Indeed, the brain-specific isoform of the sarcoglycan gene product is highly expressed in cerebellar Purkinje neurons and the dentate nucleus, with relatively lower expression in the globus pallidus (Ritz et al. 2011). Functional MRI and PET findings also support a role for the cerebellum in MDS patients (Nitschke et al. 2006; Beukers et al. 2010; Carbon et al. 2013). These findings point to the possibility that the cerebellum may play a significant role in MDS and could be a potential additional target for DBS.

DBS in Paediatric Patients With MDS

MDS often begins in childhood, with symptoms progressing into adolescence and adulthood. Historically, there has been a significant lag between diagnosis and treatment. Therefore, it is important to consider the potential benefits of performing DBS at an earlier age. To date, bilateral GPi DBS has been performed in nine paediatric patients (≤18 years) with confirmed DYT11 mutations, with reports of significant improvement in myoclonus and dystonia symptoms, similar to that described in adults (Cif et al. 2004; Gil-Robles et al. 2006; Foncke et al. 2007; Ghosh & Indulkar 2013; Kimura et al. 2014). A key issue with paediatric DBS for MDS is balancing the need for early surgery with expectant medical management. Indeed, younger age and a shorter duration of symptoms have been associated with a better response to treatment (Smith & Spindler 2015). Again, prospective data are currently lacking and the decision to operate should be individualised based on discussion between the neurosurgeon, neurologist, paediatrician, parents and, when appropriate, the older patient. In addition, target selection should also be individualised, particularly in children. The unique technical considerations for paediatric DBS include the need to perform placement of the stereotactic frame, electrode and pulse generator under general anaesthesia, a practice currently followed for performing DBS in paediatric patients with other movement disorders.

Overview of Surgical Technique

The complete DBS system consists of unilateral or bilateral intracranial electrodes connected to an internal pulse generator (IPG) typically implanted in the chest, just below the clavicle. The IPG serves as the source of electrical current and as a receiver for wireless programming and adjustment of stimulation parameters. DBS electrode placement for MDS follows the general operative technique established for other movement disorders and consists of preoperative imaging followed by placement of a stereotactic frame, DBS electrodes and IPG. In adults, we perform the electrode placement under local anaesthesia with minimal sedation if required. This allows for optimal intraoperative neuronal microelectrode recordings (MER) for neurophysiological confirmation of the target. The IPG is placed using general anaesthesia on the same or a subsequent day. Paediatric patients are implanted using general anaesthesia for all stages of the procedure in a single day.

We recommend a combination of direct targeting based on MRI as well as atlas-based indirect targeting. Coordinates are calculated using planning software and expressed relative to the anterior and posterior commissural (AC–PC) line. The optimal GPi target is located in the posteroventral pallidum approximately ±20 mm lateral, 0 mm anterior and 5 mm ventral to the AC–PC line. MERs are used to identify pallidal neuronal activity as well as to map the ventral border by identifying activity from the bordering optic tract. Microstimulation can also be used to elicit visual phosphenes to confirm the location of the optic tract. The VIM is targeted 11 mm lateral to the wall of the third ventricle or 15 mm lateral to the midline, 6–7 mm anterior to the PC and 0 mm ventral to the AC–PC line. MERs are used to identify kinaesthetic neuronal responses within the VIM and to identify its posterior border with the sensory thalamus and its inferior border with the medial lemniscus. Once the target is located, the final DBS electrode is placed under fluoroscopic guidance. Stimulation-induced side-effects are then mapped and may include paraesthesias, motor contractions, speech difficulty and visual phenomena in the case of the GPi. If necessary, data from intraoperative mapping are used to adjust the location of the DBS electrode before finalising its placement. Mapping data are also useful in guiding postoperative programming.

Postoperative Programming

Programming typically begins several weeks after surgery. The kinetics of clinical response of myoclonus-dystonia to DBS differs from that of other movement disorders. Unlike PD and essential tremor, in which symptoms typically respond to DBS within seconds, in MDS patients myoclonus responds within minutes to hours while reduction of dystonia can take several days to weeks, suggesting a role of neuronal plasticity in the response (Gruber et al. 2010). The goal of programming is to achieve the desired clinical benefit while minimising stimulation-induced side-effects. Parameter ranges reported to be effective for stimulation in MDS were as follows: for the GPi 1.5–6 V, 60–210 μs and 70–140 Hz and for the VIM 0.9–5.3 V, 60–210 μs and 130–250 Hz. In the largest case series of DBS for MDS, stimulation-induced side-effects were greater for the VIM than the GPi. Side-effects of GPi DBS included nausea and phosphenes, while VIM DBS was associated with dysarthria, dysphagia, dysguesia, worsening dystonia, headache, gait disturbance and dysaesthesias (Gruber et al. 2010). Thus, while both bilateral GPi and unilateral VIM stimulation are relatively safe, bilateral VIM stimulation carries a greater risk of speech and cognitive side-effects. In the same series, surgical adverse events included infection, haemorrhage and lead fracture, all of which were reversible (Gruber et al. 2010).

Conclusions

There is evidence that DBS may be beneficial in the treatment of severe disabling forms of MDS. Although the GPi may be the more optimal target based on its greater efficacy and lower side-effect profile, the addition of a VIM electrode may play a distinct role in refractory cases. Future prospective, randomised trials are necessary, but may be difficult due to the small number of patients involved. Additional potential targets such as the cerebellum should also be investigated. In addition, at this time, target selection should be individualised, particularly in children. DBS has been shown to be a safe and effective technique when performed properly in carefully chosen patients and should be seriously considered in severe cases of MDS. Finally, DBS provides us with the unique ability to directly study the pathophysiology of subcortical networks underlying these unusual disorders and is particularly important in developing a unified theory of how common brain networks mediate such disorders.

References

Beukers RJ, Foncke EM, van der Meer JN, Nederveen AJ, de Ruiter MB, Bour LJ, Veltman DJ, Tijssen MA. 2010. Disorganized sensorimotor integration in mutation-positive myoclonus-dystonia: a functional magnetic resonance imaging study. *Arch Neurol* 67(4):469–474.

Breakefield XO, Blood AJ, Li Y, Hallett M, Hanson PI, Standaert DG. 2008. The pathophysiological basis of dystonias. *Nat Rev Neurosci* 9(3):222–234.

Carbon M, Raymond D, Ozelius L, Saunders-Pullman R, Frucht S, Dhawan V, Bressman S, Eidelberg D. 2013. Metabolic changes in DYT11 myoclonus-dystonia. *Neurology* 80(4):385–391.

Cif L, Valente EM, Hemm S, Coubes C, Vayssiere N, Serrat S, Di Giorgio A, Coubes P. 2004. Deep brain stimulation in myoclonus-dystonia syndrome. *Mov Disord* 19(6):724–727.

Foncke EM, Bour LJ, Speelman JD, Koelman JH, Tijssen MA. 2007. Local field potentials and oscillatory activity of the internal globus pallidus in myoclonus-dystonia. *Mov Disord* 22(3):369–376.

Ghosh D, Indulkar S. 2013. Primary myoclonus-dystonia: a diagnosis often missed in children. *J Child Neurol* 28(11):1418–1422.

Gil-Robles S, Cif L, Biolsi B, Tancu C, El Fertit H, Coubes P. 2006. Neurosurgical treatment in childhood dystonias and dyskinesias. *Rev Neurol* 43 (Suppl. 1):S169–S172.

Gruber D, Kuhn AA, Schoenecker T, Kivi A, Trottenberg T, Hoffmann KT, Gharabaghi A, Kopp UA, Schneider GH, Klein C, Asmus F, Kupsch A. 2010. Pallidal and thalamic deep brain stimulation in myoclonus-dystonia. *Mov Disord* 25(11):1733–1743.

Grunewald A, Djarmati A, Lohmann-Hedrich K, Farrell K, Zeller JA, Allert N, Papengut F, Petersen B, Fung V, Sue CM, O'Sullivan D, Mahant N, Kupsch A, Chuang RS, Wiegers K, Pawlack H, Hagenah J, Ozelius LJ, Stephani U, Schuit R, Lang AE, Volkmann J, Munchau A, Klein C. 2008. Myoclonus-dystonia: significance of large SGCE deletions. *Hum Mutat* 29(2):331–332.

Kim JH, Na YC, Lee WH, Chang WS, Jung HH, Chang JW. 2014. Bilateral globus pallidus interna deep-brain stimulation in a patient with myoclonus-dystonia: a case report. *Neuromodulation* 17(8):724–728.

Kimura Y, Mihara M, Kawarai T, Kishima H, Sakai N, Takahashi MP, Mochizuki H. 2014. Efficacy of deep brain stimulation in an adolescent patient with DYT11 myoclonus-dystonia. *Neurol Clin Neurosci* 2(2):57–59.

Kinugawa K, Vidailhet M, Clot F, Apartis E, Grabli D, Roze E. 2009. Myoclonus-dystonia: an update. *Mov Disord* 24(4):479–489.

Klein C, Schilling K, Saunders-Pullman RJ, Garrels J, Breakefield XO, Brin MF, deLeon D, Doheny D, Fahn S, Fink JS, Forsgren L, Friedman J, Frucht S, Harris J, Holmgren G, Kis B, Kurlan R, Kyllerman M, Lang AE, Leung J, Raymond D, Robishaw JD, Sanner G, Schwinger E, Tabamo RE, Tagliati M. 2000. A major locus for myoclonus-dystonia maps to chromosome 7q in eight families. *Am J Hum Genet* 67(5):1314–1319.

Liu X, Griffin IC, Parkin SG, Miall RC, Rowe JG, Gregory RP, Scott RB, Aziz TZ, Stein JF. 2002. Involvement of the medial pallidum in focal myoclonic dystonia: a clinical and neurophysiological case study. *Mov Disord* 17(2):346–353.

Nitschke MF, Erdmann C, Trillenberg P, Sprenger A, Kock N, Sperner J, Klein C. 2006. Functional MRI reveals activation of a subcortical network in a 5 year old girl with genetically confirmed myoclonus-dystonia. *Neuropediatrics* 37(2):79–82.

Nygaard TG, Raymond D, Chen C, Nishino I, Greene PE, Jennings D, Heiman GA, Klein C, Saunders-Pullman RJ, Kramer P, Ozelius LJ, Bressman SB. 1999. Localization of a gene for myoclonus-dystonia to chromosome 7q21-q31. *Ann Neurol* 46(5):794–798.

Papuc E, Obszanska K, Rejdak K, Stelmasiak Z, Trojanowski T. 2014. Atypical symptomatology of myoclonus dystonia (DYT-11) with positive response to bilateral pallidal deep brain stimulation. *Mov Disord* 29(7):E3.

Popa T, Milani P, Richard A, Hubsch C, Brochard V, Tranchant C, Sadnicka A, Rothwell J, Vidailhet M, Meunier S, Roze E. 2014.

The neurophysiological features of myoclonus-dystonia and differentiation from other dystonias. *JAMA Neurol* 71(5):612–619.

Ritz K, van Schaik BD, Jakobs ME, van Kampen AH, Aronica E, Tijssen MA, Baas F. 2011. SGCE isoform characterization and expression in human brain: implications for myoclonus-dystonia pathogenesis? *Eur J Hum Genet* 19(4):438–444.

Rughani AI, Lozano AM. 2013. Surgical treatment of myoclonus dystonia syndrome. *Mov Disord* 28(3):282–287.

Schaefer KP, Wieser S. 1964. Neurophysiologische Untersuchungen zur essentiellen Myoklonie. *Archiv für Psychiatrie und Nervenkrankheiten* 205(5):571–590.

Sidiropoulos C, Mestre T, Hutchison W, Moro E, Valencia A, Poon YY, Fallis M, Rughani AI, Kalia SK, Lozano AM, Lang AE. 2014. Bilateral pallidal stimulation for sargoglycan epsilon negative myoclonus. *Parkinsonism Relat Disord* 20(8):915–918.

Smith KM, Spindler MA. 2015. Uncommon applications of deep brain stimulation in hyperkinetic movement disorders. *Tremor Other Hyperkinet Mov (NY)* 5:278.

Uruha A, Kimura K, Okiyama R. 2014. An Asian patient with myoclonus-dystonia (DYT11) responsive to deep brain stimulation of the globus pallidus internus. *Case Rep Neurol Med* 2014:937095.

van der Meer JN, Beukers RJ, van der Salm S, Caan MWA, Tijssen MAJ, Nederveen AJ. 2012. White matter abnormalities in gene-positive myoclonus-dystonia. *Mov Disord* 27(13):1666–1672.

Vidailhet M, Tassin J, Durif F, Nivelon-Chevallier A, Agid Y, Brice A, Durr A. 2001. A major locus for several phenotypes of myoclonus-dystonia on chromosome 7q. *Neurology* 56(9):1213–1216.

Volkmann J, Mueller J, Deuschl G, Kuhn AA, Krauss JK, Poewe W, Timmermann L, Falk D, Kupsch A, Kivi A, Schneider GH, Schnitzler A, Sudmeyer M, Voges J, Wolters A, Wittstock M, Muller JU, Hering S, Eisner W, Vesper J, Prokop T, Pinsker M, Schrader C, Kloss M, Kiening K, Boetzel K, Mehrkens J, Skogseid IM, Ramm-Pettersen J, Kemmler G, Bhatia KP, Vitek JL, Benecke R, DBS Study Group for Dystonia. 2014. Pallidal neurostimulation in patients with medication-refractory cervical dystonia: a randomised, sham-controlled trial. *Lancet Neurol* 13(9):875–884.

Welter ML, Grabli D, Karachi C, Jodoin N, Fernandez-Vidal S, Brun Y, Navarro S, Rogers A, Cornu P, Pidoux B, Yelnik J, Roze E, Bardinet E, Vidailhet M. 2015. Pallidal activity in myoclonus dystonia correlates with motor signs. *Mov Disord* 30(7):992–996.

Chapter 68 Deep Brain Stimulation for Tardive Dystonia

Doreen Gruber and Andreas Kupsch

Tardive dyskinesia (TDk) and tardive dystonia (TDt) are chronic disorders following exposure predominantly to neuroleptic drugs, but also to certain antiemetics (e.g. metoclopramide) or antidepressants. DSM-V diagnostic criteria for TDt or TDk include a history of more than three months cumulative exposure to dopamine receptor-blocking agents, except in elderly patients in whom one month is sufficient (American Psychiatric Association 2013), including the absence of other conditions that might produce abnormal involuntary movements.

It has been estimated that TDk has an average prevalence of 15–20 per cent (Gerlach & Casey 1988) and TDt dystonia may affect 0.04–21 per cent of neuroleptic-treated patients (Adityanjee et al. 1999). TDk and TDt may coexist in 1–4 per cent of patients (Raja 1995). TDt has commonly been considered as an acquired dystonia, although future genetic analyses may reveal genetically determined predispositions (Albanese et al. 2013).

TDk differs from TDt in epidemiology, clinical features, risk factors, pathophysiology, course, prognosis and treatment outcome (Burke et al. 1982; Adityanjee et al. 1999). TDt is characterised by generalised, segmental or focal sustained or intermittent involuntary contractions of skeletal muscles that cause abnormal positions or repetitive movements. TDt predominantly affects orofacial and cervical regions or upper limbs and may be accompanied by distal choreoathetosis of upper and lower limbs, and/or ophistotonus. For diagnosis, TDt can overlap clinically not only with TDk, but also with tardive akathisia, tardive tremor and tardive myoclonus, albeit dystonia is the most predominant disturbance (Adityanjee et al. 1999).

The clinical picture of TDt resembles segmental or generalised dystonia and may often not be readily distinguished from hereditary or idiopathic dystonic disorders, underlining the routine need to investigate potential drug exposure in the past of patients with dystonia.

The pathophysiology of TDt is complex and incompletely understood. Striatal dopamine receptor supersensitivity is thought to contribute to the development of TDt, possibly associated with an upregulation of striatal postsynaptic D2-receptors (Silvestri et al. 2000; Morigaki et al. 2016). PET studies reported increased brain activity in prefrontal and premotor frontal regions in TDt patients, which might lead to reduced motor selectivity generating abnormal involuntary movements (Thobois et al. 2008). It is likely that genetic predisposition also influences the susceptibility to develop motor disturbances (Sarro et al. 2013).

The medical treatment options of TDt/TDk comprise the gradual withdrawal of the offending medication, if tolerated (Bhidayasiri et al. 2013), and switching neuroleptic medication to atypical neuroleptics such as clozapine. Tetrabenazine, a drug that acts at the vesicular monoamine transporter and that improves chorea in patients with Huntington's disease, is probably the most efficacious drug in TDt, but it is frequently (approximately 15–20 per cent, depending on the dosage) accompanied by side-effects such as depression and symmetric parkinsonism with gait impairment, which may distinctly limit its long-term application. Other drugs that have been reported to improve TDt symptoms comprise amantadine (in combination with ongoing neuroleptic treatment), gingko biloba, levetiracetam and a newly developed tetrabenazine analogue (O'Brien et al. 2015), while vitamin E, calcium blockers and anticholinergics have shown to be not effective (cf. AAN guidelines by Bhidayasiri et al. (2013) and table 1 in review of Morigaki et al. 2016).

In general, treatment of TDt has been described to be notoriously difficult and it is often characterised by refractoriness, which may aggravate social isolation and psychiatric comorbidity (Adityanjee et al. 1999). Thus, new therapeutic options for treatment of TDt are needed. Here, we review the growing evidence of the efficacy of deep brain stimulation (DBS) in TDt.

Development of Deep Brain Stimulation for Tardive Dystonia

Although not the focus of the present review, it should be mentioned that radiofrequency lesions have been applied earlier, mainly pallidotomy or thalamotomy (Wang et al. 1997; Weetman et al. 1997; Hillier et al. 1999; Lenders et al. 2005) (for review see Thobois et al. (2011)).

Pallidal DBS was introduced for treatment of dystonia in the late 1990s (Coubes et al. 1999; Krauss et al. 1999), and its efficacy was confirmed soon thereafter in multicentre studies (Vidailhet et al. 2005; Kupsch et al. 2006).

The first case report on DBS in TDt involved a 70-year-old woman with TDt due to neuroleptic exposure (fluspirilen) for treatment of an anxiety disorder (Trottenberg et al. 2001). The patient underwent multifocal DBS in the globus pallidus internus (GPi) and the ventral intermediate (VIM) nucleus of the thalamus in one session. While GPi ameliorated dystonic symptoms by 75 per cent as assessed by the Abnormal Involuntary Movement Scale (AIMS) and the Burke–Fahn–Marsden Dystonia Rating Scale (BFMDRS), VIM-DBS neither alone nor as add-on DBS affected the dystonic symptoms. The effects of pallidal DBS were rapid (within minutes to hours) and waned rapidly as well (seconds to minutes) upon cessation of DBS. Stimulation parameters were 150 Hz, 3.0 V and 210 μsec. Over the following years several case series and case reports were published showing similar results (Table 68.1).

For the present review we searched PubMed (22 January 2017) for publications written in English language with the terms 'dystonia' and 'tardive' for case reports, clinical trials, meta-analyses, multicentre studies and reviews. Furthermore, we manually checked the reference lists of included reports and of national and international guidelines for diagnostic and therapeutic approaches of tardive dystonia.

We identified 597 publications, which were screened for content, trial design and methodological quality. Out of these, 35 case and cohort studies reported on a total of approximately 100 patients suffering from TDt or TDk treated by DBS. Ninety-five patients had pallidal DBS (for references, see Table 68.1), while four patients had subthalamic DBS (Zhang et al. 2006; Sun et al. 2007).

The studies reported a mean improvement of approximately 70 per cent of dystonia severity in the 95 patients (range 28–97 per cent; note missing improvement in two TD-patients and no available data in one TD-patient (see Krause et al. 2004) following pallidal DBS as assessed by the BFMDRS or the AIMS at the last follow-up (range: 3 (Woo et al. 2014) to 132 months (Pouclet-Courtemanche et al. 2016)). Long-term results of pallidal DBS comprise up to 7–11 years (Gruber et al. 2009; Boulogne et al. 2014; Pouclet-Courtemanche et al. 2016).

The case series are supplemented by one controlled multicentre study (so-called STARDY study) from France comprising 10 and 19 patients respectively (Damier et al. 2007; Pouclet-Courtemanche et al. 2016), with blinded video rating. Lasting benefit of approximately 50 per cent was reported. The results of a German multicentre trial with a delayed-onset design are not available yet (clinicaltrial.gov NCT00331669).

Subthalamic DBS in two Chinese TD-patients was reported to yield improvement by approximately 92 per cent at three months follow-up (Zhang et al. 2006) and a non-specified improvement of 76–100 per cent in another two patients (Sun et al. 2007). Long-term observation of stable improvement has been reported for up to 12 years (Meng et al. 2016).

Psychiatric Disorders in Patients With Tardive Dystonia Undergoing DBS

Among the 95 patients with TDk and/or TDt treated by bilateral pallidal DBS (except one case with unilateral pallidal DBS (Schrader et al. 2004)), ten patients suffered from schizophrenia, 30 patients from severe depression, partially with psychotic symptoms, eight patients from anxiety and panic disorders, ten patients from bipolar affective disorders, seven patients from psychosis, one patient from Tourette syndrome and three patients had no psychiatric disorders, but had undergone treatment with antiemetics. In the remaining patients, the indication for treatment for neuroleptics was not reported.

Only seven studies reported affective and psychiatric outcome of TDt patients following pallidal DBS (Nandi et al. 2002; Damier et al. 2007; Kosel et al. 2007; Gruber et al. 2009; Boulogne et al. 2014; Meoni et al. 2015; Pouclet-Courtemanche et al. 2016). Follow-up comprised up to 11 years, and consistently no clinically relevant worsening of mood and psychiatric symptoms was observed in either study, providing further evidence about the long-term safety of pallidal DBS in this particular population (Halbig et al. 2005; Meoni et al. 2015).

Cognitive state and quality of life were rarely assessed and have been reported to be stable or to be improved (see Table 68.1).

In the four cases with STN DBS, information on affective and psychiatric symptoms following subthalamic DBS is mostly missing. However, a stable psychiatric condition was reported in one patient during follow-up of 12 years (Meng et al. 2016).

Safety

It is difficult to arrive at a definite conclusion concerning the safety in a review of predominantly observational studies. Nevertheless, the following conclusions can be made (see also Morigaki et al. 2016). In general, GPi DBS for tardive dystonia seems to be a safe procedure with a complication rate that does not differ from other DBS indications, amounting to 5–10 per cent. Neither deaths nor suicides were reported. Misplacement of electrodes and postoperative infections have been anecdotally reported in the STARDY study and in two case series (Krause et al. 2004; Capelle et al. 2010; Pouclet-Courtemanche et al. 2016).

In the STARDY study 8/19 patients experienced transient psychiatric events during the first postoperative year, probably independent of DBS (depression, anxiety, manic state, agitation) (Pouclet-Courtemanche et al. 2016).

Future Directions

Future studies of DBS in TDt/TDk will need to assess optimisation of GPi or STN targeting (Schonecker et al. 2015). Also, electrophysiological recordings may be helpful to identify potential electrophysiological surrogate markers for TDt (Kuhn et al. 2008). For instance, the GPi in TDt is sensitive to pharmacological modulation. As it has been shown that tetrabenazine elicits parkinsonian beta-activity of the GPi in TDt patients, it remains to be established if such a sensitivity may help to further optimise GPi neuromodulation.

The possible role of the STN as a potential alternative target in TDt has so far only been explored by Chinese investigators, reporting dramatic motor improvement of TDt symptoms. With respect to the results of a Danish study (Schjerling et al. 2013), which showed similar relief of motor symptoms in generalised dystonia following either GPi or STN DBS, future studies are needed to address the question of target optimisation,

Table 68.1 Literature review of patients with TDk and TDt treated by DBS

Reference	*N*	Mean** FU in months	Type of dystonia	Mean** percentage of motor improvement of dystonia (BFMDRSm/AIMS/ESRS)	Cognitive, affective, psychiatric outcome and QoL
				GPi DBS	
Trottenberg et al. 2001, additional VIM-electrodes	1	6	seg	73/NR/NR	NR
Nandi et al. 2002	1	6	seg	Improved	Cognition improved Stable affective state
Yianni et al. 2003, including FU of 1 patient Nandi et al. 2002	1/25	12	gen	28/42/NR	NR
Eltahawy et al. 2004	1	18	gen	60/NR/NR	NR
Krause et al. 2004	3*/17	36	gen	Unchanged	NR
Schrader et al. 2004	1	5	gen	NR/55/NR	NR
Franzini et al. 2005	2	12	gen	60/NR/NR	NR
Trottenberg et al. 2005, including FU of 1 patient Trottenberg et al. 2001	5	6	seg/gen	83/78/NR	NR
Starr et al. 2006	4/23	20	seg/gen	62/NR/NR	NR
Cohen et al. 2007	2	10	gen	75/NR/NR	NR
Damier et al. 2007, STARDY study	10	6	seg/gen	NR/56/61	Cognition unchanged Depression improved (*n* = 1) Depression mildly deteriorated (*n* = 3)
Egidi et al. 2007	5/69	29	NR	47/NR/NR	NR
Kosel et al. 2007	1	18	seg	47/NR/NR	Depression improved up to six years
Magarinos-Ascone et al. 2008	1/10	12	seg	48/NR/NR	NR
Pretto et al. 2008	1/13	6	gen	80/90/NR	NR
Sako et al. 2008	6	21	NR	86/NR/NR	NR
Gruber et al. 2009, including FU of 1 patient Trottenberg et al. 2001 Trottenberg et al. 2005	9	41	seg/gen	83/79/NR	Mood and QoL improved Cognition unchanged
Katsakiori et al. 2009	1/8	12	gen	94/NR/NR	NR
Kefalopoulou et al. 2009	1	6	gen	91/77/NR	Cognition unchanged
Capelle et al. 2010	4	27	seg/gen	84/NR/NR	NR
Chang et al. 2010	5	34	seg/gen	71/NR/77	NR
Kim et al. 2011	1/10	20	NR	77/NR/NR	QoL improved
Kovacs et al. 2011	1	12	Status dystonicus	96/NR/NR	NR
Spindler et al. 2013	1	60	seg	NR/62/NR	NR
Boulogne et al. 2014	1	120	seg	NR/79/NR	Stable psychiatric state
Puri et al. 2014	1	6	seg	NR/50/NR	NR
Shaikh et al. 2015	8	36	seg/gen	85/NR/NR	NR
Trinh et al. 2014	1	18	seg	90/NR/NR	NR
Woo et al. 2014	3	3	seg/gen	76/NR/NR	QoL improved
Meoni et al. 2015	3/57	24	NR	NR/NR/NR	Stable psychiatric state
Pouclet-Courtemanche et al. 2016, including FU of ten patients Damier et al. 2007, STARDY study	19	72–132	seg/gen	NR/63/60	Cognition unchanged Mood improved in most patients (11/16) Stable psychiatric state
Sobstyl et al. 2016	2	18	gen	73/NR/NR	NR
Trezza et al. 2016	1	36	Status dystonicus	69/NR/NR	NR

Table 68.1 *(continued)*

Reference	*N*	Mean** FU in months	Type of dystonia	Mean** percentage of motor improvement of dystonia (BFMDRSm/ AIMS/ESRS)	Cognitive, affective, psychiatric outcome and QoL
			STN DBS		
Zhang et al. 2006	2/9	3	gen/ multifocal	91/NR/NR	NR
Sun et al. 2007	2/14	29	gen	89/NR/NR	NR
Meng et al. 2016, FU of 1 patient Zhang et al. 2006	1	144	gen	100/NR/NR	Stable psychiatric state

Abbreviations: AIMS, Abnormal Involuntary Movement Scale; BFMDRSm, Burke–Fahn–Marsden Dystonia Rating Scale, motor subscale; DBS, deep brain stimulation; ESRS, Extrapyramidal Symptoms Rating Scale; FU, follow-up; gen, generalised; GPi, globus pallidus internus; NR, not reported; seg, segmental; STN, subthalamic nucleus; QoL, quality of life.
*Explantation of DBS-system of one patient due to infection; **mean FU period and mean percentage improvement denote mean parameters of all patients included in case series. In column 2 (*N*) a ratio is noted if TDt/TDk patients were part of a larger case series with different dystonia subtypes.

also with respect of potentially increased psychiatric sensitivity of the STN vs GPi.

Conclusion

In summary, the above-listed results reflect level II and level III evidence for the efficacy of pallidal DBS in tardive dystonia, a disorder regularly associated with psychiatric comorbidity. Importantly, the safety profile of pallidal DBS seems to be similar to other DBS indications. Longer observation periods within controlled trials are necessary to establish the magnitude and stability of pallidal DBS in TD prior to potential recommendation as routine treatment.

References

Adityanjee, Aderibigbe YA, Jampala VC, Mathews T. 1999. The current status of tardive dystonia. *Biol Psychiatry* 45(6):715–730.

Albanese A, Bhatia K, Bressman SB, Delong MR, Fahn S, Fung VS, Hallett M, Jankovic J, Jinnah HA, Klein C, Lang AE, Mink JW, Teller JK. 2013. Phenomenology and classification of dystonia: a consensus update. *Mov Disord* 28(7):863–873.

American Psychiatric Association. 2013. *Diagnostic and Statistical Manual of Mental Disorders*. 5th edition. Arlington, VA: American Psychiatric Association.

Bhidayasiri R, Fahn S, Weiner WJ, Gronseth GS, Sullivan KL, Zesiewicz TA, American Academy of Neurology. 2013. Evidence-based guideline: treatment of tardive syndromes – report of the Guideline Development Subcommittee of the American Academy of Neurology. *Neurology* 81(5):463–469.

Boulogne S, Danaila T, Polo G, Broussolle E, Thobois S. 2014. Relapse of tardive dystonia after globus pallidus deep-brain stimulation discontinuation. *J Neurol* 261(8):1636–1637.

Burke RE, Fahn S, Jankovic J, Marsden CD, Lang AE, Gollomp S, Ilson J. 1982. Tardive dystonia: late-onset and persistent dystonia caused by antipsychotic drugs. *Neurology* 32(12):1335–1346.

Capelle HH, Blahak C, Schrader C, Baezner H, Kinfe TM, Herzog J, Dengler R, Krauss JK. 2010. Chronic deep brain stimulation in patients with tardive dystonia without a history of major psychosis. *Mov Disord* 25(10):1477–1481.

Chang EF, Schrock LE, Starr PA, Ostrem JL. 2010. Long-term benefit sustained after bilateral pallidal deep brain stimulation in patients with refractory tardive dystonia. *Stereotact Funct Neurosurg* 88(5):304–310.

Cohen OS, Hassin-Baer S, Spiegelmann R. 2007. Deep brain stimulation of the internal globus pallidus for refractory tardive dystonia. *Parkinsonism Relat Disord* 13(8):541–544.

Coubes P, Echenne B, Roubertie A, Vayssiere N, Tuffery S, Humbertclaude V, Cambonie G, Claustres M, Frerebeau P. 1999. Treatment of early-onset generalized dystonia by chronic bilateral stimulation of the internal globus pallidus. apropos of a case. *Neurochirurgie* 45(2):139–144.

Damier P, Thobois S, Witjas T, Cuny E, Derost P, Raoul S, Mertens P, Peragut JC, Lemaire JJ, Burbaud P, Nguyen JM, Llorca PM, Rascol O, French Stimulation for Tardive Dyskinesia (STARDYS) Study Group. 2007. Bilateral deep brain stimulation of the globus pallidus to treat tardive dyskinesia. *Arch Gen Psychiatry* 64(2):170–176.

Egidi M, Franzini A, Marras C, Cavallo M, Mondani M, Lavano A, Romanelli P, Castana L, Lanotte M, Functional Neurosurgery Study Group of the Italian Society of Neurosurgery. 2007. A survey of Italian cases of dystonia treated by deep brain stimulation. *J Neurosurg Sci* 51(4):153–158.

Eltahawy HA, Feinstein A, Khan F, Saint-Cyr J, Lang AE, Lozano AM. 2004. Bilateral globus pallidus internus deep brain stimulation in tardive dyskinesia: a case report. *Mov Disord* 19(8):969–972.

Franzini A, Marras C, Ferroli P, Zorzi G, Bugiani O, Romito L, Broggi G. 2005. Long-term high-frequency bilateral pallidal stimulation for neuroleptic-induced tardive dystonia: report of two cases. *J Neurosurg* 102(4):721–725.

Gerlach J, Casey DE. 1988. Tardive dyskinesia. *Acta Psychiatr Scand* 77(4):369–378.

Gruber D, Trottenberg T, Kivi A, Schoenecker T, Kopp UA, Hoffmann KT, Schneider GH, Kuhn AA, Kupsch A. 2009. Long-term effects of pallidal deep brain stimulation in tardive dystonia. *Neurology* 73(1):53–58.

Halbig TD, Gruber D, Kopp UA, Schneider GH, Trottenberg T, Kupsch A. 2005. Pallidal stimulation in dystonia: effects on cognition, mood, and quality of life. *J Neurol Neurosurg Psychiatry* 76(12):1713–1716.

Hillier CE, Wiles CM, Simpson BA. 1999. Thalamotomy for severe antipsychotic induced tardive dyskinesia and dystonia. *J Neurol Neurosurg Psychiatry* 66(2):250–251.

Katsakiori PF, Kefalopoulou Z, Markaki E, Paschali A, Ellul J, Kagadis GC, Chroni E, Constantoyannis C. 2009. Deep brain stimulation for secondary dystonia: results in 8 patients. *Acta Neurochir (Wien)* 151(5):473–478.

Kefalopoulou Z, Paschali A, Markaki E, Vassilakos P, Ellul J, Constantoyannis C. 2009. A double-blind study on a patient with tardive dyskinesia treated with pallidal deep brain stimulation. *Acta Neurol Scand* 119(4):269–273.

Kim JP, Chang WS, Chang JW. 2011. Treatment of secondary dystonia with a combined stereotactic procedure: long-term surgical outcomes. *Acta Neurochir (Wien)* 153(12):2319–2327.

Kosel M, Sturm V, Frick C, Lenartz D, Zeidler G, Brodesser D, Schlaepfer TE. 2007. Mood improvement after deep brain stimulation of the internal globus pallidus for tardive dyskinesia in a patient suffering from major depression. *J Psychiatr Res* 41(9):801–803.

Kovacs N, Balas I, Janszky J, Simon M, Fekete S, Komoly S. 2011. Status dystonicus in tardive dystonia successfully treated by bilateral deep brain stimulation. *Clin Neurol Neurosurg* 113(9):808–809.

Krause M, Fogel W, Kloss M, Rasche D, Volkmann J, Tronnier V. 2004. Pallidal stimulation for dystonia. *Neurosurgery* 55(6):1361–1368.

Krauss JK, Pohle T, Weber S, Ozdoba C, Burgunder JM. 1999. Bilateral stimulation of globus pallidus internus for treatment of cervical dystonia. *Lancet* 354(9181):837–838.

Kuhn AA, Brucke C, Schneider GH, Trottenberg T, Kivi A, Kupsch A, Capelle HH, Krauss JK, Brown P. 2008. Increased beta activity in dystonia patients after drug-induced dopamine deficiency. *Exp Neurol* 214(1):140–143.

Kupsch A, Benecke R, Muller J, Trottenberg T, Schneider GH, Poewe W, Eisner W, Wolters A, Muller JU, Deuschl G, Pinsker MO, Skogseid IM, Roeste GK, Vollmer-Haase J, Brentrup A, Krause M, Tronnier V, Schnitzler A, Voges J, Nikkhah G, Vesper J, Naumann M, Volkmann J, Deep-Brain Stimulation for Dystonia Study Group. 2006. Pallidal deep-brain stimulation in primary generalized or segmental dystonia. *N Engl J Med* 355(19):1978–1990.

Lenders M, Buschman H, Vergouwen M, Steur E, Kolling P, Hariz M. 2005. Long term results of unilateral posteroventral pallidotomy for antipsychotic drug induced tardive dyskinesia. *J Neurol Neurosurg Psychiatr* 76(7):1039.

Magarinos-Ascone CM, Regidor I, Gomez-Galan M, Cabanes-Martinez L, Figueiras-Mendez R. 2008. Deep brain stimulation in the globus pallidus to treat dystonia: electrophysiological characteristics and 2 years' follow-up in 10 patients. *Neuroscience* 152(2):558–571.

Meng DW, Liu HG, Yang AC, Zhang K, Zhang JG. 2016. Long-term effects of subthalamic nucleus deep brain stimulation in tardive dystonia. *Chin Med J (Engl)* 129(10):1257–1258.

Meoni S, Zurowski M, Lozano AM, Hodaie M, Poon YY, Fallis M, Voon V, Moro E. 2015. Long-term neuropsychiatric outcomes after pallidal stimulation in primary and secondary dystonia. *Neurology* 85(5):433–440.

Morigaki R, Mure H, Kaji R, Nagahiro S, Goto S. 2016. Therapeutic perspective on tardive syndrome with special reference to deep brain stimulation. *Front Psychiatry* 7:207.

Nandi D, Parkin S, Scott R, Winter JL, Joint C, Gregory R, Stein J, Aziz TZ. 2002. Camptocormia treated with bilateral pallidal stimulation: case report. *Neurosurg Focus* 12(2):ECP2.

O'Brien CF, Jimenez R, Hauser RA, Factor SA, Burke J, Mandri D, Castro-Gayol JC. 2015. NBI-98854, a selective monoamine transport inhibitor for the treatment of tardive dyskinesia: a randomized, double-blind, placebo-controlled study. *Mov Disord* 30(12):1681–1687.

Pouclet-Courtemanche H, Rouaud T, Thobois S, Nguyen JM, Brefel-Courbon C, Chereau I, Cuny E, Derost P, Eusebio A, Guehl D, Laurencin C, Mertens P, Ory-Magne F, Raoul S, Regis J, Ulla M, Witjas T, Burbaud P, Rascol O, Damier P. 2016. Long-term efficacy and tolerability of bilateral pallidal stimulation to treat tardive dyskinesia. *Neurology* 86(7):651–659.

Pretto TE, Dalvi A, Kang UJ, Penn RD. 2008. A prospective blinded evaluation of deep brain stimulation for the treatment of secondary dystonia and primary torticollis syndromes. *J Neurosurg* 109(3):405–409.

Puri M, Albassam A, Silver B. 2014. Deep brain stimulation in the treatment of tardive dyskinesia. *Psychiatric Annals* 44(3):123–125.

Raja M. 1995. Tardive dystonia. prevalence, risk factors, and comparison with tardive dyskinesia in a population of 200 acute psychiatric inpatients. *Eur Arch Psychiatry Clin Neurosci* 245(3):145–151.

Sako W, Goto S, Shimazu H, Murase N, Matsuzaki K, Tamura T, Mure H, Tomogane Y, Arita N, Yoshikawa H, Nagahiro S, Kaji R. 2008. Bilateral deep brain stimulation of the globus pallidus internus in tardive dystonia. *Mov Disord* 23(13):1929–1931.

Schjerling L, Hjermind LE, Jespersen B, Madsen FF, Brennum J, Jensen SR, Lokkegaard A, Karlsborg M. 2013. A randomized double-blind crossover trial comparing subthalamic and pallidal deep brain stimulation for dystonia. *J Neurosurg* 119(6):1537–1545.

Schonecker T, Gruber D, Kivi A, Muller B, Lobsien E, Schneider GH, Kuhn AA, Hoffmann KT, Kupsch AR. 2015. Postoperative MRI localisation of electrodes and clinical efficacy of pallidal deep brain stimulation in cervical dystonia. *J Neurol Neurosurg Psychiatry* 86(8):833–839.

Schrader C, Peschel T, Petermeyer M, Dengler R, Hellwig D. 2004. Unilateral deep brain stimulation of the internal globus pallidus alleviates tardive dyskinesia. *Mov Disord* 19(5):583–585.

Shaikh AG, Mewes K, DeLong MR, Gross RE, Triche SD, Jinnah HA, Boulis N, Willie JT, Freeman A, Alexander GE, Aia P, Butefisch CM, Esper CD, Factor SA. 2015. Temporal profile of improvement of tardive dystonia after globus pallidus deep brain stimulation. *Parkinsonism Relat Disord* 21(2):116–119.

Silvestri S, Seeman MV, Negrete JC, Houle S, Shammi CM, Remington GJ, Kapur S, Zipursky RB, Wilson AA, Christensen BK, Seeman P. 2000. Increased dopamine D2 receptor binding after long-term treatment with antipsychotics in humans: a clinical PET study. *Psychopharmacology (Berl)* 152(2):174–180.

Sobstyl M, Zabek M, Mossakowski Z, Zaczynski A. 2016. Deep brain stimulation of the internal globus pallidus for disabling haloperidol-induced tardive dystonia: report of two cases. *Neurol Neurochir Pol* 50(4):258–261.

Spindler MA, Galifianakis NB, Wilkinson JR, Duda JE. 2013. Globus pallidus interna deep brain stimulation for tardive dyskinesia: case report and review of the literature. *Parkinsonism Relat Disord* 19(2):141–147.

Starr PA, Turner RS, Rau G, Lindsey N, Heath S, Volz M, Ostrem JL, Marks WJ, Jr. 2006. Microelectrode-guided implantation of deep brain stimulators into the globus pallidus internus for dystonia: techniques, electrode locations, and outcomes. *J Neurosurg* 104(4):488–501.

Sun B, Chen S, Zhan S, Le W, Krahl SE. 2007. Subthalamic nucleus stimulation for primary dystonia and tardive dystonia. *Acta Neurochir Suppl* 97(Pt 2):207–214.

Thobois S, Ballanger B, Xie-Brustolin J, Damier P, Durif F, Azulay JP, Derost P, Witjas T, Raoul S, Le Bars D, Broussolle E. 2008. Globus pallidus stimulation reduces frontal hyperactivity in tardive dystonia. *J Cereb Blood Flow Metab* 28(6):1127–1138.

Thobois S, Poisson A, Damier P. 2011. Surgery for tardive dyskinesia. *Int Rev Neurobiol* 98:289–296.

Trezza A, Antonini A, Sganzerla EP, Landi A. 2016. Globus pallidus internus deep brain stimulation for the treatment of status dystonicus in tardive dystonia. *Acta Neurochir (Wien)* 158(9):1789–1791.

Trinh B, Ha AD, Mahant N, Kim SD, Owler B, Fung VS. 2014. Dramatic improvement of truncal tardive dystonia following globus pallidus pars interna deep brain stimulation. *J Clin Neurosci* 21(3):515–517.

Trottenberg T, Paul G, Meissner W, Maier-Hauff K, Taschner C, Kupsch A. 2001. Pallidal and thalamic neurostimulation in severe tardive dystonia. *J Neurol Neurosurg Psychiatry* 70(4):557–559.

Trottenberg T, Volkmann J, Deuschl G, Kuhn AA, Schneider GH, Muller J, Alesch F, Kupsch A. 2005. Treatment of severe tardive dystonia with pallidal deep brain stimulation. *Neurology* 64(2):344–346.

Vidailhet M, Vercueil L, Houeto JL, Krystkowiak P, Benabid AL, Cornu P, Lagrange C, Tezenas du Montcel S, Dormont D, Grand S, Blond S, Detante O, Pillon B, Ardouin C, Agid Y, Destee A, Pollak P, French Stimulation du Pallidum Interne dans la Dystonie (SPIDY) Study Group. 2005. Bilateral deep-brain stimulation of the globus pallidus in primary generalized dystonia. *N Engl J Med* 352(5):459–467.

Wang Y, Turnbull I, Calne S, Stoessl A, Calne DB. 1997. Pallidotomy for tardive dyskinesia. *Lancet* 349(9054):777–778.

Weetman J, Anderson I, Gregory RP. 1997. Bilateral posteroventral pallidotomy for severe antipsychotic induced tardive dyskinesia and dystonia. *J Neurol Neurosurg Psychiatr* 63(4):554–556.

Woo PY, Chan DT, Zhu XL, Yeung JH, Chan AY, Au AC, Cheng KM, Lau KY, Wing YK, Mok VC, Poon WS. 2014. Pallidal deep brain stimulation: an effective treatment in Chinese patients with tardive dystonia. *Hong Kong Med J* 20(5):455–459.

Yianni J, Bain P, Giladi N, Auca M, Gregory R, Joint C, Nandi D, Stein J, Scott R, Aziz T. 2003. Globus pallidus internus deep brain stimulation for dystonic conditions: a prospective audit. *Mov Disord* 18(4):436–442.

Zhang JG, Zhang K, Wang ZC, Ge M, Ma Y. 2006. Deep brain stimulation in the treatment of secondary dystonia. *Chin Med J (Engl)* 119(24):2069–2074.

Chapter 69

Deep Brain Stimulation for Choreoathetosis in Cerebral Palsy

Marie Vidailhet and Christian Amlang

Cerebral palsy (CP) is the most common cause of acquired dystonia in children. The prevalence of cerebral palsy is approximately 1.5–3 per 1000 live births (Koy & Timmermans 2016; Koy et al. 2016). In reality, the diagnosis of 'cerebral palsy' is an umbrella term for the neurological features that appear as a consequence of perinatal insults on an immature brain with heterogeneous aetiologies, from perinatal asphyxia, infection, trauma, metabolic brain injury, kernicterus, vascular events and, more recently, rare genetic disorders on an immature or mature (term birth) brain. Structural and functional alterations are also heterogeneous: the most affected regions are the basal ganglia (mainly pallidum and posterior putamen), the ventrolateral thalami, the sensorimotor cortex and related subcortical white matter, but more widespread grey and white matter abnormalities may be observed. From early development, children develop a variety of symptoms including abnormal and delayed developmental milestones, dystonic postures, hyperkinetic dystonic–dyskinetic movements, spasticity, axial hypotonia, ataxia, speech and swallowing difficulties, and overall abnormal motor control with maladaptive processes. Spastic CP (85 per cent of cases) and dyskinetic CP (15–20 per cent of cases) have been distinguished, although there is often some overlapping of symptoms (Koy et al. 2016).

While the estimated life expectancy of affected patients has approached that of the general population in recent years, pharmacological treatments are poorly tolerated with little or no effect, botulinum toxin injections may be used locally for dystonia, and intrathecal baclofen may be helpful against spasticity but with limited effect and risks of complications.

Therefore, as deep brain stimulation (DBS) has proved to be an excellent therapeutic option for patients suffering from primary dystonia, neurostimulation was proposed for dyskinetic CP (dystonic-choreoathetosis CP), both in children and in adults. Nevertheless, after more than a decade of DBS in CP, it is still difficult to decide, on an individual basis, to whom and when DBS should be proposed for dystonic-choreoathetosis CP patients. Movement disorder teams, experienced in DBS, have a wide range of mixed views from proactive, early-age neurostimulation, to reluctance to propose DBS for CP patients.

Indeed, 'don't throw the baby out with the bathwater': DBS is still an option to be considered in dyskinetic CP: (1) to limit, if possible, the consequences of CP during motor development (limitations of functional capacities and pain coming from dystonia, trunk and limb deformities) (Marks et al. 2011; Lin et al. 2014); (2) before the development of spinal cord complications related to severe cervical dystonia (cervical myelopathy) (Guettard et al. 2012); (3) in status dystonicus, a life-threatening complication in dystonia, including CP, as emergency surgery (DBS of the GPi) for a rapid effect on medically untreatable severe hyperkinetic movements.

Here, we briefly review the results of the literature, and then discuss the challenges and future avenues.

A Decade of DBS in Cerebral Palsy: Focus on Dystonia and Hyperkinetic Disorders

Dystonia, as Assessed by the Burke–Fahn–Marsden Rating Scale (BFMDRS)

In 2013, Koy (Koy et al. 2013) published a review paper of 20 articles on DBS surgery in CP, which included 68 patients in total. To date, this has been the most comprehensive analysis on this topic and several of its observations are worthy of mention here. For most of the 68 patients, the GPi was the target of choice. In 60 cases, bilateral GPi stimulation was carried out; three patients had unilateral GPi stimulation; and one patient received unilateral GPi stimulation with a simultaneous unilateral STN stimulation. The nucleus ventralis oralis anterior and the ventral lateral nucleus of the thalamus were alternative targets in the other four patients. The mean age at operation was 25.3, including paediatric and adult patients with an age range of 5–46 years. The outcome assessment was recorded at a median follow-up of 12 months by administering the BFMDRS motor (BFMDRS-M) and disability (BFMDRS-D) subscales. The BFMDRS-M was used for 64 patients who showed an overall improvement of 23.6 per cent. The BFMDRS-D was assessed in 60 patients and demonstrated a mean percentage improvement of 9.2 per cent. In the largest of the reviewed studies (Vidailhet et al. 2009), 13 patients with dystonia-choreoathetosis cerebral palsy due to neonatal hypoxic encephalopathy had a 24 per cent decrease in the mean BFMDRS-M 12 months after surgery. Four patients improved by 39–55 per cent, whereas four of the participating subjects did not respond (improvement <20 per cent). Only four of the 20 studies provided quality-of-life data, which is why a further meta-analysis was not feasible. A detailed review of the quality-of-life outcomes reveals that a majority of patients and caregivers reported a significant subjective improvement of symptoms that might not have been adequately reflected by the objective outcome measures. Vidailhet (Vidailhet et al. 2009) used the 36-item short form general health survey questionnaire and documented improvements in the subscores for body pain and mental health. In another study, three of five patients showed significant improvement on the Caregiver Priorities and Child Health Index of Life with Disabilities Questionnaire, and five of five patients attained improvements in performance as well as four of five in satisfaction on the Canadian Occupational Performance Measure (Gimeno et al. 2014). Krauss et al. (2003) reported that two of four CP patients felt marked improvement of symptoms on a self-rating score after DBS surgery.

When analysing possible predictors of successful DBS therapy based on the 20 reviewed studies, Koy et al. (2013) did not find any correlation between age at surgery and clinical outcome assessed by the BFMDRS. However, they observed that the more severe the dystonia was before DBS, the smaller was the postoperative percentage of improvement. Based on the data, they concluded that a preoperative BFMDRS-M of more than 85 might indicate a high risk of non-response to DBS surgery.

Six large studies have been published since Koy et al. (2013) completed their review article (Marks et al. 2013; Olaya et al. 2013; Keen et al. 2014; Kim et al. 2014; Koy et al. 2014; Romito et al. 2015). In total, 50 patients were enrolled including 18 paediatric (<18 years old) and 32 adult patients with a mean age at operation of 22.3 years and an age range of 6–47 years. In these later studies, bilateral GPi stimulation was carried out in all patients. While the overall BFMDRS-M outcome improvement of 28 per cent was similar to the meta-analysis of Koy et al., two publications stood out with a much more striking improvement rate of 49.5 per cent for severity and 39.2 per cent for disability (Romito et al. 2015). The BFMDRS-D was assessed in 39 patients. The mean percentage improvement was 13.3 per cent (16.8 per cent if we did not take into account the study by Koy et al. (2013) as those patients did not have any improvement on the disability scale). Romito et al. (2015) also used the 36-item short form general health survey questionnaire in order to assess health-related quality of life and found an improvement in most patients. As other authors before, Olaya et al. (2013) argued that the BFMDRS-D was unable to capture the subjective increased comfort levels and decided to use a subjective benefit rating scale for caregivers. Two of five patients were reported to have a good, two a minimal and one no benefit from DBS surgery. Kim et al. (2014) administered a subjective ten-point satisfaction scale, which showed an increased subjective satisfaction two years after surgery. Subjective improvement was also reported in Koy et al.'s study (Koy et al. 2014), despite no significant improvement on the BFMDRS-M and -D scales, pointing out that different outcome measures should be considered, beside the 'classical' dystonia scales, that were mainly designed for the assessment of idiopathic generalised dystonia.

Hyperkinetic Movements (Choreoathetosis/Chorea/Status Dystonicus)

As most of the studies used the BFMDRS as the primary outcome measure, which mainly focuses on dystonic symptoms and does not distinguish tonic (dystonic postures) and phasic (hyperkinetic) movements, few conclusions can be drawn about the reduction of choreoathetotic/hyperkinetic symptoms. In one study on pallidal stimulation for generalised choreoathetosis patients judged benefit as relevant when they regained their ability to improve their daily routines (Krauss et al. 2003). In the aforementioned larger cohort study with 13 adult patients, the authors highlighted a better outcome of DBS stimulation on phasic movement disorders than on tonic movements (Vidailhet et al. 2009). In contrast, a more recent study on 15 patients (13 adults and two children) challenged this finding by reporting an equivalent effect of DBS on tonic postures and phasic movements in their patients (Romito et al. 2015). A special mention should be made of status dystonicus, a life-threatening condition that combines severe tonic and hyperkinetic features. In two cases of acute status dystonicus with generalised dystonia and chorea in cerebral palsy, bilateral pallidal DBS produced immediate resolution of the hyperkinetic movement disorders (Apetauerova et al. 2010). A stronger effect of DBS on the hyperkinetic-choreoathetotic movements with only a modest improvement of dystonic symptoms was reported in another case (Gill et al. 2001).

Overall, what we have learned from a decade of DBS in cerebral palsy is that pallidal DBS, performed in emergency, can overcome life-threatening hyperkinetic movement disorders in CP, as well as in other types of dystonia. Some patients may benefit from neurostimulation, but little is known about the predictive factors of DBS outcome in dyskinetic CP: whether differences of outcome are related to clinical features heterogeneity, underlying structural or developmental lesions, selection of the target (functional alterations of the pallidum), limits of assessment tools to capture subtle effects of DBS or a combination of those remain to be disentangled.

A Different Approach: Objectives of the Patients and the Effect of DBS in CP

Different Scales to Capture the Effects of DBS on Other Symptoms?

Concerning the seemingly modest effect of DBS surgery on symptoms, several authors object that the usually administered outcome scores (above all the BFMDRS) might fail to reflect the true symptomatic improvement. Some patients reported a much better subjective improvement, especially on the functional level, than the measured improvement rate might have suggested. Other scales may be relevant for the evaluation of a wider range of movement disorders in CP: the AIMS (Abnormal Involuntary Movement Scale, that has been used for tardive dyskinesias), the Barry–Albright Dystonia Scale across time (Marks et al. 2013), the Child Health Index with Life Disabilities Questionnaire and the Canadian Occupational Performance Measure (COPM) (Gimeno et al. 2014). The COPM assesses important concerns such as pain, comfort, ability to attend school, sitting tolerance, daily care and burden to caregiver (Olaya et al. 2013), and may therefore constitute a more adequate tool to measure the postoperative outcomes. In the majority of secondary dystonias, the BFMDRS failed to demonstrate significant improvement highlighting a possible insensitivity of traditional impairment scales and a higher accuracy of the COPM and other functional assessment scales in this patient group.

Finally, the Goal Attainment Scale (GAS), already used to evaluate outcomes of surgical and non-surgical (botulinum injections) interventions may better reflect patients'/parents'/carers' aspirations, or the subjective improvement reported in some studies without over-modification of the 'classical' motor scales (Koy et al. 2014). Even subtle improvements can significantly impact quality of life and caretaking (Keen et al. 2014).

Wellbeing and Quality of Life

The CGI (Clinical Global Impression) scale may be a gross, albeit relevant measure. In addition to pain evaluation, the SF-36 general heath questionnaire may explore improvements for body pain and mental health (Vidailhet et al. 2009). Overall, there is no influence of pallidal stimulation on cognitive functions (no adverse events) or mood.

Variability of Outcome Results: Patient Related or Treatment Related, or both?

Dyskinetic Cerebral Palsy: A Very Heterogeneous Group of Individual Patients

All the studies report a wide range of different response rates in individual patients, with complete failures in some. A possible explanation for this finding is the heterogeneity of diagnosis underlying CP. Interestingly, it has be mentioned (two cases) that CP secondary to kernicterus demonstrated a particularly favourable outcome which may reinforce the idea of varying degrees of treatment responses in CP, depending on the mechanism of injury and the extent of damage to the basal ganglia. There is a great variation in the degree of white and grey matter lesions in dyskinetic CP and subsequently a higher level of difficulty, especially in children, to localise correctly the stimulation target. It has also been noted that due to these variations and abnormalities in CP patients' anatomic structures, the pallidal circuit may behave differently, which makes optimal lead placement a challenge and may reduce the efficacy of GPi stimulation (Vidailhet et al. 2009; Marks et al. 2011; Koy et al. 2013). However, no correlation could be observed between outcome improvement and MRI findings. Nevertheless, and although alternative targets (such as thalamus (Thompson et al. 2000), subthalamic nucleus and deep anterior cerebellum (Sokal et al. 2015)) have been proposed, most authors seem to agree that the GPi still seems to be the optimal target for DBS surgery in dyskinetic CP. Finally, the patterns of injury within the basal ganglia predisposing to dyskinetic cerebral palsy may have an influence: there is a consistent involvement of the lentiform nuclei in dyskinetic cerebral palsy, and two groups of patients can be distinguished in dyskinetic cerebral palsy: those with putamen-predominant damage and those with panlenticular damage involving both the putamen and the globus pallidus (Aravamuthan & Waugh 2016). In addition, multimodal MRI analysis showed decreased fractional anisotropy in the thalamocortical pathways and abnormal sensorimotor resting-state networks: whether the abnormal sensorimotor network of children with CP accounts for a poor functional prognosis after neurostimulation remains to be explored.

Deep Brain Stimulation Management: How and When?

Romito et al. (2015) reported an overall symptom improvement rate of almost 50 per cent, a result strikingly better than previous studies, with a follow-up of more than five years after surgery. It may be that long follow-up periods are needed to reach steady state in acquired dystonia related to static brain lesions, while other studies with shorter follow-up periods may have failed to capture the complete treatment effects.

A controversial question is about the best timing of DBS surgery. CP is a childhood disease that affects patients throughout their lifetime. If surgery is indicated, when would be the best moment to carry it out? Woopen et al. (2013) argue that DBS at an early stage of development might be superior compared to patients who are operated on during adulthood in terms of learning and relearning motor tasks since motor skills are probably important in all aspects of development, including cognitive function and social interactions. It has been emphasised that improvement after neuromodulation may take weeks, months and occasionally years to occur, and that cellular reorganisation has been postulated to play some role in the benefits of DBS. If this assumption is true, neurostimulation could be particularly beneficial in children as their brain is still maturing. In the same way, DBS may then be less effective in adult patients as long-standing aberrant neural plasticity may limit its effect, but some adult patients may have as good beneficial effects as those of children (Vidailhet et al. 2009). On the other hand, younger patients can have a natural progression towards an improvement of dystonic symptoms, and surgery would be unnecessary or could be harmful in their cases.

Another argument used by several authors who advocated for early intervention is that the therapeutic response may be limited by musculoskeletal contractures developing over the course of the disease in dyskinetic CP. It has also been noted that dystonia duration at the time of DBS surgery appears to inversely correlate with response following DBS. However, it is crucial to keep in mind that the only meta-analysis on DBS in CP that has been carried out thus far did not show any correlation between age and clinical outcome, but this finding should also be interpreted with caution until the results from the international registry are available.

In conclusion, from the knowledge accumulated during the past decade, DBS in dyskinetic CP should be considered with a fresh mind and no discouragement (Vidailhet et al. 2013; Cif 2015). Several steps are to be taken towards: (1) a better understanding and delineation of CP, both in term of aetiologies and in term of structural and functional abnormalities underlying the disordered movement (motor control and movement disorders); (2) a goal- and patient-oriented assessment in addition to the present motor and disability scores; (3) a different targeting method taking into account the profound reorganisation of the sensorimotor network (Papadelis et al. 2014), new approaches in the stimulation techniques more closely related to the individual physiology of each patient.

References

Apetauerova D, Schirmer CM, Shils JL, Zani J, Arle JE. 2010. Successful bilateral deep brain stimulation of the globus pallidus internus for persistent status dystonicus and generalized chorea. *J Neurosurg* 113(3):634–638.

Aravamuthan BR, Waugh JL. 2016. Localization of basal ganglia and thalamic damage in dyskinetic cerebral palsy. *Pediatr Neurol* 54:11–21.

Cif L. 2015. Deep brain stimulation in dystonic cerebral palsy: for whom and for what? *Eur J Neurol* 22(3):423–425.

Gill S, Curran A, Tripp J, Melarickas L, Hurran C, Stanley O. 2001. Hyperkinetic movement disorder in an 11-year-old child treated with bilateral pallidal stimulators. *Dev Med Child Neurol* 43(5):350–353.

Gimeno H, Tustin K, Lumsden D, Ashkan K, Selway R, Lin JP. 2014. Evaluation of functional goal outcomes using the Canadian Occupational Performance Measure (COPM) following deep brain stimulation (DBS) in childhood dystonia. *Eur J Paediatr Neurol* 18(3):308–316.

Guettard E, Ricard D, Roze E, Elbaz A, Anheim M, Thobois S, Lepeintre JF, Galanaud D, Mazel C, Vidailhet M. 2012. Risk factors for spinal cord lesions in dystonic cerebral palsy and generalised dystonia. *J Neurol Neurosurg Psychiatry* 83(2):159–163.

Keen JR, Przekop A, Olaya JE, Zouros A, Hsu FP. 2014. Deep brain stimulation for the treatment of childhood dystonic cerebral palsy. *J Neurosurg Pediatr* 14(6):585–593.

Kim AR, Chang JW, Chang WS, Park ES, Cho SR. 2014. Two-year outcomes of deep brain stimulation in adults with cerebral palsy. *Ann Rehabil Med* 38(2):209–217.

Koy A, Timmermann L. 2016. Deep brain stimulation in cerebral palsy: challenges and opportunities. *Eur J Paediatr Neurol* 21(1):118–121.

Koy A, Hellmich M, Pauls KA, Marks W, Lin JP, Fricke O, Timmermann L. 2013. Effects of deep brain stimulation in dyskinetic cerebral palsy: a meta-analysis. *Mov Disord* 28(5):647–654.

Koy A, Pauls KA, Flossdorf P, Becker J, Schonau E, Maarouf M, Liebig T, Fricke O, Fink GR, Timmermann L. 2014. Young adults with dyskinetic cerebral palsy improve subjectively on pallidal stimulation, but not in formal dystonia, gait, speech and swallowing testing. *Eur Neurol* 72(5–6):340–348.

Koy A, Lin JP, Sanger TD, Marks WA, Mink JW, Timmermann L. 2016. Advances in management of movement disorders in children. *Lancet Neurol* 15(7):719–735.

Krauss JK, Loher TJ, Weigel R, Capelle HH, Weber S, Burgunder JM. 2003. Chronic stimulation of the globus pallidus internus for treatment of non-dYT1 generalized dystonia and choreoathetosis: 2-year follow up. *J Neurosurg* 98(4):785–792.

Lin JP, Lumsden DE, Gimeno H, Kaminska M. 2014. The impact and prognosis for dystonia in childhood including dystonic cerebral palsy: a clinical and demographic tertiary cohort study. *J Neurol Neurosurg Psychiatry* 85(11):1239–1244.

Marks WA, Honeycutt J, Acosta F, Jr, Reed M, Bailey L, Pomykal A, Mercer M. 2011. Dystonia due to cerebral palsy responds to deep brain stimulation of the globus pallidus internus. *Mov Disord* 26(9):1748–1751.

Marks W, Bailey L, Reed M, Pomykal A, Mercer M, Macomber D, Acosta F, Jr, Honeycutt J. 2013. Pallidal stimulation in children: comparison between cerebral palsy and DYT1 dystonia. *J Child Neurol* 28(7):840–848.

Olaya JE, Christian E, Ferman D, Luc Q, Krieger MD, Sanger TD, Liker MA. 2013. Deep brain stimulation in children and young adults with secondary dystonia: the Children's Hospital Los Angeles experience. *Neurosurg Focus* 35(5):E7.

Papadelis C, Ahtam B, Nazarova M, Nimec D, Snyder B, Grant PE, Okada Y. 2014. Cortical somatosensory reorganization in children with spastic cerebral palsy: a multimodal neuroimaging study. *Front Hum Neurosci* 8:725.

Romito LM, Zorzi G, Marras CE, Franzini A, Nardocci N, Albanese A. 2015. Pallidal stimulation for acquired dystonia due to cerebral palsy: beyond 5 years. *Eur J Neurol* 22(3):426-e32.

Sokal P, Rudas M, Harat M, Szylberg L, Zielinski P. 2015. Deep anterior cerebellar stimulation reduces symptoms of secondary dystonia in patients with cerebral palsy treated due to spasticity. *Clin Neurol Neurosurg* 135:62–68.

Thompson TP, Kondziolka D, Albright AL. 2000. Thalamic stimulation for choreiform movement disorders in children: report of two cases. *J Neurosurg* 92(4):718–721.

Vidailhet M, Yelnik J, Lagrange C, Fraix V, Grabli D, Thobois S, Burbaud P, Welter ML, Xie-Brustolin J, Braga MC, Ardouin C, Czernecki V, Klinger H, Chabardes S, Seigneuret E, Mertens P, Cuny E, Navarro S, Cornu P, Benabid AL, Le Bas JF, Dormont D, Hermier M, Dujardin K, Blond S, Krystkowiak P, Destee A, Bardinet E, Agid Y, Krack P, Broussolle E, Pollak P; French SPIDY-2 Study Group. 2009. Bilateral pallidal deep brain stimulation for the treatment of patients with dystonia-choreoathetosis cerebral palsy: a prospective pilot study. *Lancet Neurol* 8(8):709–717.

Vidailhet M, Jutras MF, Grabli D, Roze E. 2013. Deep brain stimulation for dystonia. *J Neurol Neurosurg Psychiatry* 84(9):1029–1042.

Woopen C, Pauls KA, Koy A, Moro E, Timmermann L. 2013. Early application of deep brain stimulation: clinical and ethical aspects. *Prog Neurobiol* 110:74–88.

Chapter 70

Deep Brain Stimulation for Other Secondary Dystonias

Lars Timmermann and Anne Koy

Deep brain stimulation (DBS) has been shown to be a highly effective treatment option in a number of different dystonias. Given the impressive lasting improvements in patients with hereditary dystonias (e.g. DYT1 dystonia), there was considerable hope to improve also the larger patient cohorts with dystonias secondary to metabolic changes, trauma and hypoxia, as well as rare neurodegenerative diseases such as Huntington's disease. Unfortunately, 'secondary dystonias' tend to respond less to DBS than 'primary dystonias' (please be aware that the new nomenclature for dystonia does not have this grouping anymore; however, due to the vast majority of past papers using this term this chapter will stick to the old nomenclature). This clinical phenomenon might have two major reasons. (1) From a pathophysiological standpoint, the alteration in the interaction of different brain areas, such as after trauma, is probably much more difficult to re-establish than a progressively increasing dystonic motor output due to changes in membrane excitability, for example based on a 'channelopathy' in many hereditary forms of dystonia. (2) In an individual patient who has performed in a physiological pattern for the first years/decades of his or her life, one might assume that an intervention such as DBS might reinstall more easily a physiological interaction network than in a patient with, for example, a perinatal hypoxic brain injury who has never had a physiological brain interaction pattern before.

Deep Brain Stimulation: Results in Specific 'Secondary Dystonias'

Cerebral Palsy

Cerebral palsy (CP) is one of the most common movement disorders in the Western world: one has to assume that 2–3/1000 live births are related to mild to severe hypoxia. About 10 per cent of these patients develop a dystonic-athetotic mobile form of dystonia, often with unrestricted memory and cognition. Since pharmacological options are rather limited, DBS has been a research focus for a number of years. In a French prospective open-label multicentre trial, Vidaillhet and colleagues investigated systematically the response of adults with dystonic-choreatiform variance of CP to DBS of the globus pallidus internus (GPi) (Vidailhet et al. 2009). GPi DBS resulted in considerable improvement in the range of 20–30 per cent according to the Burke–Fahn–Marsden Dystonia Rating Scale (BFMDRS). Remarkably, a profound variability was found in the response: few patients showed a deterioration compared to the preoperative status, whereas others showed improvement in the range of patients with idiopathic dystonia at around 50 per cent. This large variability of responses is likely to reflect different pathophysiological mechanisms with resulting differences in the response to DBS. A recent meta-analysis of GPi DBS outcome until 2013 including all published patients with CP dystonia revealed a similar result (Koy et al. 2013): patients responded on average about 24 per cent compared to baseline as assessed by the BFMDRS. One might doubt whether or not the BFMDRS really catches all aspects in quality of life of patients with choreatic-dystonic CP. Furthermore, it is possible that the intervention in some adult patients might be too late. The pathophysiological interactions between different brain regions might have been damaged to such an extent that physiological states are more difficult to establish than in younger patients. To address this issue we started a prospective multicentre trial on GPi DBS in paediatric patients with CP and chorea-dystonic movement patterns (STIM-CP), which will probably end recruiting in 2017.

Posttraumatic Dystonia

After severe head trauma a number of patients develop a 'posttraumatic' dystonia. Pathophysiologically, in many patients lesions within the basal ganglia cortex loops have to be assumed. Given the very bad response of this form of dystonia to pharmacological intervention, GPi DBS has been investigated as an option for these patients (Slow et al. 2015). So far, there have been numerous cases described with improvements of dystonia in short-term intervals after GPi DBS, as well as a few cases with long-term follow-up who showed a benefit from GPi DBS after posttraumatic dystonia (Loher et al. 2000). However, systematic prospective multicentre trials are lacking, resulting in only anecdotal evidence of effectiveness in this rare indication. It is very likely that relevant and consistent success with DBS can only be achieved when individual pathophysiological aspects of the posttraumatic dystonia are reflected in customised stimulation setting and parameters.

Neurodegeneration With Brain Iron Accumulation Dystonia

An impressive, mostly generalised dystonia in early childhood occurs in patients with diseases in the spectrum of NBIA (neurodegeneration with brain iron accumulation, formerly known as Hallervorden–Spatz disease). This form of dystonia cannot be adequately treated with any pharmacological intervention or botulinum toxin alone (Koy et al. 2016), and was therefore a very early subject of investigation for the possibility of DBS. Castelnau and colleagues published a series of six patients in 2005 with the characteristic 'eye of the tiger sign' and severe dystonia due to a PKAN mutation (pantothenate kinase-associated neurodegeneration) (Castelnau et al. 2005). They described a lasting profound improvement of more than 50 per cent as measured by the BFMDRS, indicating a response in the range of patients with idiopathic generalised or segmental dystonia. This impressive result could not be observed in a number of patients in any other centre; therefore, a retrospective collection of all published and non-published cases with NBIA dystonia and GPi DBS was undertaken: this collection revealed a lasting and positive response to DBS with respect to the severity of dystonia as well as the impairment in quality of life (Timmermann et al. 2010). However, the amount of improvement shown in the single-centre data could not be reproduced. It is therefore likely that different subforms of NBIA dystonia, such as PKAN, might respond as well as some forms of hereditary dystonia, whereas other forms inducing potentially more irreversible harm to the basal ganglia cortex loops are less likely to improve after DBS. A major task for the next decade will be the identification of patient profiles with positive or negative responses as well as the individual characterisation of the pathophysiological alterations in the interaction of different brain areas.

Neuroacanthocytosis

Neuroacanthocytosis describes a range of movement disorders with dystonic, choreatic and neuropsychological features, such as McLeod syndrome or choreoacanthocytosis. Again, pharmacological treatment including botulinum toxin, as well as physical options, are limited, making it necessary to investigate surgical options including GPi DBS. Interestingly, GPi DBS in these patients has been recently demonstrated to be effective in the short term as well as over long-term follow-up in a retrospective multicentre cohort of 15 patients (Miquel et al. 2013). The author group measured choreatic movements as well as dystonia with the UHDRS (United Huntington's Disease Rating Scale) and found remarkable improvements in the short term (<6 months) by more than 50 per cent and in the long term (>6 months) by more than 40 per cent. Parkinsonism, as well as swallowing and dysarthria, did not improve in this cohort from 12 centres. The motor improvement led to a significant improvement in daily functioning as well as other disability scales. In the long run, more than 60 per cent of the patients were significantly improved. Taken together, despite lack of prospective controlled trials, the current meta-analysis indicates that major clinical deficits such as dystonia and chorea improve significantly, justifying GPi DBS in patients with neuroacanthocytosis.

Huntington's Disease

Huntington's disease (HD) is a genetically determined progressive neurodegenerative disease resulting clinically in a choreatic-dystonic movement disorder with pronounced neuropsychological deficits. The pharmacological options are rather limited, and a number of case reports indicated the potential benefit from GPi DBS. A prospective crossover single-centre pilot trial investigated whether stimulation of the internal or external part of the globus pallidus (GP) lead to differential effects in HD patients (Wojtecki et al. 2015). The authors found that patients with a 'Westphal variant' with primarily bradykinesia responded less than patients with dystonia and chorea dominating the clinical picture. Interestingly, stimulation of the GPi and the GPe was equally effective. This pilot trial served as a basis for an ongoing prospective randomised multicentre trial in Germany.

Recently, three patients with Huntington's disease undergoing GPi DBS in a French pilot trial were investigated (Delorme et al. 2016). The authors found reduced dystonia, but also deteriorated bradykinesia and dysarthria. Overall cognitive function was not altered and ventral stimulation turned out to be more successful than dorsal stimulation. The authors concluded that non-demented HD patients at early disease stages and with pronounced dystonia but little bradykinesia might be more suitable candidates for GPi DBS (Delorme et al. 2016).

Taken together, dystonia in HD patients turns out to be a promising future indication for DBS, potentially in combination with pharmacological and disease-modifying interventions.

Future Directions and Research Strategies

Individual Pathophysiological Characterisation

The current concepts of GPi DBS in patients with dystonia are using similar stimulation settings and parameters in a variety of different entities. However, one may assume that the underlying pathophysiological mechanisms are fundamentally different between various forms of dystonia, as well as between individual patients. Future attempts of DBS in different forms of dystonia should therefore work intensively on the individual characterisation of subforms and patterns of dystonia and their potentially best-suited stimulation parameters as well as on smart stimulation algorithms integrating multiple independent stimulation sites (Timmermann et al. 2015), and eventually closed-loop stimulation settings with intelligent individualised stimulation set-ups. The basis for this type of approach is a reliable, non-invasive individual characterisation of pathophysiological networks in dystonia patients – a task that has been shown to be very difficult to achieve.

Targets in Secondary Dystonias

In many secondary dystonias the GP is severely lesioned; in some diseases, such as NBIA dystonia variants, this is even part of the imaging characteristic (e.g. the 'eye of the tiger sign' as a sign of pathological structural changes of the GPi in PKAN patients). This means that the well-established target is potentially not preserved as active brain tissue and, as such, modulation of neuronal activity is potentially not effective within this target. Therefore, a number of different new targets such as the subthalamic nucleus (STN) (Ostrem et al. 2011, 2017), the subthalamic area (Pauls et al. 2014) or the thalamus could be suitable as well for positive modulation of the specific dystonia. To answer this question, randomised controlled trials with intelligent crossover designs have to test which specific target area is the best choice for different disease entities. Ideally, an individual characterisation of the pathophysiological network preoperatively would allow an individual an optimised target selection.

Registries

Many of the dystonia entities listed in this chapter are rare or even ultra-rare diseases. Performing prospective clinical multicentre trials in these indications remains a difficult task because even in high-volume centres only few patients are being operated on within a decade. Furthermore, industry funding that helped establish evidence in a number of indications for DBS is much less interested in rare diseases. Therefore, high-quality, international registries led by well-known investigators and ideally funded sustainably by public research funding or foundations are a potential solution for this problem. A great role model with respect to this approach might be the German Registry for Deep Brain Stimulation in Pediatric Movement Disorders (GEPESTIM, DRKS00006778; coordination: Anne Koy and Lars Timmermann) that is listing in a detailed way all patients with paediatric movement disorders undergoing DBS in Germany, Switzerland and Austria. This regional registry is linked to PEDI-DBS (www.pedidbs.org; PIs: Terry Sanger and Warren Marks), an international consortium to register similar populations of patients internationally.

References

Castelnau P, Cif L, Valente EM, Vayssiere N, Hemm S, Gannau A, Digiorgio A, Coubes P. 2005. Pallidal stimulation improves pantothenate kinase-associated neurodegeneration. *Ann Neurol* 57(5):738–741.

Delorme C, Rogers A, Lau B, Francisque H, Welter ML, Fernandez Vidal S, Yelnik J, Durr A, Grabli D, Karachi C. 2016. Deep brain stimulation of the internal pallidum in Huntington's disease patients: clinical outcome and neuronal firing patterns. *J Neurol* 263(2):290–298.

Koy A, Hellmich M, Pauls KA, Marks W, Lin JP, Fricke O, Timmermann L. 2013. Effects of deep brain stimulation in dyskinetic cerebral palsy: a meta-analysis. *Mov Disord* 28(5):647–654.

Koy A, Lin JP, Sanger TD, Marks WA, Mink JW, Timmermann L. 2016. Advances in management of movement disorders in children. *Lancet Neurol* 15(7):719–735.

Loher TJ, Hasdemir MG, Burgunder JM, Krauss JK. 2000. Long-term follow-up study of chronic globus pallidus internus stimulation for posttraumatic hemidystonia. *J Neurosurg* 92(3):457–460.

Miquel M, Spampinato U, Latxague C, Aviles-Olmos I, Bader B, Bertram K, Bhatia K, Burbaud P, Burghaus L, Cho JW, Cuny E, Danek A, Foltynie T, Garcia Ruiz PJ, Gimenez-Roldan S, Guehl D, Guridi J, Hariz M, Jarman P, Kefalopoulou ZM, Limousin P, Lipsman N, Lozano AM, Moro E, Ngy D, Rodriguez-Oroz MC, Shang H, Shin H, Walker RH, Yokochi F, Zrinzo L, Tison F. 2013. Short and long term outcome of bilateral pallidal stimulation in chorea-acanthocytosis. *PLoS One* 8(11):e79241.

Ostrem JL, Racine CA, Glass GA, Grace JK, Volz MM, Heath SL, Starr PA. 2011. Subthalamic nucleus deep brain stimulation in primary cervical dystonia. *Neurology* 76(10):870–878.

Ostrem JL, San Luciano M, Dodenhoff KA, Ziman N, Markun LC, Racine CA, de Hemptinne C, Volz MM, Heath SL, Starr PA. 2017. Subthalamic nucleus deep brain stimulation in isolated dystonia: a 3-year follow-up study. *Neurology* 88(1):25–35.

Pauls KA, Hammesfahr S, Moro E, Moore AP, Binder E, El Majdoub F, Fink GR, Sturm V, Krauss JK, Maarouf M, Timmermann L. 2014. Deep brain stimulation in the ventrolateral thalamus/subthalamic area in dystonia with head tremor. *Mov Disord* 29(7):953–959.

Slow EJ, Hamani C, Lozano AM, Poon YY, Moro E. 2015. Deep brain stimulation for treatment of dystonia secondary to stroke or trauma. *J Neurol Neurosurg Psychiatry* 86(9):1046–1048.

Timmermann L, Pauls KA, Wieland K, Jech R, Kurlemann G, Sharma N, Gill SS, Haenggeli CA, Hayflick SJ, Hogarth P, Leenders KL, Limousin P, Malanga CJ, Moro E, Ostrem JL, Revilla FJ, Santens P, Schnitzler A, Tisch S, Valldeoriola F, Vesper J, Volkmann J, Woitalla D, Peker S. 2010. Dystonia in neurodegeneration with brain iron accumulation: outcome of bilateral pallidal stimulation. *Brain* 133(Pt 3):701–712.

Timmermann L, Jain R, Chen L, Maarouf M, Barbe MT, Allert N, Brucke T, Kaiser I, Beirer S, Sejio F, Suarez E, Lozano B, Haegelen C, Verin M, Porta M, Servello D, Gill S, Whone A, Van Dyck N, Alesch F. 2015. Multiple-source current steering in subthalamic nucleus deep brain stimulation for Parkinson's disease (the VANTAGE study): a non-randomised, prospective, multicentre, open-label study. *Lancet Neurol* 14(7):693–701.

Vidailhet M, Yelnik J, Lagrange C, Fraix V, Grabli D, Thobois S, Burbaud P, Welter ML, Xie-Brustolin J, Braga MC, Ardouin C, Czernecki V, Klinger H, Chabardes S, Seigneuret E, Mertens P, Cuny E, Navarro S, Cornu P, Benabid AL, Le Bas JF, Dormont D, Hermier M, Dujardin K, Blond S, Krystkowiak P, Destee A, Bardinet E, Agid Y, Krack P, Broussolle E, Pollak P, French SPIDY-2 Study Group. 2009. Bilateral pallidal deep brain stimulation for the treatment of patients with dystonia-choreoathetosis cerebral palsy: a prospective pilot study. *Lancet Neurol* 8(8):709–717.

Wojtecki L, Groiss SJ, Ferrea S, Elben S, Hartmann CJ, Dunnett SB, Rosser A, Saft C, Sudmeyer M, Ohmann C, Schnitzler A, Vesper J, Surgical Approaches Working Group of the European Huntington's Disease Network (EHDN). 2015. A prospective pilot trial for pallidal deep brain stimulation in Huntington's disease. *Front Neurol* 6:177.

Chapter 71

The Subthalamic Nucleus as a Deep Brain Stimulation Target for Dystonia

Jill L. Ostrem and Kelly A. Mills

Background of DBS Therapy for Dystonia

The majority of trials evaluating the efficacy of deep brain stimulation (DBS) therapy for dystonia have used the globus pallidum internus (GPi) as the brain target. Recently, alternative brain targets have been shown to also improve dystonia. This chapter will focus on what is currently understood about the use of the subthalamic nucleus (STN) for treatment of dystonia.

Limitations of GPi DBS in Dystonia

Despite the success using pallidal DBS to treat dystonia, there are some limitations. Limited efficacy has been reported in some patients despite optimal lead placement and programming (Volkmann et al. 2012), and patients with secondary or acquired dystonia often have only modest improvement in symptoms (Vidailhet et al. 2009). Dystonia typically responds more slowly to GPi DBS than tremor or rigidity in essential tremor or Parkinson's disease (PD). GPi DBS also typically requires higher energy settings for the desired benefit compared to other traditional DBS targets, leading to more frequent battery changes or recharging. Some dystonia patients treated with GPi DBS experience new postoperative problems with gait and fine motor activities. These new motor symptoms are not attributable to spread of current to nearby corticospinal tract fibres and can best be described as bradykinetic. Stimulation-induced bradykinesia can be difficult to avoid without losing the anti-dystonic effects while programming. This bradykinetic side-effect is more likely to occur when using high stimulation frequencies (>100 Hz), but if lower-frequency stimulation (60 Hz) is used, dystonic symptoms can return (Berman et al. 2009; Schrader et al. 2011).

With these limitations in mind, an alternative brain target, the subthalamic nucleus, has emerged.

Several factors supported the rationale for STN as a possible therapeutic target for dystonia, including that STN DBS, improved early morning 'off dystonia' in PD patients. Similar brain physiology findings in dystonia and PD also suggested that STN DBS may be effective in both diseases (Schrock et al. 2009).

Subthalamic Nucleus DBS as a Target for Dystonia

Isolated (Formerly Primary) Dystonia Outcomes

Beginning in 2003, a handful of case reports or small series began to appear in the literature highlighting the use of STN in patients with various types of dystonia. Results after surgery were mixed, with some groups reporting excellent outcomes in primary generalised or primary cervical dystonia (Chou et al. 2005; Kleiner-Fisman et al. 2007; Sun et al. 2007; Pahapill & O'Connell 2010) and others reporting poor outcomes or in some cases no improvement (Detante et al. 2004; Kleiner-Fisman et al. 2007).

In 2008 the first prospective, blinded rater, clinical trial of STN DBS enrolled patients with medically refractory, isolated, predominantly cervical dystonia. STN DBS was applied to patients felt to be at the highest risk for the development of GPi DBS-induced bradykinesia given their grossly normal limb function preoperatively. The first nine patients showed a 63 per cent improvement in the total TWSTRS score one year after surgery (Ostrem et al. 2011), and in an expanded cohort of 16 a significant improvement of 65.2 per cent was seen at six months (Ostrem et al. 2014). None of the patients experienced stimulation-induced bradykinesia. Many patients could reduce medications, especially pain medications.

In 2013, the first head-to-head, crossover design, blinded video rater trial of STN or GPi DBS for generalised and cervical dystonia was published (Schjerling et al. 2013). Twelve patients were implanted with both targets and stimulated in either the GPi or STN for six months in a pseudo-randomised order. When data from the two phases were combined, the improvement in BFMDRS-M was 13.8 points (44 per cent) in the STN phase and 9.1 points (8 per cent) in the GPi phase. Some patients first stimulated with STN refused GPi treatment when they worsened during the crossover period, so these patients received simultaneous STN and GPi stimulation despite being included in the GPi group for the intention-to-treat analysis (which was not statistically significant for nucleus) (Schjerling et al. 2013).

Long-Term STN DBS in Isolated Dystonia Outcomes

Long-term follow-up on 27 patients with isolated dystonia treated with STN DBS showed an average improvement of 77 per cent and 67 per cent on the BFMDRS-M and -D scores, respectively, which persisted for 3–10 years. The degree of improvement correlated with disease duration prior to surgery, but not with the age at onset or preoperative BFMDRS-M score (Cao et al. 2013). Our group has continued to follow 14 patients annually for up to three years with sustained improvement of 66 per cent on the TWSTRS total score and a 70.4 per cent improvement on the BFMDRS-M score (Ostrem et al. 2017). Improvement at 6 months was sustained to 36 months, but four patients experienced stimulation-related dyskinesia.

STN DBS Patients With Previous Failed GPi DBS or With an Affected/Destroyed GPi Target

Having an alternative to GPi DBS available in the treatment of dystonia may be useful in cases where the underlying disease pathology or previous treatment affects the pallidum. Isolated, generalised dystonia cases previously treated with bilateral pallidotomies with dystonia recurrence have responded to subsequent STN DBS with average improvements in the BFMDRS-M ranging from 52 to 65 per cent (Fonoff et al. 2012; Dec et al. 2014). Cases of isolated segmental (Novak et al. 2008) and tardive (Fonoff et al. 2012) dystonia have also responded to STN DBS after recurrence following bilateral pallidotomy.

Non-idiopathic or combined (formerly 'secondary') causes of dystonia with structural damage to the pallidum have been treated with STN DBS in case reports and small series with mixed results. Zhang et al. reported a 90 per cent improvement in a few patients with tardive dystonia, and one case of neonatal anoxia; however, the others in the series all did poorly (Zhang et al. 2006). Other groups have reported clinically meaningful benefit with STN DBS in NBIA (Ge et al. 2011), GM1 gangliosidosis (Baizabal-Carvallo et al. 2013), methylmalonic aciduria (Chakraborti et al. 2013) and Fahr's (Ma et al. 2013) disease.

Combined Thalamic and Subthalamic DBS for Dystonia

Recently, the group in Cologne, Germany reported a series of seven dystonic head tremor patients treated with DBS targeting both the thalamic and subthalamic areas. When patients were stimulated in both areas simultaneously, there was more tremor amplitude reduction compared to stimulation of the thalamic area alone (Pauls et al. 2014). The authors concluded the degree of improvement in dystonia was on par with that of GPi DBS for cervical dystonia, but that tremor reduction was less than is typically seen with Vim DBS for essential tremor (Pauls et al. 2014).

Operative and Postoperative Considerations

Surgical Complications

When haemorrhage rates were compared between patients treated for Parkinson's disease and dystonia, the only statistically significant predictor of haemorrhage incidence was brain target (GPi (7 per cent) vs STN (2.2 per cent)) (Binder et al. 2005). In the two largest prospective trials conducted of STN DBS in dystonia, there were no reported haemorrhages. Hardware infections developed in 3 out of 18 patients requiring removal of electrodes and/or the pulse generator. In the Schjerling study, 2 out 12 patients developed infections in a protocol that involved simultaneous implantation of four electrodes (two GPi plus two STN) (Schjerling et al. 2013).

Mood

Depression after STN DBS has been reported in some individual patients with pre-existing depression, though not immediately after surgery. In studies where mood was closely monitored, measures of depression have not worsened and many patients have experienced improved depressive symptoms (Ostrem et al. 2011).

Cognition

Differences in specific cognitive outcomes after DBS in PD patients have been reported, such as decreased verbal fluency after STN DBS. In the few STN dystonia studies that have included formal neuropsychological evaluations, no areas of significant cognitive or mood decline after STN DBS have been reported (Kleiner-Fisman et al. 2007; Ostrem et al. 2011). In a study assessing cognitive function in eight STN DBS patients using a dual-task paradigm, no decline in performance was seen (Mills et al. 2015). Also, no increased impulsivity or suicide risk has been noted with the exception of one patient who was briefly suicidal after a significant life stressor (Ostrem et al. 2011, 2017).

Stimulation Parameters

Stimulation settings used in STN DBS for dystonia have been similar to those traditionally used in Parkinson's disease, using high-frequency stimulation (usually 130 Hz) with modest voltages (2–3 V) and narrow pulse widths (mostly 60 μsec) (Ostrem et al. 2011; Cao et al. 2013; Schjerling et al. 2013). One study comparing the use of low-frequency stimulation (LFS) (60 Hz) to high-frequency stimulation (HFS) (130 Hz) showed more improvement using HFS (Ostrem et al. 2014).

Possible Stimulation-Related Side-Effects

Many patients treated with STN DBS experience stimulation-induced dyskinesias when the therapy is initiated. The hyperkinetic movements can occur in all body regions and can resemble phasic dystonia or chorea and require more complex programming strategies. Dyskinesias can be minimised or avoided by slowing the rate of voltage/amplitude increase, using bipolar stimulation or sometimes adding a more dorsal STN contact (Ostrem et al. 2011, 2017; Cao et al. 2013). Transient dysarthria, dysphagia, nausea and mild hypomania have been reported and generally improved with reprogramming (Cao et al. 2013). Also, some patients have experienced weight gain (Mills et al. 2012), but in our experience the weight gain on an individual basis has been minimal.

Conclusions

Isolated dystonia can be successfully treated with bilateral high-frequency STN DBS, with an increasing number of publications in the literature supporting this claim. Patients treated with STN DBS are at risk of developing transient stimulation-induced dyskinesias/hyperkinetic movement and programming parameters may need to be carefully tailored. Until we have definitive data on which brain target might be superior in individuals with dystonia patients (GPi or STN), both targets are attractive options and target choice may largely be based on their different side-effect profiles.

References

Baizabal-Carvallo JF, Roze E, Aya-Kombo M, Romito L, Navarro S, Flamand-Rouviere C, Welter ML, Pidoux B, Bardinet E, Galanaud D, Cornu P, Vidailhet M, Pollak P, Grabli D. 2013. Combined pallidal and subthalamic nucleus deep brain stimulation in secondary dystonia-parkinsonism. *Parkinsonism Relat Disord* 19(5):566–568.

Berman BD, Starr PA, Marks WJ, Jr, Ostrem JL. 2009. Induction of bradykinesia with pallidal deep brain stimulation in patients with cranial-cervical dystonia. *Stereotact Funct Neurosurg* 87(1):37–44.

Binder DK, Rau GM, Starr PA. 2005. Risk factors for hemorrhage during microelectrode-guided deep brain stimulator implantation for movement disorders. *Neurosurgery* 56(4):722–732.

Cao C, Pan Y, Li D, Zhan S, Zhang J, Sun B. 2013. Subthalamus deep brain stimulation for primary dystonia patients: a long-term follow-up study. *Mov Disord* 28(13):1877–1882.

Chakraborti S, Hasegawa H, Lumsden DE, Ali W, Kaminska M, Lin JP, Ashkan K. 2013. Bilateral subthalamic nucleus deep brain stimulation for refractory total body dystonia secondary to metabolic autopallidotomy in a 4-year-old boy with infantile methylmalonic acidemia: case report. *J Neurosurg Pediatr* 12(4):374–379.

Chou KL, Hurtig HI, Jaggi JL, Baltuch GH. 2005. Bilateral subthalamic nucleus deep brain stimulation in a patient with cervical dystonia and essential tremor. *Mov Disord* 20(3):377–380.

Dec M, Tutaj M, Rudzinska M, Szczudlik A, Koziara H, Bonicki W, Nauman P, Mandat T. 2014. Subthalamic nucleus deep brain stimulation after bilateral pallidotomy in the treatment of generalized dystonia. *Parkinsonism Relat Disord* 20(1):131–133.

Detante O, Vercueil L, Krack P, Chabardes S, Benabid AL, Pollak P. 2004. Off-period dystonia in Parkinson's disease but not generalized dystonia is improved by high-frequency stimulation of the subthalamic nucleus. *Adv Neurol* 94:309–314.

Fonoff ET, Campos WK, Mandel M, Alho EJ, Teixeira MJ. 2012. Bilateral subthalamic nucleus stimulation for generalized dystonia after bilateral pallidotomy. *Mov Disord* 27(12):1559–1563.

Ge M, Zhang K, Ma Y, Meng FG, Hu WH, Yang AC, Zhang JG. 2011. Bilateral subthalamic nucleus stimulation in the treatment of neurodegeneration with brain iron accumulation type 1. *Stereotact Funct Neurosurg* 89(3):162–166.

Kleiner-Fisman G, Liang GS, Moberg PJ, Ruocco AC, Hurtig HI, Baltuch GH, Jaggi JL, Stern MB. 2007. Subthalamic nucleus deep brain stimulation for severe idiopathic dystonia: impact on severity, neuropsychological status, and quality of life. *J Neurosurg* 107(1):29–36.

Ma Y, Ge M, Meng F, Zhang K, Zhang J. 2013. Bilateral deep brain stimulation of the subthalamic nucleus effectively relieves dystonia secondary to Fahr's disease: a case report. *Int J Neurosci* 123(8):582–586.

Mills KA, Scherzer R, Starr PA, Ostrem JL. 2012. Weight change after globus pallidus internus or subthalamic nucleus deep brain stimulation in Parkinson's disease and dystonia. *Stereotact Funct Neurosurg* 90(6):386–393.

Mills KA, Markun LC, San Luciano M, Rizk R, Allen IE, Racine CA, Starr PA, Alberts JL, Ostrem JL. 2015. Effect of subthalamic nucleus deep brain stimulation on dual-task cognitive and motor performance in isolated dystonia. *J Neurol Neurosurg Psychiatry* 86(4):404–409.

Novak KE, Nenonene EK, Bernstein LP, Vergenz S, Cozzens JW, Rezak M. 2008. Successful bilateral subthalamic nucleus stimulation for segmental dystonia after unilateral pallidotomy. *Stereotact Funct Neurosurg* 86(2):80–86.

Ostrem JL, Racine CA, Glass GA, Grace JK, Volz MM, Heath SL, Starr PA. 2011. Subthalamic nucleus deep brain stimulation in primary cervical dystonia. *Neurology* 76(10):870–878.

Ostrem JL, Markun LC, Glass GA, Racine CA, Volz MM, Heath SL, de Hemptinne C, Starr PA. 2014. Effect of frequency on subthalamic nucleus deep brain stimulation in primary dystonia. *Parkinsonism Relat Disord* 20(4):432–438.

Ostrem JL, San Luciano M, Dodenhoff KA, Ziman N, Markun LC, Racine CA, de Hemptinne C, Volz MM, Heath SL, Starr PA. 2017. Subthalamic nucleus deep brain stimulation in isolated dystonia: a 3-year follow-up study. *Neurology* 88(1):25–35.

Pahapill PA, O'Connell B. 2010. Long-term follow-up study of chronic deep brain stimulation of the subthalamic nucleus for cervical dystonia. *Neuromodulation* 13(1):26–30.

Pauls KA, Hammesfahr S, Moro E, Moore AP, Binder E, El Majdoub F, Fink GR, Sturm V, Krauss JK, Maarouf M, Timmermann L. 2014. Deep brain stimulation in the ventrolateral thalamus/subthalamic area in dystonia with head tremor. *Mov Disord* 29(7):953–959.

Schjerling L, Hjermind LE, Jespersen B, Madsen FF, Brennum J, Jensen SR, Lokkegaard A, Karlsborg M. 2013. A randomized double-blind crossover trial comparing subthalamic and pallidal deep brain stimulation for dystonia. *J Neurosurg* 119(6):1537–1545.

Schrader C, Capelle HH, Kinfe TM, Blahak C, Bazner H, Lutjens G, Dressler D, Krauss JK. 2011. GPi-DBS may induce a hypokinetic gait disorder with freezing of gait in patients with dystonia. *Neurology* 77(5):483–488.

Schrock LE, Ostrem JL, Turner RS, Shimamoto SA, Starr PA. 2009. The subthalamic nucleus in primary dystonia: single-unit discharge characteristics. *J Neurophysiol* 102(6):3740–3752.

Sun B, Chen S, Zhan S, Le W, Krahl SE. 2007. Subthalamic nucleus stimulation for primary dystonia and tardive dystonia. *Acta Neurochir Suppl* 97(Pt 2):207–214.

Vidailhet M, Yelnik J, Lagrange C, Fraix V, Grabli D, Thobois S, Burbaud P, Welter ML, Xie-Brustolin J, Braga MC, Ardouin C, Czernecki V, Klinger H, Chabardes S, Seigneuret E, Mertens P, Cuny E, Navarro S, Cornu P, Benabid AL, Le Bas JF, Dormont D, Hermier M, Dujardin K, Blond S, Krystkowiak

P, Destee A, Bardinet E, Agid Y, Krack P, Broussolle E, Pollak P, French SPIDY-2 Study Group. 2009. Bilateral pallidal deep brain stimulation for the treatment of patients with dystonia-choreoathetosis cerebral palsy: a prospective pilot study. *Lancet Neurol* 8(8):709–717.

Volkmann J, Wolters A, Kupsch A, Muller J, Kuhn AA, Schneider GH, Poewe W, Hering S, Eisner W, Muller JU, Deuschl G, Pinsker MO, Skogseid IM, Roeste GK, Krause M, Tronnier V, Schnitzler A, Voges J, Nikkhah G, Vesper J, Classen J, Naumann M, Benecke R, DBS Study Group for Dystonia. 2012. Pallidal deep brain stimulation in patients with primary generalised or segmental dystonia: 5-year follow-up of a randomised trial. *Lancet Neurol* 11(12):1029–1038.

Zhang JG, Zhang K, Wang ZC, Ge M, Ma Y. 2006. Deep brain stimulation in the treatment of secondary dystonia. *Chin Med J (Engl)* 119(24):2069–2074.

Chapter 72

The Thalamus as a Target for Deep Brain Stimulation in Dystonia

Akshitkumar M. Mistry and Joseph S. Neimat

It is largely believed that dystonia results from imbalance within the basal ganglia-thalamo-cortical circuitry. The basal ganglia-thalamo-cortical circuitry is important in the initiation and modulation of movement as well as in the control of muscle tone. In the traditional model of basal ganglia functional organisation, this implies that reduced globus pallidus internus/substantia nigra reticulata (GPi/SNr) output via the 'direct' pathway facilitates cortically initiated, agonist muscle contraction via thalamic disinhibition. On the other hand, increased GPi/SNr output via the 'indirect' pathway inhibits antagonist muscle movements. Failure to inhibit the antagonist muscles may manifest as dystonia, a hyperkinetic movement disorder or condition resulting from sustained simultaneous co-contraction of agonist and antagonist muscles. To date, the exact pathophysiology remains unclear, but the globus pallidus and its connections to the thalamus are recognised to be important in the pathophysiology of dystonia.

Historical Perspectives: Thalamotomy for Dystonia

Historically, the main target for dystonia was the thalamus (Andrew et al. 1983; Loher et al. 2004). Cooper, a pioneer in the field of functional neurosurgery, noted in the late 1960s that stereotaxic thalamotomy in patients with Parkinson's disease relieved not only tremor but also coexisting dystonic symptoms (Cooper 1964). Based on this observation, he began to treat patients with idiopathic generalised torsion dystonia and cervical dystonia (Cooper 1964) with stereotaxic thalamotomy. He published in 1976 then the largest series of thalamotomies in 226 patients with generalised dystonia (Cooper 1976). He demonstrated improvement in up to 65 per cent of the patients at an average of eight years after surgery. His targets for dystonia were primarily VIM (ventralis intermedius), CeM (centromedian nucleus) and VCe/i (ventralis caudalis externus/internus). This ablation was extended as deemed necessary to disconnect pallidal and cerebellar afferents to the thalamus, and in refractory cases he extended the ablation to include the pulvinar. The most frequent side-effect noted was 'dysphonia' or speech disturbances. Cooper popularised thalamotomies by demonstrating remarkable improvement in patients with generalised and cervical dystonia. It was performed thereafter not only in primary dystonia but also in secondary dystonic syndromes and conditions with reportedly good outcome.

Thalamic Stimulation for Dystonia

The earliest report of thalamic stimulation for dystonia was published in German by Mundinger in 1977. His seminal paper demonstrated improvement in seven patients with cervical dystonia with stimulation of the ventro-oralis anterior (VOa) and the ventro-oralis internus (VOi) thalamic nuclei as well as the zona incerta lying beneath the thalamic nuclei in the subthalamic region (Mundinger 1977). Thalamic stimulation was also performed thereafter in a patient with hemidystonia. These reports, however, were not broadly recognised and were overshadowed by the growing popularity of pallidal targeting for dystonia. Only a handful of subsequent case reports are found in the literature, until several decades later when the Grenoble group published one of the largest case series of thalamic DBS (Vercueil et al. 2001). In this study, published in 2001, Vercueil and colleagues reported a series of 12 patients with primary generalised dystonia treated with stimulation in the VIM nucleus. Mean Burke–Fahn–Marsden Dystonia Movement Scale (BFMDRS) scores were unchanged and only five patients experienced mild-to-moderate functional improvement, primarily in limb dystonia. Axial symptoms did not demonstrate improvement. Three patients went on to receive pallidal stimulation.

Shift in the Target for Dystonia to Globus Pallidus Internus

The basal ganglia target for dystonia shifted to the pallidum, specifically the globus pallidus internus (GPi), after the observation of marked improvement of dystonic symptoms in parkinsonian patients. Pallidotomy in parkinsonian patients not only improved dyskinesias but also dystonia, with few complications from the surgery. With DBS gaining popularity, surgeons began to treat dystonia with GPi DBS and found it efficacious (Krauss et al. 1999; Coubes et al. 2000). A clear definite target with demonstrated efficacy, compared to an unclear target among the various subnuclei within the thalamus, led to the popularity of GPi DBS for treatment of dystonia.

Possible Considerations of Thalamic DBS for Dystonic Conditions: A Modern Perspective

Evidence suggests that thalamic stimulation might be useful in dystonic conditions with associated movement disorders that normally respond well to thalamic stimulation, such as dystonic tremor, primary writing tremor, writer's cramp and myoclonus-dystonia.

Tremor is one of the clinical manifestations of dystonia. Dystonic tremor or primary writing tremor demonstrates significant improvement with thalamic stimulation (Fasano et al. 2014). In virtually all refractory cases published, stimulation of Vim improved tremor. Further, reports of stimulation of the posterior portion of the ventrolateral thalamic nucleus (VLp – corresponding to Vim) also were reported to lead to improvement in dystonic arm and head tremors (Buhmann et al. 2013; Fasano et al. 2014; Pauls et al. 2014). Although the overall percentage improvement was greater on average with thalamic stimulation compared to GPi, this did not meet statistical significance in a systematic review (Fasano et al. 2014). Our own group has reported a small case series comparing Vim and GPi DBS targeting for dystonic tremor. Our findings were that tremor control was better in the patients with Vim DBS but that mild dystonic symptoms persisted (Hedera et al. 2013). While GPi DBS had limited improvement in dystonic tremor, it more markedly improved dystonic symptoms. We propose that the patients in whom dystonic tremor is the most troublesome symptom of their dystonia should be considered for Vim DBS. A combination of GPi and Vim DBS can be utilised in severe cases or cases failing to respond to stimulation at a single target.

Writer's cramp is another condition where small case series evidence exists demonstrating efficacy of targeting Vo (Taira & Hori 2003) and Vim (Fukaya et al. 2007). These publications by Drs Taira and Fukaya respectively make thalamic stimulation a viable consideration in this particular dystonia subtype. Similarly, musician's dystonia has been demonstrated to respond to stereotactic Vo thalamotomy. Horisawa and colleagues demonstrated significant mean 30-month follow-up improvement in the Tubiana Musician's Dystonia Scale in 14 out of 15 patients so treated (Horisawa et al. 2013).

Myoclonus-dystonia is characterised by myoclonic jerks and dystonia primarily of the upper extremities, and is poorly responsive to pharmacotherapy. However, it has been effectively treated with DBS, both Vim and GPi. A systemic review demonstrated at least 50 per cent improvement in myoclonus scores in 93.5 per cent of cases and BFMDRS scores in 72.7 per cent of cases (Rughani & Lozano 2013). While greater improvements in dystonia scores were noted with GPi DBS compared to Vim, similar and marked improvements were noted in both GPi and Vim DBS. The efficacy of Vim DBS in reducing myoclonic jerks is likely related to the mechanisms underlying also essential tremor, where Vim DBS is known to be efficacious. The greater improvement in dystonia scores in myoclonus-dystonia with GPi stimulation is in line with the greater effect of GPi stimulation on dystonia in general.

Lastly, secondary dystonias associated with complex constellations of subcortical brain injury have been treated with thalamic DBS. Pallidal stimulation is less efficacious in these conditions than in primary dystonias. Some have argued for a greater role and efficacy of thalamic DBS in these cases. To date, however, there is no preponderance of evidence to support one target over the other in treating these patients.

Thus far, the ideal target for thalamic DBS in dystonia has not been established (Moro et al. 2013). It remains unclear whether the Vim (VLp) or the Voa/Vop (VLa) would be the preferred location.

Conclusions

While GPi DBS has demonstrated good efficacy in primary cervical and generalised dystonia, assuming it to be the DBS target for all types of dystonic conditions may be an oversimplification of dystonic pathology and may overlook potential advantages of thalamic targets. Dystonia is a set of heterogeneous conditions; therefore, it warrants a broader therapeutic approach. Thalamic targets should be considered in patients with the specific dystonia symptoms reviewed above (dystonic tremor, writer's or musician's dystonia, and myoclonus-dystonia) and more generally in dystonias that prominently demonstrate tremulous or phasic components. The thalamic targets may also be of particular use in secondary dystonia, where the optimal target remains unclear given the unsatisfactory results of pallidal stimulation. Even cases proving refractory to GPi stimulation should be considered for the addition of thalamic stimulation. Presently, data published on thalamic DBS for dystonia do not provide guidance regarding selection of the patient and the thalamic target primarily due to lack of strong studies comparing GPi and thalamic targets or studies comparing the efficacy of various thalamic targets. These remain important areas for further investigation and may be significantly supported as our understanding of the underlying pathoneurophysiology of dystonia improves.

References

Andrew J, Fowler CJ, Harrison MJ. 1983. Stereotaxic thalamotomy in 55 cases of dystonia. *Brain* 106 (Pt 4):981–1000.

Buhmann C, Moll CK, Zittel S, Munchau A, Engel AK, Hamel W. 2013. Deep brain stimulation of the ventrolateral thalamic base and posterior subthalamic area in dystonic head tremor. *Acta Neurochir Suppl* 117:67–72.

Cooper IS. 1964. Effect of thalamic lesions upon torticollis. *N Engl J Med* 270:567–572.

Cooper IS. 1976. 20-year followup study of the neurosurgical treatment of dystonia musculorum deformans. In: Eldridge R, editor, *Advances in Neurology*. Vol. 14. New York: Raven Press.

Coubes P, Roubertie A, Vayssiere N, Hemm S, Echenne B. 2000. Treatment of DYT1-generalised dystonia by stimulation of the internal globus pallidus. *Lancet* 355(9222):2220–2221.

Fasano A, Bove F, Lang AE. 2014. The treatment of dystonic tremor: a systematic review. *J Neurol Neurosurg Psychiatry* 85(7):759–769.

Fukaya C, Katayama Y, Kano T, Nagaoka T, Kobayashi K, Oshima H, Yamamoto T. 2007. Thalamic deep brain stimulation for writer's cramp. *J Neurosurg* 107(5):977–982.

Hedera P, Phibbs FT, Dolhun R, Charles PD, Konrad PE, Neimat JS, Davis TL. 2013. Surgical targets for dystonic tremor: considerations between the globus pallidus and ventral intermediate thalamic nucleus. *Parkinsonism Relat Disord* 19(7):684–686.

Horisawa S, Taira T, Goto S, Ochiai T, Nakajima T. 2013. Long-term improvement of musician's dystonia after stereotactic ventro-oral thalamotomy. *Ann Neurol* 74(5):648–654.

Krauss JK, Pohle T, Weber S, Ozdoba C, Burgunder JM. 1999. Bilateral stimulation of globus pallidus internus for treatment of cervical dystonia. *Lancet* 354(9181):837–838.

Loher T, Pohle T, Krauss JK. 2004. Functional stereotactic surgery for treatment of cervical dystonia: review of the experience from the lesional era. *Stereotact Funct Neurosurg* 82(1):1–13.

Moro E, Gross RE, Krauss JK. 2013. What's new in surgical treatment for dystonia? *Mov Disord* 28(7):1013–1020.

Mundinger F. 1977. New stereotactic treatment of spasmodic torticollis with a brain stimulation system (author's transl.). *Med Klin* 72(46):1982–1986.

Pauls KA, Hammesfahr S, Moro E, Moore AP, Binder E, El Majdoub F, Fink GR, Sturm V, Krauss JK, Maarouf M, Timmermann L. 2014. Deep brain stimulation in the ventrolateral thalamus/subthalamic area in dystonia with head tremor. *Mov Disord* 29(7):953–959.

Rughani AI, Lozano AM. 2013. Surgical treatment of myoclonus dystonia syndrome. *Mov Disord* 28(3):282–287.

Taira T, Hori T. 2003. Stereotactic ventrooralis thalamotomy for task-specific focal hand dystonia (writer's cramp) *Stereotact Funct Neurosurg* 80(1):88–91.

Vercueil L, Pollak P, Fraix V, Caputo E, Moro E, Benazzouz A, Xie J, Koudsie A, Benabid AL. 2001. Deep brain stimulation in the treatment of severe dystonia. *J Neurol* 248(8):695–700.

Chapter 73

Dystonia Patients Non-Responsive to Deep Brain Stimulation

Amande Pauls

This chapter gives an overview of possible reasons for lack of response or reduced response to bilateral globus pallidus internus (GPi) deep brain stimulation (DBS) in dystonia, and suggests diagnostic and therapeutic approaches to these patients. The chapter focuses on GPi DBS since the majority of available data concerning DBS treatment in dystonia have been published on GPi DBS.

What Constitutes Non-Response to DBS in Dystonia?

Insufficient response to GPi DBS in dystonia can be defined in several ways. Lack of patient satisfaction with therapeutic outcome is an indicator of non-response which is difficult to quantify. In previous studies investigating effects of GPi DBS in isolated generalised and segmental dystonia, therapeutic failure was defined as a reduction in dystonia less than 25 per cent from baseline score on the Burke–Fahn–Marsden Dystonia Rating Scale Motor Score (BFMDRS-M) (Kupsch et al. 2006; Volkmann et al. 2012). A distinction is usually made as to whether there was a complete lack of postoperative improvement exceeding 25 per cent (primary therapeutic failure), or whether after initially satisfactory outcome (>25 per cent), the improvement compared to baseline falls below 25 per cent (secondary failure). A comparable value is not available for the Toronto Western Spasmodic Torticollis Rating Scale (TWSTRS), the severity scale frequently used in cervical dystonia, and for other symptom- or disease-specific scales. These considerations are particularly relevant in patients with secondary dystonias (Krauss et al. 2002).

There are several problems with this definition. First, the BFMDRS-M is a pure motor scale, and ignores factors such as pain reduction or changes in quality of life. Hence, a patient may well be satisfied with the overall therapeutic outcome despite lack of significant changes in motor status. Thus, some recent studies have moved towards more patient-centred measures such as quality of life. Second, different dystonia scales are not comparable with each other and thus, the cut-off chosen for BFMDRS-M may provide guidance, but is not transferrable to other scales such as the TWSTRS. Third, the existing scales sometimes do not adequately reflect some symptoms, such as head tremor in cervical dystonia, which can be very bothersome for the patient and frequently responds well to DBS, but is not weighted independently in the TWSTRS severity scale (Albanese et al. 2013; Jost et al. 2013). Furthermore, for many conditions with complex dystonias, no disease-specific scales are available, and for comparability, the BFMDRS-M, which was developed for isolated dystonia, is used. The BFMDRS-M has ceiling effects for severe generalised isolated and combined dystonias: for example, while independent ambulation may not be attained, ability to sit in a wheelchair (due to improvements in trunk and leg dystonia), which is very relevant for the patient, is not differentiated. Thus, improvements that are important for the patient may not be reflected in the scale.

Nevertheless, patient satisfaction and quality-of-life measures correlate with motor outcomes of DBS in dystonia and patients with little motor improvement are more likely to be dissatisfied with therapeutic results. Thus, for study purposes, improvements on BFMDRS-M below 25–30 per cent can be used as a proxy for lack of therapeutic response with the above caveats. For clinical purposes, patient satisfaction is the more important indicator that usually determines whether the patient will return frequently for further attempts at therapeutic adjustments.

Possible Causes

In a previous study investigating insufficient therapeutic response to DBS in mixed movement disorders (Parkinson's disease $n = 31$, essential tremor $n = 9$, and dystonia $n = 1$), 46 per cent had suboptimally placed electrodes, 12 per cent had diagnoses not responsive to DBS therapy, 37 per cent were inadequately programmed (due to access to programming, for example (Okun et al. 2005)) and 71 per cent required medication changes. Given the high percentage of Parkinson's patients in the cohort, the results will probably differ in dystonia (e.g. oral pharmacotherapy is frequently unsuccessful in dystonia). Also, therapeutic response to DBS in dystonia is more difficult to assess because of the more gradual onset of improvement, increasing the likelihood of pseudo non-response. In the above cohort, 51 per cent of patients could be improved via reprogramming, medication adjustments and sometimes repositioning of stimulation electrodes (Okun et al. 2005).

Device-Related Causes of DBS Non-Response

Device-related causes for lack of therapeutic response should be investigated first because they can frequently be corrected. First and foremost, a readout of the generator should be carried

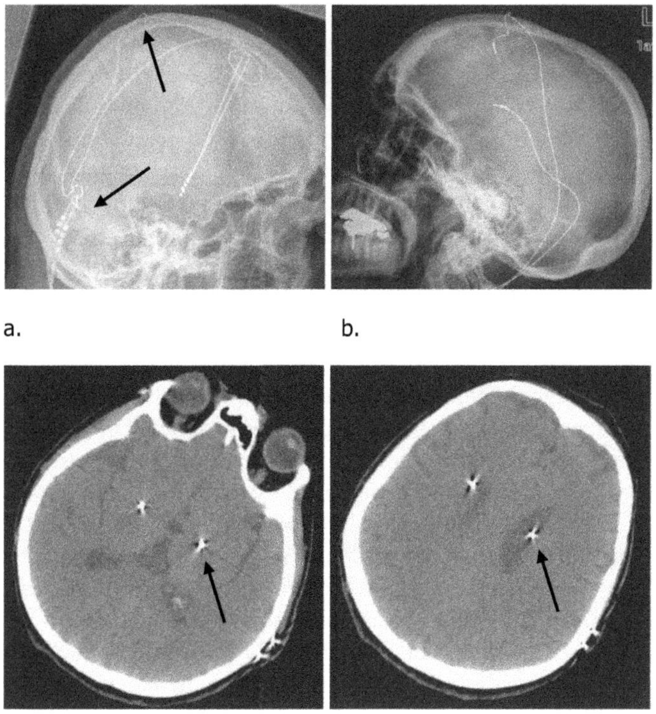

Figure 73.1 Examples for hardware problems. (a) Kinking of left electrode cable extracranially and disconnection of right electrode cable behind the ear. Increased impedances for all contacts on the right, impedances on the left were regular. Patient with severe secondary dystonia with some loss of (overall limited) DBS effect. (b). Migration of stimulation electrode into extracranial scalp due to insufficient fixation to skull. The patient complained of loss of DBS effect and local tingling of the scalp. (c)–(d) Brain CT slices showing medial displacement of left DBS electrode (c), due to entry of lead into ventricle (d). The patient, with young adult-onset generalised isolated dystonia (predominantly axial) had unexpectedly little response to GPi DBS directly postoperatively (i.e. primary DBS failure).

out to confirm the generator is switched on, the battery is sufficiently charged, and therapeutic impedances are within the normal range. Pathologically increased impedances indicate hardware-related problems such as electrode breakage, disconnection, etc., and require further investigation, usually X-rays of the entire DBS system (i.e. chest and head X-ray to visualise electrodes, cables and pulse generator and their connections). Figure 73.1a gives an example X-ray of a hardware-related DBS failure. On five-year follow-up of generalised isolated dystonia patients with GPi DBS, electrode breakage occurred in 4/40 patients (10 percent), pulse generator malfunction in 3/40 patients (7.5 per cent), partial or complete extension cable fracture in 2/40 patients (5 per cent) (Volkmann et al. 2012). In children with dystonia, 4.6 per cent (electrode breakage) and 7.7 per cent (hardware malfunction) were reported, respectively (Kaminska et al. 2016). Other surgical complications which may affect DBS function, such as tissue erosion or infections, should also be excluded.

In the case of low-frequency stimulation (<100 Hz), or pulse widths below 60 microseconds, it may be useful to try higher frequencies and longer pulse widths for at least two weeks, although some studies have shown good effects of 60 Hz stimulation (Alterman et al. 2007; Velez-Lago et al. 2012). Stimulation amplitudes can be raised to just below side-effect thresholds, which should also be tried before more invasive measures are taken. In an appropriately positioned GPi DBS electrode, the most ventral or second-most ventral electrode contacts are frequently closest to target, although this may vary. However, some patients have already received multiple adjustments to their stimulation parameters, including 'standard settings', to no avail.

Furthermore, electrode malpositioning should be excluded. Gross malpositioning or electrode migration can be visible on X-ray (Figure 73.1b; CT navigation) but usually a brain CT or MRI scan will be necessary to assess electrode positioning. Postoperative imaging is merged with preoperative brain MRIs to judge electrode position either based on individual anatomy or with respect to standard coordinate ranges. Several studies have related motor outcome to pallidal target coordinates using different technical approaches (Vayssiere et al. 2004; Starr et al. 2006; Tisch et al. 2007; Cheung et al. 2014). Starr et al. localised the active electrode contacts in the commissural plane with respect to a standardised pallidocapsular border and found no correlation between motor outcome and electrode location (Starr et al. 2006). Active electrode locations were clustered in an area in the posteroventral lateral GPi close to the plane of the commissures, 3–5 mm from the pallidocapsular border (mean 3.6 mm), and outcome >70 per cent improvement was associated with less variability in this distance (Starr et al. 2006). Tisch et al. found that more posteroventrally located active electrode contacts were associated with better motor outcome (Tisch et al. 2007), and that posteriority (y-coordinate) correlated with better outcome. Cheung and coworkers used individual MRIs and stimulation settings to calculate individual volumes of tissue activated (VTAs), which were used to construct an atlas of voxels commonly activated in patients with therapeutic outcomes >75 per cent (Cheung et al. 2014). This resulted in a relatively small common VTA located in the posterior GPi. Vayssiere et al. showed that all activated electrode contacts were in the posterolateroventral portion of the GPi, and that improvements in leg dystonia were associated with more anterior contacts, while improvements in arm dystonia were associated with more posterior contacts, pointing towards a somatotopic architecture of the posteroventral lateral GPi (Vayssiere et al. 2004).

Nevertheless, the coordinate ranges associated with good outcomes are wide and differ between studies when given. Side-effect profiles of different electrode contacts, such as very low thresholds for motor capsular effects (e.g. hand or face tension or contractions, severe dysarthria), or completely unexpected side-effects can also point towards electrode malpositioning and should be taken into account when assessing electrode positioning. An example for electrode malpositioning is given in Figure 73.1c–d.

Interestingly, repositioning electrodes deemed to be positioned suboptimally in a cohort of movement disorder patients, including four patients with dystonia, achieved mixed results (Ellis et al. 2008). The mean motor improvement in the dystonia patients was 12.8 per cent (Ellis et al. 2008). This highlights the difficulty of determining with certainty the optimal pallidal DBS target in different individuals. Thus, while severe malpositioning or electrode migration may be easy to exclude, assessing more subtle electrode positioning issues may be challenging and may depend on the assessing neurosurgeon. However, if a patient has clear electrode malpositioning with very low side-effect thresholds, inappropriate side-effect thresholds, or visible deviation from anatomical target and other causes for lack of response are excluded, electrode repositioning should be attempted.

Disease-Related Causes

Gradual worsening of dystonia over several years of an initially good response to GPi DBS points towards disease progression that can be a problem, particularly in juvenile-onset generalised dystonia (Cif et al. 2010). These patients usually have sustained effect of GPi DBS, but sometimes secondary worsening of symptoms. Some studies report successful implantation of additional GPi or subthalamic 'rescue' leads in patients with documented sustained effect of GPi DBS when reprogramming alone did not yield any improvements (Cif et al. 2010, 2012), with sometimes good results.

Limited response to GPi DBS is more frequently observed in combined dystonias, especially heredodegenerative (e.g. NBIA-dystonia) and structural dystonias (e.g. CP dystonia). An ample body of literature shows that GPi DBS motor outcomes in dystonia aetiologies associated with combined dystonias (Vidailhet et al. 2009; Timmermann et al. 2010; Koy et al. 2013; Lumsden et al. 2013) are poorer than those for isolated dystonias, such as DYT1 dystonia or idiopathic dystonia (Vidailhet et al. 2005; Kupsch et al. 2006). While the non-responder rates in isolated dystonias are typically at 15–20 per cent, the non-responder rates in the combined dystonias are frequently much higher, up to more than 50 per cent (Vidailhet et al. 2009; Timmermann et al. 2010; Koy et al. 2013), and outcomes are significantly poorer in a direct comparison (FitzGerald et al. 2014). Thus, dystonia in many combined dystonias responds less to GPi DBS, and these patients are more likely to be non-responders than patients with isolated dystonia.

Many symptoms other than dystonia that are part of combined dystonias (such as spasticity or bradykinesia) are not responsive to GPi DBS, but frequently cause significant disability and can also limit functional outcome. Tremor, especially in the dystonic limbs (e.g. head tremor in cervical dystonia), can be a part of isolated dystonia and usually responds to GPi DBS. Likewise, myoclonus in myoclonus-dystonia usually responds to GPi DBS. In special circumstances, additional symptoms can be amenable to rescue leads (Oyama et al. 2011), or other targets might be considered (Pauls et al. 2014).

Fixed dystonia can limit GPi DBS outcome in dystonia if extensive (Isaias et al. 2008). Longer disease duration is also associated with poorer outcome (Isaias et al. 2008, 2011; Lumsden et al. 2013), but whether this is related purely to fixed musculoskeletal changes or other additional factors is unknown.

Pseudo-Failure

In some cases of apparent lack of therapeutic response, pseudo-failure may be the underlying cause. This can be best assessed via comparison with preoperative video documentation, or via preoperative scores on clinical scales. The limitations of rating scales have already been discussed previously (e.g. head tremor in cervical dystonia). Preoperative video documentation and documentation of specific individual goals are useful to circumvent these limitations. Significantly reducing or turning off the stimulation for a longer period of time (hours to days, depending on response) can be useful in assessing pseudo-failure: both patient and physician can see whether DBS has effects on the severity of dystonia and associated symptoms such as pain and activities of daily living, etc.

Changes in parameters other than DBS, such as withdrawal of medication (e.g. benzodiazepines, trihexiphenidyl, baclofen) can be associated with worsening of symptoms, and reintroduction of these medications can improve dystonia. In some cases, there will be a clear (e.g. video-documented) improvement in dystonia but patient expectations are not met, or the patient is dissatisfied. This can be due to unrealistic expectations prior to surgery, but also due to other factors affecting quality of life, e.g. onset of depression, which should be treated accordingly. Furthermore, dystonia may have clearly improved, but accompanying other symptoms not responsive to GPi DBS limit outcome or quality of life (e.g. tremor, myoclonus). In these cases, addressing these additional symptoms therapeutically may help. Especially patients with unrealistic expectations, but also other pseudo non-responders can benefit from turning off DBS for some time to assess the magnitude of the therapeutic effect on dystonia.

Suggested Approach to Patients With DBS Failure

Possible diagnostic and therapeutic measures are given here and summarised in a flow chart in Figure 73.2. Problems that can be assessed and addressed more easily are listed first.

1. Check for technical device-related problems (battery status, electrode integrity, device malfunction, basic programming parameters), and address them if there is a problem (reprogram to standard parameters, try increasing stimulation amplitude to a value just below side-effect threshold, consider changing stimulation contact according to side-effect profiles and anatomy, change pulse generator/connectors/electrodes if necessary).
2. Exclude pseudo-failure by looking at preoperative video documentation or scales if available to assess preoperative symptoms and severity, check medication. If patient expectations are the problem, looking at the video together with the patient may be useful.

Consider turning stimulation off for some time. Turning off the stimulation for a day or even a couple of days if there appears to be very little improvement compared to preoperative status can help estimate the magnitude of the (remaining) therapeutic effect. In patients with generalised dystonia and in cases where the preoperative status is not known to the physician, this needs to be done with caution (i.e. in an inpatient setting), or can be

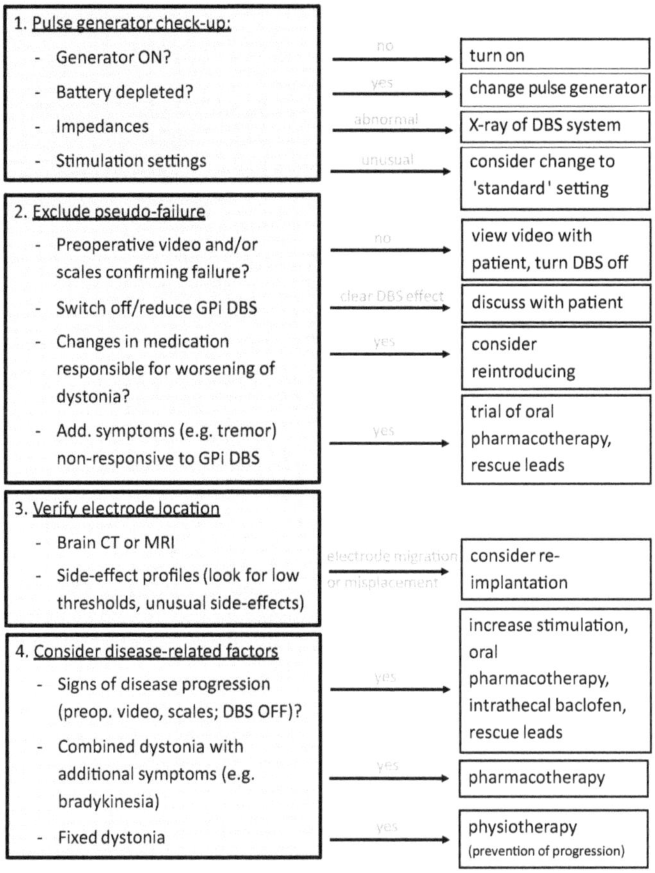

Figure 73.2 Flow chart for approaching patients with lack of therapeutic response.

preceded or replaced by a noticeable reduction in stimulation intensity (to avoid precipitating status dystonicus). Patients who are dissatisfied with the therapeutic result for other reasons (e.g. side-effects, lack of recollection of preoperative status, accompanying pseudodystonias or additional other symptoms not responsive to GPi DBS) can benefit from this procedure.

If a change in medication is the problem, consider re-introducing the medication, or try to adjust stimulation parameters. Additional botulinum toxin injection in selected muscles might also be considered, but there is a paucity of data on this approach.

3. Check for anatomical device-related problems (side-effect testing, brain MRI or CT). If this indicates dislocation or migration of electrodes, or clear misplacement compared to standard target, consider electrode repositioning (if changing to other electrode contacts is not successful).
4. Disease-related problems are more difficult to address. If there is disease progression (suggested by secondary failure, insidious worsening of dystonia after initially good outcome), increasing stimulation amplitudes or using additional electrode contacts can improve dystonia. Re-introducing or modifying oral pharmacotherapy may also help to some extent. In severe cases, a baclofen pump can provide additional relief, or additional rescue leads can be considered in special cases (Cif et al. 2010, 2012).

In some patients, limited response to pallidal DBS is caused by fixed dystonia. Therapeutic measures are scarce, but patients with generalised dystonia can still benefit from pain reduction or dystonia reduction in other body regions. In extensive fixed dystonia (e.g. spinal, ankles, knees and hips in generalised dystonia), or fixed neck dystonia in cervical dystonia, patients should be advised that this will limit functional outcome before surgery. Preventive measures, such as regular and frequent physiotherapy, and initiation of DBS early within the course of the disease have been shown to improve outcomes (Isaias et al. 2008, 2011; Lumsden et al. 2013).

Lack of therapeutic response to GPi DBS in heredodegenerative or structural dystonia is difficult to address. Additional treatment approaches for accompanying symptoms should be sought (e.g. oral or intrathecal baclofen for spasticity, dopaminergic medication for bradykinesia, supportive measures). It is also important to exclude diseases for which disease-specific treatments are available (e.g. M. Wilson, hereditary hypermanganesemia, biotin-responsive basal ganglia disease). Future studies may show that alternative anatomical targets or stimulation settings may be beneficial in some dystonias. If secondary dystonia is recognised preoperatively, expectations need to be adjusted accordingly, and more individual goals should be agreed.

If symptoms other than dystonia (such as tremor, myoclonus, bradykinesia) persist and cause disability, this can be difficult to address. A trial of treatments specific to the symptom (e.g. levodopa in parkinsonism) should be attempted. In myoclonus-dystonia, if myoclonus persists, or in persistent tremor syndromes, additional 'rescue' thalamic DBS can be considered (Oyama et al. 2011), but data on this subject are scarce and thus this approach is considered experimental.

References

Albanese A, Sorbo FD, Comella C, Jinnah HA, Mink JW, Post B, Vidailhet M, Volkmann J, Warner TT, Leentjens AF, Martinez-Martin P, Stebbins GT, Goetz CG, Schrag A. 2013. Dystonia rating scales: critique and recommendations. *Mov Disord* 28(7):874–883.

Alterman RL, Miravite J, Weisz D, Shils JL, Bressman SB, Tagliati M. 2007. Sixty hertz pallidal deep brain stimulation for primary torsion dystonia. *Neurology* 69(7):681–688.

Cheung T, Noecker AM, Alterman RL, McIntyre CC, Tagliati M. 2014. Defining a therapeutic target for pallidal deep brain stimulation for dystonia. *Ann Neurol* 76(1):22–30.

Cif L, Vasques X, Gonzalez V, Ravel P, Biolsi B, Collod-Beroud G, Tuffery-Giraud S, Elfertit H, Claustres M, Coubes P. 2010. Long-term follow-up of DYT1 dystonia patients treated by deep brain stimulation: an open-label study. *Mov Disord* 25(3):289–299.

Cif L, Gonzalez-Martinez V, Vasques X, Corlobe A, Moura AM, Bonafe A, Coubes P. 2012. Staged implantation of multiple electrodes in the internal globus pallidus in the treatment of primary generalized dystonia. *J Neurosurg* 116(5):1144–1152.

Ellis TM, Foote KD, Fernandez HH, Sudhyadhom A, Rodriguez RL, Zeilman P, Jacobson CE, Okun MS. 2008. Reoperation for suboptimal outcomes after deep brain stimulation surgery. *Neurosurgery* 63(4):754–760.

FitzGerald JJ, Rosendal F, de Pennington N, Joint C, Forrow B, Fletcher C, Green AL, Aziz TZ. 2014. Long-term outcome of deep brain stimulation in generalised dystonia: a series of 60 cases. *J Neurol Neurosurg Psychiatry* 85(12):1371–1376.

Isaias IU, Alterman RL, Tagliati M. 2008. Outcome predictors of pallidal stimulation in patients with primary dystonia: the role of disease duration. *Brain* 131(Pt 7):1895–1902.

Isaias IU, Volkmann J, Kupsch A, Burgunder JM, Ostrem JL, Alterman RL, Mehdorn HM, Schonecker T, Krauss JK, Starr P, Reese R, Kuhn AA, Schupbach WM, Tagliati M. 2011. Factors predicting protracted improvement after pallidal DBS for primary dystonia: the role of age and disease duration. *J Neurol* 258(8):1469–1476.

Jost WH, Hefter H, Stenner A, Reichel G. 2013. Rating scales for cervical dystonia: a critical evaluation of tools for outcome assessment of botulinum toxin therapy. *J Neural Transm (Vienna)* 120(3):487–496.

Kaminska M, Perides S, Lumsden DE, Nakou V, Selway R, Ashkan K, Lin JP. 2016. Complications of deep brain stimulation (DBS) for dystonia in children: the challenges and 10 year experience in a large paediatric cohort. *Eur J Paediatr Neurol* 21(1):168–175.

Koy A, Hellmich M, Pauls KA, Marks W, Lin JP, Fricke O, Timmermann L. 2013. Effects of deep brain stimulation in dyskinetic cerebral palsy: a meta-analysis. *Mov Disord* 28(5):647–654.

Krauss JK, Loher TJ, Pohle T, Weber S, Taub E, Barlocher CB, Burgunder JM. 2002. Pallidal deep brain stimulation in patients with cervical dystonia and severe cervical dyskinesias with cervical myelopathy. *J Neurol Neurosurg Psychiatry* 72(2):249–256.

Kupsch A, Benecke R, Muller J, Trottenberg T, Schneider GH, Poewe W, Eisner W, Wolters A, Muller JU, Deuschl G, Pinsker MO, Skogseid IM, Roeste GK, Vollmer-Haase J, Brentrup A, Krause M, Tronnier V, Schnitzler A, Voges J, Nikkhah G, Vesper J, Naumann M, Volkmann J, Deep-Brain Stimulation for Dystonia Study Group. 2006. Pallidal deep-brain stimulation in primary generalized or segmental dystonia. *N Engl J Med* 355(19):1978–1990.

Lumsden DE, Kaminska M, Gimeno H, Tustin K, Baker L, Perides S, Ashkan K, Selway R, Lin JP. 2013. Proportion of life lived with dystonia inversely correlates with response to pallidal deep brain stimulation in both primary and secondary childhood dystonia. *Dev Med Child Neurol* 55(6):567–574.

Okun MS, Tagliati M, Pourfar M, Fernandez HH, Rodriguez RL, Alterman RL, Foote KD. 2005. Management of referred deep brain stimulation failures: a retrospective analysis from 2 movement disorders centers. *Arch Neurol* 62(8):1250–1255.

Oyama G, Foote KD, Hwynn N, Jacobson CE, Malaty IA, Rodriguez RL, Zeilman P, Okun MS. 2011. Rescue leads: a salvage technique for selected patients with a suboptimal response to standard DBS therapy. *Parkinsonism Relat Disord* 17(6):451–455.

Pauls KA, Hammesfahr S, Moro E, Moore AP, Binder E, El Majdoub F, Fink GR, Sturm V, Krauss JK, Maarouf M, Timmermann L. 2014. Deep brain stimulation in the ventrolateral thalamus/subthalamic area in dystonia with head tremor. *Mov Disord* 29(7):953–959.

Starr PA, Turner RS, Rau G, Lindsey N, Heath S, Volz M, Ostrem JL, Marks WJ. 2006. Microelectrode-guided implantation of deep brain stimulators into the globus pallidus internus for dystonia: techniques, electrode locations, and outcomes. *J Neurosurg* 104(4):488–501.

Timmermann L, Pauls KA, Wieland K, Jech R, Kurlemann G, Sharma N, Gill SS, Haenggeli CA, Hayflick SJ, Hogarth P, Leenders KL, Limousin P, Malanga CJ, Moro E, Ostrem JL, Revilla FJ, Santens P, Schnitzler A, Tisch S, Valldeoriola F, Vesper J, Volkmann J, Woitalla D, Peker S. 2010. Dystonia in neurodegeneration with brain iron accumulation: outcome of bilateral pallidal stimulation. *Brain* 133(Pt 3):701–712.

Tisch S, Zrinzo L, Limousin P, Bhatia KP, Quinn N, Ashkan K, Hariz M. 2007. Effect of electrode contact location on clinical efficacy of pallidal deep brain stimulation in primary generalised dystonia. *J Neurol Neurosurg Psychiatry* 78(12):1314–1319.

Vayssiere N, van der Gaag N, Cif L, Hemm S, Verdier R, Frerebeau P, Coubes P. 2004. Deep brain stimulation for dystonia confirming a somatotopic organization in the globus pallidus internus. *J Neurosurg* 101(2):181–188.

Velez-Lago FM, Oyama G, Foote KD, Hwynn N, Zeilman P, Jacobson C, Wu S, Okun MS. 2012. Low-frequency deep brain stimulation for dystonia: lower is not always better. *Tremor Other Hyperkinet Mov (NY)*. doi: 10.7916/D85X27PH.

Vidailhet M, Vercueil L, Houeto JL, Krystkowiak P, Benabid AL, Cornu P, Lagrange C, Tezenas du Montcel S, Dormont D, Grand S, Blond S, Detante O, Pillon B, Ardouin C, Agid Y, Destee A, Pollak P, French Stimulation du Pallidum Interne dans la Dystonie (SPIDY) Study Group. 2005. Bilateral deep-brain stimulation of the globus pallidus in primary generalized dystonia. *N Engl J Med* 352(5):459–467.

Vidailhet M, Yelnik J, Lagrange C, Fraix V, Grabli D, Thobois S, Burbaud P, Welter ML, Xie-Brustolin J, Braga MC, Ardouin C, Czernecki V, Klinger H, Chabardes S, Seigneuret E, Mertens P, Cuny E, Navarro S, Cornu P, Benabid AL, Le Bas JF, Dormont D, Hermier M, Dujardin K, Blond S, Krystkowiak P, Destee A, Bardinet E, Agid Y, Krack P, Broussolle E, Pollak P, French SPIDY-2 Study Group. 2009. Bilateral pallidal deep brain stimulation for the treatment of patients with dystonia-choreoathetosis cerebral palsy: a prospective pilot study. *Lancet Neurol* 8(8):709–717.

Volkmann J, Wolters A, Kupsch A, Muller J, Kuhn AA, Schneider GH, Poewe W, Hering S, Eisner W, Muller JU, Deuschl G, Pinsker MO, Skogseid IM, Roeste GK, Krause M, Tronnier V, Schnitzler A, Voges J, Nikkhah G, Vesper J, Classen J, Naumann M, Benecke R, DBS Study Group for Dystonia. 2012. Pallidal deep brain stimulation in patients with primary generalised or segmental dystonia: 5-year follow-up of a randomised trial. *Lancet Neurol* 11(12):1029–1038.

Chapter 74

Akinesia Induced by Deep Brain Stimulation

Christian Blahak

In general, adverse effects induced by deep brain stimulation (DBS) for dystonia are manageable when stimulation parameters are adjusted optimally. They primarily comprise motor side-effects caused by spread of current to the corticobulbar or corticospinal tract, resulting in dysarthrophonia and tonic contraction of contralateral face and arm muscles.

General Akinesia

In a few individual patients, however, clinically relevant akinesia following DBS of the posteroventral lateral globus pallidus internus (GPi) resembling Parkinson's disease has been reported. In a patient with chronic GPi DBS for craniocervical dystonia who experienced excellent improvement of dystonia, Zauber et al. described reversible parkinsonism with shuffling, gait hesitation, turning en bloc, impaired postural reflexes, soft slurred speech and micrographia induced by DBS of the posteroventral GPi. Stimulation through dorsal contacts alleviated parkinsonism but resulted in the return of dystonia, and no stimulation parameters could alleviate the dystonia without inducing parkinsonism (Zauber et al. 2009). Tisch et al. observed in a series of 15 patients treated with GPi DBS for primary generalised dystonia two patients who developed delayed-onset akinesia with gait slowing, difficulty arising from sitting and turning in bed. In both patients the akinetic features occurred with stimulation of ventral contacts and improved by changing to more dorsal contacts (Tisch et al. 2007).

Usually, akinesia induced by DBS for dystonia is mild and only reported on enquiry. Using a patient-based questionnaire, a retrospective study revealed that 10 out of 11 patients with GPi DBS for cranial–cervical dystonia complained about at least mild hypokinetic symptoms including handwriting alterations (Berman et al. 2009). Ostrem et al. reported in their series of six patients with cranial–cervical dystonia (Meige syndrome) treated with bilateral GPi DBS that most of the patients had clear worsening of some motor function in previously normal body regions with DBS. Several patients reported slowness of walking, heaviness in their legs and subtle difficulty making turns. Others reported new difficulty with writing for long periods of time, typing or trouble getting out of a bathtub. All patients felt that these stimulation-induced adverse effects were small compared with the beneficial effect on their dystonia. The authors were not able to identify programming parameters that completely eliminated subtle motor deficits while preserving maximum relief of dystonia (Ostrem et al. 2007). Incidentally, hypokinetic symptoms including gait disturbance and impairment of fine motor activities have also been described in a patient with GPi DBS for Tourette's syndrome (Diederich et al. 2005).

Remarkably, hypokinesia and parkinsonism as a possible adverse event have not been mentioned in the large prospective multicentre trials on the effect of GPi DBS in segmental and generalised dystonia (Vidailhet et al. 2005; Kupsch et al. 2006). The often marked improvement of dystonia may mask slight bradykinesia postoperatively, thus a careful clinical examination and questionnaires focusing on these symptoms are useful.

Alterations in Hand Motor Function

Changes in handwriting represent a sensitive sign of hypokinesia. To quantify stimulation-induced handwriting, alterations were analysed in a prospective study design, in 11 patients treated with GPi DBS for segmental dystonia not affecting distal arm function. Both the maximum character height and the width of a predefined handwriting phrase were significantly reduced with DBS as compared to the preoperative recording (Figure 74.1). Furthermore, in a spiral drawing task within a given box, despite an unchanged mean spiral diameter, the number of spiral turns significantly increased postoperatively, resulting in a slightly higher winding density of the spiral turns (Blahak et al. 2011). However, only three patients in this study indicated self-perceived changes of handwriting with mild to moderate stimulation-induced micrographia. From the clinical view, very few patients report handwriting alterations by themselves, hence for the detection of mild micrographia a detailed postoperative interview and the acquisition of handwriting samples is important.

The impact of high-frequency GPi DBS on hand motor function in patients with segmental dystonia using a finger-tapping paradigm has been examined in a study by Huebl et al. In 22 patients with GPi DBS for segmental dystonia, by using a joystick button finger tapping speed was measured at four different stimulation settings: off-stimulation, 20 Hz, 50 Hz and high-frequency stimulation with the frequency used for chronic DBS before. The main finding was a frequency-specific modulation of hand motor function with deterioration during high-frequency and slight improvement during 20 Hz

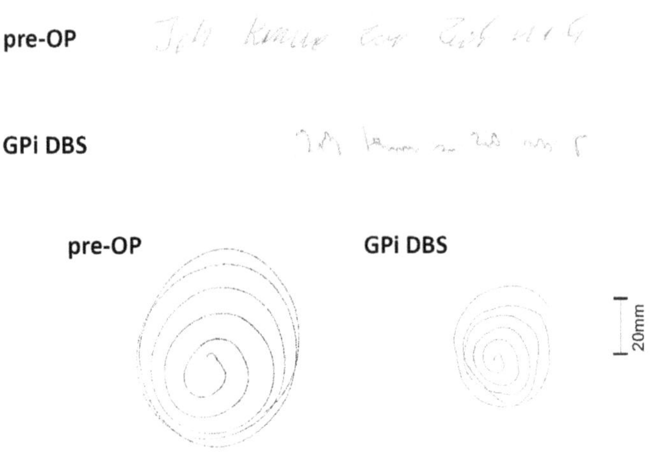

Figure 74.1 Handwriting sample and spiral drawing of a single patient who developed clear parkinsonism with almost illegible micrographia.
Source: Adapted from Blahak et al. (2011).

stimulation compared to off-stimulation. This frequency-dependent effect was more pronounced when the tapping test was performed not directly, but 60 minutes after the modification of stimulation frequency. The impairment in hand motor function under high-frequency stimulation was mirrored by the patients' observation of a deterioration in general mobility (Huebl et al. 2015).

Hypokinetic Gait Changes

Quite a few patients complain about changes in gait following GPi DBS, including the feeling of heaviness in the legs, slowing of gait and difficulty making turns.

In a retrospective study by Schrader et al., of a collective of 71 patients with dystonia, six patients presented with a new gait disorder (8.5 per cent). The spectrum ranged from mere hesitation on turning to shorter steps or start hesitation when passing narrow spaces, and finally propulsion, festination and freezing with postural instability and falls with higher amplitudes (Schrader et al. 2011). Increasing voltage can trigger, in particular, freezing of gait, sometimes worsening over a period of a few hours. It usually vanishes within minutes after ceasing DBS. Although no optimal configuration was found despite extensive testing of settings, by the reduction of pulse width from 210 to 60–90 μsec or reduction of frequency from 130 to 60 Hz a compromise between alleviating dystonia and deterioration of gait could be achieved in each case.

To better characterise already subtle changes of the gait pattern induced by bilateral GPi DBS, in another study in ten patients with segmental dystonia without involvement of the lower trunk or legs, different gait parameters were analysed and compared in detail pre- and postoperatively using a computerised gait analysis with pressure-sensitive soles (Wolf et al. 2016). Although none of the patients noticed changes in gait, the mean step length significantly decreased by about 10 per cent with GPi DBS. Due to only small changes of walking distance and gait velocity, the cadence correspondingly increased. In addition, the study revealed that the step-to-step variability of several gait parameters like the step time as well as the duration of stance phase and the swing phase significantly decreased postoperatively. The results of this study indicate that in patients with segmental dystonia, chronic DBS of the posteroventral lateral GPi is associated not only with mild hypokinesia of gait but also with a considerable decrease in gait variability. This latter aspect did not correlate with the extent of dystonic improvement with pallidal DBS, hence it was postulated that regulatory effects of basal ganglia circuits on the central control of automated gait are altered by GPi DBS.

Pathophysiological Considerations

The exact pathophysiological mechanisms of hypokinetic adverse effects of pallidal DBS are still poorly understood.

In normal non-human primates it has been shown that inactivation of the GPi can produce a mild global bradykinesia: injections of muscimol into the GPi reduced the peak velocity of arm movements to visible or remembered visual targets in monkeys (Inase et al. 1996; Wenger et al. 1999).

Likewise, observations in GPi DBS for dystonia in humans suggest that hypokinesia might be induced primarily by the stimulation of the posteroventral GPi itself. In the aforementioned case report by Zauber et al., stimulation of the GPi through the most ventral contact was associated with parkinsonism, but good control of hyperkinetic dystonic symptoms, whereas stimulation through the most dorsal contact resulted in a resolution of hypokinesia, but also increasing dystonia (Zauber et al. 2009). This might indicate that alterations of GPi output activity following chronic DBS of the posteroventral lateral GPi result in a modification of neuronal activity in ascending pallidothalamo-frontal pathways (Wichmann & DeLong 2003) and, according to recent results of electrophysiological coherence studies (Talakoub et al. 2016), in widespread striato-pallido-thalamo-cortical motor pathways.

In PD patients, distinct clinical effects on different motor symptoms could be observed when using quadripolar DBS electrodes for exploration of different sites within the GPi (Bejjani et al. 1997; Krack et al. 1998). Stimulation of the most proximal contact located in the dorsal part of the GPi considerably improved parkinsonian signs like hypokinesia and rigidity, but also resulted in an increase in levodopa-induced hyperkinesias. In contrast, by stimulation through the most distal contact located in the posteroventral part of the GPi, DBS significantly suppressed levodopa-induced hyperkinesias and still improved rigidity, but otherwise led to deterioration of hypokinesia and gait. Comparable systematic studies in dystonia are lacking.

Another hypothesis on the mechanism of hypokinesia induced by GPi DBS is based on the assumption that only GABAergic axons, but no other neuronal structures, respond to high-frequency DBS. DBS for the treatment of dystonia targets the ventrolateral part of the GPi, which contains the pallido-thalamic fibres. Thus, selective stimulation of GABAergic pallidal axons increases the GABAergic output on to the thalamus, resulting in a suppression of hyperkinetic movements. In focal and segmental forms of dystonia, hypokinetic side-effects may occur when pallidal high-frequency stimulation leads to an enhanced GABAergic output of both the inhibited dystonic neurons, but also the non-affected neurons of the GPi. In consequence, the dystonic movement disorder often is found to be suppressed quite well, but in parallel also 'normal movements' are inhibited with the result of hypokinesia in primary non-dystonic regions of the body (Amtage et al. 2013).

DBS frequency seems to be a further important factor for the occurrence of hypokinetic side-effects. The observation of an improved tapping performance at 20 Hz, no change at 50 Hz and deterioration at high-frequency stimulation >100 Hz (Huebl et al. 2015) suggests a frequency-specific activation of neuronal elements. Assuming that high-frequency DBS acts through overriding aberrant oscillatory activity (McIntyre & Hahn 2010) and in this way leads to clinical benefit, it may at the same time interfere with residual physiological activity – for example in the gamma range between 35 and 100 Hz – that is important for scaling of movement (Brucke et al. 2012; Huebl et al. 2015).

Therapeutic Consequences

How can we manage hypokinetic side-effects following pallidal DBS? Levodopa medication can be effective in some cases (Krack et al. 1998), but that's rather the exception. Usually the first choice is the reprogramming of the stimulation parameters, with the use of more ventral – that means distal – contacts and a bipolar stimulation mode. Further strategies can be reduction of the pulse width, the voltage or the frequency – for example, by trying 100 Hz stimulation. In most cases, however, a compromise between control of dystonic symptoms and the degree of hypokinetic motor impairments is necessary.

References

Amtage F, Feuerstein TJ, Meier S, Prokop T, Piroth T, Pinsker MO. 2013. Hypokinesia upon pallidal deep brain stimulation of dystonia: support of a GABAergic mechanism. *Front Neurol* 4:198.

Bejjani B, Damier P, Arnulf I, Bonnet AM, Vidailhet M, Dormont D, Pidoux B, Cornu P, Marsault C, Agid Y. 1997. Pallidal stimulation for Parkinson's disease: two targets? *Neurology* 49(6):1564–1569.

Berman BD, Starr PA, Marks WJ, Jr, Ostrem JL. 2009. Induction of bradykinesia with pallidal deep brain stimulation in patients with cranial-cervical dystonia. *Stereotact Funct Neurosurg* 87(1):37–44.

Blahak C, Capelle HH, Baezner H, Kinfe TM, Hennerici MG, Krauss JK. 2011. Micrographia induced by pallidal DBS for segmental dystonia: a subtle sign of hypokinesia? *J Neural Transm (Vienna)* 118(4):549–553.

Brucke C, Huebl J, Schonecker T, Neumann WJ, Yarrow K, Kupsch A, Blahak C, Lutjens G, Brown P, Krauss JK, Schneider GH, Kuhn AA. 2012. Scaling of movement is related to pallidal gamma oscillations in patients with dystonia. *J Neurosci* 32(3):1008–1019.

Diederich NJ, Kalteis K, Stamenkovic M, Pieri V, Alesch F. 2005. Efficient internal pallidal stimulation in gilles de la tourette syndrome: a case report. *Mov Disord* 20(11):1496–1499.

Huebl J, Brucke C, Schneider GH, Blahak C, Krauss JK, Kuhn AA. 2015. Bradykinesia induced by frequency-specific pallidal stimulation in patients with cervical and segmental dystonia. *Parkinsonism Relat Disord* 21(7):800–803.

Inase M, Buford JA, Anderson ME. 1996. Changes in the control of arm position, movement, and thalamic discharge during local inactivation in the globus pallidus of the monkey. *J Neurophysiol* 75(3):1087–1104.

Krack P, Pollak P, Limousin P, Hoffmann D, Benazzouz A, Le Bas JF, Koudsie A, Benabid AL. 1998. Opposite motor effects of pallidal stimulation in Parkinson's disease. *Ann Neurol* 43(2):180–192.

Kupsch A, Benecke R, Muller J, Trottenberg T, Schneider GH, Poewe W, Eisner W, Wolters A, Muller JU, Deuschl G, Pinsker MO, Skogseid IM, Roeste GK, Vollmer-Haase J, Brentrup A, Krause M, Tronnier V, Schnitzler A, Voges J, Nikkhah G, Vesper J, Naumann M, Volkmann J, Deep-Brain Stimulation for Dystonia Study Group. 2006. Pallidal deep-brain stimulation in primary generalized or segmental dystonia. *N Engl J Med* 355(19):1978–1990.

McIntyre CC, Hahn PJ. 2010. Network perspectives on the mechanisms of deep brain stimulation. *Neurobiol Dis* 38(3):329–337.

Ostrem JL, Marks WJ, Jr, Volz MM, Heath SL, Starr PA. 2007. Pallidal deep brain stimulation in patients with cranial-cervical dystonia (Meige syndrome). *Mov Disord* 22(13):1885–1891.

Schrader C, Capelle HH, Kinfe TM, Blahak C, Bazner H, Lutjens G, Dressler D, Krauss JK. 2011. GPi-DBS may induce a hypokinetic gait disorder with freezing of gait in patients with dystonia. *Neurology* 77(5):483–488.

Talakoub O, Neagu B, Udupa K, Tsang E, Chen R, Popovic MR, Wong W. 2016. Time-course of coherence in the human basal ganglia during voluntary movements. *Sci Rep* 6:34930.

Tisch S, Zrinzo L, Limousin P, Bhatia KP, Quinn N, Ashkan K, Hariz M. 2007. Effect of electrode contact location on clinical efficacy of pallidal deep brain stimulation in primary generalised dystonia. *J Neurol Neurosurg Psychiatry* 78(12):1314–1319.

Vidailhet M, Vercueil L, Houeto JL, Krystkowiak P, Benabid AL, Cornu P, Lagrange C, Tezenas du Montcel S, Dormont D, Grand S, Blond S, Detante O, Pillon B, Ardouin C, Agid Y, Destee A, Pollak P, French Stimulation du Pallidum Interne dans la Dystonie (SPIDY) Study Group. 2005. Bilateral deep-brain stimulation of the globus pallidus in primary generalized dystonia. *N Engl J Med* 352(5):459–467.

Wenger KK, Musch KL, Mink JW. 1999. Impaired reaching and grasping after focal inactivation of globus pallidus pars interna in the monkey. *J Neurophysiol* 82(5):2049–2060.

Wichmann T, DeLong MR. 2003. Pathophysiology of Parkinson's disease: the MPTP primate model of the human disorder. *Ann NY Acad Sci* 991:199–213.

Wolf ME, Capelle HH, Bazner H, Hennerici MG, Krauss JK, Blahak C. 2016. Hypokinetic gait changes induced by bilateral pallidal deep brain stimulation for segmental dystonia. *Gait Posture* 49:358–363.

Zauber SE, Watson N, Comella CL, Bakay RA, Metman LV. 2009. Stimulation-induced parkinsonism after posteroventral deep brain stimulation of the globus pallidus internus for craniocervical dystonia. *J Neurosurg* 110(2):229–233.

Chapter 75

Programing Deep Brain Stimulation for Treatment of Dystonia

Christos Sidiropoulos, Paul Krack and Elena Moro

Programming deep brain stimulation (DBS) devices for the treatment of dystonia can be challenging even to the experienced clinician, for several reasons. First, as opposed to essential tremor (ET) and Parkinson's disease (PD) where symptoms such as tremor and rigidity respond to stimulation within seconds to minutes, in dystonia abnormal postures may respond with a latency of hours to days, or even weeks and sometimes months to stimulation adjustments. This fact underscores the need for a diligent documentation of baseline function and subsequent changes using appropriate scales and video assessments, which requires substantial time and patience from both patient and programmer. Second, dystonia represents a much more heterogeneous group of disorders as compared to ET and PD, in terms of phenomenology and pathogenesis as well as in terms of prognosis and response to DBS, requiring considerable expertise for its interventional management. Third, expertise in dystonia programming is difficult to acquire as it is a much more rare condition than ET or PD.

For all of the above reasons, including the lack of substantially effective medical options, with the exception of botulinum toxin injections, there have been ongoing efforts to gather and codify international experience both in the early postoperative (Kupsch et al. 2011) and the late postoperative phase (Tagliati et al. 2011). Here, we will focus on programming of globus pallidus internus (GPi) stimulation, and we will briefly touch upon thalamic and STN programming.

When to Start Programming

Programming the implantable pulse generator (IPG) for DBS typically begins within a few days to a few weeks after placement of the DBS system and depends on whether the IPG is connected to the leads in a single-stage procedure or a two-stage one, as well as national healthcare reimbursement policies. Although programming can begin almost immediately after the IPG is connected to the DBS electrodes, it may make sense to delay programming until minor local cerebral oedema due to lead penetration subsides and the lesion-like effect (consisting in a transient clinical improvement of dystonia) dissipates. The latter may be less robust in dystonia as opposed to ET and PD, possibly owing to the fact that the globus pallidus internus (GPi), the most common target for DBS in dystonia, is much larger compared to the thalamus and the subthalamic nucleus (STN), the main targets for ET and PD respectively (Mann et al. 2009). This strategy may allow for better and more accurate assessment of the threshold both for side-effects and benefits during the initial programming visit. Furthermore, delaying initiation of neurostimulation does not seem to have a negative impact on motor outcomes as assessed in a recent large sham-controlled study (Volkmann et al. 2014). An exception of course is status dystonicus or dystonic storm, which can be abated by pallidal DBS immediately (Walcott et al. 2012).

Postoperative Imaging

Postoperative imaging is needed to confirm DBS electrode placement accuracy and to assess postsurgical complications such as intracranial haemorrhage. Real-time intraoperative MRI imaging is an encouraging new technique (Starr et al. 2014).

Neurostimulation Hardware

Presently several manufacturers provide DBS systems with quadripolar or octapolar lead contacts made of platinum iridium, with various intercontact distances, an extension wire and the IPG. A detailed description of the available DBS systems is beyond the scope of this chapter. However, it should be kept in mind that the basic principle of delivery of electrical energy through the currently available systems has been application of an omnidirectional field, although newer systems with current-steering options have become available (Barbe et al. 2014).

Electrical Parameters

Throughout the programming process, several stimulation settings can be changed: the active contact(s), amplitude measured in volts (V) or milliamperes (mA), pulse width measured in microseconds (μs) and frequency measured in hertz (Hz). Based on Ohm's law, current intensity (I) is defined as voltage (V) divided by tissue impedance (R), which can vary with time. Constant voltage has been used for programming of the electrical field for decades. Recently, however, constant current stimulation has become available as well (Okun et al. 2012). It remains to be seen whether this approach, based on (at least theoretical) advantages, will also be used widely in dystonia.

A Systematic Approach for the Initial Programming Phase

During the initial programming visit, each of the four contacts (or eight, depending on lead design) is assessed for side-effects and eventual rapid improvements in dystonic features, although, as discussed, there may be a considerable latency for the latter. Each contact can be set as anode (+) or cathode (−). When set as (−) either the IPG is set to (+), for a monopolar configuration, or another contact is switched to (+) for a bipolar configuration. Programming may be initiated using a single monopolar configuration, assessing each one of the lead contacts sequentially as the amplitude is gradually increased up to the point where any side-effects occur. Side-effects may include: pyramidal contractions (usually in the face or hand) due to current spread to the internal capsule; transient visual phenomena described as phosphenes due to current spread to the optic tract, especially in the most ventral contacts; dysarthria, dysaesthesia or exacerbation of dystonia/induction of chorea, likely when the globus pallidus externus (GPe) is stimulated. In terms of pulse width and frequency used, at least for the initial survey, there are different strategies. Most centres use high-frequency stimulation at 130 Hz. Reports on pulse width approaches vary, with one large clinical trial reporting 120 μs as the preferred one, based on theoretical advantages in terms of chronaxie/side-effect correlation for the GPi (Kupsch et al. 2006). The Montpellier group has used mostly high pulse widths of 450 μs with good outcomes (Coubes et al. 2000). We recommend using a low pulse width for the initial phase, such as 60 μs at 130 Hz in patients with primary generalised dystonia (Vidailhet et al. 2007). Low-frequency stimulation at 60 Hz has been used as well with the theoretical advantage of prolonged battery life based on one study in primary torsion dystonia (Alterman et al. 2007). Using the lowest needed pulse width would avoid early battery drain. Indeed, in a double-blind study in patients with cervical dystonia, pulse widths in the range of 60–120 μs were effective and well tolerated (Moro et al. 2009).

While identifying side-effects is reasonably easy for each contact, defining which one is the most clinically beneficial is a much more challenging task. Mobile or phasic dystonic features, as well as myoclonus and tremor, tend to respond more quickly to neurostimulation than tonic dystonic postures. If an initial observation of 30 min or one hour in the office is often not sufficient to clarify which contacts alleviate symptoms best, a more prolonged trial period of one day to one week may be necessary to answer this question and help establish a hierarchy of contacts that can be used as a roadmap for future programming.

If, despite best efforts, such a task remains challenging, choosing the contact just above the optic or the adjacent can be an option. For bilateral electrodes placed symmetrically in the GPi, the clinician may also elect, once the initial exploration is completed, to stimulate pairs of symmetric contacts in a bipolar configuration (Krauss et al. 2003).

As far as voltage is concerned, it should be below the threshold for side-effects (Kupsch et al. 2011), with attempts to gradually taper it down once symptoms have improved and remained stable for a period of time. On the other hand, amplitude may be increased over time to optimise clinical benefit.

The question of whether different stimulation parameters should be used based on the aetiology of dystonia has not been studied. Vercueil et al. found no differences in short-term efficacy using short vs long pulse widths in isolated generalised dystonia (Vercueil et al. 2007). In dystonia in neurodegeneration with brain iron accumulation there were no differences in outcome using either short or long pulse width at a mean follow-up of 9–15 months (Timmermann et al. 2010). In the SPIDY-2 study in patients with choreodystonic cerebral palsy, good outcomes were achieved using pulse widths of 60–150 μs. Reese et al. (2011) followed up 12 patients with Meige syndrome and GPi DBS for up to 78 months, with good improvements of dystonia. Pulse widths varied between 60 and 210 μs. In patients with myoclonus-dystonia, GPi DBS yielded robust improvement in both myoclonus and dystonia using a 60 μs/130 Hz approach and voltages ranging from 1.6 V to 4.7 V (Azoulay-Zyss et al. 2011). Gruber et al. reported significant reduction of dystonic symptoms in tardive dystonia at a mean follow-up of 41 months with a mean pulse width of 83.3 μs and a frequency of 154 Hz (Gruber et al. 2009). In the case of Huntington's disease both low (40 Hz) (Zittel et al. 2015) and high (130 Hz) frequency stimulation have been used with moderate success using a variety of pulse widths (Gonzalez et al. 2014). In a retrospective multicentre study, 10/14 patients with chorea-acanthocytosis were treated with 130–185 Hz, whereas four patients were treated with 40–60 Hz. Most patients benefited from improvement in motor outcome and quality of life, irrespective of pulse width.

One recommended algorithm is to start with standard high-frequency stimulation at 130 Hz and a pulse width of 60–120 μs. The pulse width can be gradually tapered up if clinical response is not satisfactory. The more ventral contacts might be explored first.

Subsequent Programming Sessions and Strategies

Although no evidence-based data exist on how to manage medications postoperatively, anti-dystonia drugs usually are reduced to a considerable degree when clinical improvement is robust and sustained over time. No consensus exists on the frequency of follow-up visits, but it is generally recommended that after the initial programming period, when visits can be as often as weekly or biweekly, a short-term follow-up at three months is necessary to assess the delayed response seen in dystonia. While most of the benefit is seen at 3–6 months (Volkmann et al. 2012), further reduction in dystonia can be seen up to a year and beyond. After ongoing improvement and stabilisation is adequately documented, routine follow-ups at 3–6 months may suffice. It is important to note that also due to the high settings oftentimes used in dystonia, the clinician should regularly check all electrical parameters at every office visit, including impedance and battery status to avoid unexpected battery depletion and cessation of neurostimulation.

In the case of unsatisfactory or loss of benefit, the following strategies can be used:

1. Voltage (or current intensity, if using constant current mode) is increased gradually as needed or just below the threshold for side-effects.
2. Frequency is decreased or increased. Consider a trial of low-frequency stimulation (40–60 Hz) if already using high frequency.
3. Pulse width changes. If using low to moderate pulse width (60–120 μs), consider increasing it gradually to 210–450 μs with appropriate voltage adjustment to avoid excessive charge density.
4. Double or even triple monopolar stimulation to expand the volume of activated tissue. Bipolar stimulation is an alternative.
5. Blinded assessment in off- and on-stimulation if there is doubt about the efficacy of currently used settings.
6. Interleaving stimulation, either a trial in monopolar or bipolar mode, to allow for alternating activation of two cathodal contacts with a different voltage, in order to sculpt a more refined electrical field and reduce benefit-limiting side-effects. Data are scarce but one small study provided some evidence that it can be helpful (Kovacs et al. 2012).
7. Cycling mode, providing discontinuous stimulation with adjustable periods of stimulation off and on. It has to be noted, however, that there are very limited studies reporting on its use.

Finally, giving the patient the possibility to use different groups at home for a defined period of time and document benefits/side-effects can allow for increased patient comfort.

Programming DBS in Other Targets

Significant improvements in cervical dystonia treated with STN DBS and high-frequency 130 Hz stimulation have been reported in a few patients (Ostrem et al. 2011). Contacts used were mainly in the dorsolateral sensorimotor region of the STN similar to PD. Notably, 130 Hz stimulation was more effective than 60 Hz stimulation (Ostrem et al. 2014). Schjerling et al. used 60 μs pulse width and a frequency of 130 Hz for bilateral STN DBS in dystonia (Schjerling et al. 2013). For thalamic DBS, similar stimulation settings than for pallidal DBS have been used (Pauls et al. 2014; Slow et al. 2015).

Outcome Measures and Programming

One critical aspect of DBS programming for dystonia is the criteria or variables used to assess and track outcomes of stimulation. Most studies have used well-validated dystonia rating scales such as the Burke–Fahn–Marsden Dystonia Rating Scale (BFMDRS), mainly for generalised dystonias, and the Toronto Western Spasmodic Torticollis Rating Scale (TWSTRS) for cervical dystonia. For more focal dystonias, such as blepharospasm and Meige syndrome, as well as dystonia-associated symptoms, such as myoclonus, more symptom-specific scales should be used. Visual analogue scales (VAS) may also have some value in following up subjective sensations like pain, commonly seen in cervical dystonia. Regardless of the scales used, careful documentation through videotaping at regular intervals should be applied as numbers do not always tell the whole story in dystonia and scales cannot always capture subtle but clinically meaningful improvements.

Conclusions

DBS for dystonia has become a well-established method of treatment. Programming can be challenging and time-consuming. A rational approach should always be adopted for programming DBS in order to optimise the benefit.

References

Alterman RL, Miravite J, Weisz D, Shils JL, Bressman SB, Tagliati M. 2007. Sixty hertz pallidal deep brain stimulation for primary torsion dystonia. *Neurology* 69(7):681–688.

Azoulay-Zyss J, Roze E, Welter ML, Navarro S, Yelnik J, Clot F, Bardinet E, Karachi C, Dormont D, Galanaud D, Pidoux B, Cornu P, Vidailhet M, Grabli D. 2011. Bilateral deep brain stimulation of the pallidum for myoclonus-dystonia due to epsilon-sarcoglycan mutations: a pilot study. *Arch Neurol* 68(1):94–98.

Barbe MT, Dembek TA, Becker J, Raethjen J, Hartinger M, Meister IG, Runge M, Maarouf M, Fink GR, Timmermann L. 2014. Individualized current-shaping reduces DBS-induced dysarthria in patients with essential tremor. *Neurology* 82(7):614–619.

Coubes P, Roubertie A, Vayssiere N, Hemm S, Echenne B. 2000. Treatment of DYT1-generalised dystonia by stimulation of the internal globus pallidus. *Lancet* 355(9222):2220–2221.

Gonzalez V, Cif L, Biolsi B, Garcia-Ptacek S, Seychelles A, Sanrey E, Descours I, Coubes C, de Moura AM, Corlobe A, James S, Roujeau T, Coubes P. 2014. Deep brain stimulation for Huntington's disease: long-term results of a prospective open-label study. *J Neurosurg* 121(1):114–122.

Gruber D, Trottenberg T, Kivi A, Schoenecker T, Kopp UA, Hoffmann KT, Schneider GH, Kuhn AA, Kupsch A. 2009. Long-term effects of pallidal deep brain stimulation in tardive dystonia. *Neurology* 73(1):53–58.

Kovacs N, Janszky J, Nagy F, Balas I. 2012. Changing to interleaving stimulation might improve dystonia in cases not responding to pallidal stimulation. *Mov Disord* 27(1):163–165.

Krauss JK, Loher TJ, Weigel R, Capelle HH, Weber S, Burgunder JM. 2003. Chronic stimulation of the globus pallidus internus for treatment of non-DYT1 generalized dystonia and choreoathetosis: 2-year follow up. *J Neurosurg* 98(4):785–792.

Kupsch A, Benecke R, Muller J, Trottenberg T, Schneider GH, Poewe W, Eisner W, Wolters A, Muller JU, Deuschl G, Pinsker MO, Skogseid IM, Roeste GK, Vollmer-Haase J, Brentrup A, Krause M, Tronnier V, Schnitzler A, Voges J, Nikkhah G, Vesper J, Naumann M, Volkmann J, Deep-Brain Stimulation for Dystonia Study Group. 2006. Pallidal deep-brain stimulation in primary generalized or segmental dystonia. *N Engl J Med* 355(19):1978–1990.

Kupsch A, Tagliati M, Vidailhet M, Aziz T, Krack P, Moro E, Krauss JK. 2011. Early postoperative management of DBS in dystonia: programming, response to stimulation, adverse events, medication changes, evaluations, and troubleshooting. *Mov Disord* 26 (Suppl. 1):S37–S53.

Mann JM, Foote KD, Garvan CW, Fernandez HH, Jacobson CE, 4th, Rodriguez RL, Haq IU, Siddiqui MS, Malaty IA, Morishita T,

Hass CJ, Okun MS. 2009. Brain penetration effects of microelectrodes and DBS leads in STN or GPi. *J Neurol Neurosurg Psychiatry* 80(7):794–797.

Moro E, Piboolnurak P, Arenovich T, Hung SW, Poon YY, Lozano AM. 2009. Pallidal stimulation in cervical dystonia: clinical implications of acute changes in stimulation parameters. *Eur J Neurol* 16(4):506–512.

Okun MS, Gallo BV, Mandybur G, Jagid J, Foote KD, Revilla FJ, Alterman R, Jankovic J, Simpson R, Junn F, Verhagen L, Arle JE, Ford B, Goodman RR, Stewart RM, Horn S, Baltuch GH, Kopell BH, Marshall F, Peichel D, Pahwa R, Lyons KE, Troster AI, Vitek JL, Tagliati M, SJM DBS Study Group. 2012. Subthalamic deep brain stimulation with a constant-current device in Parkinson's disease: an open-label randomised controlled trial. *Lancet Neurol* 11(2):140–149.

Ostrem JL, Racine CA, Glass GA, Grace JK, Volz MM, Heath SL, Starr PA. 2011. Subthalamic nucleus deep brain stimulation in primary cervical dystonia. *Neurology* 76(10):870–878.

Ostrem JL, Markun LC, Glass GA, Racine CA, Volz MM, Heath SL, de Hemptinne C, Starr PA. 2014. Effect of frequency on subthalamic nucleus deep brain stimulation in primary dystonia. *Parkinsonism Relat Disord* 20(4):432–438.

Pauls KA, Hammesfahr S, Moro E, Moore AP, Binder E, El Majdoub F, Fink GR, Sturm V, Krauss JK, Maarouf M, Timmermann L. 2014. Deep brain stimulation in the ventrolateral thalamus/subthalamic area in dystonia with head tremor. *Mov Disord* 29(7):953–959.

Reese R, Gruber D, Schoenecker T, Bazner H, Blahak C, Capelle HH, Falk D, Herzog J, Pinsker MO, Schneider GH, Schrader C, Deuschl G, Mehdorn HM, Kupsch A, Volkmann J, Krauss JK. 2011. Long-term clinical outcome in Meige syndrome treated with internal pallidum deep brain stimulation. *Mov Disord* 26(4):691–698.

Schjerling L, Hjermind LE, Jespersen B, Madsen FF, Brennum J, Jensen SR, Lokkegaard A, Karlsborg M. 2013. A randomized double-blind crossover trial comparing subthalamic and pallidal deep brain stimulation for dystonia. *J Neurosurg* 119(6):1537–1545.

Slow EJ, Hamani C, Lozano AM, Poon YY, Moro E. 2015. Deep brain stimulation for treatment of dystonia secondary to stroke or trauma. *J Neurol Neurosurg Psychiatry* 86(9):1046–1048.

Starr PA, Markun LC, Larson PS, Volz MM, Martin AJ, Ostrem JL. 2014. Interventional MRI-guided deep brain stimulation in pediatric dystonia: first experience with the ClearPoint system. *J Neurosurg Pediatr* 14(4):400–408.

Tagliati M, Krack P, Volkmann J, Aziz T, Krauss JK, Kupsch A, Vidailhet AM. 2011. Long-term management of DBS in dystonia: response to stimulation, adverse events, battery changes, and special considerations. *Mov Disord* 26 (Suppl. 1):S54–S62.

Timmermann L, Pauls KA, Wieland K, Jech R, Kurlemann G, Sharma N, Gill SS, Haenggeli CA, Hayflick SJ, Hogarth P, Leenders KL, Limousin P, Malanga CJ, Moro E, Ostrem JL, Revilla FJ, Santens P, Schnitzler A, Tisch S, Valldeoriola F, Vesper J, Volkmann J, Woitalla D, Peker S. 2010. Dystonia in neurodegeneration with brain iron accumulation: outcome of bilateral pallidal stimulation. *Brain* 133(Pt 3):701–712.

Vercueil L, Houeto JL, Krystkowiak P, Lagrange C, Cassim F, Benazzouz A, Pidoux B, Destee A, Agid Y, Cornu P, Blond S, Benabid AL, Pollak P, Vidailhet M, Spidy GROUP (French Pallidal Stimulation Group for Dystonia). 2007. Effects of pulse width variations in pallidal stimulation for primary generalized dystonia. *J Neurol* 254(11):1533–1537.

Vidailhet M, Vercueil L, Houeto JL, Krystkowiak P, Lagrange C, Yelnik J, Bardinet E, Benabid AL, Navarro S, Dormont D, Grand S, Blond S, Ardouin C, Pillon B, Dujardin K, Hahn-Barma V, Agid Y, Destee A, Pollak P, French SPIDY Study Group. 2007. Bilateral, pallidal, deep-brain stimulation in primary generalised dystonia: a prospective 3 year follow-up study. *Lancet Neurol* 6(3):223–229.

Volkmann J, Wolters A, Kupsch A, Muller J, Kuhn AA, Schneider GH, Poewe W, Hering S, Eisner W, Muller JU, Deuschl G, Pinsker MO, Skogseid IM, Roeste GK, Krause M, Tronnier V, Schnitzler A, Voges J, Nikkhah G, Vesper J, Classen J, Naumann M, Benecke R, DBS Study Group for Dystonia. 2012. Pallidal deep brain stimulation in patients with primary generalised or segmental dystonia: 5-year follow-up of a randomised trial. *Lancet Neurol* 11(12):1029–1038.

Volkmann J, Mueller J, Deuschl G, Kuhn AA, Krauss JK, Poewe W, Timmermann L, Falk D, Kupsch A, Kivi A, Schneider GH, Schnitzler A, Sudmeyer M, Voges J, Wolters A, Wittstock M, Muller JU, Hering S, Eisner W, Vesper J, Prokop T, Pinsker M, Schrader C, Kloss M, Kiening K, Boetzel K, Mehrkens J, Skogseid IM, Ramm-Pettersen J, Kemmler G, Bhatia KP, Vitek JL, Benecke R, DBS Study Group for Dystonia. 2014. Pallidal neurostimulation in patients with medication-refractory cervical dystonia: a randomised, sham-controlled trial. *Lancet Neurol* 13(9):875–884.

Walcott BP, Nahed BV, Kahle KT, Duhaime AC, Sharma N, Eskandar EN. 2012. Deep brain stimulation for medically refractory life-threatening status dystonicus in children. *J Neurosurg Pediatr* 9(1):99–102.

Zittel S, Moll CK, Gulberti A, Tadic V, Rasche D, Baumer T, Fellbrich A, Bruggemann N, Engel AK, Tronnier V, Hamel W, Munchau A. 2015. Pallidal deep brain stimulation in Huntington's disease. *Parkinsonism Relat Disord* 21(9):1105–1108.

Chapter 76

Complications of Deep Brain Stimulation for Dystonia

Marwan Hariz and Gun-Marie Hariz

Since the pioneering of the modern era of deep brain stimulation (DBS) for dystonia by Krauss et al. and Coubes et al., both in 1999 (Coubes et al. 1999; Krauss et al. 1999), DBS has become the first-line surgical procedure for medically refractory dystonias, especially in patients with primary generalised, segmental and cervical dystonia, and increasingly in other types of dystonia (Andrews et al. 2010; Moro et al. 2013). The main established and evidence-based target for DBS in dystonia has remained the posteroventral globus pallidus internus (GPi) (Vidailhet et al. 2005; Volkmann et al. 2012), although other targets in various parts of the motor thalamus and the subthalamic nucleus (STN) are being targeted (Ostrem et al. 2011). These other brain targets are being used in some dystonia patients either for *de novo* DBS, or as additional targets to DBS in the GPi, in staged surgical sessions, or in the same session (Wohrle et al. 2012).

Even though DBS for dystonia is a safe surgical procedure, and notwithstanding the variable but generally positive effect of the stimulation on the symptoms (depending, among other factors, on the type of dystonia), complications and side-effects of DBS may and do happen. Dystonia patients, unlike Parkinson's disease (PD) patients, exhibit a larger heterogeneity of symptoms due to great variations in phenotype, body distribution and aetiology of dystonia. Additionally, dystonia patients are in general younger than PD patients, and they may have higher expectations from DBS surgery than PD patients. Patients with dystonia have a long life expectancy; they are at an age where they may be, or wish to be, working and leading an active life; women with dystonia may wish to become pregnant and have children (Paluzzi et al. 2006). Other aspects that differentiate dystonia patients from PD patients are that dystonia patients do not have an efficient medication (like dopaminergic drugs) to fall back on, and will be very much depending on the good maintenance of DBS for the rest of their long life. For all these reasons, possible complications and side-effects of DBS have to be known and as much as possible avoided and properly managed if they appear.

General complications of DBS in dystonia, especially those related to the surgery itself, share many common features with surgical complications of DBS for PD. Complications and side-effects of DBS are usually grouped into three categories: those related to the surgery itself, those related to the hardware, and those related to the chronic stimulation. It goes without saying that in many respects a complication in one category may have negative implications on other categories: a poor surgical technique can result in hardware-related complications (breakage of wires, skin erosion, etc.), and a poor surgical targeting with misplacement of the DBS leads can result in relevant side-effects upon stimulation, aside from no effect on the symptoms. Notwithstanding this, it is convenient from a didactic point of view to describe complications and side-effects according to each category.

Complications Related to Surgery

A poor knowledge of anatomy of the target area in the brain will certainly result in a misplacement of the electrode. For example, it was stated in a Continuous Medical Education publication that 'The GPi and GPe are anatomically adjacent, separated by the internal capsule' (Shrivastava & Germano 2001). GPi targeting should ensure that at least one contact of the DBS electrode should lie in the posteroventral third of the GPi, close to the lamina medullaris interna, because it is here that the sensorimotor part lies, and the best effects are obtained (Tisch et al. 2007).

The most dreadful – and fortunately rare – complication of DBS surgery is intracerebral haemorrhage (ICH). Employing too many exploratory tracks of microelectrode recording (MER) may increase the risk of ICH, especially when the pallidum is the target, as evidenced in an analysis of risk factors of haemorrhage during MER-guided DBS implantation in various deep brain targets by the San Francisco group (Binder et al. 2005). On the other hand, employing a magnetic resonance imaging (MRI) guided and verified DBS surgery without MER can virtually eliminate that risk (Maldonado et al. 2009; Zrinzo et al. 2012). Epileptic seizures can happen rarely in the immediate postoperative period, but this has practically never led to epilepsy in dystonia patients (Volkmann et al. 2012).

Complications Related to the Hardware

It has been said that hardware-related complications such as migration or dislocation of leads, and breakage of leads or cables are more common in dystonia patients because of the sometimes violent movements (Falowski et al. 2012). These, and other hardware-related complications such as skin erosion over the neurostimulator or cables, bowstringing of cables, twiddler syndrome, formation of seroma in the pocket around the neurostimulator and, of course, infections of hardware may happen. Almost all these complications will require surgical revisions, or removal of hardware, which can, in patients who have been really dependent on stimulation, lead to a dangerous and difficult-to-treat status dystonicus, when the successful DBS therapy is abruptly withdrawn (Falowski et al. 2012; Volkmann et al. 2012).

Complications Related to the Stimulation

As in any movement disorder treated with bilateral DBS targeting the basal ganglia and the motor thalamus, 'complications' related to high-frequency stimulation in those areas can lead to bothersome adverse events, especially – but not exclusively – in cases where the electrodes are misplaced in the target area. Since some of these adverse events may be managed by changes in stimulation parameters, they are better labelled 'side-effects' than true complications. Hence, this section will deal with possible side-effects in the setting of DBS for dystonia. These stimulation-induced side-effects may affect speech articulation, which is probably the most common side-effect. Of course, if the active contact of the DBS electrode is close to the internal capsule or to the optic tract, capsular or visual side-effects may happen, especially if the stimulation parameters are high. In general dystonia patients require higher stimulation intensities than PD patients, which is important when planning the DBS targeting to be not too close to the internal capsule or the optic tract. Swallowing may be negatively affected if the bilateral leads are too close to the internal capsule.

A peculiar side-effect of chronic stimulation in dystonia, first described by Tisch et al. (2007) and later confirmed by others (Schrader et al. 2011; Huebl et al. 2015), is the appearance of parkinsonian features such as gait initiation difficulties, gait shuffling, micrography and general hypokinesia in some patients. These phenomena do not develop immediately after surgery but appear gradually over months or years of stimulation. It is not clear what exactly is the mechanism here, whether it is an 'overshoot' in the changes of brain plasticity due to chronic DBS, or whether it is due to a long-standing slight affection of nearby capsular fibres by the stimulating electrical current. It is of interest to note that this 'overshoot' of the good effect of the DBS on the all too mobile components of the dystonic symptom may result in some patients in a state of hypo-mobility replacing the previous hyper-mobility that was the hallmark of their dystonic phenotype, and for which they were treated with DBS in the first place. Some have attempted to alleviate this side-effect by activating more dorsal contacts of the DBS electrode, but stimulation in these areas that lie more rostral in the pallidum are in general not as efficient as contacts in the posteroventral sensorimotor internal pallidum (Tisch et al. 2007).

Another possible side-effect of stimulation in dystonia patients is negative affection of mood: although depression has been relatively well described in some PD patients treated by DBS of the STN, especially in relation to a too radical decrease of dopaminergic medication, depression in DBS-treated dystonia patients may seem less frequent. Nevertheless, mood problems and even suicide attempts or suicide have been reported (Foncke et al. 2006; Volkmann et al. 2012).

Complications Due to Arrest of DBS

As mentioned above, a sudden arrest of stimulation in some dystonia patients successfully treated by chronic DBS can result in a malignant life-threatening condition, a dystonic crisis or status dystonicus, necessitating intensive care. This may be due to a sudden depletion of the battery of the implantable pulse generator (IPG) and will necessitate an emergency replacement of the IPG. Therefore, dystonia patients have to be monitored closely and the IPG should be replaced pre-emptively, before its battery is completely flat. The condition is not easily managed in cases where the stimulation arrest is due to removal of hardware following an infection. In these cases, the IPG cannot be replaced before some months later, when the infection is cured, and in the meantime it may be difficult to manage the patient outside an intensive care unit. One strategy could be performing a unilateral pallidotomy, which can be quite efficient in controlling dystonia in the meantime (Marras et al. 2014). When suggesting DBS for dystonia, it is important to inform the patient about the need to monitor the battery, and especially about the need for several replacements over the remainder of their life. These replacements may be more frequent than in DBS for PD, since on the one hand dystonia patients are generally younger, and on the other hand stimulation parameters are generally higher than in DBS for PD. Also, this may have economic implications for patients in countries where DBS is not reimbursed by social security. There are tragic examples where patients desperately needing an IPG replacement could not afford to pay for it, leading to a state in which their condition is worse than before surgery. A rechargeable IPG that lasts longer may be a solution, but even that will eventually need to be replaced, aside from the fact that it is more expensive than a non-rechargeable one.

'Complications' Due to False Expectations From and Difficult Coping With DBS

In patients with dystonia, especially younger patients who may not have experienced a life without dystonia, expectations from DBS may be very high (Hariz et al. 2011; Okun & Foote 2012). After DBS, patients may face new difficulties and new challenges, and may need support and counselling to cope with and re-orientate into, their new life situation, and reach a new psychosocial adjustment. Patients may not obtain the full improvement in symptoms that they expected from DBS. Even so, patients will become dependent on DBS both physically and emotionally, which may cause anxiety. They will have to accept some possible unwanted effects such as slurred speech, and mood swings (Hariz et al. 2011). For all these reasons, one way to temper the expectations and decrease the negative perception of eventual complications and side-effects of stimulation is to have a thorough discussion about what DBS entails with the patients and the families prior to surgery, and to tell them what can be expected. Equally important is to maintain close contact with patients after surgery to monitor not only their hardware and clinical somatic status, but also their emotional status and assist them in coping with their new situation by providing help and support from all members of the multidisciplinary DBS team.

Conclusions

Dystonia patients submitted to DBS are generally young, with a long life expectancy. Complications and side-effects of DBS in dystonia patients are not very common, but also not very rare. As such, they need to be understood, pre-empted as much as possible, and managed properly if they occur. They may occur at different levels and with variable severity, and they may be related not only to the surgical technique, the hardware and the chronic stimulation per se. They may also depend on the selection of the patient for surgery, on the age of the patient, on the aetiology of dystonia, on the phenotype, whether fixed or mobile, on the choice of brain target, on the expectations of the patient and on the care and support of the patient after surgery, both the neurological somatic care and the psychological and emotional support.

A good selection of, and honest information provided to, dystonia patients for DBS according to their symptoms and the likelihood of those symptoms to respond to stimulation, together with a meticulous surgery and a comprehensive management of stimulation, and an empathic physical and emotional follow-up and support after surgery, are mandatory to minimise complications and side-effects of DBS.

Acknowledgements

MH is supported by The Monument Trust and Parkinson Appeal UK.

GMH is supported by the Swedish Research Council.

References

Andrews C, Aviles-Olmos I, Hariz M, Foltynie T. 2010. Which patients with dystonia benefit from deep brain stimulation? A metaregression of individual patient outcomes. *J Neurol Neurosurg Psychiatry* 81(12):1383–1389.

Binder DK, Rau GM, Starr PA. 2005. Risk factors for hemorrhage during microelectrode-guided deep brain stimulator implantation for movement disorders. *Neurosurgery* 56(4):722–732.

Coubes P, Echenne B, Roubertie A, Vayssiere N, Tuffery S, Humbertclaude V, Cambonie G, Claustres M, Frerebeau P. 1999. Treatment of early-onset generalized dystonia by chronic bilateral stimulation of the internal globus pallidus: apropos of a case. *Neurochirurgie* 45(2):139–144.

Falowski S, Ooi YC, Smith A, Verhargen Metman L, Bakay RA. 2012. An evaluation of hardware and surgical complications with deep brain stimulation based on diagnosis and lead location. *Stereotact Funct Neurosurg* 90(3):173–180.

Foncke EM, Schuurman PR, Speelman JD. 2006. Suicide after deep brain stimulation of the internal globus pallidus for dystonia. *Neurology* 66(1):142–143.

Hariz GM, Limousin P, Tisch S, Jahanshahi M, Fjellman-Wiklund A. 2011. Patients' perceptions of life shift after deep brain stimulation for primary dystonia: a qualitative study. *Mov Disord* 26(11):2101–2106.

Huebl J, Brucke C, Schneider GH, Blahak C, Krauss JK, Kuhn AA. 2015. Bradykinesia induced by frequency-specific pallidal stimulation in patients with cervical and segmental dystonia. *Parkinsonism Relat Disord* 21(7):800–803.

Krauss JK, Pohle T, Weber S, Ozdoba C, Burgunder JM. 1999. Bilateral stimulation of globus pallidus internus for treatment of cervical dystonia. *Lancet* 354(9181):837–838.

Maldonado IL, Roujeau T, Cif L, Gonzalez V, El-Fertit H, Vasques X, Bonafe A, Coubes P. 2009. Magnetic resonance-based deep brain stimulation technique: a series of 478 consecutive implanted electrodes with no perioperative intracerebral hemorrhage. *Neurosurgery* 65(6 Suppl.):196–201.

Marras CE, Rizzi M, Cantonetti L, Rebessi E, De Benedictis A, Portaluri F, Randi F, Savioli A, Castelli E, Vigevano F. 2014. Pallidotomy for medically refractory status dystonicus in childhood. *Dev Med Child Neurol* 56(7):649–656.

Moro E, Gross RE, Krauss JK. 2013. What's new in surgical treatment for dystonia? *Mov Disord* 28(7):1013–1020.

Okun MS, Foote KD. 2012. Setting realistic expectations for DBS in dystonia. *Lancet Neurol* 11(12):1014–1015.

Ostrem JL, Racine CA, Glass GA, Grace JK, Volz MM, Heath SL, Starr PA. 2011. Subthalamic nucleus deep brain stimulation in primary cervical dystonia. *Neurology* 76(10):870–878.

Paluzzi A, Bain PG, Liu X, Yianni J, Kumarendran K, Aziz TZ. 2006. Pregnancy in dystonic women with in situ deep brain stimulators. *Mov Disord* 21(5):695–698.

Schrader C, Capelle HH, Kinfe TM, Blahak C, Bazner H, Lutjens G, Dressler D, Krauss JK. 2011. GPi-DBS may induce a hypokinetic gait disorder with freezing of gait in patients with dystonia. *Neurology* 77(5):483–488.

Shrivastava RK, Germano IM. 2001. Deep brain stimulation for the treatment of Parkinson's disease. *Contemp Neurosurg* 23(16):1–9.

Tisch S, Zrinzo L, Limousin P, Bhatia KP, Quinn N, Ashkan K, Hariz M. 2007. Effect of electrode contact location on clinical efficacy of pallidal deep brain stimulation in primary generalised dystonia. *J Neurol Neurosurg Psychiatry* 78(12):1314–1319.

Vidailhet M, Vercueil L, Houeto JL, Krystkowiak P, Benabid AL, Cornu P, Lagrange C, Tezenas du Montcel S, Dormont D, Grand S, Blond S, Detante O, Pillon B, Ardouin C, Agid Y, Destee A, Pollak P, French Stimulation du Pallidum Interne dans la Dystonie (SPIDY) Study Group. 2005. Bilateral deep-brain stimulation of the globus pallidus in primary generalized dystonia. *N Engl J Med* 352(5):459–467.

Volkmann J, Wolters A, Kupsch A, Muller J, Kuhn AA, Schneider GH, Poewe W, Hering S, Eisner W, Muller JU, Deuschl G, Pinsker MO, Skogseid IM, Roeste GK, Krause M, Tronnier V, Schnitzler A, Voges J, Nikkhah G, Vesper J, Classen J, Naumann M, Benecke R, DBS Study Group for Dystonia. 2012. Pallidal deep brain stimulation in patients with primary generalised or segmental dystonia: 5-year follow-up of a randomised trial. *Lancet Neurol* 11(12):1029–1038.

Wohrle JC, Blahak C, Capelle HH, Fogel W, Bazner H, Krauss JK. 2012. Combined pallidal and subthalamic nucleus stimulation in sporadic dystonia-parkinsonism. *J Neurosurg* 116(1):95–98.

Zrinzo L, Foltynie T, Limousin P, Hariz MI. 2012. Reducing hemorrhagic complications in functional neurosurgery: a large case series and systematic literature review. *J Neurosurg* 116(1):84–94.

Section X

Emerging Therapies for Dystonia

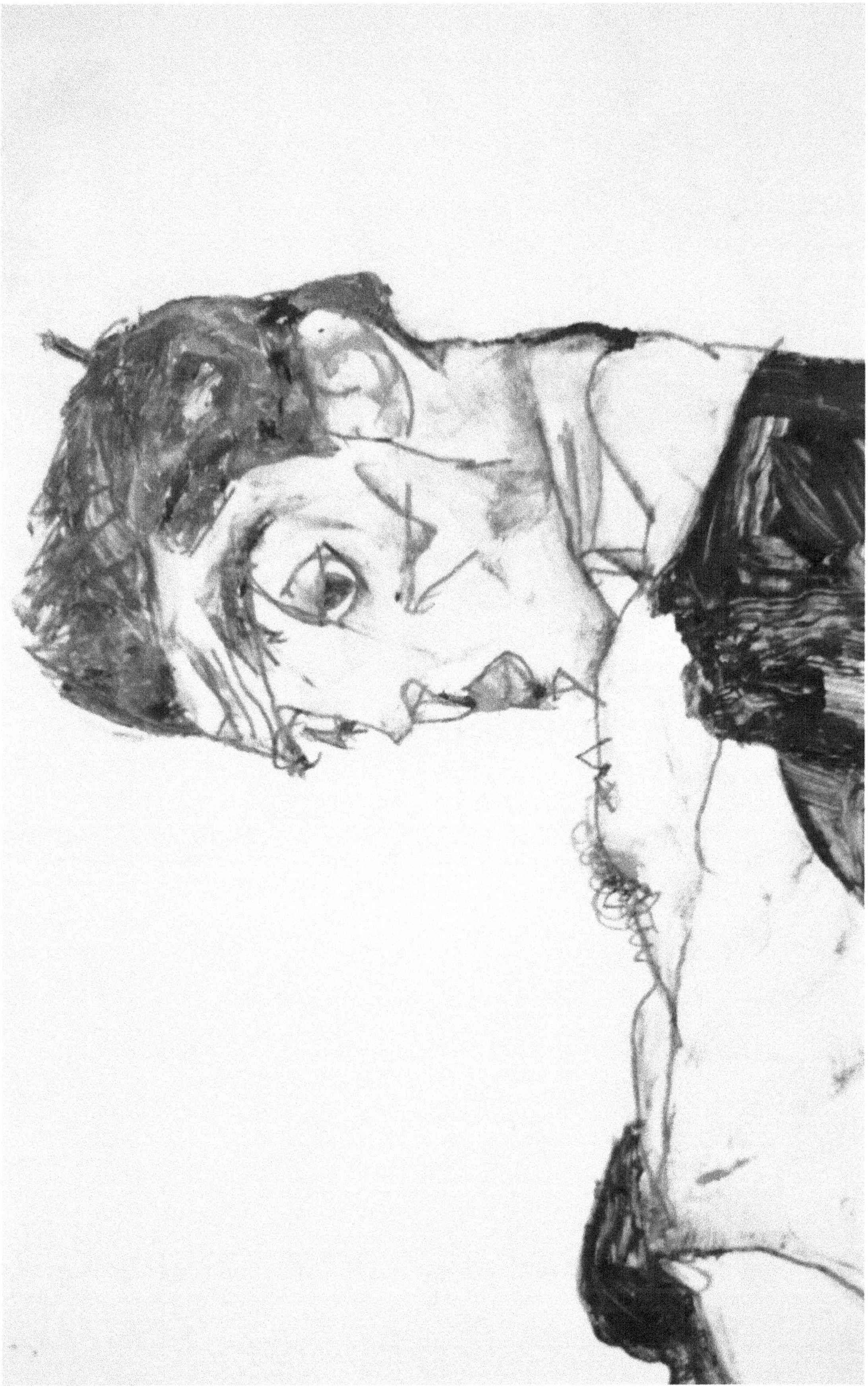

Chapter 77

Experimental Occupational Therapies for Writer's Cramp

Arne Knutzen and Kirsten E. Zeuner*

The Clinical Picture

In writer's cramp, the dystonic co-contraction triggered with writing may be painful. The abnormal posturing includes involuntary finger flexion/extension in combination with wrist flexion/extension. As a result of the dystonic movements, secondary postures such as extension of the wrist or abduction of the shoulder may occur. Most patients initially present with dystonic symptoms occurring only triggered by writing (simple writer's cramp), and may progress to develop symptoms with multiple fine motor tasks (complex writer's cramp).

Reverse Abnormal Sensory Processing

Background

Although routine sensory examination in patients with dystonia is usually normal, several neurophysiological and imaging studies have shown impaired perception, sensorimotor integration (Hallett 2006; Zeuner & Molloy 2008) and abnormal homuncular organisation of the finger representation in the primary somatosensory cortex in patients with writer's cramp (Hallett 2006; Zeuner & Molloy 2008). The performance in tactile spatial acuity and spatial discrimination are impaired predominantly in the affected hand (Hallett 2006; Zeuner & Molloy 2008). Since the sensory system is the major driving force behind the motor system, abnormalities could be relevant in causing motor dysfunction. Therefore, attempting to reverse abnormalities in the sensory system may be a potential experimental treatment approach.

Treatment Studies

Sensory Training

Braille reading has been evaluated as sensory training in ten patients with writer's cramp compared to normal controls with the aim to reverse abnormal somatosensory cortical dysfunction (Zeuner et al. 2002; McKenzie et al. 2009). All individuals were trained in Braille reading (grade 1) for eight weeks, for a duration of 30–60 minutes daily. Further practice involved reading with each finger individually. Sensory discrimination, measured with the Johnson–van-Boven–Phillips domes, improved in both patients and controls and ameliorated motor function in writer's cramp patients (Zeuner et al. 2002). However, only continuous training for one year produced sustained improvement in writing in some patients (Zeuner & Hallett 2003). Sensory training in other studies included identifying objects and surfaces such as number and configuration of dots on dominoes or textures, shapes, small plastic letters and numbers (McKenzie et al. 2009). However, those training techniques were part of a complex training programme, as discussed below.

Biofeedback

Visual or auditory biofeedback was performed using surface electromyography (EMG) electrodes recording from the wrist flexors. In most studies it was either combined with other training methods (Cottraux et al. 1983; Baur et al. 2009a) or applied exclusively (Deepak & Behari 1999; Berger et al. 2007). Patients were instructed to reduce either the EMG sound (Deepak & Behari 1999) or to maintain the motor unit amplitude at the minimum possible level (Berger et al. 2007) while writing exercises. After daily practice for 5–10 minutes for 1–6 months (Deepak & Behari 1999) the decrement of the motor unit amplitude was associated with improved writing (Deepak & Behari 1999; Berger et al. 2007) and normalisation of striatal D2-binding as assessed by [123I]IBZM SPECT (Berger et al. 2007). In a different biofeedback technique a pen with force sensors distributed across its surface was used. Seven patients with writer's cramp practised writing exercises that were accompanied by auditory grip force feedback in seven sessions each lasting 50 minutes, complemented by 10 minutes without feedback. The feedback contained a continuous low-frequency tone that was raised incrementally in four pitches for grip force level of 5–10 N, 10–20 N, 20–30 N and more than 30 N. Patients attempted to reduce the grip force such that they heard a low-frequency tone (Baur et al. 2009a). A third biofeedback method included a brain–computer interface system. Two patients were trained with EEG feedback twice per week for five months. They performed a tonic contraction, a right-hand extension and a writing task, while the integrated EMG

* We would like to thank Dr Fiona M. Molloy, consultant neurologist and neurophysiologist, clinical director of the Clinical Neurophysiology Department, Beaumont Hospital, Dublin, Ireland, for her valuable comments on the manuscript.

recorded the activity from the right extensor carpi radialis muscle (Hashimoto et al. 2013). The authors describe improved writing paralleled by improved event-related desynchronisation and synchronisation in one of the two patients.

KinesioTaping

One study evaluated the treatment effect of KinesioTaping of the forearm muscles compared to sham taping. In a randomised crossover pilot study in ten writer's cramp patients, KinesioTaping over a 14-day period induced a 19 per cent subjective pain relief, while disease severity showed no change in the writer's cramp rating scale (Pelosin et al. 2013). The sensory discrimination threshold decreased selectively in the taped area.

TENS

TENS has been investigated in ten writer's cramp (Tinazzi et al. 2007) and nine primary writing tremor patients (Meunier et al. 2011). In patients with writer's cramp, TENS was delivered to the forearm flexor muscles for two weeks by an electrostimulator and had a beneficial therapeutic effect that lasted three weeks. In contrast, primary writing tremor remained unchanged using TENS at 5 and 25 Hz. At 50 Hz, tremor even worsened and cortical excitability increased (Meunier et al. 2011).

Reverse Abnormal Excitability

Background

There is converging evidence that task-specific dystonia is associated with abnormal patterns of activity in cortical and subcortical areas during sensorimotor tasks (Hallett 2006). The inhibitory activity at multiple levels within the sensorimotor system is decreased. Based on these findings, novel therapeutical approaches have aimed at retuning the abnormal excitability of the motor cortex and restoring the de-differentiation of sensorimotor representations (Zeuner & Molloy 2008). Immobilisation of the affected limb and motor training with and without splints have been investigated.

Immobilisation

The rationale behind sensory and motor deprivation using a forearm splint for four weeks in combination with a retraining programme was to unlearn a fixed motor programme and re-learn non-dystonic movement strategies (Zeuner et al. 2005, 2008; Zeuner & Molloy 2008). After immobilisation, ten patients conducted specific or non-specific motor training programmes and demonstrated improvement in writing pressure and fluency as measured with kinematic handwriting analysis (Zeuner et al. 2008).

Training With Finger Splints

Patients trained successfully with individually manufactured splints and orthoses (Zeuner et al. 2005, 2008).

With finger and wrist splints, involuntary dystonic movements were restricted and thus co-contraction prevented. Patients wore finger splints while practising each individual finger. They trained either non-task-specific exercises (Zeuner et al. 2008) such as clockwise and counter-clockwise circles, the letters ll, zz and mm on a piece of paper or writing exercises (Waissman et al. 2013).

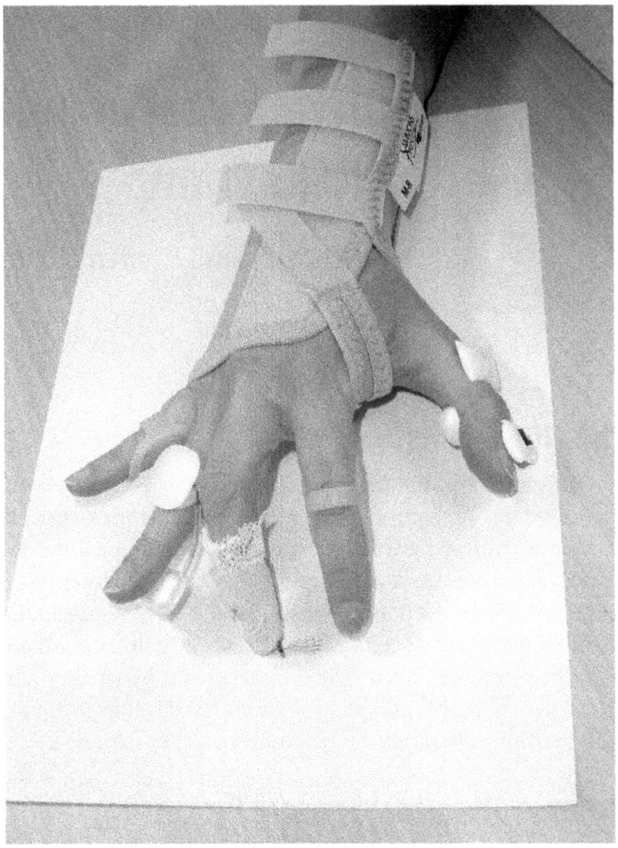

Figure 77.1 Training with finger splints.

Training With Therapeutical Putty

Therapeutical putty is a valuable tool to practice fine motor movements, improve force control, train individual finger movements and strengthen hand muscles. Patients adjusted speed and power to their dystonic symptoms so that no dystonic co-contraction occurred. The training was based on standardised and generally established putty exercises (Zeuner et al. 2008) such as finger flexion, rotation, abduction, adduction and extension against resistance. An eight-week period of daily motor training with putty improved task-specific dystonia, global hand function and movement kinematics in patients with WC in the same way as training with splints. The task-specific and non-task-specific retraining programme required the training of individual finger movements, and this may be the critical feature that mediates therapeutic efficacy (Zeuner et al. 2008).

Handwriting Training

The handwriting training of 50 patients consisted of several different steps. In a first step, undisturbed movements were analysed and supported (Mai & Marquardt 1999; Schenk et al. 2004). The second step included exercises containing single movements (finger, wrist, arm) and progressed to more complex movements. In a third step, the training started with writing short characters or words and progressed to sentences. The training procedure requires several important aspects: first, the sheet of paper should be blank to allow ample space for writing movements; second, handwriting should be performed without excessive control of the writing movements; third, the pen should be lifted frequently to relax finger and hand muscles without disrupting the flow.

The writing was simplified using a mixture of cursive and block, and thus supported ergonomic movements. Different ways of gripping the pen were tested to reduce dystonic movements and to improve the range of motion (Baur et al. 2009b). Additionally, the occupational therapist tested strategies in patients with writer's cramp to reduce the writing pressure and encouraged them to change writing postures, such as writing on a clipboard or while standing (Schenk et al. 2004; Zeuner et al. 2005, 2008; Baur et al. 2009b). The average training lasted approximately one hour per day for four months. A similar training programme was combined with botulinum toxin injections in a retrospective study and indicated that a short structured occupational therapy programme might further improve the effect of botulinum toxin treatment in some patients with writer's cramp (Berg & Naumann 1999).

Complex Interventions

Complex interventions (CI) included a combination of different treatment approaches. Therefore they were not based solely on a certain aspect of the pathophysiology. Complex interventions included sensory, motor, cognitive training and physical fitness.

In practice, occupational and physical therapists consider CI as an ideal way to address the complexity of writer's cramp. However, it remains unclear which treatment part finally led to the improvement.

There are three different programmes with CI:

The **first two CIs** with 13 patients each included exercises for mental imagery, biofeedback, mirror-therapy, sensory discrimination, inhibition of abnormal movements and physical fitness. Training was once per week supervised and otherwise home-based for eight weeks. The first study established a learning-based sensorimotor training (LBSMT), computerised memory training (software program BrainFit) and fitness exercises (Byl et al. 2009). In the LBSMT, patients learned positive thinking, to intentionally normalise the muscle tone, grading and fine motor training. An extended programme was evaluated in the second study and comprised stretching exercises, passive mobilisation of tightened tissues, strengthening of hand muscles, relaxation techniques, the adaptation of writing aids and finger splinting (McKenzie et al. 2009). The improvement could be demonstrated for musculoskeletal (physical) parameters, sensory processing and fine motor control.

In the first part of the **second CI** programme, 11 patients practised a home-based training programme with weekly supervision for 2–12 months (average of 5.5 months) (Bleton et al. 2010). Part of their training programme included special relaxation techniques in which patients were advised to deliberately switch between work and relaxation while movements and muscle tone were corrected. They continued with drawing and writing exercises of increasing complexity, while dexterity, pressure, sensory control and pen grip were adjusted. The purpose of the applied handwriting techniques was to unravel the dystonic motor programme and re-establish synergies between proximal and distal muscles (Bleton et al. 2010). Patients improved their writing, and the enlarged S1 representation measured with the magnetencephalography (MEG) somatosensory map of the cortex normalised after the training (Bleton et al. 2010).

In the **third CI** programme, 12 patients with writer's cramp took part in a body awareness training programme in two phases each lasting four weeks (Waissman et al. 2013). The purpose of phase I was to improve body awareness and postural re-education and therefore comprised stretching, relaxation and postural correction. During the supervised and home-based phase II, writing was trained with splints for the wrist and the primary dystonic finger to inhibit dystonic movements. Patients learned to differentiate hand and shoulder movements. The exercises proceeded from simple drawing to complex writing exercises. Additionally, games were employed to optimise motor coordination and concentration. After the rehabilitation, dystonic posture and pressure and motor control improved. Table 77.1 provides an overview of the studies discussed.

Common Aspects in All Studies

Most training programmes share some common components. These components include: (a) relaxation and stretching to reduce the muscle tone (this has been part of the biofeedback treatment (Deepak & Behari 1999; Berger et al. 2007; Baur et al. 2009a) and other complex interventions (Schenk et al. 2004; Tinazzi et al. 2007; Baur et al. 2009a; McKenzie et al. 2009); (b) reduction of the writing speed (Zeuner et al. 2005, 2008; Byl et al. 2009; Bleton et al. 2010; Waissman et al. 2013); and (c) splinting and wrist immobilisation during the training to reduce dystonic posturing (Zeuner et al. 2005, 2008; Mckenzie et al. 2009; Waissman et al. 2013). Several studies start with simple writing or drawing exercises and progress to more complex writing (Zeuner et al. 2005, 2008; Baur et al. 2009b; Byl et al. 2009; McKenzie et al. 2009; Bleton et al. 2010; Waissman et al. 2013). Finally, long-term training is required to maintain the improvement (Zeuner & Hallett 2003; Zeuner et al. 2005, 2008; Waissman et al. 2013).

While some studies used objective parameters such as the kinematic handwriting programme (Mai & Marquardt 1999; Schenk et al. 2004; Zeuner et al. 2005, 2008; Baur et al. 2009b), others rely on subjective measurements. The functional outcome in daily life for patients is not clear in most studies. Therefore we propose to define individual goals for each patient prior to training.

Ergonomic Devices

The purpose of the investigated writing devices was to use shoulder movements for writing similar to writing on a blackboard. The writing posture may change, which may improve dystonic co-contraction (Ranawaya & Lang 1991; Singam et al. 2013). However, daily usage of these awkward devices in public is limited (Singam et al. 2013).

Table 77.1 Overview of occupational therapy performed

Training methods	Relaxation stretching	Slowing down	Splinting/ immobilisation	Writing/drawing exercises	Non-task-specific sensorimotor training	Biofeedback
Sensory						
Zeuner et al. 2002					X	
Biofeedback						
Baur et al. 2009a				X		X
Cottraux et al. 1983	X					X
Deepak & Behari 1999						X
Berger et al. 2007						X
Hashimoto et al. 2013						X
KinesioTaping						
Pelosin et al. 2013			Taping			
TENS						
Tinazzi et al. 2007						X
Meunier et al. 2011						X
Finger splints						
Zeuner et al. 2008; Zeuner et al. 2005		X	X	X	X	
Therapeutical putty						
Zeuner et al. 2008		X			X	
Handwriting						
Mai & Marquardt 1999	X			X		X
Schenk et al. 2004	X			X		X
Baur et al. 2009b	X			X		X
Berg & Naumann 1999				X		
Complex interventions						
McKenzie et al. 2009	X		X	X	X	X
Byl et al. 2009		X		X	X	X
Bleton et al. 2010		X		X	X	
Waissman et al. 2013	X		X	X	X	

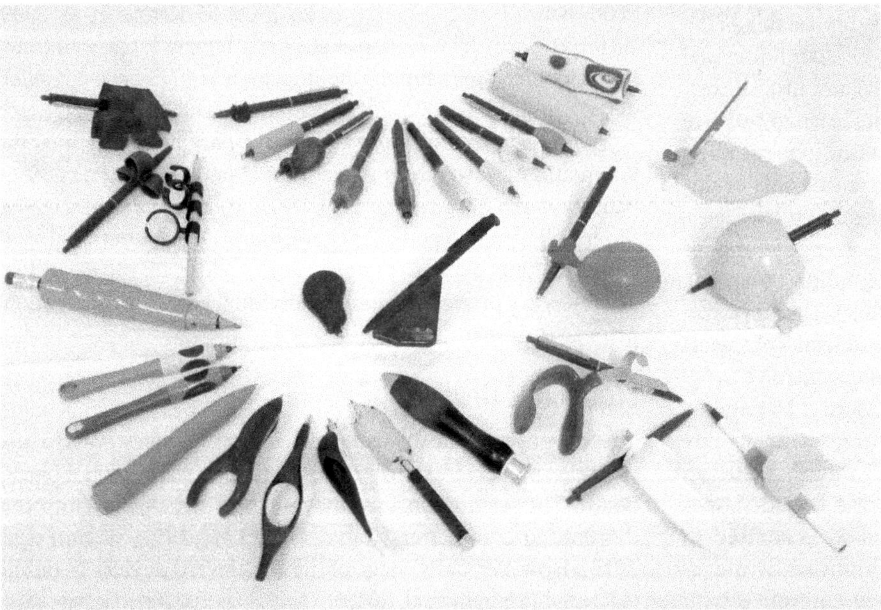

Figure 77.2 Examples of writing aids.

Summary

In summary, there is evidence that occupational therapy can improve writing in some patients with WC. There are different aspects that have been investigated: biofeedback, sensory training using Braille reading or identifying objects had some effect. Task-specific and non-task-specific motor training were compared, and there was no difference between the two training methods. In conclusion, training should include several different aspects. One could start with sensory training and therapeutic putty and move on to task-specific programmes described by Baur and Schenk (Schenk et al. 2004; Baur et al. 2009b). It is desirable that training programmes are designed for long-term practice at home and should ideally involve no more than 30 minutes of practice each day.

References

Baur B, Furholzer W, Jasper I, Marquardt C, Hermsdorfer J. 2009a. Effects of modified pen grip and handwriting training on writer's cramp. *Arch Phys Med Rehabil* 90(5):867–875.

Baur B, Furholzer W, Marquardt C, Hermsdorfer J. 2009b. Auditory grip force feedback in the treatment of writer's cramp. *J Hand Ther* 22(2):163–170.

Berg D, Naumann M. 1999. Therapeutic strategies in writer's cramp. *Neurol Rehabil* 4(5):199–205.

Berger HJ, van der Werf SP, Horstink CA, Cools AR, Oyen WJ, Horstink MW. 2007. Writer's cramp: restoration of striatal D2-binding after successful biofeedback-based sensorimotor training. *Parkinsonism Relat Disord* 13(3):170–173.

Bleton JP, Vidailhet M, Bourdain F, Ducorps A, Schwartz D, Delmaire C, Lehéricy S, Renault B, Garnero L, Meunier S. 2010. Somatosensory cortical remodelling after rehabilitation and clinical benefit of in writer's cramp. *J Neurol Neurosurg Psychiatry* 82(5):574–547.

Byl NN, Archer ES, McKenzie A. 2009. Focal hand dystonia: effectiveness of a home program of fitness and learning-based sensorimotor and memory training. *J Hand Ther* 22(2):183–197.

Cottraux JA, Juenet C, Collet L. 1983. The treatment of writer's cramp with multimodal behaviour therapy and biofeedback: a study of 15 cases. *Br J Psychiatry* 142:180–183.

Deepak KK, Behari M. 1999. Specific muscle EMG biofeedback for hand dystonia. *Appl Psychophysiol Biofeedback* 24(4):267–280.

Hallett M. 2006. Pathophysiology of writer's cramp. *Hum Mov Sci* 25(4–5):454–463.

Hashimoto Y, Ota T, Mukaino M, Ushiba J. 2013. Treatment effectiveness of brain–computer interface training for patients with focal hand dystonia: a double-case study. *Conf Proc IEEE Eng Med Biol Soc* 2013:273–276.

Mai N, Marquardt C. 1999. *Schreibtraining in der neurologischen Rehabilitation*. 2nd edition. Dortmund: Borgmann Publishing.

McKenzie AL, Goldman S, Barrango C, Shrime M, Wong T, Byl N. 2009. Differences in physical characteristics and response to rehabilitation for patients with hand dystonia: musicians' cramp compared to writers' cramp. *J Hand Ther* 22(2):172–181.

Meunier S, Bleton JP, Mazevet D, Sangla S, Grabli D, Roze E, Vidailhet M. 2011. TENS is harmful in primary writing tremor. *Clin Neurophysiol* 122(1):171–175.

Pelosin E, Avanzino L, Marchese R, Stramesi P, Bilanci M, Trompetto C, Abbruzzese G. 2013. Kinesiotaping reduces pain and modulates sensory function in patients with focal dystonia: a randomized crossover pilot study. *Neurorehabil Neural Repair* 27(8):722–731.

Ranawaya R, Lang A. 1991. Usefulness of a writing device in writer's cramp. *Neurology* 41(7):1136–1138.

Schenk T, Bauer B, Steidle B, Marquardt C. 2004. Does training improve writer's cramp? An evaluation of a behavioral treatment approach using kinematic analysis. *J Hand Ther* 17(3):349–363.

Singam NV, Dwivedi A, Espay AJ. 2013. Writing orthotic device for the management of writer's cramp. *Front Neurol* 4:2.

Tinazzi M, Farina S, Bhatia K, Fiaschi A, Moretto G, Bertolasi L, Zarattini S, Smania N. 2005. TENS for the treatment of writer's cramp dystonia: a randomized, placebo-controlled study. *Neurology* 64(11):1946–1948.

Waissman FQ, Orsini M, Nascimento OJ, Leite MA, Pereira JS. 2013. Sensitive training through body awareness to improve the writing of patients with writer's cramp. *Neurol Int* 5(4):e24.

Zeuner KE, Hallett M. 2003. Sensory training as treatment for focal hand dystonia: a 1-year follow-up. *Mov Disord* 18(9):1044–1047.

Zeuner KE, Molloy FM. 2008. Abnormal reorganization in focal hand dystonia: sensory and motor training programs to retrain cortical function. *Neuro Rehabil* 23(1):43–53.

Zeuner KE, Bara-Jimenez W, Noguchi PS, Goldstein SR, Dambrosia JM, Hallett M. 2002. Sensory training for patients with focal hand dystonia. *Ann Neurol* 51(5):593–598.

Zeuner KE, Shill HA, Sohn YH, Molloy FM, Thornton BC, Dambrosia JM, Hallett M. 2005. Motor training as treatment in focal hand dystonia. *Mov Disord* 20(3):335–341.

Zeuner KE, Peller M, Knutzen A, Hallett M, Deuschl G, Siebner HR. 2008. Motor re-training does not need to be task specific to improve writer's cramp. *Mov Disord* 23(16):2319–2327.

Chapter 78

Transcranial Electric and Magnetic Stimulation for Dystonia

Ulf Ziemann

Rationales for Non-Invasive Brain Stimulation to Treat Dystonia

Functional magnetic resonance studies demonstrated that the primary sensorimotor cortex and other nodes of the motor network such as the dorsal premotor cortex (PMd) may be overactive during dystonic voluntary motor activation (Pujol et al. 2000; Delnooz et al. 2013). The concept of exaggerated motor cortical excitability was supported further by transcranial magnetic stimulation (TMS) studies. Resting motor threshold and motor-evoked potential (MEP) size, a marker of corticospinal excitability, were similar in FHD and healthy controls in a resting hand muscle, but during voluntary contraction of that hand muscle, MEP facilitation was significantly stronger in FHD, indicating motor cortical hyperexcitability during voluntary activation (Mavroudakis et al. 1994; Ikoma et al. 1996). The duration of the cortical silent period (CSP), a marker of gamma-aminobutyric acid type B ($GABA_B$) receptor-mediated postsynaptic inhibition, did not change with increasing levels of contraction of the non-affected hand, but abnormally shortened with contraction level in the dystonic hand, indicating a deficient function of inhibitory control in the primary motor cortex (M1) representing the dystonic hand (Filipovic et al. 1997). Also, the short-interval intracortical inhibition (SICI), a paired-pulse TMS measure of $GABA_A$ receptor-mediated postsynaptic inhibition in M1, was reduced in FHD (Ridding et al. 1995; Stinear & Byblow 2004a). Short-latency afferent inhibition, tested by median nerve electrical stimulation followed at around 20 ms by TMS of the contralateral M1 was normal in FHD, but a later facilitatory input, probably reflecting the long-latency reflex II was exaggerated, pointing to abnormally facilitated sensorimotor signal transmission in FHD (Kessler et al. 2005). Long-latency afferent inhibition at an interstimulus interval of 200 ms showed paradoxical MEP facilitation in FHD (Abbruzzese et al. 2001). Surround inhibition, i.e. the MEP inhibition in surround muscles (e.g. the abductor pollicis brevis), during preparation for and execution of a focal voluntary activation of a target hand muscle (e.g. the first dorsal interosseous) was reduced in writer's cramp (Sohn & Hallett 2004; Beck et al. 2008, 2009; Houdayer et al. 2012; Veugen et al. 2013), supporting the idea that disturbed surround inhibition is a relevant pathophysiological mechanism of dystonia. Finally, paired-coil TMS studies demonstrated abnormal effective connectivity between PMd and M1 (Pirio Richardson et al. 2014), between ventral premotor cortex and M1 (Beck et al. 2009; Houdayer et al. 2012), between the M1 of the non-affected hemisphere to the M1 of the affected (dystonic) hemisphere (Nelson et al. 2010), and between the contralateral cerebellum and the affected M1 (Brighina et al. 2009).

In addition to employing TMS for testing abnormal sensorimotor excitability, several studies have used repetitive TMS (rTMS) protocols to change motor excitability in order to test for abnormal plasticity in FHD. A first study demonstrated that short-term plasticity induced by 1 Hz rTMS of M1 was highly abnormal in FHD, showing a pathological MEP increase rather than the MEP decrease of the healthy control subjects (Siebner et al. 1999b). Low-intensity 1 Hz rTMS of M1 also decreased MEP amplitude and lengthened CSP duration in healthy controls, but failed to alter these measures in FHD (Stinear & Byblow 2004b). Similarly, short-term plasticity in the form of increased MEP amplitude induced by a short 5 Hz rTMS train was exaggerated in magnitude and duration in FHD compared to healthy controls (Gilio et al. 2007). Also, the long-term potentiation (LTP)-like MEP increase induced by paired associative stimulation (PAS_{LTP}) was abnormally enhanced in FHD, with loss of topographical specificity, i.e. the LTP-like MEP increase was not limited to the target muscle but was also strongly expressed in a non-stimulated hand muscle (Quartarone et al. 2003; Weise et al. 2006; Belvisi et al. 2013). On the other hand, LTP-like MEP increase induced by intermittent theta-burst stimulation in healthy controls was absent in FHD (Belvisi et al. 2013), indicating that the observed abnormalities (i.e. exaggeration vs deficiency) in LTP-like plasticity in the M1 of FHD may depend on the specific non-invasive brain stimulation (NIBS) induction protocol. Finally, homeostatic metaplasticity in M1, a fundamental principle to maintain synaptic weight in neuronal networks in a physiological range (Hulme et al. 2013), was deficient in FHD when testing the interaction between two subsequent NIBS protocols (Quartarone et al. 2005) or one priming NIBS protocol and a subsequent motor learning task (Kang et al. 2011), and the degree of this abnormality correlated with the clinical severity of dystonia (Kang et al. 2011). In a similar vein, priming PAS_{LTP}-induced LTP-like plasticity in M1 by continuous or intermittent theta-burst stimulation of the contralateral lateral cerebellum resulted in an enhancement or blockade, respectively, of the PAS_{LTP} effect in healthy controls but not in FHD (Hubsch et al. 2013). This loss of cerebellar control over motor cortical plasticity may contribute to building up an incorrect (dystonic) motor programme during intensive practice of motor tasks such as writing, and may imply the cerebellum, in addition to the classical sensorimotor network of M1, PMd and the primary somatosensory cortex (S1) as a target for therapeutic NIBS.

In summary, these data provide consistent evidence that the sensorimotor cortex in FHD is hyperexcitable, in particular during voluntary activation, and exhibits exaggerated degrees of plasticity induction and deficient control mechanisms, such as homeostatic metaplasticity. These abnormalities provide the basis for employing NIBS techniques to FHD patients in order to normalise these abnormalities, with the hope that this will extend towards improvement of the clinical signs of dystonia.

Non-Invasive Brain Stimulation Protocols

Non-invasive brain stimulation protocols to change motor cortical excitability have been reviewed extensively elsewhere (e.g. Ziemann et al. 2008). Therefore, it should be mentioned here only that specific NIBS protocols have been developed that typically increase or decrease excitability of the stimulated brain network. This has most extensively been demonstrated for M1, with changes in MEP size as the standard readout. In brief, low-frequency (≤1 Hz) regular rTMS typically results in long-term depression (LTD)-like MEP decrease (Chen et al. 1997), while high-frequency (≥5 Hz) regular rTMS leads to an LTP-like MEP increase (Pascual-Leone et al. 1994). Continuous vs intermittent theta-burst stimulation (cTBS, iTBS) results in LTD- vs LTP-like MEP change, respectively (Huang et al. 2005). Paired associative stimulation (i.e. repeated pairs of median nerve electrical stimulation followed by TMS of contralateral M1) at short interstimulus intervals (around 10 ms) vs longer intervals (around 25 ms) result in LTD- vs LTP-like MEP change, respectively (Stefan et al. 2000; Wolters et al. 2003). Finally, cathodal vs anodal transcranial direct current stimulation (tDCS) of M1 also leads to LTD- vs LTP-like MEP change, respectively (Nitsche & Paulus 2001; Nitsche et al. 2003). Therefore, it appears that several NIBS protocol options are available to treat abnormal motor cortical excitability in FHD. However, at least two caveats should be noted: (1) recent evidence pointed out that the dichotomy of the effects of the NIBS protocols as summarised above (one particular protocol results in an LTD-like MEP decrease, the other one results in an LTP-like MEP increase) is no longer tenable as there seems to be very large intersubject variability of these effects, even in healthy subjects, with not much or even no MEP change in the grand average across all subjects (Müller-Dahlhaus et al. 2008; Hamada et al. 2013; Lopez-Alonso et al. 2014; Wiethoff et al. 2014); (2) as reviewed above, FHD patients may respond abnormally to NIBS protocols so that it is difficult to predict to what extent the desired response (i.e. a decrease in motor cortical excitability) will actually occur in these patients. It might be a reasonable possibility for future therapeutic trials to use markers such as motor cortical excitability or motor network functional connectivity at baseline to predict clinical responses to a given therapeutic NIBS intervention (Bharath et al. 2015; Kimberley et al. 2015).

Review of NIBS Treatment Effects in Focal Hand Dystonia

All of the reviewed studies in this text are also indicated in more detail in Table 78.1.

Stimulation of Primary Motor Cortex (M1)

The first study in this field demonstrated that 1 Hz rTMS of primary motor cortex (M1) increased SICI and decreased vertical writing pressure in writer's cramp patients. In addition, 6 of 16 patients self-reported improvement in hand function (Siebner et al. 1999c). One hertz M1 rTMS during scribbling resulted in decrease of MEP amplitude, increase of SICI, decrease of vertical writing pressure and increase in drawing regularity in writer's cramp, and 10/12 patients noted an improvement of handwriting lasting for ~1 day (Siebner et al. 1999a). Cathodal tDCS of M1 had no effect on clinical, kinematic or TMS excitability measures in a sham-controlled parallel design (Benninger et al. 2011). In patients with musician's dystonia (professional guitarists), a single session of cathodal tDCS of the affected M1 did not improve the performance of guitar playing (Buttkus et al. 2010). Also, in patients with musician's dystonia (pianists) a single session of cathodal or anodal tDCS of the affected M1 combined with simultaneous retraining consisting of slow, voluntarily controlled movements on the piano did not result in any improvement of dystonia (Buttkus et al. 2011). In contrast, cathodal tDCS of the affected M1 and simultaneous anodal tDCS of the unaffected M1 in musician's dystonia (pianists) resulted in improvement in the rhythmic accuracy of sequential finger movements with the affected hand, but only if concurrently bimanual mirrored finger movements were performed (Furuya et al. 2014). This improvement was retained four days after the intervention. Neither the reversed montage of electrodes (anodal tDCS of the affected M1, cathodal tDCS of the unaffected M1) nor unilateral anodal tDCS of the unaffected M1 or sham stimulation yielded any improvement (Furuya et al. 2014). Furthermore, the amount of motor improvement correlated directly with the severity of the symptoms, i.e. the most severely affected patients benefited most from the intervention. These findings suggest a therapeutic potential of behavioural training assisted by bihemispheric and polarity-specific tDCS in restoring fine motor control in musician's dystonia (Furuya et al. 2014).

Stimulation of the Dorsal Premotor Cortex (PMd)

Use of 0.2 Hz rTMS of dorsal premotor cortex (PMd) led to an increase of CSP duration, a decrease in vertical writing pressure and a decrease of tracking error in a circle-drawing task (Murase et al. 2005). These effects were specific to PMd stimulation and did not occur with 0.2 Hz rTMS of M1 or the supplementary motor area (SMA) (Murase et al. 2005). One hertz

Table 78.1 Summary of the NIBS studies for treatment of FHD

Patients	Protocol duration intensity	Stimulation site	Significant effects	Reference
7 WC off treatment 7 HC	1 Hz rTMS 30 min (1.800 P) 90% RMT	M1	SICI ↑ APP ↓	Siebner et al. 1999c
12 WC	1 Hz rTMS 10 × 1 min (600 P) 95% AMT	M1, sham	MEP ↓ SICI ↑ APP ↓ Drawing regularity ↑	Siebner et al. 1999a
2 × 6 WC (ctDCS vs sham) off treatment	ctDCS 20 min 2 mA	M1, sham	No effects on clinical, kinematic or TMS excitability measures	Benninger et al. 2011
10 MC (guitarists)	ctDCS 20 min 2 mA	M1	No effect on video-documented guitar playing performance	Buttkus et al. 2010
9 MC (pianists)	ctDCS, atDCS, sham 20 min 2 mA	M1	No effect on rhythmic accuracy of sequential finger movements	Buttkus et al. 2011
10 MC (pianists) 10 healthy pianists	ctDCS AH + atDCS UH atDCS AH + ctDCS UH atDCS UH sham 24 min 2 mA	M1	Rhythmic accuracy of sequential finger movements of the affected hand ↑ (ctDCS AH + atDCS UH)	Furuya et al. 2014
9 WC 7 HC	0.2 Hz rTMS 200 P 80% RMT	PMd, M1, SMA, sham	CSP ↑ (PMd) APP ↓ (PMd) Tracking error in circle-drawing task ↓ (PMd)	Murase et al. 2005
3 WC 3 MC 9 HC	1 Hz rTMS 900 P over five days 90% RMT	PMd, sham	CSP ↑ Pen velocity ↑	Borich et al. 2009
9 WC off treatment 9 HC	cTBS 300 or 600 P 80% AMT	PMd	SICI ↑ (cTBS 600) RI ↑ (cTBS 600) Spiral maze drawing task performance ↑	Huang et al. 2010
2 × 9 WC (cTBS vs sham) 10 HC	cTBS 600 P over five days 80% AMT	PMd, sham	SICI ↑ MEP ↓ (after day five) Spiral maze drawing task performance (↑)	Huang et al. 2012
Sham: 3 WC, 2 MC rTMS: 9 WC, 3 MC	1 Hz rTMS 1,200 P over five days 90% RMT	PMd, sham	CSP ↑ APP ↓	Kimberley et al. 2013
15 WC 10 HC	cTBS 600 P 70% RMT	PMd	No change in SI Writing speed ↑	Veugen et al. 2013
1 MC	1 Hz rTMS 2 × 600 P over five days 90% RMT	PMd	80% improvement in capability to play the violin	Kieslinger et al. 2013
20 WC	1 Hz rTMS 30 min over five days	S1, sham	Handwriting ↑	Havrankova et al. 2010
5 WC 5 HC	5 Hz rTMS 1250 P 90% RMT	S1, sham	No effect on tactile discrimination accuracy	Schneider et al. 2010
5 WC, 3 MC, all treatment naïve, 8 HC	atDCS, ctDCS, sham 20 min 2 mA	Lateral cerebellum	CBI ↓ (atDCS) APP ↓ (atDCS, ctDCS)	Bradnam et al. 2015

Abbreviations: AH = affected hemisphere; APP = axial pen pressure; atDCS = anodal transcranial direct current stimulation; CBI = cerebellar–brain inhibition; ctDCS = cathodal transcranial direct current stimulation; HC = healthy control; M1 = primary motor cortex; MC = musician's cramp; P = pulses; PMd = dorsal premotor cortex; RI = third phase of spinal reciprocal inhibition; RMT = resting motor threshold; S1 = primary somatosensory cortex; SI = surround inhibition; SICI = short-interval intracortical inhibition; SMA = supplementary motor area; UH = unaffected hemisphere; WC = writer's cramp; ↓ decrease; ↑ increase or improvement.

rTMS of PMd over five consecutive days in a sham-controlled study increased CSP duration and either increased pen velocity (Borich et al. 2009) or decreased vertical writing pressure (Kimberley et al. 2013). These changes were still observable at follow-up ten days after the NIBS intervention (Borich et al. 2009). A single case study reported in a therapy-refractory patient with musician's dystonia (professional violinist) that 1 Hz rTMS of the PMd over five consecutive days resulted in an 80 per cent improvement of this condition that persisted for four months (Kieslinger et al. 2013). cTBS of the PMd increased SICI and the third phase of spinal reciprocal inhibition that were abnormally reduced compared to healthy controls at baseline, and decreased completion time and error score in a spiral maze drawing test (Huang et al. 2010). In another study by the same group, cTBS of the PMd over five consecutive days increased SICI, decreased MEP amplitude (but only after day 5) and improved performance in the spiral maze drawing test (Huang et al. 2012). This study, therefore, suggested that some of the remodelling effects of PMd stimulation may develop only if stimulation has continued over a sufficient period of time. Also, cTBS of the PMd improved writing speed but did not alleviate the abnormally reduced surround inhibition in writer's cramp (Veugen et al. 2013), suggesting that PMd is an effective target for therapeutic NIBS but questions the involvement of the PMd in the loss of surround inhibition, and possibly also the direct link between abnormally reduced surround inhibition and dystonia.

Stimulation of the Primary Somatosensory Cortex (S1)

Only two studies have tested this target. In a sham-controlled study, 1 Hz rTMS of S1 over five consecutive days improved handwriting performance in writer's cramp patients and increased the BOLD signal bilaterally in S1, the posterior parietal cortex and in the supplementary motor area during hand activation in a functional MRI experiment (Havrankova et al. 2010), indicating significant remodelling of large-scale network activity as a consequence of this intervention. In another study, 5 Hz rTMS of S1, that in healthy subjects led to improvement in tactile discrimination accuracy associated with task-related increases in the BOLD signal in the stimulated S1, and bilateral premotor cortex and basal ganglia, failed to improve deficient tactile discrimination performance in writer's cramp patients and to increase the task-related BOLD signal in the basal ganglia that was already abnormally high before the NIBS intervention (Schneider et al. 2010). These nil findings may reflect abnormal basal ganglia to S1 signal processing, and/or compensatory basal ganglia hyperactivation at baseline that was saturated and could not be further improved by rTMS.

Stimulation of the Lateral Cerebellum

Anodal tDCS of the lateral cerebellum resulted in a decrease in cerebellar–brain inhibition and a decrease of writing pressure in FHD, but these changes in effective connectivity between cerebellum and M1 and motor function were not related to each other (Bradnam et al. 2015). Nevertheless, this is the first therapeutic trial that suggests that NIBS of the lateral cerebellum may have therapeutic potential in FMD.

Summary and Outlook

The therapeutic application of NIBS in FHD is based on thorough evidence of abnormal sensorimotor excitability and plasticity in this disorder. However, as it stands, NIBS treatment of FHD is currently still experimental. The available studies summarised in Table 78.1 are all small scale with typically less than ten patients. Accordingly, no recommendation on rTMS efficacy was given in a recent evidence-based guidelines paper commissioned by the International Federation of Clinical Neurophysiology (Lefaucheur et al. 2014). Given the still preliminary positive evidence for therapeutic effects, larger-scale randomised controlled trials are clearly warranted. To make significant progress, future trials will need to take into consideration important questions, such as the target(s) of stimulation (including novel targets such as the lateral cerebellum, and concomitant stimulation of more than one node in the motor network), predictive markers for a therapeutic response, dose and duration of the NIBS protocol, combination with specific motor retraining procedures and more sophisticated treatment protocols (e.g. state-dependent or even closed-loop stimulation).

References

Abbruzzese G, Marchese R, Buccolieri A, Gasparetto B, Trompetto C. 2001. Abnormalities of sensorimotor integration in focal dystonia: a transcranial magnetic stimulation study. *Brain* 124:537–545.

Beck S, Richardson SP, Shamim EA, Dang N, Schubert M, Hallett M. 2008. Short intracortical and surround inhibition are selectively reduced during movement initiation in focal hand dystonia. *J Neurosci* 28:10363–10369.

Beck S, Houdayer E, Richardson SP, Hallett M. 2009. The role of inhibition from the left dorsal premotor cortex in right-sided focal hand dystonia. *Brain Stimul* 2:208–214.

Belvisi D, Suppa A, Marsili L, et al. 2013. Abnormal experimentally- and behaviorally-induced LTP-like plasticity in focal hand dystonia. *Exp Neurol* 240:64–74.

Benninger DH, Lomarev M, Lopez G, Pal N, Luckenbaugh DA, Hallett M. 2011. Transcranial direct current stimulation for the treatment of focal hand dystonia. *Mov Disord* 26:1698–1702.

Bharath RD, Biswal BB, Bhaskar MV, et al. 2015. Repetitive transcranial magnetic stimulation induced modulations of resting state motor connectivity in writer's cramp. *Eur J Neurol.* doi: 10.1111/ene.12653.

Borich M, Arora S, Kimberley TJ. 2009. Lasting effects of repeated rTMS application in focal hand dystonia. *Restor Neurol Neurosci* 27:55–65.

Bradnam LV, Graetz LJ, McDonnell MN, Ridding MC. 2015. Anodal transcranial direct current stimulation to the cerebellum improves handwriting and cyclic drawing kinematics in focal hand dystonia. *Front Hum Neurosci* 9:286.

Brighina F, Romano M, Giglia G, et al. 2009. Effects of cerebellar TMS on motor cortex of patients with focal dystonia: a preliminary report. *Exp Brain Res Experimentelle Hirnforschung* 192:651–656.

Buttkus F, Weidenmüller M, Schneider S, et al. 2010. Failure of cathodal direct current stimulation to improve fine motor control in musician's dystonia. *Mov Disord* 25:389–394.

Buttkus F, Baur V, Jabusch HC, et al. 2011. Single-session tDCS-supported retraining does not improve fine motor control in musician's dystonia. *Restor Neurol Neurosci* 29:85–90.

Chen R, Classen J, Gerloff C, et al. 1997. Depression of motor cortex excitability by low-frequency transcranial magnetic stimulation. *Neurology* 48:1398–1403.

Delnooz CC, Helmich RC, Medendorp WP, Van de Warrenburg BP, Toni I. 2013. Writer's cramp: increased dorsal premotor activity during intended writing. *Hum Brain Map* 34:613–625.

Filipovic SR, Ljubisavljevic M, Svetel M, Milanovic S, Kacar A, Kostic VS. 1997. Impairment of cortical inhibition in writer's cramp as revealed by changes in electromyographic silent period after transcranial magnetic stimulation. *Neurosci Lett* 222:167–170.

Furuya S, Nitsche MA, Paulus W, Altenmuller E. 2014. Surmounting retraining limits in musicians' dystonia by transcranial stimulation. *Ann Neurol* 75:700–707.

Gilio F, Suppa A, Bologna M, Lorenzano C, Fabbrini G, Berardelli A. 2007. Short-term cortical plasticity in patients with dystonia: a study with repetitive transcranial magnetic stimulation. *Mov Disord* 22:1436–1443.

Hamada M, Murase N, Hasan A, Balaratnam M, Rothwell JC. 2013. The role of interneuron networks in driving human motor cortical plasticity. *Cereb Cortex* 23:1593–1605.

Havrankova P, Jech R, Walker ND, et al. 2010. Repetitive TMS of the somatosensory cortex improves writer's cramp and enhances cortical activity. *Neuro Endocrinol Lett* 31:73–86.

Houdayer E, Beck S, Karabanov A, Poston B, Hallett M. 2012. The differential modulation of the ventral premotor–motor interaction during movement initiation is deficient in patients with focal hand dystonia. *Eur J Neurosci* 35:478–485.

Huang Y-Z, Edwards MJ, Rounis E, Bhatia KP, Rothwell JC. 2005. Theta burst stimulation of the human motor cortex. *Neuron* 45:201–206.

Huang YZ, Rothwell JC, Lu CS, Wang J, Chen RS. 2010. Restoration of motor inhibition through an abnormal premotor–motor connection in dystonia. *Mov Disord* 25:696–703.

Huang YZ, Lu CS, Rothwell JC, et al. 2012. Modulation of the disturbed motor network in dystonia by multisession suppression of premotor cortex. *PLoS One* 7:e47574.

Hubsch C, Roze E, Popa T, et al. 2013. Defective cerebellar control of cortical plasticity in writer's cramp. *Brain* 136:2050–2062.

Hulme SR, Jones OD, Abraham WC. 2013. Emerging roles of metaplasticity in behaviour and disease. *Trends Neurosci* 36:353–362.

Ikoma K, Samii A, Mercuri B, Wassermann EM, Hallett M. 1996. Abnormal cortical motor excitability in dystonia. *Neurology* 46:1371–1376.

Kang J-S, Terranova C, Hilker R, Quartarone A, Ziemann U. 2011. Deficient homeostatic regulation of practice-dependent plasticity in writer's cramp. *Cereb Cortex* 21:1203–1212.

Kessler KR, Ruge D, Ilic TV, Ziemann U. 2005. Short latency afferent inhibition and facilitation in patients with writer's cramp. *Mov Disord* 20:238–242.

Kieslinger K, Höller Y, Bergmann J, Golaszewski S, Staffen W. 2013. Successful treatment of musician's dystonia using repetitive transcranial magnetic stimulation. *Clin Neurol Neurosurg* 115:1871–1872.

Kimberley TJ, Borich MR, Arora S, Siebner HR. 2013. Multiple sessions of low-frequency repetitive transcranial magnetic stimulation in focal hand dystonia: clinical and physiological effects. *Rest Neurol Neurosci* 31:533–542.

Kimberley TJ, Borich MR, Schmidt RL, Carey JR, Gillick B. 2015. Focal hand dystonia: individualized intervention with repeated application of repetitive transcranial magnetic stimulation. *Arch Phys Med Rehabil* 96:S122–S128.

Lefaucheur JP, Andre-Obadia N, Antal A, et al. 2014. Evidence-based guidelines on the therapeutic use of repetitive transcranial magnetic stimulation (rTMS). *Clin Neurophysiol* 125:2150–2206.

Lopez-Alonso V, Cheeran B, Rio-Rodriguez D, Fernandez-Del-Olmo M. 2014. Inter-individual variability in response to non-invasive brain stimulation paradigms. *Brain Stimul* 7:372–380.

Mavroudakis N, Caroyer JM, Brunko E, Zegers de Beyl D. 1994. Effects of diphenylhydantoin on motor potentials evoked with magnetic stimulation. *Electroencephal Clin Neurophysiol* 93:428–433.

Müller-Dahlhaus JF, Orekhov Y, Liu Y, Ziemann U. 2008. Interindividual variability and age-dependency of motor cortical plasticity induced by paired associative stimulation. *Exp Brain Res Experimentelle Hirnforschung* 187:467–475.

Murase N, Rothwell JC, Kaji R, et al. 2005. Subthreshold low-frequency repetitive transcranial magnetic stimulation over the premotor cortex modulates writer's cramp. *Brain* 128:104–115.

Nelson AJ, Hoque T, Gunraj C, Ni Z, Chen R. 2010. Impaired interhemispheric inhibition in writer's cramp. *Neurology* 75:441–447.

Nitsche MA, Paulus W. 2001. Sustained excitability elevations induced by transcranial DC motor cortex stimulation in humans. *Neurology* 57:1899–1901.

Nitsche MA, Nitsche MS, Klein CC, Tergau F, Rothwell JC, Paulus W. 2003. Level of action of cathodal DC polarisation induced inhibition of the human motor cortex. *Clin Neurophysiol* 114:600–604.

Pascual-Leone A, Valls-Sole J, Wassermann EM, Hallett M. 1994. Responses to rapid-rate transcranial magnetic stimulation of the human motor cortex. *Brain* 117:847–858.

Pirio Richardson S, Beck S, Bliem B, Hallett M. 2014. Abnormal dorsal premotor–motor inhibition in writer's cramp. *Mov Disord.* doi: 10.1002/mds.25878.

Pujol J, Roset-Llobet J, Rosines-Cubells D, et al. 2000. Brain cortical activation during guitar-induced hand dystonia studied by functional MRI. *NeuroImage* 12:257–267.

Quartarone A, Bagnato S, Rizzo V, et al. 2003. Abnormal associative plasticity of the human motor cortex in writer's cramp. *Brain* 126:2586–2596.

Quartarone A, Rizzo V, Bagnato S, et al. 2005. Homeostatic-like plasticity of the primary motor hand area is impaired in focal hand dystonia. *Brain* 128:1943–1950.

Ridding MC, Sheean G, Rothwell JC, Inzelberg R, Kujirai T. 1995. Changes in the balance between motor cortical excitation and inhibition in focal, task specific dystonia. *J Neurol, Neurosurg, Psychiatr* 59:493–498.

Schneider SA, Pleger B, Draganski B, et al. 2010. Modulatory effects of 5Hz rTMS over the primary somatosensory cortex in focal dystonia: an fMRI–TMS study. *Mov Disord* 25:76–83.

Siebner HR, Auer C, Ceballos-Baumann A, Conrad B. 1999a. Has repetitive transcranial magnetic stimulation of the primary motor hand area a therapeutic application in writer's cramp? *Electroencephalogr Clin Neurophysiol Suppl* 51:265–275.

Siebner HR, Auer C, Conrad B. 1999b. Abnormal increase in the corticomotor output to the affected hand during repetitive transcranial magnetic stimulation of the primary motor cortex in patients with writer's cramp. *Neurosci Lett* 262:133–136.

Siebner HR, Tormos JM, Ceballos-Baumann AO, et al. 1999c. Low-frequency repetitive transcranial magnetic stimulation of the motor cortex in writer's cramp. *Neurology* 52:529–537.

Sohn YH, Hallett M. 2004. Disturbed surround inhibition in focal hand dystonia. *Ann Neurol* 56:595–599.

Stefan K, Kunesch E, Cohen LG, Benecke R, Classen J. 2000. Induction of plasticity in the human motor cortex by paired associative stimulation. *Brain* 123:572–584.

Stinear CM, Byblow WD. 2004a. Elevated threshold for intracortical inhibition in focal hand dystonia. *Mov Disord* 19:1312–1317.

Stinear CM, Byblow WD. 2004b. Impaired modulation of corticospinal excitability following subthreshold rTMS in focal hand dystonia. *Hum Mov Sci* 23:527–538.

Veugen LC, Hoffland BS, Stegeman DF, van de Warrenburg BP. 2013. Inhibition of the dorsal premotor cortex does not repair surround inhibition in writer's cramp patients. *Exp Brain Res Experimentelle Hirnforschung* 225:85–92.

Weise D, Schramm A, Stefan K, et al. 2006. The two sides of associative plasticity in writer's cramp. *Brain* 129:2709–2721.

Wiethoff S, Hamada M, Rothwell JC. 2014. Variability in response to transcranial direct current stimulation of the motor cortex. *Brain Stimul* 7:468–475.

Wolters A, Sandbrink F, Schlottmann A, et al. 2003. A temporally asymmetric Hebbian rule governing plasticity in the human motor cortex. *J Neurophysiol* 89:2339–2345.

Ziemann U, Paulus W, Nitsche MA, et al. 2008. Consensus: motor cortex plasticity protocols. *Brain Stimul* 1:164–182.

Section X Emerging Therapies for Dystonia

Chapter 79

Cannabinoids in Dystonias

Eckart Altenmüller and Andrè Lee

Introduction

Dystonias are mainly regarded as the result of basal ganglia (BG) dysfunction (Berardelli 1998; Breakefield et al. 2008) with a loss of inhibition (Hallett 2006, 2011). Recent research, however, suggests a network problem including cerebellar pathways (Neychev et al. 2008; Argyelan et al. 2009). It is known that in both the BG and the cerebellum, CB1-cannabinoid receptors are expressed at a particularly high density (Herkenham et al. 1991; Llano et al. 1991; Matsuda et al. 1993). The localisation of CB1 receptors at presynaptic synapses implies that they have a modulating effect on synaptic function (Iversen 2003). Two mechanisms have been described by which the modulating effect occurs: depolarisation-induced suppression of inhibition (Llano et al. 1991; Pitler & Alger 1992) and depolarisation-induced suppression of excitation (Kreitzer & Regehr 2001). The modulatory effect on inhibitory and excitatory pathways in the BG was investigated by Sañudo-Peñja et al. (1999). They were able to show that hyperkinesia through dopamine D1 receptor agonists in the striato-nigral pathway could be reversed after administration of a cannabinoid. This was explained by the cannabinoid-induced presynaptic inhibition of GABA release in the substantia nigra pars reticularis, leading to a disinhibition of the thalamocortical pathway, resulting in the observed inhibition of movement. Another study showed an increase in locomotor activity after treatment with a CB1-receptor antagonist (Compton et al. 1996). These results are also supported by animal models of dystonia, where an anti-dystonic effect of CB1-receptor agonists was reported in mice with dystonic symptoms (Richter & Löscher 1994, 2002).

Results of Case Reports and Clinical Research in Treatment of Dystonia With Cannabinoids

The above-mentioned results of preclinical research have led to the suggestion that cannabinoid agonists may be used for the treatment of dystonia. A recent review by Kluger et al. (2015) summarised outcomes of case studies and clinical trials. This review produced a mixed picture with regard to effectiveness and safety of treatment of dystonias using cannabinoids.

In an early study, Consroe et al. applied cannabidiol (CBD) in an oral dosage between 100 and 600 mg to five patients suffering from dystonia secondary to diverse causes. These authors found an improvement of dystonic symptoms in all five patients, but reported marked side-effects (Consroe et al. 1986). In a case study in a patient with blepharospasm, an improvement in symptoms and, consequently, in the patient's social life, was reported under treatment with Dronabinol®, a CB1 and CB2 agonist (Gauter et al. 2004). In an impressive case study by Jabusch et al., a reduction in dystonia-induced impairment of piano playing in a professional pianist after application of THC in a dosage of 5 mg was found, whereas no improvement was observed after application of placebo. Importantly, no effect of THC on motor precision of the unaffected hand was noticeable (Jabusch et al. 2004) (Figure 79.1).

There are other cases reporting improvement of smoked cannabis for generalised dystonia in Wilson's disease (Uribe Roca et al. 2005) and idiopathic hemidystonia (Chatterjee et al. 2002). A small (n = 13) randomised double-blind placebo-controlled crossover trial tested a single dose of 0.03 mg/kg nabilone, a synthetic cannabinoid that mimics THC, on patients with medication refractory focal or generalised dystonia using the Burke–Fahn–Marsden dystonia scale (Fox et al. 2002). When comparing nabilone to placebo, they reported no significant differences between groups at 60, 120 or 180 minutes, including when separating generalised from segmental patients. Four patients reported a subjective improvement lasting three days after nabilone and two patients withdrew after hypotension and sedation. This negative result was discussed as possibly being due to an insufficient dosage or to the heterogeneity of the patients, since patients were suffering from both generalised and segmental dystonia. Finally, it was discussed whether lack of improvement was due to an erroneous understanding of the pathogenesis of primary dystonias. A second small (n = 7) randomised placebo-controlled crossover trial assessed 7.5 mg Dronabinol®, given twice daily for two weeks, in patients with cervical dystonia. These authors used the Toronto Western Hospital Spasmodic Torticollis Rating Scale (TWSTRS) to assess improvements (Zadikoff et al. 2011). There were no significant differences noted on TWSTRS (total or subscales) or subjective ratings. One subject withdrew due to insomnia and sensations of heart racing, and all but one subject reported mild side-effects including lightheadedness, hypotension, vertigo and dry mouth.

Adverse Effects and Risk of Addiction

Generally cannabinoids appear to be well tolerated when used in small dosages. However, adverse effects (AEs) are clearly a

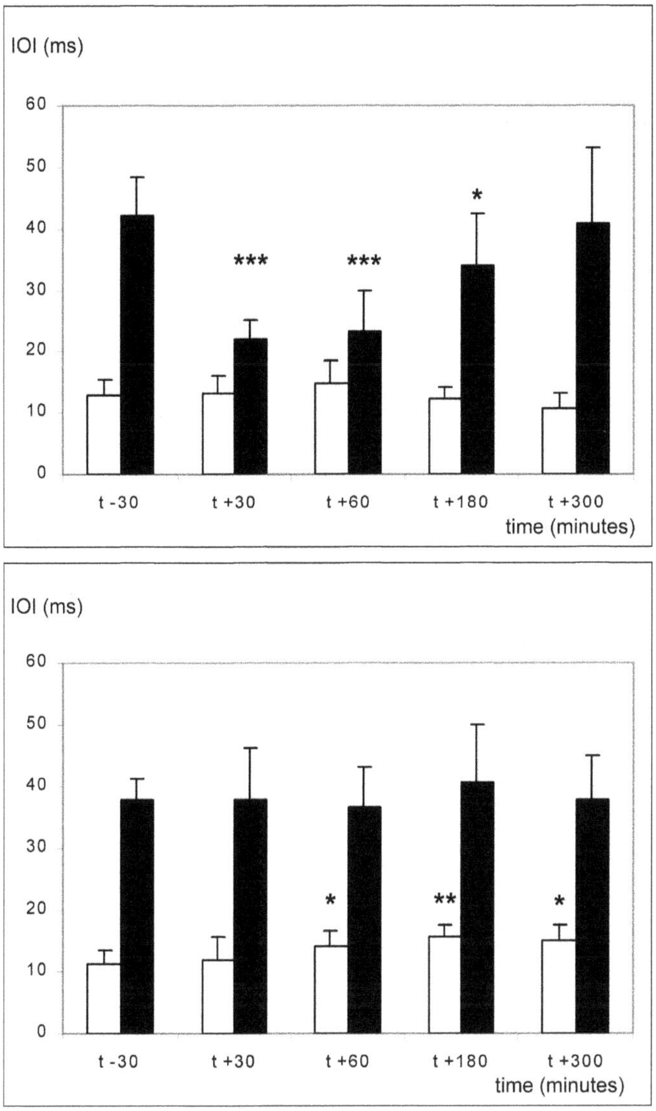

Figure 79.1 IOI values in a pianist with focal hand dystonia after THC (top) and after placebo (bottom). Black bars: IOI of affected hand; open bars: IOI of unaffected hand; t: time since THC/placebo intake (minutes); range of normality: IOI = 13.7 ms.; level of significance after alpha-adjustment (Mann-Whitney U-test): * $p < 0.05$ vs $t - 30$ of respective hand; ** $p < 0.01$ vs $t - 30$ of respective hand; *** $p < 0.001$ vs $t - 30$ of respective hand; IOI: mean standard deviation of inter-onset intervals.

major concern and widely discussed in the medical community. In the systematic review of CB studies conducted by the AAN, 6.9 per cent (95 per cent CI 5.7–8.2 per cent) of participants stopped their medication due to AEs (Koppel et al. 2014). AEs include ataxia, nausea, impaired short-term memory, cognitive impairment, dry mouth, suicidal ideation, hallucinations, dizziness, fatigue, behavioural or mood changes, impaired motor skills, increased weakness, heart rate and increased appetite (Riedel & Davies 2005; Moreira et al. 2009; Koppel et al. 2014). Marijuana use is also associated with an increased risk of trait anxiety disorder, depression and psychosis, although presently it is unclear whether CB use is the cause or the result of mood disorder and pre-psychotic depression (Volkow et al. 2014a).

Clearly, side-effects and therapeutic effects vary depending on the cannabinoid formulation, concentration and/or ratio of cannabinoid formulations. For example, 100 microlitres of Sativex-Spray® contains 2.7 mg delta-9-tetrahydrocannabinol (THC) and 2.5 mg cannabidiol, which seems to be relatively well tolerated when administered in a slowly increasing dosage, as announced in the patient's information documentation (Borgelt et al. 2013). The advantage of the combined use of THC and CBD is a synergistic effect, while AEs are reduced (Russo & Guy 2006). Smoking cannabis has been associated with lung cancer risk, which is not only related to the tobacco agents, but also to carcinogenic substances in the cannabis plant. These may be the more detrimental, as usually the drug is administered through deep inhalation (Martinasek et al. 2016). Therefore future trials should focus on other methods of ingestion. Oral administration is also problematic due to deposition of cannabinoids into fatty tissue, from which they are released slowly, causing variability in plasma concentrations (Lile et al. 2013).

As reflected in the public health discussion on the use of cannabinoids in medical treatment, there is also some risk of abuse with marijuana and cannabis-based drugs (Haberstick et al. 2014). Studies of marijuana outside of the medical context estimate between 9 and 16 per cent of persons using cannabis may become addicted and experience symptoms of withdrawal after quitting the drug (Warner et al. 1995; Richter et al. 2016). The mechanism of abuse in marijuana users is still not well understood. However, according to Kluger et al. (2015), the abuse mechanism may involve blunted dopamine reactivity. This is supported by the observation that marijuana abusers, compared to healthy controls, showed markedly reduced dopamine responses when methylphenidate was administered. Furthermore, in PET scans using [11C] raclopride, a D2 ligand, dopamine concentration in the ventral striatum of marijuana abusers was inversely correlated with addiction severity and craving (Volkow et al. 2014b). It is probable that patients using medical formulations are at lower risk, since usually lower doses are applied. However, at present no systematic data are available in CB users with medical conditions (Trigo et al. 2016). Finally, epidemiological studies suggest that cannabis may be a 'gateway drug', as its use is associated with later use of other illicit substances (Secades-Villa et al. 2014). Therefore, it seems important for future clinical trials to monitor for current and subsequent use of other illicit substances when applying cannabis in medical conditions such as dystonia.

Discussion and Directions for Future Research

As Kluger et al. (2015) point out, there are marked gaps in our knowledge about the effects of cannabinoids on motor pathways. There are also marked discrepancies and conflicting results in preclinical studies, including the precise effects of cannabinoids on neurotransmission and cellular mechanisms of neuroprotection. Future studies should address not only motor and behavioural effects of cannabinoids but, because of their proven effects on the sensory system, also explore their effects on sensorimotor integration, a problem which is increasingly recognised as an aspect of dystonia (Altenmüller and Jabusch 2010). Conflicting preclinical results

Table 79.1 Sativex-Spray® dosing scheme in musicians with dystonia

Day	Morning sprays between waking up and 12 noon	Evening sprays between 4 p.m. and bedtime	Total sprays each day
Day 1	0	1	1
Day 2	0	1	1
Day 3	0	2	2
Day 4	0	2	2
Day 5	1	2	3
Evaluation			
Day 6	1	3	4
Day 7	1	4	5
Day 8	2	4	6
Day 9	2	5	7
Day 10	3	5	8
Following days	Modify dosage timing according to needs, rehearsals, concerts		

may be caused by cannabinoids interacting with a wide range of pharmacological targets. The complex localisation of cannabinoid receptors at different sites in basal ganglia circuits and the broad array of formulations and doses used in preclinical and clinical studies may also help explain contradictory results (Koppel et al. 2014). Therefore, future clinical trials should be adequately powered, employ appropriate methodology and outcome measures for the specific movement disorder being studied, and assess blinding adequacy. According to our own, unpublished observations in musicians suffering from focal hand dystonia, it seems that there are 'responders' and 'non-responders' in a ratio of about one to three. Unfortunately, no prospective randomised clinical trials are underway, and several grant applications in Germany have been declined. In musician's dystonia (MD), it seems reasonable to try a treatment with Sativex-Spray® according to the dosing scheme in Table 79.1 in order to define whether the patient belongs to the 'responder' group. This is most important for embouchure dystonia, since there are few other treatment options, and botulinum toxin injections are not appropriate for this form of MD.

After a titration period of five days, Sativex-Spray® should be applied at the dosage of three sprays per day. This will result in a maximum dosage of 8.1 mg THC per day (1 spray = 100 µl ≙ 2.7 mg THC). This maximum dosage is recommended for two reasons. First, it has been found that doses lower than 10 mg/day are safe and do not influence neuropsychological performance (Müller-Vahl et al. 2003). Second, in the study by Jabusch et al. (2004), a dosage of 5 mg/day was found to have an effect on MD. After reaching this maintenance dosage, behavioural assessments should be done to find out whether treatment is efficient or not. If it is efficient, patients can be considered 'responders'. Subsequently, dosage can be increased to a maximum as indicated in Table 79.1. Final dosage should not exceed eight sprays per day. Musicians may modify the timing of sprays according to professional needs, such as rehearsal times or concerts, taking a spray about 30 minutes prior to performance to benefit from a maximum therapeutic effect.

Acknowledgement

We want to thank Prof. Dr Hans-Christian Jabusch for the courtesy to publish Figure 79.1 (previously unpublished), which illustrates the data published in Jabusch et al. 2004.

References

Altenmüller E, Jabusch H-C (2010) Focal dystonia in musicians: phenomenology, pathophysiology, triggering factors, and treatment. *Med Probl Perform Art* 25:3–9.

Argyelan M, Carbon M, Niethammer M, Ulug AM, Voss HU, Bressman SB, Dhawan V, Eidelberg D (2009) Cerebellothalamocortical connectivity regulates penetrance in dystonia. *J Neurosci* 29:9740–9747.

Berardelli A (1998) The pathophysiology of primary dystonia. *Brain* 121:1195–1212.

Borgelt LM, Franson KL, Nussbaum AM, Wang GS (2013). The pharmacologic and clinical effects of medical cannabis. *Pharmacotherapy* 33:195–209.

Breakefield XO, Blood AJ, Li Y, Hallett M, Hanson PI, Standaert DG (2008) The pathophysiological basis of dystonias. *Nat Rev Neurosci* 9:222–234.

Chatterjee A, Almahrezi A, Ware M, Fitzcharles MA (2002) A dramatic response to inhaled cannabis in a woman with central thalamic pain and dystonia. *J Pain Symptom Manage* 24:4–6.

Compton DR, Aceto MD, Lowe J, Martin BR (1996) In vivo characterization of a specific cannabinoid receptor antagonist (SR141716A): inhibition of delta 9-tetrahydrocannabinol-induced responses and apparent agonist activity. *J Pharmacol Exp Ther* 277:586–594.

Consroe P, Sandyk R, Snider SR (1986). Open label evaluation of cannabidiol in dystonic movement disorders. *Int J Neurosci* 30:277–282.

Fox SH, Kellett M, Moore AP, Crossman AR, Brotchie JM (2002) Randomised, double-blind, placebo-controlled trial to assess the potential of cannabinoid receptor stimulation in the treatment of dystonia. *Mov Disord* 17:145–149.

Gauter B, Rukwied R, Konrad C (2004) Cannabinoid agonists in the treatment of blepharospasm: a case report study. *Neuro Endocrinol Lett* 25:45–48.

Haberstick BC, Young SE, Zeiger JS, Lessem JM, Hewitt JK, Hopfer CJ (2014) Prevalence and correlates of alcohol and cannabis use disorders in the United States: results from the national longitudinal study of adolescent health. *Drug Alcohol Depend* 136:158–161.

Hallett M (2006) Pathophysiology of writer's cramp. *Hum Mov Sci* 25:454–463.

Hallett M (2011) Neurophysiology of dystonia: the role of inhibition. *Neurobiol Dis* 42:177–184.

Herkenham M, Lynn AB, Johnson MR, Melvin LS, de Costa BR, Rice KC (1991) Characterization and localization of cannabinoid receptors in rat brain: a quantitative in vitro autoradiographic study. *J Neurosci* 11:563–583.

Iversen L (2003) Cannabis and the brain. *Brain J Neurol* 126:1252–1270.

Jabusch H-C, Schneider U, Altenmüller E (2004) Delta9-tetrahydrocannabinol improves motor control in a patient with musician's dystonia. *Mov Disord* 19:990–991.

Kluger B, Triolo P, Jones W, Jankovic J (2015) The therapeutic potential of cannabinoids for movement disorders. *Mov Disord* 30:313–327.

Koppel BS, Brust JC, Fife T, Bronstein J, Youssof S, Gronseth G, Gloss D (2014) Systematic review: efficacy and safety of medical marijuana in selected neurologic disorders – report of the Guideline Development Subcommittee of the American Academy of Neurology. *Neurology* 82:1556–1563.

Kreitzer AC, Regehr WG (2001) Retrograde inhibition of presynaptic calcium influx by endogenous cannabinoids at excitatory synapses onto Purkinje cells. *Neuron* 29:717–727.

Lile JA, Kelly TH, Charnigo RJ, Stinchcomb AL, Hays LR (2013) Pharmacokinetic and pharmacodynamic profile of supratherapeutic oral doses of Delta(9)-THC in cannabis users. *J Clin Pharmacol* 53:680–690.

Llano I, Leresche N, Marty A (1991) Calcium entry increases the sensitivity of cerebellar Purkinje cells to applied GABA and decreases inhibitory synaptic currents. *Neuron* 6:565–574.

Martinasek MP, McGrogan JB, Maysonet A (2016) A systematic review of the respiratory effects of inhalational marijuana. *Respir Care* 61:1543–1551.

Matsuda LA, Bonner TI, Lolait SJ (1993) Localization of cannabinoid receptor mRNA in rat brain. *J Comp Neurol* 327:535–550.

Moreira FA, Grieb M, Lutz B (2009) Central side-effects of therapies based on CB1 cannabinoid receptor agonists and antagonists: focus on anxiety and depression. *Best Pract Res Clin Endocrinol Metab* 23:133–144.

Müller-Vahl KR, Prevedel H, Theloe K, Kolbe H, Emrich HM, Schneider U (2003) Treatment of Tourette syndrome with delta-9-tetrahydrocannabinol (delta 9-THC): no influence on neuropsychological performance. *Neuropsychopharmacol* 28:384–388.

Neychev VK, Fan X, Mitev VI, Hess EJ, Jinnah HA (2008) The basal ganglia and cerebellum interact in the expression of dystonic movement. *Brain* 131:2499–2509.

Pitler TA, Alger BE (1992) Postsynaptic spike firing reduces synaptic GABAA responses in hippocampal pyramidal cells. *J Neurosci* 12:4122–4132.

Richter A, Löscher W (1994) (+)-WIN 55,212-2, a novel cannabinoid receptor agonist, exerts antidystonic effects in mutant dystonic hamsters. *Eur J Pharmacol* 264:371–377.

Richter A, Löscher W (2002) Effects of pharmacological manipulations of cannabinoid receptors on severity of dystonia in a genetic model of paroxysmal dyskinesia. *Eur J Pharmacol* 454:145–151.

Richter L, Pugh BS, Ball SA (2016) Assessing the risk of marijuana use disorder among adolescents and adults who use marijuana. *Am J Drug Alcohol Abuse* 13:1–14.

Riedel G, Davies SN (2005) Cannabinoid function in learning, memory and plasticity. *Handb Exp Pharmacol* 168:445–477.

Russo E, Guy GW (2006) A tale of two cannabinoids: the therapeutic rationale for combining tetrahydrocannabinol and cannabidiol. *Med Hypotheses* 66:234–246.

Sañudo-Peña MC, Patrick SL, Khen S, Patrick RL, Tsou K, Walker JM (1998) Cannabinoid effects in basal ganglia in a rat model of Parkinson's disease. *Neurosci Lett* 248:171–174.

Secades-Villa R, Garcia-Rodriguez O, Jin CJ, Wang S, Blanco C (2014) Probability and predictors of the cannabis gateway effect: a national study. *Int J Drug Policy* 26:135–142.

Trigo JM, Lagzdins D, Rehm J, Selby P, Gamaleddin I, Fischer B, Barnes AJ, Huestis MA, Le Foll B (2016) Effects of fixed or self-titrated dosages of Sativex on cannabis withdrawal and cravings. *Drug Alcohol Depend* 161:298–306.

Uribe Roca MC, Micheli F, Viotti R (2005) Cannabis sativa and dystonia secondary to Wilson's disease. *Mov Disord* 20:113–115.

Volkow ND, Baler RD, Compton WM, Weiss SR (2014a) Adverse health effects of marijuana use. *N Engl J Med* 370:2219–2227.

Volkow ND, Wang GJ, Telang F, Fowler JS, Alexoff D, Logan J, Jayne M, Wong C, Tomasi D (2014b) Decreased dopamine brain reactivity in marijuana abusers is associated with negative emotionality and addiction severity. *Proc Natl Acad Sci* 111:3149–3156.

Warner LA, Kessler RC, Hughes M, Anthony JC, Nelson CB (1995) Prevalence and correlates of drug use and dependence in the United States: results from the National Comorbidity Survey. *Arch Gen Psychiatry* 52:219–229.

Zadikoff C, Wadia PM, Miyasaki JM, Chen R, Lang, AE, So J, Fox SH (2011) Cannabinoid, CB1 agonists in cervical dystonia: failure in a phase IIa randomized controlled trial. *Basal Ganglia* 1:91–95.

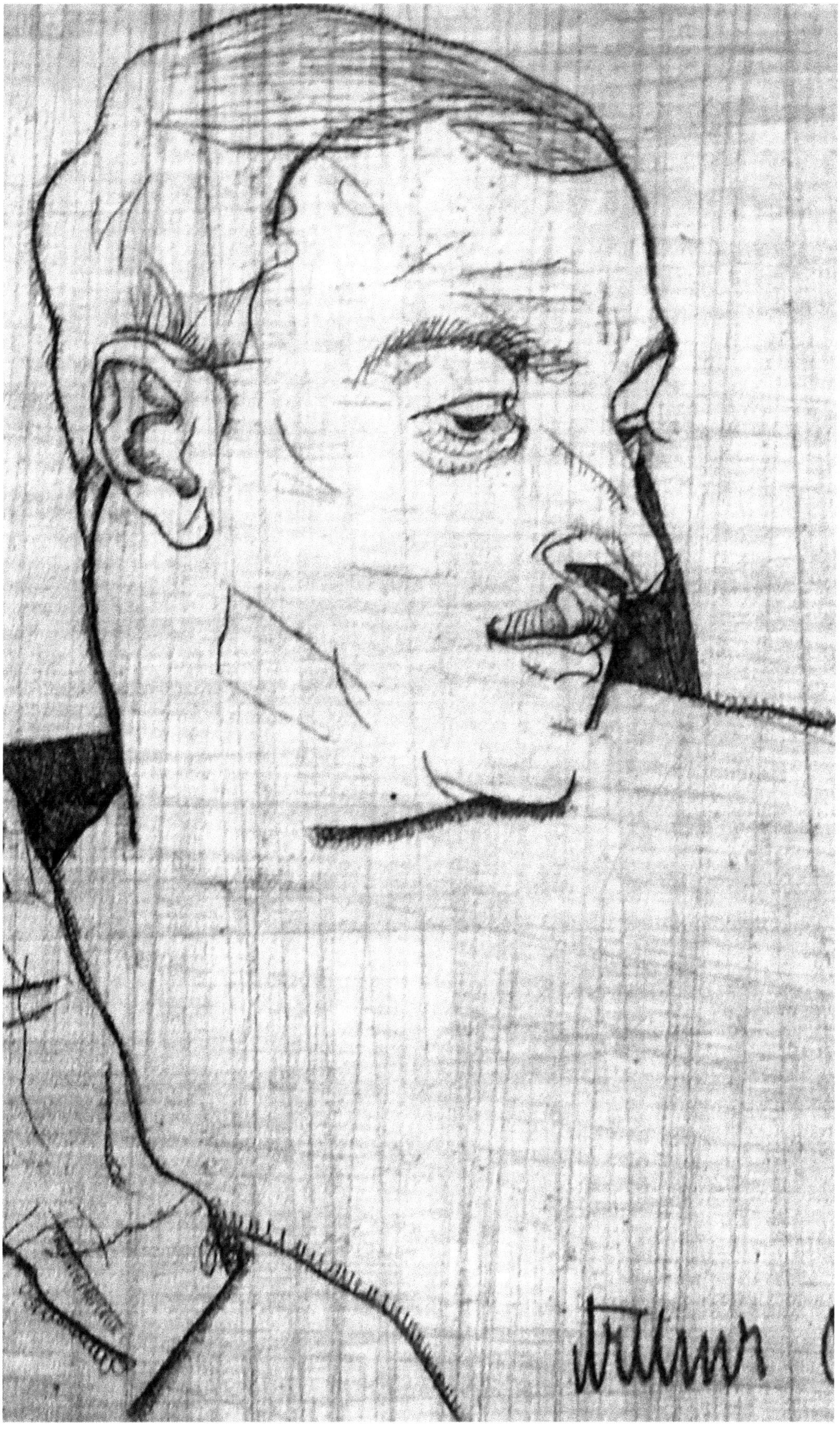

Chapter 80

Future Trends in Dystonia Research

Dirk Dressler, Eckart Altenmüller, Thomas Gasser, Mark Hallett* and Joachim K. Krauss

Introduction

Ever since the current concept of dystonia was introduced by Stanley Fahn and C. David Marsden, the field of dystonia has developed rapidly: botulinum toxin therapy and deep brain stimulation emerged as new treatment options and new insight was generated by neurophysiology and genetics. This chapter explores how this field may develop in the future. For this, experts in the main fields of dystonia research share their views.

Thomas Gasser on the Future of Genetics

In his seminal paper on 'dystonia musculorum deformans' of 1911, Hermann Oppenheim described two siblings of Jewish ancestry presenting during childhood with dystonia in the legs and suggested that dystonia was a hereditary disease (Oppenheim 1911). Eventually, the cause for this disorder, now known as primary torsion dystonia, was identified in 1997: an in-frame deletion of a single GAG-codon in the torsinA (TOR1A) gene (Ozelius et al. 1997). At the same time, this important discovery suggested aetiologic heterogeneity of dystonia, as only a small subset of patients with a specific phenotype, usually with onset during adolescence in a limb and rapidly progressing to generalised dystonia, is caused by this mutation. The subsequent identification of, at latest count, more than 20 dystonia genes in rare Mendelian forms of the disease, mostly by pursuing a classic 'positional cloning' approach in large multi-case families, proved this point (Klein 2014).

While discovery of these genes has opened up a window into the complex molecular underpinnings of dystonias, their understanding is far from complete. The function of only a few of these genes can be placed easily within the context of our current knowledge of the pathophysiology of dystonia. For example, corroborating the prominent role of the dopaminergic system, as several genes are involved in dopamine synthesis, most prominently GTP-cyclohydrolase (GCH1), but also tyrosine hydroxylase (TH) and sepiapterine reductase (SR), have been found to underlie different forms of dopa-responsive dystonia (DRD, DYT5). For many of the other mutated genes, including TOR1A and ε-sarcoglycan (SGCE), the gene for myoclonus-dystonia syndrome (M-D, DYT11), it is still unknown how they cause the specific network dysfunction which clinically presents as dystonia. A better understanding of these mechanisms is certainly one of the major challenges of dystonia research in the coming years and genetic research may in fact continue to play a pivotal role in this process.

Only a small fraction of all cases with dystonia can be explained by mutations in presently known genes. This applies in particular to common forms of focal dystonia with onset in mid to late adulthood, although a genetic contribution to their aetiology has been suggested (Fletcher et al. 1990).

Two recent advances in molecular genetic technology, genotyping arrays as the basis for genome-wide association studies (GWAS) and whole-exome or whole-genome sequencing (WES or WGS) technology are likely to provide an even deeper insight into the genetic underpinnings of dystonia syndromes.

In many complex diseases, including neurodegenerative diseases such as Alzheimer's disease or Parkinson's disease, GWAS have uncovered dozens of common genetic variants (usually so-called single nucleotide variants or SNPs), which increase or decrease the risk of developing the disorder. Although their individual effect is small (odds ratios for SNPs are usually in the order of 1.1–1.5), collectively they explain up to 15–20 per cent of the total population risk for the diseases. In the dystonias, the success of GWAS has so far been limited (Lohmann et al. 2014; Mok et al. 2014). This could be due to the fact that the genetic architecture of the dystonias is different from that of neurodegenerative diseases, but it could also simply mean that current studies have not been sufficiently powered.

While GWAS are designed to detect common (>5 per cent in the population) genetic variants which usually reside in non-coding (presumably regulatory) regions of the genome, WES targets (usually rare) coding variants. The coding sequence of the human genome, the sum of all exons, together about 50 million base pairs (the 'exome'), harbours several million rare to very rare variants from the consensus sequence, more than half of them altering the encoded proteins (Lupski et al. 2011) and many of them suspected to lead to functional changes of the encoded proteins. It is likely that a substantial proportion of the so far 'missing heritability' in sporadic cases of complex disorders can be accounted for by these variants and their almost innumerable combinations. However, the more or less complete mapping of these variants

* MH was supported by the NINDS Intramural Program.

is a daunting task. Their low frequency (<1 per cent of the population) requires the study of large patient cohorts and the fact that their effect strength is only moderate (in other words: their penetrance is reduced, which is why the disease appears to be sporadic) means that they can also be detected, although at even lower frequencies, in asymptomatic individuals. Sophisticated bioinformatic analyses taking into account existing knowledge of functional gene networks will be necessary to make sense of the enormous amounts of data generated by WES.

So far, WES has already successfully facilitated the discovery of several new rare Mendelian dystonia genes (Klein 2014). However, this also highlights a challenge for future research: at least two of the recently reported genes, CIZ1, found in a family with predominantly cervical dystonia (Xiao et al. 2012), and CACNA1B, found to be mutated in a patient with myoclonus-dystonia syndrome (Groen et al. 2015), could not be confirmed by other groups (Dufke et al. 2015; Mencacci et al. 2015). It is likely that over the coming years, dozens, maybe hundreds of genes will be nominated as potential disease or risk genes for dystonia. Their functional validation will be a major challenge for the neurosciences. They will form an increasingly complex network that promises to eventually not only provide a better understanding of the causes of dystonia, hopefully leading to new and better treatments, but may help us to understand the functions of sensorimotor integration of the human brain on a molecular level.

Mark Hallett on the Future of Neurophysiology

In order to understand and treat a disorder like dystonia, it is necessary to deal with issues from basic aetiologies such as genetics and environment to clinical phenomenology. Neurophysiology sits somewhere in the middle, translating the molecular biology to specific signs and symptoms. Moreover, current neurophysiological tools can modify brain function, as well as analyse it, and therefore can be used for therapy. Although drugs like the benzodiazepines were discovered serendipitously, it has been the neurophysiological findings of loss of inhibition that have made clear the probable reasons for their efficacy. The use of brain stimulation methods to increase inhibition has followed the discovery of loss of inhibition.

Clearly, more neurophysiological understanding is needed (Quartarone & Hallett 2013). What is the precise mechanism for loss of inhibition? What is the role of GABA, glycine, acetylcholine and dopamine in the inhibition? Some of this information can be obtained with pharmacological interventions combined with clinical neurophysiology and some combined with neuroimaging; it would be beneficial to be able to work with relevant animal models. There is some progress with animal models for DYT1 (Pappas et al. 2015), but none for the more common adult-onset isolated dystonias.

In all studies, it is crucial to keep in mind that all dystonias are not necessarily the same (Hallett 2015). Childhood-onset generalised isolated dystonia may differ from adult-onset focal isolated dystonia and the adult-onset dystonias may differ from each other. It will be critical going forward to be clear on which abnormality is identified in which disorder; this will not only be helpful by itself, but will likely shed some light on how an abnormality is relevant.

Exactly how does loss of inhibition contribute to the clinical manifestations (Hallett 2011)? While on the face of it, it seems simple – loss of inhibition leads to excess movement – the detail is not so clear. First, the loss of inhibition is seen in asymptomatic body parts of patients with dystonia and might even be abnormal in asymptomatic relatives (Kimmich et al. 2014). Perhaps that means that the loss of inhibition is only an endophenotype that by itself has no phenotypic consequence. Can a specific type of loss of inhibition be identified that will correlate with the dystonia itself? Second, loss of surround inhibition, which has promise to explain overflow movements, is only a somewhat weak phenomenon that also does not correlate well with the amount of dystonia in a body part. Moreover, surround inhibition is present only during the phasic phase of a quickly begun tonic movement, and it is not clear how the lack of overflow movement is maintained during the tonic phase (Beck et al. 2008). It has been pointed out that the timing of surround inhibition correlates with the transient increase in excitability of the spinal cord at the onset of movement – the Jendrassik effect. Hence, surround inhibition seems needed particularly during this period, but still some mechanism would seem valuable for tonic movements.

There must be more understanding also of the problems with brain plasticity. In many physiological measures, plasticity is increased. Yet, motor learning, if anything, is deficient (Quartarone & Hallett 2013). If learning depends on plasticity, how can these two findings be reconciled? Moreover, plasticity has many different features, including, importantly, homeostatic plasticity. The identified loss of homeostatic plasticity could well be a critical feature for long-term maladaptive plasticity in the dystonic brain, but this will require study, likely with a longitudinal investigation.

One area that will be critical in our neurophysiological advancement is functional (psychogenic) dystonia. It is more than a little curious that many of the features of loss of inhibition are also seen in functional dystonia (Espay et al. 2006). Its meaning is not clear for the loss of inhibition or for the pathophysiology of the condition. Could it be that loss of inhibition is a contributing factor to functional dystonia in a similar way as to organic dystonia? Could it be that the loss of inhibition is a product of the dystonia and not the other way round? There are some data suggesting that one differentiating test of inhibition is the blink reflex recovery curve (Schwingenschuh et al. 2011). How is this test different from the others? There are also data indicating that plasticity is normal in functional dystonia. This needs further study. Clarity regarding this problem will likely shed light on both dystonia and the nature of functional disorders.

Separation of organic and functional dystonia also are critical for appropriate therapy. Already, for example, a number of patients with functional dystonia have received deep brain stimulation (Ramos et al. 2015). This is certainly not optimal therapy and is wasteful of resources.

As the basic genetic and cellular biology advances, neurophysiology should be able to see how these observations can be translated. For example, recent work on DYT1, including the development of an apparently highly relevant animal model, points to critical abnormalities of the cholinergic system (Pappas et al. 2015). The role of cholinergic mechanisms has also been studied in animal models (Eskow Jaunarajs et al. 2015), but how this plays out in humans needs further study. We know empirically that anticholinergic agents can be valuable, but the link between the animal models and the pharmacological influence is not yet established. Understanding of this might lead to better ways of using anticholinergic therapy and also possibly aid drug development of improved agents.

Neurophysiological interventions might also be improved going forward. Such interventions are now rather simply based on increasing inhibition local to the brain stimulation. Might we be able to do better with more information? Can we modulate circuits? If we understood sensory tricks better (Ramos et al. 2014), could this lead to innovative therapy? Would it be sensible to combine brain stimulation with certain types of pharmacology or physical therapy rather than to do brain stimulation alone? Also, might superficial brain stimulation be helpful in making decisions about (or even improving) deep brain stimulation?

There is much more to learn about dystonia and neurophysiology can play a critical role, including in advancing therapy.

Dirk Dressler on the Future of Botulinum Toxin Therapy

Botulinum Toxin (BT) therapy started in ophthalmology, but soon expanded into neurology. Neurological indications have been the core indications for BT therapy ever since, especially when adult cerebral palsy, blepharospasm, spasticity, chronic migraine and hyperhidrosis are included. Only aesthetic use as such may have larger volumina in the number of patients treated and the amount of BT used. Within all neurological indications, dystonia is still the largest indication. Only spasticity may have the potential to surpass dystonia. Within dystonia, new patients groups have now become candidates for BT therapy as BT high-dose therapy was recently introduced (Dressler et al. 2014) and allows treatment of patients with more severe and more widespread dystonia. With the availability of low-antigenicity BT drugs, shorter injection intervals can now also be used to improve treatment algorithms, therapy outcome and patient satisfaction (Dressler et al. in press). Use of ultrasound or electromyography may facilitate BT application in critical body parts such as the forearms. New technologies are now trying to combine ultrasound and electromyography. New neurological indications for BT therapy may emerge in pain treatment, but are less likely in movement disorders. Nevertheless, BT manufacturers should be encouraged to formally register more dystonia indications to resolve reimbursement problems associated with off-label use.

BT drugs have not changed since they were introduced some 30 years ago. BT type B was tried but failed to succeed due to antigenicity and adverse effect problems. The introduction of incobotulinumtoxinA, a BT drug with removed complexing proteins and advanced quality of its botulinum neurotoxin component, has reduced antigenicity and with this allowed new treatment algorithms. Several new BT drugs with removed complexing proteins are currently being developed. Attempts are underway to allow transdermal BT application by binding botulinum neurotoxin to carrier substances. For dystonia, transdermal BT application may be interesting in patients with blepharospasm. Modifications of BT's duration of action, either as reduced duration of action or as prolonged duration of action, may be interesting in certain clinical situations. Apparently, these research projects have been initiated by some BT manufacturers. Routes to success, however, remain unclear. Increasing BT's affinity to the target tissue may help to reduce BT volumes applied and thus reduce antigenicity. Projects to provide ready-made liquid preparation of the existing BT drugs are primarily driven by marketing considerations. Providing a fixed dilution would reduce the injector's choice, especially as a wide range of different dilutions is used even for dystonia indications. Raising temperature restrictions for storage and handling of BT drugs, as in incobotulinumtoxinA, may simplify logistics, reduce costs and increase availability.

The number of BT manufacturers is steadily growing, with new products coming out of China, Korea and Russia. Although the quality of their products is not independently evaluated and registrations in major countries are lacking, new manufacturers will eventually aim for worldwide distribution and, thus, increase competition further. Subsequently, drug costs are likely to fall. On the one hand, this may help to increase the availability of BT therapy. However, at the same time, reduced profits will also reduce funding necessary for raising awareness of dystonia and for BT therapy.

A primary goal for the future is to make BT therapy available to all patients needing it. Manufacturers, together with the medical community, should reach out to introduce BT therapy in as many countries as possible.

Joachim K. Krauss on the Future of Surgical Treatment

Surgical treatment, in particular deep brain stimulation (DBS), has attracted remarkable attention over the past two decades and it has become a cornerstone in the contemporary repertoire of therapeutic options for dystonia. Most likely its range will increase in the near future and with a better understanding of the pathophysiology of dystonia we will explore alternative targets, apply advanced technology and investigate new indications. The randomised sham-controlled trials with blinded delayed-onset stimulation have unequivocally proven the efficacy of pallidal DBS both for primary (inherited and idiopathic) generalised and segmental dystonia as well as for cervical dystonia (Kupsch et al. 2006; Volkmann et al. 2014). More studies with similar designs are needed also for other manifestations of dystonia where pilot studies have indicated beneficial outcomes. The challenge is, however, that due to the rarity of some types of dystonia, transnational or even transcontinental efforts may be necessary to reach this goal.

The posteroventral lateral globus pallidus internus (GPi) has become the most frequent and widely accepted 'standard' target for DBS in dystonia, just like the subthalamic nucleus in Parkinson's disease. Certainly, there is also the strongest evidence for the efficacy of pallidal DBS as compared to other possible targets. GPi stimulation provides solid improvement in many manifestations of dystonia with a low frequency of side-effects. The more recently discovered appearance of bradykinesia and gait problems, in particular in adult patients with segmental dystonia who achieve a good response to DBS, has not been fully understood yet, but is has opened new views on the function of the basal ganglia (Blahak et al. 2011; Schrader et al. 2011). Fortunately, these side-effects can generally be managed by a compromise between maximal stimulation benefit and the occurrence of these symptoms. Yet, what will be the long-term sequelae (if any) of these emergences?

Considering that GPi-DBS does not work in all manifestations of dystonia and given the widespread dysfunction in the network circuitry of the basal ganglia, other targets also need to be taken into account. Despite promising results of subthalamic DBS for dystonia, however, there is still relatively little experience with its use thus far (Ostrem et al. 2017). Another interesting target would certainly be the sensorimotor thalamus, especially as it once was the 'standard target' for dystonia in the times of radiofrequency lesioning (Loher et al. 2004; Pauls et al. 2014). One challenge for future research will be to determine which region in the ventrolateral thalamus would be the better target: its anterior portion (i.e. the Voa according to Hassler) or its posterior portion (the Vim), or even the intermediate region (the region formerly termed Vop). Recent concepts on possible cerebellar involvement in the pathophysiology of dystonia suggest that cerebellar neuromodulation might also be of interest in the future. Another option that has been explored only to a limited extent is multi-target stimulation. Obviously, both the application and the evaluation of multi-target stimulation are complex and time-consuming. Algorithms need to be developed to further explore this option.

It is unclear why dystonia patients with a similar genetic background develop different phenotypes of dystonia. It is even more puzzling what determines that patients with cervical dystonia either turn their head to the right or to the left and how the dystonic pattern affects various sets of muscles which may even change over time in the same patient (Münchau et al. 2001). A deeper understanding of the causes of such variability along with a more solid knowledge of the somatotopy in the GPi probably would allow determination of specific 'sweet spots' in the GPi to optimise chronic DBS in individual patients.

We are only beginning to understand how DBS works in dystonia and why the improvement of the tonic elements of dystonia occurs often with a delay of several months (Ruge et al. 2011). While we know now that the complex interplay between modification of maladaptive plasticity, altered inhibition and pathologic oscillatory activity in the basal ganglia circuitry is relevant, there are still several unclear points to be solved. Long-term outcome of chronic DBS is characterised often by progressive improvement with stable stimulation settings. It is intriguing to see that while dystonia recurs within minutes to hours after stimulation has been switched off within the first two years of chronic DBS (Grips et al. 2007), withdrawal of stimulation after DBS of several years might not result in an imminent deterioration of the clinical benefit that has been achieved (Ruge et al. 2014). Considering the possible mechanisms of DBS in dystonia it might well be that DBS can act as a true disease-modifying treatment and with that regard it might be justified to consider offering DBS earlier in the course of disease, and not only when conservative treatment either is not available or is poorly effective. Given the safety profile of pallidal DBS, the time for an 'early stim' study in dystonia has come.

How could new technology for DBS be applied in dystonia? Would there be a place for adaptive stimulation as it has been postulated for Parkinson's disease regarding the impact of DBS on local beta field potential activity? There is indeed preliminary evidence that high-frequency stimulation reduces the mean power in the 4–12 Hz band of local field potential recordings from the GPi thought to be characteristic for dystonia (Barow et al. 2014).

Future outcome measures need to consider not only the improvement of specific dystonia severity scales. In addition to changes in disability and quality of life, also patient-specific characteristics are to be respected. Particularly, in acquired dystonia 'success' or 'failure' of therapy needs to be redefined (Gimeno & Lin 2017).

We also must remember that DBS is not the only surgical alternative in dystonia. DBS is a valuable, but also costly treatment and it is not available to large segments of the population in underdeveloped countries. Measures have to be taken such that the art of performing peripheral selective denervation will not be lost (Krauss 2017). Also, new treatment options are on the horizon such as focused ultrasound ablation (Elias et al. 2016). There is no experience in dystonia yet, but certainly we will see progress here soon as well.

Eckart Altenmüller on the Future of Pharmacotherapy, Rehabilitation and Electrophysiological Treatments

Pharmacotherapy

Besides the relatively well-established drugs, such as trihexyphenidyl, tetrabenazine, dopaminergics and benzodiazepines, a case report demonstrated robust effects of cannabinoids in focal hand dystonia (Jabusch et al. 2004). However, several controlled studies yielded mixed results and were overall disappointing (review in Koppel et al. 2014; Kluger et al. 2015). This may be due to the heterogeneity of dystonias and their underlying pathophysiology and possible genetic differences in cannabinoid receptors within the basal ganglia (see Chapter 79). Future controlled trials should a priori separate responders from non-responders. Another potentially interesting group of drugs, which has to date not been systematically assessed, are selective serotonin-reuptake inhibitors. Clinical experience suggest their usefulness to directly reduce muscle hyperactivity and to indirectly reduce depression and thus improve quality of life.

Rehabilitation

Conventional rehabilitation including stretching, strengthening exercises, manual therapy and splinting are frequently used when patients are referred for physical or occupational therapy. However, their effects are mostly not evaluated in rigorous scientific studies (Byl & McKenzie 2000; Byl et al. 2004; Kimberley et al. 2015). The effectiveness of these therapies is mirrored in pain reduction and improved wellbeing (Altenmüller & Jabusch 2010). However, controlled prospective studies in larger populations are still needed. In limb dystonia, investigators have proposed intensive motor training to recover voluntary motor control. This primarily motor approach has been frequently explored in treating musician's dystonia using the methods known as 'sensorimotor retraining' (see Chapter 51). Others focused on the reorganisation of cortical somatosensory or motor maps by using methods such as Braille training (Byl et al. 2009) or 'learning-based sensorimotor training' (Kimberley et al. 2015). Similar to constraint-movement therapy – a method often used in stroke rehabilitation – some investigators have approached unaffected joints in limb dystonia to decrease compensatory movements (Candia et al. 1999). Despite different theoretical approaches, studies on rehabilitation of limb dystonia suggest positive outcomes (Delnooz et al. 2009; Van Vugt et al. 2014), but are limited by usually small-scale trials, lack of control groups, inappropriate blinding and lack of true randomisation. Additionally, trials have not been sufficiently long, given how long it generally takes to produce dystonia in the first place. Also, there have not been comparative studies, so little is known about which approach is best. Given the nascent stage of rehabilitation research in focal dystonias, full-scale clinical trials have yet to be conducted. Thus, definitive conclusion regarding efficacy and clinical implementation of a particular methodology cannot yet be made.

A major future challenge is to determine appropriate controls and to clearly specify the interventions to improve reproducibility. The hallmark of rehabilitation is that it requires active participation of the patient and that it is tailored to each patient's unique needs. For a control group to be effective, it must mimic the true intervention, but should not contain components of the experimental intervention. Blinding and controls are essential for future studies, as care from a therapist may impart benefits secondary to feeling cared for in addition to a pure placebo effect. Consequently, future investigations in limb dystonia need to carefully address this issue by comparing different treatment strategies with similar frequency, duration and interaction between patient and therapist.

Electrophysiological Treatments

Non-invasive brain stimulation techniques, such as rapid transcranial brain stimulation (rTMS) and transcranial direct-current stimulation (tDCS), have been applied in both basic research and therapeutic trials of hand dystonia (for a review, see Cho & Hallett 2016). Both methods can alter brain excitability in sensorimotor networks, which can be used to reduce abnormal excitation in the sensorimotor cortex. The precise neurophysiological mechanisms underlying this change in excitability are not fully understood. However, high-frequency rTMS and anodal tDCS are able to reduce the resting potential in cortical pyramidal cells, resulting in increased excitability in the upper neuronal layers of the sensorimotor cortex. Low frequency rTMS and cathodal tDCS produce inhibitory effects.

With respect to therapeutic trials, inhibitory low-frequency rTMS has been examined in several controlled trials (Havrankova et al. 2010). Studies typically included less than ten mostly writer's cramp patients and most used a crossover design with stimulation targeting the hemisphere contralateral to the dystonic hand. Siebner et al. (1999) found that motor cortex (M1) stimulation had some beneficial effects in focal hand dystonia. However, Murase et al. (2005) showed that premotor cortex (PMC) was a better target to modulate writer's cramp than M1 and supplementary motor area. Subsequently, more studies used PMC as a target and showed promising results either by physiologic or behavioural measures (Borich et al. 2009). However, the results of these small-scale clinical trials with low-frequency rTMS have been mixed and routine clinical application cannot be recommended. Here, much larger studies carefully variating parameters such as frequency and stimulation site are still needed.

In the last years, tDCS has gained popularity, partly due to its simple application combined with its low cost and low risk for adverse events. Cathodal tDCS of the affected M1 and simultaneous anodal tDCS of the unaffected M1 in dystonic pianists resulted in improvement in the rhythmic accuracy of sequential finger movements of the affected hand, but only if concurrent bimanual mirrored finger movements were performed (Furuya et al. 2014). This improvement was retained for four days after the intervention. These findings suggest therapeutic potential in behavioural training assisted by bihemispheric and polarity-specific tDCS in restoring fine motor control in musician's dystonia. Again, there is a lack of research concerning (1) responder vs non-responder characteristics, (2) effects of long-term stimulation and (3) effects of parametric variations, such as current intensity, stimulation duration and accompanying rehabilitation programme.

References

Altenmüller E, Jabusch HC (2010) Focal dystonia in musicians: phenomenology, pathophysiology, triggering factors, and treatment. *Med Probl Perform Art* 25:3–9.

Barow E, Neumann WJ, Brücke C, Huebl J, Horn A, Brown P, Krauss JK, Schneider GH, Kühn AA (2014) Deep brain stimulation suppresses pallidal low frequency activity in patients with phasic dystonic movements. *Brain* 137:3012–3024.

Beck S, Richardson SP, Shamim EA, Dang N, Schubert M, Hallett M (2008) Short intracortical and surround inhibition are selectively reduced during movement initiation in focal hand dystonia. *J Neurosci* 28:10363–10369.

Blahak C, Capelle HH, Baezner H, Kinfe TM, Hennerici MG, Krauss JK (2011) Micrographia induced by pallidal DBS for segmental dystonia: a subtle sign of hypokinesia? *J Neural Transm* 118:549–553.

Borich M, Arora S, Kimberley TJ (2009) Lasting effects of repeated rTMS application in focal hand dystonia. *Restor Neurol Neurosci* 27:55–65.

Byl NN, McKenzie A (2000) Treatment effectiveness for patients with a history of repetitive hand use and focal hand dystonia: a planned, prospective follow-up study. *J Hand Ther* 13:289–301.

Byl NN, Archer ES, McKenzie A (2009) Focal hand dystonia: effectiveness of a home program of fitness and learning-based sensorimotor and memory training. *J Hand Ther* 22:183–197.

Candia V, Elbert T, Altenmuller E, Rau H, Schafer T, Taub E (1999) Constraint-induced movement therapy for focal hand dystonia in musicians. *Lancet* 353:342.

Cho HJ, Hallett M (2016) Non-invasive brain stimulation for treatment of focal hand dystonia: update and future direction. *J Mov Disord* 2:55–62.

Delnooz CC, Horstink MW, Tijssen MA, van de Warrenburg BP (2009) Paramedical treatment in primary dystonia: a systematic review. *Mov Disord* 24:2187–2198.

Dressler D, Adib Saberi F (2016) Immunological safety of incobotulinumtoxinA (Xeomin®) therapy with reduced interinjection intervals. *J Neural Transm* (Epub).

Dressler D, Adib Saberi F, Kollewe K, Schrader C (2014) Safety aspects of incobotulinumtoxinA high dose therapy. *J Neural Transm* 122:327–333.

Dufke C, Hauser AK, Sturm M, Fluhr S, Wächter T, Leube B, Auburger G, Ott T, Bauer P, Gasser T, Grundmann K (2015) Mutations in CIZ1 are not a major cause for dystonia in Germany. *Mov Disord* 30:740–743.

Elias WJ, Lipsman N, Ondo WG, Ghanouni P, Kim YG, Lee W, Schwartz M, Hynynen K, Lozano AM, Shah BB, Huss D, Dallapiazza RF, Gwinn R, Witt J, Ro S, Eisenberg HM, Fishman PS, Gandhi D, Halpern CH, Chuang R, Butts Pauly K, Tierney TS, Hayes MT, Cosgrove GR, Yamaguchi T, Abe K, Taira T, Chang JW (2016) A randomized trial of focused ultrasound thalamotomy for essential tremor. *N Engl J Med* 25(375):730–739.

Eskow Jaunarajs KL, Bonsi P, Chesselet MF, Standaert DG, Pisani A (2015) Striatal cholinergic dysfunction as a unifying theme in the pathophysiology of dystonia. *Prog Neurobiol* 127–128:91–107.

Espay AJ, Morgante F, Purzner J, Gunraj CA, Lang AE, Chen R (2006) Cortical and spinal abnormalities in psychogenic dystonia. *Ann Neurol* 59:825–834.

Fletcher NA, Harding AE, Marsden CD (1990) A genetic study of idiopathic torsion dystonia in the United Kingdom. *Brain* 113(Pt 2):379–395.

Furuya S, Nitsche MA, Paulus W, Altenmuller E (2014) Surmounting retraining limits in musicians' dystonia by transcranial stimulation. *Ann Neurol* 75:700–707.

Gimeno H, Lin JP (2017) The International Classification of Functioning (ICF) to evaluate deep brain stimulation neuromodulation in childhood dystonia-hyperkinesia informs future clinical & research priorities in a multidisciplinary model of care. *Eur J Paediatr Neurol* 21:147–167.

Grips E, Blahak C, Capelle HH, Bäzner H, Weigel R, Sedlaczek O, Krauss JK, Wöhrle JC (2007) Patterns of reoccurrence of segmental dystonia after discontinuation of deep brain stimulation. *J Neurol Neurosurg Psychiatry* 78:318–320.

Groen JL, Andrade A, Ritz K, Jalalzadeh H, Haagmans M, Bradley TE, Jongejan A, Verbeek DS, Nürnberg P, Denome S, Hennekam RC, Lipscombe D, Baas F, Tijssen MA (2015) CACNA1B mutation is linked to unique myoclonus-dystonia syndrome. *Hum Mol Genet* 24:987–993.

Hallett M (2011) Neurophysiology of dystonia: the role of inhibition. *Neurobiol Dis* 42:177–184.

Hallett M (2015) The dystonias: a heterogeneous collection. *Eur J Neurol* 22:741–742.

Havrankova P, Jech R, Walker ND, Operto G, Tauchmanova J, Vymazal J, Dusek P, Hromcik M, Ruzicka E (2010) Repetitive TMS of the somatosensory cortex improves writer's cramp and enhances cortical activity. *Neuro Endocrinol Lett* 31:73–86.

Jabusch, HC, Schneider U, Altenmüller E (2004) Delta9-tetrahydrocannabinol improves motor control in a patient with musician's dystonia. *Mov Disord* 19:990–991.

Kimberley TJ, Schmidt RL, Chen M, Dykstra DD, Buetefisch CM (2015) Mixed effectiveness of rTMS and retraining in the treatment of focal hand dystonia. *Front Hum Neurosci* 9:385.

Kimmich O, Molloy A, Whelan R, Williams L, Bradley D, Balsters J, Molloy F, Lynch T, Healy DG, Walsh C, O'Riordan S, Reilly RB, Hutchinson M (2014) Temporal discrimination, a cervical dystonia endophenotype: penetrance and functional correlates. *Mov Disord* 29:804–811.

Klein C (2014) Genetics in dystonia. *Parkinsonism Relat Disord* 20 (Suppl. 1):S137–S142.

Kluger B, Triolo P, Jones W, Jankovic J (2015) The therapeutic potential of cannabinoids for movement disorders. *Mov Disord* 30:313–327.

Koppel BS, Brust JC, Fife T, Bronstein J, Youssof S, Gronseth G, Gloss D (2014) Systematic review: efficacy and safety of medical marijuana in selected neurologic disorders. *Neurology* 82:1556–1563.

Krauss JK (2017) Selective peripheral denervation for cervical dystonia. In: *Youmans and Winn Neurological Surgery*, 7th edition. Winn HR (ed.). Elsevier, Amsterdam: 672–677.

Kupsch A, Benecke R, Müller J, Trottenberg T, Schneider GH, Poewe W, Eisner W, Wolters A, Müller JU, Deuschl G, Pinsker MO, Skogseid IM, Roeste GK, Vollmer-Haase J, Brentrup A, Krause M, Tronnier V, Schnitzler A, Voges J, Nikkhah G, Vesper J, Naumann M, Volkmann J, Deep-Brain Stimulation for Dystonia Study Group (2006) Pallidal deep-brain stimulation in primary generalized or segmental dystonia. *N Engl J Med* 355:1978–1990.

Loher TJ, Pohle T, Krauss JK (2004) Functional stereotactic neurosurgery for treatment of cervical dystonia: review of the experience from the lesional era. *Stereo Funct Neurosurgery* 82:1–13.

Lohmann K, Schmidt A, Schillert A, Winkler S, Albanese A, Baas F, Bentivoglio AR, Borngräber F, Brüggemann N, Defazio G, Del Sorbo F, Deuschl G, Edwards MJ, Gasser T, Gómez-Garre P, Graf J, Groen JL, Grünewald A, Hagenah J, Hemmelmann C, Jabusch HC, Kaji R, Kasten M, Kawakami H, Kostic VS, Liguori M, Mir P, Münchau A, Ricchiuti F, Schreiber S, Siegesmund K, Svetel M, Tijssen MA, Valente EM, Westenberger A, Zeuner KE, Zittel S, Altenmüller E, Ziegler A, Klein C (2014) Genome-wide association study in musician's dystonia: a risk variant at the arylsulfatase G locus? *Mov Disord* 29:921–927.

Lupski JR, Belmont JW, Boerwinkle E, Gibbs RA (2011) Clan genomics and the complex architecture of human disease. *Cell* 147:32–43.

Mencacci NE, R'bibo L, Bandres-Ciga S, Carecchio M, Zorzi G, Nardocci N, Garavaglia B, Batla A, Bhatia KP, Pittman AM, Hardy J, Weissbach A, Klein C, Gasser T, Lohmann E, Wood NW (2015) The CACNA1B R1389H variant is not associated with myoclonus-dystonia in a large European multicentric cohort. *Hum Mol Genet* 24:5326–5329.

Mok KY, Schneider SA, Trabzuni D, Stamelou M, Edwards M, Kasperaviciute D, Pickering-Brown S, Silverdale M, Hardy J, Bhatia KP (2014) Genomewide association study in cervical dystonia demonstrates possible association with sodium leak channel. *Mov Disord* 29:245–251.

Münchau A, Bahlke G, Allen PJ, Quinn NP, Lees AJ, Rothwell JC, Palmer JD, Bhatia KP (2001) Polymyography combined with time-locked video recording (video EMG) for presurgical assessment of patients with cervical dystonia. *Eur Neurol* 45:222–228.

Murase N, Rothwell JC, Kaji R, Urushihara R, Nakamura K, Murayama N, Igasaki T, Sakata-Igasaki M, Mima T, Ikeda A, Shibasaki H (2005) Subthreshold low-frequency repetitive transcranial magnetic stimulation over the premotor cortex modulates writer's cramp. *Brain* 128:104–115.

Oppenheim H (1911) Über eine eigenartige Krampfkrankheit des kindlichen und jugendlichen Alters (Dysbasia lordotica progressiva, Dystonia musculorum deformans). *Neurol Centralblatt* 30:1090–1107.

Ostrem JL, San Luciano M, Dodenhoff KA, Ziman N, Markun LC, Racine CA, de Hemptinne C, Volz MM, Heath SL, Starr PA (2017) Subthalamic nucleus deep brain stimulation in isolated dystonia: a 3-year follow-up study. *Neurology* 88:25–35.

Ozelius LJ, Hewett JW, Page CE, Bressman SB, Kramer PL, Shalish C, de Leon D, Brin MF, Raymond D, Corey DP, Fahn S, Risch NJ, Buckler AJ, Gusella JF, Breakefield XO (1997) The early-onset torsion dystonia gene (Dyt1) encodes an ATP- binding protein. *NatGenet* 17:40–48.

Pappas SS, Darr K, Holley SM, Cepeda C, Mabrouk OS, Wong JM, LeWitt TM, Paudel R, Houlden H, Kennedy RT, Levine MS, Dauer WT (2015) Forebrain deletion of the dystonia protein torsinA causes dystonic-like movements and loss of striatal cholinergic neurons. *eLife* 2015;4.

Pauls KA, Hammesfahr S, Moro E, Moore AP, Binder E, El Majdoub F, Fink GR, Sturm V, Krauss JK, Maarouf M, Timmermann L (2014) Deep brain stimulation in the ventrolateral thalamus/subthalamic area in dystonia with head tremor. *Mov Disord* 29:953–959.

Quartarone A, Hallett M (2013) Emerging concepts in the physiological basis of dystonia. *Mov Disord* 15(28):958–967.

Ramos VF, Karp BI, Hallett M (2014) Tricks in dystonia: ordering the complexity. *J Neurol Neurosurg Psychiatry* 85:987–993.

Ramos VF, Pillai AS, Lungu C, Ostrem J, Starr P, Hallett M (2015) Intraoperative neurophysiology in deep brain surgery for psychogenic dystonia. *Ann Clin Transl Neurol* 2:707–710.

Ruge D, Cif L, Limousin P, Gonzalez V, Vasques X, Hariz MI, Coubes P, Rothwell JC (2011) Shaping reversibility? Long-term deep brain stimulation in dystonia: the relationship between effects on electrophysiology and clinical symptoms. *Brain* 134:2106–2115.

Ruge D, Cif L, Limousin P, Gonzalez V, Vasques X, Coubes P, Rothwell JC (2014) Longterm deep brain stimulation withdrawal: clinical stability despite electrophysiological instability. *J Neurol Sci* 342:197–199.

Schrader C, Capelle HH, Kinfe TM, Blahak C, Bäzner H, Lütjens G, Dressler D, Krauss JK (2011) GPi-DBS may induce a hypokinetic gait disorder with freezing of gait in patients with dystonia. *Neurology* 77:483–488.

Schwingenschuh P, Katschnig P, Edwards MJ, Teo JT, Korlipara LV, Rothwell JC, Bhatia KP (2011) The blink reflex recovery cycle differs between essential and presumed psychogenic blepharospasm. *Neurology* 76:610–614.

Siebner HR, Tormos JM, Ceballos-Baumann AO, Auer C, Catala MD, Conrad B, Pascual-Leone A (1999) Low-frequency repetitive transcranial magnetic stimulation of the motor cortex in writer's cramp. *Neurology* 52:529–537.

van Vugt FT, Boullet L, Jabusch HC, Altenmüller E (2014) Musician's dystonia in pianists: long-term evaluation of retraining and other therapies. *Parkinsonism Relat Disord* 20:8–12.

Volkmann J, Mueller J, Deuschl G, Falk D, Kuehn A, Kupsch A, Kivi A, Schneider G, Schnitzler A, Südmeyer M, Voges J, Wittstock M, Wolters A, Müller JU, Poewe W, Eisner W, Hering S, Vesper J, Prokop T, Pinsker M, Krauss JK, Schrader C, Kloss M, Kiening K, Boetzel K, Mehrkens J, Skogseid IM, Ramm-Pettersen J, Timmermann L, Kemmler G, Bhatia KP, Vitek J, Benecke R (2014) Pallidal neurostimulation in patients with medication-refractory cervical dystonia: a sham-controlled randomized trial. *Lancet Neurol* 13:875–884.

Xiao J, Uitti RJ, Zhao Y, Vemula SR, Perlmutter JS, Wszolek ZK, Maraganore DM, Auburger G, Leube B, Lehnhoff K, LeDoux MS (2012) Mutations in CIZ1 cause adult onset primary cervical dystonia. *Ann Neurol* 71:458–469.

Appendix I: Dystonia Medical Research Foundation: 40 Years of Patient Advocacy and Stimulating Research

Janet Hieshetter and Jessica Feeley

Introduction

Samuel and Frances Belzberg founded the Dystonia Medical Research Foundation (DMRF) in 1976 in partnership with John H. Menkes, the first scientific director. At the time, most of the medical community mistakenly categorised dystonia as a marginal psychogenic phenomenon. A small group of pioneering neurologists was publishing early descriptions of generalised dystonia; patient resources were virtually non-existent.

The initial goals were straightforward: motivate investigators to study dystonia, and provide information and support for patients. Recognising the necessity of a global effort, the DMRF adopted a borderless strategy for stimulating dystonia research through relationships and collaboration. The Belzbergs believed in the importance of a strong relationship between the lay Board of Directors and the Medical & Scientific Advisory Council – a value that influences the DMRF to this day.

Patient advocacy groups such as the DMRF serve several important functions: supporting research, promoting public awareness of rare disorders, and supporting and educating populations impacted by chronic disease and disability. Patient groups help mitigate the intense feelings of isolation so commonly reported by those diagnosed with serious illnesses.

Stimulating Research

Early on, the DMRF realised there was a need for consensus in the medical community on the fundamental characteristics of dystonia. In 1984, the DMRF assembled a committee of movement disorder specialists to draft a clinical definition and classification that became the accepted dystonia description for decades. Several revised classification systems have since been proposed. The DMRF supported an international consensus update to the clinical definition and classification initiated by Alberto Albanese and published in 2013.

Founding members of the DMRF created the International Dystonia Symposia, the definitive series of international dystonia meetings. The fifth and latest International Dystonia Symposium was a joint effort among the DMRF, Dystonia Europe and the Dystonia Coalition.

Scientific workshops convening experts from around the world have addressed advanced translational topics: genetics, RNA interference, proteins, pathways, drug development, surgical advancements, imaging, rating scales, designing clinical trials. Additional meetings have focused on animal models, nuclear envelope, myoclonus-dystonia, musician's dystonia and integrative collaborations. Meetings inevitably inspire new projects and collaborations. In recent years each workshop preceded a request for proposals.

DMRF research funding helps fill opportunity gaps left by government agencies and industry companies; the goal is often to provide seed funding that leads to more robust government grants. The DMRF has offered various research funding mechanisms: grants, contracts, fellowships and young investigator awards. Over 500 projects have been funded. The identification of the DYT1 dystonia gene by DMRF-funded investigators in 1997 preceded a groundswell of progress that continues to this day in uncovering novel dystonia genes and proteins. Decades of investment in basic research have yielded opportunities for clinical applications, including sophisticated genetic studies and drug development. International private–public partnerships have identified novel drug targets and compounds poised for clinical trials.

The Dystonia Study Group is an international group of physicians who are experienced in the care of dystonia patients and dedicated to clinical research. The DSG partnered with the DMRF to establish a network of physicians and patients that can be mobilised for clinical trials.

Investing in young investigators and creating opportunities for physicians to establish careers in movement disorders are stated DMRF priorities. A number of funding awards have focused on young investigators and career development. A clinical fellowship training programme supports training of physicians in preparation for a career in movement disorders with special expertise in dystonia.

Patient-Centred Collaborations

The DMRF works collaboratively with other dystonia patient organisations. Relationships with Dystonia Europe and national societies have led to patient- and research-focused initiatives. The DMRF provides administrative support for the Dystonia Advocacy Network (DAN), a collective of five American organisations that addresses legislative and policy needs – this includes advocating for federal funding sources for dystonia investigators including the US National Institutes of Health. DAN advocates have kept dystonia on the list of conditions eligible for study through the US Department of Defense Congressionally-Directed Medical Research Program every year since 2010, resulting in millions of dollars of new dystonia research funding. The DAN has addressed a number of domestic issues including protecting and increasing overall federal research spending, physician reimbursement for services, follow-on biologics, and protecting patient access to all treatments approved by the US Food and Drug Administration, including botulinum toxins and deep brain stimulation.

Multiple community-based research efforts depend on the DMRF for administrative support. These include the Dystonia Study Group, Dystonia Brain Collective, Global Dystonia Registry and Dystonia Coalition.

Public Awareness and Patient Resources

Despite being among the most common movement disorders, overall public awareness of dystonia is limited. Misdiagnosis, even among neurologists, remains common. Results from an international survey of cervical dystonia patients suggest that individuals need to be better informed about the disorder, treatments and expected outcomes from treatment. And yet the path of a newly diagnosed patient to become informed about dystonia is littered with obstacles. Incorrect information is pervasive online, in media stories, and even from sources that claim to be authorities on dystonia.

The DMRF's educational resources help time-pressed physicians inform patients about the disorder and prescribed treatments. The DMRF offers newsletters, medically reviewed brochures, educational meetings and a website.

The annual *Dystonia Moves Me* campaign mobilises the international dystonia community to promote greater awareness on grassroots and national levels. The DMRF has supported award-winning documentary films such as *Twisted* (2006) and *Changing Keys: Billy McLaughlin and the Mysteries of Dystonia* (2011).

Attendance at dystonia support group meetings is high. Web-based technology allows patients across the globe to communicate. The DMRF helps patients and families on a case-by-case basis connect with one another for coping support.

Future Directions

Scientific progress in dystonia is limited only by the imaginations of the world's investigators and funding available to invest. The DMRF will continue to stimulate research progress by directly addressing the most pressing areas in dystonia and expanding the global network of collaborators. New and emerging web-based technologies provide unique opportunities to reach patients and foster a sense of community among individuals and families regardless of geography. The leadership of the DMRF believes the most important service it can provide its constituents is to work tirelessly towards more effective treatments and a cure, while working equally hard to improve daily life for patients who need relief now.

Sources

Albanese A, Bhatia K, Bressman SB, DeLong MR, Fahn S, Fung VSC, Hallett M, Jankovic J, Jinnah HA, Klein C, Lang AE, Mink JW, Teller JK. Phenomenology and classification of dystonia: a consensus update. *Mov Disord* 2013;28:863–873.

Comella C, Bhatia K. An international survey of patients with cervical dystonia. *J Neurol* 2015;262(4):837–848.

Fahn S, Marsden, CD, Calne DB. Classification and investigation of dystonia. In: Marsden CD, Fahn S, editors. *Movement Disorders 2*. London. Butterworth; 1987.

Ozelius LJ, Hewett JW, Page CE, Bressman SB, Kramer PL, Shalish C, de Leon D, Brin MF, Raymond D, Corey DP, Fahn S, Risch NJ, Buckler AJ, Gusella JF, Breakefield XO. The early-onset torsion dystonia gene (DYT1) encodes an ATP-binding protein. *Nat Genet* 1997;17:40–48.

Appendix II: Dystonia Europe: Developing Partnerships in the Dystonia Community

Alistair Newton

Dystonia Europe (DE) is the international platform at the European level, whose goal is 'Connecting people for dystonia'. Our aim is to create links and facilitate collaborations among the stakeholders in dystonia across Europe and beyond, helping to develop worthwhile and successful connections between scientists and society in the dystonia community (www.dystonia-europe.org).

As the understanding of dystonia and the options for effective treatment have expanded over the past 20 years, DE's strategy to achieve its aim has adjusted to meet the changes in the dystonia landscape.

The Early Years: Exploring Political Lobbying in Brussels; Developing Partnerships With Dystonia Specialists; Epidemiological Study of Dystonia in Europe

DE was founded in 1993 as the 'European Dystonia Federation' – an alliance of national dystonia patient organisations trying to find ways of influencing the timescale of diagnosis and the effectiveness of treatment of dystonia. Although 'health' is supposedly an issue for national governments within the European Union (EU), it was becoming obvious even in 1993 that decisions in the three EU institutions (Council of Ministers, Parliament and Commission) were becoming increasingly important in the 'public health agenda'.

In those early years, too, DE's instigation and funding of the 'Epidemiological Study of Dystonia in Europe' (2000) – led by Prof. David Marsden and Prof. Tom Warner – fostered links with dystonia researchers and clinicians across Europe.

This period of development in pan-European patient advocacy helped to encourage medical professionals to discover that working in partnership with this new generation of patient-led organisations could be beneficial.

- Patient meetings offer the opportunity to inform patients more fully about the illness generally, away from the time restrictions of the clinic.
- Possible access to more support for small-scale research projects, including easier recruitment of patient subjects.
- When health service or insurance reimbursement of treatment costs becomes difficult, well-organised groups representing large numbers of patients can help to inform the decisions of the paying authorities more effectively than scientists alone. Increasingly, appeals like this and project applications to government and other medical research funding bodies are expected to involve patient organisations as well as scientists and clinicians.

Working With Medical Specialists and Organisations: MDS, EFNS (EAN) and BMJ; Creating Broader Alliances for Neurology and 'the Brain': Where Dystonia Europe has Been Active

- **DE information booths** – at annual congresses of the Movement Disorder Society (MDS) and European Federation of Neurological Societies (EFNS, now EAN – European Academy of Neurology).
- **DE representation** on the EFNS Education and European Liaison Committees.
- **DE representation** on the British Medical Journal (BMJ) Ethics Committee.
- The **European Federation of Neurological Associations** (EFNA – www.efna.net) was founded in 1997. An 'umbrella' organisation for pan-European federations in the individual neurological illnesses, with the intention of influencing EU policy in neurology.
- Simply, politicians prefer to deal with one organisation which represents many illnesses, rather than deal individually with all of them. DE has been very actively represented in the work of EFNA.
- **European Brain Council** – in 2003, the principal pan-European clinical and research organisations in neurology and psychiatry came together with EFNA and the Psychiatric Patient Alliance, to form the European Brain Council (EBC – www.europeanbraincouncil.org). The aim is to inform EU institutions more effectively on issues on brain research. DE has been centrally involved on the EBC Board.

Focus Directly on Dystonia: Encouraging the Interest of Younger Clinicians and Researchers; Contributing to Greater Understanding of the Illness; Organising International Scientific Meetings Solely on Dystonia; Actively Supporting Research Networking

DE has encouraged more direct interest in dystonia by activity in areas such as:

- **The David Marsden Award**

  DE established the **David Marsden Award** as a €10 000 biennial prize for the best dystonia research paper submitted by a young scientist. The award and the winning paper have been presented on several occasions at the movement disorders session during EFNS congresses.
- **Hannover congresses 2010 and 2013 – 'Treatment of Dystonia'**

  DE has hosted an information booth at both congresses, and presented an award for the best poster on a dystonia rehabilitation topic.
- **Publications on dystonia guidelines**

  DE representative – joint author of 'A systematic review on the diagnosis and treatment of primary (idiopathic) dystonia and dystonia plus syndromes: report of an EFNS/MDS-ES Task Force' (Albanese et al. 2006) and 'EFNS guidelines on diagnosis and treatment of primary dystonias' (Albanese et al. 2011).
- **Organising scientific congresses solely on dystonia.**

  Hamburg – Dystonia Europe 2008: 192 participants from 25 countries; organised and funded by DE.

  Barcelona 2011 – 5th International Dystonia Symposium: 560 participants from 39 countries; organised and funded by DE, in partnership with Dystonia Medical Research Foundation and the Dystonia Coalition.

Since the Barcelona symposium, DE has held smaller-scale two-day international meetings each year for scientists and patients in various European capital cities.

- **European Dystonia Research Network**

  In 2011, Dystonia Europe took part in a joint action with many dystonia specialists and researchers, to form a research network in Europe – with funding from COST (www.cost.eu). DE was also appointed by the scientists to take the legal and financial responsibilities as Grantholder of the Network. Alongside a number of research collaborations, and the development of a dystonia registry and biobank over four years, more than 150 young dystonia specialists have benefited from grants to attend one of the three training

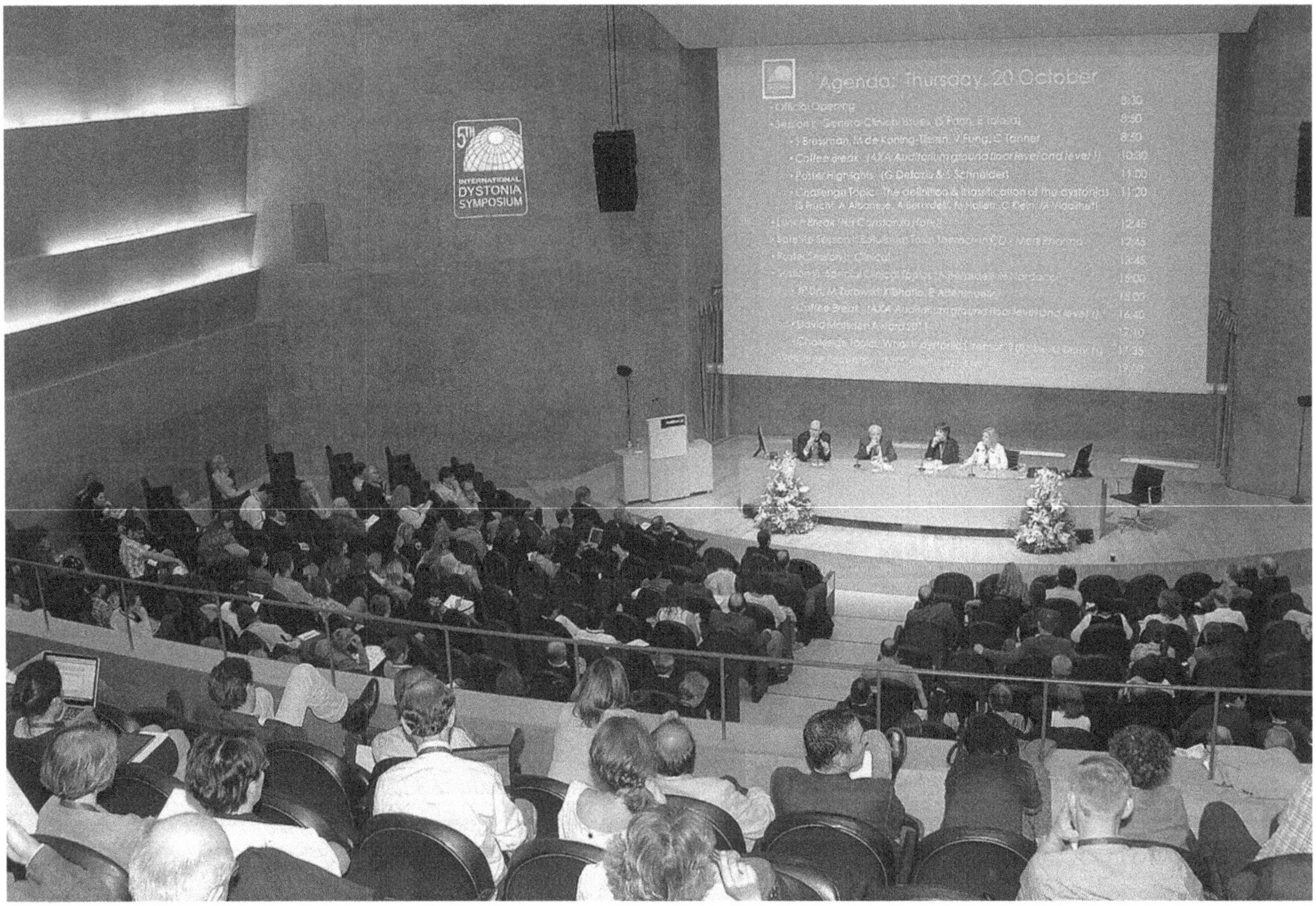

Figure II.1 Barcelona 2011 – question time with international experts.

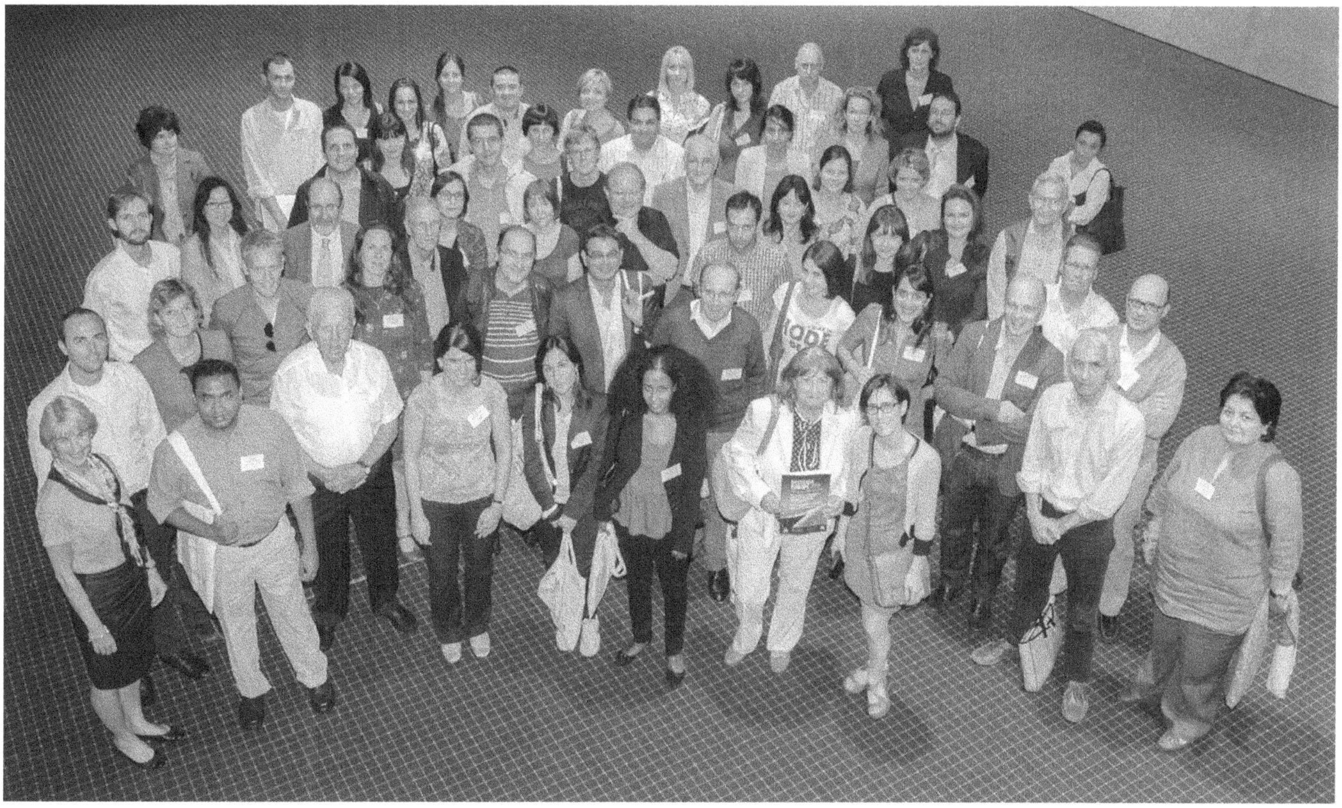

Figure II. 2 European Dystonia Research Network – Bol, Croatia 2012. Trainers and trainees.

schools and more than 30 received support for short-term research periods in laboratories in other countries (Epidemiological Study of Dystonia in Europe (ESDE) Collaborative Group 2000).

- ***Other projects linked to clinicians and researchers***

Dystonia Stories – for DE's 20th anniversary in 2013, 20 short video interviews were produced, featuring the views and reflections of patients as well as eminent dystonia specialists. These showed clearly how scientific interest in the illness, and joint activities involving scientists and Dystonia Europe had developed strongly (https://dystonia-europe.org/media/dystonia-stories). **MyDystonia** – an app has been developed to allow patients to record many features of their dystonia symptoms on a daily basis, providing them and their clinicians with better data to use in assessing treatment outcomes. Many dystonia specialists have already expressed considerable interest in this initiative (www.mydystonia.com).

The Dystonia Community in Europe: A Continuum, Changing Over time

Dystonia Europe's objective is to contribute to the efforts of the greater dystonia 'community' to improve the lives of the people – present and future – who live with dystonia. That community itself has been greatly developed over the past 20 years by our efforts and activities to bring people together for dystonia, and by the efforts of so many other individuals and organisations, especially among the clinicians and researchers. Real partnerships have been created and sustained and will go on changing in the years ahead. New projects, and advances in scientific knowledge and approach, will bring new directions for these partnerships and, we hope, even more beneficial results for dystonia patients.

References

Albanese A, Barnes MP, Bhatia KP, Fernandez-Alvarez E, Filippini G, Gasser T, Krauss JK, Newton A, Rektor I, Savoiardo M, Valls-Solè J. A systematic review on the diagnosis and treatment of primary (idiopathic) dystonia and dystonia plus syndromes: report of an EFNS/MDS-ES Task Force. *Eur J Neurol* 2006;13(5):433–444.

Albanese A, Asmus F, Bhatia KP, Elia AE, Elibol B, Filippini G, Gasser T, Krauss JK, Nardocci N, Newton A, Valls-Solé J. EFNS guidelines on diagnosis and treatment of primary dystonias. *Eur J Neurol* 2011;18(1):5–18. doi: 10.1111/j.1468-1331.2010.03042.x.

Epidemiological Study of Dystonia in Europe (ESDE) Collaborative Group. Epidemiological Study of Dystonia in Europe. *J Neurol* 2000;247(10):787–792.

Appendix III: The Dystonia Coalition

Ami R. Rosen and Hyder A. Jinnah*

Introduction

Dystonia research historically has faced two big challenges. The first is that dystonia is uncommon, making it difficult for any single centre to collect enough patients for meaningful studies rapidly. The second is that different forms of dystonia often are seen by different subspecialists. The Dystonia Coalition (DC) was created to address some of these challenges. It currently focuses on isolated dystonias (previously called primary dystonias), including cervical dystonia, blepharospasm and other craniofacial dystonias, laryngeal dystonia, musician's dystonias, limb dystonias such as writer's cramp, and others. It also addresses various combinations of segmental dystonia, multifocal dystonia, hemidystonia and generalised dystonia.

The DC is a collaboration of medical researchers and patient advocacy groups (PAGs) supported by the Office of Rare Diseases Research (ORDR) in the National Center for Advancing Translational Sciences (NCATS) and the National Institute for Neurological Diseases and Stroke (NINDS) at the National Institutes of Health (NIH) in the United States (www.rarediseasesnetwork.org/dystonia/). Over 43 academic medical centres and private practices are participating (Table III.1). These centres are located in the USA, Canada, Europe and Australia. The DC has an open-door policy that allows new centres to join the effort at any time.

Integral to the DC's mission is the participation and support of many associated PAGs that are based in the USA, Canada and Europe. There are currently 14 PAGs affiliated with the DC (Table III.2). Each PAG participates in a manner that suits its particular mission. Many attend the yearly DC meeting, some help to support the pilot projects and training programmes, and one, very importantly, helps in the overall administration of the DC.

The rationale for the DC is that strength and synergy in rare diseases research comes from a broadly collaborative and inclusive approach, rather than one that relies on competition. Inclusion of many sites provides access to larger numbers of patients with varying types of dystonia than normally achievable at a single centre. Investigators benefit from having access to larger numbers of patients, and patients benefit by having investigators more openly share findings and progress.

Organisational Plan and Projects

The DC consists of many separate programmes and projects. The administrative unit (PI: H. A. Jinnah, Emory University, Atlanta GA) is in charge of the overall direction of research, communications with other investigators, facilitating projects that are selected and financial management.

The DC has four main clinical projects, each organised at a different site. Project 1 (PI: Joel Perlmutter, Washington University in St. Louis, MO) is a Natural History and Biorepository study that involves the collection of clinical data and DNA from subjects with any of the isolated dystonias. As of September 2015 this project had accrued 2261 subjects. Project 2 (PI: Cynthia Comella, Rush University, Chicago, IL) is a study designed to develop comprehensive evaluation tools for cervical dystonia. This project has completed subject enrolment of 209 subjects with one manuscript published (Comella et al. 2014) and others in preparation. Project 3 (PI: Christy Ludlow,

* This work was supported in part by a grant to the Dystonia Coalition (U54 NS065701/TR001456), a consortium of the Rare Diseases Clinical Research Network (RDCRN) that is supported by the Office of Rare Diseases Research (ORDR) at the National Center for Advancing Clinical and Translational Studies (NCATS) in collaboration with the National Institute for Neurological Diseases and Stroke (NINDS). Dr Jinnah serves on the Scientific Advisory Boards for the Dystonia Medical Research foundation, Tyler's Hope for a Cure, the Lesch–Nyhan Syndrome Children's Research Foundation and Lesch–Nyhan Action France. Dr Jinnah serves as PI of the Dystonia Coalition, which receives the majority of its support through NIH grant NS065701 from the Office of Rare Diseases Research, NCATS and National Institute of Neurological Disorders and Stroke. The Dystonia Coalition receives additional material or administrative support from industry sponsors (Allergan Inc. and Merz Pharmaceuticals) as well as private foundations (The Benign Essential Blepharospasm Foundation, Cure Dystonia Now, Dystonia Inc., Dystonia Ireland, the Dystonia Medical Research Foundation, the European Dystonia Federation, the Foundation for Dystonia Research, the National Spasmodic Dysphonia Association, the National Spasmodic Torticollis Association, Tyler's Hope for a Dystonia Cure). Ami Rosen reports nothing to disclose.

Table III.1 Participating centres

	Site Name	Site principal investigator
1	Baylor College of Medicine	Joseph Jankovic
2	Beth Israel Deaconess Medical Center	Ludy Shih
3	Beth Israel Medical Center	Lawrence Severt
4	Booth Gardner PD Care Center	Pinky Agarwal
5	Emory University	H. A. Jinnah
6	Hadassah Medical Center	David Arkadir
7	James Madison University	Christy Ludlow
8	Johns Hopkins University	Zoltan Mari
9	Lahey Clinic	Julie Leegwater-Kim
10	Mayo Clinic, Arizona	Charles Adler
11	Medical College of Wisconsin	Joel Blumin
12	Mount Sinai School of Medicine	Steven Frucht
13	NINDS Intramural Program	Mark Hallett
14	PD and Movement Center of Maryland	Stephen Grill
15	PD and Movement Disorders Institute	Daniel Truong
16	Rush University	Cynthia Comella
17	Hôpital de la Salpêtrière	Emmanuel Flamand-Roze/Marie Vidailhet
18	Sanford Health	Tanya Harlow
19	U College London	Kailash Bhatia
20	U of Alabama, Birmingham	Natividad Stover
21	U of Alberta	Oksana Suchowersky
22	U of Bari	Giovanni DeFazio
23	U of California, San Diego	Fatta Nahab/David Peterson
24	U of Chicago	Tao Xie
25	U of Cincinnatti	Alberto Espay
26	U of Colorado, Denver	Brian Berman
27	U of Florida	Irene Malaty
28	U of Iowa	Ergun Uc
29	U of Luebeck	Christine Klein
30	U of Maryland	Stephen Reich
31	U of Minnesota	Teresa Kimberley/Andrew Harrison
32	U of Montreal	Sylvain Chouinard
33	U of New Mexico	Sarah Pirio Richardson
34	U of Rochester	Richard Barbano
35	U of Rome	Alfredo Berardelli
36	U of Tennessee	Mark LeDoux
37	U of Texas	William Ondo
38	U of Texas Southwestern	Neepa Patel
39	U of Toronto	Susan Fox
40	Virginia Commonwealth University	Claudia Testa
41	Wake Forest University	Allison Brashear
42	Washington University in St. Louis	Joel Perlmutter
43	Westmead Hospital	Victor Fung

Table III.2 Patient advocacy groups associated with the Dystonia Coalition

	Name	Location
1	Action for Dystonia, Diagnosis, Education, and Research (ADDER)	England, UK
2	Beat Dystonia	Texas, USA
3	Benign Essential Blepharospasm Research Foundation (BEBRF)	Texas, USA
4	Cure Dystonia Now (CDN)	New York, USA
5	ST/Dystonia	Wisconsin, USA
6	Dystonia Europe	Belgium
7	Dystonia Ireland	Ireland, UK
8	Dystonia Medical Research Foundation (DMRF)	Illinois, USA
9	Dystonia Medical Research Foundation – Canada (DMRFC)	Ontario, Canada
10	The Dystonia Society	England, UK
11	Dystonie-Qc	Quebec, Canada
12	National Spasmodic Dysphonia Association (NSDA)	Illinois, USA
13	National Spasmodic Torticollis Association (NSTA)	California, USA
14	Tyler's Hope for a Dystonia Cure (TH)	Florida, USA

James Madison University, Harrisonburg, VA) involves establishing a novel diagnostic and severity scale for spasmodic dysphonia. This project also has completed enrolment of ~200 subjects, and results are being assembled for manuscripts. Project 4 (PI: Mark Hallett, NINDS, Bethesda, MD) is a new study aimed at testing a novel diagnostic and severity scale for blepharospasm recently developed in Italy (Defazio et al. 2013, 2015).

In addition to its four large clinical research projects, the DC also supports studies through its Pilot Project Programme. The goal of the programme is to foster the most promising clinical and translational studies relevant to the isolated dystonias, with a short timeline of 1–2 years. Applications are typically accepted once or twice per year, and they are competitively reviewed by a rotating committee of individuals from the DC, scientific representatives from PAGs and representatives from the NIH. Thirteen applications have been funded so far (Table III.3).

The DC also supports a Career Development Program, where the goal is to facilitate career advancement for junior investigators interested in clinical and translational dystonia research. So far, 11 awards have been made (Table III.4). A related opportunity is the Travel Stipend, which has been supported by PAGs. These stipends provide junior investigators with travel funds to attend the DC annual meeting, and 62 have been granted already.

Most of the financial support for all of these activities comes from the NIH. However, some support also comes from PAGs, the Dystonia Study Group or the pharmaceutical industry. The various projects are supported using a 'fee for service' model

Table III.3 Funded pilot projects

Title	Principal investigator (PI)	PI institution/location
THAP1 Sequence Variants in Dystonia	Mark LeDoux	University of Tennessee USA
Development and Validation of Clinical Diagnostic Guidelines and a Novel Severity Rating Scale for Primary Blepharospasm*	Giovanni DeFazio	University of Bari Italy
DYT6 Dystonia: A Window to the Mechanisms of Primary Dystonia?	Kailash Bhatia	University College of London England, UK
Cerebellum and Cortical Plasticity: The Case of Focal Dystonia	Emmanuel Roze	Salpêtrière Hospital France
Characterization of Endophenotypes in Focal Task-Specific Dystonia	Christine Klein	University of Lbeck Germany
Increasing CERTainty in Blepharospasm Rating Scales	David Peterson	University of California San Diego USA
A New Rating Scale for Focal Task-Specific Dystonia of the Musician's Hand	Steven Frucht	Mount Sinai School of Medicine USA
Item Response Theory: An Individualized Approach to Evaluating a Comprehensive Cervical Dystonia Rating Scale	Sheila Eichenseer	Rush University USA
An Investigation of the Neuropathology, Clinical Phenotype and Expression Characteristics of Brain Tissue with *THAP1* and *TOR1A* Mutations	Henry Houlden	University College of London England, UK
Dystonia Coalition iPS Resource**	H. A. Jinnah	Emory University USA
Targeted Sequencing and Copy Number Assays in Primary Dystonia Genes	Mark LeDoux	University of Tennessee USA
Functional Connectivity in Spasmodic Dysphonia and Muscle Tension Dysphonia	Scott Norris	Washington U in St. Louis USA
Unravelling Novel Genetic Causes in Alcohol-Responsive Dystonia by Exome Sequencing	Katja Lohmann	University of Lbeck Germany

* Funded in partnership with the Benign Essential Blepharospasm Research Foundation.
** Co-funded by the Bachmann–Strauss Dystonia and Parkinson's Foundation.

in which individual investigators are paid for specific activities such as recruiting patients for a large clinical project or directing their own local pilot project. This financial model allows each site to determine how much effort it wants to expend on different projects.

Dystonia Coalition Meetings

The DC holds a two-day meeting every year. The first day focuses on the research priorities of one of the types of isolated dystonia (Jinnah et al. 2013). Previous meetings have focused on cervical dystonia, blepharospasm, laryngeal dystonia and generalised dystonia. The second day focuses on progress and questions related to DC projects and programmes. This meeting is open to anyone who wishes to attend, including those who are not officially affiliated with the DC. There are an average of 100 attendees, including DC leadership and investigators, study coordinators, investigators who received pilot project or development awards, travel stipend awardees and representatives from PAGs, the NIH and pharmaceutical companies.

In addition to its annual meeting, DC investigators have facilitated or participated in several other meetings devoted to dystonia, including workshops focusing on the genetics or neurobiology of dystonia, or development of novel treatments (Galpern et al. 2013).

Past Progress and Future Goals

The DC has supported the publication of 45 peer-reviewed articles and 39 reviews or commentaries. It has facilitated six independent grants by its investigators. Project 1 now has clinical data and DNA samples for 2261 subjects with various forms of dystonia. However, true progress is challenging to measure when the real goal is to build a collaborative spirit, develop consensus where it is lacking and create resources for future clinical and translational studies.

One of the enduring areas of progress for the DC involves obtaining international consensus on several items of central importance, such as the core definition of dystonia (Albanese et al. 2013; Jinnah & Albanese 2014) and the classification of its many subtypes (Fung et al. 2013). Other important areas of progress include the development of formal diagnostic criteria where expert consensus has been lacking, such as laryngeal dystonia or blepharospasm (Ludlow et al. 2008; Ludlow 2011; Defazio et al. 2013). And they include more comprehensive and rigorously evaluated rating tools to monitor severity, such as cervical dystonia (Comella et al. 2014) and blepharospasm (Defazio et al. 2015). These advances in clinical and translational research do not directly advance our scientific knowledge of the biological basis for dystonia, but they are

Table III.4 Funded career development awards

Title of project*	Awardee
Sensorimotor Network Activity as a Functional Imaging Marker for Dystonia	Maren Carbon-Correll, The Feinstein Institute for Medical Research USA
Sensory and Emotional Processing in Psychogenic Dystonia: A Functional Magnetic Resonance Imaging Study	Alberto Espay, University of Cincinnati USA
Dystonia Coalition: Psychiatric Assessment	Mateusz Zurowski, University of Toronto Canada
Determining the Efficacy of Synergistic Intervention in Focal Hand Dystonia with rTMS and Sensorimotor Retraining	Teresa Kimberley, University of Minnesota USA
GPi Induced Plasticity in Primary Cervical Dystonia	Morvarid Karimi, Washington U in St. Louis USA
Functional Connectivity of the Basal Ganglia in Primary Focal Dystonia: A Pilot Study	Brian Berman, University of Colorado, Denver USA
STN DBS in Primary Cervical Dystonia: A Pathophysiological Insight	Aparna Wagle Shukla, University of Florida USA
Effects of Cerebellar Theta-Burst Stimulation on Arm and Neck Movement Kinematics in Patients with Primary Dystonia	Matteo Bologna, Sapienza, University of Rome Italy
The Contribution of Blinks and Spasms to Blepharospasm Severity	David Peterson, University of CA, San Diego USA
Identification of Optimal Stimulation Site for Cervical Dystonia Symptoms: An Exploratory Study	Sarah Pirio Richardson, University of New Mexico USA
Reinforcement Learning in DYT1	David Arkadir, Hadassah Medical Center Israel

* All funded in partnership with the Dystonia Medical Research Foundation.

essential prerequisites for obtaining clearly defined populations of patients for all types of studies, and for measuring success in clinical trials.

The DC will continue to build on its created synergies and resources. Two of its large clinical research projects are nearing completion, but a new one is starting. The Natural History and Biorepository Project data are being accessed more frequently now that its numbers have grown. The DC PAGs and scientific community will continue to work towards the common goal of improving treatment and care for people with isolated dystonia.

References

Albanese A, Bhatia K, Bressman SB, DeLong MR, Fahn S, Fung VSC, Hallett M, Jankovic J, Jinnah HA, Klein C, Lang AE, Mink JW, Teller JK. 2013. Phenomenology and classification of dystonia: a consensus update. *Mov Disord* 28:863–873.

Comella CL, Fox SH, Bhatia KP, Perlmutter JS, Jinnah HA, Zurowski M, McDonald WM, Marsh L, Rosen AR, Waliczek T, Wright LJ, Galpern WR, Stebbins GT. 2014. Development of the comprehensive cervical dystonia rating scale: methodology. *Mov Disord Clin Pract.* doi: 10.1002/mdc3.12131.

Defazio G, Hallett M, Jinnah HA, Berardelli A. 2013. Development and validation of a clinical guideline for diagnosing blepharospasm. *Neurology* 81:236–240.

Defazio G, Hallett M, Jinnah HA, Stebbins GT, Gigante AF, Ferrazzano G, Conte A, Fabbrini G, Berardelli A. 2015. Development and validation of a clinical scale for rating the severity of blepharospasm. *Mov Disord* 30:525–530.

Fung VS, Jinnah HA, Bhatia K, Vidailhet M. 2013. Assessment of the patient with dystonia: an update on dystonia syndromes. *Mov Disord* 28:889–898.

Galpern WR, Coffey CS, Albanese A, Cheung K, Comella CL, Ecklund DJ, Fahn S, Jankovic J, Kieburtz K, Lang AE, McDermott MP, Shefner JM, Teller JK, Thompson JL, Yeatts SD, Jinnah HA. 2013. Designing clinical trials for dystonia. *NeuroRx* 11:117–127.

Jinnah HA, Albanese A. 2014. The new classification for the dystonias: why was it needed and how was it accomplished? *Mov Disord Clin Pract* 1:280–284.

Jinnah HA, Berardelli A, Comella C, Defazio G, DeLong M, Factor S, Galpern WR, Hallett M, Ludlow CL, Perlmutter JS, Rosen AR; Dystonia Coalition Investigators. 2013. The focal dystonias: current views and challenges for future research. *Mov Disord* 7:926–943.

Ludlow CL. 2011. Spasmodic dysphonia: a laryngeal control disorder specific to speech. *J Neurosci* 31:793–797.

Ludlow CL, Adler CH, Berke GS, Bielamowicz SA, Blitzer A, Bressman SB, Hallett M, Jinnah HA, Juergens U, Martin SB, Perlmutter JS, Sapienza C, Singleton A, Tanner CM, Woodson GE. 2008. Research priorities in spasmodic dysphonia. *Oto Head Neck Surg* 139:495–505.

Appendix IV: DystonieNet: A Dutch Approach for Optimising the Treatment of Cervical Dystonia

Maria A. J. de Koning-Tijssen and Joost van den Dool

DystonieNet

Cervical dystonia (CD) involves abnormal postures and/or involuntary movements of the head and is the most common form of adult-onset focal dystonia (Epidemiologic Study of Dystonia in Europe (ESDE) Collaborative Group 2000; Jankovic et al. 2007). It is estimated that around 8000 people suffer from CD in the Netherlands. Patients are referred to a neurologist for diagnosis and treatment. The first line of treatment are injections of the affected neck muscles with botulinum toxin (BTX) to decrease the severity of abnormal postures and/or involuntary movements and pain (Costa et al. 2005). Successful BTX treatment depends on many factors, like proper identification and injection of the affected muscles, determination of the right dose and the experience of the physician administering the BTX.

In addition to BTX treatment, many CD patients are referred for physical therapy (PT) to overcome problems with activities of daily living. The evidence towards the effectiveness of PT, however, is lacking and currently there is no consensus on the rehabilitative strategies to use in clinical practice (Delnooz et al. 2009). An additional problem is the relative rarity of the condition. Therefore, most physical therapists are not familiar with dystonia, and the small number of patients per PT limits the possibility to gain enough experience to provide optimal care for CD patients.

In 2010, the Movement Disorders working group of the Dutch Neurological Society recognised these problems and asked four university hospitals to initiate DystonieNet (University Medical Centres of Groningen, Amsterdam, Leiden and Nijmegen) together with the PT department of the Amsterdam University of Applied Sciences (Tijssen et al. 2013). The main goal of DystonieNet is to optimise the treatment for CD patients by facilitating collaboration between specialised neurologists and physical therapists in local networks, with the aim to educate healthcare providers and to facilitate research in CD.

To achieve the DystonieNet goals, a website was developed that serves as a digital platform for healthcare providers (Tijssen et al. 2013). This website gives information on regional meetings, focused skills workshops, (inter)national meetings on dystonia and ongoing research studies on dystonia.

A special feature of the website is the search tool, which allows medical doctors, physical therapists and patients to find the nearest participating neurologist for treatment with BTX based on their zip code. The DystonieNet website is linked to the website of the Dutch dystonia patient association so patients have access to the search tool and information on ongoing studies (Dystonievereniging 2015). In addition to the website, a digital newsletter is sent to all participating neurologists, nurses and physical therapists twice per year with the latest news on the developments of DystonieNet and ongoing studies. The newsletter also enables recruitment of patients via their neurologist for research projects. To date, 84 neurologists from 58 hospitals across the country participate, and 171 physical therapists are willing to work in DystonieNet (Figure IV.1).

Another way to achieve the DystonieNet goals are the regional meetings organised by the four university hospitals to discuss issues related to dystonia for groups of movement disorder (dystonia) neurologists, nurses and physical therapists. On a national level, a skills workshop is organised twice per year with the focus on the treatment of CD and blepharospasm. These local multidisciplinary meetings and national workshops enable collaboration of healthcare providers on important issues in CD. Recently, national BTX treatment recommendations were developed for physicians and specialised nurses. In addition, a nationwide study towards the effectiveness of a standardised PT programme in CD was initiated with the aim to develop evidence-based PT treatment recommendations (van den Dool et al. 2013).

BTX Treatment Recommendations

The Dutch BTX treatment recommendations were developed in 2012 based on a literature search on the latest evidence towards BTX treatment. If there was no available literature on a certain topic, consensus was reached during one of the three consensus meetings with a group of experienced neurologists. Practical diagrams and photo illustrations are added to help determine the proper muscles, dose and location for injection in the different subtypes of CD. The Dutch version of the recommendations can be downloaded from www.dystonienet.nl (Tijssen et al. 2013). The Dutch recommendations come with a free application for iPhone, iPad and Android platforms that is

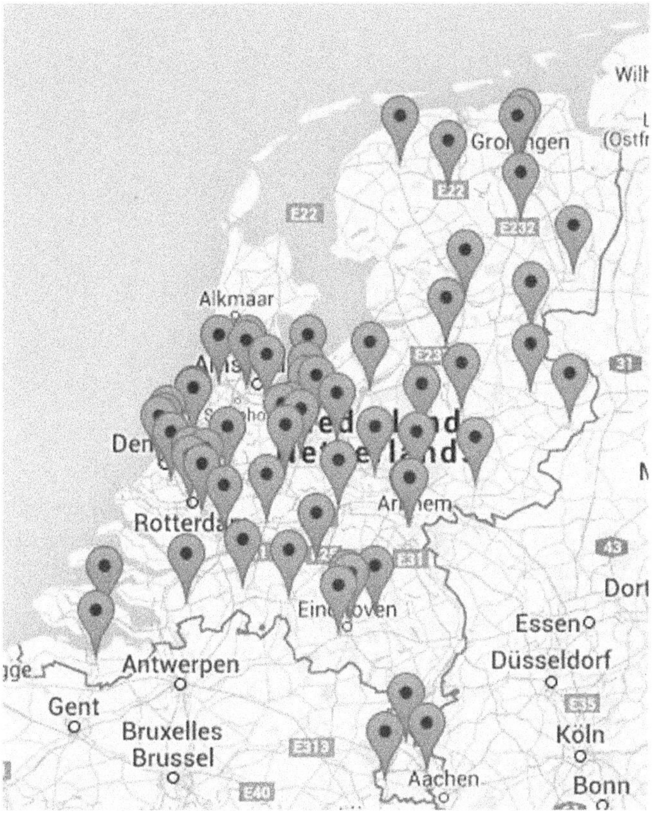

Figure IV.1 Overview of participating hospitals (www.dystonienet.nl/component/zorgzoeker/?view=zorgzoeker&id=1&Itemid=117).

easy to use in the outpatient clinics. The application is available in the Apple App store and the Google Play Store.

Physical Therapy Treatment Recommendations

Due to the lack of good-quality class A studies towards the effectiveness of PT interventions and the lack of consensus towards the use of rehabilitative strategies in CD, it was not possible to create evidence-based PT treatment recommendations. Therefore, a new standardised physical therapy programme was developed together with experienced physical therapists and neurologists during three consensus meetings (van den Dool et al. 2013) The (cost-) effectiveness of this standardised physical therapy programme in addition to BTX treatment is currently being studied in a single-blind, randomised controlled trial to provide class A2 evidence towards the effectiveness of PT interventions in CD (van den Dool et al. 2013). The results of this study will form the basis for a best evidence/best practice treatment recommendation. The study will be finished by the end of 2016 and the treatment recommendations are expected to be available in 2017. After that, special training courses will be given to physical therapists participating in DystonieNet. Therapists who have completed the training course will be added to the physiotherapy search tool on the DystonieNet website so physicians and patients can easily find a nearby specialised therapist online.

Future Directions

For now, the main focus of DystonieNet has been on the BTX and PT treatment of CD. In the (near) future other allied health disciplines like occupational therapy and psychology will also be involved. Furthermore, other forms of dystonia will be included in DystonieNet. Currently, the DystonieNet concept is being introduced in Europe: DystoniaNet. The website will be translated into different languages so it can be used as a digital platform for dystonia in different EU countries. The national websites will be linked to national patient associations and the European patient association, Dystonia Europe, for easy access. The ultimate goals are to develop and implement best evidence treatment recommendations on a Europe-wide scale, to combine knowledge on dystonia and give uniformity of treatment among healthcare providers and use the DystoniaNet for collaborative studies throughout Europe.

In conclusion, DystonieNet/DystoniaNet is a practical approach to improving care for (cervical) dystonia patients, but can also serve as a tool for (international) collaboration in care, education and research for patients with dystonia.

Acknowledgements

The authors would like to thank the DystonieNet collaborators Dr J. H. T. M. Koelman (Academic Medical Centre Amsterdam), Dr B. P. C. van de Warrenburg (Radboud University Medical Centre), Prof. Dr J. J. van Hilten (Leiden University Medical Centre) and Dr B. Visser (Amsterdam University of Applied Sciences) for their comments on the manuscript.

References

Costa J, Espirito-Santo C, Borges A, Ferreira JJ, Coelho M, Moore P, Sampaio C. 2005. Botulinum toxin type A therapy for cervical dystonia. *Cochrane Database Syst Rev* 1:CD003633.

Delnooz CC, Horstink MW, Tijssen MA, van de Warrenburg BP. 2009. Paramedical treatment in primary dystonia: a systematic review. *Mov Disord* 24(15):2187–2198.

Dystonievereniging. 2015. Dystonie Vereniging. Available from www.dystonievereniging.nl.

Epidemiologic Study of Dystonia in Europe (ESDE) Collaborative Group. 2000. A prevalence study of primary dystonia in eight European countries. *J Neurol* 247(10):787–792.

Jankovic J, Tsui J, Bergeron C. 2007. Prevalence of cervical dystonia and spasmodic torticollis in the United States general population. *Parkinsonism Relat Disord* 13(7):411–416.

Tijssen MAJ, Dool van den J, Hillten van JJ, Warrenburg van der BPC. 2013. DystonieNet. Available from: www.dystonienet nl.

van den Dool J, Visser B, Koelman JH, Engelbert RH, Tijssen MA. 2013. Cervical dystonia: effectiveness of a standardized physical therapy program – study design and protocol of a single blind randomized controlled trial. *BMC Neurol* 13:85.

Appendix V: Musicians With Dystonia

Glen Estrin

Musicians are subject to a wide range of occupational injuries. Problems typically recognised easily by specialists include muscle injuries (such as tendinitis), nerve entrapments (carpal tunnel syndrome, to name one) and overuse syndrome, where chronic repetitive use of certain muscles can lead to pain. Task-specific focal dystonia, the neurological movement disorder that presents in musicians, is extremely difficult to diagnose, and was a true mystery until the last two decades of the twentieth century.

The prominent American-born pianists Leon Fleisher and Gary Graffman were both stricken with unexplained involuntary, painless spasms of the fingers of their right hands when attempting to play, Mr Fleisher in the 1960s and Mr Graffman over ten years later. They were among the most respected pianists of their time, so the mysterious thwarting of their tremendous instincts and abilities was beyond comprehension. Due to their tenacity in seeking a correct diagnosis and searching worldwide for answers for many years, it was finally determined by Fred Hochberg, MD, a neurologist at Massachusetts General Hospital, that the strange problem was not muscular, but neurological. Why couldn't musicians be afflicted with a fine motor skill dystonia, which can shut down so many tasks and has been known for a century under the terminology 'writer's cramp?' Musicians finally had an answer to their 'losing their chops!'

Leon Fleisher and Gary Graffman became the 'grandfathers' of musician task-specific focal dystonia as a diagnosis. Thousands of musicians throughout the years had either ended their careers, or, when possible, continued performing with tremendous difficulty, despite lack of an explanation as to what was occurring. Documentation regarding strange, unexplained problems of musicians that were most certainly dystonia date back to composer/pianist Robert Schumann in the 1830s.

Fortunately for afflicted musicians, the disorder is focal and typically affects only the part of the body used for performing. Pianists, guitarists and string players are afflicted in their fingers, hands or even bow arms. Brass players develop dystonia in their embouchure (lip and mouth position). Woodwind players are in double jeopardy as they can be victimised in the hands or mouth. The disorder is typically painless, and in most cases is task-specific to attempting to play the instrument. In the words of Leon Fleisher, when comparing musician dystonia to the other extremely painful and debilitating forms of the disorder, 'We are the lucky ones! If we don't play, we are fine!'

Specialty of Performing Arts Medicine is Founded

Performing arts medicine as a specialty was initiated over 30 years ago by the late Alice Brandfonbrener, MD, of The Rehabilitation Institute of Chicago at Northwestern University Hospital, and Richard Lederman, MD, PhD, a neurological movement disorder specialist at the Cleveland Clinic. These two inspiring physicians determined the substantial need for diagnosis and treatment for musicians, singers and dancers. Similar to sports medicine facilities, Drs Brandfonbrener and Lederman created and founded the two most renowned performing arts medicine clinics in the USA at their institutions. They also founded the international Performing Arts Medicine Association in 1989, which is dedicated to promoting the highest quality of care for all performing artists and recognising their special needs.

The leading institution in the world for musician health was started on a small scale in 1974 at the Hannover University for Music, Drama and Media in Germany. Prof. Dr med. Eckart Altenmuller became the head of the institute in 1994, and the centre was renamed The Institute of Music Physiology and Musicians' Medicine. This magnificent and comprehensive facility for treating musicians has grown exponentially since Dr Altenmuller was appointed, and patients from around the world seek their care. Most of the cutting-edge research involving musicians is performed at the institute, and many of the top specialists treating musicians throughout the world have trained here.

Exciting news is upon us in the USA at this time: neurologist Alexander Pantelyat, MD, is launching the Johns Hopkins Center for Music and Medicine as a joint venture with the Peabody Institute of Music (the Conservatory that is also part of Johns Hopkins University) and their musician wellness and guitar expert, Serap Bastepe-Gray, MD. The centre will involve the collaboration of multiple departments at Hopkins Medicine and Peabody Conservatory pertaining to issues of performing artists within one clinical setting. Research will be strongly promoted, and, very interestingly, the centre will also focus on studying the effects of music- and dance-based therapies for patients with a wide range of disorders, including Parkinson's disease, Alzheimer's disease and stroke.

Musicians With Dystonia Program

The arduous road to correct diagnosis of musician focal task-specific dystonia is extremely frustrating and can take years. Musicians suffering from dystonia typically describe their symptoms in musical terms, complaining of a progressive loss of control in playing their instruments. Initially they may feel that they need to expend more energy or thought to play passages that were previously routine. Specific tasks, such as stretching on a keyboard or legato brass playing, may be exclusively involved. With time, automatic movements become difficult, and there may be a sense that the involved body part is weak.

The case history most familiar to me is my own. The retelling here will certainly elucidate why the founding of Musicians With Dystonia was so imperative.

I enjoyed a wonderful career as a French horn player for over 20 years, performing and recording with everyone from the Chicago Symphony to Frank Sinatra, who I toured the world with for the last 12 years of his career. While maintaining a very busy schedule as a New York City freelance musician, I started to notice my lower lip was not as responsive as usual. This led to muscle spasms throughout the lips, tongue and jaws, and within six months even the most rudimentary tasks while playing the horn were nearly impossible. The symptoms occurred only when attempting to play, which created further mystery for me and all of the healthcare practitioners I visited.

I was treated by internists, dentists, oral surgeons, massage therapists, acupuncturists and myofunctional therapists. Diagnoses included everything from TMJ to trismus and cervicocranial disorder, and most of the doctors suggested the problems were 'in my head' and I should seek psychiatric care. This was almost a natural conclusion, since I couldn't do my job and there were no evident symptoms.

Fifteen months after the unbelievable and constant search for answers began, and nine months after I had to end my career, I finally visited a neurologist. After relating my story, he promptly diagnosed focal dystonia. I then flew to Chicago to visit the aforementioned guru Dr Brandfonbrener to confirm the diagnosis. She did, and recommended treatment at Columbia Presbyterian Hospital in my home city, New York.

The Neurological Institute at Columbia is renowned, and the Movement Disorders division under Stanley Fahn, MD, is one of the great centres in the world. My first visit there was extremely serendipitous, as I was treated by the brilliant and wonderful neurologist Steven Frucht, MD. Dr Frucht was very interested in musician issues as he is an incredibly accomplished violinist and has studied at The Juilliard School and the Tanglewood Music Festival. I was immediately diagnosed with dystonia, and when relating my absurd quest for answers Dr Frucht explained that this was the norm. Many of his musician dystonia patients had searched for correct diagnoses for five to ten years!

Dr Frucht suggested we find a way together to create some awareness in the musician community. After many sessions of brainstorming, the Musicians With Dystonia Program was born in 1999. In our plan, Dr Frucht would comprehensively handle the medical needs, and I would be the contact point for musicians. Dr Fahn then suggested we operate with the Dystonia Medical Research Foundation, as they had been looking for a conduit to the musical population for many years. When hearing our proposal, the Foundation invited us to become a programme entity of this largest dystonia foundation in the world. We provide information, support and medical referrals, as we have amassed a worldwide network of neurologists that specialise in musicians.

We have published dozens of articles in musical and medical journals since 2000, and have presented on musician dystonia at symposia throughout the world. Dr Frucht has treated hundreds of musicians at Columbia (now New York-Presbyterian), Mount Sinai Medical Center in New York, and in his current home as Director of NYU Langone's Division of Movement Disorders. The Foundation's awareness drive has been so wonderfully successful that we can proudly relate that typical diagnosis time for musicians is now down to weeks after the onset of symptoms, and the first visit is to a movement disorder specialist!

The tremendous success of Musicians With Dystonia has stimulated similar groups being founded, such as the Hannover collaboration of Drs Eckart Altenmuller and Hans-Christian Jabusch with their programme, Musiker Mit Dystonie. We also work jointly with most of the dystonia foundations across the globe, including Dystonia Europe and the National Spasmodic Dysphonia Association, and musician treatment organisations such as the Performing Arts Medicine Association.

Contact Information

The website of the Dystonia Medical Research Foundation is www.dystonia-foundation.org

Email contacts are musicians@dystonia-foundation.org or gsestrin@aol.com

Appendix VI: Funding for Dystonia Research: Trends and Challenges

Jan K. Teller

Introduction

There can be no new effective treatments of diseases without adequately conducted and financially supported medical research. Research funding is often described in economic terms as an investment. One can also call it a moral obligation of a civilised society. These approaches and interpretations are not mutually exclusive as long as the final outcome is an effective and sustained sustenance of disease-oriented research. In this short section I will attempt to review and comment on current trends and challenges in dystonia research funding.

Principles and funding patterns that apply to medical research in general also apply to funding of research on dystonia as a disease as well as a biological phenomenon underlying this condition. As in other disease-oriented research areas, financial incentives to conduct basic and clinical investigations are driven by the desire to understand the disease process and its mechanisms in order to provide rationally developed treatments. In this case, the variety of dystonias is an obstacle and, at the same time, an opportunity to develop new therapeutics thanks to numerous mechanistic overlaps and possibilities of targeting common symptomatology. Moreover, although the dystonias are recognised as unique clinical entities, there are numerous 'overlaps' with other movement disorders like Parkinson's disease, Huntington's disease and others. From a research funding point of view this creates inherent difficulties in analysing the dystonia funding landscape, the major frustration being that there is still limited and inadequate cross-talk, both in terms of research and funding initiatives, between closely related movement disorders.

Why Do We Fund Research on Dystonia?

Certainly, we do it 'because it is there', to paraphrase rock climbers. The disease affects many people. One can claim there is a growing number of people diagnosed with dystonia. This is mostly thanks to advances in genetics, which unequivocally defined new forms of dystonia, and due to dramatically improved clinical diagnoses that put dystonia distinctly on the map of neurological movement disorders. Somewhat paradoxically, dystonia is such a complex and neurophysiologically subtle condition that solving its mysteries may provide deeper insight into brain functioning in general. This provides additional incentive to fund pioneering research on dystonia.

How Do We Do It?

Like in other medical research areas, mechanisms of funding are varied and range from research project grants, individual research or clinical fellowships, and large collaborative and infrastructure initiatives to clinical trials. If there is an emerging principle here it is an appreciation of the fact that dystonia is a rare disease and, considering the scarcity of resources, only collaborative efforts can significantly speed up progress in tackling this disease.

What Do We Fund?

Quick inspection of available information about dystonia research projects reveals several major trends. Genetic forms of dystonia, although numerically a minority, attract a lot of attention and funding. Clearly, identifying new genes leads to better understanding of dystonia and identifies potentially feasible therapeutic targets. Substantial funding supports functional analysis of dystonia at diverse levels: from non-invasive interventions and deep brain stimulation studies, brain imaging in different forms of dystonia and neurophysiological studies of patients, to attempts to understand functional and pathophysiological changes in the basal ganglia and the cerebellum of humans and animals. Recent genetic discoveries have stimulated and inspired several lines of research, often unexpectedly, where the molecular basis of the dystonias is directly studied. Significant funding is also directed towards training of an incoming cadre of movement disorder neurologists specifically concentrating on dystonia. Finally, a number of projects have recently been funded to investigate novel drug candidates that target various brain receptors implicated in dystonia.

Who Is Funded?

It is interesting to note that over the last several decades there has been a dramatic shift in who is funded in the dystonia field. Early formative studies, primarily limited to dystonia patients, were typically conducted by clinical neurologists. Attempts to study dystonia in animals or *in vitro* were very limited. The advent of genetics allowed for multiple models of dystonia that can conveniently be studied in the lab. This drew new investigators into the field, many who had never heard about this disease. This trend continues and provides hope that many experts will join the effort to solve dystonia's secrets. Increasingly, more emphasis is placed on attracting and recruiting young researchers so they can commit to dystonia research.

Who Funds It?

Traditionally, at least in the USA, three major sectors provide funding for medical research: the government agencies, the pharmaceutical and medical devices industry and private foundations. Contributions from each of these entities vary widely depending on the specific disease and current state of the economy. In case of dystonia, the National Institutes of Health (NIH) have played a leading role in funding dystonia-related projects. In the last few years, the US Department of Defense (DoD) added dystonia to its list of studied conditions. As a result, several dystonia-focused grants have been awarded. As the government funding information is readily available, the level of interest and financial involvement of industry is extremely difficult to assess. Several clinical trials are being conducted or initiated, which provides funding not only to evaluate novel treatments but also to gain valuable clinical knowledge about dystonia. Industry collaborates with several dystonia foundations to provide grants that have established dystonia clinical fellowships and supported very much needed dystonia-focused meetings and workshops. The foundations themselves have championed the dystonia cause for many years, providing critical funding primarily to support high-risk projects that, whenever successful, transition to the NIH-supported projects. Although this brief analysis is heavily US-biased, there is substantial and outstanding dystonia research activity in Europe, where funds also originate from the three major sources mentioned above.

How Much Support Goes to Dystonia Research?

Again, due to the limited access to sources, the quantification provided here is US-biased. Over the last five years the NIH supported dystonia-related research at a relatively steady level of \$12–14 million per year. This includes traditional grant funding (so-called R01 and R21 grants) as well as intramural (NIH) projects and larger collaborative research projects. It is projected that this level will remain the same in the next two years. If we assume that at least 250 000 people in the USA suffer from some form of dystonia, the NIH funding amounts to approximately \$50 per patient per year spent on dystonia research – not a very impressive number. During the last few years, the DoD came to the rescue, offering sizeable grants to support dystonia projects.

As stated before, quantification of the industry contribution is difficult; however, several companies that offer products that help dystonia patients systematically support the dystonia research field and patient organisations. Funding offered by dystonia foundations, which hovers most likely around \$1–2 million per year worldwide, is easier to follow, although the scale of it is dwarfed by the NIH figures. Nonetheless, foundations' grants, often no more than \$50 000 per year, provide vital support for high-risk explorations that historically have led to major dystonia discoveries.

What Next?

If the NIH funding remains steady (even after adding the DoD contribution), and industry is not going to pursue dystonia more aggressively, most of the burden of supporting dystonia research will fall on private foundations. With their limited resources they will have to continue to be creative and trailblazing champions of dystonia research. Extensive collaborations among all the entities involved will be the only option to provide innovative and cost-effective solutions to support dystonia research. In the end, it is not only about research – suffering dystonia patients are waiting for treatments.

Sources

www.projectreporter.nih.gov/reporter.cfm
www.cdmrp.army.mil/funding/prmrp.shtml
www.dystonia-foundation.org
www.rarediseasesnetwork.org/dystonia

Index

Locators in **bold** refer to tables; those in *italic* to figures
Abbreviations used in subheadings
BT = botulinum toxin; DBS = deep brain stimulation

For EU product safety concerns, contact us at Calle de José Abascal, 56–1°,
28003 Madrid, Spain or eugpsr@cambridge.org.

www.ingramcontent.com/pod-product-compliance
Ingram Content Group UK Ltd.
Pitfield, Milton Keynes, MK11 3LW, UK
UKHW052040110226
467941UK00009B/142

* 9 7 8 1 1 0 7 1 3 2 8 6 3 *